CHILD DEVELOPMENT

CHILD DEVELOPMENT

Mary Tudor, R.N., M.N.
Clinical Nurse Specialist, Development Disabilities
Jefferson County Health Department and
Division of Developmental Disabilities
Jefferson County, Washington

Advisors:

Margaret E. Armstrong, R.N., M.S.
Visiting Professor, College of Nursing
University of Utah
Salt Lake City, Utah

Marie Scott Brown, R.N., Ph.D.
Associate Professor, School of Nursing
University of Colorado Medical Center
Denver, Colorado

Sally M. O'Neil, R.N., Ph.D.
Professor and Chairperson
Department of Maternal Child Nursing
School of Nursing
University of Washington
Seattle, Washington

McGraw-Hill Book Company

New York St. Louis San Francisco Auckland Bogotá Guatemala Hamburg
Johannesburg Lisbon London Madrid Mexico Montreal New Delhi
Panama Paris San Juan São Paulo Singapore Sydney Tokyo Toronto

CHILD DEVELOPMENT

Copyright © 1981 by McGraw-Hill, Inc. All rights reserved. Printed in the United States of America. No part of this publication may be reproduced, stored in a retrieval system, or transmitted, in any form or by any means, electronic, mechanical, photocopying, recording, or otherwise, without the prior written permission of the publisher.

1 2 3 4 5 6 7 8 9 0 HDHD 8 9 8 7 6 5 4 3 2 1

This book was set in Palatino by Bi-Comp, Incorporated.
The editors were David P. Carroll, Abe Krieger, and Tricia K. Geno;
the designer was Joan E. O'Connor;
the production supervisor was Jeanne Skahan.
The drawings were done by J & R Services, Inc.
Halliday Lithograph Corporation was printer and binder.

Library of Congress Cataloging in Publication Data
Main entry under title:

Child development.

    Bibliography: p.
    Includes indexes.
    1. Child development. 2. Pediatric nursing.
I. Tudor, Mary. [DNLM: 1. Child development—
Nursing texts. WY159 C534]
RJ131.C53   612'.65'024613   80-14835
ISBN 0-07-065412-3

To the children: past, present, and future:
"If anything at all in life is true,
there is a miracle in you."

Tom T. Hall

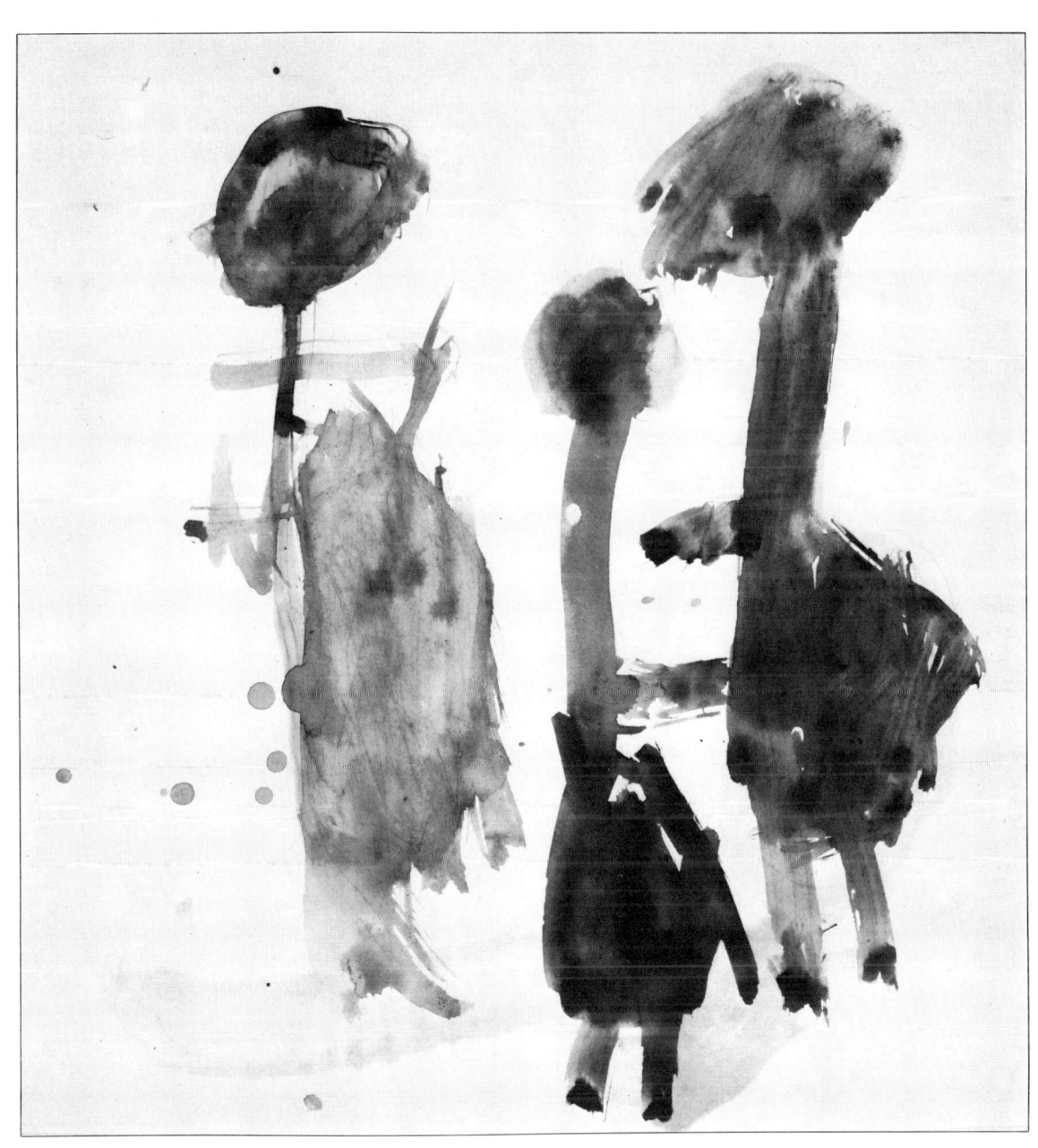

CONTENTS

	List of Contributors	xiii
	Preface	xvii

PART ONE

	CHAPTER 1	THE NURSING PROFESSION AND THE DEVELOPING CHILD	3
Kathryn E. Barnard		The Nursing Role in Promotion of Child Development	3
Marie Scott Brown		The Nursing Process in Provision of Services to Promote Child Development	8
Mary Tudor		Child Development: What, Why, When	11

	CHAPTER 2	PHYSICAL DEVELOPMENT	21
	SECTION 1	*Processes of Physical Development*	21
Wilma Peterson		General Considerations of Physical Development: Growth and Maturation	21
Veronica M. Ladensack Young		Human Genetics: Blueprint for Development	47
Veronica M. Ladensack Young		General Considerations of Physical Development: Cellular Growth, Differentiation, and Morphogenesis	62
	SECTION 2	*Principles of Development of Organ Systems*	71
Mary Tudor		Calvarium and Face	71
Mary D. Guthrie		Nervous System	74
Anna M. Tichy		Sensory System	75
Sherrilyn Passo		Musculoskeletal System	75
Mary Tudor		Cardiovascular System	79
Virginia J. Neelon		Respiratory System	80
Anna M. Tichy and Dianne Chong		Gastrointestinal System	84
Norma J. Briggs		Endocrine System	84
Nancy Reame		Reproductive System	85
Ida M. Martinson and Nancy V. Rude		Urinary System	87
Mary Tudor		Integumentary System	88
	SECTION 3	*Assessment of Physical Development and Status*	90
Mary Alexander Murphy		Physical Assessment	90
Andrea Netten Sechrist		Nutrition Assessment	96

CHAPTER 3		**BEHAVIORAL DEVELOPMENT**	107
SECTION 1		*Principles of Behavioral Development*	107
	Ruth Hepler	General Considerations of Behavioral Development	107
	Marion H. Rose	Effect of Parenting on Behavioral Development	115
	Mary Jane Amundson	Child-Development Theories	117
SECTION 2		*General Considerations of Behavioral Development*	129
	Veronica A. Binzley	Perceptual Development	129
	Fay F. Russell and Beverly R. Richardson	Gross Motor Development	132
	Barbara Newcomer McLaughlin and Nancy L. Morgan	Fine Motor Development	134
	Virginia Pidgeon	Cognitive Development	135
	Shirley Joan Lemmen	Language Development	139
	Doris Julian	Self-Help Skill Development and Independent Functioning	141
	Susan Blanch Meister	Social Development	143
SECTION 3		*Assessment of Behavioral Development*	149
	Ruth Hepler	Behavioral Assessment	149
CHAPTER 4		**PARENTING AND THE DEVELOPING CHILD**	163
	Marion H. Rose	The Parent-Child Relationship	163
	Marcene Powell Erickson	Assessment of the Child's Environment	176
	Jeanene B. Brown	Child-Care and Development Theorists: Resources for Parents	184

PART TWO

CHAPTER 5		**THE EMBRYO AND FETUS: CONCEPTION TO BIRTH**	199
SECTION 1		*Development of the Embryo: The Period of Organogenesis*	200
	Mary Tudor	Conception through Establishment of Body Form	200
	Mary Tudor	Development of the Face	222
	Mary D. Guthrie	Development of the Central Nervous System	225
	Anna M. Tichy	Development of the Sensory System	230
	Sherrilyn Passo	Development of the Musculoskeletal System	234
	LaNelle E. Geddes	Development of the Cardiovascular System	237
	Virginia J. Neelon	Development of the Respiratory System	244
	Anna M. Tichy and Dianne Chong	Development of the Gastrointestinal System	247
	Norma J. Briggs	Development of the Endocrine System	250
	Nancy Reame	Development of the Reproductive System	252
	Ida M. Martinson and Nancy V. Rude	Development of the Urinary System	256
	Mary Tudor	Development of the Integumentary System	260
	Mary Tudor	Dysmorphology	261

SECTION 2	*The Fetal Period: The Period of Elaboration and Growth*	264
Mary Tudor	Fetal Development	264
Mary Tudor	Prenatal Behavior	274
Margot Edwards	Labor and Birth	282

CHAPTER 6	**THE NEONATE: BIRTH TO 1 MONTH**	293
SECTION 1	*Physical Development*	294
Jean A. Foster	Physical Status and Development of the Neonate	294
Holly E. Miner	Maturation and Growth Deviation in the Neonate	297
Holly E. Miner	Development of Organ Systems	304
Mary D. Guthrie	Nervous System	305
Anna M. Tichy	Sensory System	305
Sherrilyn Passo	Musculoskeletal System	307
LaNelle E. Geddes	Cardiovascular System	308
Virginia J. Neelon	Respiratory System	312
Anna M. Tichy and Dianne Chong	Gastrointestinal System	315
Norma J. Briggs	Endocrine System	321
Nancy Reame	Reproductive System	322
Ida M. Martinson and Nancy V. Rude	Urinary System	324
Judith Anne Ritchie	Development of Body Concept and Concepts of Illness and Wellness	326
SECTION 2	*Behavioral Development*	328
Mary Tudor	The Neonate: Awakening	328
Clarissa Beardslee	Sleep	330
Veronica A. Binzley	Perceptual Development	333
Fay F. Russell and Beverly R. Richardson	Gross Motor Development	337
Barbara Newcomer McLaughlin and Nancy L. Morgan	Fine Motor Development	345
Virginia Pidgeon	Cognitive Development	347
Shirley Joan Lemmen	Language Development	350
Susan Blanch Meister	Social Development	350
Judith Anne Ritchie	Perception of Behavioral Competency and Development of Self-Esteem	351

CHAPTER 7	**THE INFANT: 1 MONTH TO 12 MONTHS**	359
SECTION 1	*Physical Development*	360
Marilyn A. Chard and Martha Underwood Barnard	Physical Development of the Infant	360
Mary Tudor	Calvarium and Face	366
Mary D. Guthrie	Central Nervous System	366
Anna M. Tichy	Sensory System	367
Sherrilyn Passo	Musculoskeletal System	368
Anna M. Tichy and Dianne Chong	Gastrointestinal System	368
Norma J. Briggs	Endocrine System	370
Judith Anne Ritchie	Development of Body Concept and Concepts of Illness and Wellness	370

SECTION 2 — Behavioral Development — 373

Author	Topic	Page
Mary Tudor	The Infant: Outward and Upward	373
Veronica A. Binzley	Perceptual Development	374
Fay F. Russell and Beverly R. Richardson	Gross Motor Development	377
Barbara Newcomer McLaughlin and Nancy L. Morgan	Fine Motor Development	387
Virginia Pidgeon	Cognitive Development	393
Shirley Joan Lemmen	Language Development	396
Doris Julian	Self-Help Skill Development	398
Susan Blanch Meister	Social Development	401
Judith Anne Ritchie	Perception of Behavioral Competency and Development of Self-Esteem	403

CHAPTER 8 — THE TODDLER: 1 YEAR TO 3 YEARS — 409

SECTION 1 — Physical Development — 410

Author	Topic	Page
M. Colleen Caulfield	Physical Development of the Toddler	410
Mary Tudor	Calvarium and Face	415
Anna M. Tichy	Sensory System	416
Sherrilyn Passo	Musculoskeletal System	417
Anna M. Tichy and Dianne Chong	Gastrointestinal System	417
Judith Anne Ritchie	Development of Body Concept and Concepts of Illness and Wellness	418

SECTION 2 — Behavioral Development — 422

Author	Topic	Page
Mary Tudor	The Toddler: Demanding Recognition	422
Veronica A. Binzley	Perceptual Development	423
Fay F. Russell and Beverly R. Richardson	Gross Motor Development	425
Barbara Newcomer McLaughlin and Nancy L. Morgan	Fine Motor Development	427
Virginia Pidgeon	Cognitive Development	430
Shirley Joan Lemmen	Language Development	432
Doris Julian	Self-Help Skill Development	436
Susan Blanch Meister	Social Development	439
Judith Anne Ritchie	Perception of Behavioral Competency and Development of Self-Esteem	441

CHAPTER 9 — THE PRESCHOOL CHILD: 3 YEARS TO 5 YEARS — 449

SECTION 1 — Physical Development — 450

Author	Topic	Page
M. Colleen Caulfield	Physical Development of the Preschool Child	450
Anna M. Tichy	Sensory System	451
Judith Anne Ritchie	Development of Body Concept and Concepts of Illness and Wellness	452

SECTION 2 — Behavioral Development — 457

Author	Topic	Page
Mary Tudor	The Preschool Child: "Here I Am!"	457
Veronica A. Binzley	Perceptual Development	458
Fay F. Russell and Beverly R. Richardson	Gross Motor Development	460

Barbara Newcomer McLaughlin and Nancy L. Morgan	Fine Motor Development	461
Virginia Pidgeon	Cognitive Development	461
Shirley Joan Lemmen	Language Development	464
Doris Julian	Self-Help Skill Development	467
Susan Blanch Meister	Social Development	469
Judith Anne Ritchie	Perception of Behavioral Competency and Development of Self-Esteem	471
CHAPTER 10	**THE SCHOOL-AGE CHILD: 5 YEARS TO PUBERTY**	477
SECTION 1	*Physical Development*	478
Maija S. Ljunghag	Physical Development of the School-Age Child	478
Mary Tudor	Puberty	485
Mary Tudor	Calvarium and Face	485
Sherrilyn Passo	Musculoskeletal System	486
Nancy Reame	Reproductive System and Pubertal Changes	487
Judith Anne Ritchie	Development of Body Concept and Concepts of Illness and Wellness	496
SECTION 2	*Behavioral Development*	502
Mary Tudor	The School-Age Child: Age of Achievement	502
Veronica A. Binzley	Perceptual Development	503
Fay F. Russell and Beverly R. Richardson	Gross Motor Development	504
Barbara Newcomer McLaughlin and Nancy L. Morgan	Fine Motor Development	506
Virginia Pidgeon	Cognitive Development	507
Doris Julian	Self-Help Skill Development	510
Susan Blanch Meister	Social Development	512
Judith Anne Ritchie	Perception of Competency and Development of Self-Esteem	514
	Indexes	519
	Name Index	
	Subject Index	

LIST OF CONTRIBUTORS

MARY JANE AMUNDSON, R.N., Ph.D.
Assistant Professor, Mental Health Nursing Graduate Program and Acting Chairperson,
Department of Professional Nursing
University of Hawaii School of Nursing
Honolulu, Hawaii
CHILD-DEVELOPMENT THEORIES

KATHRYN E. BARNARD, R.N., Ph.D.
Professor of Nursing
Maternal Child Nursing Department
School of Nursing and Affiliate, Child Development and Mental Retardation Center
University of Washington
Seattle, Washington
THE NURSING ROLE IN PROMOTION OF CHILD DEVELOPMENT

MARTHA UNDERWOOD BARNARD, R.N., M.N.
Ph.D. Candidate
Faculty/Clinical Specialist
School of Nursing and School of Medicine
Departments of Pediatrics
University of Kansas College of Health Sciences and Hospital
Kansas City, Kansas
PHYSICAL DEVELOPMENT OF THE INFANT

CLARISSA BEARDSLEE, R.N., Ph.D.
Associate Professor, Nursing Care of Children
School of Nursing
University of Pittsburgh
Pittsburgh, Pennsylvania
SLEEP

VERONICA A. BINZLEY, R.N., Ph.D.
Director, Program Support Services
Warrensville Center
Ohio Department of Mental Health and Mental Retardation
Warrensville Township, Ohio
PERCEPTUAL DEVELOPMENT

NORMA J. BRIGGS, R.N., Ph.D.
Assistant Professor
School of Nursing
University of Wisconsin—Eau Claire
Eau Claire, Wisconsin
DEVELOPMENT OF THE ENDOCRINE SYSTEM

JEANENE B. BROWN, R.N., M.S.
Family Child Nurse Specialist and Coordinator, Family Nurse Practitioner Program
University of Kansas School of Nursing Outreach
Hays, Kansas
CHILD-CARE AND DEVELOPMENT THEORISTS: RESOURCES FOR PARENTS

MARIE SCOTT BROWN, R.N., Ph.D.
Associate Professor
School of Nursing
University of Colorado Medical Center
Denver, Colorado
THE NURSING PROCESS IN PROVISION OF SERVICES TO PROMOTE CHILD DEVELOPMENT

M. COLLEEN CAULFIELD, R.N., M.N.
Instructor, Maternal Child Nursing
School of Nursing
University of Washington
Seattle, Washington
PHYSICAL DEVELOPMENT OF THE TODDLER
PHYSICAL DEVELOPMENT OF THE PRESCHOOL CHILD

LIST OF CONTRIBUTORS

MARILYN A. CHARD, R.N., Ed.D.
Professor, School of Nursing and
Assistant Professor, School of Medicine
University of Kansas College of Health Sciences
Kansas City, Kansas
PHYSICAL DEVELOPMENT OF THE INFANT

DIANNE CHONG, B.S., B.A., M.S.
Research Associate, Maternal Child Nursing
College of Nursing
University of Illinois at the Medical Center
Chicago, Illinois
DEVELOPMENT OF THE GASTROINTESTINAL SYSTEM

MARGOT EDWARDS, R.N., M.A.
Childbirth Educator
Pacific Grove, California
LABOR AND BIRTH

MARCENE POWELL ERICKSON, R.N., M.N.
Ph.D. Candidate
University of Utah
Salt Lake City, Utah
ASSESSMENT OF THE CHILD'S ENVIRONMENT

JEAN A. FOSTER, R.N., B.S.N., M.S.N.
Unit Director, Parent Education and Preparation Unit
James Whitcomb Riley Hospital for Children
Indiana University Medical Center
Indianapolis, Indiana
PHYSICAL STATUS AND DEVELOPMENT OF THE NEONATE

LaNELLE E. GEDDES, R.N., Ph.D.
Professor, Department of Nursing
Purdue University
West Lafayette, Indiana
DEVELOPMENT OF THE CARDIOVASCULAR SYSTEM

MARY D. GUTHRIE, R.N., Ph.D.
Professor, Department of Anatomy
School of Medicine
University of Texas
San Antonio, Texas
DEVELOPMENT OF THE NERVOUS SYSTEM

RUTH HEPLER, R.N., Ph.D.
Assistant Professor
Social Sciences Division
Kennesaw College
Marietta, Georgia
GENERAL CONSIDERATIONS OF BEHAVIORAL DEVELOPMENT
BEHAVIORAL ASSESSMENT

DORIS JULIAN, R.N., M.N.
Associate Professor, School of Nursing
University of Oregon Health Sciences Center
Portland, Oregon
SELF-HELP SKILL DEVELOPMENT AND INDEPENDENT FUNCTIONING

SHIRLEY JOAN LEMMEN, R.N., M.Ed.
Director, Pediatric Disabilities Treatment Center
Providence Hospital
Everett, Washington
LANGUAGE DEVELOPMENT

MAIJA S. LJUNGHAG, R.N., M.S.N., S.N.P.
Assistant Professor
University of Colorado Medical Center and
School Nurse Practitioner
Jefferson County Schools
Lakewood, Colorado
PHYSICAL DEVELOPMENT OF THE SCHOOL-AGE CHILD

IDA M. MARTINSON, R.N., Ph.D., F.A.A.N.
Professor and Director of Research
School of Nursing
University of Minnesota
Minneapolis, Minnesota
DEVELOPMENT OF THE URINARY SYSTEM

BARBARA NEWCOMER McLAUGHLIN, R.N., B.S.N., M.N.
Formerly, Program Nurse Consultant and
District Perinatal Coordinator
Improved Pregnancy Outcome Project
South Carolina Department of Health and Environmental Control
Aiken, South Carolina
FINE MOTOR DEVELOPMENT

SUSAN BLANCH MEISTER, R.N., M.S.N.
Ph.D. Candidate
Clinical Nursing Research

School of Nursing
University of Michigan
Ann Arbor, Michigan
SOCIAL DEVELOPMENT

HOLLY E. MINER, R.N., M.S.N.
University of Massachusetts Medical Center
Worcester, Massachusetts
DEVELOPMENT OF ORGAN SYSTEMS
MATURATION AND GROWTH DEVIATION
  IN THE NEONATE

NANCY L. MORGAN, R.N., B.S.N., M.A.T.
Director, Staff Development
Henrietta Egleston Hospital for Children
Atlanta, Georgia
FINE MOTOR DEVELOPMENT

MARY ALEXANDER MURPHY, R.N., M.S.
Instructor, Department of Pediatrics
School of Medicine
University of Colorado
Denver, Colorado
PHYSICAL ASSESSMENT

VIRGINIA J. NEELON, R.N., Ph.D.
Assistant Professor, Nursing and Physiology
School of Nursing
University of North Carolina
Chapel Hill, North Carolina
DEVELOPMENT OF THE RESPIRATORY SYSTEM

SHERRILYN PASSO, R.N., M.S.N.
Instructor, School of Nursing
Indiana University
Indianapolis, Indiana
DEVELOPMENT OF THE MUSCULOSKELETAL
  SYSTEM

WILMA PETERSON, R.N., Ph.D.
Associate Professor, School of Nursing
University of Oregon Health Sciences Center
Portland, Oregon
GENERAL CONSIDERATIONS OF PHYSICAL
  DEVELOPMENT: GROWTH AND MATURATION

VIRGINIA PIDGEON, R.N., Ph.D.
Associate Professor, College of Nursing
University of Illinois at the Medical Center
Chicago, Illinois
COGNITIVE DEVELOPMENT

LIST OF CONTRIBUTORS **XV**

NANCY REAME, R.N., Ph.D.
Assistant Professor
School of Nursing
Wayne State University
Detroit, Michigan
DEVELOPMENT OF THE REPRODUCTIVE SYSTEM

BEVERLY R. RICHARDSON, R.N., B.S.N.
Child Development Center
University of Tennessee Center for the Health Sciences
Memphis, Tennessee
GROSS MOTOR DEVELOPMENT

JUDITH ANNE RITCHIE, R.N., Ph.D.
Associate Professor, Graduate Program
School of Nursing
Dalhousie University
Halifax, Nova Scotia
DEVELOPMENT OF BODY CONCEPT AND
  CONCEPTS OF ILLNESS AND WELLNESS
PERCEPTION OF BEHAVIORAL COMPETENCY AND
  DEVELOPMENT OF SELF-ESTEEM

MARION H. ROSE, R.N., Ph.D.
Associate Professor
Maternal Child Nursing Department
School of Nursing and
Director, Handicapped Child Care Project
Child Development and Mental Retardation Center
University of Washington
Seattle, Washington
EFFECTS OF PARENTING ON BEHAVIORAL
  DEVELOPMENT
THE PARENT-CHILD RELATIONSHIP

NANCY V. RUDE, R.N., M.S.
Research Associate
School of Nursing
University of Minnesota
Minneapolis, Minnesota
DEVELOPMENT OF THE URINARY SYSTEM

FAY F. RUSSELL, R.N., M.N.
Associate Professor
College of Nursing and
Chief of Nursing, Child Development Center
University of Tennessee Center for the Health Sciences
Memphis, Tennessee
GROSS MOTOR DEVELOPMENT

ANDREA NETTEN SECHRIST, M.S.
   Nutrition Consultant
   Alta California Regional Center
   Sacramento, California
   NUTRITION ASSESSMENT

ANNA M. TICHY, R.N., Ph.D.
   Associate Professor, Maternal-Child Nursing
   College of Nursing
   University of Illinois at the Medical Center
   Chicago, Illinois
   DEVELOPMENT OF THE SENSORY SYSTEM
   DEVELOPMENT OF THE GASTROINTESTINAL SYSTEM

MARY TUDOR, R.N., M.N.
   Clinical Nurse Specialist,
      Developmental Disabilities
   Jefferson County Health Department and
   Division of Developmental Disabilities
   Jefferson County, Washington
   CHILD DEVELOPMENT: WHAT, WHY, WHEN
   DEVELOPMENT OF THE CALVARIUM AND FACE

CARDIOVASCULAR SYSTEM
DEVELOPMENT OF THE INTEGUMENTARY SYSTEM
CONCEPTION THROUGH ESTABLISHMENT OF BODY FORM
DEVELOPMENT OF THE FACE
DYSMORPHOLOGY
FETAL DEVELOPMENT
PRENATAL BEHAVIOR
THE NEONATE: AWAKENING
THE INFANT: OUTWARD AND UPWARD
THE TODDLER: DEMANDING RECOGNITION
THE PRESCHOOL CHILD: "HERE I AM!"
PUBERTY
THE SCHOOL-AGE CHILD: AGE OF ACHIEVEMENT

VERONICA M. LADENSACK YOUNG, R.N., B.S.N., Ph.D.
   Assistant Professor
   School of Nursing
   University of California
   San Francisco, California
   HUMAN GENETICS: BLUEPRINT FOR DEVELOPMENT
   GENERAL CONSIDERATIONS OF PHYSICAL DEVELOPMENT: CELLULAR GROWTH, DIFFERENTIATION, AND MORPHOGENESIS

PREFACE

From its inception, the goal of this textbook has been to present development of the complete child, for it is the undivided child who is the recipient of nursing care. Childhood is defined as beginning with conception and ending with completion of sexual maturation at puberty. Development encompasses *physical and behavioral* change over time. The developmental picture presented is seen as expected or *normal*, the goal for all children in the United States of America. We start with this as a common base in order to understand health as well as variation and deviation.

Physical development is a primary accomplishment of childhood and, yet, developmental anatomy and physiology have been overlooked too long as a major focus of study. This book responds to that void. Morphogenesis, growth, and maturation are critical concepts discussed.

Behavioral development has been a significant component of nursing education for some time, but it is often borrowed from other professions and unrelated to physical development which is the very substrate for increasing adaptive function. The emphasis of this textbook is not to describe developmental milestones plotted against time but to explore why as well as how behavior unfolds. Presentation of motor, cognitive, language, social, and self-help areas completes the picture of the whole child.

Physical and behavioral development are, of course, not separate within the child but are integrated into one phenomenon of change. This change is initiated and directed by the internal and external environment: the genetic legacy, nutrition and health status, self-concept, parenting, and provision of appropriate experiences.

The major goal of presenting the whole child dictated a unique design for a contributed textbook. The development of the child is presented by age group in Chapters 5 through 10 as the embryo and fetus, neonate, infant, toddler, preschool child, and school-age child. Chapters 2, 3, and 4 present theoretical foundations for the age-group chapters and discuss environmental factors which influence development, especially parenting. Chapter 1 presents concepts of nursing practice relative to child development.

The breadth and depth of this textbook could only be obtained by multiple authorship. Each of the 40 authors was selected to write within her area of expertise as reflected in previous publications as well as practice, research, and teaching. Their enthusiasm and competence are evident in the text; these nurse professionals are an inspiration for more in-depth study of specific areas of development. Each chapter, then, is a blending of contributed manuscripts brought together to present a unified framework of development. Each author's topic(s) is noted below her name and credentials in the front of the textbook. In addition, the table of contents lists specific authors and contributed manuscripts.

It is hoped that *Child Development* will be used as a foundation for practice as well as a stimulus for further study. In health maintenance and in treatment of illness and disability, practice based on thorough knowledge of normal development will enable the nurse to provide complete, integrated, and effective care to the total child and to the adult who is the product of his or her childhood.

To avoid a confusion of pronouns, this book consistently refers to the infant, toddler, etc., as *he* and to the nurse as *she*. The former is done for ease of reading and is intended to indicate female and male children. The author and contributors acknowledge the many men who are also active and successful in nursing practice and do not intend to exclude them through the use of the traditional pronoun.

Acknowledgments

This book is the product of the contributors and so thanks must first go to them. Their willingness to write manuscripts to fit into a unified whole made this endeavor possible.

I wish to thank Peg Armstrong, R.N., M.S.; Marie Scott Brown, R.N., Ph.D.; and Sally O'Neil, R.N., Ph.D., who served as ever-patient and always helpful advisors in review of the initial book outlines and final reading of the manuscript.

Peggy Chinn, R.N., Ph.D., professor, school of nursing, Wright State University; Marcene Powell Erickson, R.N., M.N., doctoral candidate, University of Utah; and Mary D. Guthrie, R.N., Ph.D., professor, University of Texas, San Antonio served as final book manuscript reviewers and I am very grateful for their assistance.

I also wish to thank Dr. David W. Smith, professor of pediatrics, school of medicine, University of Washington, Seattle for review of the manuscripts: "Physical Development: Growth and Maturation," "Calvarium and Face," "Dysmorphology," and "Factors Influencing Fetal Growth."

Thanks also goes to the following persons for review and advice in manuscript preparation: Gilbert Gottlieb, psychology laboratory, Dorthea Dix Hospital, Raleigh, North Carolina for review of "Prenatal Behavior;" Joseph L. Harris, M.D., fellow, maternal-fetal medicine, University of California, San Francisco for review of "General Concepts of Prenatal Development," "Development of the Placenta and Fetal Membranes," and "The Fetal Period;" Nancy Reame, R.N., Ph.D., for review of "Gametogenesis;" and Trent D. Stephens, Ph.D., research associate, central laboratory for human embryology, University of Washington, Seattle for review of "Development of the Embryo: Period of Organogenesis."

I am grateful to all who shared words of faith, encouragement, and enthusiasm: you kept me going. Special thanks goes to Randy Jacobs, my husband, who at age 5 created the art on the dedication page; to my parents for their love; to David Carroll, nursing editor; and to Debi Tudor, the only green-faced typist in captivity in the summer of '79.

Finally, special thanks go to the "special" children. The impetus to know normal child development and thus the stimulus for this book is the desire to aid in their development. "I'll help you where you're going while I love you as you are."

Mary Tudor

CHILD DEVELOPMENT

PART ONE

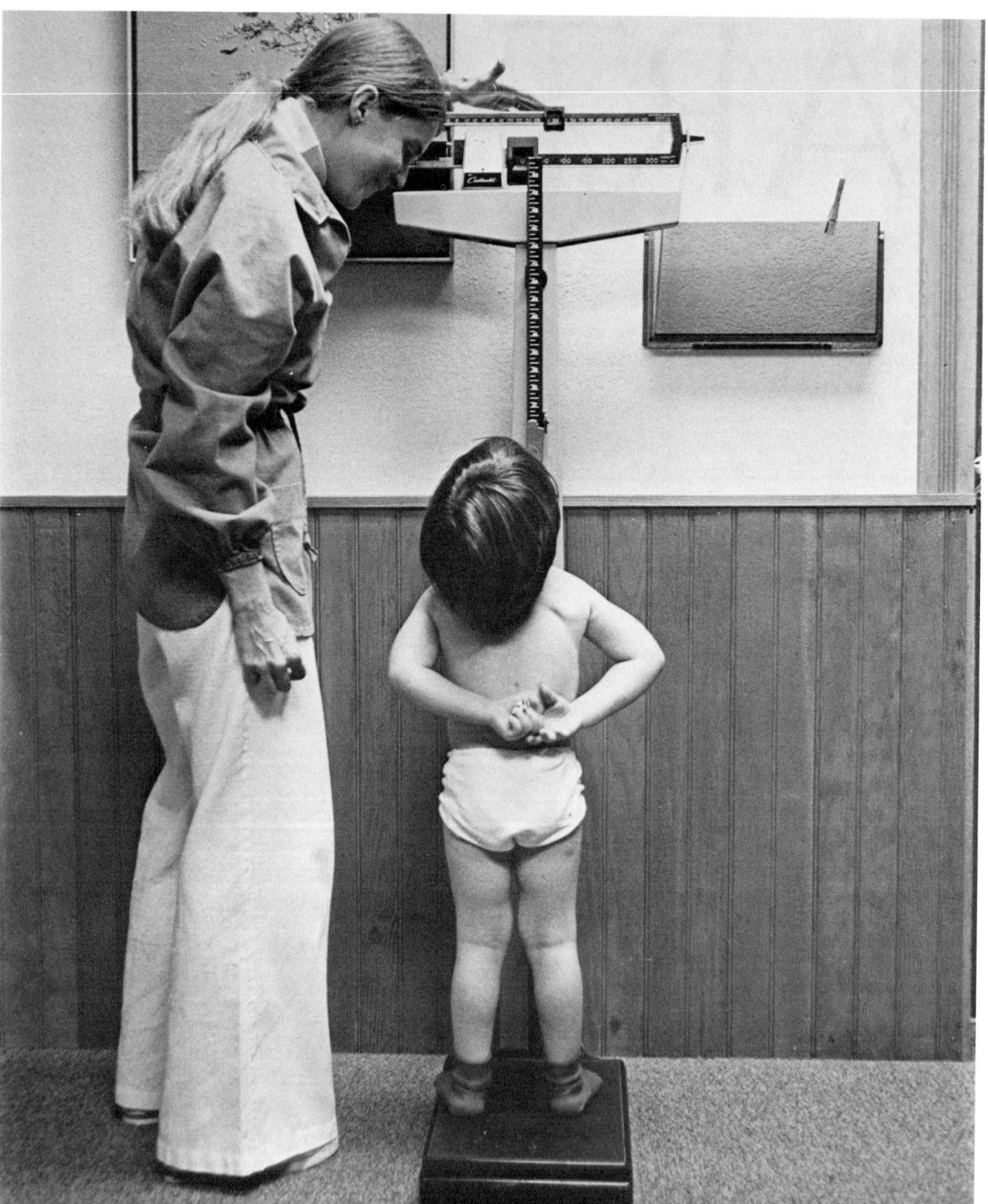

CHAPTER 1

The Nursing Profession and the Developing Child

The nursing role in promotion of child development Kathryn E. Barnard

A PERSPECTIVE ON CHILD-DEVELOPMENT THEORIES

Many theorists have offered notions of how the newborn infant changes to become an independent human being. Some ideas have emphasized the role of *genetic potential,* such as the work of Arnold Gesell (Gesell and Thompson, 1938). As Gesell and his colleagues at Yale University watched children grow, they charted a "natural unfolding" of motor skills, language, and general adaptive behavior. They felt that the general nature of this unfolding was genetically programmed and therefore little could be done to influence the course of development. Gesell set out to prove this in twin studies where one twin was provided motor training for undeveloped skills while the other twin was not trained. The results suggested no effect on eventual attainment of the skill, although the twin with training developed it slightly ahead of schedule.

Other theorists have emphasized the role of the *nurturing environment.* B. F. Skinner (1971) was noted for his research which demonstrated the dramatic influence of reinforcement of behavior to promote and maintain selected behaviors. Sidney Bijou and Donald Baer (1961) are credited with extending the theories of operant conditioning to explain how the child's environment did influence the development of skills and behavior. The young infant learning to verbalize, according to these theories, was influenced by having the sounds he made reinforced either with imitations of the sounds, new sounds, or some other forms of attention. The theories of operant conditioning have been widely applied in developmental studies and found to be highly successful in treating children or adults with developmental problems such as conditions of mental retardation and autism.

A compromise began to emerge in the 1950s and 1960s that focused on an interaction between the genetic potential of the organism and his environment. Jean Piaget's (1953) work on cognitive development typifies this framework. Like Gesell, Piaget based his ideas on detailed observations of children, his own. You can read from his works the precise recordings he made of how his children both acted on and reacted to the events of their environment. Likewise from a psychoanalytic framework, the thinking of Erik Erikson (1950) became popular in explaining the emotional growth of the human being. In describing the first stage, "trust versus mistrust," Erikson cites that the first evidence of the infant's trusting is maintaining an extended sleep period. Emotionally the baby is able to do this when the care giver has repeatedly demonstrated that needs of hunger, warmth, comfort, and attention will be consistently met. Both Piaget and Erikson have had a significant impact on shaping present developmental perspectives.

Just as the predominant perspective in development in the 1960s was basically one of nature-nurture interaction, in the 1970s Michael Lewis and T. Berry Brazelton (Lewis and Rosenblum, 1974) popularized theoretical ideas which suggested that the infant played a much more determining role in shaping his development than previously suspected. Researchers working on infants were proving that the infant was quite capable of seeing, hearing, processing information, and responding. In fact, a whole series of reports were published in 1974 by Michael Lewis and Leonard Rosenblum in *The Effect of the Infant on Its Caregiver.* As these editors point out, the first tasks in understanding the effect of the infant on the care giver are to (1) know the features of each partner and (2) know what happens when they are together.

Currently researchers are studying what naturally occurring behaviors the infant has, such as arousal level, motor activity, and irritability, and how these behaviors are responded to by the care giver. Studies are also in progress which seek to modify the care-giving response and then observe the influence on behavior. As developmental theory has come to place more importance on the child's environment and care giving, the nurse's role has emerged with renewed importance as a force in influencing the health and well-being of children.

It will be important for you as a nurse to think about your perspective of development since the view you have

FIGURE 1-1.

will regulate the questions you ask, the observations you make, and the actions you take. If, for instance, you are convinced that development and health are largely determined by genetic factors, then you would be primarily interested in making assessments of the individual, whereas if you are persuaded that there is an interaction between the organism and the environment, then your assessment strategies must extend to the environment. You should seriously study the past and present theoretical perspectives for yourself. Ask questions of these theories, and in the end elaborate your own developmental perspective. While what will be most useful to you is the personal synthesis you achieve, it is important to have a model to work from. Although the previous theories all have considerable merit, it is well to keep in mind that they have originated from the thinking of biologists, ethologists, psychologists, anthropologists, and/or sociologists. It is natural that their theories are oriented to explaining the phenomena from their perspectives of understanding of the innate behavior of human beings, the social behavior of human beings, and so forth. It is important to introduce additional propositions and assumptions and eventually arrive at theories which are oriented to explaining human development from the perspective of nursing. Nursing seeks to understand human beings in relation to their environment and then learn how this interaction influences health and development.

The area of pediatric nursing has always had a developmental orientation. The writings of Florence Blake in *The Child, His Parents and the Nurse* (1954) clearly describe the importance of the child's environment in influencing subsequent developmental status. Her thinking was greatly influenced by the stages of development and psychoanalytical models. With each developmental stage there are characteristic behaviors, problems, and opportunities. Her stated assumptions went beyond considering the features of the child to considering the environmental context, the developmental tasks, and the care giver's contribution. In speaking about the infant between 3 and 12 months she says, "The infant needs a mother who provides optimal physical health, has respect for the developmental progress and interest in his need to explore and provides the tools he requires for development" (Blake, 1954, p. 119).

This historical tradition in nursing has advanced our thinking and practice so that developmental theories are considered in both general nursing and subspecialty fields. When nursing advances a developmental perspective, it is important for you to remember that this involves an understanding, not only of the individual, the environment, and the care giver, but also of the dynamic interaction between these elements. Human development is a process whereby the individual achieves increasingly complex and integrated functional ability. As studies with prematurely born infants have shown, the infant, due to central nervous system immaturity, lacks basic coordination of sucking, swallowing, and breathing, whereas the mature infant integrates these behaviors and can go beyond this integration to achieve visual and motor integration. This integration continues throughout one's lifetime. Recent life-span orientations, made popular by such publications as Gail Sheehy's *Passages* (1976), speak to this continual process of organized function and stability alternating with a transitional period marked by instability. In striving to promote growth, the nurse must understand the organization and integration of behavior.

ORGANIZATION AND TRANSITIONS IN DEVELOPMENT

Traditionally the theories have directed us to consider the development of major systems, such as the physical, mental, social, and sexual ones. Early studies recorded in *The Measurement of Man* (Harris, Jackson, Paterson, and Scammon, 1930) demonstrate a pattern concerning the velocity of growth in systems. Mental growth, as reflected in both the increase in size and the functional ability of the central nervous system, was shown to be most rapid during the first 4 years. Physical growth occurs rapidly during the first 18 months and then again during pubescence. Growth of sexual organs and function occurs most rapidly at adolescence. The fourth system detailed was the growth of the lymphatic system. This system's growth is quite rapid during the preschool to school years; then there is a decrease in size. The exposure of the child to a larger world of people, and therefore to new organisms, at 3 years is aided by this highly functional lymph system.

Social-behavioral systems have not been thought of as having the same velocity characteristics as the biological systems. We become convinced, however, by observing behavior that the social behavior of the child is highly influenced by his biological time clock. Sigmund Freud developed a stage theory that has been widely accepted: the oral, anal, and phallic stages of psychosexual development. These basic concepts were used by Erik Erikson (1950) in his "eight stages of man" theory. The stage of trust and mistrust relates to Freud's oral stage; the stage of shame versus autonomy and doubt relates to the anal stage. Throughout this book you will be introduced to the specifics of these stages.

THE NURSING ROLE IN PROMOTION OF CHILD DEVELOPMENT 5

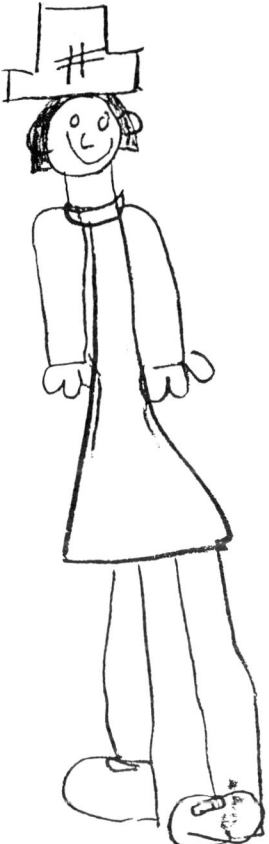

FIGURE 1-2. "Nurse" by Monica, 7 years old.

The reason it is important for you to understand the hallmarks of development is that to understand any one child or group of children you must know what growth and development has been achieved, what is in progress, and what features or tasks are yet to come. You can only make a judgment about the behavior you observe if you are aware of the developmental context. By this is meant whether the developmental phenomena you are observing are well established or just emerging. For instance, if you are observing one 12 month old child walk, you might find that the gait was wobbly and wide-based, while another 12-month-old child walked with smoother, more regulated movements. The functional difference in motor ability in these two children is probably a function of skill development. Sure enough, in obtaining a history from the children's mothers it was established that the first infant had been walking for only 2 weeks, whereas the second child started walking at 10 months. Therefore the better-quality motor coordination in the second child is a result of practice, and the wobbly gait of the first child is from lack of practice. A skilled performance is often the result of well-developed and stable behavior. Poor-quality behavior or highly variable performance is most frequently associated with immaturity.

Parallel to the importance of whether a behavior is developed or emerging is evidence that in the normal course of development not all systems are changing and developing simultaneously or at the same speed. Therefore when the child is putting great effort into fine hand-eye coordination, the changes in language performance may be slower. This is still another reason for understanding the context of the developmental features you are observing. While it requires some memory work to know the basic developmental landmarks in expected weight-length increments, sitting, walking, speaking real words and sentences, riding a tricycle and bicycle, and using self-help skills, you will find this knowledge useful as these landmarks serve to give you a first approximation of where a particular child may be functioning. While these behaviors are influenced by both the genotype and the environmental context, they characteristically occur in orderly sequences, and most normal children demonstrate the skills, given the opportunity. These behaviors are in contrast to behavioral styles that are typical of personality in individuals; for example, some children are more active than others. Thomas, Chess, Birch, and Hertzig (1960), in studies of what makes up personality and hence individual differences, found that these temperament characteristics are relatively stable features of the individual and do not show the same developmental progression as language or motor development. The nine temperament characteristics they identified are quality of mood; activity level; approach-withdrawal from new situations; persistence, or attention span; rhythmicity; distractibility; intensity of response; adaptiveness to new or altered situations; and response threshold.

Therefore, to understand development, the elements you should be aware of are as follows:

- The level of growth and the development of systems that show developmental progression, such as the physical and mental systems
- The tasks of particular developmental periods as they relate to behavioral and social development, such as developing a sense of trust or entering the oral stage
- Whether the observed features are representative of a stable, well-established organization or of an emerging skill

- The consistent, personal characteristics of the individual child, such as general body tempo or activity level
- The environmental context of the child, including his care-giving situation and the amount and type of stimulation he receives
- The functional abilities of the individual in activities of daily living, including eating, sleeping, elimination, locomotion, playing, working, and communicating.

This last element, functional ability, is often referred to as the individual's adaptive capacity, typically a focus for nursing. Most often your purpose in understanding the development of the child will be to assist the child in attaining an optimal functional adaptive capacity.

PROMOTING CHILD DEVELOPMENT

A historic nursing leader, Florence Nightingale (1860), in describing nursing, indicated that the nurse's responsibility was to put the patient in the best condition for nature to act. In stating this belief, she definitely classified herself as an interactional theorist, since this philosophy emphasizes the interaction between the individual organism and the environment. This belief has become a strong part of nursing philosophy. Nursing knowledge is concerned with individual capacities and characteristics and how the environment or nature supports the individual. Contemporary nursing is strongly oriented toward this interactional view of human development and function.

There are many ways that nurses become involved in influencing the development of children. Except for unusual situations where the nurse becomes the child's only care giver, most of the nurse's influence on the child will be in assisting others, primarily the child's family, to provide the nurture and support the child needs to flourish. Nurses are involved in many health-service settings, providing care for children and their families. While it is typical to recognize the nurse's role in the care of the hospitalized child, this is only one example of the many opportunities. Prenatal clinics, parent classes, day-care programs, community-health nursing, schools, and churches are representative of the types of agencies and programs which focus on care of children.

In all these settings the nurse assumes an important role in providing an assessment of the child's development, functional capacities, and care-giving environment. Mary Neal (1977) classifies this nursing function as that of surveillance. In her discussion of nursing as a regulatory process, surveillance is the act of keeping a constant watch and taking a positive action when necessary; this positive action in the Neal construct could be any one of eight regulatory processes: administration, alteration, confrontation, displacement, ministration, modification, negotiation, and reinforcement. How does all this relate to promoting child development, you ask? There is an answer, simple to state and deceptively complex in interpretation. Basically the nurse functions to promote child development by knowing what it is and how it is influenced—by being able to assess the individual child's characteristics and then determine what environmental conditions will best promote optimal integration and organization of that child.

In studies at the University of Washington, nursing researchers have been asking questions about the environmental conditions that will best promote the infant's growth. In the situation where an infant is born before 35 weeks gestational age, the infant's ability to maintain a regular pattern of quiet sleep (i.e., rapid eye movement or REM sleep) is hampered by his central nervous system's immaturity. The higher brain center controls are not well established before 35 to 36 weeks of age, and the infant can characteristically maintain only a short quiet-sleep period. If the baby were still in utero, as nature planned, the mother's activity patterns would serve as regulators of the baby's sleep and activity. For a baby without the maternal regulators and lacking mature central nervous system regulators, can environmental conditions be created which promote the organization of sleep patterns? In a series of experimental studies done since 1970 (Barnard, 1973), the answer is emerging that by providing the infant with a soothing and temporally regulated pattern of stimulation the premature infant's capacity to maintain a pattern of quiet sleep is improved. The mechanism used was a rocking bed built into the incubator and a heartbeat tone, both of which turned on automatically every hour. Providing a comforting stimulus at regularly timed intervals helped the baby shut out other disturbing stimuli and learn to discriminate a repeated and consequently familiar stimulus. With our knowledge of the biological importance of quiet sleep for promoting growth (since growth hormone is produced during that stage of sleep and all body systems function optimally during that stage), we can see how important it is to determine what conditions of the environment could promote sleep. Answers about the appropriate environmental conditions come from understanding how the central nervous system processes information and how repeated, familiar nonarousal stimuli could teach the infant not to attend, or habituate. Barnard's research illustrates that as infants learn to entrain their behavior to the environmental stimuli, optimal sleep patterns are fostered. This typifies how repeatedly you, as a nurse, will be engaged in observing the individual's function and then asking how the environment does or does not assist the individual in maintaining or improving functional ability.

While studies (Barnard and Douglas, 1974; Barnard and Eyres, 1979) have repeatedly shown that the young child's environment is more predictive of later development than information about the child's own development, we are just beginning to understand the specifics of how the environment influences the child. Socioeconomic factors and the educational level of the parents are positively correlated with the child's later cognitive development. These factors, money and education, are not the direct cause of the child's eventual attainment. We are now learning about the specific qualities of the parent-child interaction that are important and the type of stimulation and discipline a child needs. As we understand more of the relationships between the individual child and his environment, we will be in a stronger position to advocate for children. There is increasing certainty that the quality of family life, the parent-child relationships, and the resources available to the family are of critical importance.

There are unfortunately a high percentage of children with health and developmental problems. Chronic illnesses are a fact in the lives of over 25 percent of children under 18 years of age. Respiratory conditions, both chronic and acute, account for the major incidence of illness. In school-age children, over 61 percent of school absences due to illness are caused by respiratory problems. The morbidity and mortality of accidents in children is significant, accounting for further chronic conditions, and a leading cause of death. Other major health and developmental problems include mental retardation, physical handicaps, dental problems, child abuse and neglect, chemical dependency, teenage pregnancies, and lack of communicable-disease immunization (U.S. Department of Health, 1979).

Statistics in the 1970s show that of children born in 1977 over 45 percent will live part of their childhood in one-parent families and that in over 50 percent of those families where a female is the "one parent" the family lives below the poverty level. The incidence of divorce has created more family instability, which adds at least episodic stress to the parents and children. While most children live with their biological parents, approximately 25 percent do not; this represents the need for alternative care giving such as adoption, foster care, and institutional care (U.S. Department of Health, 1979).

Health care of children must address these major problems. The focus must continually be oriented to understanding the factors of the child, parent, and environment that interact to support optimal health.

A major feature found in children and families that thrive is their pattern of relationships. In parent-child interaction the parental qualities that are important are the following:

- Sensitivity to child cues
- Ability to alleviate distress of the child
- Ability to provide social and emotional growth-fostering opportunities
- Ability to provide cognitive growth-fostering opportunities

Likewise, the clarity of the child's cues and the responsiveness of the child to the parent are qualities which are important in fostering the parent-child relationship (Barnard, 1975). Observations of parent-child interaction qualities have shown that when these qualities are present, the relationship thrives and the child demonstrates good mental, motor, and language development.

In families where parents have been identified as abusers, the parents have been observed to be less sensitive to the child's cues and provide a less-than-optimal growth-fostering environment. In these families the child is also less responsive to the care giver, thus indicating how a problem like abuse of the child affects the whole system, the relationship and qualities of the dyad (Nursing Child Assessment, 1979).

The concern for maintaining optimal care giving of children is an important responsibility of the nursing profession. Knowledge about growth and development becomes the basis for optimal care giving. An increasing role for the nurse will be educating parents and health education for school-age children. Nurses will continue to have a vital role in all health programs for children since more than in any other profession the nurses' education prepares them to bridge the link between the biological and social nature of human existence.

8 THE NURSING PROFESSION AND THE DEVELOPING CHILD

The nursing process in provision of services to promote child development Marie Scott Brown

THE NURSING PROCESS
The nurse's role in promotion of healthy child development is really no different from the nurse's role in relation to any other aspect of health or illness. The nursing process (data gathering, assessment, diagnosis, prescription or implementation, and evaluation) is as applicable to this area of practice as to any other.

As in all phenomena of human experience, health can be viewed as a continuum ranging from an optimal sense of well-being to almost complete dysfunction (see Fig. 1-3). Specifically related to development, one end of the continuum can be characterized as the optimally vital growth and unfolding of the child's potential and the other end as stagnation (the most typical example of which is infantile marasmus).

CONSIDERATIONS OF CHILD DEVELOPMENT
There are three concepts to be considered when applying the nursing process to promotion of healthy child development:

- The child's health status and development
- Factors which are currently or potentially hindering this development (both internal and external)
- Factors which are currently or potentially facilitating this development (both internal and external)

Each of these three aspects of development must be considered when working with a child and his family. They are first considered in relation to each area of development and then in relation to the totality of the child's health and development. As knowledge in this field increases, we as nurses become aware of what should be considered. There is a vast and challenging amount of knowledge related to healthy maturation in many aspects of child development: perceptual development, cognitive development, social and emotional development, moral development, artistic development, motor development, neurological development, physical growth, and more.

As the field of child development grows, more data will give more scientific knowledge concerning other areas of normal development (for example, cultural development, development of coping styles, development of interpersonal skills). It is crucial that the nurse working with children keep abreast of current research on these topics.

How the nurse might apply this model to one specific area of development—language—in one child, Alicia, will be examined.

STAGE I: DATA GATHERING

The child's health status and development In the initial stage of the nursing process, data relevant to the above three concepts of the child's development must be gathered. Data gathering is also referred to as assessment in later sections of the text. Data related to the child's actual development can be obtained in two basic ways.

In some cases, data will be collected and recorded in a descriptive fashion when taking and recording health histories. These data yield qualitative data as contrasted to quantitative information about the child. Not only whether he ties his shoes, but how he ties his shoes is

FIGURE 1-3. A model for using the nursing process with child development.

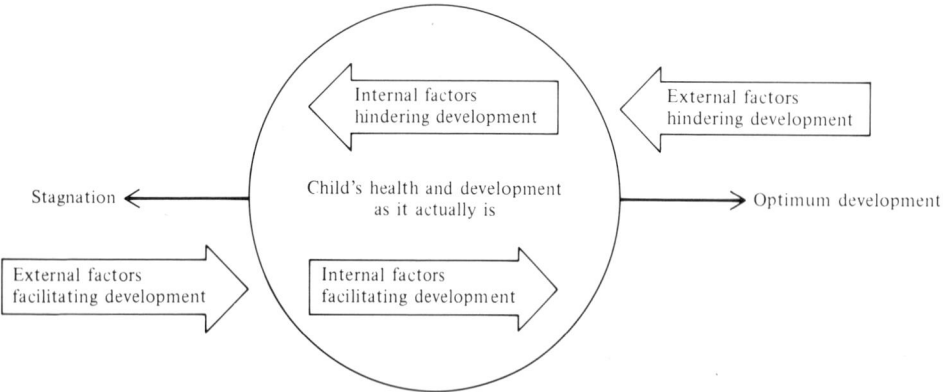

determined. The data are facts about the skills he does have and more importantly facts about what kind of person he is and is becoming. Descriptive data tap areas of his development which the second type of data gathering (standardized tests) cannot: how he copes with stress; his preferences in social interactions; and his style of thinking, responding, and reacting. This type of data gathering has the advantage of being the most holistic approach; however, it needs to be supplemented by the second approach to data gathering, that of using standardized developmental tests.

In standardized tests, only that data are gathered which can then be compared with what is known about many other children of similar chronological age. Examples of this are both the developmental assessment tests, which test specific skills in depth such as perceptual or motor skills, and the more generalized screening tests such as the Denver Developmental Screening Test, which attempts to get a more overall measure of the child's progress. It is important to remember that the vast majority of such screening tests are constructed to detect children who are falling far toward the negative end of the developmental continuum; the purpose of the tests is to detect dysfunctional development rather than to point out ways to foster optimal development. They give little information regarding the quality of the individual child's development but only compare relatively objective measures of development against those of other children. Combining both sources of information is important. The developmental screening tools are useful for early detection of children with relatively severe forms of dysfunctional or nonadaptive behaviors. They are also important because they supply a relatively objective measure of the child's development.

The more descriptive health history is important in rounding out the picture and in helping the individual family to appreciate and facilitate the child's health as well as his unique style of development and to foster the child's maximal potential.

Factors currently or potentially hindering the child's health and development As Fig. 1-3 shows, factors hindering the child's health and development can be both internal and external. Data gathering from both sources is important. Again, data gathering can be done both by a complete, holistic type of health-history interview and by a more objective, but less complete, set of screening tests. As discussed above, it is important to use both to obtain the most information.

The health history must include a discussion of symptoms indicating internal factors that might now or later lead to a less-than-optimum development. This requires a very sound background of physiological and psychosociocultural knowledge. For example, it would be easy, but tragic, to dismiss the young child's symptoms of constant constipation without further investigation if the nurse were not well versed in the signs and symptoms of hypothyroidism. There are also some very important screening tests which can help detect physiological factors that might hinder a child's health and development. Screening tests for poor vision or a hearing deficit, and a variety of laboratory screening tests for other inborn problems (sickle cell disease, phenylketonuria or PKU, anemia) are invaluable for ensuring that internal factors are not overlooked.

The history should also include information related to possible external hindering factors, such as lack of home stimulation, and environmental hazards, for example, lead paint. A few screening tests are available to assess the external environment, in order to discover any factors which might hinder the child's development.

Factors currently or potentially facilitating health and development Similarly, it is important to detect the child's internal and external strengths which will foster development. Whether these are innate strengths, such as intelligence, physical prowess, or musical talents, or whether they are external strengths, such as a strong cultural heritage, extended family, or loving parents, it is important that they be assessed. There are many fewer screening tests available to discover strengths than to determine weakness. Although some, like the Caldwell HOME Inventory, are available, it would seem that development of tools to determine areas of strength is an important area for further investigation by nursing research.

The data-gathering process is demonstrated in a hypothetical case, Alicia, about whose health and development Ms. Gonzales, the nurse, is gathering data. Alicia is a 3-year-old child who obtains well-child care from the nurse. Because the parents are particularly worried about Alicia's language development, the nurse has begun to systematically gather a complete data base about Alicia. Ms. Gonzales uses both a health history and a variety of linguistic screening devices. The health history reveals some important information relevant to Alicia's linguistic development:

1 She is a twin.
2 There is a history of rubella in her mother's fourth

month of pregnancy; otherwise the pregnancy was uneventful.
3 There were no apparent difficulties at delivery.
4 Her growth has been within normal parameters.
5 She has had no major illnesses or hospitalizations.
6 Her diet is basically adequate but low in sources of calcium.
7 Her family is bilingual.
8 She interacts with few other children except her twin brother. They have a language of their own: the two of them can understand each other, but no one else can understand them.
9 She can, however, speak English and German, both of which are entirely understandable to her parents.

A complete physical examination is carried out. In addition, the screening tests the nurse chooses to do in this situation are the following:

- An audiometric sweep test to gather data about any possible internal problems which might hinder her language development. This was particularly important because of the question of rubella in the pregnancy.
- The Peabody Picture Vocabulary Test to determine her English vocabulary at this time and to get an estimate of intelligence (an internal factor which might facilitate or inhibit her language ability).
- A Denver Articulation Screening Exam to gather data about how developmentally appropriate her articulation is at this time.
- The Caldwell HOME Inventory to gather data about factors in the home environment which might facilitate or inhibit language development.

STAGE II: ASSESSMENT OF THE DATA

Once these data are gathered, they are assessed. The data-gathering process is simply that: gathering data; in the assessment process, the nurse takes these data and analyzes and synthesizes the information into a more complete picture of the child's health and function in particular areas of development. This is where the assessment model is helpful (see Fig. 1-4). The results of each test are computed, and information elicited in the health history is evaluated against the nurse's knowledge of physical and psychosociocultural factors relevant to language development.

In considering Alicia's language development, it is recognized that bilingualism is a disadvantage because it means that fewer words in a specific language are spoken; however, it is also an advantage. Because of Ms. Gonzales' knowledge base, she knows that most bilingual children have a larger number of total words and a broader scope of thought process since they have experiences in two psycholinguistic worlds.

Not only are the strengths and weaknesses in each specific area of development weighed against and compared with each other, but the areas of development are related to one another so that a picture of the whole child and his relationship to his environment emerges. The facts related to linguistic development are assessed in relation to all other types of development.

In assessing Alicia's language development, Ms. Gonzales found that Alicia's articulation skills as measured by the Denver Articulation Screening Exam are age appro-

FIGURE 1-4. Alicia's language development.

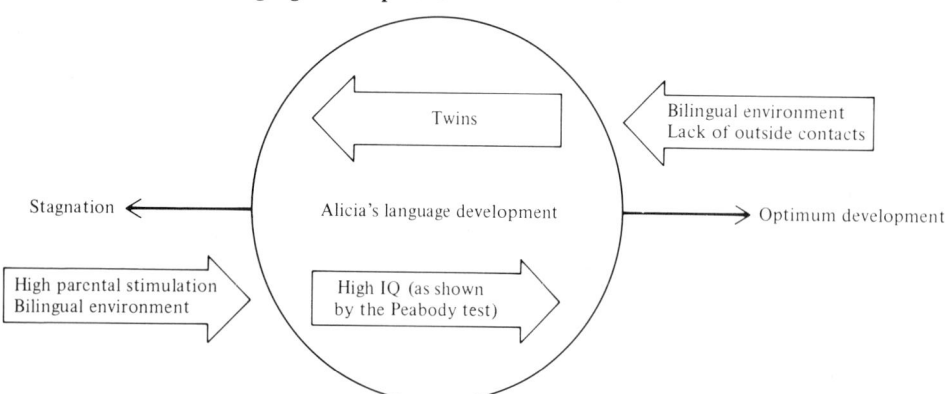

priate. Her vocabulary in English is comparable to an average 2½-year-old's, but her syntax development was advanced for her age. The Caldwell HOME Inventory indicated that her home environment was appropriate in providing the stimuli necessary for her optimal development. Ms. Gonzales diagramed her assessment as shown in Fig. 1-4.

STAGE III: DIAGNOSIS
Once the data have been gathered and assessed, it is important that a decision be made; this decision is the nursing diagnosis. It is not merely a statement that the child is delayed or advanced in acquisition of a particular developmental skill. Rather it is a statement indicating where this child is on the continuum of development in relation to where his potential could allow him to be.

In the case of Alicia, for example, the nurse decided that the development of language was appropriate at this time; no delay was indicated, even though the vocabulary test alone indicated a lag. The nurse was able to make this decision because she had the data from the other tests and from the health history. Especially important was the nurse's knowledge about language development of bilingual children, specifically vocabulary attainment, and how it differs from that of monolingual children. The diagnosis also included determining which of the factors in the external and internal environment were or were not helpful in moving Alicia toward a higher level of functioning. These decisions are indicated by the arrows shown in the model applied to Alicia's linguistic development (see Fig. 1-4). These diagnoses are crucial to the next stage, the prescription.

STAGE IV: PRESCRIPTION
This step in the nursing process involves making a decision about what should or should not be changed in the diagnosis and how that should be done. The prescription (or nursing intervention) is arrived at jointly by the nurse and the family. In the case of Alicia, Ms. Gonzales chose to prescribe some changes in the environmental factors and not to change, but to support, others. Her prescription involved the following:

1 Recommending that the parents provide opportunities for Alicia to socialize with children other than her twin
2 Giving the parents feedback on the very stimulating environment they were providing to Alicia and explaining how this was important to her linguistic development
3 Reassuring them that although bilingualism might be viewed as a detriment to attaining vocabulary in the early years, this disadvantage could be offset by other advantages
4 Recommending dietary changes to increase calcium intake, necessary for normal growth. Alicia's family agreed with all four prescriptions.

STAGE V: EVALUATION
The nursing process requires that the nursing prescription and/or intervention and the results be evaluated. In the case of Alicia, Ms. Gonzales asked the family to return in 3 months to repeat the data-gathering process (both the health history and the screening tests) so that she and the parents could mutually evaluate the results of the steps taken.

This is an overview of the nurse's role in relation to the child's healthy development—a role of data gathering, assessing, diagnosing, prescribing, and evaluating. The following chapters will provide a knowledge base necessary to carry out the nursing process with children as they develop.

Child development: What, why, when
Mary Tudor

Child development is a concept that is understood by all, defined by many, and agreed upon by few. Knowingly adding to a substantial selection of differing definitions, another viewpoint is presented, encompassing many of these definitions, as the orientation to this textbook.

WHAT
To begin, a translation of child development is offered. These themes are seen in observation of children and recur in the literature describing them:

Child = activity
Development = change

These two concepts can be considered the first question, the "what" of child development, and initiate the composition of a true definition. The child as activity personified and development as a change process are areas of study in this textbook.

WHY
The "why" of child development (also the "how") relates to the third and fourth areas of study of the textbook: the genetic basis and the environmental support and modifi-

cation. Why does a child develop? What is the stimulus for this progression? At this stage of the science, the nature-nurture controversy is behind us. The need to ask, "Which commands development?" has been set aside. Credit is given to both factors in percentages depending on the background of the creditor, and the debate goes on. However, it is not simply a matter of dual domination but of the impact of a complex interaction.

Both the directing force of heredity and the molding influences of environment play important roles in development. These two factors are, however, unlike in quality. Actually, both are components of a common interacting system, and to argue which is the more important is meaningless. To weigh the value of one against the other is to lose sight of the integrated process of development as a whole; each is essential and important. All of the developmental effects are produced cooperatively by interactions between genic and environmental factors. (Arey, 1965, pp. 6–7)

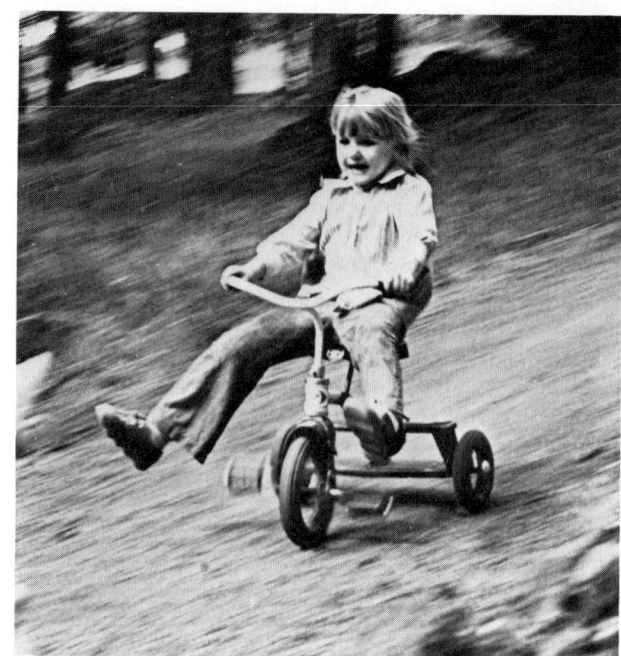

FIGURE 1-5. (*Courtesy of Betsy Smith.*)

WHEN

And finally, the "when": The time frame or duration of development is asked. Human development is a continuum beginning at conception and stopped by death. Child development, as presented in this text, begins at conception and ends with passage through puberty and into another era: adolescence.

ACTIVITY CREATES CHANGE

The essence of childhood is dynamic: activity, dissipating energy. To paraphrase biologists (Berrill and Karp, 1976), the child is not an object; he is a happening. The futility of describing an energetic happening in static, lifeless, ink-on-paper words is apparent. However, these words will hopefully cause recall of past observations of children in their daily lives and stimulate further observations. Through these images and observations, the reader can then capture the essence of the concepts described in the text.

"Developmental changes are a product of the child's activity" (Mussen, Conger, and Kagan, 1974, p. 37). Four concepts are presented relating to qualities of this activity or energy of childhood as it creates change (see Table 1-1). The first concept is that the activity or energy is progressive, resulting in evolutionary change. This is perhaps the essence of the concept of development. Development is an upward spiral; the child is constantly becoming. "As structures or processes grow or evolve, new totalities come into being not only by a simple adding together of what has been present and observable before but also by a creation of truly novel items which have genuinely new properties" (Carmichael, 1970, p. 449).

The second concept is that the activity is directed; the energy follows a course. Although the source of this energy continues to be unidentified, the progression is recognized. Directed activity results in systematic change.

TABLE 1-1 Child development concepts

Activity	Change
Progressive	Evolutionary
Directed	Systematic
Constant	Predictable
Variable	Unique

Spatial direction of the developmental change is a familiar concept and generally holds true across all development. It is as follows:

Cephalad to caudad
Ventral to dorsal
Proximal to distal

The systematic changes in the child follow, according to these directional "laws."

The third concept of activity is its constancy resulting in a predictable pattern of change. Children are similar in their development relative to each other and across the continuum of time. If this were not so, this book could not have been written.

Fourth, in contrast to but standing with the above, the activity of childhood and thus development is variable from child to child and is also variable from time to time in the same child. Thus, there are no absolutes but a range in the predictability. This *variability* of activity results in the unique pattern of development of every child.

> In a given (characteristic), such as height, or intelligence, a child may, over a period of years, shift from high to average, to low, and back to average again, as compared to his age peers. The very frequency of these shifts leads us to assume that, for the most part, they are normal and healthy patterns of growth. . . . We find that individual patterns are the rule. (Bayley, 1956, p. 45)

CHANGE THAT IS DEVELOPMENT

The primary purpose of this textbook is to describe the developing child as a whole. The reason is clear: The nursing profession is responsible, in its application of knowledge and skills, to the whole child and to the adult who is the product of his childhood.

This description, considered above as the what, why, and when of child development, involves material covering many scientific areas of development, primarily the organismic (embryology, developmental physiology) and the behavioral, or psychological. The organismic sciences are concerned primarily with structure and function, formation, evolution, and reproduction of the organism, in this case the human. The behavioral sciences are interested in the integrated activity (behavior) of the human. The sciences of human genetics and ecology also come into play as the forces programming and directing human development.

To pull all these sciences and their concepts into a unifying whole recognizable as the developing child is the endeavor of these nurse authors. The problem of the endeavor is obvious: "The organism as a whole, though clearly recognizable, is practically indefinable" (Berrill and Karp, 1976, p. 3). Describing a whole without naming its parts might be compared to attempting to sing a song in one tone.

However, the alternative reductionist tack of identifying parts in order to describe this change that is child development reduces it to somewhat less than it is. "The properties of the whole emerge as a result of the organization of the parts, the whole being neither comprehensible nor predictable from knowledge of the individual parts" (Berrill and Karp, 1976, p. 3).

DEVELOPMENT: PHYSICAL AND BEHAVIORAL

With recognition of this unresolvable conflict, development is described as two equally important, interacting, and indivisible components:

Physical development
Behavioral development

Remember, however, that "we cannot separate mind and body, structure and function. They are inextricably woven into the system" (Gordon, 1977, p. 9).

For every behavior there is a physiological substrate, a physical effector. "Every psychological occurrence is itself a biological occurrence, that is, it is correlated with organismic events" (Bijou and Baer, 1961, pp. 9–10). Conversely, behavior directly affects and modifies physical status and well-being:

Physiology ↔ behavior

More than that, physiological substance *is* behavior; behavior *is* physiological substance.

Physiology ⇄ behavior

Of course, behavior has an effect on further behavior; physiological events result in physiological events.

Physiology ⇄ behavior

Even these diagrams do not fully describe the participatory effect of one on the other, which is inescapable. This

14 THE NURSING PROFESSION AND THE DEVELOPING CHILD

theory of the active, developing child is schematically presented in Fig. 1-6.

PHYSICAL DEVELOPMENT

Physical development is integrated differentiation and growth leading to maturation and eventually to aging. Physical development of the child occurs on seven levels. The levels of physical development are the following:

- Intracellular (chromosomal)
- Intercellular
- Tissue
- Organ
- System
- Body segment
- Whole body

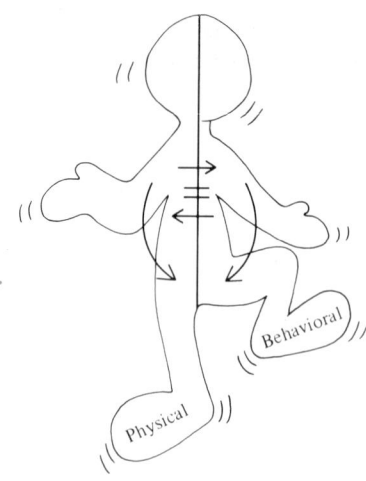

FIGURE 1-6. Schematic representation of the developing child as activity and interaction of physical and behavioral development.

Changes on every level affect every other level. As noted above, those changes resulting in development are genetically programmed and environmentally produced and molded.

Physical development begins at conception; a majority of it is completed by birth. This textbook presents embryological as well as postnatal physical development, encompassing five processes of physical development which occur on all seven levels. These processes are as follows:

- Differentiation
- Growth
- Integration
- Maturation
- Aging

Differentiation Differentiation, genetically directed, takes place on two levels. *Histogenesis* is differentiation of cellular structure and function resulting in cell specialization. Histogenesis leads to *morphogenesis*, which is defined as progressive attainment of structures and bodily form. Through differentiation the zygote becomes the highly complex neonate; he is larger, yes, but also entirely changed.

Growth Growth is quantitative change, an increase in size. Growth occurs through two processes generally observed at the cellular level: *hyperplasia*, increase in cell number, and *hypertrophy*, increase in cell size. Growth also occurs as increase in amount of intercellular material. Although most growth results in increase in size, regrowth occurs in renewal, repair, and regeneration, a necessary component of the developmental process.

Growth of the child is differential, thus giving form and change in form. Falkner and Tanner, considering the processes of growth and differentiation as one, state, "Differential growth creates form: external form through growth rates which vary from one part of the body to another and one tissue to another; and internal form through the series of time-entrained events which build up in each cell the specialized complexity of its particular function" (1978, p. ix).

Both growth and differentiation follow the rules of cephalad to caudad, proximal to distal, and ventral to dorsal. However, there are some known exceptions to these rules. One is that, in the central nervous system, lower brain centers are dominant at the time of birth; higher centers gradually assume control. Also, in skeletal growth during late childhood, the distal portions of the limbs enter the growth spurt of puberty before the proximal portions.

Integration The processes of growth and differentiation must be integrated. Without the integrative processes of developmental change, a harmonious whole would not result. In addition, integration of the seven physiological levels must occur. Primary responsibility for this integration originates in the genetic code. Ongoing integration on a higher level is the result of endocrine and nervous system activity.

Maturation Maturation, the fourth process of physical development, in one sense encompasses the previous three. It also refers to elaboration of the form and function which resulted from growth and differentiation. Prenatally, the embryonic systems move from a prefunctional to a functional state. In postnatal development, a continuing increase in efficiency results from maturational change in the developing child. Maturation describes the qualitative changes which occur after morphogenesis is completed (prenatally) in harmony with the quantitative changes of growth.

Aging Ironically, aging and cell death are integral to the change process of development. In the embryological period, cell death is necessary for morphogenesis. Tissues and structures of the developing child age and die: epithelial lining of the intestines, epidermis, hair, and nails. Yet in comparison with the other process of development, aging plays a minor role until full maturity is reached.

Change from physical processes Physical development, the change which occurs through these processes, is (as noted above) evolutionary, systematic, predictable, and unique. The changes, in more detail, are as follows:

- Less to more specialized
- Smaller to larger
- Simple to more complex
- Less to more organized
- Less to more efficient
- More to less "plastic," or malleable

Exceptions to this description will be reviewed where appropriate in following sections.

BEHAVIORAL DEVELOPMENT

Behavioral development is the attainment and integration of skills leading to independent, adaptive functioning. As physical development is said to occur on seven physiological levels, behavioral development is likewise described in six functional areas:

- Motor: gross motor and fine motor
- Cognitive
- Language
- Perceptual
- Social-emotional
- Self-help

Like the seven physiological levels, the areas of behavioral development in the developing child are not independent or discreet. Behavior in any area is causal to, affected by, and an indicator of behavior in any other area. Division is strictly for the purpose of discussion, as evidenced by the many alternative divisions: perceptual-motor, psychosocial, psychomotor, fine motor–adaptive, and others. This division is only a means to an end for study of child development.

Physical development is discussed first for the reason that, on the whole, it precedes and allows behavioral development. "Behavior is rooted in the brain and in the sensory and motor systems" (Knobloch and Pasamanick, 1960, p. 3). This is most clearly demonstrated in the discussion of prenatal behavior.

Reflecting this physiological basis, four processes of behavior development can be seen as theoretically similar to those of physical development. They are the following:

- Growth
- Differentiation
- Maturation
- Integration

"Growth" of behavioral skills In comparative observations of an infant and a preschool child, one notes a quantitative increase in motor, language, and all other skills. This view of quantitative increase in adaptive functioning is a simplistic, but important, first consideration. It is an initial characterization of basic change that occurs with behavioral development. The older child *can*, in a sense, do *more*. (As a 4-year-old child said about his infant sibling, "He don't even do nutten'.") On closer observation, one notes that, rather than simple change in one dimension, behavioral development involves integrated and qualitative change, which is inherent in this increase in skills. Definition of any one absolute "skill," however, will vary among observers.

Differentiation Qualitative change occurs through behavioral differentiation. Through development of form and structure, behavior becomes less restricted and more diversified and elaborated. Differentiation leads to the evolution of more complex, adaptive functioning. It is differentiation of behavior and increasing specialization that is studied most often by the child-development student.

Maturation Maturation of the basic, differentiated form of behavior is movement from predominantly reflexive to voluntary behavior, refinement and elaboration of higher levels of functioning, and establishment of objectives and goals for behavior leading to eventual independence. Differentiation of skills dominates in younger children; maturation of behavior may also begin early but is notable in late childhood and through maturity.

Integration The above processes leading to adaptive functioning are not possible without their integration by the central nervous system. Behavioral skills are integrated, resulting in a different structure of performance. Integration involves all body systems and parts in addition to all areas of development.

Behavioral development, the change which occurs through these processes, is also evolutionary, systematic, predictable, and unique. Looking at this change, eight descriptors emerge:

- Less skilled to more skilled
- Reflexive to volitional
- Random to purposeful
- General to specific
- Gross to refined
- Simple to complex
- Homogenous to heterogenous
- Ineffectual to effectual

ENVIRONMENTAL IMPACT

Although the above section may appear to define child development adequately, it does not. "Development is a process of transaction between organism and environment" (Gordon, 1974, p. 4). Thus, all developmental processes in both physical and behavioral realms must be considered within their environmental context, both animate and inanimate, internally and externally applied.

Genetic control guarantees variability as well as sameness in children; however, the environment is the great modifier—the great unequalizer. The environment impacts on physical development and on behavioral development; more accurately, it impacts on the interactive processes of physiological processes and behavior.

The general growth of structure and function always occurs in an organism that is in an environment. Organisms do not live or grow in a physical or biological vacuum. From the first cell division in the developing individual, each process of structural and functional modification is, moreover, to be considered as a complex resultant of activities. Some of these determinants are intrinsic in the cell and are, indeed, in the correct sense of the term hereditary, but such intrinsic determinants always act in a dynamic system which is also a resultant of these two sets of forces working interdependently. (Carmichael, 1970, p. 533)

The environment provides fuel for development: food, maintenance of health and prevention of disease, oppor-

FIGURE 1-7. Schematic representation of the developing child and the major influences on development. The genetic basis for development comes from the child's parents. Environmental input—both negative and positive, animate (parents) and inanimate (represented by sun, cloud, and rain)—molds the child's development. The child, seen as active and changing, in turn influences the environment, animate and inanimate.

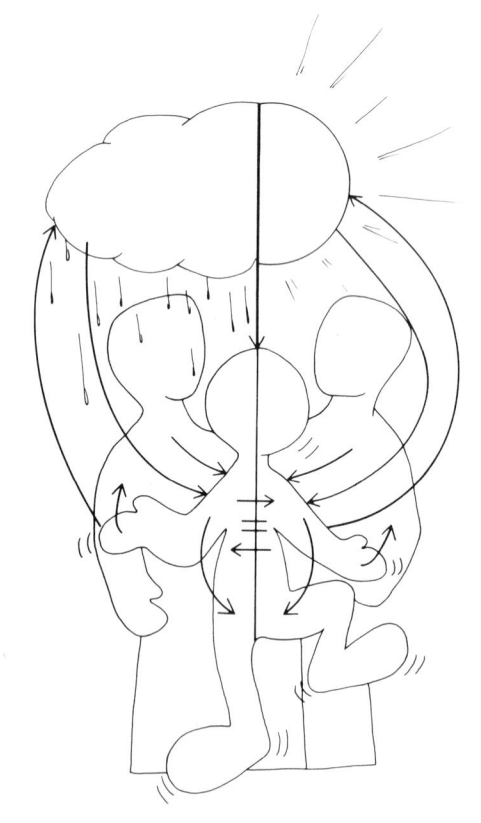

tunities for mobility, positive parenting, social and cultural input, sensory stimulation, and provision of tools. The environment allows, enables, and creates development. However, the environment can also prevent, hinder, and destroy development. Thomas and Chess, following the work of L. J. Henderson, describe the positive-negative continuum of environmental effect, "goodness of fit" between child and environment.

> Goodness of fit results when the properties of the environment and its expectations and demands are in accord with the organism's own capacities, characteristics, and style of behaving. When this *consonance* between organism and environment is present, optimal development in a progressive direction is possible. Conversely, poorness of fit involves discrepancies and *dissonances* between environmental opportunities and demands and the capacities and characteristics of the organism, so that distorted development and maladaptive functioning occur. (1977, p. 11)

As the environment impinges on the child, the child also seeks environmental input. As the child is changed by the environment, the environment is changed by the child. Illustrated in Fig. 1-7 are these concepts.

The process of child development, physical and behavioral, in all its numerous facets, beginning in and directed by biochemical messages from the genes of one cell and molded by all aspects of the environment over time, results in an independent, skilled, and biologically efficient human being.

Bibliography

THE NURSING ROLE IN PROMOTION OF CHILD DEVELOPMENT

Barnard, K. E.: The effect of stimulation on the sleep behavior of the premature infant. In M. V. Batey (Ed.), *Communicating nursing research* (Vol. 6). Boulder, Colorado: Western Interstate Commission for Higher Education, 1973.

―――: Trends in nursing care and prevention of developmental disabilities. *Amer. J. Nurs.*, October 1975.

――― and H. B. Douglas (Eds.): *Child health assessment part 1: A literature review.* U.S. Department of Health, Education, and Welfare Publication No. 1741-00082, 1974.

――― and S. J. Eyres (Eds.): *Child health assessment part 2: The first year of life.* U.S. Department of Health, Education, and Welfare Publication No. 017-041-00131-9, 1979.

Bijou, S. W., and D. M. Baer: *Child development* (Vol. 1). New York: Appleton-Century-Crofts, 1961.

Blake, F. G.: *The child, his parents and the nurse.* Philadelphia: Lippincott, 1954.

Brazelton, T. B.: Neonatal behavior assessment scale. *National Spastics Society Monograph.* London: Heinemann, 1974.

―――, B. Koslowski, and M. Main: The origins of reciprocity: The mother-infant interaction. In M. Lewis and L. A. Rosenblum (Eds.), *The effect of the infant on its caregiver.* New York: Wiley, 1974.

Erikson, E. H.: *Childhood and society.* New York: Norton, 1950.

Gesell, A., and H. Thompson: *The psychology of early growth.* New York: Macmillan, 1938.

Harris, J. A., C. M. Jackson, D. G. Paterson, and R. E. Scammon: *The measurement of man.* Minneapolis: University of Minnesota Press, 1930.

Lewis, M., and L. A. Rosenblum (Eds.): *The effect of the infant on its caregiver.* New York: Wiley, 1974.

Neal, M. (Ed.): A conceptual basis for maternal child health nursing practice. *Proceedings of a Perinatal Conference, University of Maryland, March, 1976.* Baltimore: University of Maryland, School of Nursing, 1977.

Nightingale, F.: *Notes on nursing: What it is, and what it is not.* New York: Appleton, 1860.

Nursing Child Assessment Satellite Training: *NCAST project report.* (Unpublished manuscript, University of Washington, School of Nursing, 1979.)

Piaget, J.: *The origins of intelligence in the child.* London: Routledge, 1953.

Sheehy, Gail: *Passages.* New York: Bantam, 1976.

Skinner, B. F.: *Beyond freedom and dignity.* New York: Bantam, 1971.

Thomas, A., H. Birch, S. Chess, and M. E. Hertzig: A longitudinal study of primary reaction patterns in children. *Compr. Psychiat.*, 1960, *1* (2), 103–112.

U.S. Department of Health, Education, and Welfare, *Health, United States 1978.* U.S. Department of Health, Education, and Welfare Publication No. (PHS) 78-1232, 1979.

CHILD DEVELOPMENT: WHAT, WHY, WHEN

Arey, L. B.: *Developmental anatomy.* Philadelphia: Saunders, 1965.

Bayley, N.: Individual patterns of child development. *Child Develop.*, 1956, *27*, 45–74.

Berrill, N. J., and G. Karp: *Development.* New York: McGraw-Hill, 1976.

Bijou, S. W., and D. M. Baer: *Child development I; A systematic and empirical theory.* New York: Appleton-Century-Crofts, 1961.

Carmichael, L.: Onset and early development of behavior. In P. H. Mussen (Ed.), *Carmichael's manual of child psychology* (Vol. I). New York: Wiley, 1970.

Falkner, F., and J. M. Tanner: *Human growth 1, Principles and prenatal development.* New York: Plenum, 1978.

Gordon, I. J.: *Human development, a transactional perspective.* New York: Brunner/Mazel, 1977.

Henderson, L. J.: *The fitness of the environment.* New York: Macmillan, 1913.

Horowitz, F. D.: *Review of child development research.* Chicago: University of Chicago Press, 1975.

Knobloch, H., and B. Pasamanick: Environmental factors affecting human development before and after birth. *Pediatrics,* 1960, *26,* 210–218.

—— and ——: *Gesell and Amatruda's developmental diagnosis* (3d ed.). Hagerstown, Maryland: Harper & Row, 1974.

Mussen, P. H., J. J. Conger, and J. Kagan: *Child development and personality.* New York: Harper & Row, 1974.

Thomas, A., and S. Chess: *Temperament and development.* New York: Brunner/Mazel, 1977.

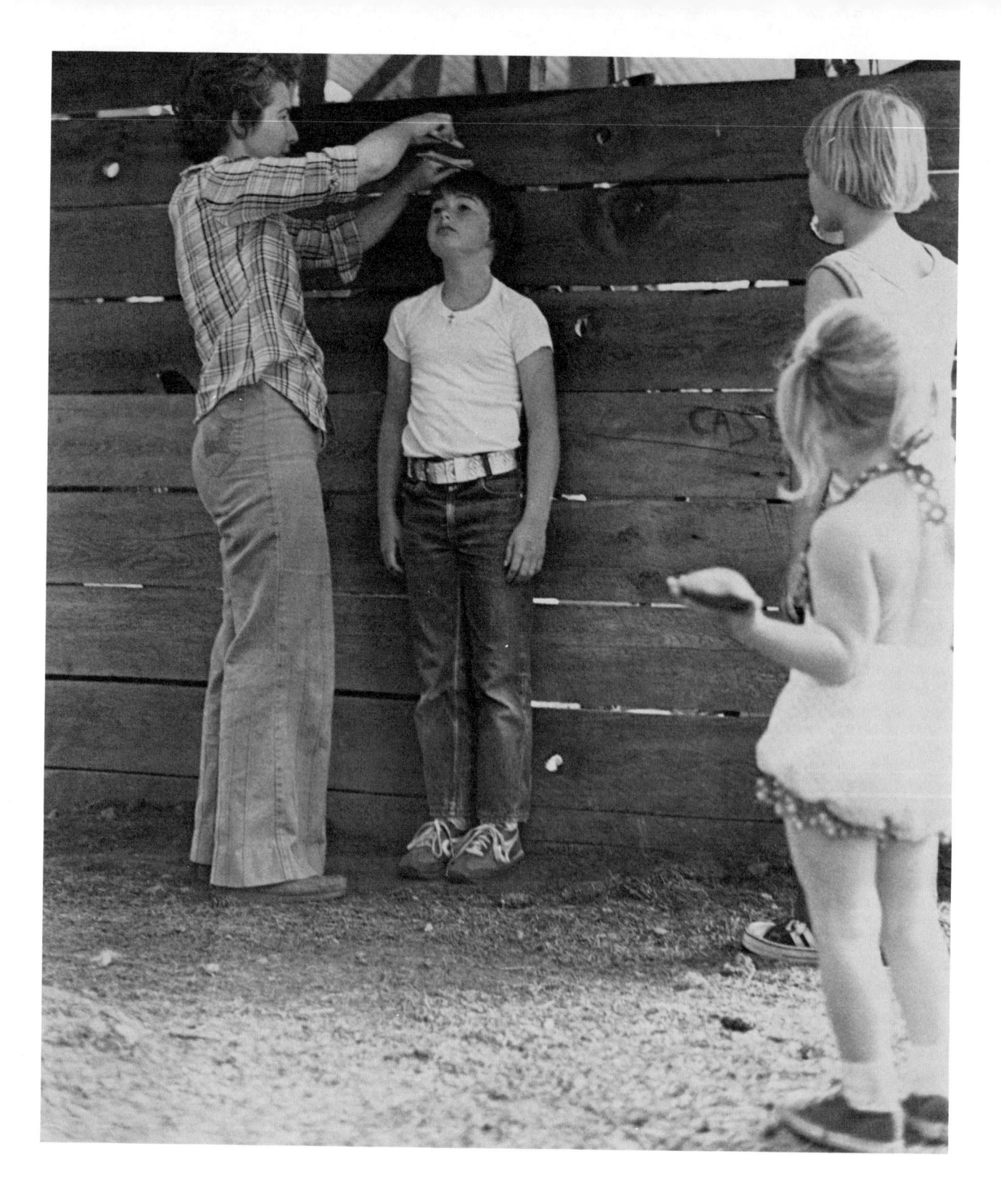

CHAPTER 2
Physical Development

SECTION 1

Processes of Physical Development

Physical development, a major task of childhood, is defined as integrated differentiation and growth leading to maturation and enabling independent function. The blueprint for physical development is found in the genotype. Through the developmental processes of differentiation, growth, and maturation the one-cell zygote is directed in its transformation into a mature individual. The processes and principles governing these changes are presented in this chapter.

General considerations of physical development: Growth and maturation — Wilma Peterson

INTRODUCTION

Physical growth is defined as increase in cell size and number resulting in enlarged mass. It has the distinct quality of lending itself to measurement. Maturation, however, implies changes in function, generally toward a more complex level. Because these two processes proceed simultaneously and are so intricately related, they are regarded as a unit implying magnitude and quality of physical development.

Growth in length, or height, and weight is a sensitive reflection of the normalcy, health, and well-being of an individual child or the population at large. It has been noted that larger mothers generally have larger infants who are better equipped for life. This asset coupled with quality nutrition and continued good health allows the child to reach genetic potential. Measurement of growth in height reflects these hereditary traits and may also be used to indicate problems of a chronic nature.

Weight reflects acute changes, but its values are difficult to interpret since all tissues are included. Head circumference is an indicator of the size and growth of the brain. The majority of brain growth and growth of associated structures occurs prenatally and in the first 2 years of postnatal life. This indicates the significance of the need for quality nutrition and health maintenance during this critical time of development.

PRINCIPLES OF PHYSICAL DEVELOPMENT

Growth in the healthy child is individualized. It is an intrinsically complex, highly organized, and regulated process. Because of these qualities, it is a valuable index of health and well-being. The physiological basis for growth is determined by genetic factors, which are integrated by all systems of the body and influenced by the environment.

Five phenomena of physical development have been identified: *canalization, heterochronism, compensatory growth, sensitive periods,* and *homeostasis.* These phenomena form a foundation for understanding growth and maturation.

FIGURE 2-1. *(Photo courtesy of Betsy Smith.)*

CANALIZATION

The child's growth pattern has been likened to the trajectory of a rocket (Tanner, 1963). The control system is the individual's genetic endowment, and this is empowered by the environment. An adverse environment, such as acute malnutrition or severe illness, deflects the child from his trajectory, retarding growth.

However, a restorative force develops as soon as adequate nutrients are consistently provided or recovery from the disease occurs (see Fig. 2-2). Initially the growth rate is rapid, as the growth pattern returns to its original curve. The growth rate then decreases progressively so that when growth reaches its regular pattern, the rate is adjusted to the original path (Tanner, 1963).

The term canalization is used to describe the tendency of growing organisms to return to their original genetically determined path of growth once the cause of the deviation has been corrected. The term catch-up growth refers to the rapid growth which returns the child to the original growth curve (Prader, Tanner, and vonHarnack, 1963).

Though the mechanisms of canalization are poorly understood, certain factors relating to the phenomenon have been established, and there is evidence to suggest other important relationships. It has been established that female children are better canalized than males and show less growth retardation as a result of malnutrition or disease. It appears that the principle of canalization applies to brain growth and the development of mental ability, particularly at the time that the brain is developing rapidly.

The phenomenon of catch-up growth occurs physiologically following the transitory weight loss seen in the neonatal period. It has been noted to be greater for small than for large infants, and though it involves both length and weight, it probably is greater in terms of length. Fetal growth is controlled by uterine factors. This allows a female of only average or small size to give birth to an infant genetically programmed for largeness. Catch-up growth permits this child to establish his genetically determined percentile ranking (channel) during infancy if provided an environment conducive to growth. The genetically small child needs little or no catch-up growth in the neonatal period, while the constitutionally large child requires a greater degree of catch-up growth to reach his growth channel. (This process is discussed in more detail in Chap. 8.)

Malnutrition studies with newborn rats demonstrate that in this animal model there are critical periods of rapid growth. When early starvation is induced followed by adequate feeding, the growing rat pups respond with a degree of catch-up growth but never reach full adult size. Starvation induced following weaning does not alter adult size (Widdowson, Mavor, and McCance, 1964; Widdowson and McCance, 1960). Because of the short gestational period of the rat, it has been inferred that this period of severe malnutrition can be compared to starvation in utero in the human.

This supports the finding that some full-term neonates with abnormally low birth weight and length fail to catch up after birth and remain small throughout life. However, most small-for-gestational-age infants show catch-up growth postnatally. It therefore appears that the degree of catch-up growth is influenced by both the normal rate of growth for the individual at the time of the insult and the duration of the undernutrition. This suggests that the amount of unmet growth potential is critical to the outcome.

During catch-up growth there is uniform increase of body size consistent with chronological age implying that the stimulus to growth is systemic. It has been postulated that the signal to initiate or arrest growth may arise in the hypothalamus. It in turn activates or inhibits pituitary secretion of somatotropin (growth hormone), adrenocorticotropic hormone, thyrotropin, and thyroid hormone. Each body cell then must have the characteristic of a "target" for growth and must carry a code for its own maturity.

An alternative theory suggests central receptor sites for regulation of growth in the brain. The degree of inhibition is determined by the complexing of inhibitor with receptor sites, while the number of receptor sites varies with the degree of maturity of the specific central nervous system centers.

A theory for tissue-growth control at the local level suggests that inhibitors are produced within specific tissues, diffuse, and circulate to similar tissues to inhibit growth. This simple theory may explain control of growth for specific tissues such as muscle and bone.

HETEROCHRONISM AND DISHARMONIC DEVELOPMENT

A simplified analogy can be drawn between early embryological development and an assembly line. In embryologic development there are many highly complex, genetically influenced mechanical and chemical reactions occurring that enable the unicellular zygote to undergo growth and development resulting in a unique multicellular neonate. This process requires cell differentiation

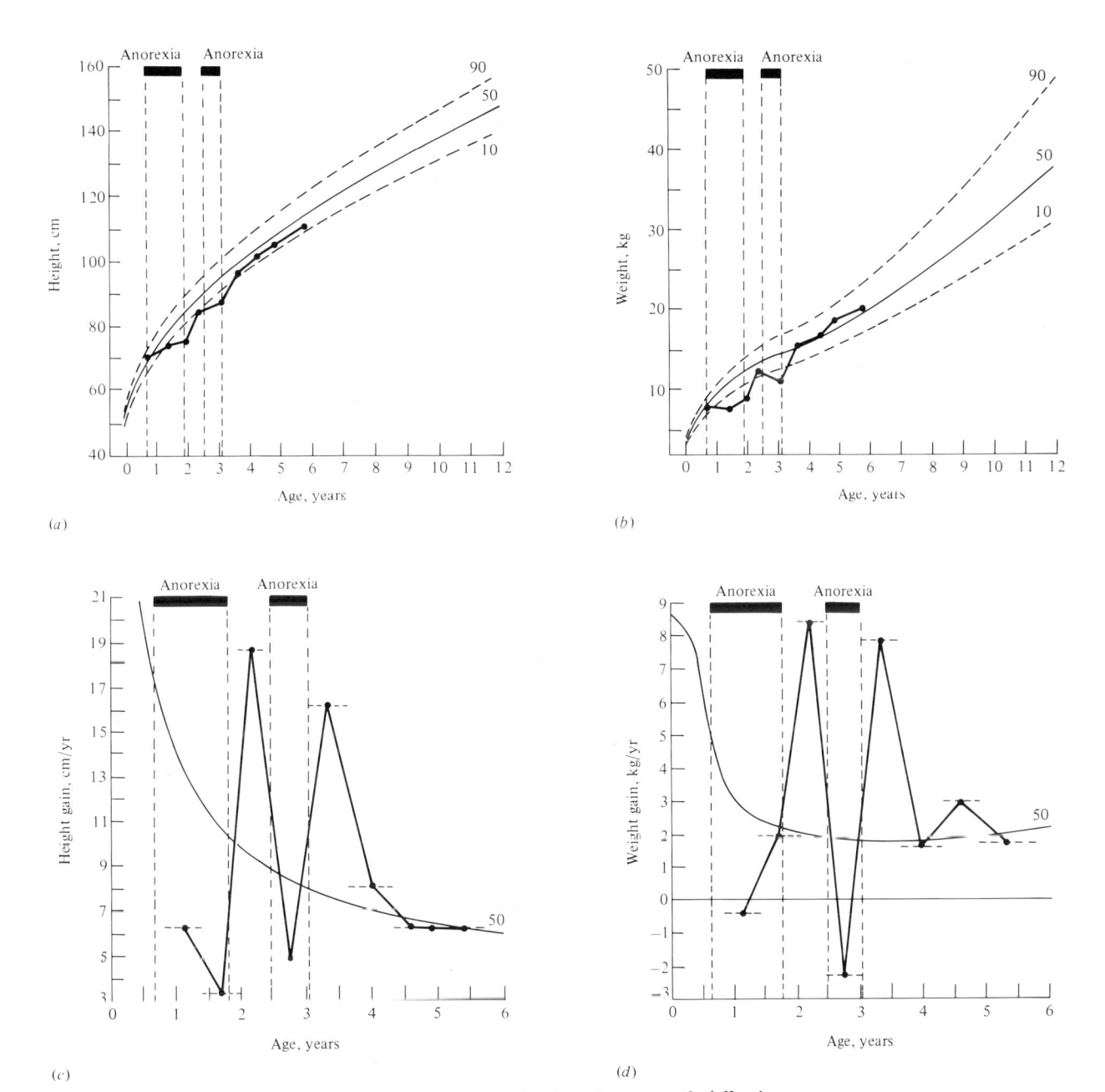

FIGURE 2-2. Demonstration of canalization: two periods of catch-up growth following episodes of anorexia nervosa in a young child. (*a*) and (*b*) Height and weight distance charts; (*c*) and (*d*) height and weight velocity charts. [*Adapted from A. Prader, J. M. Tanner, and G. A. von Harnack, Catch-up growth following illness or starvation: An example of developmental canalization in man. J. Pediat., 1963, 62(5), 646–659. Reprinted with permission of the C. V. Mosby Company.*]

and growth of tissues, organs, structures, and body systems that are functionally efficient within the neonate. As the coordination functions of a systems engineer are important to efficiency of manufacturing, likewise precision and timing of developmental events are critical to the outcomes of pregnancy. (Cell differentiation and tissue growth are discussed later in this section.)

An illustration of the need for precision relates to development of the eye. Visual acuity depends upon the ability of the eye to focus light rays on the retina, and this ability depends upon harmonized growth of the lens and depth of the eyeball. The many people who require corrective lenses indicates the frequency with which a degree of disharmony of eye growth occurs. There is evidence which indicates that growth of facial and skull features are controlled by genes that also influence growth in other parts of the body. Initially, discrete facial structures grow at their own unique rate; later overall regulatory forces appear to coordinate growth rates and the fusion of the parts into an acceptable whole. On occasion the regulatory forces for harmonizing the growth velocity of various parts are not successful, and normal development does not occur.

Variation in the speed of development of different tissues and functions is termed *heterochronism*. This process underlies many individual differences in body structure. Established standards for the weights of organs at various ages indicate that these tissues generally follow characteristic growth velocity patterns designated as follows:

- Lymphoid
- Neural
- General
- Genital

A graphic illustration of these types of growth according to age is shown in Fig. 2-3. Note the precocity of neural growth. The general type of somatic growth is represented by an *S*, or sigmoid, curve. Skeletal muscle growth follows this general type of growth curve. Cardiac muscle, proportionately large to body size in early life, later follows the general type of growth. The thymus appears to follow the general pattern during the first 5 years of postnatal life; then it maintains a steady state with involution at puberty. As a result of these different growth curves, the various organs have achieved a different percentage of their mature weight at a given point in time (see Fig. 2-4).

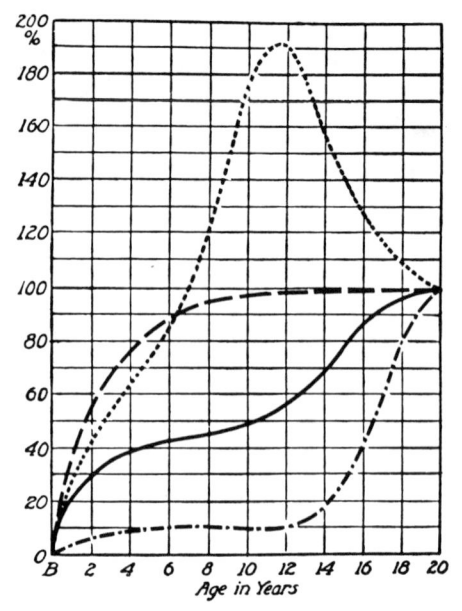

FIGURE 2-3. Growth curves for the four main types of growth in humans: general, lymphoid, neural, and genital. General growth (solid curve) includes the body as a whole, external dimensions (except head and neck), respiratory organs, digestive organs, kidneys, aorta and pulmonary trunks, spleen, musculature as a whole, skeleton as a whole, and blood volume. Lymphoid growth (dots) includes the thymus, lymph nodes, and intestinal lymphoid masses. Neural growth (dashes) includes the brain, dura, spinal cord, optic apparatus, and overall head dimensions. Genital growth (dashes and dots) includes the ovary, uterine tube, testis, epididymis, prostate, prostatic urethra, and seminal vesicle. [Adapted from R. E. Scammon, The measurement of the body in childhood. In J. A. Harris, C. M. Jackson, D. G. Paterson, and R. E. Scammon (Eds.), *The measurement of man*. Minneapolis: University of Minnesota Press, 1930. Reprinted with permission of the publisher.]

COMPENSATORY GROWTH

The term compensatory growth is used to describe growth of organs or other body parts, that is, the process of replacement or regeneration. Regrowth of a part can be demonstrated easily in lower forms of life, as in the planaria, while in mammals the most obvious example is in wound healing and scar formation. Tissues that are capable of cell division will demonstrate compensatory growth by hyperplasia. This is seen in the increase in the number of cells in hepatic and blood cell regeneration. Other tissues, such as the kidney, undergo compensatory growth through an increase in cell size. For example, when one kidney is removed, the remaining kidney undergoes hypertrophy.

Mechanisms initiating and regulating compensatory

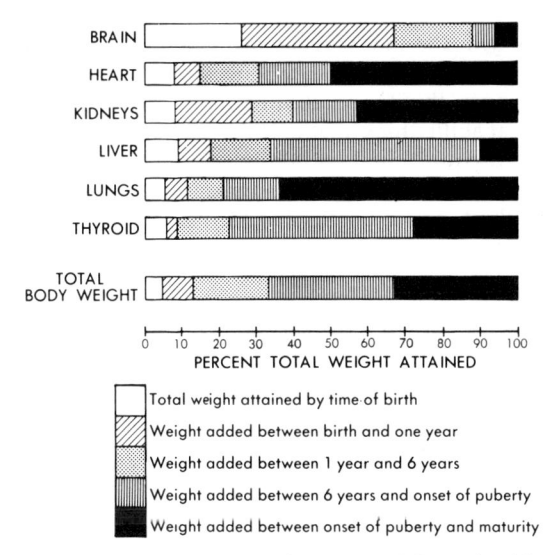

FIGURE 2-4. Percentage of mature weight attained by selected organs at specified ages. (*From D. V. Whipple, Dynamics of development: Euthenic pediatrics. New York: McGraw Hill, 1966. Reprinted by permission of the publisher.*)

growth remain unresolved at the present time. Research has focused on the relation of two factors underlying the regulation of the process: the role of mass versus the role of function. In embryological development it is clear that tissue mass and rate of differentiation precede functional competence of both tissues and organs. The functional demands placed upon tissues and organs in the mature individual may impose qualitatively different requirements from those operating in utero. Thus, understanding from the embryological environment cannot be applied directly to the mature individual.

SENSITIVE PERIODS

Sensitive periods are times during which a particular influence or stimulus from another part of the developing organism or from the environment evokes a specific response. Since the event begins gradually, reaches a peak, and decreases by degrees, the term sensitive period is more accurate in describing the event than the designation critical period and is receiving more general usage.

Because of rapid cell division and differentiation during the embryonic stage, there are many sensitive periods between the fifth day after fertilization and the end of the eighth week. Indeed, this period is the most important in human development because the beginnings of all major external and internal structures are laid. In addition, exposure of the embryo to teratogens during this crucial time of development may cause major congenital malformations (Moore, 1977).

In the embryo a tissue is said to show competence to a specific stimulus at a definite time. Should the stimulus not be presented at this time, the prescribed developmental event fails to occur. In the human male embryo the action of the genes on the Y chromosome cause the undifferentiated gonad to become recognizable as a testis at the seventh week conceptual age. By the ninth week, Leydig cells appear and increase rapidly in number until the twenty-second week. This is a true sensitive period. Thereafter there is no increase in the volume of these cells until after birth. Leydig cells produce testosterone or a related substance which acts on the undifferentiated external genitals to begin the progressive growth of the penis and scrotum.

It has been suggested, based on animal studies, that the sensitive period for brain development occurs at the time the largest number of enzyme systems are being activated and the growth rate is at its highest. It is thought that there may be sensitive periods related to maturation of the structures of the brain and that learning readiness may be related to this competence in the brain.

Sensitive periods in postnatal somatic growth are not well defined. It has been shown that unless a congenital cataract is removed or esotropia corrected by a certain age, the child will not develop sight in the affected eye. Other sensitive periods of physical development may be operating postnatally but elude the present body of knowledge.

HOMEOSTASIS

The concept of a relatively constant, regulated *milieux interieur* was described by the noted French physiologist, Claude Bernard, in 1845. Since then the concept has been enlarged and validated by several scientists. Walter Canon first used the word homeostasis to indicate the sum total of all physiological changes necessary to combat internal and external challenges. He pointed out the contribution of the sympathetic nervous system and its neurotransmitters to the adaptive response of the body. More recently, Hans Selye added a further dimension as he recognized the central role of the hypothalamic-pituitary-adrenocortical system in the response of the individual to environmental influences. He coined the term general adaptation syndrome.

Homeostatic mechanisms are necessary to maintain the dynamic equilibrium that must exist between the growing child and his environment. The interaction of child and environment begins as the hereditary material lodged within the fertilized ovum becomes implanted in the uterine wall. From this point on, the interactions become increasingly complex as the embryo changes the surroundings and in turn is changed by the maternal environment. Thus the hereditary material and environment become interwoven in the child in an inseparable way.

These interactions continue throughout life in physiological processes such as the ingestion of food or in respiration. The child assimilates some of the environment and in so doing is changed by it while at the same time altering the environment. In spite of the sometimes extensive changes brought about by the interactions with the outside world, the healthy child is able to maintain a relative constancy within the internal environment. Immediately upon birth, the neonate must maintain relative constancy of blood glucose, oxygen, carbon dioxide, and electrolyte levels, along with other processes such as temperature regulation. These are accomplished by the combined, complex functioning and interaction of body systems. The physiological processes whereby homeostasis is maintained in the human neonate are not fully developed, and he requires a protected environment while the body systems mature to the point that they can maintain equilibrium.

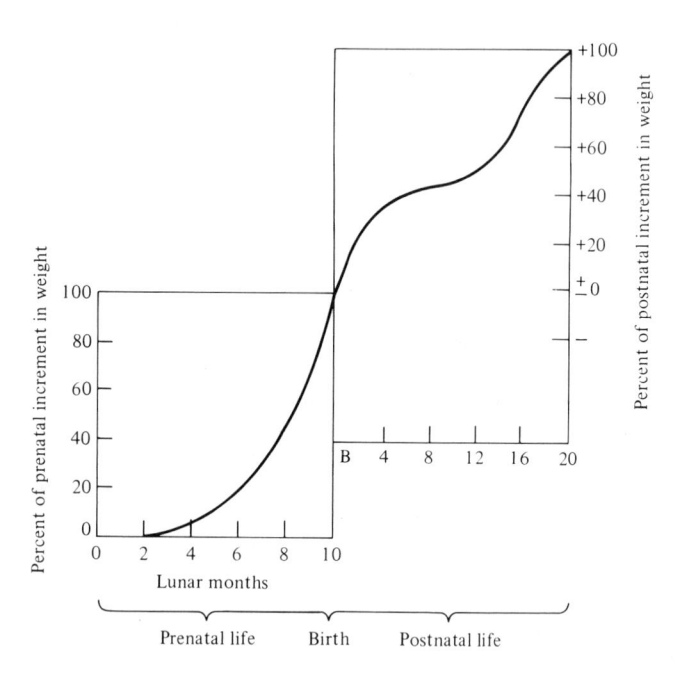

Coupled with the mechanisms of homeostasis, which regulate such processes as sleep and waking states, motor activity, hunger, thirst, and elimination in the infant, is the innate capability for growth. The infant demonstrates nutritional disequilibrium by bodily activity and crying, and in being fed ingests nutrients to restore equilibrium within the fluid compartments and the cells as well as to promote growth.

New cells become a part of the body that must be maintained, and so the cycles of equilibrium-disequilibrium associated with growth and development continue. The changes within the individual are sometimes so gradual that they are imperceptible from day to day but can be detected as physical development when the observations are plotted against previous values.

PROCESSES OF GROWTH AND MATURATION

Increasing size, growth, is one of the most obvious changes in infancy and childhood. Increase in mass is reflected in greater weight and length, or height. Growth is particularly rapid during the last half of gestation and during the first 2 years. During the remainder of childhood, changes in height and weight are so gradual that they may go unnoticed unless frequent measurements are made. Accelerated growth is then seen in the pubertal growth spurt with a final deceleration and eventual end to increase in overall size (see Fig. 2-5). Deviation from the normal rate of physical growth is significant as an indica-

FIGURE 2-5. Pre- and postnatal weight curve. [*Adapted from R. E. Scammon, The measurement of the body in childhood. In J. A. Harris, C. M. Jackson, D. G. Paterson, and R. E. Scammon (Eds.), The measurement of man. Minneapolis: University of Minnesota Press, 1930. Used with permission of the publisher.*]

tion of malnutrition, disease, deprivation, or other negative environmental influence.

Anthropometric measurement is a means of "expressing quantitatively the form of the body" (Cameron, 1978, p. 35). It is systematic measurement of the human body along different parameters. Anthropometric measurement of a growing individual has been termed *auxological anthropometry* by Cameron (1978, p. 35).

Multiple anthropometric measurements are possible, as illustrated in Fig. 2-6. Measurements more commonly used in clinical practice are weight, recumbent length (crown-heel), crown-rump length (recumbent sitting), standing height (stature), sitting height, head circumference, and chest circumference.

FIGURE 2-6. Major surface measurements. (1) Recumbent (crown-heel) length or stature; (2) crown-rump length or sitting height; (3) occipital-frontal circumference; (4) chest circumference; (5) upper-arm circumference; (6) upper-thigh circumference; (7) calf circumference; (8) upper-arm length (from lateral border of acromion to head of radius); (9) forearm length (from head of radius to distal end of radius); (10) hand length (from distal end of radius to longest fingertip); (11) tibial length (from proximal-medial border of the tibia to the distal border of medial malleolus); (12) biacromial diameter; (13) bi-iliac diameter. [*Adapted from N. Cameron, The methods of auxological anthropometry. In F. Falkner and J. M. Tanner (Eds.), Human growth 2, Postnatal growth. New York: Plenum, 1978.*]

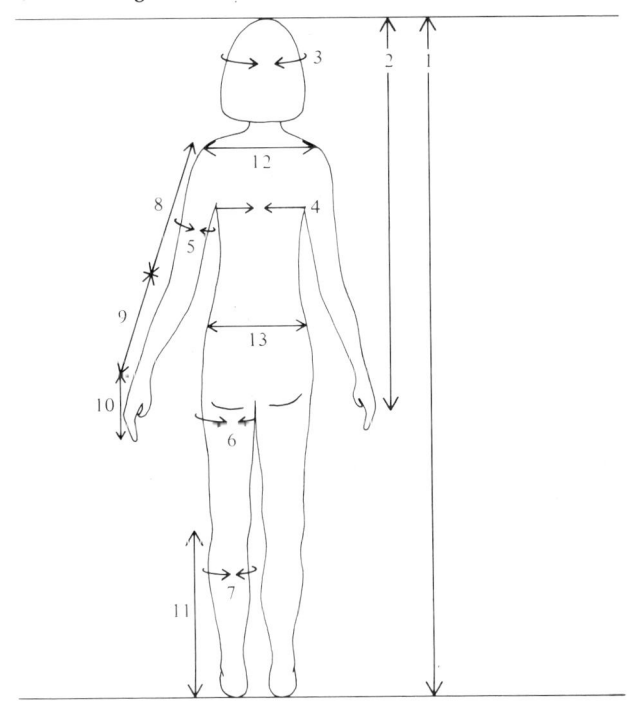

GROWTH STANDARDS

Data sampling In order to determine standards of growth, anthropometric measurement is done on large numbers of children. This data sampling can be done in different ways. Growth data may be longitudinal, that is, collected on the individual child over a number of years, or cross-sectional, using a one-time measurement from a group of children. *Mixed longitudinal study* designates data collected over a prolonged period of time where children who leave the study are replaced by other subjects. Both cross-sectional and longitudinal data are useful in assessing growth; however, they do not yield the same information and cannot be used in the same way.

Cross-sectional data are relatively easy and inexpensive to collect on a large number of subjects. In contrast, longitudinal studies are carried out over a long period of time, are laborious to conduct, and require high standards of measurements to reduce error. Cross-sectional data provide information on a distance curve (see below) but do not show individual differences in growth rates or the rate of particular events. Knowledge of individual growth rate, that is, how fast the chld is growing, is necessary to study genetic control of growth and to correlate physical growth to psychological development, social behavior, or educational achievement.

Distance and velocity curves The earliest longitudinal study of growth to be reported occurred from 1759 to 1777 when Count Philibert de Montbeillard measured and recorded the height of his son every 6 months from birth to 18 years (Tanner, 1962). The curve obtained by plotting data of height attained at successive ages provides a distance curve, which allows comparison to previous years and shows how much the child has grown. In contrast, when increments in height per year are plotted against age, a velocity curve is obtained. This reveals how fast the child has grown and may be stated as the rate of growth per year.

The growth rate is a more useful value as it reflects the child's state at any one particular time; for example, it indicates the deceleration of growth that occurs during the first 2 years of life. The differences between a distance and a velocity curve are clearly seen in Fig. 2-7.

Tanner, Whitehouse, and Takaishi (1965) contend that

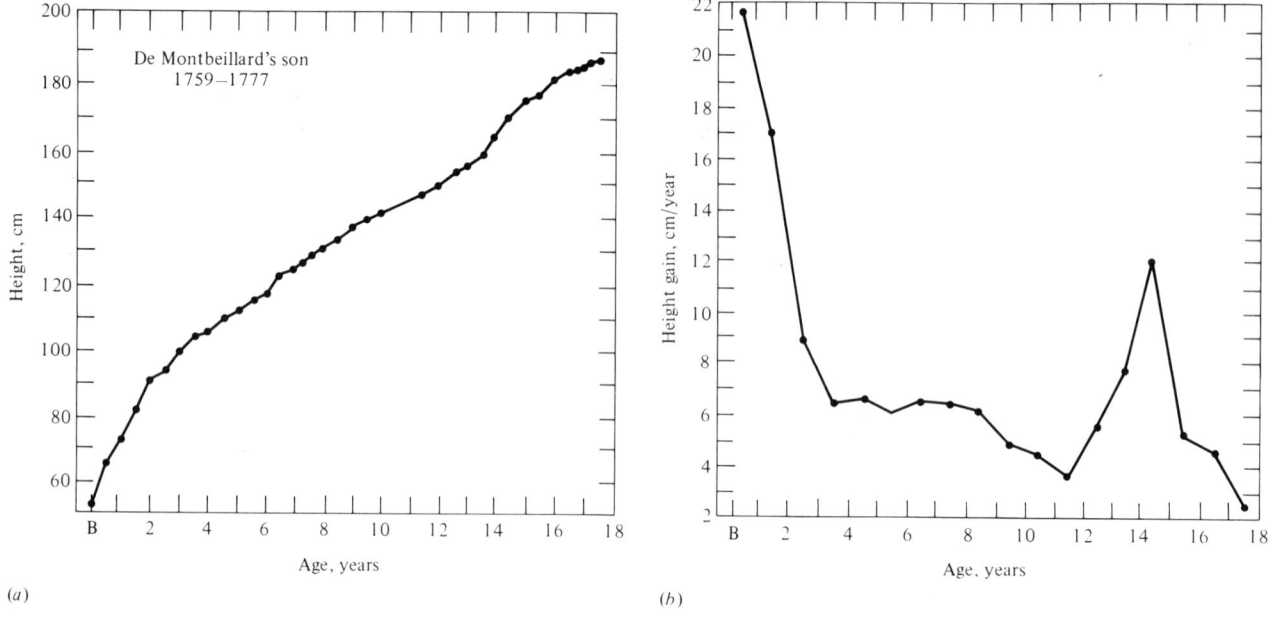

FIGURE 2-7. Growth in stature of Count Philibert de Montbeillard's son. (a) Distance curve: height attained at each age; (b) velocity curve: annual increments of height. [*From J. M. Tanner, Growth at adolescence (2d ed.). Oxford, London: Blackwell Scientific Publications, 1962. Reprinted with permission of the publisher.*]

growth in general is a very regular process with gradual growth-velocity changes from one age to another, in contrast to those who believe that growth occurs by fits and starts. Tanner et al. base this belief on the fact that carefully collected measurements at the bodily level, including x-ray measurements of individual bones, show complete continuity. This does not rule out the possibility that growth at the cellular level may be discontinuous.

CURRENT GROWTH CURVES

Growth charts are used to graph anthropometric data to assess a child's growth status. Two of the growth (anthropometric) charts which had extensive use were developed by Stuart and Meredith in Boston and by Jackson in Ohio in the 1940s. In 1974, as a result of problems in analyzing data obtained from the Ten-State Nutritional Survey, the National Academy of Science urged the compilation of new growth charts based on current data (Committee on Nutrition, 1974; Owen, 1974). In response, the National Center for Health Statistics (NCHS) prepared new percentiles for assessing the physical growth of children in the United States.

Distance growth curves The National Institute of Child Health and Human Development sponsored a workshop in 1975 to discuss ethnic differences in growth. The participants determined that "although appreciable anthropometric differences have been demonstrated among certain ethnic groups living under similar environmental conditions in other parts of the world, the use of one standard in the United States for height and weight would be unlikely to cause serious error" (Roche and McKigney, 1976, p. 62). The new charts are based on measurements obtained in more recent national surveys and are representative of all children in the United States, not middle-class, Caucasian children, as were previous charts.

The NCHS growth charts are 14 distance curves that plot the growth of children and adolescents from birth to age 18 years with separate curves for females and males (see Figs. 2-8 to 2-13 and 2-16 to 2-23):

- Female: Birth to 3 years
  Length
  Weight
  Occipital-frontal circumference
  Weight for length
- Male: Birth to 3 years
  Length
  Weight
  Occipital-frontal circumference
  Weight for length
- Female: 2 to 18 years
  Height
  Weight
- Male: 2 to 18 years
  Height
  Weight
- Female: Prepubescent
  Weight for height
- Male: Prepubescent
  Weight for height

Each curve presents seven percentiles: 5th, 10th, 25th, 50th, 75th, 90th, and 95th. The last two tables were developed because weight-for-stature percentiles are assumed to be age independent before pubescence and are not applicable after the appearance of secondary sex characteristics. Thus, these charts are used until about age 10 years.

The child's weight, head circumference, and length or height are plotted against age. The percentile ranking provides data for assessment of physical growth and indicates how a child compares in size in relation to contemporary United States children of the same age and sex. If a child's measurements fall within the central or intermediate range of the percentiles, his growth is considered within current standards. However, if the child's measurements lie beyond the extreme percentiles, it is considered an indication of a genetic, endocrine, nutritional, or other problem.

Velocity growth curves Velocity curves were developed from measurements of British children by Tanner, Whitehouse, and Takaishi. Although not used in the clinical setting in this country, they give a visual description of growth in stature, weight, and head circumference for

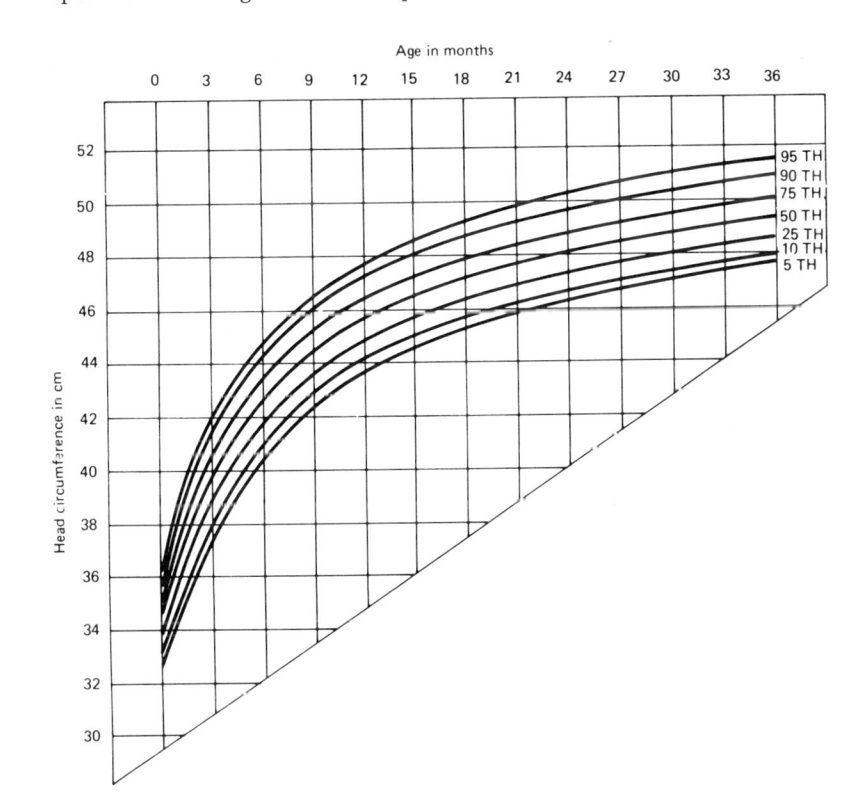

FIGURE 2-8. Head-circumference–by–age percentiles for girls age birth to 36 months. (From P. V. N. Hamill et al., NCHS growth charts. Hyattsville, Maryland: U.S. Department of Health, Education, and Welfare, 1977.)

girls and boys. The height and weight curves are birth to postpuberty and the head circumference curve from birth to age 3 years.

The height and weight velocity curves show the rapid decrease in rate of growth until the pubertal growth spurt, when the curve gain increases and decreases for the final time (see Fig. 10-9). Rate of head growth shows a striking downward movement during the first year with a continued but less dramatic deceleration of rate in the second and third years.

PARAMETERS OF GROWTH

Monitoring physical growth of well children by measuring height, weight, and head circumference for comparison with standard normal values is an essential screening procedure. Comparing the individual child with standard values presumes that the child who deviates from the typical growth patterns is more likely to have a nutrition or health-related problem and should be agnosis. The degree of sensitivity of this screening is greater during infancy than during succeeding years of growth. Serial observations are more meaningful than individual measures as they permit calculation of growth over a defined time, or velocity of growth, while a one-time measure yields information only as it relates to size.

It is generally accepted that variables to be routinely monitored for the assessment of physical growth are head circumference, length or height, and weight. The recommended schedule for obtaining measurements include at birth; at discharge from the hospital; at 1, 2, 4, and 6 months of age; and thereafter at 6-month intervals through the third year. Beyond 3 years of age, height and weight are measured annually. Recumbent length measures are recommended through the third year of life; thereafter standing height is measured. To obtain accurate measurement examiners should be trained in the use of quality equipment, which is recalibrated at scheduled intervals. Recommended techniques for obtaining reliable measurements are described in "Physical Assessment."

Head circumference Occipital-frontal circumference (OFC) is a particularly significant measurement because

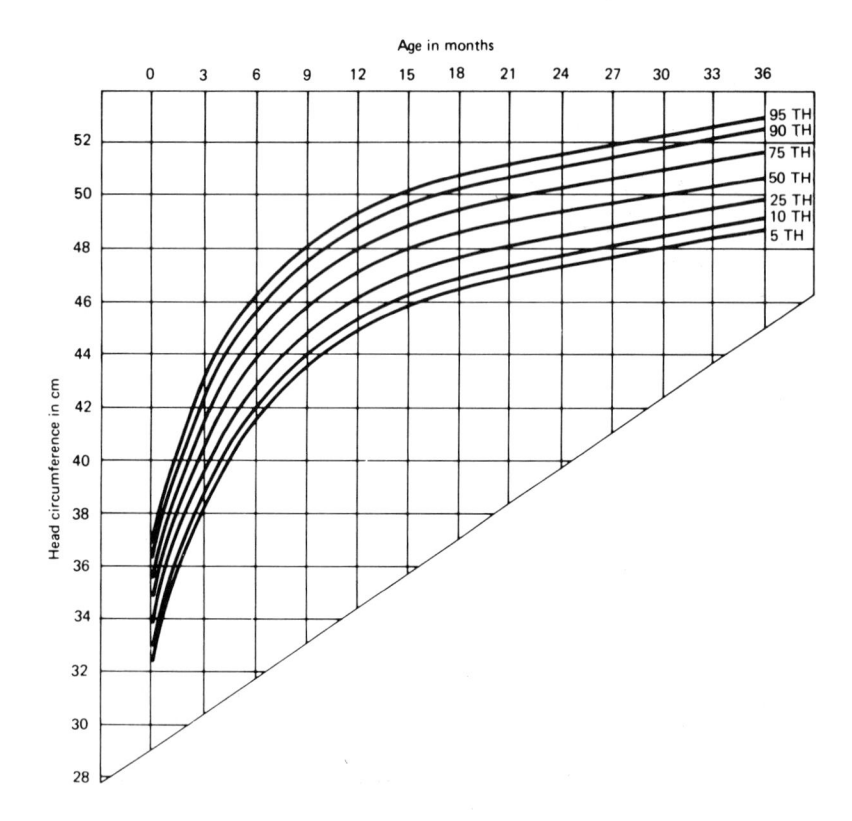

FIGURE 2-9. Head-circumference-by-age percentiles for boys age birth to 36 months. (From P. V. N. Hamill et al., NCHS growth charts, 1977.)

of the high correlation between increase in brain mass and head circumference. The head grows rapidly during the fetal period and the first year of life, achieving two-thirds of adult size. By 2 years of age the head is four-fifths of adult size (see Figs. 2-8 and 2-9).

Median head circumference at birth is larger in males than females; however, as the values are so similar for the two sexes, the mean is often used for clinical appraisals. Variations of 4 cm (1.5 in) are considered to be within normal range. By 1 year there is an average increase of 12 cm (4.75 in), an increase of over 30 percent.

Whether there is predictable correlation of head circumference and body size has been difficult to determine. However, some clinicians state that OFC correlates well with weight for the first 6 months of extrauterine life in both sexes (Illingworth, 1975a; Illingworth and Eid, 1971). Thus, in evaluating head size, it has been recommended that OFC be related to weight of the infant, not just to its percentile rank on growth charts. The suggestion is made that OFC in the 50th percentile, for example, may indicate relative microcephaly in an infant whose weight is in the upper percentiles. Occipital-frontal circumference and height are reported to be not highly correlated in this age group. This question remains unresolved, however (see "Calvarium and Face"). Even less information is available on the correlation of OFC to body size in older children.

Height Height (length) reflects the individual's genetic endowment and is influenced by the environment. It is a particularly useful growth variable as it is not as sensitive to negative environmental influences as weight. The maximum growth rate for length occurs during the fourth month of intrauterine life (see Fig. 2-14). Thereafter annual increments continue to decrease from birth to maturity, except for the rapid increase in height during puberty (see Figs. 2-10 to 2-13).

The male median birth length is greater than that of the female neonate. Because of the rapid growth during the first 6 months, these values increase significantly. By the end of the first year the median lengths have increased approximately 50 percent. Growth rate, which was decelerating in late infancy, continues to decrease in velocity during the second year and then remains relatively steady throughout the preschool years. The pubertal growth spurt occurs in girls beginning about 10 to 11 years of age and in boys about 12 to 13 years.

Birth length has not been found to be a reliable value for predicting adult height because the intrauterine environment overrides genotype in determining size of the fetus. In contrast, the height at 3 years shows a fairly reliable correlation to adult height and enabled Tanner, Whitehouse, and Takaishi to derive a formula for predicting height at maturity from midparental height (see Chap. 8). For a quick calculation, Illingworth (1975b, p. 50) suggests that adult height will equal twice the stature at age 2 years.

Body proportions Body proportions undergo characteristic changes during physical development from fetal to adult life. Prenatal and postnatal changes have been portrayed graphically in Fig. 2-14. These changes in body proportions are the result of the different growth rates of various organs and body parts. The most striking changes are early brain growth with the resultant large head size relative to body length and short extremity length relative to total body length.

The head of the 2-month-old fetus constitutes one-half of total body length, while the still relatively large head of the neonate accounts for one-quarter of body length. As growth progresses, the trunk and extremities increase in size at a more rapid rate; head growth rate begins to decrease after the first 2 years, and the child moves gradually toward adult body proportions. The term cephalocaudal describes this preponderance of growth and early elaboration of function of the cephalad portion of the body followed by growth of the more caudal portions.

Crown-rump length of the neonate represents 70 percent of the body length, while at 3 years it represents only 57 percent. The lower part of the body undergoes significant growth during the school-age years and accounts for the greatest percentage of increase in stature during this time. In the adult, sitting (crown-rump) height is approximately one-half of total stature (see Fig. 2-15).

These characteristic changes in body proportions alter the midpoint of stature in the infant versus that of the older child or adult. In the neonate the midpoint lies at the level of the umbilicus. It gradually shifts to the level of the pubic symphysis by adulthood. This redistribution of the midpoint of stature affects weight distribution and is reflected in the increasing gracefulness of body movement that accompanies growth.

There is a difference in upper- and lower-extremity–to–trunk ratio in males compared with females and in Negroes compared with Caucasians. Men have longer arms and legs relative to the trunk than women; this is also found in the comparison of Negroes to Caucasians.

Weight Weight is a primary indicator of nutrition and health both pre- and postnatally and, to a lesser degree, an indicator of developmental maturation. It may be use-

32 PHYSICAL DEVELOPMENT

ful in early detection of deviations in normal growth patterns. It has the advantage of being readily measured, and the margin of error is low.

Fetal weight is more sensitive than length to maternal environment and shows greater variability than length, which is influenced by both hereditary and environmental factors. Many maternal factors influence birth weight including parity, height, weight gain during pregnancy, nutritional status, health status, and complications of pregnancy such as toxemia, chronic disease, infections, smoking, and multiple births.

Median birth weight is greater in male than female infants. Infants usually double their weight by 5 months, though some normal infants now achieve this milestone at an even earlier age (Neumann and Alpaugh, 1976). Birth weight is generally tripled by the end of the first year and is quadrupled by the end of the second year. Weight gain continues at a slower but steady rate from 3 years through the early school years. Variation in weight among normal children increases with age. This is particularly true as they enter the pubertal growth spurt, which also results in difference between the sexes. Unlike stature, weight does not stabilize after puberty (see Figs. 2-16 to 2-19).

Weight for height Comparing weight and length or height to each other describes the "leanness" or "fatness" of a child and offers more information on the child's

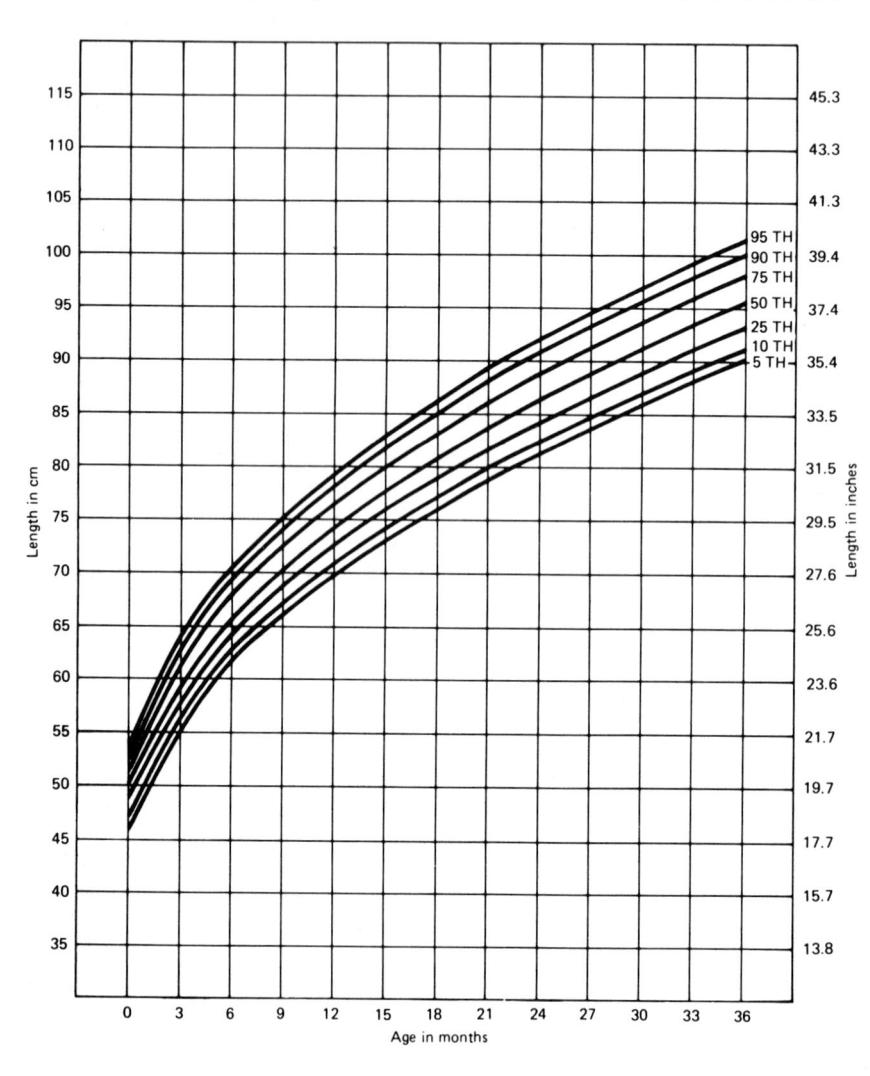

FIGURE 2-10. Length-by-age percentiles for girls age birth to 36 months. (*From P. V. N. Hamill et al., NCHS growth charts, 1977.*)

growth pattern and nutritional status. The *ponderal index* (height cubed over weight) has been used as a comparison of height and weight. However this index is limited as it differs between girls and boys and at different ages (National Center, 1977).

An alternative means of calculation is through the use of the NCHS percentile distributions of body weights by sex for a given length or stature. Weight for length is graphed for children birth to 3 years and weight for height is graphed for prepubescent children (see Figs. 2-20 to 2-23). There are separate curves for girls and boys. In these graphs, weight and length are plotted against each other independently of age.

Weight-to-height relation and body proportions change dramatically as puberty begins, and these changes invalidate the charts. Thus, if the beginning of puberty can not be determined, it is recommended that the charts be used, for girls, only to age 10 years or to 137 cm in height and, for boys, only to age 11½ years or to 146 cm in height (National Center, 1977). The interpretation of findings on these curves is discussed later in this chapter.

Physique Each child has an innate growth potential closely related to height and weight that is expressed in body form, referred to as physique. Three classic somatotypes have been identified and named *ectomor-*

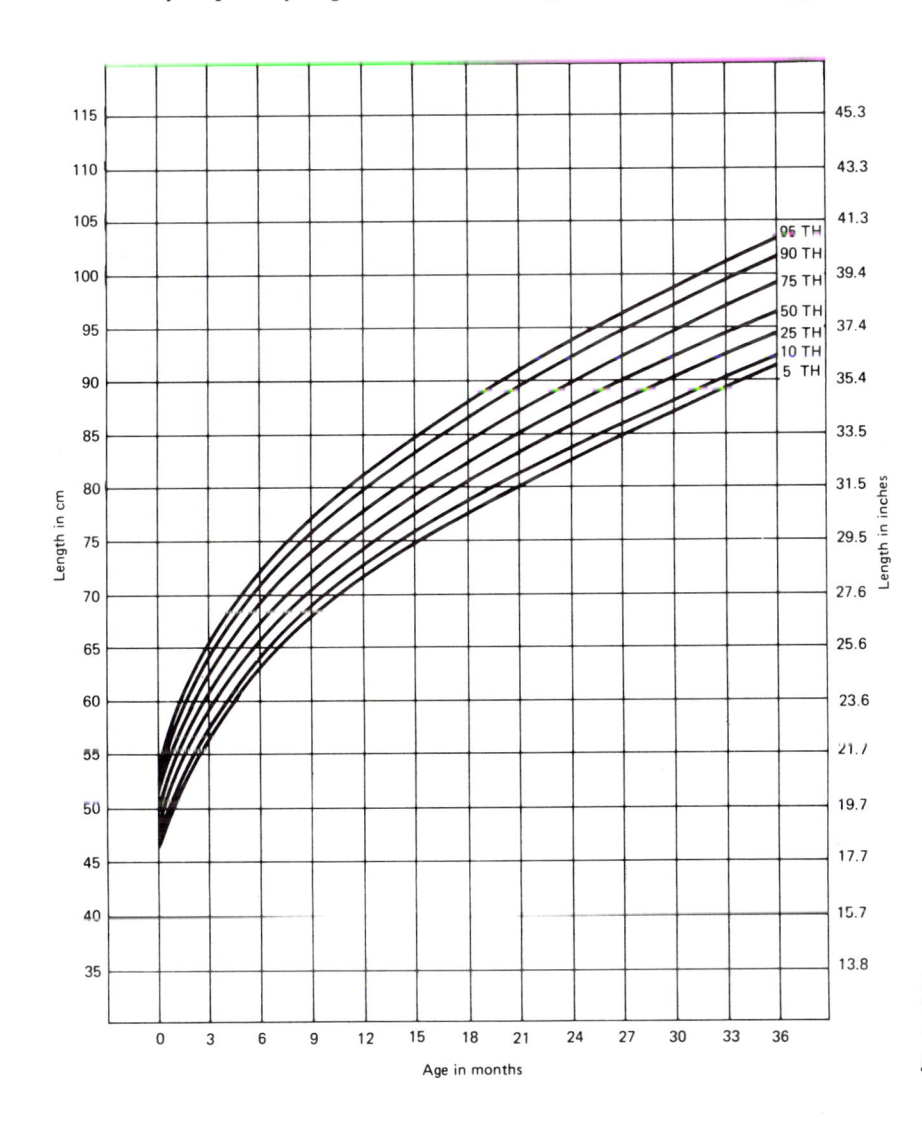

FIGURE 2-11. Length-by-age percentiles for boys age birth to 36 months. (*From P. V. N. Hamill et al., NCHS growth charts, 1977.*)

phic, mesomorphic, and *endomorphic* (Sheldon, 1940) after the three primary germ layers of the embryo: ectoderm, mesoderm, and endoderm.

Endoderm gives rise primarily to the epithelial portions of major body systems. The physique termed endomorphy has characteristic qualities of body roundness: short neck; increased abdominal adipose tissue; large trunk and thighs; and small, seemingly tapering extremities.

Mesoderm gives rise to the muscular and skeletal systems. The characteristics of mesomorphy are an overall rectangular outline with a tendency toward predominance of muscles, bones, and connective tissue.

Ectoderm gives rise to the nervous and integumentary systems. A delicate appearance suggests ectomorphy, characterized by thin muscles, minimal subcutaneous tissue, large body surface to weight, and increased length.

The child with endomorph characteristics appears to grow and mature earlier and thus during late childhood tends to be taller than the child with ectomorph characteristics. However, this difference is reduced when the latter reaches maturity.

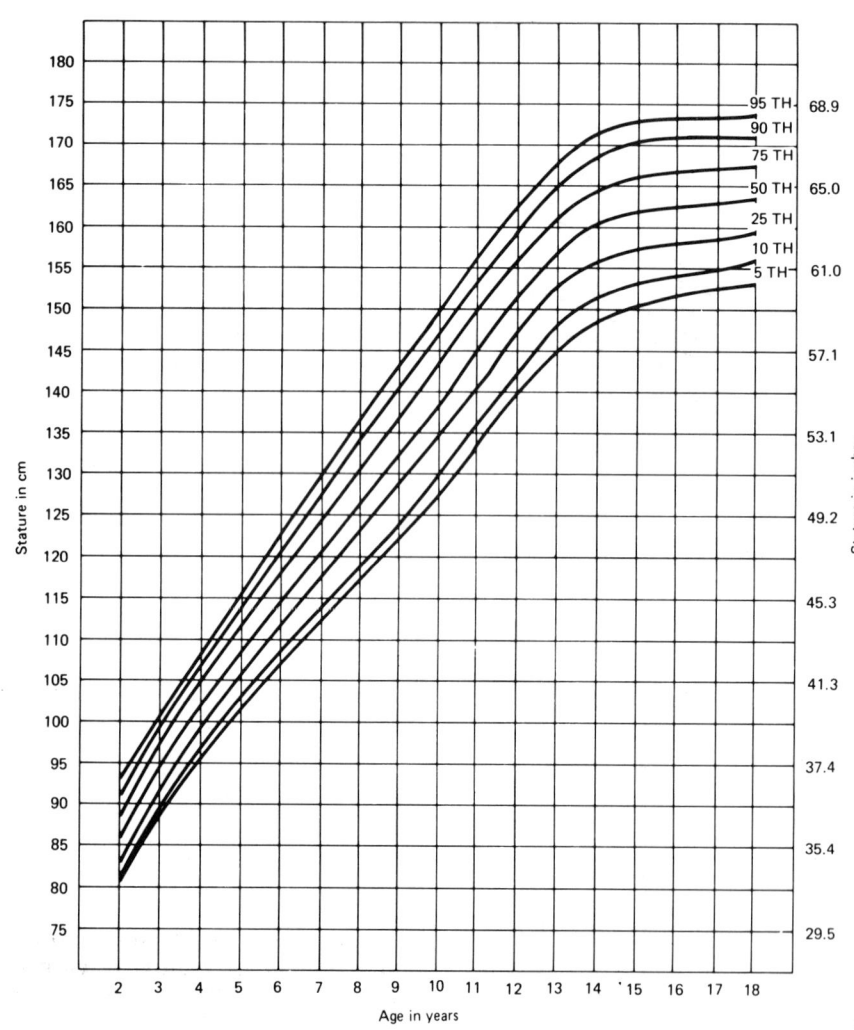

FIGURE 2-12. Stature-by-age percentiles for girls age 2 to 18 years. (*From P. V. N. Hamill et al., NCHS growth charts, 1977.*)

Body composition Normal growth and maturation is accompanied by qualitative and quantitative changes in the components of the tissues, such as changes in intracellular and extracellular fluid volume, lean body mass, and amount of adipose tissue. Estimates of these changes in body composition have been done through chemical analyses of bodies and tissues, indirect measurements of water and electrolytes, excretion studies, and estimations of fatness (see Table 2-1).

Water is the main solvent for organic compounds from foods and metabolic products and for inorganic salts, and these constitute the internal environment. Total body water expressed as a percentage of body weight is highest during the early prenatal period with the largest portion of fluid being extracellular. At birth, total body water is approximately 75 to 80 percent of body weight and will decrease throughout infancy to reach the adult level of 60 percent. Total body water content has been found to vary inversely to body fat and directly to lean body mass. Thus the decreasing water content seen in infancy can be related to the deposition of fat that is occurring (Timaris, 1972). The decrease in body water during infancy is al-

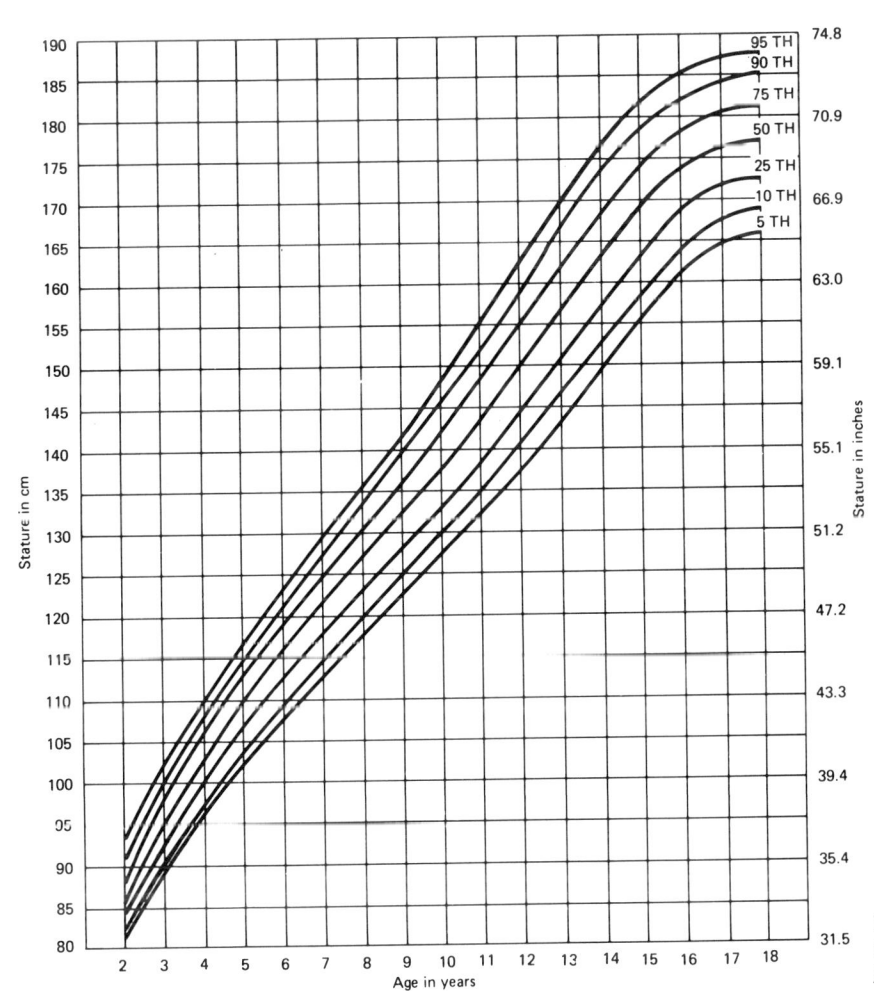

FIGURE 2-13. Stature-by-age percentiles for boys age 2 to 18 years. (*From P. V. N. Hamill et al., NCHS growth charts, 1977.*)

most entirely from the extracellular compartment and represents a reduction of fluid from 44 to 26 percent of total body weight.

The decrease in extracellular fluid volume arises from such discrete tissues as muscle, heart, and brain and is replaced by intracellular fluid and cell solids. Intracellular water and total body potassium continue to rise relative to body weight throughout the growing period but particularly from birth to 8 years. This corresponds to the increase in muscle mass and its transition into a high-potassium tissue.

After 8 years of age, total potassium relative to body weight decreases in girls, an event that coincides with increase in adipose tissue, an early indication of puberty. In boys at 8 years of age, there is also a temporary decrease in total body potassium, which is followed by an increase during puberty. These changes in water and potassium reflect the changes in body composition in terms of lean body mass: percentage of bone, muscle, and fat. To a lesser extent, they also reflect the maturation of those tissues themselves (Timaris, 1972).

Taller children of the same sex have a greater amount of lean body mass than their peers who are shorter in stature. A linear relation exists between height and lean body mass for children of any age, with sex differences apparent in the early years, while an exponential relationship exists between lean body mass, height, and age groups (Forbes, 1972).

Lipids have a wide distribution throughout the body and are an integral part of the nervous system, bone marrow, and cell membranes. Lipids are also stored in adipose tissue sites. Lipids serve a variety of functions, are a metabolically active tissue, and are responsible for the greatest differences in body composition among children of both sexes in all age groups.

Appreciable fetal fat does not appear until the third trimester when it begins to increase rapidly so that by birth total body fat averages 16 percent of body weight. Fat is laid down rapidly during the first 9 months of life; between 2 and 6 months the increase in adipose tissue is

TABLE 2-1 Body composition at different stages of growth

Subject and age, years	Height, cm	Body weight, kg	Σ organ weight*	Muscle mass†	Body fat‡	ECF volume§
Low birth weight		1.1	21	<10	3	50
Newborn	50	3.5	18	20	12	40
Child 0.25	60	5.5	15	22	11	32
Child 1.5	80	11.0	14	23	20	26
Child 5	110	19.0	10	35	15	24
Child 10	140	31.0	8.4	37	15	25
Male 14	160	50	5.7	42	12	21
Male adult	180	70	5.2	40	11	19
Female 13	160	45	4.8	39	18	19
Female adult	162	55	4.4	35	20	16

* Sum of brain, liver, heart, and kidney (Holliday, 1971).
† Derived from creatinine excretion (Holliday, 1971).
‡ Interpolated values from literature (Widdowson and Dickerson, 1964; Friis-Hansen, 1971).
§ Average of bromide space (Gamble, 1946) and thiosulfate space (Cheek, 1961; Friis-Hansen, 1957).
Source: M. A. Holliday, Body composition and energy needs during growth. In F. Falkner and J. M. Tanner (Eds.), *Human growth 2, Postnatal growth.* New York: Plenum, 1978, p. 123. Reprinted by permission of Plenum Press.

twice as great as the increase in muscle volume (Fomon, 1974). Female infants deposit a greater percentage of weight as fat than males.

Yearly increments of fat decrease steadily during childhood with some children showing a prepubertal spurt. A sex difference has been noted in fat deposition during accelerated linear growth. In girls undergoing rapid increase in height, the deposition of fat is reduced, while in boys there is an actual loss of fat during accelerated growth velocity.

Measurement of skinfold thickness provides a useful assessment of percentage of a child's subcutaneous fat when compared with established reference standards. Values are particularly useful as an adjunct to recommended growth variables to clarify the relationship between height and weight. For instance, a child who has well-developed muscles may appear overweight or obese for height and weight when he actually has appropriate subcutaneous tissue.

Racial differences have been noted and must be considered in interpretation of skinfold-thickness data. Puerto Rican children have greater skinfold thickness than North American Negro or Caucasian children, and Negro infants through 4 years of age have greater subcutaneous fat measurements than Caucasian infants and children. After 4 years, however, these values are reversed.

A special caliper calibrated to provide constant tension is used to measure subcutaneous fatness. The triceps skinfold (also termed fat fold) is the site of choice as it is representative of body fatness and is easy to measure. The subscapular skinfold can also be measured. The recommended technique for obtaining the triceps skinfold-thickness measurement is described in "Nutrition Assessment."

INDICES OF MATURITY

Because ossification of the skeleton follows a predictable order during development, bone age has been established as the best index of general maturity, especially before puberty. Roentgenogram (x-ray) studies of various ossification centers have been used to establish standards for bone age. These standards from children followed in longitudinal surveys appear in classical volumes of pediatric medicine. The most widely used standards are those of Greulich and Pyle (1959) for the hand and Reynolds and Asakawa (1951) for the lower extremity and head of the humerus in early infancy.

Girls are more advanced in bone age than boys, and thus it has been necessary to establish separate values for the sexes. Skeletal ossification is also more advanced in Negroes than in Caucasians at birth (see "Musculoskeletal Development" for further discussion).

Bone age is used to assess physiological maturity in a child whose linear growth appears to be progressing at a slower or more rapid rate than his chronological age indicates. Skeletal ossification is closely linked to nutritional

FIGURE 2-14. Change in body proportions from 2 months gestational age to adulthood. *(From C. E. Corliss, Patten's human embryology. New York: McGraw-Hill, 1976. Reprinted by permission of the publisher.)*

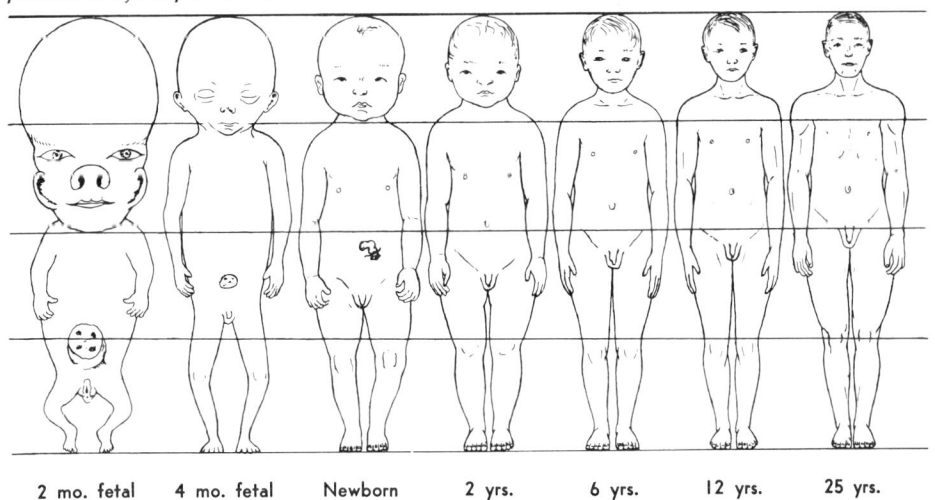

2 mo. fetal   4 mo. fetal   Newborn   2 yrs.   6 yrs.   12 yrs.   25 yrs.

status. Inadequate caloric intake will slow bone growth and delay calcification of the ossification centers, and the bone may appear thinner. Inadequate and/or poor-quality protein results in reduced bone growth, delay in appearance of ossification centers, and possible alterations in the ossification sequence. It is of interest that obese children have been found to have advanced skeletal age.

ENVIRONMENTAL FACTORS INFLUENCING PHYSICAL DEVELOPMENT

Just as growth in all other living forms responds to the surrounding environment, so physical development of the human is influenced by many factors in the environment. Optimal physical development is promoted when environmental factors vary within definable limits and in relation to each other. Factors influencing prenatal development are discussed in Chap. 5; influences on postnatal development are discussed below.

HEALTH STATUS AND DISEASE

An intricate relation exists between health status and physical development. The health of the individual child has a major influence upon physical development; therefore, growth and maturation are monitored in well-child examinations and used as an index of health status.

It is apparent that there are varying degrees of health ranging from optimal to poor and that these degrees of health influence physical development. Though measured grossly as growth and maturation, ultimately health is determined and maintained at the cellular and organ level of organization. Optimal health is dependent upon such factors as genetic endowment; an adequate nutrient intake to promote growth, function, and repair of body structures; freedom from disease and infection; and a psychological environment conducive to development.

Disease conditions vary in timing, length, and degree, and these factors influence the specific effect upon growth. Acute minor illnesses, such as influenza or antibiotic-treated middle-ear infections, may cause temporary weight loss, but growth rate is not perceptibly retarded in well-nourished children. Chronic infection also results in reduced growth rates. The precise mechanism

FIGURE 2-15. Changes in body proportions and stance in girls, 1½ to 12 years, and boys, 1½ to 14 years. (*Adapted from L. M. Bayer and N. Bayley, Growth diagnosis. Chicago: University of Chicago Press, 1959. By permission of University of Chicago Press.*)

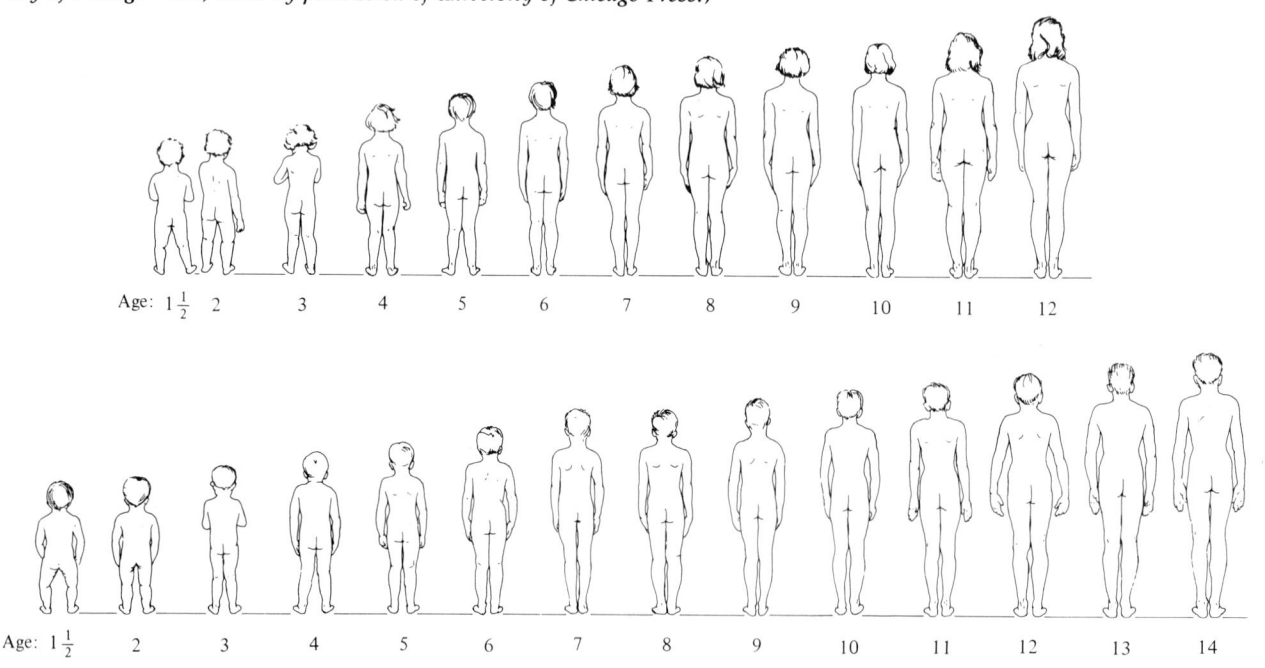

that produces growth deficiency is unknown, but diminished mitotic rate and decreased cell numbers have been demonstrated. Less-than-optimal growth may result from defective enzyme systems, as in phenylketonuria (PKU) and malabsorption syndromes.

Major illnesses that require hospitalization and lengthy convalescence are associated with utilization of energy for repair rather than for growth and with reduced activity. These factors may cause considerable slowing of growth, which is compensated by catch-up growth upon recovery. The mechanism of the growth retardation probably varies with the disease. It has been suggested that an increased secretion of cortisol may reduce growth rate (Tanner, 1970). Diminished growth rates are noted in diseases resulting in reduced hemoglobin and in some kidney diseases. This slowed growth is no doubt related to reduced oxygen supply to cells, reduced ability to synthesize vitamin A, and reduced ability to excrete metabolic waste products.

It has been suggested that reduced stature, which often accompanies both mild and chronic disease or malnutrition, is the result of reduced cartilage formation. The rate of cartilage formation, or growth, is thought to be slowed while ossification of cartilage, or maturation, continues at its usual rate, thus creating an imbalance and reduced height (Acheson, 1966).

Thus health and disease influence physical development in complex, interrelated, and sometimes little-

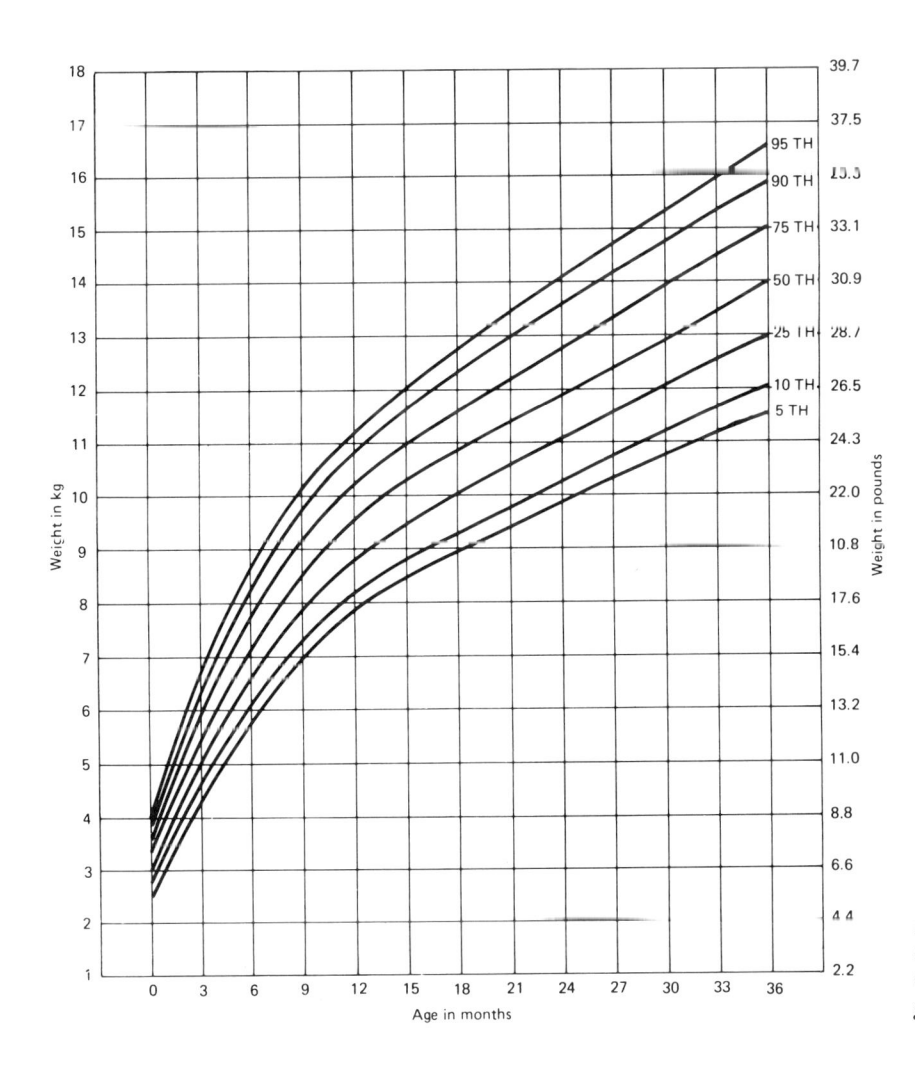

FIGURE 2-16. Weight-by-age percentiles for girls age birth to 36 months. (*From P. V. N. Hamill et al., NCHS growth charts, 1977.*)

understood ways. Growth and maturation are used as indexes of health, and health in turn influences growth and maturation.

NUTRITIONAL FACTORS

It is necessary for a child to have nutrient intake which will support metabolic processes for the capture of energy and the synthesis and support of new and existing tissues. Nutritional influences upon physical development exert both positive and negative effects. When influences have such a negative effect as to be disruptive to normal physical growth and maturation, the degree of impact is directly related to the degree and duration of the insult.

The effects of famine resulting from war have been documented twice within this century for German school children. There was a uniform drop in height during the later years of both world wars as the food supplies decreased (Tanner, 1970). Though children will recover from acute starvation, chronic undernutrition results in reduced adult stature because of its effect upon skeletal ossification. The deficient caloric intake slows bone growth and calcification of ossification centers. Protein undernutrition results in reduced bone growth and in delay in development of the ossification centers (Garn, 1966).

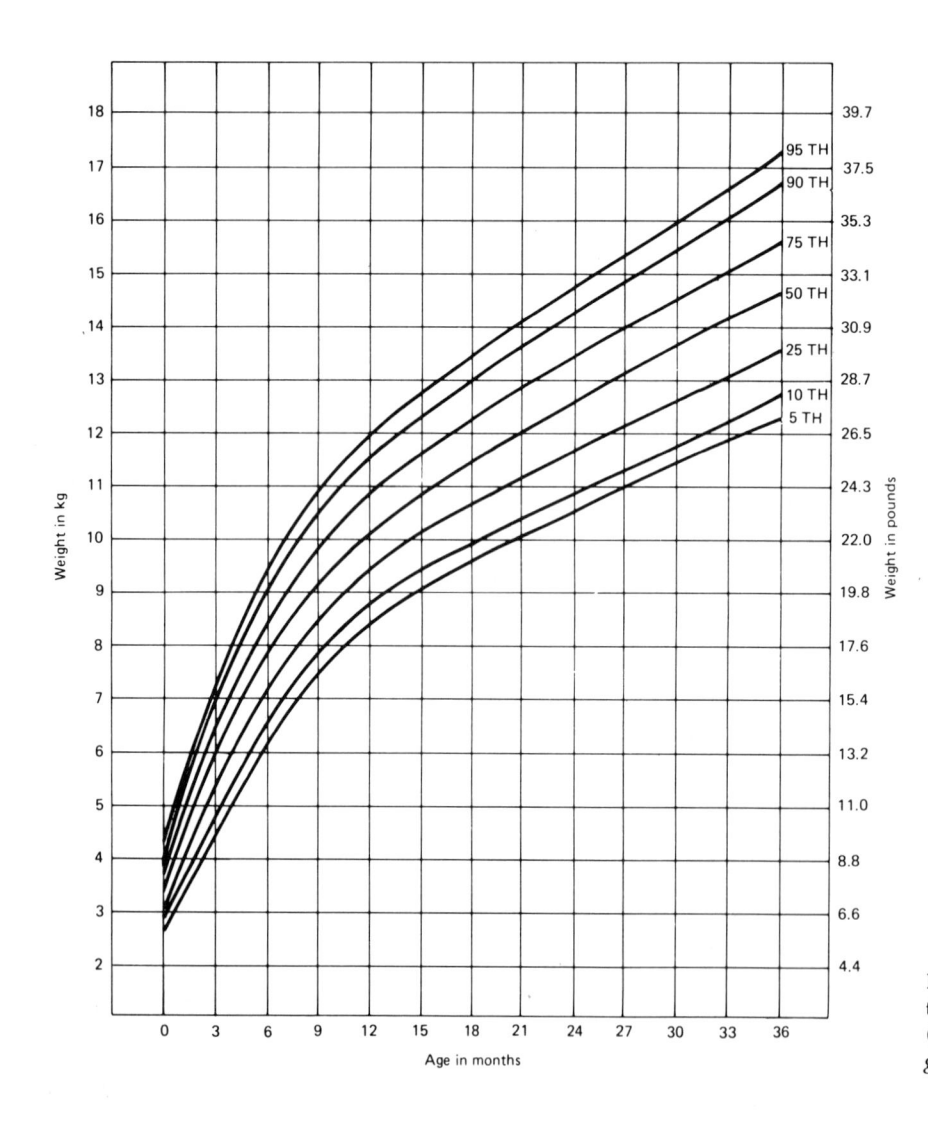

FIGURE 2-17. Weight-by-age percentiles for boys age birth to 36 months. (From P. V. N. Hamill et al., NCHS growth charts, 1977.)

The timing of the nutritional deficit is even more important in determining long-term effects. Startling evidence regarding the effects of undernutrition upon brain growth during the first year of life has been documented. In pathology studies of tissues from marasmic and normal infants who died during the first year of life, there was found to be a significant reduction in the overall weight of the brain and in the amount of protein and DNA in the brain tissues (Winick, Rosso, and Waterlon, 1970). It has been determined that human brain cells do not increase in number after the first 15 months of life; thus it may be inferred that undernutrition during the prenatal period and first year of life have irreversible disruptive effects upon neurological development.

SOCIOECONOMIC FACTORS

Socioeconomic factors as well as health influence physical development. Findings from several studies conducted under the auspices of the World Health Organization have shown a relation between mean birth weight and socioeconomic status: the result of the interaction of multiple environmental factors. (Because the studies represented groups in which the caste system was practiced, assortive mating may be assumed to have contributed a strong hereditary influence.)

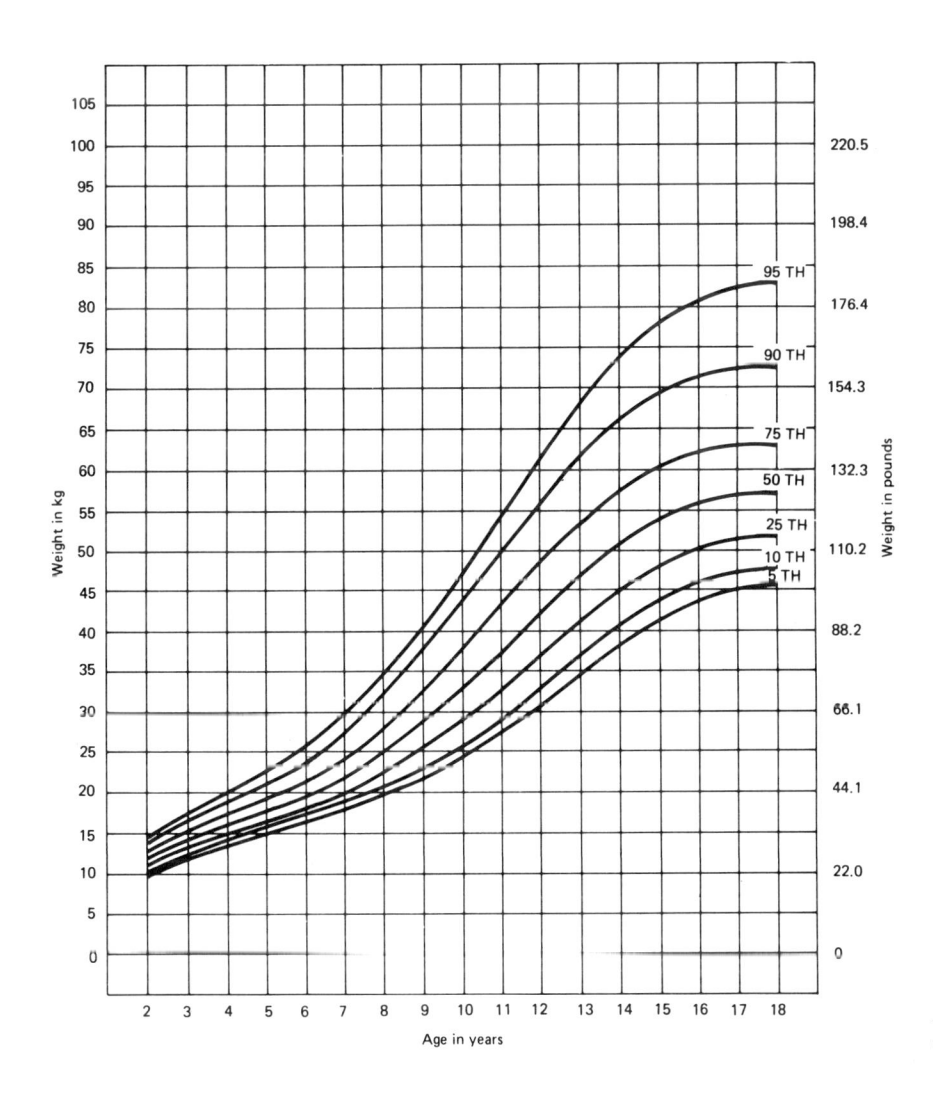

FIGURE 2-18. Weight-by-age percentiles for girls age 2 to 18 years. (*From P. V. N. Hamill et al., NCHS growth charts, 1977.*)

It has been found that birth weight tends to be lower in the least-favored sections of any community, but it has also been found that the relation between the various factors was not a simple one. In the United States, social class tends to vary within a family and is markedly unstable over generations; thus mean birth weight is a doubtful measure in biological studies. In addition, it has been noted that two or more generations are required to undo the effects of adverse childhood environmental circumstances upon the childbearing females who did not achieve their full growth potential.

Traditionally, overall body size of all age groups of children has been strongly correlated with the father's occupation irrespective of the number of children in the family. In Britain, a height differential of 2.5 to 5 cm (1 to 2 in) was reported between children of professional parents versus children of the lower socioeconomic class. While most of the earlier data showed a difference in age of menarche of approximately 2 to 4 months, relative to socioeconomic class, in more recent studies the difference has disappeared.

Many complex, interrelated factors influence growth differentials associated with socioeconomic conditions. Of these factors, home conditions, which are a reflection of the parents' intelligence and personality, exert a greater influence on growth than do economic circumstances. Growth differential associated with number of children in the family appears to be closely related to nutritional factors. As the number of children increase, there tends to be a decrease in both the quantity and the quality of care provided.

CULTURAL INFLUENCES

The significant role of cultural factors upon the developing child was recognized by Gesell and Ilg (1949, p. 61). However, the specific influences of culture upon physical growth and development are not as well described in the literature.

Cultural prescription may determine selection of individuals for marriage, selection of a mate, and selection of individuals permitted to live. Indirectly, these cultural determinants affect the gene pool and hence the characteristics favored to remain. For example, if in a certain cultural group the characteristic of light skin is favored in selection for marriage, the gene pool will be strengthened in the direction of lightly pigmented skin. Further, if individuals with genetically linked diseases are not selected for marriage, the gene pool for those conditions will be reduced.

In a now-classic study, Frank (1938) identified specific, well-organized physiological processes for which the infant surrenders functional autonomy to cultural control. Each of these processes is directly dependent upon physical development, especially upon maturation of the nervous system. The infant must learn to transform hunger into appetite, that is, to become progressively more dependent upon the external situation to arouse the desire for food in place of the intraorganic stimuli. Further, the infant must learn to give up the intimacy of body contact with the mother and the satisfaction of suckling needs and to substitute auditory approval for tactile sensations. The child also must learn to recognize increased pressure in the bladder and bowel and to control the automatic sphincter release according to external circumstances and cultural requirements.

Patterns of child care are cultural influences that are thought to affect physical development, though results from studies are not conclusive. In groups where swaddling is practiced, the infant is denied the opportunity for

TABLE 2-2 Major causes of death of children in the United States, by age (1975)*

Cause of death	Age, years <1	1–4	5–14
Accidents	43.3 (4)	28.2 (1)	18.1 (1)
Neonatal conditions; birth injuries, anoxia, etc.	863.4 (1)	0.1	—
Congenital anomalies	278.7 (2)	8.9 (3)	2.0 (3)
Infectious illnesses	161.6 (3)	9.0 (2)	2.0 (3)
Neoplasms, malignant and benign	6.0	5.9 (4)	5.1 (2)
Cardiovascular diseases	26.4 (5)	2.6 (5)	1.5 (5)

* Rates per 100,000 estimated population in specified age group are given. Numbers in parentheses indicate the rank order for the five leading causes of death in each age group.
Source: Adapted from data presented in National Center for Health Statistics Monthly Vital Statistics Reports, 1976, 25(10) and 1977, 25(11). Also adapted from I. Barry Pless, Current morbidity and mortality among the young. In R. A. Hoekelman et al. (Eds.), *Principles of pediatrics: Health care of the young.* New York: McGraw-Hill, 1978, p. 1876.

flexion or extension of his extremities in space. However, studies have shown that, on release from swaddling at the end of the first year, the infants are physically intact and in a matter of hours develop motor skills comparable to infants who had been free to move their limbs. However, other studies report that when permissiveness is the custom and children are encouraged to explore their environment, there is an increase in the development and control of the maturing neuromuscular system.

The adult value system is reflected in practices of daily living. When food resources are limited, a culture that places higher value on males will offer meat to males while females receive broth. If children in such groups are given low food priority, their degree of malnutrition may become severe. Hence, the nutritional status will vary within the members of the group, depending upon the value system.

Some cultural groups equate "bigness" with health. Within such a system parents may overfeed children in order to conform to cultural pressure. Some cultures may equate bigness with masculinity or maleness with involvement in competitive sports and encourage physical

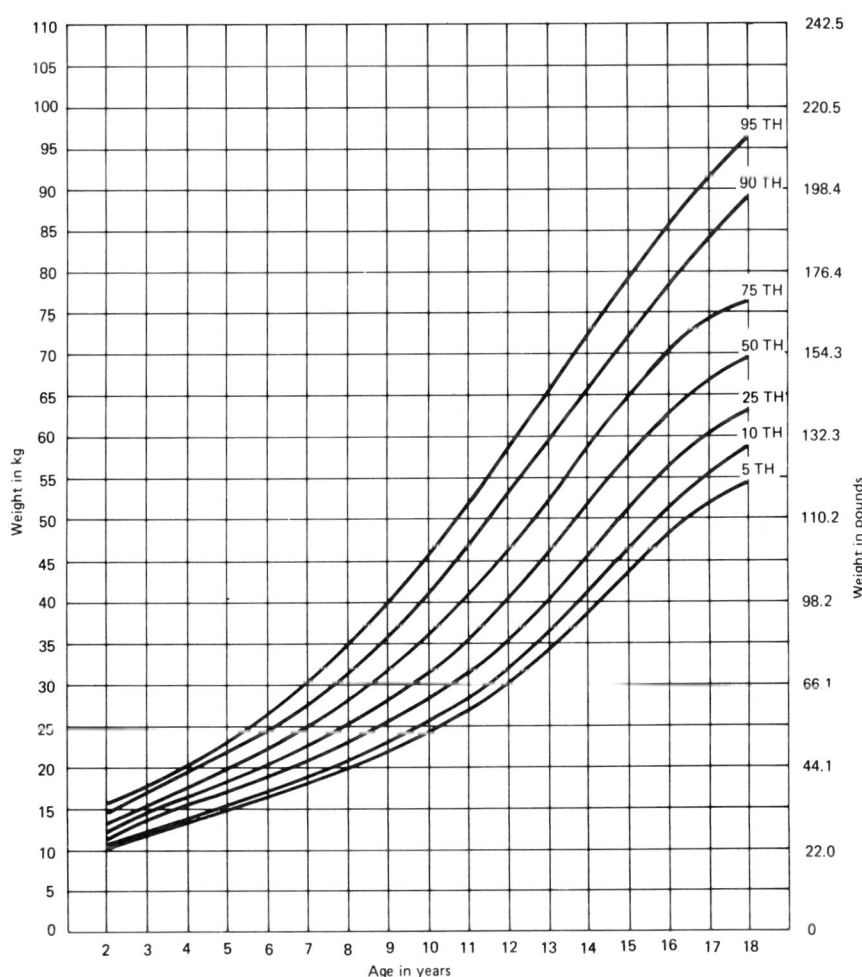

FIGURE 2-19. Weight-by-age percentiles for boys age 2 to 18 years. (*From P. V. N. Hamill et al., NCHS growth charts, 1977.*)

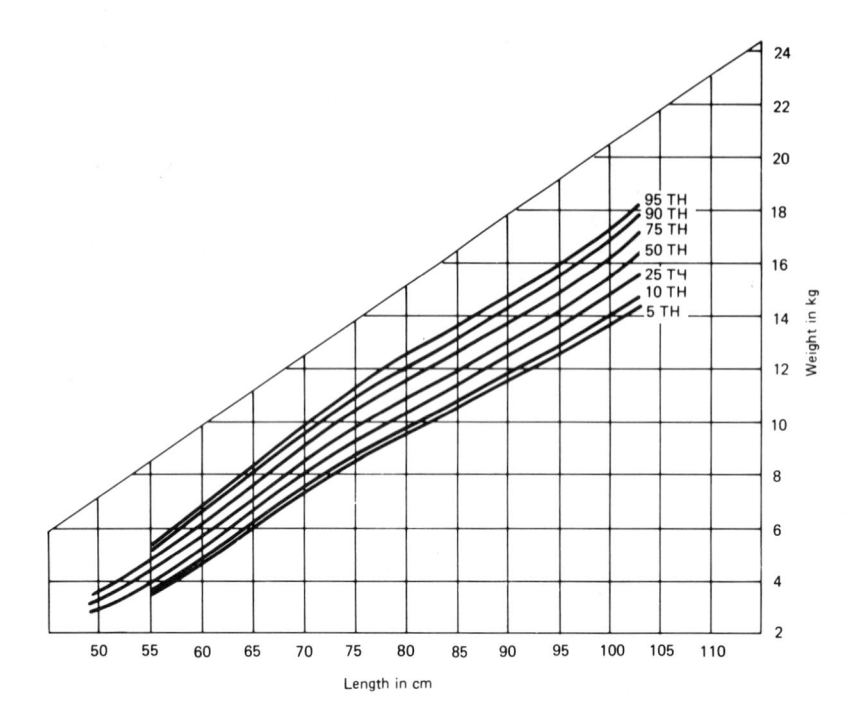

FIGURE 2-20. Weight-by-length percentiles for girls age birth to 36 months. (*From P. V. N. Hamill et al., NCHS growth charts, 1977.*)

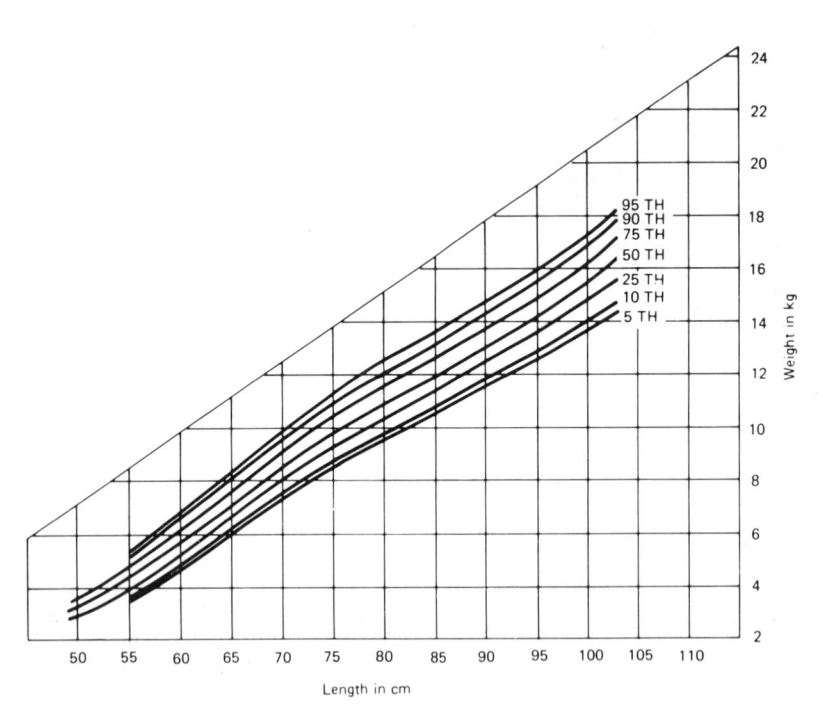

FIGURE 2-21. Weight-by-length percentiles for boys age birth to 36 months. (*From P. V. N. Hamill et al., NCHS growth charts, 1977.*)

activity in males, thus affecting physical strength and coordination as well as self-expectations.

STIMULATION VERSUS DEPRIVATION

The impact of institutionalization upon children was brought to the attention of such researchers as Bowlby, Spitz, and Goldfarb. Studies showed that children exposed to a deprived environment from early infancy were likely to demonstrate an overall delay in motor and mental development. The mechanisms responsible for this growth delay are not fully understood (Silver and Finkelstein, 1967).

It has also been documented that emotional deprivation retards physical development. The effects of deprivation upon physical development are noticeably evident in the failure-to-thrive syndrome. Within this overall term, two specific conditions have been identified (Whitten and Krieger, 1977). In maternal deprivation syndrome, infants are undergrown and show varying degrees of developmental retardation, emotional disturbance, and altera-

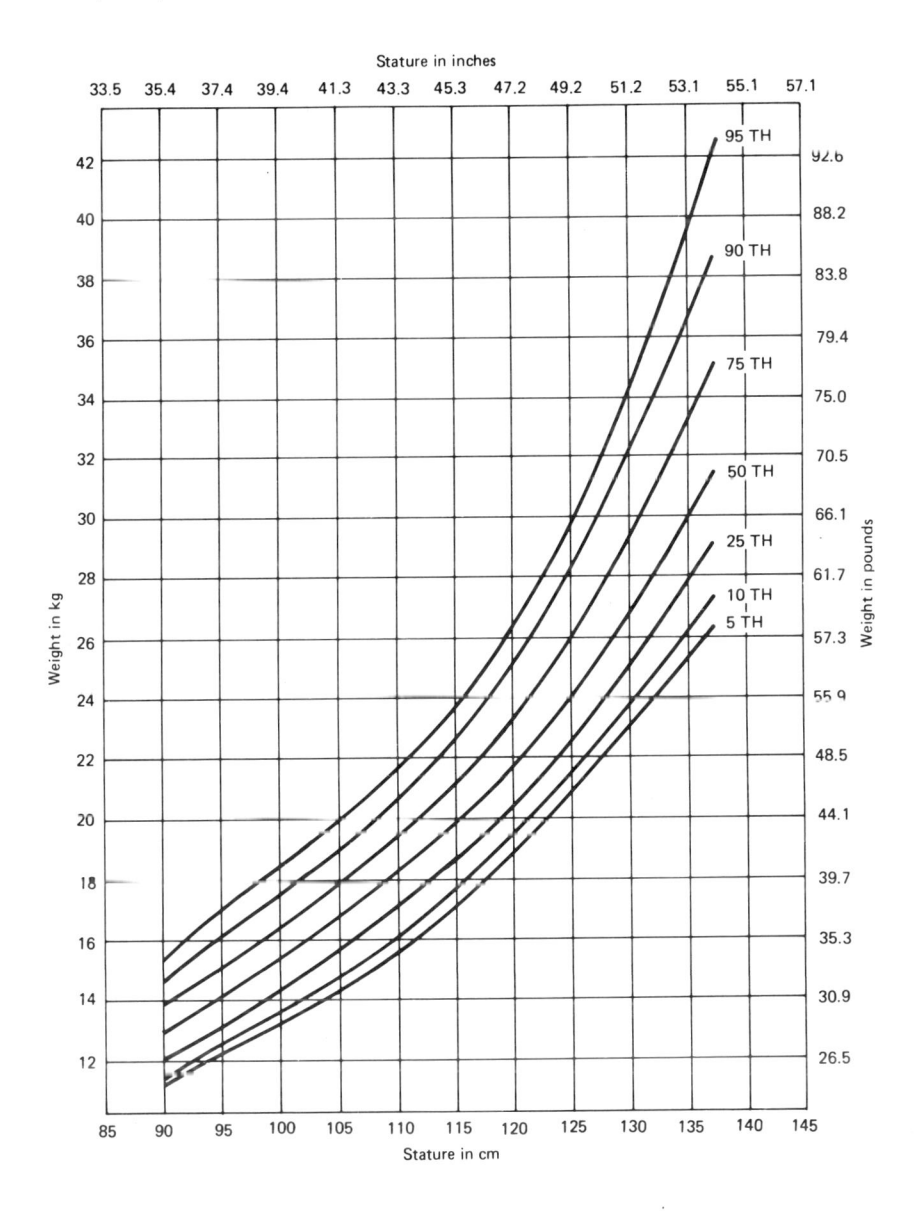

FIGURE 2-22. Weight-by-stature percentiles for prepubertal girls. (From P. V. N. Hamill et al., NCHS growth charts, 1977.)

46 PHYSICAL DEVELOPMENT

tions in affect, supposedly from lack of mothering. Some postulate that all symptoms are actually secondary to malnutrition.

The term psychosocial dwarfism refers to older children who show growth failure and bizarre eating habits from adverse parenting. The growth failure associated with parental deprivation is initially manifested in failure to gain weight followed by linear growth failure. Some infants demonstrate endocrine changes, such as decreased thyroxine, increased basal metabolic rates, and increased cortisol secretion (Krieger and Good, 1970; Krieger and Tagi, 1975; Powell, Brasel, Raiti, and Blizzard, 1967). In psychosocial dwarfism there is deficient growth hormone. Severe psychological stress appears to be capable of retarding growth by "switching off" the release or synthesis of growth hormone. It has been noted that these small children eat excessive amounts of food, sleep poorly, and learn slowly. When they are removed from the traumatic

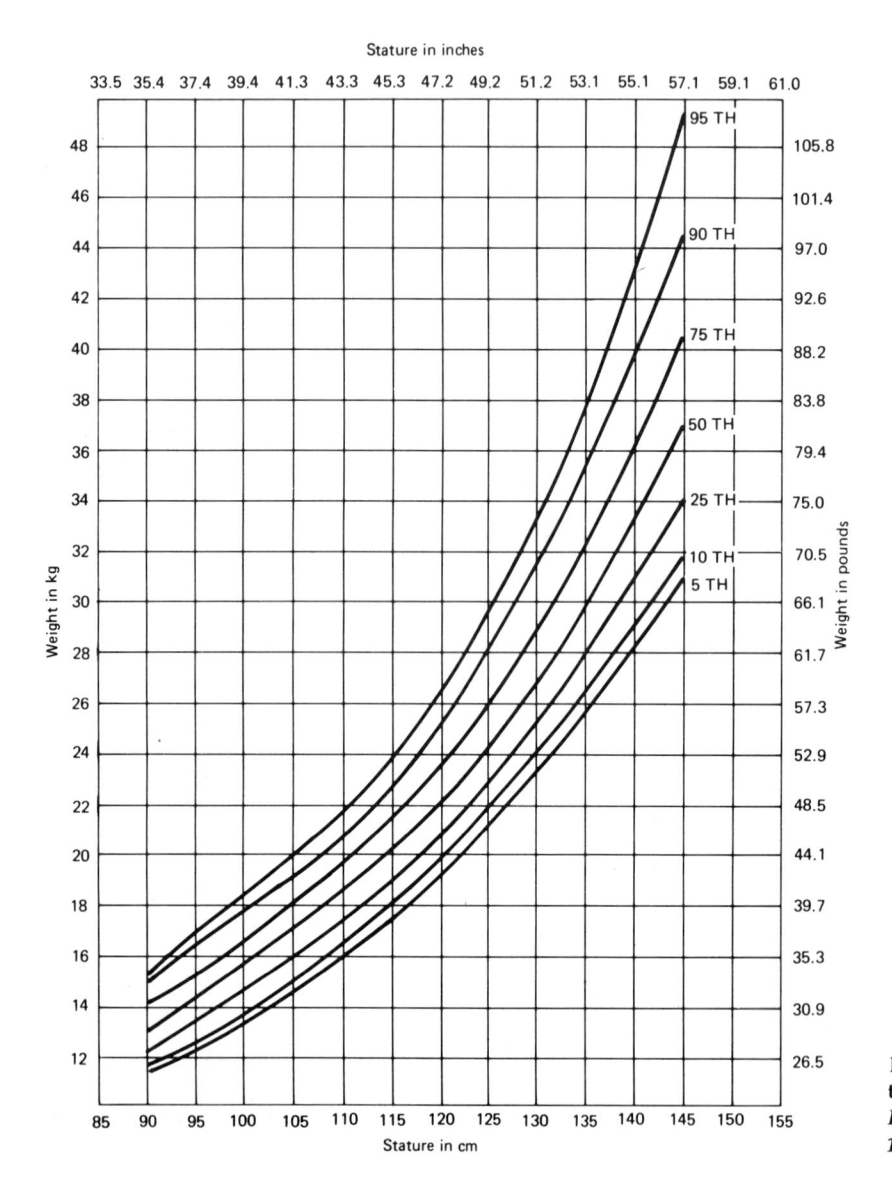

FIGURE 2-23. Weight-by-stature percentiles for prepubertal boys. (*From P. V. N. Hamill et al., NCHS growth charts, 1977.*)

environment, they show catch-up growth and a return to the production of normal levels of growth hormone.

A challenge to further research is appropriate in the light of the lack of definitive information regarding the effect of stimulation upon later growth and maturation. Studies on the effect of stimulation upon the infant and child should be geared to investigating the outcomes of all aspects of physical development.

Human genetics: Blueprint for development Veronica M. Ladensack Young

Genetics plays a major role in growth and development, because it establishes the biochemistry necessary to maintain the growth and the living state of the embryo, child, and adult. Genetics is the science of inherited traits. Genetic information is encoded in deoxyribonucleic acid (DNA), which determines the polypeptide structure of proteins. The DNA is transcribed through the synthesis of another macromolecule, *ribonucleic acid* (RNA). There are three types of RNA. *messenger RNA* (mRNA), *ribosomal RNA* (rRNA), and *transfer RNA* (tRNA). The RNA and the linear amino acid sequences in the polypeptides are precisely determined by the base sequences of genes in DNA.

The most impressive attribute of cells is their ability to transmit hereditary information to the next generation. The physical basis of heredity was not understood until the twentieth century, when the chromosomal theory of inheritance was established (Watson, 1976).

CHROMOSOME THEORY OF INHERITANCE

Chromosomes control hereditary traits because they are the physical and cellular locations of *genes*. Genes were first discovered by Gregor Mendel in 1886, but their importance was not realized until the start of the 1900s. Mendel proposed that a gene for each hereditary trait is given by each parent to its offspring. The physical basis for this is in the distribution of maternal and paternal homologous chromosomes. In each person's makeup, there are chromosomes from the mother and corresponding *homologues* from the father. Homologues are chromosomes which are morphologically and structurally similar to each other. During meiosis and gamete formation, one of each pair of homologous chromosomes, with the genes contained on it, is randomly distributed to each sex cell.

DEFINITION OF TERMS

The word gene comes from the Greek suffix *-genēs*, meaning born. In modern genetic terminology, the gene is the *cistron*. The essential idea is that the gene is the biological unit of heredity, consisting of DNA, which codes for a specific amino acid sequence in a polypeptide (protein), and the gene is located on a definite *locus* (position) on a particular chromosome. At conception, each person receives a set of genes that will determine the pattern of development and the physical and physiological traits. Each gene can exist in a variety of different forms called *alleles*. A given population may have many alleles; two are carried by a given individual. The *genotype* makes each person unique and is the pattern of all the alleles at every loci on the chromosomes. External appearance is the *phenotype*, determined by both genotype and environmental factors.

A chromosome is a body of nucleic acid that is tightly bound by proteins. Chromosomes are found in the cell's nuclei and contain the gene-carried information for the metabolic control of growth, development, and the continuity of the species. Through chromosomes, the hereditary characteristics are transmitted from one generation to the next. Chromosomes always exist in pairs (homologues); humans have 46 chromosomes in 23 pairs. The members of each pair are identical in their sequence of genes; for example, the Rh gene is located in the same chromosomal position, on the short arm in both the maternal and paternal homologues.

Mitosis is cell division to produce two identical cells, which contain the same quantity and type of DNA as the original cell. Somatic cells are produced by mitosis; these cells are *diploid*, which means they contain 46 chromosomes. (Mitosis is further discussed later in this chapter.) In contrast, *meiosis* is a special cell division which reduces the original 46 chromosomes by half to a *haploid* number of 23. Gametes are the only cells produced by meiosis and contain the reduced or haploid number of 23 chromosomes.

As a genetic term, *inheritance* means the acquisition of traits or characteristics by transmission of genes from parents to children. *Heredity* indicates the genetic constitution of an individual and the genetic transmission of a particular trait or quality from parent to offspring. One's genetic background represents the diversity and contributions of *all* ancestors. *Pedigree* is the family tree diagramed to represent many generations.

Family is a group of individuals descended from a common ancestor and sharing the same genetic background. The term familial seems to be confused with genetic terms; familial refers to a trait that occurs in or affects more family members than would be expected by chance. Families do share the same genetic background, but familial traits are not necessarily due to this genetic similarity. Family studies account for one criterion in determining if a trait is genetic, but they will not supply sufficient data by themselves. Familial is not synonymous with genetic.

Chromosome aberrations are changes in the number or structure of chromosomes. They can be detrimental and even fatal to the embryo or fetus. Chromosomes can be changed in many ways, including breaks, deletions, translocations, and lags in cell division (nondisjunctions).

CHROMOSOME MORPHOLOGY

Human chromosomes were described in the cell nucleus in the 1870s, but it was not until 1956 that the normal diploid human chromosome number was correctly identified as 46. These 46 chromosomes occur as 23 homologous pairs (maternal and paternal pairs). Twenty-two pairs (44 total chromosomes) are *autosomes*. The twenty-third pair is made up of sex chromosomes: X and X, female, or X and Y, male.

An analysis of chromosomes is done by preparing a karyotype usually of peripheral blood lymphocytes. The lymphocytes are grown in tissue culture flasks, stopped at the metaphase stage of mitosis, and placed on chromosome slides. Under the microscope, the chromosomes appear as small letter X's (see Fig. 2-24). They are grouped and defined by their size and centromere position (see Table 2-3).

Centromeres are primary constrictions in the chromosome and are used to define the chromosome's shape. *Metacentric* chromosomes have the centromere in the middle of the chromosome, creating p and q arms of equal length. *Submetacentric* chromosomes have a centromere closer to one end, creating a short p arm and a longer q arm. *Acrocentric* chromosomes have a secondary constriction above to the p arm, creating a short chromosome stalk (see Fig. 2-25).

CHROMOSOME BANDING

In 1968, the first significant work on chromosome identification was performed using quinacrine mustard, a fluorescing chemical. Quinacrine mustard applied to metaphase and prometaphase cells shows varying degrees of fluorescent intensity along the length of the genome. By photographing and comparing the fluorescent regions, or *bands* of fluorescence, the chromosomes can be distinguished from one another. An advantage of

TABLE 2-3 Normal human chromosomes by group, size, description

Group	Chromosome no.	Size	Description
Group A	1	Largest	Metacentric
	2		Submetacentric
	3		Metacentric
Group B	4	Large	Submetacentric
	5		Submetacentric
Group C	6–11,X	Medium	Submetacentric
	12		Submetacentric
Group D	13–15	Medium small	Acrocentric
Group E	16	Medium small	Metacentric
	17		Submetacentric
	18		Submetacentric
Group F	19,20	Very small	Metacentric
Group G	21,22,Y	Smallest	Acrocentric

distinguishing chromosomes from each other is that they can be matched with their proper homologue: The maternal chromosome number 1 can be paired and matched with the paternal chromosome number 1, for example.

CLINICAL USE OF CHROMOSOME BANDING

Clinical use of quinacrine staining (Q staining) has been readily applied. The most exciting clinical application was the identification of Down syndrome as trisomy of the twenty-first chromosome. By the late 1960s the entire human chromosome complement could be identified. Due to various complications, however, most clinical and research laboratories had not begun to use quinacrine mustard as a laboratory tool in human karyotype analysis.

GIEMSA STAINING

By accident and astute observation, Pardue and Gall (1970) observed the differential binding of Giemsa blood stain on the centromeres of mouse chromosomes. The chromosomes stained in a differential way, hypothesized to be short, repeated base sequences in the DNA. Other workers quickly modified the Giemsa stain (G stain) techniques and applied them to human chromosomes (Arrighi and Hsu, 1971; Jones, 1970). Giemsa staining techniques are easier and less costly than those of Q staining to implement in a laboratory, and chromosomes retain the stain during long-term storage of slides. With the use of G-staining techniques, laboratories worldwide

FIGURE 2-24. The complete chromosome complement of the human female and male includes 46 chromosomes in each, but 1 of the 23 pairs, the sex chromosomes, differs between the two sexes. The female has two X chromosomes; the male has one X and one Y chromosome. (*From D. O. Woodward and V. W. Woodward, Concepts of molecular genetics. New York: McGraw-Hill, 1977, p. 341. Reprinted by permission of the publisher.*)

began using chromosome banding for karyotype analysis. A variation of the process that gives reverse bands is called R staining.

Bands were defined by the National Foundation–March of Dimes–sponsored Paris Conference in 1971 as "parts of a chromosome which are clearly distinguishable from its adjacent segments by appearing darker or lighter with Q-, G-, R-staining methods. Bands that stain darkly with one method may stain lightly with other methods. The chromosomes are visualized as consisting of a continuous series of light and dark bands" (see Fig. 2-26). The impact of banding on clinical cytogenetics has truly been remarkable. It has served to confirm chromosome patterns previously hypothesized and to establish the diagnosis of new chromosome rearrangements, translocations, deletions, and gene locations.

Clinical application of Giemsa chromosome-banding techniques includes a more sophisticated karyotype analysis, possible because homologues of each chromosome can be matched. Maternal and paternal chromosomes therefore will show the same chromosome-banding patterns. Particular attention is paid to the chromosome arms, *chromatids*, and the longitudinal dark and light band patterns. The patterns on each chromosome number 1 will match, but be distinctly different from, the patterns on any other chromosome. Natural differences between chromosomes, *polymorphisms*, do occur consistently for certain chromosomes.

ARRANGEMENT OF GENES ON CHROMOSOMES

Through family studies, pedigree analysis, and especially the laboratory techniques called somatic cell hybridization, nearly 100 genes have been assigned to specific sites, or loci, on human chromosomes. For example, chromosome number 1 contains Rh genes. The estimated number of genes in the human genome is 100,000.

GENE ACTION

DEOXYRIBONUCLEIC ACID

Genes are specific base sequences of DNA, arranged in a linear manner in chromosomes. The backbone of DNA, or 2-deoxyribonucleic acid, is composed of alternating sugar and phosphate with bases that project inward from the backbone. The genetic information is carried in the sequence of these four nitrogenous bases: *adenine* (A) and *guanine* (G), which are *purines*, and *thymine* (T) and *cytosine* (C), which are *pyrimidines*. An infinite number of genetic messages can be coded with the four letters, A, G, T, C, of the nucleic acid alphabet. The number of se-

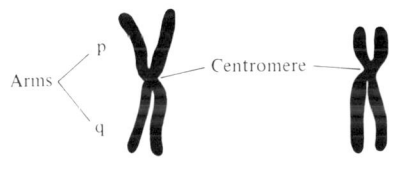

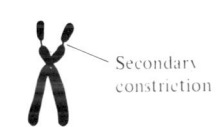

FIGURE 2-25. An example of metacentric, submetacentric, and acrocentric chromosomes.

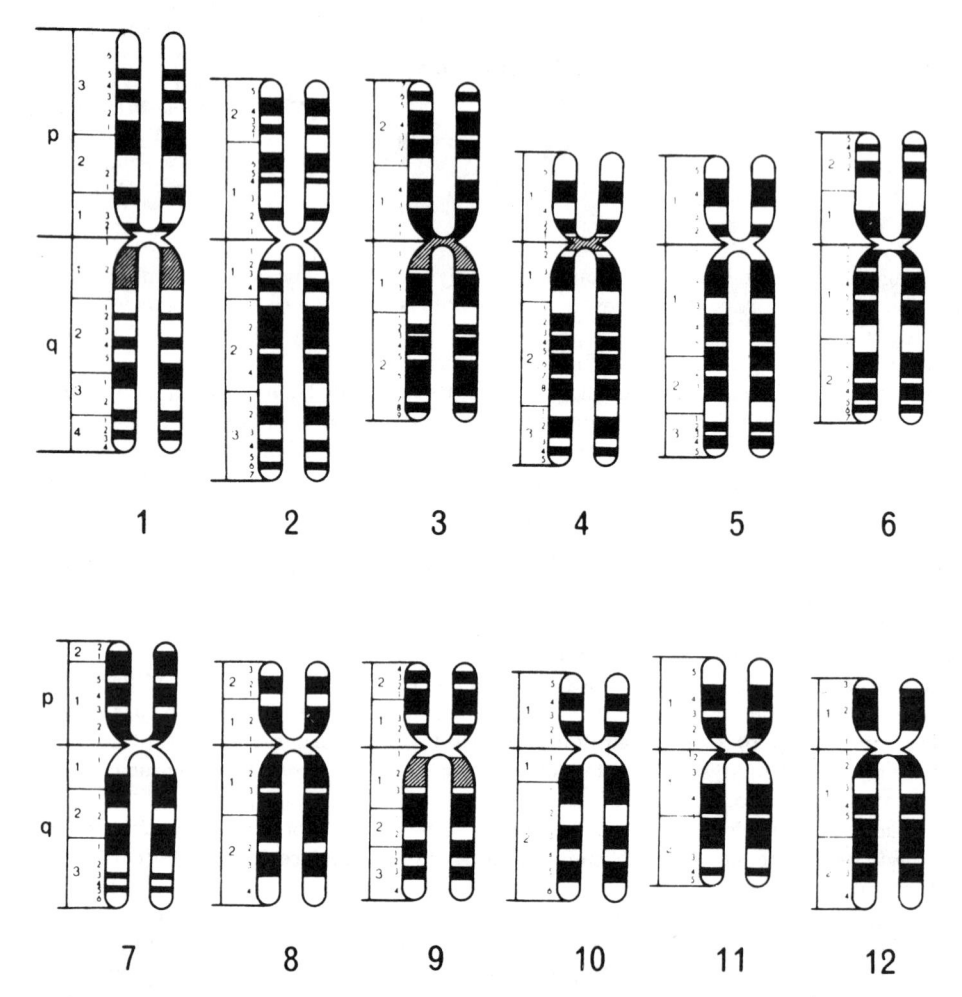

FIGURE 2-26. Chromosome bands: Diagrammatic representation of chromosome bands as observed with the Q-, G-, and R-staining methods. [*From D. Bergsma (Ed.), Paris Conference, 1971: Standardization in human cytogenetics. Birth Defects Original Article Series, 8(7). White Plains: National Foundation—March of Dimes, 1972. Reprinted with permission of the National Foundation—March of Dimes.*]

PROCESSES OF PHYSICAL DEVELOPMENT   51

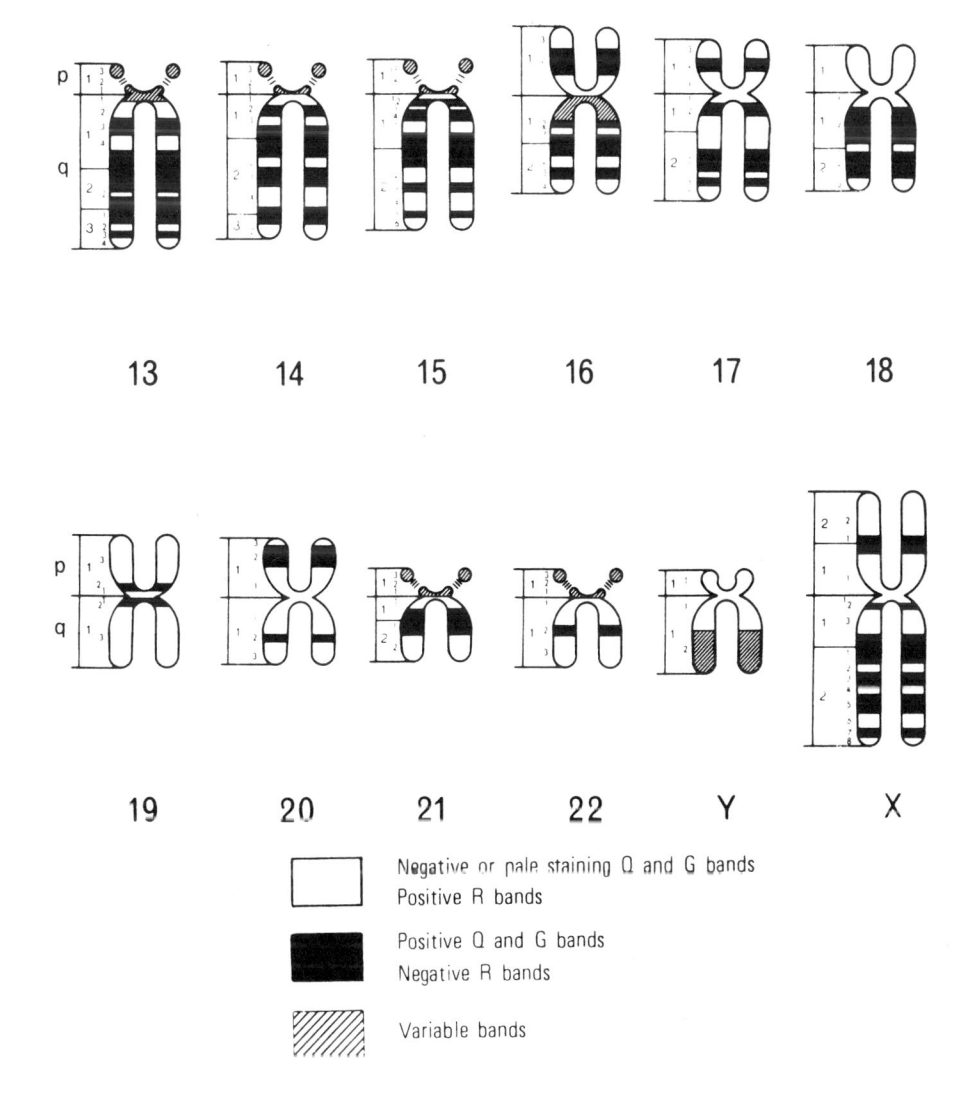

13   14   15   16   17   18

19   20   21   22   Y   X

☐ Negative or pale staining Q and G bands
  Positive R bands

■ Positive Q and G bands
  Negative R bands

▨ Variable bands

quence permutations is 4^n, where n is the number of bases in the nucleotides in a molecule.

DNA contains two strands of polynucleotides (many nucleotides with bases) wound around each other into the form of a *double helix*. The two strands are complementary, which means that the adenine bases in one strand are always paired with thymine in the other strand. Guanine pairs with cytosine. Base pairing will often be referred to as A-T and G-C pairing (see Fig. 2-27). The order of the purine and pyrimidine bases is variable depending on the gene it makes up. The two strands are joined by hydrogen bonds between the inside pair of bases.

DNA REPLICATION

When DNA duplicates in cell division, the hydrogen bonds between the bases break, and the strands replicate as they unwind. Each DNA strand functions as a template, or model, for the newly forming DNA chains. The new chains are complementary to the unwound DNA template, which means that the new bases must obey the A-T and G-C base-pair rules. The replication of DNA forms two new chains from the single initial DNA double helix (see Fig. 2-28). The daughter cells which receive the newly formed DNA are guaranteed of receiving the same genetic information contained in the parent cell. The Watson and Crick model for DNA (Fig. 2-28) represents the two-stranded DNA helix (Watson and Crick, 1963).

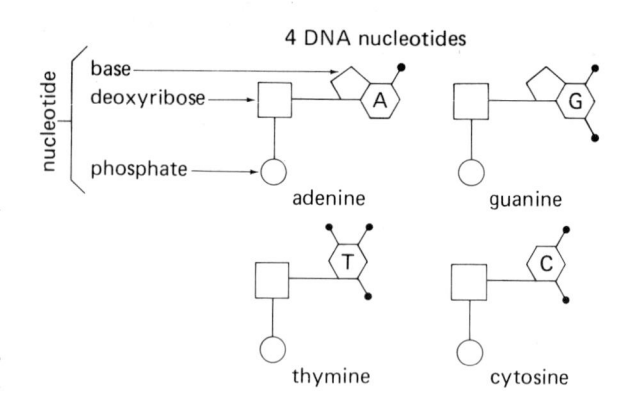

The unwound DNA strands do not function alone as templates but require enzymes to catalyze the synthesis of the new long-chain polymers of DNA. The cellular enzyme which catalyzes the reaction of new DNA replication is DNA polymerase.

PROTEINS, THE PRIMARY GENE PRODUCT

The primary product of genes is proteins. The central dogma of genetics is the following:

DNA $\xrightarrow{\text{transcribes}}$ RNA $\xrightarrow{\text{translates}}$ protein

Proteins are important because they are part of the cells' functional parts. Myelin sheaths or neurons, all enzymes, the globulins, cell membranes, and the three-dimensional structure of chromosomes all have proteins as an integral part. Proteins consist of a combination of the essential and nonessential amino acids linked together with strong peptide bonds into single chains. Proteins can take on more complex forms when the primary structure (single chains of amino acids) folds, twists, and bends back upon itself. The larger, convoluted forms are the secondary and tertiary structures of proteins. Quaternary protein structures can be formed when several proteins combine.

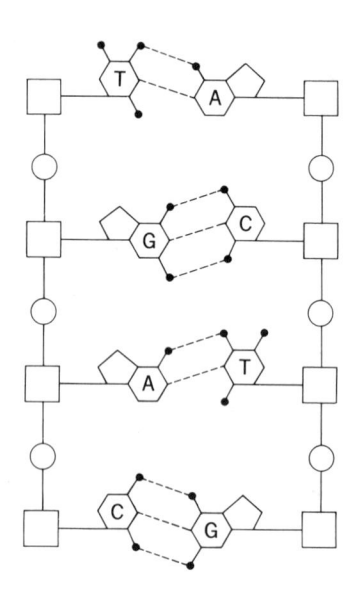

In a person with sickle cell disease, the DNA that is transcribed and translated into the hemoglobin molecules has been altered. A single nitrogenous base in DNA was

FIGURE 2-27. Double-helical structure of DNA showing thymine-adenine and guanine-cytosine pairing. (*From D. S. Luciano, A. J. Vander, and J. S. Sherman, Human function and structure. New York: McGraw-Hill, 1978. Reprinted with permission of the publisher.*)

changed, and therefore the RNA transcribed from that gene was altered. Likewise the protein translated from the altered messenger was formed with the amino acid sequence altered resulting in sickle cell hemoglobin, which is less stable inside the red blood cell.

GENE FUNCTION, CONTROL OF GENES

It is known that genes transmit the hereditary information from one generation of cells to another and from one generation of people to the next. Daughter cells resemble the original cell because of the messages coded in the genes. Also it is known that genes function by directing the metabolism of every living cell. But how does the DNA → RNA → protein dogma direct differentiation of the embryo? In the growing embryo, cellular differentiation of the *morula* is the first chemical step indicating that DNA directs the production of enzymes and proteins. Unwound DNA transcribes information to an mRNA in the transcription process. The mRNA leaves the nucleus, passes into the rough endoplasmic reticulum of the cytoplasm, and associates with a ribosome.

Translation of RNA into proteins needs the two other types of RNA: transfer and ribosomal. Ribosomal RNA is located in the ribosomes. Transfer RNA is complexed with a specific amino acid and an activating enzyme. The amino acid–tRNA complex attaches to specific coding sites on the mRNA. After the tRNA is positioned on the mRNA, the bonds between the amino acid and the tRNA are broken. The amino acids are transferred and bonded with a peptide bond to the growing chain of polypeptides (translation). As the polypeptide chain grows, the newly forming protein moves away from the ribosome into the cytoplasm (see Fig. 2-29).

Differential transcription of DNA is ultimately responsible for the normal sequence of tissue and organ growth in the embryo. Not all DNA is transcribed and translated in every living cell. For instance, only red blood cells produce hemoglobin, and only fetuses and neonates produce fetal hemoglobin. Bile is produced normally in the liver and nowhere else in the body. Therefore some genes must be derepressed, or induced (turned on), or repressed (turned off) during the course of a day or a lifetime. The control of genes is central to cell processes like differentiation, hormone action, and even the abnormal process of cancer cell formation.

Since the cell's genetic information is in the sequence of nucleotides in the DNA, its control must be coordinated with the transcription process. Current research suggests

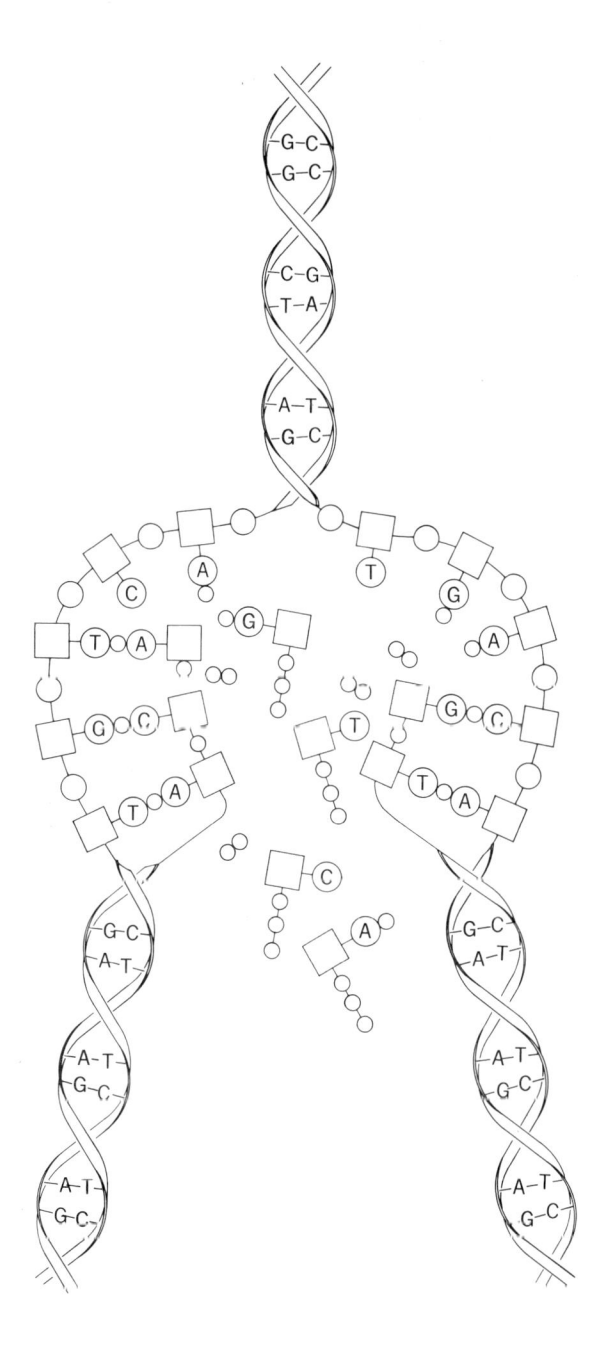

FIGURE 2-28. Replication of DNA: The two strands of the DNA double helix separate. Bases of free nucleotides pair with the exposed bases of the old DNA strands. Two identical double-helical molecules of DNA result, each containing one old and one new nucleotide strand. (From D. S. Luciano, A. J. Vander, and J. S. Sherman, *Human function and structure.* New York: McGraw-Hill, 1978. Reprinted with permission of the publisher.)

that the chromosomal proteins, called *histones,* are responsible for genes being repressed. Histones are proteins rich in the amino acids arginine and lysine and have a positive charge overall. Research suggests that histones block transcription by binding with DNA (Huang and Bonner, 1962). DNA that is combined with histones is repressed and will not be transcribed into RNA, and so the genes are considered turned off.

Acidic proteins, a large group of proteins which range in their molecular weight, are found inside cells sometimes in close proximity of chromosomal DNA. At least some of the acidic proteins, or *nonhistones,* are involved in the regulation of specific gene activity. Nonhistone proteins vary greatly between animal species and even vary within the same organism depending on the tissue being examined. This would be expected, since proteins would change when the gene activity changed.

Nonhistones associate with the cell's DNA-histone complex and become phosphorylated (which means that negatively charged phosphate groups are added to the DNA-histone–acidic protein complex). After phosphorylation, the DNA is freed of the histone–acidic protein–phosphate complex. The DNA is then free to carry on RNA synthesis, by transcribing its base sequences of genes into the three forms of ribonucleic acid (mRNA, tRNA, and rRNA). In other words, the phosphorylation of nonhistone proteins is associated with cellular differentiation and the activation of genes. In the laboratory, the

FIGURE 2-29. Protein synthesis: the central dogma of genetics. (*a*) The formation of mRNA. The DNA strands separate in one area; a strand of RNA is built up as shown and then leaves the nucleus. (*b*) The mRNA becomes associated with ribosomes. Molecules of tRNA are then assembled on the mRNA strand in a sequence complementary to it. Each tRNA bears an amino acid. In this way the amino acid sequence of the finished protein is determined. (*From E. P. Solomon and P. W. Davis, Understanding human anatomy and physiology. New York: McGraw-Hill, 1978. Reprinted with permission of the publisher.*)

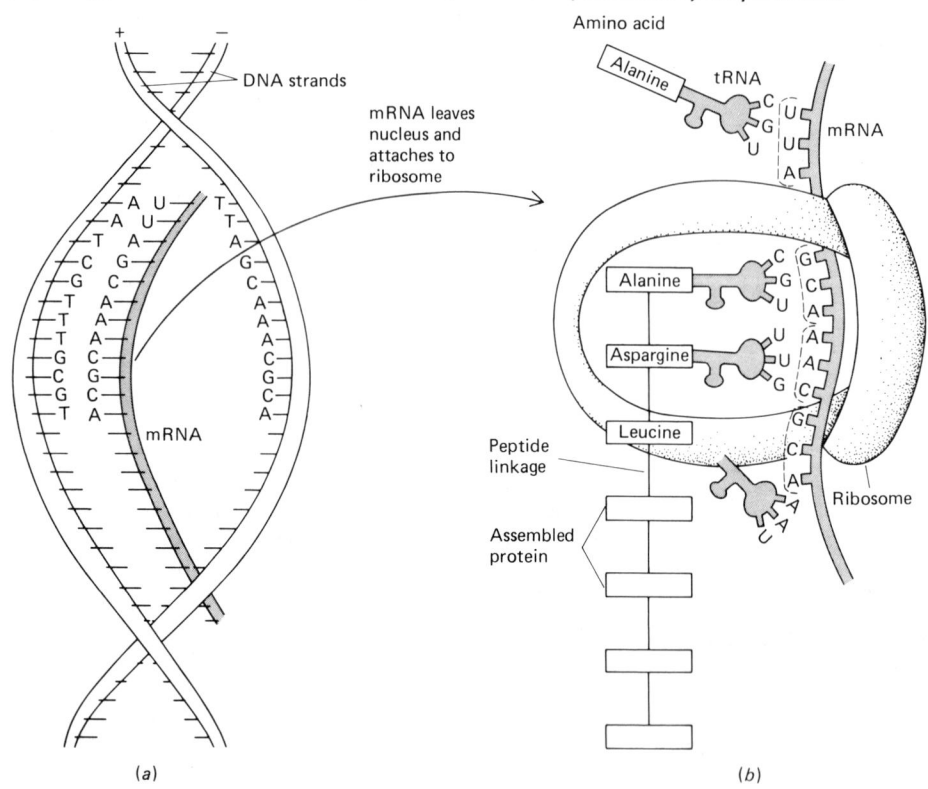

ability of nonhistone proteins to stimulate RNA synthesis in cell-free systems has been shown to be dependent on phosphorylation. Therefore, the addition of phosphate to nonhistone proteins may somehow be involved in the mechanism by which these molecules regulate gene transcription.

Although the central dogma of genetics is understood and the cellular control of genes is being analyzed, there is little understanding of how newly translated proteins affect the tissue and organ development of the fertilized ovum. The only cell-surface protein that is specifically known to cause cells to form an organ is the one responsible for the primary sex determination of male fetuses.

GENETIC CONTROL OF PRIMARY SEX DETERMINATION

The basic embryonic plan of the human is inherently feminine. The embryonic indifferent gonad shows an automatic tendency to develop into ovaries. Müllerian ducts differentiate to fallopian tubules and the uterus. The urogenital sinus differentiates to a vulva and a vagina. All growing fetuses will develop into females unless male-forming steps intervene.

Y chromosome Presence of a Y chromosome in the male embryo directs the embryonic indifferent gonadal ridge to develop and organize a testis. Once the testis is organized, the Leydig cells synthesize and secrete testosterone. Testosterone is an effective hormone that induces all the external masculine development.

Testosterone induces the differentiation of (1) Wolffian ducts to masculine reproductive tracts and the accessory glands and (2) urogenital sinus areas to the penis and scrotum. Sertoli cells of the Y-organized fetal testis are thought to produce a factor that causes the regression of the Müllerian ducts. The testis-organizing role of the Y chromosome is apparently due to the presence of a gene located on the long arm of the Y chromosome: the H-Y–activating gene.

H-Y antigen and male determination In the presence of a Y chromosome, the H-Y–activating gene is transcribed and translated into a protein on the plasma membrane. The plasma protein is detectable as an H-Y antigen and is responsible for the primary sex determination in the male embryo because it organizes the indifferent gonad into a testis. The H-Y antigen is important because any male that lacks this gene will automatically develop as a female. The H-Y antigen is the first cell-surface protein known to specifically cause organogenesis (Ohno, 1976, 1978).

MEIOSIS

Meiosis, two cell divisions with a single duplication of the chromosome complement, reduces the number of chromosomes in each cell from the usual diploid number (46) to the haploid number (23). The *spermatocyte* and *oocyte* are two highly specialized haploid cells, or gametes, that combine to create a new individual. *Gametogenesis*, the process of gamete production, has one meiotic phase that reduces the chromosome number from diploid ($2n$) to haploid (n). Each gamete, either sperm or ovum, will then contain 22 autosomes and a single sex chromosome.

To accomplish the special function of reducing and dividing the chromosome number in half, gonadal *stem* (totipotential) cells undergo two separate cell cycles: meiosis I and meiosis II (see Fig. 2-30). Each cell cycle has the following phases: *prophase, metaphase, anaphase, telophase,* and *interphase,* the same as in mitosis (see "Mitosis" later in this section). The fundamental purpose of meiosis is to reduce the parental number of chromosomes by half in the gametes.

MEIOSIS I

The first meiotic phase, prophase, has five distinct phases of its own.

1. *Leptotene:* Chromosomes appear for the first time as fine threads. Duplication of the chromosomes has occurred during the interphase just before leptotene.
2. *Zygotene:* Homologous chromosomes, homologues, pair (synapse) side by side in a close association. The pairing process is not random. There is an exact point-to-point lineup of homologous sections of the chromosomes. The centromeres of the chromosomes never fuse, but the chromosomes are visible as 23 tightly joined pairs (bivalents).
3. *Pachytene:* Chromosome coiling increases, and chromosomes appear thicker. While synapsed, maternal and paternal chromosomes can exchange genetic segments by *crossing-over*.
4. *Diplotene:* The chromosome pairs become even more densely coiled and shorter, while they begin to separate longitudinally. The synapsed chromosomes do not separate completely because many segments are still in crossover and exchanging pieces.
5. *Diakinesis:* Homologues appear to repulse each other, and the synapsed areas look like X's that have slipped to the chromosome ends.

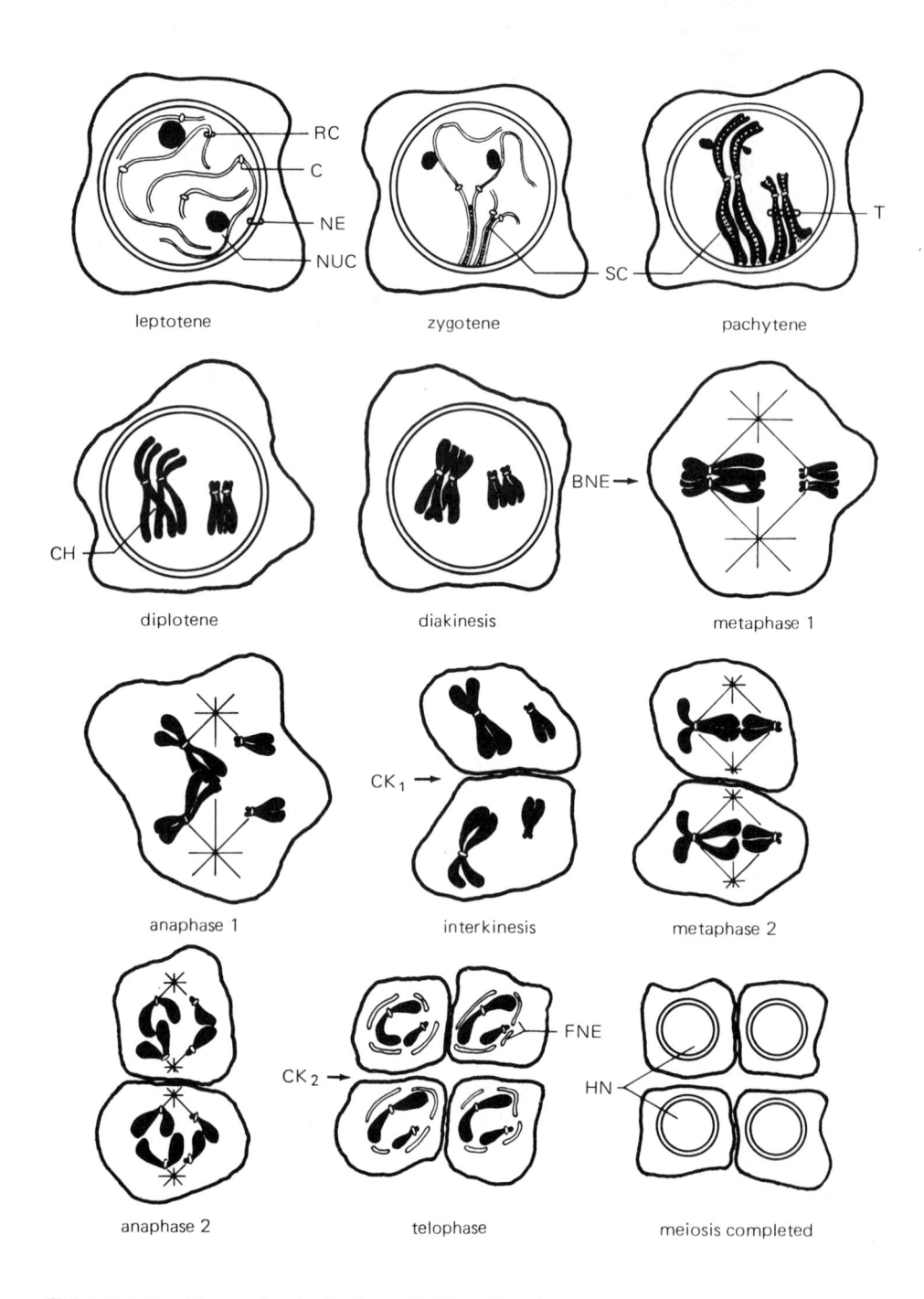

FIGURE 2-30. Stages of meiosis. *(From N. J. Berrill and G. Karp, Development. New York: McGraw-Hill, 1976. Reprinted with permission of the publisher.)*

The first prophase of meiosis I results in separation of the homologous chromosomes that were paired during the previous zygotene stage. Maternal and paternal chromosomes have exchanged some genetic segments and separated, and the number of chromosomes in each resultant cell is reduced from the original diploid ($2n$) to the haploid (n) number.

MEIOSIS II

Meiosis II results in a separation of duplicated sister chromatids and in centromere separation. Meiosis II proceeds through prophase, metaphase, anaphase, telophase, and interphase resulting in haploid gametes. Gametogenesis is discussed in full in Chap. 5.

DNA CHANGES

Crossing-over Genetic DNA can be altered in parent cells by several mechanisms. During meiosis, crossing-over during the pachytene stage of prophase I changes the alleles linked together on a single chromosome. Chromatids from maternal and paternal chromosomes lie close to each other (synapse of chromosomes) and can cross over and twist around each other. If they break, the broken chromatid ends rejoin but not necessarily with the original piece. If broken ends from different chromatids join together, then a genetic exchange occurred between maternal and paternal chromosomes. Crossing-over is a normal process, and it does not change the number of genes the embryo inherits. The loci or position of the genes is exactly the same as before crossing-over, but the genetic code is altered. Crossing-over increases genetic variation in embryos more than simple independent recombination.

Linkage Genes on the same chromosome are linked together. *Linkage* is the tendency for these genes, or this linkage group, to be inherited together. The strength of linkage depends on the distance between the genes. Genes near each other have a less likely chance of being separated during crossing-over in meiosis. Genes which are always inherited together are "tightly linked" and probably have genetic loci so close to each other that there is little space for crossing-over. If loci are very far apart, then crossing-over is likely to separate them. The inheritance pattern of the far-apart loci is similar to independent loci, which are on different chromosomes.

Translocations *Translocations* are segments of chromosomes which are detached and rejoined onto another part of a homologous or nonhomologous chromosome. A balanced translocation results in the same amount of DNA, although a chromosome piece has been shifted to a different chromosome. Chromosome-banding techniques could be utilized to analyze the exact segment which was broken and translocated. Although individuals with balanced translocations are phenotypically normal, they have an increased risk of having multiple spontaneous abortions and abnormal children with chromosome deletions.

Deletions Deletions are chromosome deficiencies, or lost segments. Deletions can occur during meiosis, when rejoining does not occur, or during mitosis, when chromosomes are broken and fail to repair. Any broken chromosome segment which lacks a centromere (acentric) will be lost. Acentric fragments can not be pulled toward a spindle pole during daughter cell formation. Daughter cells with deletions, no matter how small, are deficient in DNA. Deletions are always abnormal because they result in the loss of many genes.

MENDELIAN LAWS

The term *Mendelian inheritance* is named for the Austrian monk, Gregor Mendel, and his recognition of patterns of inheritance. Mendel crossbred pea plants and then studied the patterns of physical traits appearing in the next generation. Mendel worked with the only thing that was visible to him, the phenotype of the plants. *Dominant* and *recessive* inheritance patterns are based on phenotypic appearance and measurements, called the level of ascertainment. This is an important concept, and the dominance of a gene ultimately depends on what is being measured and the criteria used in measurement. Analysis of the physical traits in the first and second generations led Mendel to conclude that there must be some orderly processes occurring. The laws of inheritance are *segregation, independent assortment,* and *dominance*.

SEGREGATION

Segregation is the orderly separation of allelic genes, or alleles, in the formation of gametes. Separation of maternal and paternal chromosomes during reduction division occurs during gametogenesis. A maternal chromosome contains one allele for a genetic loci, while the paternal chromosome contains the other allele. The alleles segregate in a random combination of gametes. The *punnet square* allows analysis of the possible offspring from the combination of different parental gametes (see Fig. 2-33 and 2-34).

INDEPENDENT ASSORTMENT

The law of independent assortment states that there is independent inheritance of genes that govern separate traits. Genes which are located on separate chromosomes (not linked) will be inherited separately from each other and not be influenced by each other's alleles. For example, genes on chromosome number 1 undergo segregation, crossing-over, and recombination in gametogenesis and are not influenced by genes on other chromosomes.

LAW OF DOMINANCE

When defining the effect of a pair of genes, if one member of the pair exerts its effect greater than the other, the gene is dominant. The dominant gene will exert its effect on the phenotype when it is present in the homozygous form (two dominant genes) or in the heterozygous form (one dominant gene and one recessive gene). Recessive genes must be present in the homozygous form to elicit an effect on the phenotype. In the punnet square, a capital letter represents dominance, and a lower case letter represents recessive.

PEDIGREE ANALYSIS

Construction and interpretation of pedigree charts are done to study inheritance in an extended family. The symbols used are illustrated in Figs. 2-31 and 2-32. Generations are numbered with Roman numerals. Vertical lines extending from marital lines represent the children. Children within a generation are numbered with script numbers from left to right in birth order. The black arrow is the propositus, also called index case of proband. This is the person under study in a clinical situation.

AUTOSOMAL DOMINANT INHERITANCE

Pedigrees of families with an autosomal dominant trait will generally have the following characteristics:

- If a trait appears in the first and third generations, it must be present in the second; it cannot "skip" generations.
- Males and females will be affected in the same ratio: there is no sexual bias for autosomal dominant traits.
- Over several generations, approximately one-half the offspring will display the phenotype.
- Only persons with the gene can transmit the trait to their children. (However, spontaneous mutations can occur.)
- If one parent is heterozygous for the trait, then each child will have a 50 percent chance of inheriting the trait.
- If one parent is homozygous for the trait, all children will inherit the trait.
- If both parents have the trait, then each child has a 75 percent chance of inheriting the trait (see Fig. 2-33).

AUTOSOMAL RECESSIVE INHERITANCE

Recessive genes must be present in the homozygous form for an autosomal recessive trait to be expressed. Some of the characteristics of autosomal recessive traits in families will be as follows:

- The trait will usually not be phenotypically present in every generation but will appear to skip generations. In some families there may only be one individual who displays the recessive phenotype even though the pedigree includes four or more generations.

FIGURE 2-31. Symbols for pedigree charts.

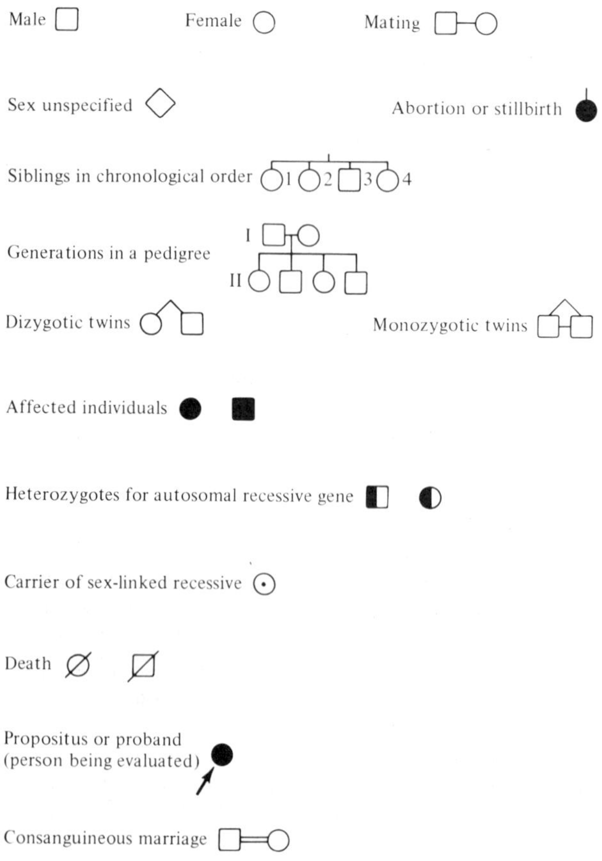

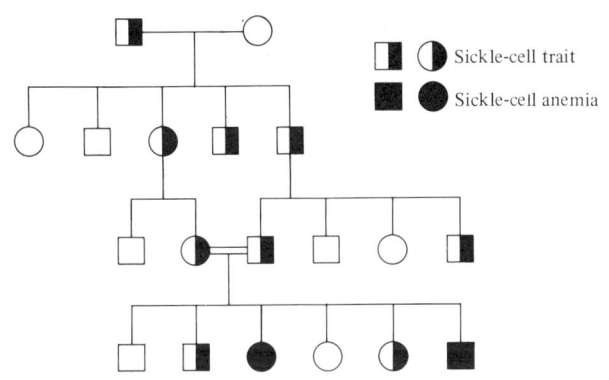

FIGURE 2-32. Pedigree of a family with sickle cell anemia. [*From V. A. McKusick, Human genetics (2d ed). Englewood Cliffs, New Jersey: Prentice-Hall, 1969, p. 55. Reprinted by permission of the publisher.*]

- A parent who is a *carrier*, heterozygous for a recessive trait, can have affected children only if the other parent is also a heterozygote or is a homozygote for the same trait.
- A carrier may be unaware of being a heterozygote unless tests are performed or the carrier has a child with a recessive phenotype. For example, carriers for Tay-Sachs disease or the sickle cell trait are healthy individuals who are unaware of their genetic background unless laboratory tests are performed to detect their heterozygosity. Cystic fibrosis carriers do not have a conclusive test to detect their recessive gene and will only know of their carrier status if they produce a child with cystic fibrosis.
- *Consanguinity* (inbreeding) is likely to be a factor when children have a recessive trait that is very rare in a population. For instance, the child of a person with a recessive gene has a greater probability of inheriting the same gene from an ancestor than from someone in the general population if the carriers in the population are very rare.
- If both parents are heterozygotes, or carriers, then there is a 25 percent chance that each child will be homozygous and display the recessive trait. There is a 50 percent chance that each child will be a carrier, not displaying the trait, there is a 25 percent chance that each child will not have the recessive gene at all (see Fig. 2-34a).
- If one parent is a carrier and the other parent does not

(a)

	D	d
d	Dd	dd
d	Dd	dd

50% heterozygous (Dd): trait present phenotypically
50% homozygous (dd): trait absent genotypically and phenotypically

(b)

	D	D
d	Dd	Dd
d	Dd	Dd

100% heterozygous (Dd): trait present phenotypically

(c)

	D	d
D	DD	Dd
d	Dd	dd

25% homozygous (DD): trait present phenotypically
50% heterozygous (Dd): trait present phenotypically
25% homozygous (dd): trait absent genotypically and phenotypically

FIGURE 2-33. Dominant inheritance patterns. (*a*) One parent is heterozygous (Dd). (*b*) One parent is homozygous, dominant (DD). (*c*) Both parents are heterozygous (Dd).

have the recessive gene (homozygous dominant), then no children are at risk for the recessive trait; 50 percent will be carriers (see Fig. 2-34b).
- If one parent is heterozygous and one homozygous displaying the trait, there is a 50 percent chance that each child will be a heterozygote (carrier) and a 50 percent chance of being homozygous for the recessive gene displaying the trait (see Fig. 2-34c).
- If a child displays the recessive trait that neither parent displays (parents are carriers), then his siblings displaying the dominant trait will have a two-thirds chance of being carriers.

X-LINKED INHERITANCE

Genes that are located on the X chromosomes are transmitted by *X-linked inheritance*. Females inherit an X chromosome from both their mother and father and thus have a pair of X chromosomes: XX. Males inherit one X chromosome from their mother and the Y chromosome from their father; they have a pair of sex chromosomes, but the set is an unmatched pair: XY. Genes located on the X chromosome will have the same properties of being dominant or recessive, as on the autosomes, but the pattern of inheritance will be different in males and females due to the single X chromosome in the male.

Pedigrees of families with an X-linked recessive trait will display the following patterns:

- The X-linked trait is expressed in half the sons but none of the daughters when the mother is a carrier (heterozygous) and the father is not affected. Half the daughters will be carriers themselves (see Fig. 2-35).
- Even though the gene is recessive, all males who carry the gene will express it in their phenotype as there is no corresponding gene on a second chromosome.
- Females will only express the recessive phenotype if they are homozygous for the recessive gene. X-linked traits are rarely seen in females.

FIGURE 2-34. Recessive inheritance patterns. (a) Both parents are heterozygous, carriers (Rr). (b) One parent is heterozygous, carrier (Rr), and one parent is homozygous, dominant (RR). (c) One parent is heterozygous, carrier (Rr), and one parent is homozygous recessive, affected (rr).

	R	r
R	RR	Rr
r	Rr	rr

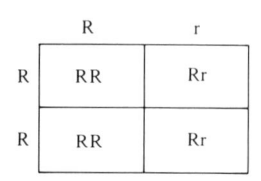

25% homozygous (RR): trait absent genotypically and phenotypically
50% heterozygous (Rr, carriers): trait present genotypically but not phenotypically
25% homozygous (rr): trait present genotypically and phenotypically

(a)

	R	r
R	RR	Rr
R	RR	Rr

50% homozygous (RR): trait absent genotypically and phenotypically
50% heterozygous (Rr, carriers): trait present genotypically but not phenotypically

(b)

	R	r
r	Rr	rr
r	Rr	rr

50% heterozygous (Rr, carriers): trait present genotypically but not phenotypically
50% homozygous (rr, affected): trait present genotypically and phenotypically

(c)

	X^r	X
X	X^rX	XX
Y	X^rY	XY

DAUGHTERS
50% X^rX (carriers)
50% XX

SONS
50% X^rY (trait observed)
50% XY

FIGURE 2-35. X-linked recessive inheritance where mother is a carrier (XX) and father is not affected (XY).

POLYGENIC INHERITANCE

Polygenic inheritance is the type of heredity for which many genes contribute to a particular trait. Stature, eye color, hair color, and fingerprint patterns are all examples of characteristics controlled by several pairs of genes, but the exact number of genes involved is not known. Since the inheritance patterns of most physical traits are very complicated, polygenic inheritance, or multiple genes, is the most common form of inheritance in humans.

Environmental factors can greatly affect the growth of cells; genetic factors and environmental influences acting together constitute *multifactorial inheritance.*

GENETIC INFLUENCES ON BEHAVIOR

Evidence is growing that there are genetic and biological factors that have an effect on behavior. Behavior is a response brought about by a stimulation of the central nervous system. Since the primary product of genes is the production of proteins and enzymes, how does the genotype affect the phenotype and the eventual outward display of behavior?

Behavior geneticists are interested in such psychological behaviors as perception, cognition, learning, and some forms of mental illness. Behavior genetics is an area of study that strives to determine a genetic origin of behaviors and to describe behaviors which are displayed in certain gene or chromosome abnormalities.

Genes produce proteins, but no proof exists that proteins are responsible for mental health or mental illness. Considerable evidence does exist, however, for a genetic predisposition to affective disorders, to schizophrenia, and for some cognitive abilities. Through investigation of abnormal behavior and possible genetic implications, more can be learned regarding genetic effects on normal behavior.

AFFECTIVE DISORDERS

The National Institute of Mental Health's section on psychogenetics reviewed data on affective disorders, mania and depression (Gershon, Targum, Kessler, Mazure, and Bunney, 1977). Tests included twin studies, family studies, adoption studies, chromosomal linkage markers, and tests on the transmission of physiological and biochemical deficits.

Twin studies for affective disorders revealed a concordance rate for monozygotic (MZ) twins of 69.2 percent, compared with 13.3 percent for dizygotic (DZ) twins. To understand how much environment contributes to this behavior, MZ twins that were raised apart were also studied, and the concordance rate was 67 percent. This is suggestive of a genetic component for affective behavior disorders.

Family studies have reported a higher incidence of affective illness in first-degree relatives of persons with affective illness when compared with the general population. The mode of inheritance has been postulated to be a dominant gene on the X chromosome. But data are not consistent between research centers, and the frequency is too low to conform to simple Mendelian inheritance patterns.

Biochemical and physiological tests have revealed some important variations in families with affective disorders. In the biochemical pathway converting tyrosine to catecholamines, the enzyme catecholorthomethyltransferase (COMT) is responsible for conversion of norepinephrine and epinephrine to the metanephrines. Increased COMT activity is found to segregate with the bipolar form of affective disorders (both mania and depression). Therefore, COMT could be a physiological marker and possibly indicate the susceptibility of family members to this form of mental illness.

SCHIZOPHRENIA

Schizophrenia is a controversial mental illness. The phenotype has been difficult to define, and its definition varies among clinicians and nations. Twin studies help to support the hypothesis that there is a genetic cause of schizophrenia. Comparisons of MZ and DZ twins show an MZ concordance rate of 15 to 85 percent and a DZ concordance rate of 2 to 10 percent. Family studies reveal that parents of schizophrenic children have a 2 to 5 percent rate of schizophrenia, and the siblings have a 6 to 10 percent chance of developing the illness. In families where one child and one parent are affected, the siblings have a greater chance (10 to 20 percent) of developing schizophrenia. In contrast, schizophrenia in the general population is about 1 percent.

Biochemical theories for schizophrenia suggest a blocked metabolic pathway and the resultant accumulation of chemical by-products. It is thought that the accumulated by-products are responsible for increased abnormal behavior. Monoamine neurotransmitters are under study, and research has included the synthesis, secretion, transport, reabsorption, and degradation of monoamine oxidase (MAO). People with chronic schizophrenia have less than one-half the normal level of MAO in their platelets. Even discordant twins reflect this reduced level of MAO, but normal levels of MAO are present in platelets of persons with acute schizophrenia. This information is not yet understood, and further study is required before schizophrenia can be classified as a genetic disease on the basis of biochemical data.

COGNITIVE AND OTHER ABILITIES
The psychometric tests used by behavior geneticists measure cognitive and perceptual capabilities, not genotypes. One of the main problems with any behavioral study is there is no clear relation between genetic synthesis of polypeptides and the ultimate change in behavior which is thought to deviate from normal.

Evidence of a heritable component in normal reading ability has been provided by several relatively large-scale twin studies. Data from 113 twin pairs (48 MZ and 65 DZ) indicate that MZ twins have 90 percent concordance and DZ twin pairs have 35 percent concordance for reading ability (DeFries, Vandenberg, and McClearn, 1976).

Numerous other conditions have been hypothesized to have a genetic origin including spatial abilities, IQ, hyperactivity, aphasia, narcotic addiction, and alcoholism. Data are not conclusive for a genetic cause, but some familial tendencies have been reported.

GENETIC VARIATION TO DRUG DISPOSITION
It is well documented that there is genetic variation to the absorption, distribution, biotransformation, excretion, and interaction of drugs with the receptor sites on cell membranes (Vesell, 1972). In addition, there is a genetic variation to drugs which affect behavior; the tricyclic antidepressents are one example (Alexanderson and Sjoqvist, 1971).

SUMMARY
In conclusion, it can be stated that the human brain is an extremely complex and delicate organ. The early development of the central nervous system is effected by a host of genetic (as well as environmental and maternal) factors. Since the brain controls responses to external stimuli, any damage to or hindrance of brain functions could appear as inappropriate behavior. Behavior, however, is a blend of perception, experience, learning, memory, and conditioning to stimuli.

General considerations of physical development: Cellular growth, differentiation, and morphogenesis
Veronica M. Ladensack Young

GROWTH AND DIFFERENTIATION AT THE CELLULAR LEVEL
Tremendous growth occurs between the time an ovum is fertilized and an adult matures. Most of this growth occurs because of the production of new cells. The mature adult has 10^{14} cells, or 100 quadrillion cells, which is an astonishing increase from the original single-cell zygote.

MITOSIS
New cell production arises from other cells by a process of division: mitosis. The growth cycle of an average cell involves a gradual increase to twice its initial size, followed by a division process producing two identical daughter cells (see Fig. 2-36).

The cell membrane is 75 to 100 Å thin and is the limiting boundary of the cell. Through the membrane, the cell receives oxygen, electrolytes, hormones, and many other substances and eliminates waste products and carbon dioxide. If cell mass becomes too large in volume, it can not efficiently diffuse substances to meet cellular needs. Although the cell membrane is increasing in size, it is not proportional to the significantly larger increase in cytoplasmic volume. Thus, cell division becomes necessary.

Mitosis has five phases: prophase, metaphase, anaphase, telophase, and interphase. Cell synthesis, cell growth, and cell division are accomplished in the five phases of mitosis.

Prophase Prophase is the first phase of mitosis. Chromosomes are visible for the first time within the cell. The nuclear membrane disappears, and centrioles (achromatic spindles) appear as the growing cell develops polar bodies. Chromosomes will be pulled down and

FIGURE 2-36. Mitosis. (From E. P. Solomon and P. W. Davis, Understanding human anatomy and physiology. New York: McGraw-Hill, 1978. Reprinted with permission of the publisher.)

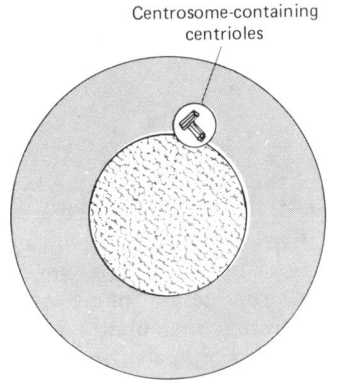

Interphase. The cell is carrying out its normal life activities.

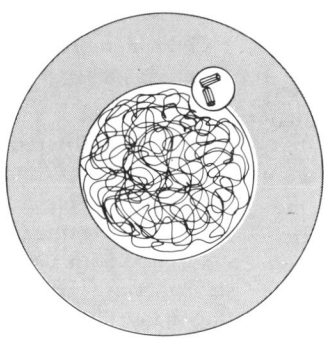

Centrosome-containing centrioles

Late interphase. Sensitive instruments detect doubling of the hereditary material (chromatin) of the nucleus.

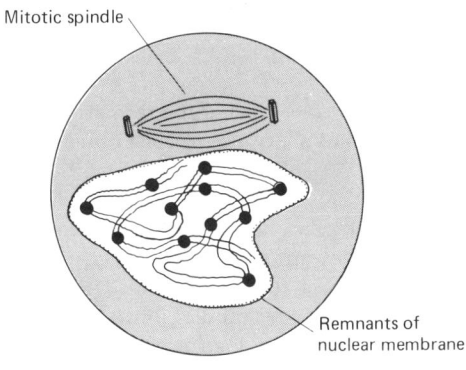

Early prophase. Nuclear membrane and nucleolus disappear. Long, threadlike bodies of chromatin become evident and begin to condense into the form of chromosomes.

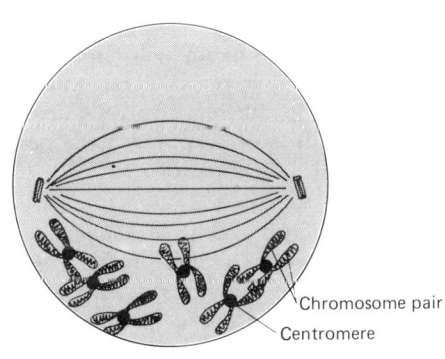

Mitotic spindle

Remnants of nuclear membrane

Late prophase. Chromosomes attain their definitive form though they continue to shorten and thicken. Spindle forms between the centrioles, which have moved to the poles of the cell.

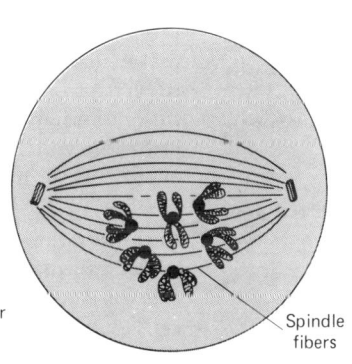

Chromosome pair
Centromere

Prometaphase. Spindle fibers attach to the centromeres of the chromosomes.

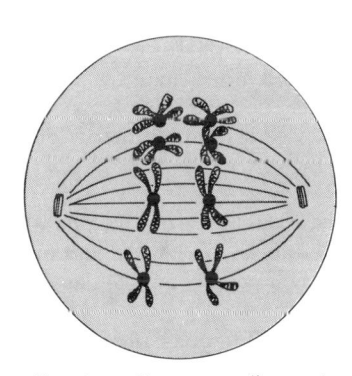

Spindle fibers

Metaphase. Chromosomes line up at the equator, and as the next stage of cell division begins, the centromeres divide, permitting duplicate members of chromosome pairs to be separated.

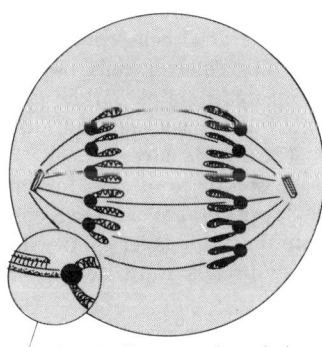

Spindle fibers are microtubules perhaps interconnected with cross bridges as in cilia

Anaphase. Chromosomes move toward the poles but no actual cell division (cytokinesis) has yet occurred.

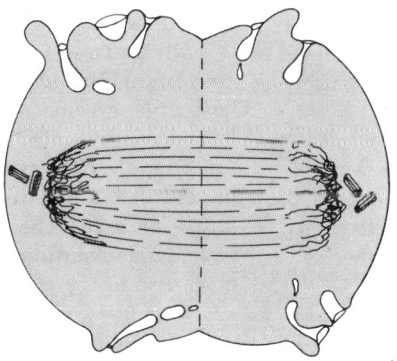

Telophase. The events of prophase are reversed, with the nuclei reforming, and physical cell division taking place so as to produce two daughter cells. Extensive pinocytosis often occurs at this stage of cell division. Centrioles duplicate.

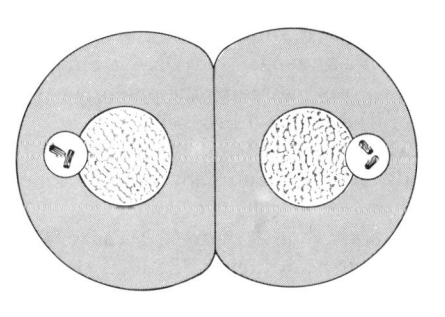

Daughter cells are formed, genetically (and usually physically) identical to parent cell except for size.

drawn to the centrioles during the formation of daughter cells. The centrioles are opposite each other, forming two polar bodies.

Metaphase Metaphase is the phase of mitosis when the chromosomes are arranged at the equatorial plate. Chromosomes appear to be "lined up" in the middle of the cell. The centriole, or spindle, forms asters, which are rays of protein fibers growing from the spindle. The rays attach to the centromere, or the middle of the chromosome. This is an important step, and any chromosomes which do not have a ray attaching them to the mitotic spindle apparatus at each pole cannot be pulled into the dividing cells.

Anaphase Anaphase is the phase when chromatids separate and move along the protein fibers of the spindle apparatus. Each chromatid is a new chromosome and moves toward the pole that is pulling it with a spindle aster.

Telophase Telophase is the phase during which the new daughter nuclei are formed and the cytoplasm is pinched off into two new, complete daughter cells.

Interphase Interphase for the two daughter cells is the time for DNA and protein synthesis. The chromosomes are not visible, and the cell incorporates molecules and substrates, which are necessary for the next round of mitosis. The nuclear membrane reappears.

Through mitosis, each new cell receives identical complements of all chromosomes in the original cell so that all the somatic or mitotic cells in the body contain the same chromosomes, genes, and DNA from the first fertilized ovum. Mitosis maintains the parental chromosome number (46) in every dividing cell.

The one-cell zygote undergoes 44 generations of mitosis to produce a newborn infant and only 4 more to reach the adult number of cells. Of course the 48 generations of mitosis are average figures, because some cells reach maturity early and never divide again, while other cells continue to replace damaged or destroyed cells.

CRITICAL CELLULAR EVENTS
Development at the cellular level depends on four critical cellular events. These events primarily occur prenatally and result in the ultimate formation of a full-term neonate:

- Cell proliferation
- Cell migration
- Cell differentiation
- Cell death

Early cell proliferation After the first division, the zygote undergoes a series of divisions called *cleavage*. Cleavage is a rapid mitotic division without growth, or cellular enlargement. Cleavage of the fertilized ovum is associated with a change in cell proportions: The cell loses its spherical shape; the cell-limiting membrane arches unequally; and the cytoplasm is incorporated into new cells but has not increased in volume greatly. Cleavage may be a means of restoring the nuclear/cytoplasmic ratio, which was heavily cytoplasmic during oogenesis.

Cleavage distributes the nuclear DNA to successively smaller cells: *blastomeres*. The blastomeres adhere to each other, probably by living connections and not merely physical adhesion (Blechschmidt and Gasser, 1978). Cell metabolism at the surface of the ovum will already be different from the interior, where oxygen will not enter as freely. Perhaps this beginning difference in cell-surface diffusion will help the dividing cells approach the next events of cell migration and differentiation.

Cell migration Cell migration is growth and movement of cells to other positions over the embryo mass. Rapid cell division is characteristic of the embryo, and when cells grow and move, a difference is established in gradients of cell metabolites. Metabolism and surface area also change rapidly during cell migration. Migrating cells are probably not differentiated cells, but their movement and growth will help establish different metabolic and kinetic fields across the embryo's surface, which may initiate the differentiation process.

After cleavage, the zygote is called a morula. A morula is a solid mass of cells, with superficial cells completely enveloping the internal cells. The interior cells have a basophilic cytoplasm, which means it stains darkly with basic dyes (pyronine, toluidine blue); basic staining indicates rapid RNA synthesis. The inside layer of cells is important because it is the major source of cells for the future embryo. The outside layer, or enveloping cells, have a pale-staining cytoplasm, and this layer eventually gives rise to the embryonic membranes and placenta.

Cell differentiation Differentiation is a process leading to a specialized cell type. The transition from an embryonic cell to a differentiated cell is a gradual process that involves increased complexity in growing cells. This increased complexity involves the differential transcription and translation of nuclear DNA and the progressive specialization of cells. The differentiated cell may display altered cell organelle ratios (increased mitochondria), organelle size, appearance of additional cell structures, and unequal or allometric growth patterns. All the changes are the result of preferential synthesis and the destruction of cell membrane proteins, structural proteins, and cellular enzymes. Cell differentiation should therefore be attributable to the transcription of DNA to form mRNA and the translation of mRNA in the formation of proteins.

Differentiation is a cellular process that indicates that a cell acquires new morphological and functional properties that make it different from other cells. The morphological changes in size, staining, and appearance are visible alterations which are most likely controlled by changes in the expression of the cell's genetic material, or genome. *Primordium* is a cellular beginning of a future tissue or part even before it acquires the gross features or characteristics of the differentiated tissue, organ, or part.

MOLECULAR BASIS FOR GENETIC CONTROL OF DIFFERENTIATION Gene expression is regulated during cleavage and embryo differentiation by transcription of DNA regions into RNA. The mechanisms of control are not known, but they are hypothesized (Davidson and Britten, 1979):

1. Genes could be regulated by specific interactions occurring at repetitive sequences in the DNA genome.
2. Differentiation is based on diverse and specific cytoplasmic mRNA sequences.
3. Cells have specific mRNA that result from structural genes being transcribed in cell-specific patterns.

RIBONUCLEIC ACID IN THE NUCLEUS Nuclear RNA is synthesized in genes from DNA. The DNA is known to contain regions that have highly repetitive sequences which could reflect the types of mRNA produced. It is also known that there are significant differences in the nuclear RNA in different cell types. The cytoplasm of the fertilized ovum is thought to have different rates and types of repetitive transcribed RNA, and this could give rise to early differential patterns of gene expression.

During differentiation and cell specialization, genes are activated (turned on) and repressed (turned off). In each of the ultimate cell types (neurons, alveoli, etc.), only a certain combination of genes is transcribed, or expressed, in accordance with the cell's specific function. For example, in muscle cells the structural genes coding for myoglobin are turned on. In the islet of Langerhans in the pancreas, the gene which transcribes insulin is activated. And yet, the DNA in each of these specialized cell types is the same. In general, less than 10 percent of the total genetic information is expressed at any one time. Differential genetic expression is the major cellular control over embryo differentiation.

DIFFERENTIATION, AN IRREVERSIBLE PROCESS Cell differentiation usually occurs during the gastrula stage, and the cell cannot revert to an embryonic cell once it has differentiated. Therefore it is important to note that embryonic development involves a series of progressive determinations and progressive restrictions of developmental capacity. Cell forms and functions change, which allows the human to contain cells specializing in all operations necessary to its survival. Cells vary in size, shape, and component. Specialized cells are capable of energy transfer, synthesis of complex molecules, electrical conduction, and reproduction.

Embryonic differentiation hypotheses The main question in embryonic development is this: How is differential DNA transcription initiated and directed to ultimately cause new cellular phenotypes? Numerous models to understand the concept of differentiation have been proposed and have been grouped into the following categories (Brunner, 1977):

1. Differentiation as a product of asymmetrical replication of the genome (Dierstmann and Holtzer, 1975; Heyden and Heyden, 1973; Holtzer, Weintroub, Mayne, and Mochan, 1972; Kauffman, 1967; Steward, 1972). Nuclear DNA is thought to be selectively activated or repressed by the chromosomal proteins, histones, and acidic proteins.
2. Differentiation arising from the existence of gradients across the cell (Babloyantz and Hiernanz, 1974; Gilbert, 1968; Runnstrom, 1967). Water and oxygen are thought to create pressure gradients across the cell's cytoplasm and affect the membrane and DNA.
3. Differentiation based on changes in concentration of internal metabolites (Baserga, 1974; Epel, 1979; McMahon, 1974; Wangenheim, 1976). Intracellular levels of calcium, sodium, and hydrogen ions are thought to raise pH levels. These ions may alter transport properties of the membrane, protein synthesis in the cytoplasm, and DNA synthesis and chromosome condensation in the nucleus.
4. Differentiation arising from differential transcription (Bonner, 1965; Davidson and Britten, 1971; Gierrer,

1974; Riley, 1973). Mechanisms acting on the transcription level include regulator genes that control operons, proteins which act as repressor and effector operator genes, and small molecules that function as inducers.
5. Differentiation controlled by chromosomal structure (Cook, 1973; Crick, 1971; Shapiro, Ganse, and Zakharov, 1974; Sutton, 1972; Zuckerkandle, 1974). Highly repetitive sequences of DNA and darkly staining DNA (heterochromatin) are hypothesized to have a role in differentiation and chromosome replication in eukaryotic cells (cells with a true nucleus).
6. Cybernetic and other theoretical models (Edelstein, 1972; Kauffman, 1971; Lindenmayer, 1971; Robertson and Cohen, 1972; Wassermann, 1972; Wolpert and Lewis, 1975). Mechanical action of cell movement is hypothesized to initiate and sustain the differentiation process.
7. Differentiation based on an "outside-inside" concept (Blechschmidt and Gasser, 1978; Brunner, 1977). Differentiation is directed primarily from outside the cell, not inside the cell's nucleus. Outside forces exert an effect on the cell's limiting membrane, which then acts as a regulatory control point by transducing signals from the outside to the inside. The DNA exerts its effect on the transcription and translation of proteins only after receiving outside messages via the cell membrane. Differentiation is theorized to begin always from the outside and proceed inward. The microenvironment of the cell is thought to direct, to modulate, and ultimately to effect the expression of the nuclear DNA. The outside-inside concept will be used to develop ideas of induction, primary germ layer formations, and the formation of metabolic fields.

Outside-inside concept of cell differentiation The cell's nucleus and membrane cannot act without each other because they are kinetically related to each other by the cytoplasm. Growth occurs with the absorption of materials which can migrate from the membrane to the nucleus. Nuclear DNA, the genetic information of the cell which responds to external stimuli, can then give rise to growth processes in the interior of the cell and on the membrane of the newly dividing cells.

Induction is a concept that involves two tissues: (1) an "organizer" tissue and (2) a "competent" tissue. The competent tissue is induced to differentiate by the organizer tissue. The outside-inside concept of induction maintains that, during cell proliferation and cell overgrowth, metabolic fields are initiated. A metabolic field is a region of ordered and metabolic movements. For example, the surface growth of the ectoderm in the newly forming embryo is not equal. The ectoderm shows a greater mitosis, or cell proliferation, on the outside free surfaces. The endodermal surface does not have as rapid a growth rate as the ectoderm, and because of this unequal growth rate, the distance between the ectoderm and endoderm increases. Mesoderm will arise as an aggregation of cells in the space between the rapidly growing ectoderm and the slowly growing endoderm. As the mesoderm grows, it exudes its cellular catabolites into the cellular interspaces, and a biological and mechanical pressure field is established.

Cell death The embryo loses many cells by cell death. As many as 33 to 50 percent of the embryonic cells and 8 percent of the spinal and neural tube cells die.

Cell death may be caused by a lack of nourishment and adequate waste removal. The ultimate effect of cell death is necrosis, a defect in the tissue, and finally clearance by macrophages. Cell death should be thought of as a normal process, critical to embryogenesis. Death of cells may directly contribute to the rise and diversity of new cell types by exposing new spaces and allowing cell layers to come close and exchange secretions.

Compression of the epithelial layers establishes the metabolic field known as a corrosion field (Blechschmidt and Gasser, 1978, p. 184). A corrosion field is first established when two epithelial cell layers are pressed together by other growing cells and a thin, double-walled membrane is formed. For example, the neural folds contact each other; compression of the epithelial cells occurs; inner tissue loses nutrients; and neural fold cells die and necrose, leaving a neural tube.

Developing blood vessels display the principle of corrosion fields. The dorsal aortas are paired in the growing embryo, and the medial walls contact while they are still approximately capillary size. The two adjoining medial walls compress, necrose the lumina of the vessels, and establish an open space.

Cell death is thought to cause the disappearance of the human embryonic tail (Fallon and Simandl, 1978). The tail develops in the third week of embryogenesis and persists only through the sixth week, when the embryo is 8 to 10 mm in length. The tail consists of undifferentiated mesenchyme, somites, extensions of the neural tube, notochord, and gut. The gut is thought to lose vascularization first, necrose, set up an open space, and cause tail regression. Cell death is therefore a common developmental mechanism to remove transient structures and to remodel structures that persist into adult life.

DIFFERENTIATION AND GROWTH AT THE TISSUE AND ORGAN LEVEL

HISTOGENESIS

Cell specialization, or histogenesis, resulting in tissue formation, involves the aggregation, functional formation, and integration of many similar cells. Structure does not form because of a functional demand. Function and structure develop simultaneously. At any particular moment during development, an embryo functions according to the features its organs have attained at that time. Organs are able to function postnatally only if they established a function during the prenatal period. In other words, all developing organs will have some function prenatally, no matter how minor, if they will eventually secrete, absorb, or excrete after birth.

The more specialized the tissue, the less ability it has to regenerate; therefore, increased specialization leads to decreased mitosis. Deep secondary burns will destroy specialized cells of hair follicles and sweat glands, which cannot regenerate as skin heals. Epithelial cells which are less specialized will regenerate.

MORPHOGENESIS

Morphogenesis results in organ formation from layers of cells by changes in cell position, movement, migration, and arrangement. In contrast, growth is mainly accomplished by cellular growth and proliferation, involving assimilation of nutrients, DNA synthesis, and mitosis. Morphogenesis is a result of cell migration (morphogenetic movements), allometric (unequal) growth rates, and cell death (see Fig. 2-37).

It is convenient to define tissues as aggregations of cells and organs as groups of tissues, but morphogenesis does not proceed in this stepwise fashion. Two of the first morphogenetic events are the formation of symmetry and polarity. Symmetry in humans is the mirror-image formation of the left and right sides of the body. Polarity is the orientation of cellular components to the axis of the growing embryo as a whole. First, the anterior and posterior axis develops; then the dorsal and ventral axis forms. In development, the general body plan is formed; then rudimentary organs form from tissue aggregates; and gradually cells proliferate and aggregate within the organs.

TYPES OF CELL POPULATIONS

Tissues and organs develop from cells which vary in functions, growth rates, and renewal rates, depending on specialization. The three types of cell populations which characterize the majority of organs are (1) renewing cell populations, (2) expanding cell populations, and (3) static cell populations (Leblond and Walker, 1956).

Renewing cell populations Cell mitosis in some organs, like gastrointestinal epithelium and mucosal cells, divide rapidly but do not increase the size of the cell layer. Although there is rapid cell renewal, cells are lost by constant sloughing; these cell populations are called renewing cell populations. Rapid cell division is seen in stem cells, which are the least differentiated cells of a tissue. Examples of renewing cell populations include the hematopoietic stem cells, which give rise to formed elements of the blood, red blood cells (RBC), and white blood cells (WBC).

Stratified squamous epithelium is the main protection epithelium. The mitotic activity of the cells in the lower layers is high. The mitotic activity is partly related to the

FIGURE 2-37. Stereogram illustrating morphogenetic processes: (1) cell migration; (2) cell aggregation; (3) localized growth; (4) fusion and splitting; (5) folding; and (6) bending. (*Adapted from L. B. Arey, Developmental anatomy. Philadelphia: Saunders, 1965. Used with permission of the publisher.*)

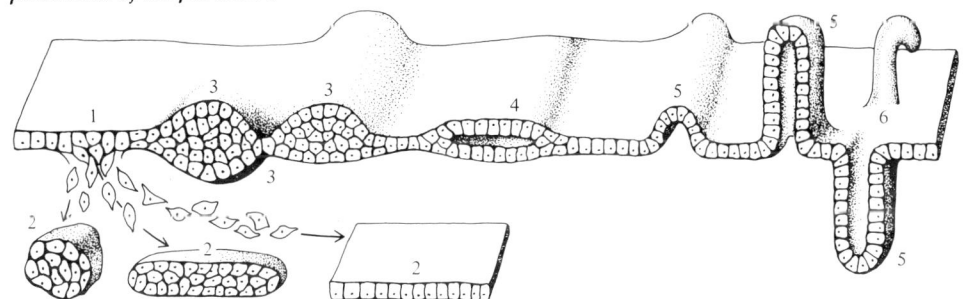

rich underlying capillary bed that provides oxygenation, nutritive substances, and waste removal. As more epithelial cells are formed, the lower, or basal, cells are pressed upward away from the capillaries and die when vascularization is lost. Cells are continuously cast off from these epithelial layers.

Expanding cell populations Cell populations that continue to proliferate after birth have been called expanding cell populations. Kidney cells and pancreatic cells continue to grow and mature after birth for a limited time by increasing the cell number, overall dimension of the organ, and length and function of the tissue. In the kidney, the nephron is immature and has a short loop, making the neonate unable to form concentrated urine. As the infant grows, the nephron loop increases in length and surface area and therefore increases its function in the reabsorption of water and the production of concentrated urine.

Static cell populations Many cell populations have reached the final and total cell number about the time of birth; they are static cell populations. They undergo their last mitoses, or proliferations, at the time of birth. The regenerative ability of static cell populations is minimal or nonexistent. Mitosis in the central nervous system (CNS) stops shortly after birth, and so there is little increase in cell number postnatally. Growth of the CNS and increased function is possible by the growth of interaxon myelinated tracts, the proliferation of glial cells, and an increase in neuron size (Leblond, 1964). Proliferative regrowth of several axons after injury is seen in the autonomic nervous system, only slightly seen in the somatic peripheral nervous system, and hardly ever seen in the CNS, where Schwann cells are lacking.

Cardiac muscle has little or no regeneration of mitotic capacity following injury. Scar formation is the method of healing. Heart growth during childhood is by an increase in myofiber size, not by an increase in cell numbers (Copenhaver, Bunge, and Bunge, 1971).

Extraordinary cell populations The three types of cell populations (static, renewing, and expanding) do not characterize all possible cell tissue and organ types in the body. Some organs are capable of increasing in size while decreasing cell number.

Liver cells have a great capacity to regenerate due to their fourfold nuclear content. Damaged hepatic cells will regenerate and will not have the same overall organ architecture but maintain the majority of organ function. The ovary increases in size during development but has decreased cell number and increased organ function.

TISSUES DERIVED FROM PRIMARY GERM LAYERS
The blastula cells, called blastoderm, give rise to the multilayered system of ectoderm, endoderm, and mesoderm, the primary germ layers (see Fig. 2-38).

Ectoderm The ectoderm is the external cell layer which gives rise to skin, hair, nails, and the entire nervous system.

Endoderm The primitive gut is formed from endoderm, as are most of the advanced organs including the pharynx, trachea, lungs, esophagus, stomach, duodenum, liver, thyroid, pancreas, intestines, and urinary bladder.

Mesoderm Mesodermal tissue is the third cell layer to develop and ultimately forms somatic muscles, the skeleton and connective tissues, cardiac muscle tissue, the adrenal cortex, blood cells, and endocardium.

REGULATION OF TISSUE-ORGAN GROWTH BY METABOLIC FIELDS
Later in embryonic development, during tissue and organ formation, late metabolic fields are established (Blechschmidt and Gasser, 1978). Biochemical and histochemical changes are taking place during organ and tissue growth. Cell microenvironment, growth, and pressure establish eight late-metabolic fields (Blechschmidt and Gasser, 1978). The eight metabolic fields are *corrosion, densation, contusion, distusion, retention, dilation, parathelial loosening,* and *detraction.*

Corrosion fields A corrosion field results from compression of epithelial layers into a thin, double-layered membrane, until cell death creates an open space. Corrosion fields are one example of cell death allowing increased organ differentiation.

Densation fields Densation fields are seen when spherical mesenchymal cells establish a cartilage condensation area and give rise to the appearance of skeleton. Densation fields may very well be the kinetic explanation for the induction concept. They are metabolic zones and areas of mesenchymal cells that have little intercellular fluids between cells.

An example is in differentiation of the ribs. After the heart and liver mass increase in the embryo, the thoracic region and all the mesenchymal tissue between the spinal

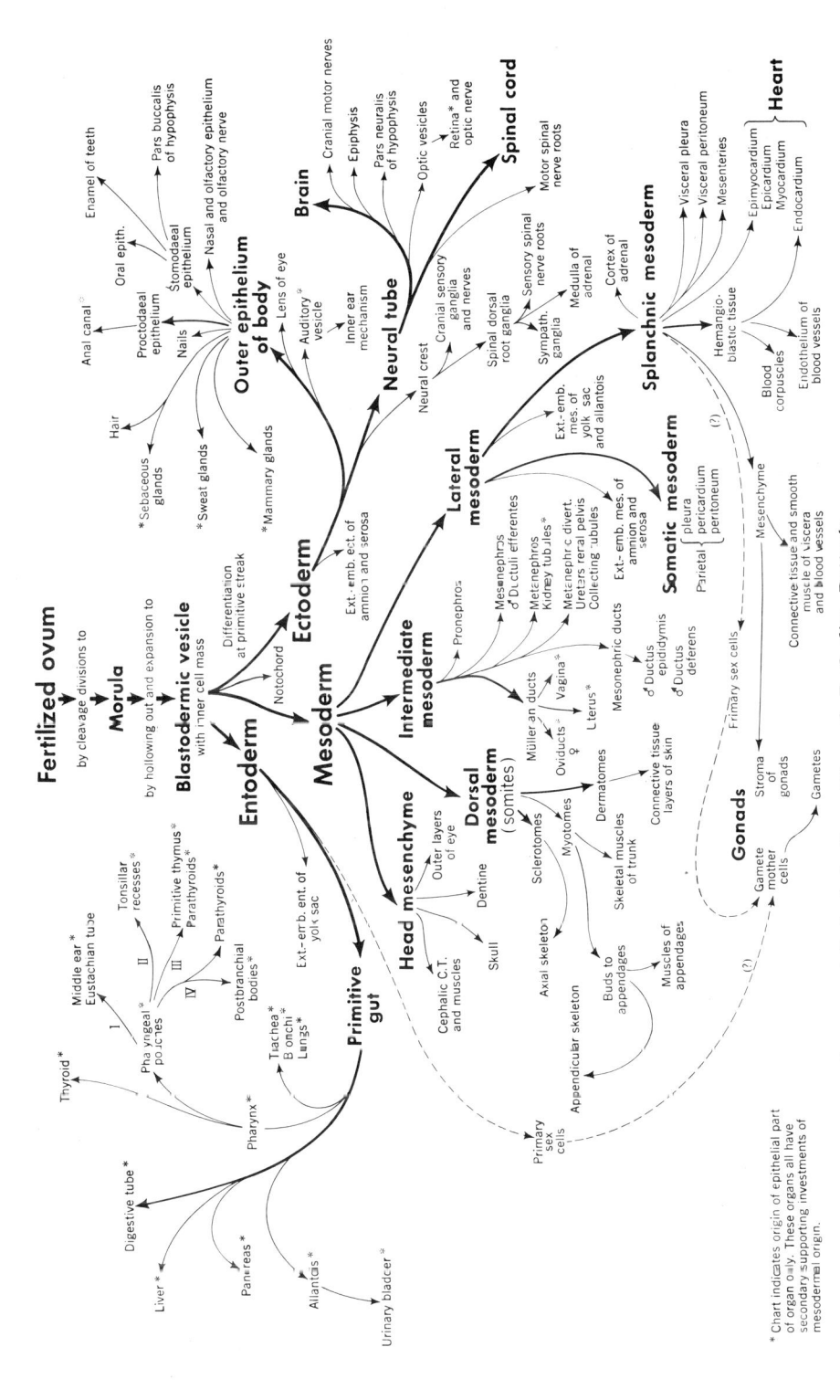

FIGURE 2-38. Primary germ layers and their derivatives. *(From C. E. Corliss, Patten's human embryology. New York: McGraw-Hill, 1976. Reprinted by permission of the publisher.)*

*Chart indicates origin of epithelial part of organ only. These organs all have secondary supporting investments of mesodermal origin.

69

nerves in the thoracic wall are stretched, curved, and straightened and form a spherical mesenchymal mass. This spherical mass is the precursor of skeletal ribs.

Contusion fields Contusion fields are zones of compression where cells have flattened. As cells become compressed from one dimension, they widen in another. Contusion field cells become disk-shaped and are seen in examples of cartilage cells.

Distusion fields Distusion fields are zones of pressure created from fluid-absorbing cartilage cells. The swelling of cartilaginous tissue also decreases water content around the distusion field, and a hardened capsule forms around the cells. The movement of water from the intercellular spaces is so intense that gradual calcification occurs. Distusion fields spatially rely on neighboring cell differentiations. The distusion field concept emphasizes that future organ shape is actually determined by the inner embryonic structure development. For example, the embryonic cartilaginous tibia has the functional structure of the adult bone before ossification occurs.

Often it is thought that growth of an adult organ is determined by the workload that it will bear in adult life. The distusion fields do not clarify this concept but seem to imply that embryonic growth and functional structure is the precursor, not formation on the basis of functional demand.

Retention fields Retention fields are created when unspecialized mesenchymal tissue is stretched to form fibrous connective tissue. Inner tissue that is stretched during embryonic stages generally remains short (Blechschmidt and Gasser, 1978, p. 213). As inner tissue is stretched, intercellular fluid is extruded from between the stressed cells. Liquid precollagen is first observed between the slenderized cells, and their precollagen solidifies to form the collagen fibers. Retention fields help in formation of ligaments, tendons, and aponeuroses.

Dilation fields Dilation fields result when unrestricted mesenchyme is stretched and no transverse compression is present. Dilation fields are present during the formation of precursors for skeletal, cardiac, and smooth muscle fibers.

Parathelial loosening fields Loosening fields are caused by the congestion of released cellular fluids and secretions trapped in inner tissues. Fluid vesicles gradually blend together creating areas that can differentiate into blood vessels, endocrine glands, and exocrine glands.

Detraction fields As mesenchymal cells slide on an acute angle over osseous tissue, the ossification process increases until the underlying tissue is quite hardened. Because the groups of mesenchymal cells create friction on the underlying tissue as they slide past them, fluid is lost from the osseous ground substance, and it hardens.

General concepts of differentiation have been presented. Differentiation on the cellular and tissue level gives rise to organ systems, each unique in its morphogenesis, growth, and maturation as well as function. An overview of these differences will be discussed in Sec. 2 in preparation for discussion of specific age-related changes.

SECTION 2
Principles of Development of Organ Systems

Each organ system differentiates and grows somewhat autonomously and yet in harmony with the whole. General principles of organ differentiation and maturation of specific organ systems are presented in this section.

Calvarium and face Mary Tudor

The face, perhaps more than any other physical feature save stature, tells of the maturation of the human from infancy to maturity; age is often correctly estimated by facial characteristics.

The skull is composed of two sections: the *neurocranium,* or *calvarium,* which encloses the brain, and the *viscerocranium,* or face. The neurocranium develops (except for the base of the skull) in harmony with the central nervous system (CNS). In contrast the face, originating from the branchial arches, follows more general somatic growth and thus lags behind the neurocranium in growth. This cephalocaudal development results in the characteristic infantile appearance of a large head relative to small facial size. From birth to adulthood, the neurocranium volume will increase four times, while the facial area will increase 12 times (Sullivan, 1978). In the 1-month-old infant, calvarium-to-face ratio is 6:1; in the adult the ratio is 2.5:1 (Israel, 1978).

Growth of the neurocranium and especially the viscerocranium is a complex process of continuous remodeling along with increase in size. Whether by intramembranous or endochondral ossification, shaping (deposition and resorption) of bone is necessary to maintain relative position of facial parts and to attain final mature shape.

Environmental as well as genetic factors appear to interact in the growth and formation of the face and calvarium. Environmental factors include mechanical forces, or stress; pressure stimulates bone resorption, and tension causes deposition. Skeletal muscles of mastication, including mouth and tongue, influence facial formation. The stress of the growing brain stimulates growth of the calvarium (Enlow, 1975; Sullivan, 1978).

All bones of the skull are probably under some genetic influence; but each bone must also respond to stresses exerted by other sections of the skull, secondary mechanical forces, to achieve a unified configuration.

CALVARIUM
Because growth of the calvarium is directly related to brain growth, if brain development slows prematurely or stops, growth of the skull stops as well. Bone formation is primarily intramembranous: bone is laid down in the dura. (Endochondral ossification occurs at the base of the skull.)

Postnatal growth of the calvarium occurs primarily by deposition of bone on the outer surface of the skull with simultaneous resorption from the interior surface (see Fig. 2-39). The sutures are fibrous joints separating the bones of the calvarium. It has been theorized that intramembranous ossification at the sutures is secondary growth to the outward appositional growth of the individual bones of the neurocranium.

The major portion of growth of the CNS, and thus the calvarium, is achieved by 10 to 12 years; final size is essentially achieved by 16 to 18 years; however, growth does not cease, and the skull continues to increase in size by about 1 percent per decade for life (Israel, 1978). Cessation of rapid calvarium growth does not necessarily herald closure of sutures. The metopic suture separating the frontal bones is the first to close, during the first 10 years of life. However, the sagittal, coronal, and lambdoid sutures may not close until 30 or 40 years of age.

Although the base of the skull develops by endochondral ossification, it is somewhat related in its growth to the neurocranium and brain development. The anterior cranial base grows in accordance with the frontal brain. Its development is also thought to be related to and affected by muscles of mastication. Growth results in increased skull length and breadth and forward mandibular movement.

FACE
Facial development is complex and involves interrelated growth and the contour change of several separate and somewhat autonomous segments. The increasing length of the face, relative to head size, changes the childlike appearance to that of an adult.

The upper face grows downward and forward with development. As the neonate's eyes are nearly adult size, the orbits are large relative to the nasomaxillary portion. The eyes appear more widely spaced relative to the rest of the face.

Mandibular growth is especially significant postnatally and is accomplished later than the upper face in development. Mandibular growth contributes a major portion to the vertical and forward growth of the face. As with the maxilla, growth must accommodate the increasing alveolus and the developing dentition. However, dental formation and facial development are relatively autonomous.

Considering the complexity and relative autonomy of cranial and facial growth, it is surprising that a remarkably harmonious product usually results. This complex process of facial development, however, explains the particular vulnerability of the face to minor and major malformations. However, these factors also allow the endless individuality of the human face.

TOOTH FORMATION

Teeth begin as buds in embryonic gums at 7 weeks conceptual age. A total of 52 teeth, 20 deciduous and 32 permanent, will develop during prenatal life and the first 6 to 7 years of postnatal life (see Fig. 2-40). Timing of tooth formation and eruption is primarily under genetic influence; each tooth also has a separate, genetically determined schedule of development. Variation in dentition development is seen between individuals as well as racial groups. Negro children have more advanced dental de-

FIGURE 2-39. (a) Growth of the calvarium. (1) Appositional growth. Deposition of bone takes place on the outer surface of the skull, while resorption takes place on the inner surface, maintaining the thickness of the calvarium and allowing brain growth. (2) Growth at the suture. The amount of fibrous tissue increases and is invaded by ossification from adjacent bones. [From D. Sinclair, Human growth after birth (3d ed.). London: Oxford University Press, 1978. Reprinted by permission of the publisher.] (b) Radial movement of the calvarial bones in response to brain growth. Compensatory sutural growth is shown in black. Note the relatively small size of the viscerocranium of the neonate. [Adapted from P. G. Sullivan, Skull, jaw and teeth growth patterns. In F. Falkner and J. M. Tanner (Eds.), Human growth 2, Postnatal growth. New York: Plenum Press, 178. Also adapted from D. Sinclair, Human growth after birth (3d ed.). London: Oxford University Press, 1978.]

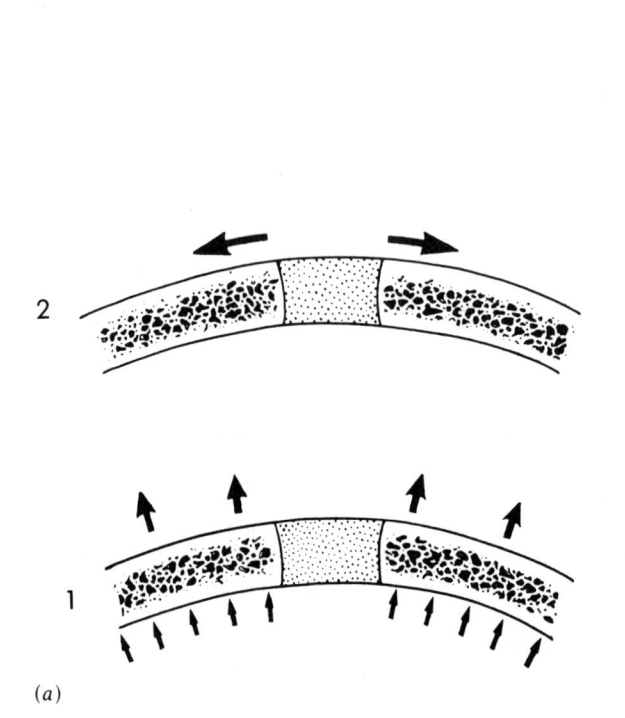

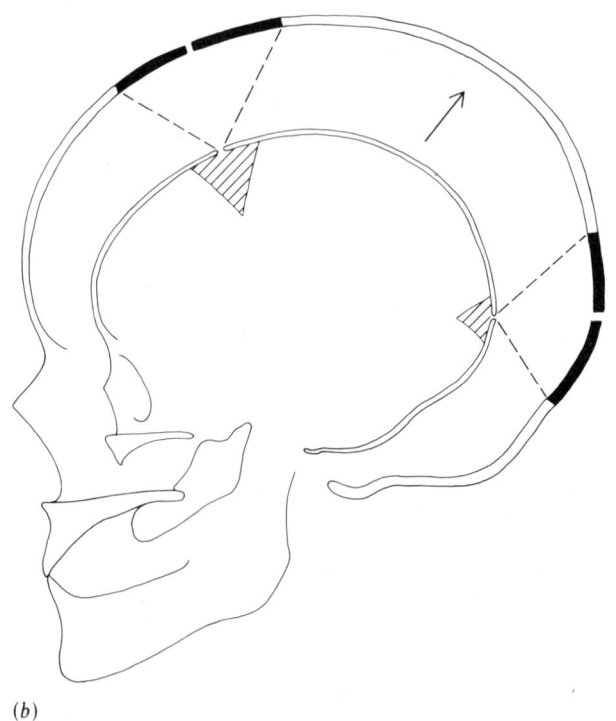

PRINCIPLES OF DEVELOPMENT OF ORGAN SYSTEMS **73**

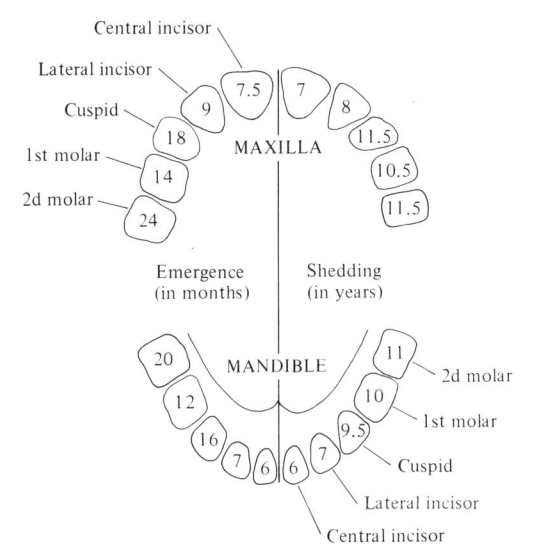

FIGURE 2-40. Emergence (in months) and shedding (in years) of deciduous teeth.

the tooth pierces the gum to appear in the oral cavity. In actuality, eruption is a much longer process during which the tooth passes through the alveolar bone of the mandible or maxilla, through the gum tissue, and to the occlusal level. Tooth "emergence" may be a more accurate term to describe piercing the gum to emerge in the oral cavity (Demirjian, 1978).

Dental development is considered relatively independent from other major growth parameters including skeletal age. In fact, dental emergence is more highly correlated with chronological age than with bone age (Lacey, 1973). Because of this, dental age can be used to assess maturity. In the past, emergence of a tooth into the oral cavity was used as a criterion. There are several disadvantages to this, however. As noted, there is variability among children and populations; environmental factors influence emergence as well. Using emergence of the tooth, one must base the level of maturity on one tooth; considering the variability between teeth, this can also lead to inaccuracies. Between the ages of $2\frac{1}{4}$ and 6 years and after age 13, few or no teeth are emerging, limiting the time such a system can be used.

Dental calcification is known to be a more precise and

velopment than Caucasian children (Demirjian, 1978). There are probably no sex differences in eruption of deciduous teeth, but girls are 1 to 6 months advanced in eruption of permanent teeth.

Tooth "eruption" is commonly used to refer to the time

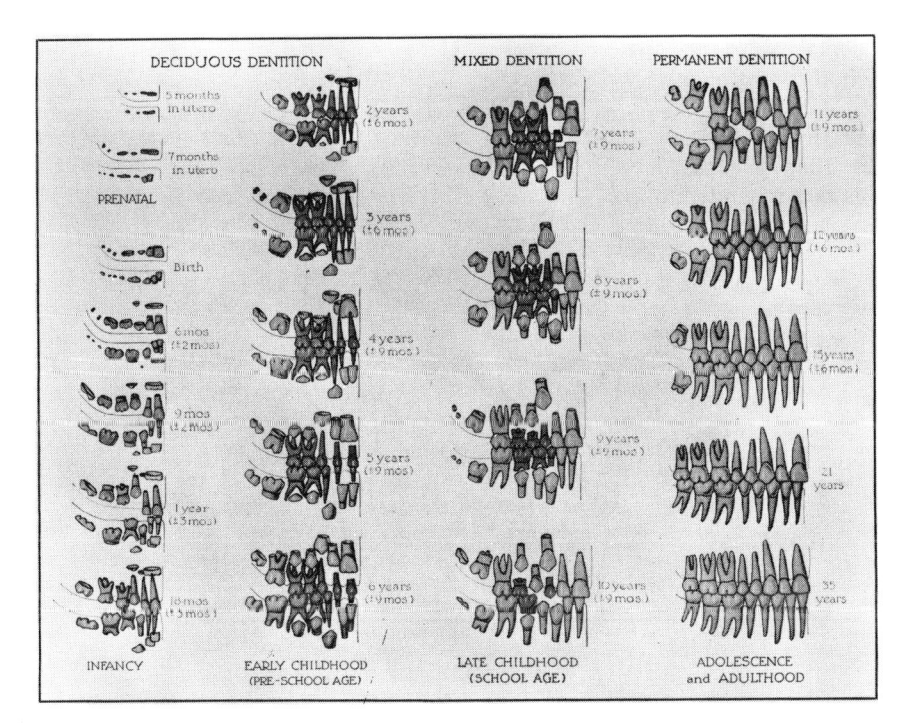

FIGURE 2-41. Development of human dentition. (*From I. Schour and M. Massler, Development of human dentition. J. Am. Dent. Assoc., 1941, 28, 1154. Copyright by the American Dental Association. Reprinted by permission.*)

continuous method of determining dental age. Calcification (formation) of deciduous teeth occurs between 3 months gestation and 3 years postnatally; calcification of permanent teeth occurs between 6 months postnatally and 14 to 15 years, excluding the third molars (see Fig. 2-41). Calcification begins at what will be the occlusal surface, the crown, and ends with closure of the apex of the tooth at the root. Radiographs showing full tooth calcification within the jaws as well as calcification of those already emerging into the oral cavity allow better assessment of dental age based on full dentition.

Calcification stage does not specifically correlate with emergence of the tooth through the gum. Deciduous tooth emergence begins at about 6 months postnatally and is completed by about 2 years of age. Permanent-tooth emergence occurs from about age 6 years to the end of the twelfth year. An exception is the third permanent molar, which may emerge at about 18 years or after or may never emerge. The mandible precedes the maxilla in eruption; however, there is synchrony between the two halves of each jaw with eruption occurring in an anterior-to-posterior pattern.

Environmental factors can affect tooth formation prenatally and postnatally as well as affect the timing of eruption. Adequate fluoride during calcification is important to tooth formation and resistance to dental caries. A fluoride concentration of 1 part per million (ppm) or 1 mg/L in drinking water reduces incidence of dental caries by 40 to 60 percent (Nelson, Vaughn, and McKay, 1975). Fluoride over 2 ppm, however, causes mottling. In areas with nonfluoridated water, 0.5 mg/day is recommended for children under 3 years of age; 1.0 mg/day for ages 3 to 12 or 13.

Early extraction of a deciduous tooth delays the eruption of the underlying permanent tooth. The degree of crowding of permanent teeth, due to dental arch size, affects their position. Tooth decay and periodontal disease can cause loss of permanent teeth and subsequent resorption of the alveolar processes.

Nervous system Mary D. Guthrie

Much of present-day knowledge of the embryology of the nervous system comes from late-nineteenth-century studies of avian embryos. With the increase of facilities and technology in this century there has been added information pertinent to mammalian embryology. One must be very careful when extrapolating the animal experiments and observations to the human fetus. For example, glial cell production in the mouse brain is completed at one-half of the gestation period, whereas the human glial cells are produced until the end of the second year after birth.

The central nervous system (CNS) is one of the first systems to initiate development in the embryo. This is a property inherent in the embryonic cells and under genetic control; it is not dependent on outside influence. This continued precocity in development compared to other systems is demonstrated in Fig. 2-42.

Not all the development of this system is under genetic control, however. The amount of cellular response, when there is exposure to nongenetic factors, differs according to the stage of development of the nervous system. In addition to malnutrition, placental insufficiency, and radiation, factors such as infections, toxins, hyperthermia, and trauma may be the cause of CNS developmental defects. At the present time, when one-half the world's population suffers from malnutrition, especially protein deficiency, it is of concern that the period of maximal brain development is affected by this factor. Reduced pro-

FIGURE 2-42. Neonate and adult reconstructed to the same height showing the precocious development of the central nervous system. (*From Corliss, Patten's human embryology. New York: McGraw-Hill, 1976, p. 121. Reprinted by permission of the publisher.*)

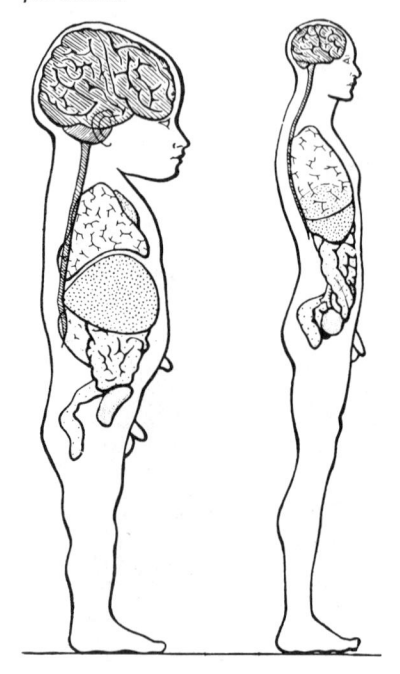

tein intake in the mother causes lowered brain weight and retardation in the child and is effective into the second year of life of the infant. The other nongenetic factors that experimentally cause CNS defects are usually species and agent specific.

Sensory system   Anna M. Tichy

Development of sense organs, which keep the child informed of conditions within the body and in the external environment, begins early in prenatal life in harmony with and as part of the CNS. An awareness of and successful adaptation to the world is contingent upon the physiological mechanisms involved in constant information processing. Sensory input, which is picked up by the appropriate nerve endings, the receptors, is coded into neural activity indicating the intensity, location, quality, and duration of the stimulus.

This coded information is conveyed to the brain, where interpretation or processing of the afferent information takes place. This process enables an appropriate response to sensory stimuli to occur. Traditionally, five special senses are classified: vision, audition, olfaction, gustation, and tactile.

The sensory system is functional, although to an imperfect degree, in late fetal life. Thus, the neonate sees, hears, smells, tastes, and feels. Although all systems are functional prenatally, postnatal maturation of the sensory receptors and myelinization of corticospinal pathways and cortex are responsible for further refinement. The visual system is the least mature, needing 6 or 7 years to reach adult visual acuity, primarily due to the shape of the globe. Refractive power, however, changes throughout life (see Fig. 2-43).

Through the sensory system, the child "takes in" his environment and receives the stimulation that promotes development.

Musculoskeletal system   Sherrilyn Passo

The musculoskeletal system is composed of bones, muscles, joints, tendons, and ligaments. Together, these structures allow active movement, provide support, protect vital organs, and are active in hematopoiesis. This highly visible, supporting system is generally viewed as the indicator of somatic growth. Height is almost synonymous with growth. Certainly, more studies of growth have used the skeletal system, not only in terms of absolute size, but also radiographically to evaluate maturation.

Growth of the musculoskeletal system follows the general growth pattern (see Fig. 2-3). Unlike other systems, the growth of the musculoskeletal system is under mechanical as well as genetic control. Thus, for these supporting tissues, local rather than systemic control is critical in growth and development. Mechanical forces, such as tension from muscle movement, gravity, and physical activity, stimulate growth of the musculoskeletal system.

SKELETAL SYSTEM

The skeleton is divided into two sections, the axial skeleton (skull, vertebrae, ribs, and sternum) and the appendicular skeleton (long bones of the limbs, pectoral girdle, and pelvic girdle). The bones that comprise the skeleton vary in their structure, function, and growth. Long bones provide support, short bones allow greater motion, and flat bones function mainly to protect delicate tissues and organs. The spine serves as the axis of the body.

Skeletal growth, a result of the interplay of genetic and environmental factors, begins in embryonic development. Development and growth of bone involves formation of the bony tissue; growth in length, width, diameter, and density; and changes in shape, or remodeling. Bone length and, to some extent, shape are genetically determined. Nutrition has a major effect on bone development, as in vitamin D deficiency and rickets.

Mechanical force plays an important role in bone growth and shape, affecting lateral growth (thickness of

FIGURE 2-43. Age trends in refractive power. (*From E. V. L. Brown, Net average yearly changes in refraction of atropinized eyes from birth to beyond maturity. Arch. Ophthal., 1938, 19, 719. Reprinted by permission of the American Medical Association.*)

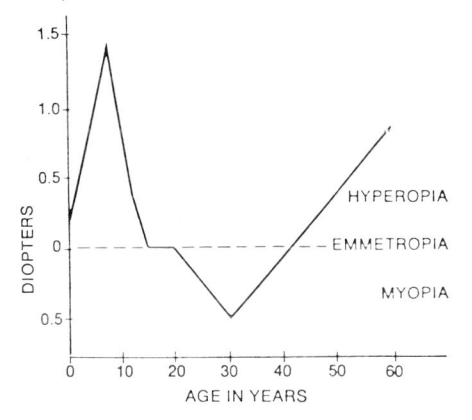

shaft) as well as density. Weight bearing on long bones as well as muscle tension of movement stimulates growth in diameter and increased density. There is conflicting evidence as to extent of long-bone growth from exercise. It is known, however, that inactivity results in decreased diameter and density.

Prenatally and postnatally, skeletal weight and total body weight are positively correlated; however, increase in height results in an increase of skeletal weight per centimeter. This increase in skeletal weight relative to height is more marked in males due to increased density. Overall, males have increased skeletal weight for size, especially after puberty (see Chap. 10).

BONE FORMATION

Bone forms by one of two processes: endochondral or intramembranous ossification. In endochondral ossification, mesenchymal tissue differentiates into a cartilage model of the bone. The cartilage grows by interstitial growth and, more importantly, by appositional growth, during which more cartilage is laid down on the surface. The cartilage, in turn, is invaded by blood vessels carrying *osteoblasts* and *osteoclasts* and is replaced by bone. Almost all bones of the body are formed by this process.

Intramembranous ossification takes place without the cartilage model; instead, mesenchymal tissue is replaced directly by bone. This method of ossification is seen primarily in the skull. As important as bone deposition by the osteoblasts in bone formation is bone removal by the osteoclasts, which results in shaping and remodeling of the bone. This is especially true in growth of facial bones. Thus, bone growth results from simultaneous appositional growth and resorption, resulting in remodeling as well as increased size.

Short-bone growth Short-bone growth begins with a central core of ossification inside the cartilaginous model. As this cartilaginous model grows, the osseous core grows faster, overtaking and replacing the cartilage (see Fig. 2-44).

Long-bone growth In long-bone growth, a special plate of growing cartilage, the *epiphyseal plate* (growth plate) separates the *diaphysis,* or shaft of the long bone, from the end segment of the bone, the *epiphysis.* The primary ossification center of long bones is in the midportion of the diaphysis. The secondary ossification center is in the epiphysis. At the epiphyseal plate, continuous growth in length of the bone takes place (see Fig. 2-45).

Growth occurs more rapidly at one end of the long bones. In the upper long bones, the shoulder and wrist are the more active ends; in the lower extremities, the more active ends are all at the knee. Thus, injury to the epiphyseal plates on the active end of a long bone will result in a more significant growth problem. Interstitial growth in length does not occur in long bones. Where bone growth is rapid, as in the ends of long bones, spongelike honeycomb bone is produced. Where growth is slow, the bone formed is dense. In long bones, this is in the midportion of the diaphysis.

Increased diameter results from the activity of osteoblasts in the periosteum covering the bone. Simultaneously, beginning at the primary ossification site, osteoclasts remodel the bone and produce a cavity which will store bone marrow. Formation of the cavity parallels bone growth, maintaining approximately the same relative size to bone. However, cortical thickness does increase somewhat with growth.

Vertebral growth Growth of the spinal column—the vertebrae and intervertebral disks—is a significant element in total body height. Different sections of the spinal column grow at different rates. At birth the lower sections, lumbar and sacral, are smallest, reflecting—as the pelvis and legs—the cephalocaudal direction of growth and maturation.

The spinal column continues to grow well into adulthood, until approximately 25 years (Sinclair, 1978). The

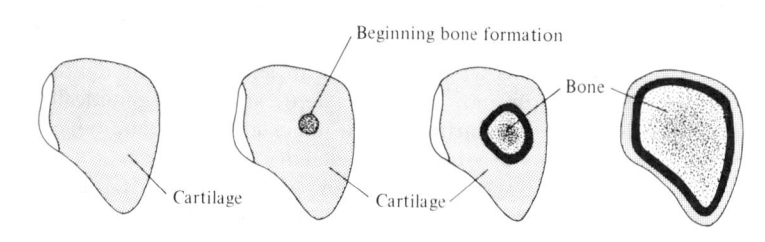

FIGURE 2-44. Maturation of a carpal bone (overall size has been kept constant) demonstrating short-bone growth. [*Modified from A. F. Roche, Bone growth and maturation. In F. Falkner and J. M. Tanner (Eds.), Human growth 2, Postnatal growth. New York: Plenum, 1978. Also modified from D. Sinclair, Human growth after birth (3d ed.). London: Oxford University Press, 1978.*]

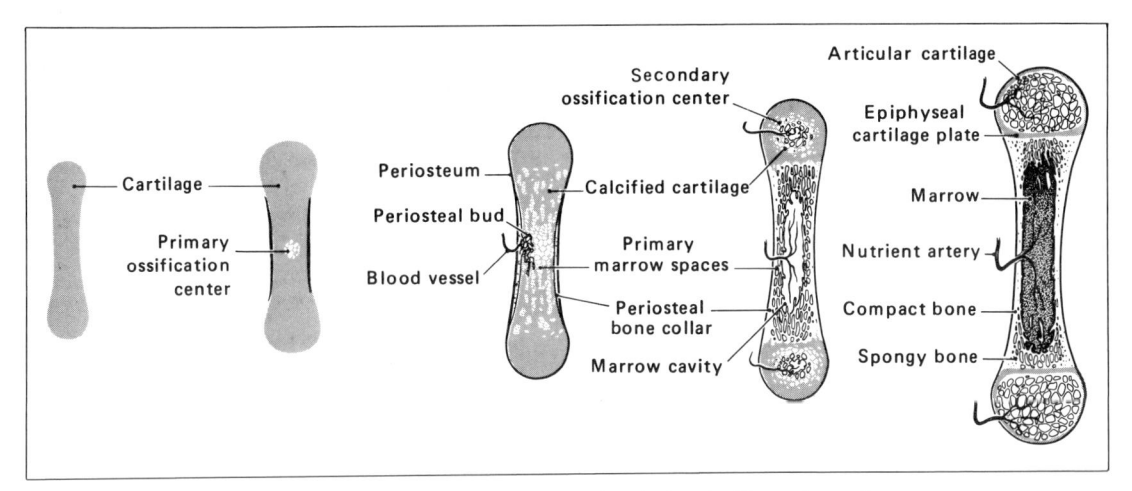

FIGURE 2-45. Long-bone maturation and growth: stages of endochondral bone formation. Shading indicates extent of cartilage. Note the persistence of cartilage at the epiphyseal plate and on articular surfaces. (From L. L. Langley, I. R. Telford, and J. B. Christensen, *Dynamic anatomy and physiology.* New York: McGraw Hill, 1974. Reprinted by permission of the publisher.)

individual vertebra grows in diameter and height; each vertebra has an epiphysis on each end, which fuses to the main vertebral body when growth ceases.

SKELETAL MATURATION

Development of the skeletal system from the embryonic cartilage model to the fully ossified bones of the adult takes approximately 20 years in the female and 23 years in the male. Three stages are described which make up these 20-plus years:

1. Ossification of diaphyses of long and short bones
2. Osteogenesis in long-bone epiphyses and in short bones
3. Bony fusion of the epiphyses and diaphyses, which completes growth

Stage 1 is nearly completed by the end of the prenatal period, stage 2 is completed by puberty, and stage 3 is completed by 20 to 23 years (Acheson, 1966).

Cartilage formation begins during the fifth week after conception; ossification begins at the end of the embryonic period, about 9 weeks postconception. At birth, ossification is incomplete. Bone growth is rapid during childhood, and remodeling of the bone is a continuous process as bone is deposited and resorbed.

The human body contains about 270 bones. Some of these fuse during infancy, reducing the total number. But as the epiphyses and the bones of the carpus and tarsus appear, there is a steady increase in the number. When the epiphyses and diaphyses fuse, growth ceases. The turnover of bone tissue continues during adulthood but at a much slower rate. The time frame for formation of the epiphyses in the fetus and child and for fusion of the epiphyses, mainly during adolescence and young adulthood, is presented in Fig. 2-46.

By puberty, the total number of separate bony masses has increased to 350, and this number increases even further during adolescence. At that point, fusion of the epiphyses has begun, and when fusion is complete during adulthood, the total number of bones is reduced to 206. The skeleton then makes up 14 percent of total body weight.

SKELETAL AGE

Changes in the skeletal system serve as references in assessing the growth of the child. Growth of the brain is reflected in skull growth. Determination of skeletal age and dental age are two commonly used methods to determine a child's physiologic development distinct from his chronological age.

Skeletal age is determined by taking an x-ray of specific parts of the skeletal system. Usually a single radiograph is made of the left hand and wrist (see Fig. 2-47). Other areas may be studied in the child less than 1 year of age or over 12 to 13 years of age. In the neonate, a radiograph of the foot and knee is more useful. In the infant between 3 and 12 months, the shoulder is preferred. The older child, ages 12 to 14 years, may require radiographs of the elbow and hip.

The number, shape, and size of the epiphyses are noted and compared with published radiographic standards appropriate for the age and sex of the child. There is a range of variability allowed for the child. This range varies at different ages. Between 1 and 2 years of age, this standard deviation is 2 to 4 months, and the standard deviation gradually increases to 12 months for the child over 8 years of age.

Several factors influence the determination of skeletal age. Sexual differences are most important. Skeletal age is more advanced for chronological age and is also less variable in females than in males. Genetic factors also cause variation; the time of appearance of some epiphyses may be familial. In the United States, black children of average height have a more mature skeletal age than white children of the same age, which in all probability represents polygenic differences.

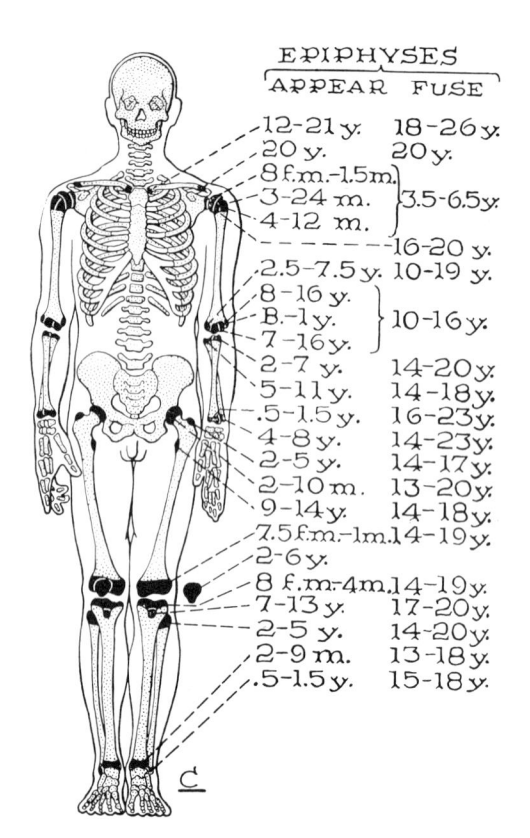

FIGURE 2-46. Appearance and fusion of the epiphyses: f.m. is fetal months (menstrual age); m. is postnatal months; y. is years. [*From J. P. Schaeffer, Morris' human anatomy (11th ed.). New York: McGraw-Hill, 1953. Reprinted by permission of the publisher.*]

BONE MARROW

Bone marrow begins to function in production of red blood cells during the latter part of gestation, taking over this function from the liver, spleen, and lymph nodes. All bones of the body produce red blood cells until age 5 years. At this time, the marrow of the long bones begins to develop fatty tissue and, except for the proximal portions of the humeri and tibiae, produces no more red

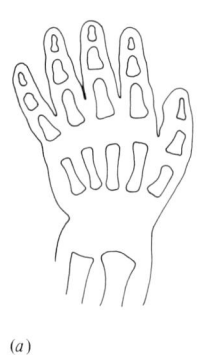

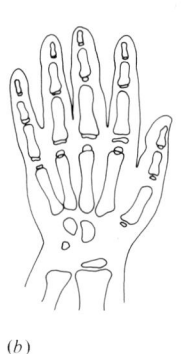

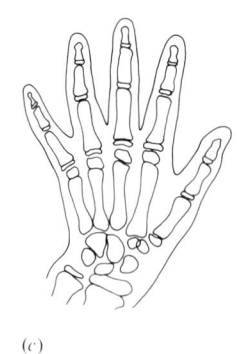

FIGURE 2-47. Progressive ossification with development of the epiphyses at (*a*) birth, (*b*) 3 years, and (*c*) 7 years. [*Adapted from L. B. Arey, Developmental anatomy (7th ed.). Philadelphia: Saunders, 1965, p. 388.*]

blood cells after approximately 20 years of age. Beyond this age, the marrow of the membranous bones, including the vertebrae, sternum, ribs, and pelvis, contributes most to red blood cell production. Even these bones become less productive with age. Unusual stimuli during the life span can cause hyperplasia of those marrow areas which are actively producing red blood cells and can stimulate inactive marrow to once again become productive.

Bone marrow is also involved in formation of white blood cells. The polymorphonuclear cells, or granulocytes, as well as the monocytes and megakaryocytes are normally formed only in the bone marrow.

MUSCULAR SYSTEM

MUSCLE GROWTH

Muscle mass is the largest component of the body composition representing 45 percent in the young adult. Beginning muscle formation is evident by 5 weeks after conception. Muscle tissue develops and grows by hyperplasia and hypertrophy both prenatally and during the first few postnatal months. After that, increase in muscle mass is thought to be achieved by hypertrophy only, defined as an increase in the diameter, length, and also nuclei of each muscle fiber. Thus, each muscle fiber is a multinucleated cell, with the number of nuclei increasing with age. In girls, this number increases tenfold between birth and maturity, while in boys the increase is fourteenfold. Recently, however, there has been some evidence that reopens the possibility that hyperplasia of muscle fibers occurs in the early postnatal years.

Generally, muscle mass increases in linear relation to age and body size, although variation does occur between muscles according to their function. Muscle mass is also the most variable of all components of body weight. Muscle growth is dependent on nutrition as well as on tension from both bone elongation and nervous stimulation or movement.

As the bone grows, the muscle is stretched between its points of attachment, there is a separation of tendon from bone, and the muscle correspondingly lengthens. Lengthening of muscle fiber is also governed by the tension from the amount and range of movement of a limb. Thus, enlargement of a muscle after sustained physical exercise is a result of hypertrophy of existing cells, not an increase in cell number.

There is not a significant difference between girls and boys in muscle size (of the same body weight) until after puberty.

There is a spurt of muscle growth correlating with the pubertal growth spurt which is more pronounced and prolonged in males. Adult muscle diameter is reached between 12 and 15 years of age. Muscle mass accounts for about 24 percent of body weight at birth, 35 percent at 5 years, and 45 percent in young adults. After growth stops, however, many factors affect muscle mass such as sex, age, metabolism, nutrition, and physical exercise.

Cardiovascular system Mary Tudor

The cardiovascular system provides the means for circulating nutrients and waste products to and from individual cells in the human body. Due to rapid growth and the relatively insignificant food supply contributed by the human oocyte and yolk sac, implantation and establishment of a primitive placental "circulation," or exchange by diffusion, occurs very early, 10 to 12 days after conception. In the embryo, fetus, child, and adult the cardiovascular system provides the means for circulating nutrients and waste products to and from the individual cells in the human body from a few hundred initially to 10^{14}.

The cardiovascular system begins to differentiate on the eighteenth to twentieth day after conception, is the first system to become functional, and normally remains fully functional until death. The heart evolves from a tube-shaped structure to a two- and then four-chambered organ by the eighth week after fertilization (8 weeks conceptual age). Contractions begin on the twenty-second day after conception, starting circulation which is first an embryonic, then fetal, and finally postnatal pattern. The cardiovascular system not only evolves gradually in form and function, but also, with the respiratory system, makes sudden, significant structural and functional changes at birth.

The heart, arteries, and veins grow in parallel with overall body growth and demands of the fetus and child. The heart-weight–to–body-weight ratio changes during fetal and early postnatal life. During the first trimester the heart-weight–to–body-weight ratio is 1:68; it decreases during the third trimester to 1:138 at term. The final ratio of 1:200 is reached by 6 months of postnatal life, and this remains fairly constant under normal conditions through maturity (Brasel and Gruen, 1978). There is a growth spurt of weight and transverse diameter of the heart during adolescence, correlating with the overall pubertal growth spurt, which is of equal magnitude for both sexes (Marshall, 1978).

Cardiac growth is achieved prenatally by an increase in the number of myocardial fibers. This hyperplastic growth also continues during early postnatal development. Hypertrophic growth occurs as well; the diameter of ventricular fibers doubles from infancy to adulthood. After growth of the heart stops, increased work load can cause hyperplastic growth, increasing fiber length as well as diameter (Brasel and Gruen, 1978). Thus, after birth, when the left side of the heart must work harder due to the shift from fetal to neonatal circulation, the left ventricle becomes and remains larger than the right.

Position of the heart also changes markedly during embryogenesis, fetal life, and childhood. Developing initially outside the embryo proper, the heart comes to lie within the chest cavity during fetal life. At term, the heart is higher in the chest and is more horizontal in comparison with that of the adult. Thus, in external cardiac massage the compression is higher, at midsternum, in infants. With growth, the heart assumes a position lower in the chest cavity and a more oblique lie.

As heart size increases during development, heart rate falls and blood pressure increases through adolescence (see Figs. 2-48 and 2-49). Blood volume increases in linear correlation with body weight during childhood and adolescence.

Hematologic values also change during development (see Table 2-4). Embryonic hemoglobin is produced initially, then fetal, and, by 6 to 12 months postnatally, adult hemoglobin is fully present.

Respiratory system Virginia J. Neelon

While the primary function of the mature lung is gas exchange, in the prenatal lung the major considerations are organization of growth, surfactant synthesis, and establishment of respiration at birth. Nevertheless, it is toward the end of efficient gas exchange in the face of varying demands that growth and development of the lung are directed. An understanding of the factors important to the lung's physiological functions allows greater appreciation of the process of its growth.

Exchange of oxygen and carbon dioxide involves gas flow within the respiratory system; diffusion across the air-blood barrier; and diffusion and chemical reactions within the plasma, red blood cells, and tissues. These processes are dependent on normal lung structure and growth.

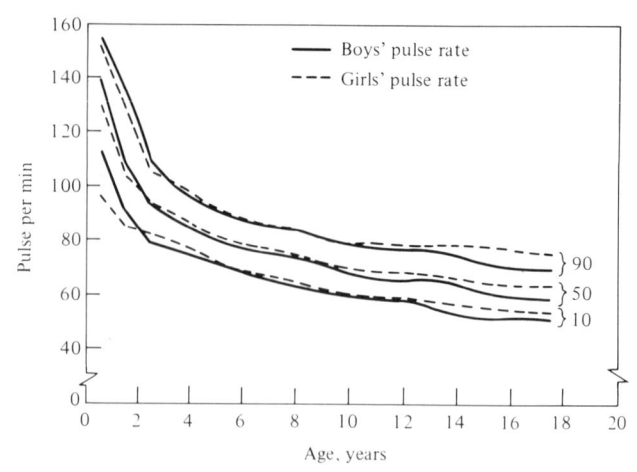

FIGURE 2-48. The 10th, 50th, and 90th smoothed percentile zones of pulse rates for children between 2 months and 18 years of age. [*From A. Iliff and V. Lee, Pulse rate, respiratory rate, and body temperature of children between two months and eighteen years of age. Child Develop., 1952, 23(4), 239. Reprinted by permission of The Society for Research in Child Development, Inc.*]

The respiratory tract consists of structural components for the exchange of gas with the outside environment and respiratory components for the exchange of gas between the alveolus and the capillary. The upper portion of the respiratory tract—the nose, pharynx, larynx, and upper part of the trachea—warm, moisten, and filter the inspired air. Development and growth of the lower portion—the distal trachea, bronchi, bronchioles, and alveoli—are reviewed.

LUNG DEVELOPMENT

Embryological development of the lung begins about the twenty-fourth day after conception; development and growth of the lung continues throughout the period of body growth. The trachea divides into two primary bronchi; the basic branching of the bronchial tree in each lung occurs by division of the parent branch, each branch decreasing in diameter. Each group of branches is one generation. Eighteen generations develop before birth and six generations after birth.

The conducting airways—trachea, bronchi, and nonrespiratory bronchioles—are generations 1 through 19. Their smallest airway diameter in the adult is 0.7 mm and in the newborn 0.3 mm (Scarpelli, 1975). The conducting airways move air between the external environment and the distal sites of gas exchange and also serve to clear particles from inspired air.

The terminal respiratory units (acini) include the respiratory bronchioles and the alveolar components, generations 20 through 27. The smallest alveolar diameter in the adult is about 0.3 mm and in the neonate only 0.05 mm (Scarpelli, 1975).

The volume of the airways from the mouth to the distal branches is about 150 mL in the adult and 7 to 8 mL in the neonate and represents the anatomic dead space. The portion of inspired air which remains in this dead space (conducting airways) is not available for gas exchange with the blood. However, the space does permit inspired air to be warmed, saturated with water vapor, and filtered. Alveolar exchange can also be diminished due to inadequate or ineffective perfusion by the pulmonary circulation resulting in alveolar dead space. Diseases states, such as respiratory distress syndrome (RDS) in the neonate, increase the alveolar dead space and greatly compromise the exchange of oxygen and carbon dioxide (Fraser and Paré, 1977; Murray, 1976).

LUNG GROWTH

Lung growth itself occurs mostly by increasing respiratory airways tenfold; increasing alveolar diameter fivefold and number fifteenfold; increasing lung surface area thirtyfold; and increasing lung weight tenfold (Scarpelli, 1975). While growth is most rapid during the embryonic and fetal periods, significant growth occurs after birth, particularly with respect to specific functional capacities. Growth during the first 3 months is limited by the chest wall, but after that time chest wall growth exceeds the growth of the lung.

The first year of life is the period of rapid alveolar growth. Around 5 years of age, conductance shows a dramatic change indicating a significant increase in airway cross-sectional area. Finally, as one approaches

FIGURE 2-49. Blood pressure change for (a) girls and (b) boys from 2 to 18 years of age. [*From Recommendations of the task force on blood pressure control in children, Pediatrics, 1977, 59, 797–820 (suppl.).*]

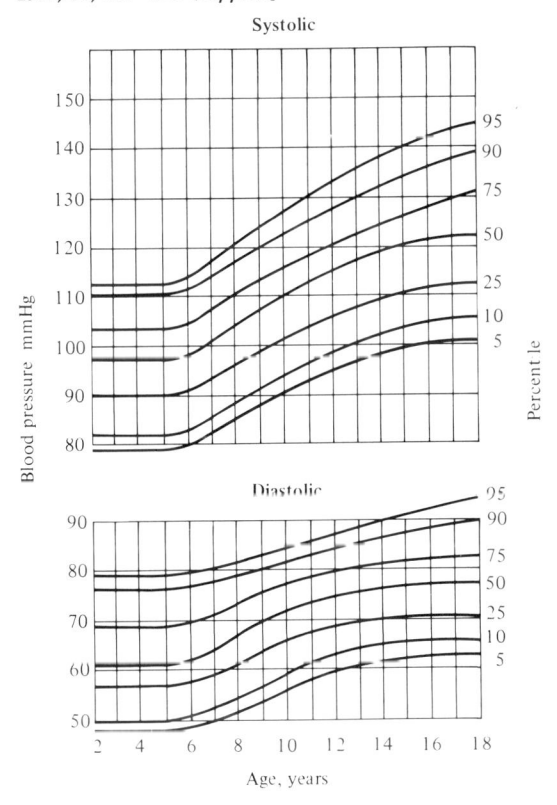

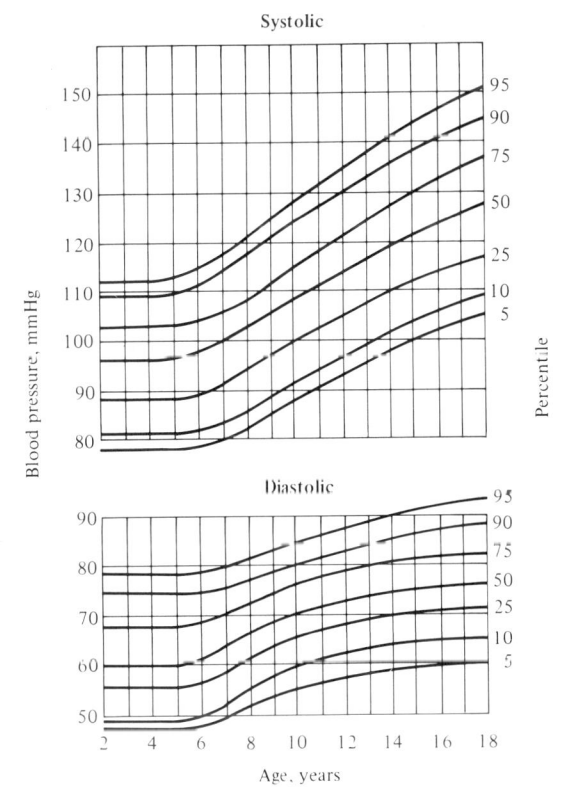

(a)

(b)

maturity, collateral pathways for ventilation develop between alveolar walls (pores of Kohn). Thus, in the very young, because of small peripheral airways which limit conductance and because of a lack of collateral ventilation, any obstruction results in a more severe respiratory functional loss (Hogg, 1977).

Growth and development of the lungs normally ceases when somatic growth stops. From this time on, the lung shares with other organs the consequences of aging. Nevertheless, in the absence of disease the lung with its large reserve capacity is capable of accommodating normal demands throughout life.

MECHANICS OF THE RESPIRATORY SYSTEM

Lung airflow is caused by active motion of the chest wall. Four groups of muscles are important in the adult for inspiration: diaphragm, external intercostal, scalenus (anterior neck muscles), and sternocleidomastoids. During infancy and early childhood the mechanical work of respiration is done mostly through action of the diaphragm. At 5 to 7 years of age the thoracic muscles take on a more significant function. When inspiration is marked in the infant, the sternocleidomastoid muscles are the most important accessory muscles and are responsible for the characteristic prominence of the sternum observed in acute respiratory distress. For the infant with RDS, the sternum may actually appear depressed due to poorly developed chest wall cartilage and limited lung compliance.

LUNG FUNCTION

Respiratory rate decreases with development; the most significant decrease occurs during the first 2 years postnatally. There is little difference between girls and boys, and the overall normal range is relatively narrow (Iliff and Lee, 1952) (see Fig. 2-50).

Pulmonary function measurements for the most part are unchanged when related to standard references of body weight or surface area. This constancy is not surprising since respiration and gas exchange are dictated by metabolic needs of the body at any age. In the developing child, pulmonary function values relate more to stature than to chronological age.

Lung function and effective gas exchange are most commonly evaluated by measurement or calculations of lung volumes, lung capacities, and blood-gas tensions. Lung capacities are illustrated in Fig. 2-51 for the normal neonate and adult.

Tidal volume (TV) is a measure of the amount of gas moving in and out of the lung with each respiratory cycle. Like all lung volumes, TV is related to size and is correlated with the height of the child. In the neonate, however, body weight is more appropriate than length.

TABLE 2-4 Hematology values from birth to 12 years

Age	Hemoglobin, g	% hematocrit	WBC/mm^3	% polys.	% retics.
1 day	16–22*	53–73*	18,000 (7000–35,000)	45–85	2.5–6.5
1 week	13–20*	43–66*	10,000 (4000–20,000)	30–50	0.1–4.5
1 month	16	53	10,000 (6000–18,000)	30–50	0.1–1.0
3 months	11.5	38	10,000 (6000–17,000)	30–50	0.7–3.0
6 months	12	40	10,000 (6000–16,000)	30–50	0.7–2.3
1 year	12	40	10,000 (6000–15,000)	30–50	0.6–1.7
2–6 years	13	43	9000 (7000–13,000)	35–55	0.5–1.0
7–12 years	14	46	8500 (5000–12,000)	40–60	0.5–1.0

Absolute eosinophil count: 100–600/mm^3; average, 250.

* Under the age of 1 month, capillary hemoglobin and hematocrit exceed venous, the average difference being 3.6 g at 1 h, 2.2 g at 5 days, and 1.1 g at 3 weeks.
Source: R. A. Hoekelman et al. (Eds.), *Principles of pediatrics.* New York: McGraw-Hill, 1978, p. 1940. Reprinted by permission of McGraw-Hill Book Company.

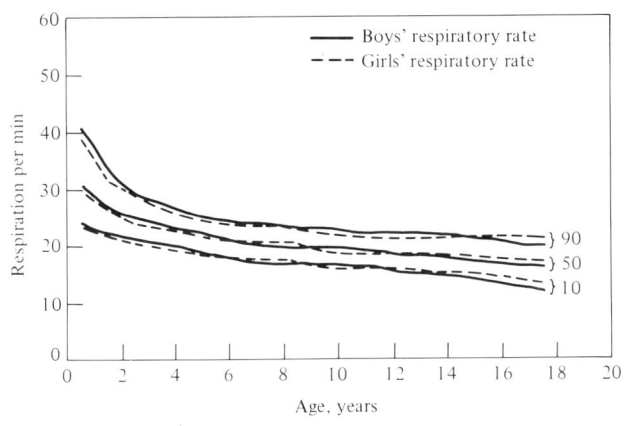

FIGURE 2-50. Respiratory rate change between 2 months and 18 years of age. The 10th, 50th, and 90th percentile zones are given for girls and boys. [*From A. Iliff and A. V. Lee, Pulse rate, respiratory rate and body temperature of children between two months and 18 years of age. Child Develop., 1952, 23(4), 241. Reprinted by permission of The Society for Research in Child Development.*]

Inspiratory reserve volume (IRV) is the maximal amount of gas that can be inspired beyond normal tidal inspiration, while expiratory reserve volume (ERV) is the maximal volume that can be expired after a normal tidal expiration. The volume of gas remaining in the lungs at the end of maximal expiration is the residual volume (RV) and is the only one of the lung volumes that cannot be measured directly.

The four lung capacities each include two or more of the lung volumes described above. Total lung capacity (TLC) is the amount of gas in the lung at the end of a maximal inspiration. Vital capacity (VC) is the maximal volume of gas that can be expelled after maximal inspiration. Inspiratory capacity (IC) is the maximal volume of gas inspired from the resting expiratory state. Functional residual capacity (FRC) is the volume of gas remaining in the lungs at the resting expiratory level.

There is a wide range of normal values in the healthy child. Measurements show a negative correlation with age; this may reflect, not only the effect of age, but also the fact that young people are significantly taller. Differences can also be attributed to sex, ethnic origin, physical activity, smoking habits, and environmental factors. Given these considerations, a functional loss of less than 20 percent is probably not significant in the adult (Fraser and Paré, 1977).

A critical step in the development of the respiratory system in readiness for extrauterine life is the production

FIGURE 2-51. Lung function. (a) Adult lung volumes in mL; (b) lung function of a normal, 3-kg neonate. [*Adapted from several sources, including Avery, 1975; Scarpelli, 1975; Ross, 1978; as adapted from J. H. Comroe, Physiology of respiration (3d ed.). Chicago: Year Book, 1974.*]

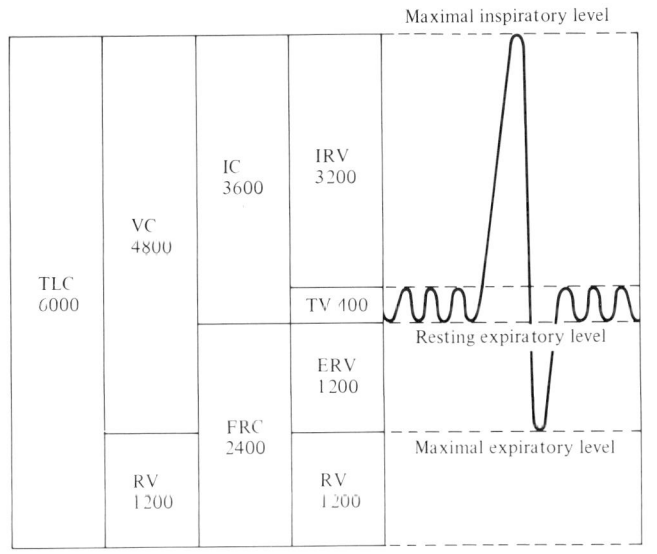

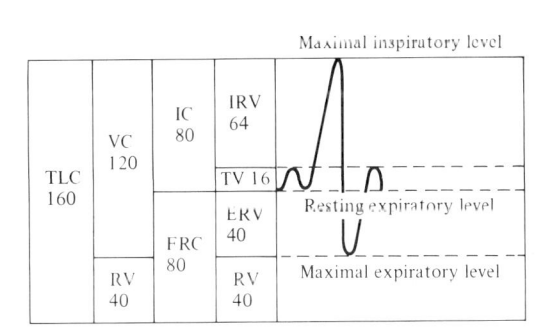

(a)

(b)

of surfactant. Because of certain properties of molecules at an air-liquid interface, the alveoli exhibit a surface tension which tends to contract the surface area of the alveolar space. Surfactant acts to stabilize the lung, lowering resistance to inflation yet preventing collapse (see Chap. 6).

GAS EXCHANGE

The exchange of oxygen and carbon dioxide involves three distinct steps: the flow of molecules within the air spaces of the respiratory units, diffusion across the air-blood barrier, and diffusion and chemical reactions within the plasma and red blood cells. Diffusing capacity increases during growth and decreases gradually with age from the third decade on. The most important factors affecting diffusing capacity are changes in pulmonary blood flow and changes in the alveolar-membrane surface.

OTHER LUNG FUNCTIONS

During development and throughout life, the lungs are vulnerable from both sides of their structural surfaces. On the capillary side they act as a filter for the venous outflow of all other organs and are subject to acute systemic insults. In contrast, the external surface of lung suffers more from chronic insults, beginning in infancy. However, the lung manifests resistance afforded by structural factors and significant cellular defense mechanisms.

The lung acts as a reservoir of blood, normally containing about 10 percent of the total blood volume. The lung also acts as an excretory organ, eliminating the end products of metabolic overloads, including acetone, ammonia, and alcohol. Finally, the vascular surface of the lung is involved in the activation (angiotension) and inactivation (serotonin) of several vasoactive substances (Murray, 1976).

Gastrointestinal system Anna M. Tichy and Dianne Chong

GROWTH OF THE GASTROINTESTINAL SYSTEM

Organs of the gastrointestinal system perform the complex functions of ingestion, digestion, absorption, and egestion. Development of the organs of the alimentary canal progresses from cephalad to caudad beginning early in prenatal life. Numerous anatomical changes, such as growth, recanalization, and positioning of organs as well as the establishment of limited physiologic function, occurs during gestation. Though gastrointestinal tract functioning in utero is not essential for life, many of the microscopic glands within the walls of the digestive organs are capable of assuming their role.

Between conception and 1 year of age, the child's gastrointestinal system achieves the major portion of its development. However, changes in size, structure, position, and function continue throughout childhood. The surface area of the gastrointestinal tract increases fourfold between birth and adulthood, and the related musculature undergoes structural and functional maturation. There is adequate capacity of the system to nourish the child from birth, but development also reflects the progression in the form of nutrients from milk to solid food.

DEVELOPMENT OF FUNCTION

The function of suck and swallow are fully developed during the first few days of life in a full-term neonate. The relation to respiratory activity is important in preventing aspiration during feeding. Esophageal and gastric peristalsis in the first few days is usually nonpropagative. The wave activity of the small and large intestine motility resembles that of the adult; however, the activity of the small intestine is only one-third that of the adult.

While salivary enzymes are found in the fetus, development of the salivary glands is not complete until after birth. The concentration of electrolytes in the saliva is high in infants and decreases markedly during the first week and less sharply over the first 2 years. The gastric alkalinity found in neonates, probably due to ingested saliva and amniotic fluid, disappears a few hours after birth. Acidity rises to the level of the adult between the third and fourth year. Pepsin secretion is an adult level at 2 years and intrinsic factor at 3 months.

Digestion and absorption of fat is not completely developed in the neonate. Adult levels of absorption are reached at 8 to 12 months. With the exception of amylase, the enzymes necessary for the digestion of carbohydrates are well developed at birth. Proteolytic enzyme activity is present at the fifth month of gestation. Transport of amino acids is probably similar to that of adults.

Significant variances in absorption, motility, and protective immunological mechanisms have been identified between the young child and adult. However, despite these differences the healthy child is able to adequately ingest, digest, and absorb the nutrients essential for normal growth and development and eliminate the waste materials of these processes.

Endocrine system Norma J. Briggs

The endocrine system is comprised of a variety of glands and tissues which play important roles in maintaining the internal environment of the developing as well as of the mature human. The discussion of the endocrine system includes the adenohypophysis, neurohypophysis, hypothalamus, pineal, thyroid, parathyroids, thymus, pancreas, adrenals, and placenta.

Some of these glands and tissues are functional during the prenatal period, such as the thyroid gland, and others are not; it is recognized that the placenta is a prenatal endocrine organ. After birth, however, all endocrine glands and tissues in the neonate are activated to regulate growth as well as to maintain temperature, water, electrolyte, mineral, and glucose balance. Change in body temperature with development is shown in Fig. 2-52.

Physical development is affected by both internal factors, such as genetic and endocrine influences, and external factors, such as diseases and nutrition. Growth of the fetus is regulated primarily by maternal, genetic, and nutritional factors. Hormonal effects on the growth of the developing fetus are more indirect.

From the neonatal period until puberty, *somatotropin* (growth hormone) and thyroid hormones are seen as more directly related to growth than other hormones. Somatotropin (STH) has a generalized or systemic effect on the body. STH affects protein anabolism, which makes it possible for all types of tissue to respond to the hormone. STH also affects long-bone growth, which contributes to an increase in linear growth.

Thyroid hormones affect growth through their genetic control of RNA and protein synthesis. Since growing cells need nutrients, any hormones which affect mineral transport and balance will also affect growth.

Two important aspects of the endocrine system are considered in regard to function. One aspect is the interrelations of endocrine and nonendocrine tissue functions, and the other is the feedback control mechanisms which maintain the functions of the system within normal ranges.

In the development and function of the human endocrine system, both the developmental stage of a specific endocrine tissue and the maternal influences on the endocrine tissue must be kept in perspective. For while a specific endocrine gland or tissue is developing prenatally, its functional role may be entirely or partially suppressed by maternal influences which effect primarily the feedback control mechanisms.

After birth, any hormonal dysfunction in the child may cause marked alterations in the pattern of growth and development. Hormonal deficits and subsequent growth failures only become apparent in the growing child. However, an allowance for normal variation in growth and development is always kept in perspective.

Reproductive system Nancy Reame

The reproductive system is composed of a group of organs, glands, and tissues which communicate via nervous and hormonal pathways for the conception, development, and delivery of a new human being. The reproductive system in the child does not have a purposive function until the onset of puberty, although changes in hormonal activity may begin as early as age 8 or 9 years. Even earlier events must have taken place in the brain to trigger the hormonal changes; thus, puberty may be more closely associated with child development than currently assumed.

Although the organs of the genital tract are essential for reproduction, the most important component of the reproductive system is the brain. It not only influences reproductive behavior but also plays a central role in the hormonal regulation of gametogenesis, fetal develop-

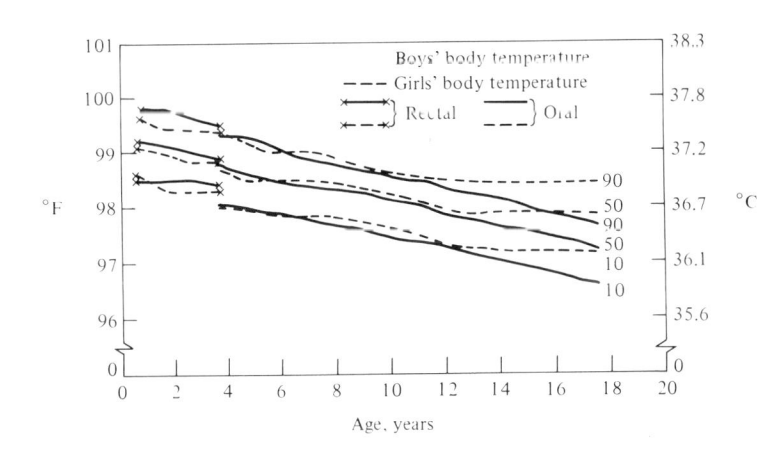

FIGURE 2-52. Body temperature change between 2 months and 18 years of age for girls and boys. [*From A. Iliff and V. A. Lee: Pulse rate, respiratory rate and body temperature of children between two months and 18 years of age. Child Develop., 1952, 23(4), 243. Reprinted by permission of The Society for Research in Child Development.*]

ment, parturition, lactation, and puberty. Without the brain, especially the hypothalamus and its underlying target gland, the pituitary, none of these reproductive processes would be possible.

HORMONAL CONTROL

The hypothalamus secretes a releasing hormone in both males and females throughout life that stimulates the secretion of gonad-specific *gonadotropic hormones* from the pituitary gland, which controls growth, maturation, and the hormone secretion of the gonads. This hormonal relay system in the female is specifically referred to as the *hypothalamic-pituitary-ovarian axis,* and in the male it is the *hypothalamic-pituitary-testicular axis* (see Fig. 2-53).

In the female, the gonadotropic hormones of the pituitary are *luteinizing hormone* (LH) and *follicle-stimulating hormone* (FSH). Both LH and FSH are controlled by a single hormone from the hypothalamus called *gonadotropin-releasing hormone* or sometimes gonadotropin-releasing factor (GnRF). Ovulation is dependent upon pituitary hormones to stimulate maturation of an oocyte and ovulation, and for formation of the corpus luteum for the production of progesterone. In prepubescent girls, the cyclic secretory pattern for LH and FSH does not exist although even the fetal brain is capable of producing very low levels of gonadotropins. Puberty, then, is not an awakening of dormant glands but a change in the level of activity of the already actively functioning hypothalamic-pituitary-ovarian axis.

In the male, the gonadotropic hormones from the pituitary are FSH, which stimulates spermatogenesis, and *interstitial cell–stimulating hormone* (ICSH), which acts on the interstitial cells of the testis to stimulate the production of testosterone. The functions of prolactin and oxytocin in the male are not known.

PATTERN OF GROWTH OF REPRODUCTIVE ORGANS

The rate of growth of the reproductive organs after birth follows the genital pattern of growth (see Fig. 2-3) with an initial rise in early childhood followed by a leveling off between the ages of 5 and 10 years and then finally ending in a pubertal growth spurt (see Chap. 10). The initial rise in the genital growth curve is much less marked than growth in general, and the upsurge at puberty is much more dramatic. Although the reproductive tract of a

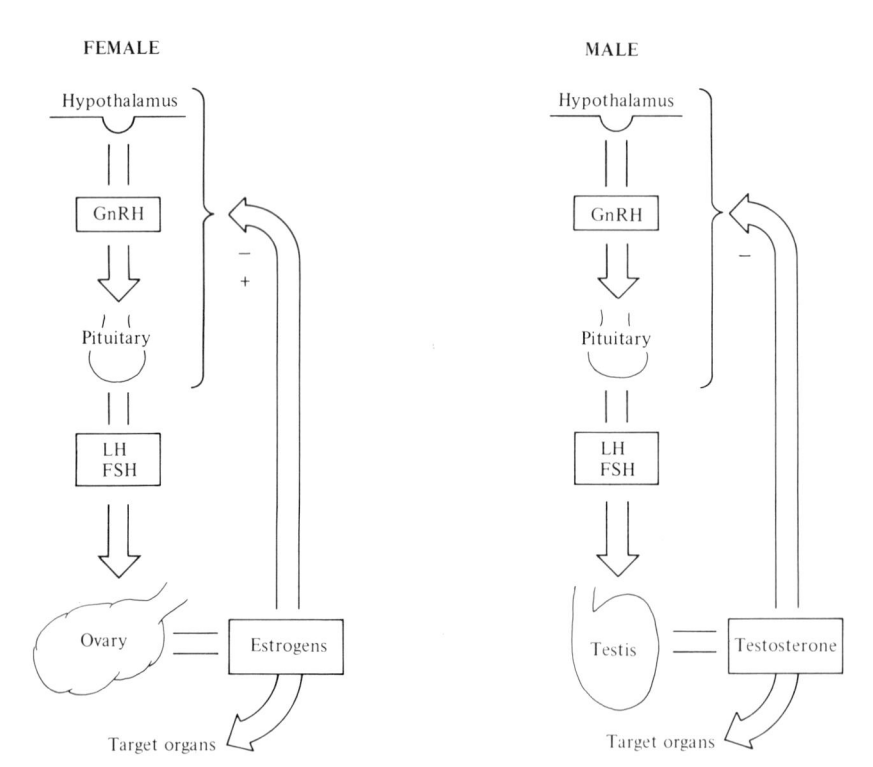

FIGURE 2-53. Schematic representation of the differences in gonadal control mechanisms for LH and FSH secretion in the adult female and male.

9-year-old girl is not much larger than it was at 1 year of age, between the ages of 9 and 16 years, the ovaries increase fourfold in weight.

Until puberty, the cervix is larger than the body of the uterus. The uterus and ovaries are higher in the child's pelvic cavity, but with increased length and growth of the pelvis by adolescence, they are in the adult position. The vagina grows very little until puberty.

In boys, the largest growth spurt occurs in the testes and prostate gland between the ages of 13 and 20 years. In contrast, postnatal neural development is much more rapid and complete so that, by age 10, the nervous system organs, including the brain, have to gain only 5 percent of their adult size and do not have a pubertal growth spurt. This advanced neural maturation makes sense physiologically, since the CNS appears to trigger the pubertal events of other systems, especially of the reproductive system.

Even though the reproductive system is the last to mature and begin functioning, it is one of the first to affect the development and function of other systems. Of more importance is the impact of the reproductive system on psychological and sociocultural development.

SEX DIFFERENCES IN GENERAL GROWTH AND DEVELOPMENT

The sex of the developing child has a distinct effect on physical growth and maturation. Full-term male neonates are on the average heavier and longer than full-term female neonates. Skeletal differences also exist at birth. Girls have shorter forearms, longer index fingers, and larger pelvic measurements. Female infants are slightly ahead of boys in bone development and accumulate fat at a faster rate from birth onward. The effects of gonadal hormones on reproductive organ development and on growth in general during puberty are discussed in following chapters.

Urinary system   Ida M. Martinson and Nancy V. Rude

The primary role of the kidney is to maintain a stable composition and volume of the extracellular environment through maintenance of a proper balance of water and extracellular substances. A secondary yet very important role of the kidney is the maintenance of a proper pH balance. The body's pH is essentially determined by hydrogen ion and bicarbonate ion concentrations, in which the kidney plays a major role in excretion.

Each kidney is estimated to have over 1 million nephrons, the basic unit of the kidney, which are all present by birth. The number of nephrons does not increase after birth. Each nephron consists of a renal corpuscle and a renal tubule. The renal tubule, which adjusts the composition and volume of the urine, becomes more efficient as the child develops. Filtration occurs at the glomerulus, a network of capillaries of the renal corpuscle.

The composition and volume of urine is equal to filtration minus reabsorption plus secretion. Filtration, reabsorption, and secretion are necessary processes to maintain the composition of body fluids. Antidiuretic hormone (ADH) and aldosterone are present and effective from birth.

DEVELOPMENT OF THE URINARY SYSTEM

The urinary system appears early in the developing embryo, during the third week. Excretory organs appear and disappear. It is only the third set of excretory units that remain and begin to function in a manner similar to the adult kidney. While the previous, primitive organ only filtered plasma, the final organ begins regulating the internal fluid of the fetus about the third month of gestation. Urine begins to be excreted at this time, contributing to the amniotic fluid. However, the fetal kidney is relatively dormant as the placenta is the primary regulatory and excretory organ.

URINARY SYSTEM GROWTH

While all units of the kidney are present at birth, they undergo further development throughout childhood until natural levels of glomerular filtrate appear around the end of puberty. Kidney weight increases approximately 10 times from birth to maturity primarily due to increase in renal tubular mass. Glomerular enlargement also occurs, increasing GFR.

Kidney growth postnatally is highly dependent on the demands placed on the system. Adult size is generally attained by adolescence; however, as an expanding tissue, cell division as well as increase in cell size remain possible throughout life. This hyperplasia and hypertrophy will increase the size of existing nephrons, but new nephrons are not formed. Thus, the kidney can, after final growth is achieved, respond with compensatory growth to reduction in mass and/or increase in workload.

Bladder size, and thus bladder capacity, also increases from birth through adolescence. As other muscular tissue, the bladder grows in response to tension. Increased bladder capacity, which occurs with development, results from hypertrophy following stretching of the bladder walls. In infancy, the bladder is within the abdominal cavity, but with growth it becomes a pelvic organ. During this time of descent, the bladder changes from a more cylindrical organ to the adult, pyramidal shape (see Fig. 2-54).

The urinary system develops in close association with the genital system. Indeed some structures first function as urinary structures only later to become functional within the genital system. Thus, in following chapters references are made to the related development of reproductive structures although the primary focus will be on development of the urinary system.

Integumentary system Mary Tudor

A three-layered structure, the integument is composed of the *epidermis, dermis,* and a subcutaneous *fatty layer.* It provides protection from trauma and bacterial invasion, and it effects and regulates metabolic rate and heat loss for thermoregulation. Vitamin D is synthesized on the skin surface and absorbed into underlying tissue. The integument also allows tactile input from the environment, especially important for the child.

The integument must respond to growth of all body systems collectively. During growth and throughout life the outermost, keratinized, dead layer of the epidermis, as well as hair and nails, grows, is shed, and regenerates. The germinative basal layer of the epidermis is responsible for regeneration of new cells, which become part of the outer, horny layer by 12 to 14 days (Sinclair, 1978). The accumulation of intercellular keratin causes cell death.

Skin thickens with growth; the two-layered organ is 1 to 2 mm thick in the neonate, increases only 0.25 mm in childhood, and is 2 to 4 mm thick in the mature adult (Whipple, 1966). Maturation of the integument with decrease in percentage of water content occurs steadily during childhood with a rapid spurt of growth, maturation, and sweat gland function in puberty.

Immaturity of the integument, including increased permeability, increased pH, and decreased pigment and sebum formation, results in increased sensitivity to chemical, bacterial, and ultraviolet assault. Evaporation of sebum and sweat results in a skin pH of 4.5 to 6.5 in the adult, making the integument relatively bacteriocidal. As secretion of sebum and sweat is minimal in infancy and early childhood, the pH is higher during early years.

The integument is measured as the body surface area which changes radically during growth. At birth, the surface area is approximately 2200 cm^2; due to significant growth, surface area doubles by 12 months of age and has increased seven times by maturity (Arey, 1974). Surface area decreases relative to weight, however. In the neonate, surface area is 800 cm^2/kg. As weight increases from birth to maturity by about 20 times and surface area only 7 times, the relative surface area of an adult is 300 cm^2/kg (Arey, 1974).

Surface area is highly significant in evaluating metabolism and nutritional needs. Water and electrolyte requirements correlate with body surface area over the period of growth. Surface area is also important in determin-

FIGURE 2-54. Comparison of (*a*) neonatal and (*b*) adult bladders. Note the difference in shape and position relative to other organs.

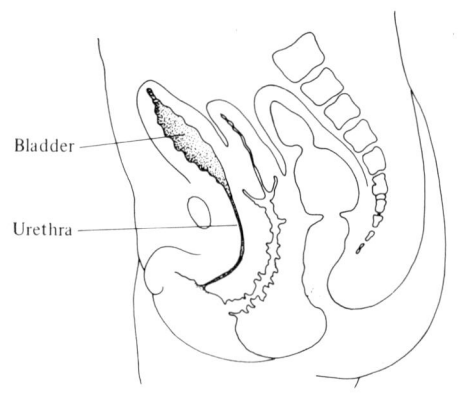

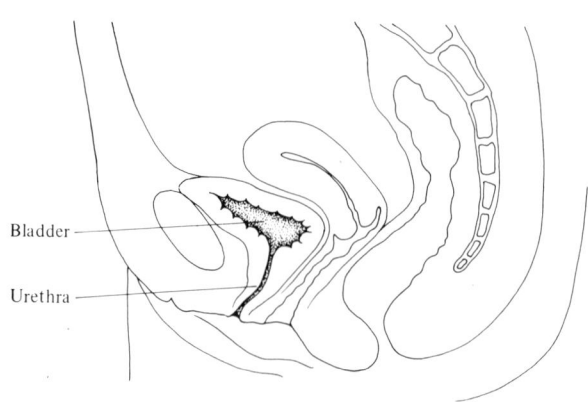

(*a*)   (*b*)

ing dosage of certain medications. Surface area can be calculated for a child based on his weight and height by use of a nomogram.

Areas of integument subject to wear regenerate more rapidly; thus the areas of the body differ in rate of mitotic regeneration. Hair is shed and regenerated throughout life also. Infants lose their scalp hair during the first 6 postnatal months, and new permanent hair growth follows. Scalp hair darkens and thickens during childhood with particularly noticeable changes during puberty. Axillary and pubic hair growth is the result of hormonal changes of puberty (see Chap. 10).

SECTION 3
Assessment of Physical Development and Status

An understanding of the process of physical development on all levels, from intracellular to whole child, and across time, from conception through childhood, serves as a foundation for pediatric nursing. Physical assessment, as part of the nursing process, is presented in this section as an application of this knowledge. Nutrition assessment, critical in consideration of physical status and growth, is also presented.

Physical assessment Mary Alexander Murphy

GENERAL CONSIDERATIONS

Physical examination is a process which helps the nurse gather data about a specific child. Physical growth, maturity, and wellness are assessed by examination. It is not a set of complex, esoteric maneuvers but an organized evaluation process. It is a systematic method by which nurses use their senses acutely. Before actually beginning the physical assessment, the nurse will want to consider several factors involved with data gathering.

SETTING

While a physical examination can be done anywhere and under a variety of conditions, the most data and the most benefits will be derived if some preplanning is done. Privacy is not essential but definitely adds to the comfort of the child and parent and allows a freer exchange of information.

If the examination is conducted in an examining room, comfortable chairs, an examination table, a writing table, space for needed equipment, good lighting, and handwashing facilities are basic considerations. The nurse should be aware of the temperature before undressing a child in a chilly room. Extras that make the atmosphere more enjoyable to children include mirrors on the wall next to the examining table, a box of toys and books, colored pictures or mobiles, and a rug on the floor.

If the child is examined during a home visit, the nurse will need to modify the approach based on the furniture and lighting in the home. An infant can be examined on the kitchen or dining table; the older child, either sitting upright in a straight-backed chair or lying on a couch or bed. The nurse may have to secure privacy by sending siblings and neighbors to another part of the home. If lighting is a problem, table lights can be brought into use, or the child could be examined near a large window if this affords enough light. The nurse should not hesitate to employ or move any furniture or other household items to obtain the best examination setting.

The physical atmosphere sets some of the tone for the examination, but the examiner is the most important aspect. A few minutes spent in setting a positive tone and approach will pay off fully as the history and physical examination proceed.

HOW TO EXAMINE

Once the setting is appropriate, the nurse decides how each child will be examined. Careful observation during the first minutes of the meeting and a background of growth and development will help the nurse decide how each child will be comfortable and cooperative. A newborn infant easily adapts to any system selected.

A toddler may not object to having clothing removed as long as he is sitting on the parent's lap, but he may protest being placed on an examination table. It will probably be best to perform most of the examination on the parent's lap. The 2-year-old may be more difficult as he generally does not like to be undressed by anyone, does not like the examiner, does not like to be touched, does not want to sit on the parent's lap or the examining table, and may spend the entire time crying and protesting.

The 3- to 5-year-old child is usually delightful to examine. He is interested in the room, toys, nurse, and equipment. He can be examined almost anywhere: lying on a table, sitting in a parent's lap, standing in front of the nurse, or sitting beside the parent. Most 6- to 12-year-old children conform and will dutifully perform as told but may or may not be interested in the procedure. Some need privacy; most are very interested in their own bodies. Applying general growth and development knowledge to the situation can help the nurse make the appropriate decision for each patient.

The process of examining children can be delightful, but it is up to the sensitive, observant nurse to bring a good background in growth and development to the situation and to control the situation so that parent, child, and nurse find the time spent together successful as well as pleasurable.

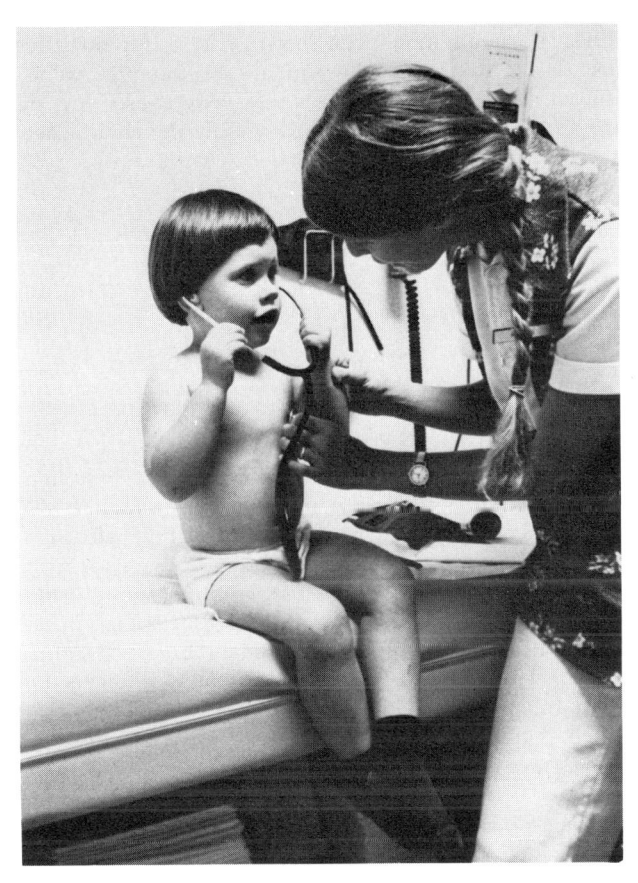

ASSESSMENT OF PHYSICAL DEVELOPMENT AND STATUS

FIGURE 2-55.

PHYSICAL ASSESSMENT

Physical assessment is, in actuality, a tool used to collect objective data in a pediatric examination. Several tools, techniques, or methods are used to look at the child and assess how he is developing. Every physical evaluation of a child contains four basic components:

- Subjective data: The history of the child's health and development to the present time
- Objective data: Information gathered through observation and inspection of the child and by performing certain tests or procedures
- Assessment of the data: The impression or diagnosis the nurse makes after considering both subjective and objective data
- A plan: How the data will be used, or what action will be taken

SUBJECTIVE DATA

Most often, an examination begins with obtaining the child's health history. This information is obtained from the parent, with the older child assisting. It is best if the parent can tell the story of the child's life, but to save time and gather the most pertinent information, the nurse organizes the questions and leads the parent in giving the information. The questions can be read rote fashion, or the nurse can use a combination of direct and indirect questioning, such as, "Have you been well?" "Can you tell me about these allergies?" The following is one form of the problem-oriented method of history taking which would give base-line data. For every child, the first "problem" considered is well-child care, which includes evaluation of health and development.

Problem 1: Subjective data for well-child care
Past history
   Birth: Prenatal, natal, postnatal
   Growth patterns
   Allergies
   Accidents
   Operations
   Hospitalizations
   Well-child care including immunizations
Family history
   Family members
   Family diseases
   Social
Review of systems
Habits
   Eating
   Bowels
   Sleep
Development and activities

Each of these sections can be expanded or reduced depending on child, place, family, and time. Once the base-line data is recorded, the nurse need review only what has happened to the child since the last visit. The reader will note that this sequence follows the child's life. The beginning sections inquire about past life; but the last sections, habits and development, describe the child today.

OBJECTIVE DATA

Objective data include both the physical examination and all screening data. Generally screening is done first; if it takes time to get laboratory results, they will be ready once the nurse has finished the physical examination and is ready to compile the data.

Screening Screening, as defined by the World Health Organization, is "The presumptive identification of unrecognized disease or defects by the application of tests, examinations, or other procedures which can be applied rapidly. Screening tests sort out apparently well persons who probably do not have the disease from those who probably do have the disease. A screening test is not intended to be diagnostic" (Frankenburg and Camp, 1976, p. 1).

The screening procedure must be valid yet economical in cost, time, and effort. Screening should be applied only to indicate those conditions for which some treatment or management will help to minimize or cure the condition. Any condition positively screened must have proper follow-up. The child is referred for further, more specific and extensive evaluation. Some problems discovered on health screening can be promptly and directly aided. For example, if it is found that an infant has a low weight, low hematocrit, and poor diet, the nurse may take steps to improve the diet.

Developmental (behavioral) screening is also done in conjunction with physical assessment. It includes simple procedures to indicate the child's general range of skill development. Developmental screening is discussed in the following chapter of this part. A child who fails a developmental screening test may or may not be developmentally delayed. He must be referred for specific, more extensive developmental assessment.

Vision screening is also done and should include acuity, farsightedness, near-point vision, heterophoria, color blindness, and visual fields. Hearing screening is difficult to perform on infants but should nevertheless be included in newborn screening, infant screening, and childhood screening.

There are many laboratory screening tests, and the nurse must decide which are appropriate according to population, cost effectivenesses, laboratory equipment, personnel, and available follow-up. Blood tests generally include hematocrit, hemoglobin, glucose-6-phosphate dehydrogenase, Dextrostix, glactosemia, hypothyroid, sickle cell, and lead-poison screening. Urine testing includes Phenistix for phenylketonuria (PKU) and specific gravity and dipsticks for urine pH, protein, ketones, glucose, blood, and bilirubin.

Physical examination The second part of the objective data deals with the actual examination of the child's physical status. Essentially it means measuring, observing, inspecting, feeling, smelling, and hearing the child! There are six basic techniques employed when examining the body:

- Measurement
- Observation
- Inspection
- Palpation
- Auscultation
- Percussion

Anthropometric measurements are usually done first. Then the child as a whole is observed: posture, physique, stature, symmetry, how he moves, overall tone, alertness, and other observations are important general descriptions. Inspection is closer observation of body parts. Sometimes instruments are used to see better or farther. Palpation is feeling, touching, and probing. The nurse must feel every part of the body. The nurse's fingers and palms must be developed into sensitive instruments of touch. Auscultation is listening either with the naked ear or, at other times, with the stethoscope, which is usually used for listening to the heart and lung. Percussion is tapping a surface and listening for the returning sound.

Anthropometric measurements One of the major characteristics of childhood is growth, and growth is measurable. A child's measurements are critical in evaluating growth, and yet, despite the simplicity of obtaining such measurements, they are often overlooked. This is particularly true if a child is examined only during acute-illness episodes and is not seen for the purpose of well-child evaluation. Weight is often the only measurement obtained, and yet it is the least indicative of growth and maturation.

Anthropometric measurements are taken at each well-child visit; it is recommended that length, weight, and occipital-frontal (head) circumference be obtained at birth and at 1, 2, 4, 6, 12, 18, 24, 30, and 36 months of age. Height and weight are then obtained at yearly intervals through completion of growth after puberty. It is difficult to obtain accurate measurements in the home setting. Unless the nurse has portable anthropometric equipment, it is advised that the child be measured in the clinic setting.

Data obtained through measurement should be plotted on standardized growth grids as soon as the measurements are taken. The appropriate grid for measurement (length or height, weight, height/weight ratio, head circumference), for age (birth to 36 months or 2 to 18 years), and for sex is selected. Care must be taken in plotting data so that the correct age line as well as the correct value line is determined. Premature infants are plotted using the corrected age: chronological age minus weeks of prematurity, until 24 months. (The examiner may want to use corrected age until 3 years for consistency until changing growth grids.)

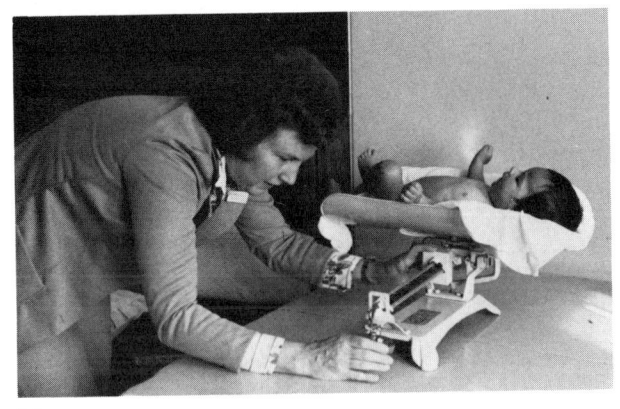

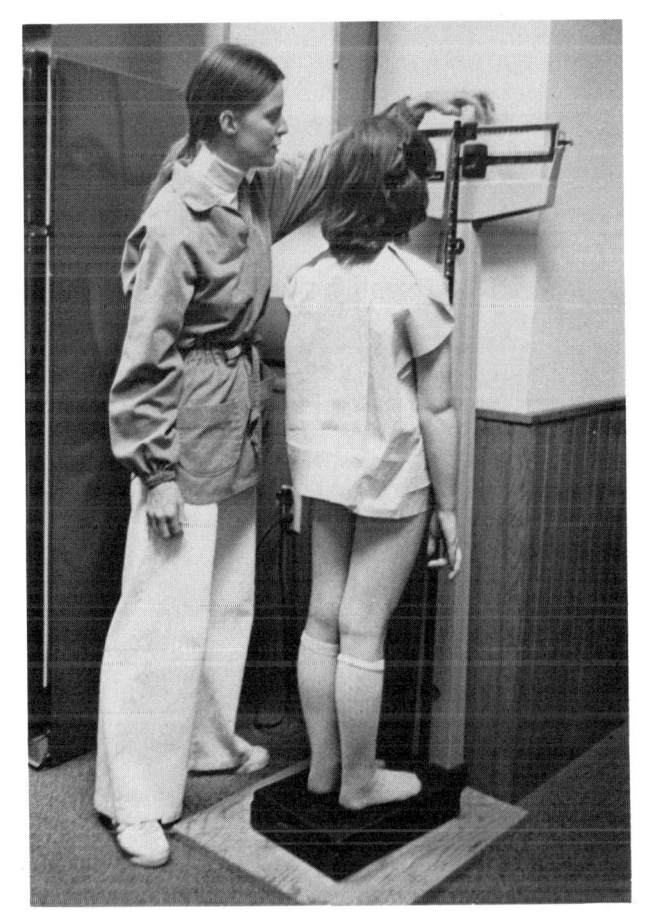

WEIGHT Weight is a good indication of a child's nutritional status and health and should be measured at each well-child examination. Weight is simple to obtain, but the instrument must be accurate. A scale of the balance-arm design is preferred. Weight is obtained nude for children under 3 years of age and with a minimum of underwear or an exam gown (no shoes) thereafter (see Fig. 2-56).

LENGTH/HEIGHT Accuracy in length and height measurements is difficult but critical, especially in the first few months, to monitoring growth. Recumbent crown-heel length is obtained until 3 years of age. It is preferable to plot 2- to 3-year-old children on the birth- to 36-months graph utilizing recumbent length rather than on the 2- to 18-years graph utilizing standing height. First, the birth-to 36-months graph is more accurate in that age range. Second, many 2- to 3-year-olds are difficult or impossible to measure accurately in standing (Fomon, 1974).

Length marked on paper on an uneven examination table is bound to be inaccurate. The appropriate apparatus must be used for accurate measurement. One person holds the child's head against the headboard of a recumbent-length instrument with his face directed upward. Keeping the child's back flat and straight and his knees extended, a second person places the footboard on the soles of the child's feet, which are at a 45° angle (see Fig. 2-57a).

Crown-rump length may be obtained in the same age group under special circumstances to evaluate body proportions. The same general technique is used, however; the footboard is placed next to the buttocks and thighs with the thighs vertical (see Fig. 2-57b).

Standing height is obtained on children 3 years of age and older. Shoes are removed, and the child is asked to stand as "tall" as possible with back, buttocks, and heels in contact with the scale. The child should look straight ahead with shoulders relaxed, legs straight, and feet to-

FIGURE 2-56. Measurement of body weight. (*a*) Infant; (*b*) older child.

gether. The arm of the scale is then lowered to press firmly on the child's head (see Fig. 2-58a).

Sitting height is the upright equivalent of crown-rump length. Sitting height is difficult to measure without special equipment and is not commonly used in well-child examinations. The child is measured from the surface he is sitting on to the top of his head. His back is again in contact with the vertical part of the scale, and he is instructed to "sit tall" and look straight ahead (see Fig. 2-58b).

HEIGHT/WEIGHT RATIO After height and weight are plotted on the appropriate growth grids, each measurement is also plotted on the weight-for-length or weight-for-height grid. There is a grid for each sex from birth to 36 months and for prepubertal girls (below age 10 years) and prepubertal boys (below age 11.5 years). This correlation, unlike the other measurements, is not plotted against age; the measurements are plotted against each other. The resulting percentage relates to weight-for-length or -height. It is useful in determining obesity or underweightedness. (See "Nutrition Assessment" later in this section for a discussion of skinfold-thickness measurement, another measure to indicate nutritional status.)

HEAD CIRCUMFERENCE Often the first indication of a central nervous system abnormality is abnormal head circumference, or abnormal rate of growth of the head. Thus, frequent, accurate head-circumference measurements are very important in the first 3 years. A nonstretchable tape measure, preferably metal, should be used. The tape is placed around the head across the most anterior (frontal) protuberance and the most posterior (occipital) protuberance (see Fig. 2-59). The circumference is noted, the tape removed, and the procedure repeated twice. The occipital-frontal circumference (OFC) is the largest of the three measurements. The tape will probably not be horizontal but will slope downward toward the occiput. It is important to compress the hair against the scalp to reduce error.

CHEST CIRCUMFERENCE Chest circumference is important in the first 2 years relative to OFC. Chest circumference is smaller than OFC at birth but is approximately equal at 12 months and larger thereafter. The tape is placed around the chest at the level of the nipple line in a horizontal plane.

(a)

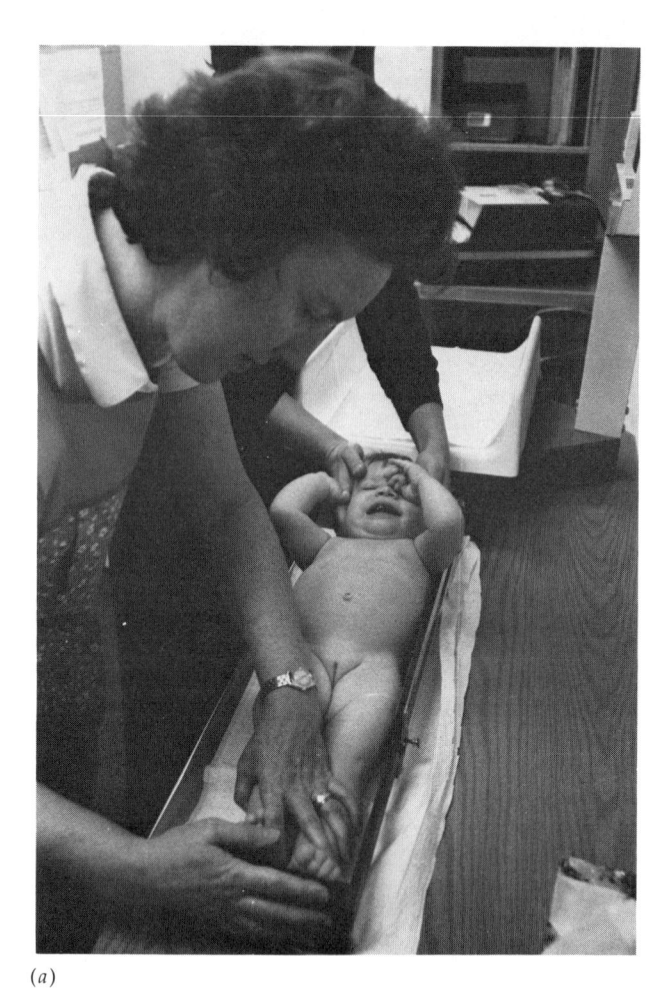

FIGURE 2-57. Measurement of length, age birth to 3 years: (a) Crown-heel (recumbent) length; (b) crown-rump length measurement.

INTERPRETATION If a significant discrepancy is noted from measurements taken at the last visit or if there is a significant discrepancy between height and weight percentiles, one should first check to see if age and data were correctly plotted. If they were correctly plotted, the child should be remeasured.

Height, length, weight, and OFC measurements between the 25th and 75th percentiles are generally interpreted to represent normal growth. Measurements between the 10th to 25th and 75th to 90th percentiles should be suspect, and all other information from the physical assessment should be noted.

Measurements below the 10th and above the 90th are highly suspect, and referral is probably warranted. Referral is recommended for measurements below the 5th and above the 95th percentiles. Referral is also recommended

(b)

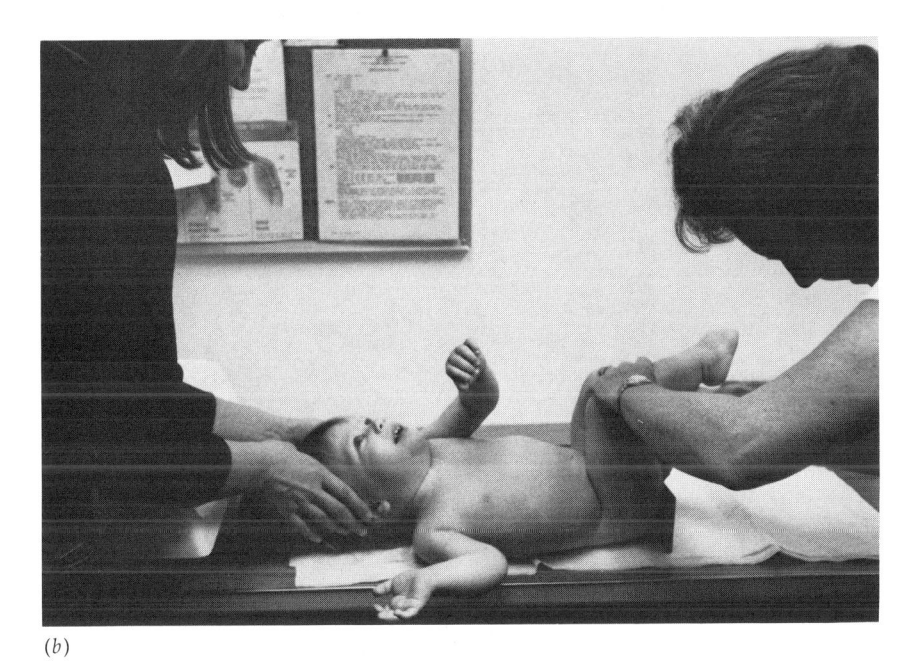

FIGURE 2-57. (*Continued*)

when a child shows more than a 25-percentile difference on any measurement from one visit to the next.

Weight-for-length or -height above the 75th or below the 25th percentile indicates a need for nutrition screening. Weight-for-length or -height above the 95th percentile is considered evidence of obesity (Fomon, 1976). It is recommended for children over age 9 years, however, that skinfold thickness be used to determine obesity because of lack of satisfactory height/weight ratio data; use of weight only is not satisfactory.

Illingworth has stated that head circumference correlates best with weight. At this time, however, most interpretations of OFC are based on chest-head circumference comparison until 12 months of age and then on percentile ranking of head measurement alone (Illingworth and Eid, 1971, p. 336).

Passive and active manipulation The child's body is not a solid, immovable mass but an active, moving object. The child's activity may be evaluated with each body part or all at once at the end of the examination. If the infant cannot move on command, the nurse can help him, to ascertain whether full movement is possible. To do so, gently roll his head from side to side to watch and feel the full, smooth rotation. From the beginning of the exam, watch his spontaneous movements. Older children can demonstrate active manipulation by being asked to perform certain movements. The body must not only look normal in an inactive state but must move fully, smoothly, and symmetrically.

System review sequence Each nurse will develop a personal variation of the physical examination. Some begin at the feet and work upward, start at the head and work downward, or start in the middle and work outward. But the exam must be organized, detailed, and routine. Once certain of the system, the nurse can modify it according to the age and development of the child.

The above is an overview of physical assessment. (For a detailed discussion, refer to pediatric physical-assessment textbooks.) Once the subjective-data and objective-data collection is complete, the nurse comes to some conclusions (analysis, impression, or diagnosis) about the child's growth, physical status, and health. This is shared with the parents and, when appropriate, the child as well. Any plan should be explained to them to gain their cooperation and mutual participation. Maintaining a healthy physical status for optimal growth and maturation are all important tasks of childhood and warrant careful monitoring by the nurse.

Nutrition assessment Andrea N. Sechrist

OBJECTIVES OF NUTRITION ASSESSMENT
The main objectives of nutrition screening and assessment are to identify existing or potential nutritional disorders and to intervene as early as possible to prevent serious health and development problems. Nutrition screening and assessment should be an integral part of routine, comprehensive well-child care. The number of nutritionists and dietitians is limited at this time; therefore, other members of the health care team, particularly nurses, are important in identifying children in need of specialized nutrition intervention.

Nutrition screening and assessment involve four major components: clinical observations, biochemical indices, anthropometric measurements, and dietary and social information. All four areas are necessary to provide meaningful nutrition information about a child.

Growth reflects the interaction of genetic, environmental, and nutritional factors, as well as general state of health. Nutrition evaluation should consider the influence these variables have on each other. Optimal nutrition provides all nutrients in sufficient amounts to meet daily needs and needs for growth and body reserves.

Dietary deficiencies of one or more nutrients result in depletion of body reserves, though overt signs of deficiency may not be apparent for some time. Following an extended period of dietary deficiency, biochemical abnormalities become apparent. By this time, the deficiencies may become severe enough to interfere with growth and resistance to disease. Finally, prolonged deficiencies may become so severe that growth and tissue integrity are compromised. Overt physical signs of tissue deterioration become visible. Malnutrition of sufficient severity and duration results in death, either from damage to body structure and function or from lowered resistance to infection.

CLINICAL OBSERVATIONS
The child's general appearance and state of health is observed. The child is then examined for overt signs of nutritional deficiency. It can be noted whether the child is tired, listless, and apathetic.

BIOCHEMICAL INDICES
Nutrition screening routinely requires a fasting blood sample for serum cholesterol, hematocrit, and hemoglobin. Both hematocrit and hemoglobin are good indicators

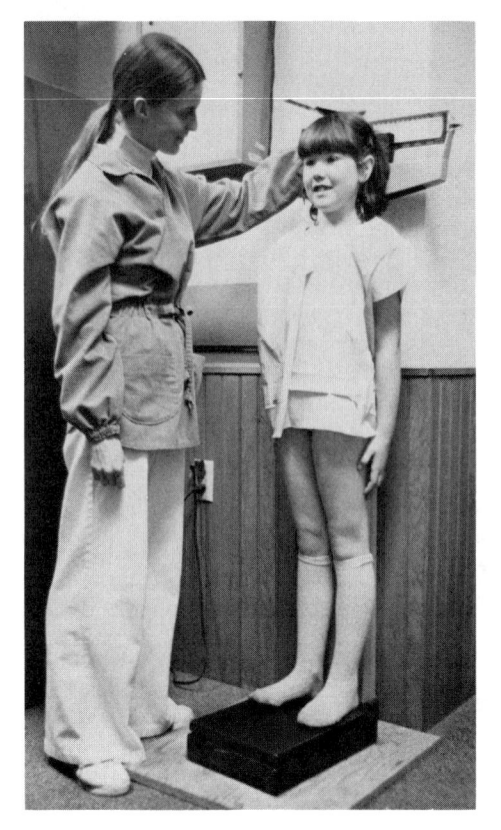

(a)

FIGURE 2-58. Measurement of height, age 3 to 18 years: (a) Stature; (b) sitting height. (b. from Cameron, 1978, p. 72. Reprinted by permission of Plenum Press.)

of overall nutrition, since production of normal red blood cells requires several nutrients (iron, folic acid, copper, nickel, cobalt, vitamin C, vitamin B_{12}, and pyridoxine). In the presence of anemia, additional physical and dietary information may be required in order to distinguish between diet-related iron-deficiency anemia and anemia of other etiology.

ANTHROPOMETRIC MEASUREMENTS

HEIGHT AND WEIGHT
Satisfactory increase in height and weight, continuing in the same approximate percentile, is a good gross indication of adequate nutrition. Minimum screening should consist of carefully executed height and weight measurements and head circumference (if the child is under 3 years of age). Serial measurements are essential for evaluation of the child's overall growth pattern. This gives in-

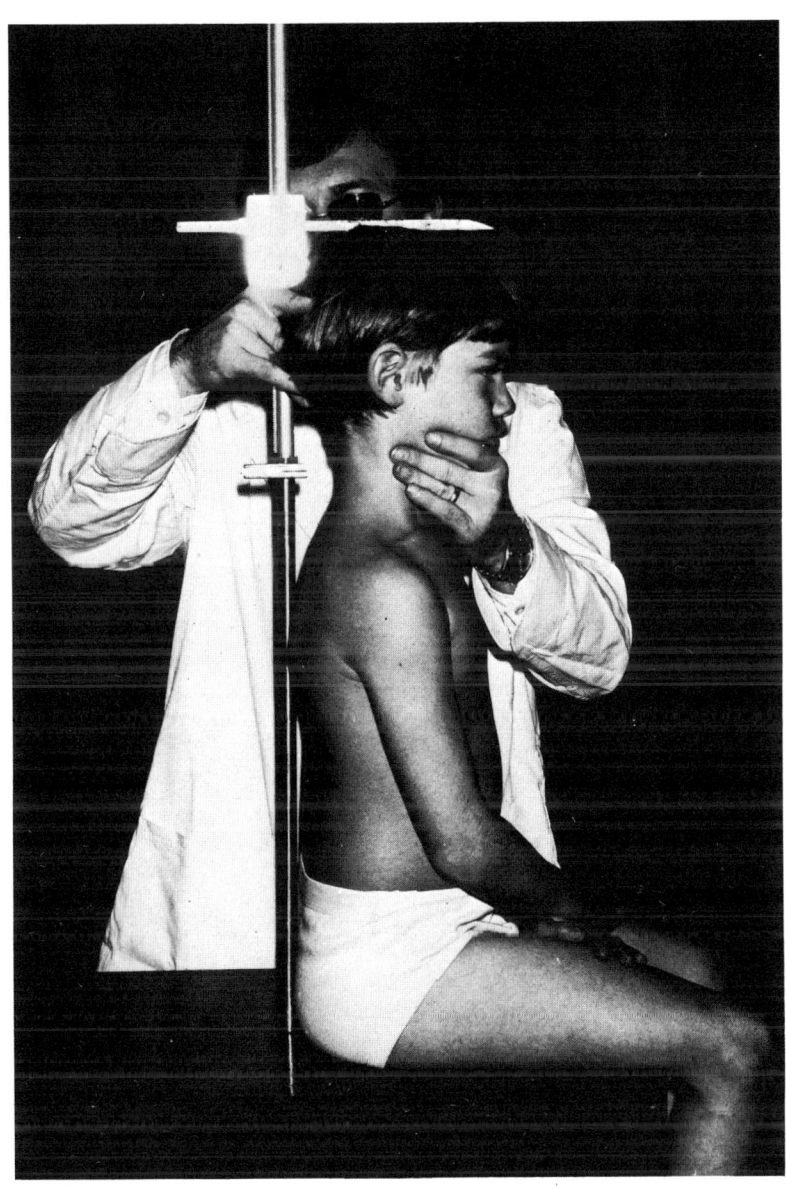

FIGURE 2-58. (*Continued*)

(b)

formation about trends in growth and adequacy of nutrition. Single-point measurements can be misleading; they fail to show long term dropping off of height or weight growth. Once an undesirable change in growth trend is spotted, one can investigate possible dietary circumstances in operation at the time of deviation. (Of course, physical, social, and other variables are also investigated.)

Significant nutrition deficiencies are reflected in a slowing or cessation of growth. This is first reflected in weight and, when more severe, in length. Head circumference, reflecting brain growth, is not affected unless the child is malnourished to a life-threatening degree.

98 PHYSICAL DEVELOPMENT

In nutrition assessment, neither height nor weight alone provides meaningful data, but rather the two must be evaluated together. It must be determined whether weight is appropriate for height as well as whether height is appropriate for age. This can be evaluated on one visit; however, an even more meaningful comparison is the relation between the height-growth *trend* and weight-growth *trend*. Again, single-point measurements can be extremely misleading.

SKINFOLD THICKNESS

In addition to height and weight, triceps and/or subscapular skinfold-thickness and midarm-circumference measurements are advised in nutrition screening. Skinfold thickness refers to the measurement of subcutaneous fat deposits with skinfold calipers. The procedure is quick, easy, and painless.

Triceps measurement is simplest to obtain and more commonly utilized. Accurate calipers are required which meet the recommendations of the Committee on Nutritional Anthropometry (Fomon, 1974). The measurement requires precise technique as well as practice to obtain a reliable reading; there is, as with height, a large potential for error by utilizing improper technique.

The examiner should make certain the child is relaxed. The child's left arm is used, held in a position that depends on age. When measuring an infant, he is held in the parent's lap with the left arm relaxed, flexed at 90°, and the palm directed medially. An older child is measured standing with his arm hanging freely, the elbow extended.

The examiner palpates the acromial and olecranon processes and marks them with a pen. The midpoint between these marks is measured and marked on the posterior aspect of the arm. Then the examiner sweeps, with left index finger and thumb, over the surface of the child's arm to grasp the skin and subcutaneous tissue in a longitudinal fold 1 cm above the midpoint mark. The examiner must be careful not to grasp underlying muscle. The left hand maintains this fold throughout the measurement.

Next the examiner places the caliper jaws over the skinfold at the midpoint mark and releases (or presses) the calipers so that they exert the standardized pressure (see Fig. 2-60). The calipers' reading is then noted and the skinfold released. The child's arm circumference is obtained next by placing a tape around the child's arm at the same midpoint mark, again with the arm relaxed.

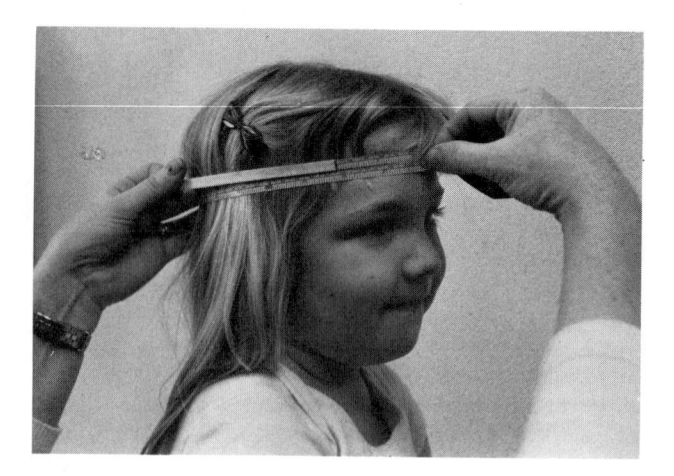

FIGURE 2-59. Measurement of occipital-frontal head circumference.

FIGURE 2-60. Measurement of triceps skinfold. (*Photo courtesy of Andrea Netten Sechrist.*)

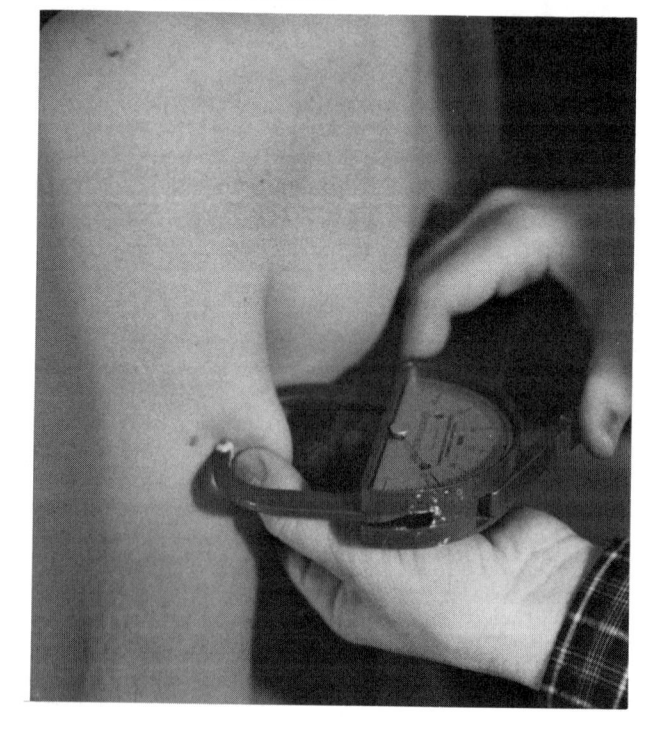

Triceps skinfold measurement is then compared with midarm circumference, and an estimate of body composition, proportion of fat to muscle mass, is made.

Triceps skinfold-thickness and arm-circumference percentiles through 12 years are reported in Frisancho (1974). It should be noted that skinfold measurement has questionable value under 2 years of age since no highly reliable charts for comparison have yet been developed for infants and young children.

There are racial differences in skinfold thickness. Negro children from birth through 4 years of age have greater skinfold-thickness measurements than Caucasian children. Between 4 years and adolescence, however, the reverse is true; Caucasian children have greater measurements (Pipes, 1977). The percentiles in Frisancho (1974) were constructed based on measurement of Caucasian children only.

When skinfold thickness is above the 85th percentile, one should consider counseling and monitoring for weight control. It is recommended that children with a measurement above the 95th percentile be referred for treatment and counseling for obesity (Fomon, 1974). However, it should be remembered that height, weight, and height/weight ratio as well as body composition should be used when evaluating possible obesity or underweight. Evaluation of any of these measurements alone may be misleading.

Skinfold thickness correlates better with height/weight ratio than with height alone or weight alone. For example, if a child is at the 5th percentile for height and 5th percentile for weight but height/weight ratio is at the 50th percentile, skinfold thickness would be expected to be at about the 50th percentile also.

DIETARY AND SOCIAL INFORMATION

Dietary screening procedures enable the nurse to identify children at risk for nutritional problems and to intervene with dietary modifications before growth and resistance to disease are compromised. Screening includes exploration of dietary factors as well as the child's socioeconomic environment.

PROCEDURES FOR DIETARY SCREENING

Current nutrient intake Dietary intake is evaluated to determine whether a child is consuming foods which supply major sources of nutrients in adequate amounts and in forms appropriate for his level of feeding skills. Dietary assessment helps to identify children who receive excessive amounts of vitamin and/or mineral supplements (several are toxic in large doses). Nutrient deficiencies rarely occur in isolation but instead are more likely to reflect a generally inadequate diet. This may occur, for instance, if a child refuses a whole food group.

The following are commonly used techniques for evaluation of dietary intake:

- 24-h recall: The parent reports the child's intake of the past 24 h and notes whether this was a typical day. The intake is then evaluated for major sources of essential nutrients. This form is frequently used in basic nutrition screening.
- Food-frequency cross-check: Food-frequency cross-checks are used with the 24-h recall to estimate how many times a week various foods (major nutrient sources) are eaten. This provides a clearer picture of the general meal pattern, variety of food and texture, and amounts the child consumes.
- 3- to 4-day diet records: An exact record is kept of all foods and amounts of each food which the child eats or drinks during a specified period. This can be analyzed in detail for exact nutrient content. Instructions must be given carefully since the final analysis is only as accurate as the original record. This method is time-consuming for both nurse and parent and is usually reserved for a detailed nutrition assessment.

Dietary history and feeding milestones It is helpful to obtain a brief summary of the child's feeding history (feeding experiences, feeding skills, problems). Early feeding problems often develop into more severe difficulties. Timely intervention can minimize future problems. Dietary history also gives the nurse insight into family food patterns and food beliefs which influence the child's intake.

Adequate nutrition, critical for normal health, growth, and maturation, should be monitored carefully and maintained for every child during the child's developing years.

Bibliography

GENERAL CONSIDERATIONS
OF PHYSICAL DEVELOPMENT: GROWTH
AND MATURATION

Acheson, R. M.: Maturation of the skeleton. In F. Falkner (Ed.), *Human development.* Philadelphia: Saunders, 1966.

Bouchard, J. C.: Physical growth and development. In K. E. Barnard and H. E. Douglas (Eds.), *Child health as-*

sessment, part I, literature review. U.S. Department of Health, Education, and Welfare Publication No. (HRA) 75-30, 1974.

Bowlby, J.: *Maternal care and mental health monograph series* (No. 2). Geneva: World Health Organization, 1951.

Cameron, N.: The methods of auxological anthropometry. In F. Falkner and J. M. Tanner (Eds.), *Human growth 2, Postnatal growth.* New York: Plenum, 1978.

Committee on Nutrition: Comparison of body weights and lengths or heights of groups of children. *Nutr. Rev.*, 1974, *32*, 284.

Dahlmann, N., and K. Peterson: Influences of environmental conditions during infancy on final body stature. *Pediat. Res.*, 1977, *11*(5), 675–700.

Fomon, S. J.: *Infant nutrition.* Philadelphia: Saunders, 1974.

Forbes, G. B.: Relation of lean body mass to height in children and adolescents. *Pediat. Res.*, 1972, *6*, 32.

Frank, L. K.: Cultural control and physiological autonomy. *Amer. J. Orthopsychiat.*, 1938, *8*, 662–666.

Friis-Hansen, B.: Body composition during growth. *Pediatrics*, 1971, *47*, 264.

Garn, S. M.: Malnutrition and skeletal development in the preschool child. In *Preschool child nutrition, primary deterrent to human progress.* National Academy of Science Publication No. 1282: Washington D.C., 1966.

Gessel, A., and F. L. Ilg: *Child development, An introduction to the study of human growth.* New York: Harper & Row, 1949.

Gruelich, W. W., and S. I. Pyle: *Radiographic atlas of skeletal development of the hand and wrist.* Stanford, California: Stanford University Press, 1959.

Hamill, H. V. V., and W. M. Moore: Contemporary growth charts: Needs, construction and application. *Pediat. Curr.*, August 1976 (special issue).

Harris, J. A., C. M. Jackson, D. G. Paterson, and R. E. Scammon: *The measurement of man.* Minneapolis: University of Minnesota Press, 1930.

Holliday, M. A.: Metabolic rate and organ size during growth from infancy to maturity. *Pediatrics*, 1971, *47*, 169.

Illingworth, R. S.: *The development of the infant and young child: Normal and abnormal* (6th ed.). New York: Churchill Livingstone, 1975a.

———: *The normal child* (6th ed.). New York: Churchill Livingstone, 1975b.

———, and E. E. Eid: The head circumference in infants and other measurements to which it may be related. *Acta Paediat. Scand.*, 1971, *60*(3), 333–339.

Kaplan, S. L., C. A. L. Abrams, J. J. Bell, et al.: Growth and growth hormone. *Pediat. Res.*, 1968, *2*, 43.

Krieger, I., and M. Good: Adrenocortical and thyroid function in the deprivation syndrome. *Amer. J. Dis. Child.*, 1970, *120*, 95.

———, and R. C. Mellinger: Pituitary function in the deprivation syndrome. *Amer. J. Pediatr.*, 1971, *79*, 216.

———, and Q. Taqi: Free serum thyroxine level and basal metabolic rate. *Amer. J. Dis. Child.*, 1975, *129*, 830.

Lowery, G. H.: *Growth and development of children* (7th ed.). Chicago: Year Book, 1978.

Marshall, W. A.: Puberty. In F. Falkner and J. M. Tanner (Eds.), *Human growth 2, Postnatal growth.* New York: Plenum, 1978.

Moore, K.: *The developing human* (2d ed.). Philadelphia: Saunders, 1977.

National Center for Health Statistics: NCHS growth curves for children 0–18 years. *United States Vital Health Statistics* (Series II, No. 165). Washington: Government Printing Office, 1977.

Neumann, C. G., and M. Alpaugh: Birthweight doubling time, A fresh look. *Pediatrics*, 1976, *57*, 469.

Owen, G. M.: The assessment and recording of measurements of growth of children: Report of a conference. *Pediatrics*, 1974, *51*(3), 461–466.

Powell, G. F., J. A. Brasel, S. Raiti, and R. M. Blizzard: Emotional deprivation and growth retardation stimulating idiopathic hypopituitarism. II. Endocrinologic evaluation of the syndrome. *New Engl. J. Med.*, 1967, *276*, 1279.

Prader, A., J. M. Tanner, and G. A. vonHarnack: Catch-up growth following illness or starvation: An example of developmental canalization in man. *J. Pediat.*, 1963, *62*(5), 646–659.

Reynolds, E. L., and T. Asakawa: Skeletal development in infancy: Standards for clinical use. *Amer. J. Roentgen.*, 1951, *62*, 403m.

Roche, A. F., and J. I. McKigney: Physical growth of ethnic groups comprising the U.S. population. *Amer. J. Dis. Child.*, 1976, *130*, 62.

Sheldon, W. H.: *The varieties of human physique.* New York: Harper, 1940.

Silver, H. K., and M. Finkelstein: Deprivation dwarfism. *J. Pediat.*, 1967, *70*, 317.

Sinclair, D.: *Human growth after birth* (3d ed.). London: Oxford University Press, 1978.

Smith, D. W.: *Growth and its disorders* (Vol. XV): *Major problems in clinical pediatrics.* Philadelphia: Saunders, 1977.

———: Shifting linear growth during infancy: Illustrations of genetic factors in growth from fetal life through infancy, *J. Pediat.*, 1976, *89*, 225–230.

Tanner, J. M.: *Growth at adolescence.* Oxford, England: Blackwell, 1962.

———: Physical growth. In P. H. Mussen (Ed.), *Carmichael's manual of child psychology* (3d ed.). New York: Wiley, 1970.

———: The regulation of human growth. *Child Develop.*, 1963, *34*, 817–847.

———, R. H. Whitehouse, and M. Takaishi: Standards from birth to maturity for height, weight, height velocity and weight velocity, British children. *Arch. Dis. Child.*, 1965, *41*, 454–469.

Thompson, R. G., A. Parra, R. B. Schultz, and R. M. Blizzard: Endocrine evaluation in patients with psychosocial dwarfism. *Amer. Fed. Clin. Res.*, 1969, *17*, 592 (abstract).

Timiras, P. S.: *Developmental physiology and aging.* New York: Macmillan, 1972.

Widdowson, E. M., and R. A. McCance: Some effects of accelerating growth. I. General somatic development. *Proc. Roy. Soc. Brit.*, 1960, *152*, 188–206.

———, W. O. Mavor, and R. A. McCance: The effect of undernutrition and rehabilitation on the development of the reproductive organs: Rats. *J. Endocr.*, 1964, *29*, 119–126.

Wingerd, F., I. L. Soloman, and E. J. Schoen: Parent-specific height standards for preadolescent children of three racial groups, with method for rapid determination. *Pediatrics*, 1973, *52*(4), 555–560.

Winick, M., P. Rosso, and J. Waterlon: Cellular growth of cerebrum, cerebellum and brain stem in normal and marasmic children. *Exp. Neurol.*, 1970, *26*, 393.

HUMAN GENETICS: BLUEPRINT FOR DEVELOPMENT

Ad Hoc Committee on Genetic Counseling: Genetic counseling. *Amer. J. Hum. Genet.*, 1975, *27*, 240–242.

Alexanderson, B., and F. Sjoqvist: Individual differences in the pharmacokinetics of monomethylated tricyclic antidepressants: Role of genetic and environmental factors and clinical importance. *Ann. N. Y. Acad. Sci.*, 1971, *179*, 739–751.

Arrighi, F. E., and T. C. Hsu: Localization of heterochromatin in human chromosomes. *Cytogenetics (Basal)*, 1971, *10*, 81–86.

Caspersson, T., G. Lomakka, and L. Zech.: The 24 fluorescence patterns of the human metaphase chromosomes—Distinguishing characters and variability. *Hereditas (Lund)*, 1971, *67*, 89–102.

Chicago Conference: Standardization in human cytogenetics. *Birth Defects: Original Article Series*, 1966, *2*(2).

Childs, B., J. M. Finucci, M. S. Preston, and A. E. Pulver: Human behavior genetics. In H. Harris and K. Hirschhorn (Eds.), *Advances in human genetics.* New York: Plenum, 1976.

Defries, J. C., S. G. Vandenberg, and G. E. McClearn: Genetics of specific cognitive abilities. *Ann. Rev. Genet.*, 1976, *10*, 179–207.

Epstein, C., R. P. Erickson, B. D. Hall, and M. Golbus: The center-satellite system for the wide-scale distribution of genetic counseling services. *Am. J. Hum. Genet.*, 1975, *27*, 322–332.

Gershon, E. S., S. D. Targum, L. R. Kessler, C. M. Mazure, and W. E. Bunney, Jr.: Genetic studies and biologic strategies in the affective disorders. In A. G. Steinberg, A. G. Bearn, A. G. Motulsky, and B. Childs (Eds.), *Progress in medical genetics* (Vol. II). Philadelphia: Saunders, 1977.

Huang, R. C., and J. Bonner: Histone, A suppressor of chromosomal RNA synthesis. *Proc. Nat. Acad. Sci. U.S.A.*, 1962, *48*, 1216–1222.

Jones, K. W.: Chromosomal and nuclear location of mouse satellite DNA in individual cells. *Nature (London)*, 1970, *225*, 912–915.

Kucherlapati, R. S., and F. H. Ruddle: Advances in human gene mapping by parasexual procedures. In *Progress in medical genetics, New series* (Vol. I). Philadelphia: Saunders, 1976.

Lewontin, R. C.: Genetic aspects of intelligence. *Ann. Rev. Genet.*, 1975, *9*, 387–405.

McKay, R. D. G., M. Bobrow, and J. H. Cooke: The identification of a repeated-DNA sequence involved in the karyotype polymorphism of the human Y chromosome. *Cytogenet. Cell Genet.*, 1978, *21*, 19–22.

McKusick, V. A.: *Mendelian inheritance in man. Catalogs of autosomal dominant, autosomal recessive and X-linked phenotypes* (4th ed.). Baltimore: Johns Hopkins University Press, 1975.

MacLean, N.: *Control of gene expression.* London: Academic, 1976.

McMichael, A., and H. McDivitt: The association between the HLA system and disease. In *Progress in medical genetics, New series* (Vol. II). Philadelphia: Saunders, 1977.

Murphy, E. A., and G. A. Chase: *Principles of genetic counseling.* Chicago: Year Book, 1975.

Ohno, S.: Major regulatory genes for mammalian sexual development. *Cells*, 1976, *7*, 315–321.

———: The role of H-Y antigen in primary sex determination. *J. A. M. A.*, 1978, *239*, 217–220.
Pardue, M. L., and J. Gall: Chromosomal localization of mouse satellite DNA. *Science*, 1970, *168*, 1356–1358.
Paris Conference: Standardization in human cytogenetics. *Birth Defects: Original Article Series,* 1972, *8*(7).
Sahin, S. T.: The multifaceted role of the nurse as genetic counselor. *Amer. J. Maternal Child Nurs.*, 1976, *1*, 211–216.
Vesell, E. S.: Pharmacogenetics. *New Engl. J. Med.*, 1972, *287*, 904–909.
Watson, J. D.: *Molecular biology of the gene* (3d ed.). Menlo Park, California: W. A. Benjamin, 1976.
———, and F. H. Crick: A structure for deoxyribose nucleic acid. *Nature* (London), 1963, *171*, 737–738.

GENERAL CONSIDERATIONS OF PHYSICAL DEVELOPMENT: CELLULAR GROWTH, DIFFERENTIATION AND MORPHOGENESIS

Babloyantz, A., and J. Hiernanz: Models for positional information and positional differentiation. *Proc. Natl. Acad. Sci. U.S.A.*, 1974, *71*, 1530.
Baserga, R.: The control of cell proliferation in mammalian cells. In E. Mihich (Ed.), *Drugs and cell regulation.* New York: Academic, 1974.
Blechschmidt, E., and R. F. Gasser: *Biokinetics and biodynamics of human differentiation.* Springfield, Illinois: Charles C Thomas, 1978.
Bonner, J.: *The molecular biology of development.* Oxford: Clarendon, 1965.
Brunner, G.: Membrane impression and gene expression. Towards a theory of cytodifferentiation. *Differentiation,* 1977, *8*(2), 123–132.
Cook, P. R.: Hypothesis on differentiation and the inheritance of gene expression. *Nature* (London), 1973, *245*, 23.
Copenhaver, W. M., R. P. Bunge, and M. B. Bunge: *Bailey's textbook of histology* (16th ed.). Baltimore: Williams & Wilkins, 1971.
Crick, F.: General model for the chromosomes of higher organisms. *Nature* (London), 1971, *234*, 25.
Davidson, E. H.: *Gene activity in early development* (2d ed.). New York: Academic, 1976.
———, and R. J. Britten: Note on the control of gene expression during development. *J. Theor. Biol.*, 1971, *32*, 123.
——— and ———: Regulation of gene expression: Possible role repetitive sequences. *Science,* 1979, *204*, 1052–1059.
Dienstmann, S. R., and H. Holtzer: Myogenesis: A cell lineage interpretation. In J. Reinert and H. Holtzer (Eds.), *Cell cycle and cell differentiation.* New York: Springer, 1975.
Edelstein, B. B.: The dynamics of cellular differentiation and associated pattern formation. *J. Theor. Biol.*, 1972, *37*, 221.
Epel, D.: The triggering of development as fertilization. In J. D. Eberg and T. S. Okada (Eds.), *Mechanism of cell change.* New York: Wiley, 1979.
Fallon, J. F., and B. K. Simandl: Evidence of a role for cell death in the disappearance of the embryonic human tail. *Amer. J. Anat.*, 1978, *152*(1), 111–130.
Gierer, A.: Molecular models and combinatorial principles in cell differentiation and morphogenesis. *Cold Spring Harbor Symposium in Quantitative Biology,* 1974, *38*, 951.
Gilbert, D. A.: Differentiation, oncogenesis and cellular periodicities. *J. Theor. Biol.*, 1968, *21*, 113.
Heyden, H. W., and D. Heyden: Differentiation and cell growth by symmetrical and asymmetrical mitosis: A hypothesis. *Perspect. Biol. Med.*, 1973, *16*, 348.
Holtzer, H., H. Weintraub, R. Mayne, and B. Mochan: The cell cycle, cell lineages and cell differentiation. *Curr. Top. Develop. Biol.*, 1972, *7*, 229.
Kauffman, S. A.: Sequential DNA replication and the control of differences in gene activity between sister chromatids—A possible factor in cell differentiation. *J. Theor. Biol.*, 1967, *17*, 483.
———: Gene regulation networks: A theory for their global structure and behaviors. *Curr. Top. Develop. Biol.*, 1971, *6*, 145.
Leblond, C. P.: Classification of cell populations on the basis of their proliferation behavior. *National Cancer Institute Monograph,* 1964, *14*, 119.
——— and B. E. Walker: Renewal of cell populations. *Physiol. Rev.*, 1956, *36*, 255.
Lindenmayer, A.: Development systems without cellular interactions: Their languages and grammars. *J. Theor. Biol.*, 1971, *30*, 455.
McMahon, D.: Chemical messengers in development: A hypothesis. *Science,* 1974, *185*, 1012.
Riley, P. A.: The principles of sequential dependence in cellular differentiation. *Differentiation,* 1973, *1*, 183.
Robertson, A., and M. H. Cohen: Control of developing fields. *Ann. Rev. Biophys. Bioenerg.*, 1972, *1*, 409.
Runnstrom, J.: The mechanism of control of differentiation in early development of the sea urchin: A tentative discussion. *Exp. Biol. Med.*, 1967, *1*, 52.
Shapiro, J. M., G. G. Ganse, and A. F. Zakharov: A model

of the mechanism regulating the timing of chromosome replication in eucaryotic cells. *Differentiation,* 1974, *2,* 125.

Steward, C. R.: Asymmetric replication and cellular differentiation. *J. Theor. Biol.,* 1972, *36,* 639.

Sutton, W. D.: Chromatin packing, repeated DNA sequences and gene control. *Nature (London),* 1972, *237,* 70.

Vogel, F. A.: A preliminary estimate of the number of human genes. *Nature (London),* 1964, *201,* 847.

Wangenheim, K. H.: A mechanism for the endocellular control of cell differentiation and cell proliferation. *J. Theor. Biol.,* 1976, *59,* 205.

Wassermann, G. D.: *Molecular control of cell differentiation and morphogenesis: A systematic theory.* New York: Marcel Dekker, 1972.

Wolpert, L., and J. H. Lewis: Towards a theory of development. *Fed. Proc.,* 1975, *34,* 14.

Zuckerkandel, E.: A possible role of "inert" heterochromatin in cell differentiation. Action of and completion for "locking" molecules. *Biochemistry,* 1974, *56,* 937.

CALVARIUM AND FACE

American Academy of Pediatrics Committee on Nutrition: Flouride as a Nutrient. *Pediatrics,* 1972, *49,* 456.

Corliss, C. E.: *Patten's human embryology.* New York: McGraw-Hill, 1976.

Demirjian, A.: Dentition. In F. Falkner and J. M. Tanner (Eds.), *Human growth 2, Postnatal growth,* New York: Plenum, 1978.

Enlow, D. H.: *Handbook of facial growth.* Philadelphia: Saunders, 1975.

Garn, S. M., and S. M. Bailey: Genetics of maturational processes. In F. Falkner and J. M. Tanner (Eds.), *Human growth 1, Principles and prenatal growth.* New York: Plenum, 1978.

Israel, H.: The fundamentals of cranial and facial growth. In F. Falkner and J. M. Tanner (Eds.), *Human growth 2, Postnatal growth.* New York: Plenum, 1978.

Lacey, K. A.: Relationship between bone age and dental development. *Lancet,* 1973, *2,* 736.

Nelson, W., V. Vaughn, and R. McKay: *Textbook of pediatrics* (10th ed.). Philadelphia: Saunders, 1975.

Schour, I., and M. Massler: Development of human dentition, *J. Amer. Dent. Ass.,* 1941, *28,* 1153–1160.

Sinclair, D.: *Human growth after birth* (3d ed.). London: Oxford University Press, 1978.

Sullivan, P. G.: Skull, jaw, and teeth growth patterns. In F. Falkner and J. M. Tanner (Eds.), *Human growth 2, Postnatal growth.* New York: Plenum, 1978.

SENSORY SYSTEM

Arey, L. B.: *Developmental anatomy* (7th ed.). Philadelphia: Saunders, 1965.

Bordley, J. E., and W. G. Hardy: The special senses. In R. E. Cooke (Ed.), *The biologic basis of pediatric practice.* New York: McGraw-Hill, 1968.

Moore, K. L.: *The developing human* (2d ed.). Philadelphia: Saunders, 1977.

MUSCULOSKELETAL SYSTEM

Acheson, R. M.: Maturation of the skeleton. In F. Falkner (Ed.), *Human development.* Philadelphia: Saunders, 1966.

Arey, Leslie B.: *Developmental anatomy* (7th ed.). Philadelphia: Saunders, 1974.

Garn, S. M., and S. M. Bailey: Genetics of maturational processes. In F. Falkner and J. M. Tanner (Eds.), *Human growth 1, Principles and prenatal growth.* New York: Plenum, 1978.

Goss, R. J.: Adaptive mechanisms of growth control. In F. Falkner and J. M. Tanner (Eds.), *Human growth 1, Principles and prenatal growth.* New York: Plenum, 1978.

Hilt, N., and E. W. Schmitt: *Pediatric orthopedic nursing.* St. Louis: Mosby, 1975.

Malina, R. M.: Growth of muscle tissue and muscle mass. In F. Falkner and J. M. Tanner (Eds.), *Human growth 2, Postnatal growth.* New York: Plenum, 1978.

Passo, S.: The musculoskeletal system. In G. Scipien, M. Barnard, M. Chard, J. Howe, and P. Phillips (Eds.), *Comprehensive pediatric nursing* (2d ed.). New York: McGraw-Hill, 1979.

Roche, A. F.: Bone growth and maturation. In F. Falkner and J. M. Tanner (Eds.), *Human growth 2, Postnatal growth.* New York: Plenum, 1978.

Rudolph, A. M. (Ed.): *Pediatrics* (16th ed.). New York: Appleton-Century-Crofts, 1977.

Sinclair, D.: *Human growth after birth* (3d ed.). London: Oxford University Press, 1978.

Sullivan, P. G.: Skull, jaw, and teeth growth patterns. In F. Falkner and J. M. Tanner (Eds.), *Human growth 2, Postnatal growth.* New York: Plenum, 1978.

CARDIOVASCULAR SYSTEM

Brasel, J. A., and R. K. Gruen: Cellular growth: Brain, liver, muscle, and lung. In F. Falkner and J. M. Tanner (Eds.), *Human growth 2, Postnatal growth.* New York: Plenum, 1978.

Iliff, A., and V. A. Lee: Pulse rate, respiratory rate and

body temperature of children between two months and 18 years of age. *Child Develop.*, 1952, *23*(4), 237–245.

Marshall, W. A.: Puberty. In F. Falkner and J. M. Tanner (Eds.), *Human growth 2, Postnatal growth*. New York: Plenum, 1978.

Moore, K.: *The developing human*. Philadelphia: Saunders, 1977.

———: Recommendations of the task force on blood pressure control in children. *Pediatrics*, 1977, *59*(5), 797–820 (supplement).

Shock, N.: Physiological growth. In F. Falkner (Ed.), *Human development*. Philadelphia: Saunders, 1966.

Sinclair, D.: *Human growth after birth*, (3d ed.). London: Oxford, 1978.

RESPIRATORY SYSTEM

Avery, G. B.: *Neonatology*. Philadelphia: Lippincott, 1975.

Fraser, R., and J. Paré: *Organ physiology: Structure and function of the lung* (2d ed.). Philadelphia: Saunders, 1977.

Hogg, J. C.: Age as a factor in respiratory disease. In E. L. Kendig, Jr., and V. Chernich (Eds.), *Disorders of the respiratory tract in children*. Philadelphia: Saunders, 1977.

Horsfield, K., and G. Cummings: Morphology of the bronchial tree man. *J. Appl. Physil.*, 1968, *24*, 373.

Iliff, A., and V. A. Lee: Pulse rate, respiratory rate and body temperature of children between two months and 18 years of age. *Child Develop.*, 1952, *23*(4), 237–245.

Kendig, E. L., Jr., and V. Chernich (Eds.): *Disorders of the respiratory tract in children*. Philadelphia: Saunders, 1977.

Murray, J. F.: *The normal lung*. Philadelphia: Saunders, 1976.

Scarpelli, E.: Pulmonary physiology of the fetus, newborn, and child. Philadelphia: Lea & Febiger, 1975.

Youmans, W., and A. Siebens: Respiration. In J. R. Brobeck (Ed.): *Best and Taylor's physiological basis of medical practice* (9th ed.). Baltimore: Williams & Wilkins, 1973.

GASTROINTESTINAL SYSTEM

Cunningham, D. J.: *Cunningham's manual of practical anatomy*. New York: Oxford University Press, 1977.

Davenport, H. W.: *Physiology of the digestive tract*. Chicago: Year Book, 1977.

Guyton, A. C.: *Textbook of medical physiology*. Philadelphia: Saunders, 1971.

Schade, J. P.: *Introduction to functional human anatomy*, Philadelphia: Saunders, 1974.

ENDOCRINE SYSTEM

Williams, R. H.: *Textbook of endocrinology* (5th ed.). Philadelphia: Saunders, 1974.

REPRODUCTIVE SYSTEM

Barnett, H. L., and A. H. Einhorm: *Pediatrics* (15th ed.). New York: Appleton-Century-Crofts, 1972.

Marshall, W. A.: Puberty. In F. Falkner and J. M. Tanner (Eds.), *Human growth 2, Postnatal growth*. New York: Plenum, 1978.

Tanner, J. M.: Puberty. In A. McLaren (Ed.). *Advances in reproductive physiology* (Vol. 2). London: Academic, 1967.

URINARY SYSTEM

Goss, R. J.: Adaptive mechanisms of growth control. In F. Falkner and J. M. Tanner: *Human growth 1, Principles and prenatal growth*. New York: Plenum, 1978.

INTEGUMENTARY SYSTEM

Arey, L. B.: *Developmental anatomy* (7th ed.). Philadelphia: Saunders, 1974.

Langley, L. L., I. R. Telford, and J. B. Christiansen: *Dynamic anatomy and physiology* (4th ed.). New York: McGraw-Hill, 1974.

Sinclair, D.: *Human growth after birth* (3d ed.). London: Oxford University Press, 1978.

Whipple, D. V.: *Dynamics of development: Euthenic pediatrics*. New York: McGraw-Hill, 1966.

PHYSICAL ASSESSMENT

Alexander, M. M., and M. S. Brown: *Pediatric physical diagnosis for nurses*. New York: McGraw-Hill, 1974.

American Academy of Pediatrics: *Standards of child health care* (3d ed.). Evanston, Illinois: American Academy of Pediatrics, 1975.

Barness, L. A.: *Manual of pediatric physical diagnosis*. Chicago: Year Book, 1972.

Bates, B.: *A guide to physical examination*. Philadelphia: Lippincott, 1974.

Chinn, P. L., and C. J. Leitch: *Handbook for nursing assessment of the child*. Salt Lake City: University of Utah Printing Service, 1973.

Fomon, S. J.: *Nutritional disorders of children*. U.S. Department of Health, Education, and Welfare Publication No. (HSA) 76-5612, 1976.

———: *Infant nutrition*. Philadelphia: Saunders, 1974.

Frankenburg, W. K., and B. W. Camp: *Pediatric screening tests*. Springfield, Illinois: Charles C Thomas, 1976.

Garb, S.: *Laboratory tests in common use.* New York: Springer, 1971.

Hervada, A. R.: Nursery evaluation of the newborn. *Amer. J. Nurs.*, 1967, *67*(8), 1669–1671.

Hurst, W. J., and H. K. Walker: *The problem-oriented system.* New York: Medcom, 1972.

Illingworth, R. S., and E. E. Eid: The head circumference in infants and other measurements to which it may be related. *Acta Paediat. Scand.*, 1971, *60*(3), 333–339.

Northern, J. L., and M. Downs: *Hearing children.* Baltimore: Williams & Wilkins, 1974.

Tudor, M.: Developmental screening. *Compr. Pediat. Nurs.*, 1977, *2*(2), 1–13.

NUTRITION ASSESSMENT

Fomon, S. J.: *Infant nutrition.* Philadelphia: Saunders, 1974.

Frisancho, A. R.: Triceps skinfold and upper arm muscle size norms for assessment of nutritional status. *Amer. J. Clin. Nutr.*, 1974, *27*, 1052–1058.

Nutritional assessment in health programs. *Amer. J. Public Health*, 1973, *63* (supplement).

Nutritional disorders of children, prevention, screening, follow up. U.S. Department of Health, Education, and Welfare Publication No. (HSA) 76-5612, 1976.

Pipes, P. L.: *Nutrition in infancy and childhood.* St. Louis: Mosby, 1977.

Zerfas, A., F. Shorr, and C. Neumann: Office assessment of nutritional status. *Pediat. Clin. N. Amer.*, 1977, *24*(1).

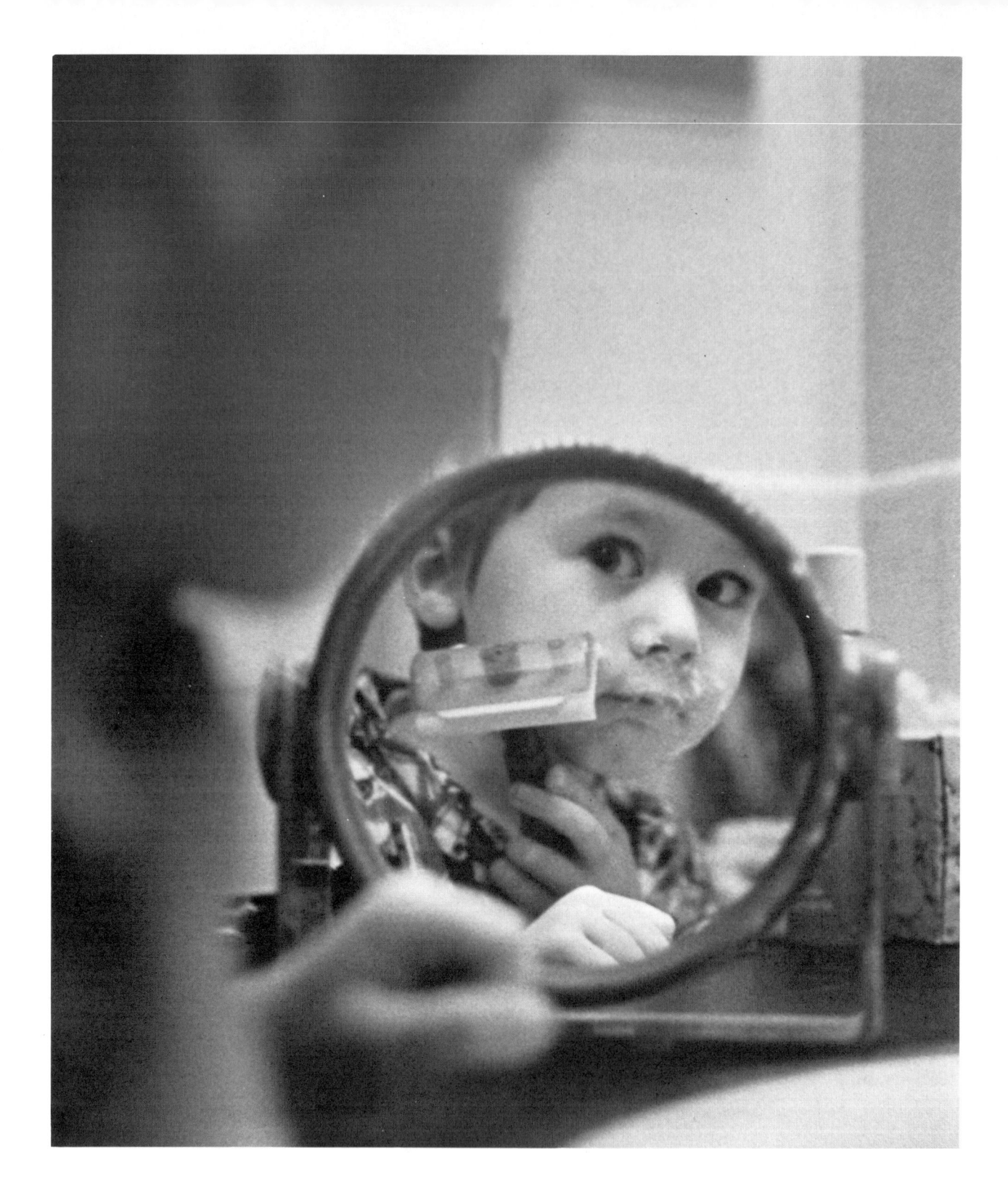

CHAPTER 3
Behavioral Development

SECTION 1
Principles of Behavioral Development

Behavioral development is the attainment and integration of skills leading to independent, adaptive functioning. Concepts of physical development, the substrate and effector of behavior, have been presented. Theoretical concepts of the behavioral change observed in childhood are presented in this chapter.

General considerations of behavioral development   Ruth Hepler

An infant grasps a surprised parent's finger. A group of preschoolers play "doctor." A schoolchild joins a "secret club." These observations are a small sample indicating that the behavioral repertoire of the human organism is a vast array of observable responses occurring in an endless variety of circumstances. In an effort to facilitate understanding of the formation of this immense repertoire, investigators of behavior have watched for patterns in behavioral development that can be identified as principles, or basic propositions, to explain a variety of behaviors. It can thus be observed that whether a theoretical explanation of behavior is presented in the terms of a simple stimulus-response paradigm or in more complex terms ascribing growth to a psychological drive for self-actualization, common underlying principles of development can be identified.

FIGURE 3-1. *(Photo courtesy of William E. Boyson.)*

PRINCIPLES OF DEVELOPMENT

DIFFERENTIATION

Among the various principles of behavioral development are those that have achieved wide acceptance as providing a valid and reliable base for organization of observed data. One of these principles is that of differentiation. According to this principle, behavior develops on a continuum from relatively restricted, repetitive forms to more elaborated and fluid ones. Various comparative terms have been used to describe this continuum: simple to complex, general to specific, and homogenous to heterogenous. Whatever the descriptive terms, however, differentiation of behavior is the basic observation. An example of general-to-specific differentiation is seen in the behavior of an infant in reaction to stress. Early stress reactions are described as generalized, diffuse, fretful behaviors. As the infant's stress-induced behavior develops, however, more specific response patterns are observed that can be identified as being related to such experiences as hunger, pain, anger, or loneliness.

FUNCTIONAL SUBORDINATION

A second, related principle is that of functional subordination. This principle divides the differentiation of singular, isolated experiences or behaviors (functions) into different levels of application resulting finally in the development of higher-level experience. The progression observed in hammering behavior is illustrative of functional subordination: the older infant and toddler engage in indiscriminate hammering behavior (a function); the preschooler hammers nails into a board (function assumes some purpose); the 10-year-old hammers to produce a birdhouse (function now subordinate to the experience and skill of production).

STAGE FORMATION

Observations of behavioral development have resulted in the formulation of a principle that such development occurs in identifiable stages. A developmental stage is defined as a period during which certain behaviors are given a priority that is different from behavioral priorities observed at other periods. Observations of development of social behavior in children exemplifies the principle of stages. The infant's almost total preoccupation with self gives way to the beginning awareness and acceptance of other children, seen in the parallel play of the toddler. This stage of socialization is then replaced by group play characteristic of preschoolers, which is also subsequently replaced by the peer society developed by school-age children.

CRITICAL OR SENSITIVE PERIODS

Studies of development of young animals have yielded the observation of a behavioral phenomenon known as *imprinting*. Imprinting is operationally defined as learning to fix on a certain object and develop behaviors specific to that object, e.g., "fixing" on a mother object and developing a behavior such as following. Continued observation of this phenomenon resulted in the translation of an important principle of physical (embryonic) development into behavioral terms as it became clear that such behavior could only be developed in a specific time period.

This physical-behavioral principle of critical or sensitive periods indicates that there are definite time periods during which a particular feature of development is most responsive to cultivation, trauma, or neglect. In studies of development of attachment behavior in infants the occurrence of a critical period has been identified. It is reported that if formation of close social attachments is delayed much beyond 6 months of age in an infant's experience, impairment of the child's ability ever to form such attachments can occur.

READINESS

The principle of *readiness*, developed on the basis of observations that certain maturational changes are prerequisite for development of certain behaviors, stresses the correlation of physical and behavioral development. The behavior of walking, for example, cannot be achieved until the child has reached appropriate stages of motor development and spatial orientation.

SCHEMATIZATION OF EXPERIENCE

The work of Swiss psychologist Jean Piaget in the area of cognitive development in childhood has had many implications for general behavioral development. The principle of *schematization of experience* is illustrative of this. In terms of cognitive development, children develop ideas, or concepts, about what a thing is like; in other words they develop a schema (plural, schemata) of that thing. In behavioral studies the stranger anxiety demonstrated by infants has been interpreted in terms of this principle. The infant is described as developing a schema of familiar people. When a stranger, someone not part of the schema "familiar people," appears, the infant experiences discomfort, which is manifest in such behaviors as crying and clinging to the familiar person. In older children the principle of schematization of experience has been employed in explaining development of behaviors such as those related to prejudice.

GROWTH AMBIVALENCE

Behaviors indicating an apparent conflict between a progressive, risk-taking urge and a more cautious, safety-oriented urge are identified as demonstrating the principle of *growth ambivalence*. The toddler's autonomous strivings to "do it myself," alternating with periodic regressions to dependent, infantile behaviors, are examples of growth ambivalence.

COMPETENCE MOTIVATION VERSUS DISEQUILIBRIUM

The principle that behavior develops in response to strivings toward a goal or curiosity and excitement about new experiences has been called *competence motivation*. A somewhat controversial principle, competence motivation contrasts sharply with principles which ascribe behavioral development to the child's awareness of *disequilibrium,* or felt needs or imbalances.

ACCUMULATION

A final principle of behavioral development presented, the principle of *accumulation* also has supporters and critics from varying theoretical orientations. The principle of accumulation implies an ongoing continuity of behavioral development to the extent that childhood experiences are identified as primary influences on subsequent adult behavior. Well-controlled longitudinal studies are needed to validate this principle.

From independent observations of isolated developmental incidents, patterns in development can be observed which then give rise to principles of development. Studies of behavioral development have resulted in the formulation of such principles as differentiation, functional subordination, stage formation, critical or sensitive periods, readiness, schematization of experience, growth ambivalence, competence motivation, and accumulation.

ENVIRONMENTAL FACTORS INFLUENCING BEHAVIORAL DEVELOPMENT

STIMULATION VERSUS DEPRIVATION

Studies of the effects of institutional rearing, such as those reporting the important work of René Spitz and John Bowlby, emphasize the significance of the influence of stimulation versus deprivation on child development. The literatures of developmental and comparative psychology contain numerous reports of studies of both animal and human infants whose behavior appears to be related to varying degrees of stimulation or deprivation experienced during early, formative periods of life.

Stimulation It has been observed in a variety of studies that young organisms, both animal and human, provided with a rich—i.e., stimulating—early environment demonstrate more positive growth curves in such areas of functioning as social and exploratory behavior and the use of motor skills than do those without such stimulation.

Effective stimulation of the developing child may be achieved in various ways. Manipulation of the infant's physical (inanimate) environment offers an obvious means of providing stimulation. Visual objects, such as toys and mobiles, and auditory stimuli, such as recorded music, have been used effectively in facilitating development of desired behaviors in infants. Social (animate) forms of stimulation, such as touching, rocking, looking at, or talking to the infant, have also been identified as important components of a growth-fostering early environment.

Positive effects of stimulation have been observed in numerous settings including the home, child-care institutions, and hospital units providing care for premature infants. Cross-cultural studies have provided still further information on the effects of stimulation. In one study, Gerber (1958) describes the precocious motor development—head control, sitting, prehension—demonstrated by Ugandan infants as compared with their European counterparts. This development is attributed by Gerber to the massive stimulation Ugandan infants receive from the constant mother-infant contact characteristic in this culture.

Deprivation Evidence of the detrimental effects of deprivation on behavioral development has been demonstrated both experimentally and through ex post facto observations of behavior of infants reared in deprived environments. Experimental deprivation is demonstrated in animal studies. In a series of studies summarized by Sackett (1967), infant monkeys were exposed to four different conditions of deprivation; (1) total social isolation for periods of 3, 6, or 12 months; (2) partial isolation in which seeing and hearing but not touching other monkeys was permitted; (3) peer contact only (no mothers present); and (4) contact with both peers and mothers. Tests conducted throughout the development of these monkeys indicated that total isolation (extreme deprivation) for periods of 6 to 12 months resulted in apparently irreversible deficits in behavior related to socialization as well as in the development and persistence of negative, nonsocial behaviors. Variations in the extent of deprivation experienced resulted in varying degrees of deficient behavior—appropriate behaviors increasing as depriving conditions decreased. The variable of peer contact was identified as a particularly potent socializing influence.

Deprivation as a deterrent to behavioral development of human infants has been identified in the behavior of infants reared in situations lacking sufficient environmental and/or social stimulation, as in some group homes or hospitals. Conditions such as lack of play materials or inadequate or inconsistent contact with care givers are considered depriving to the young infant. Adequate physical care may or may not be a feature of a depriving setting.

Children reared in such conditions demonstrate inadequate behavioral development through such behaviors as absence of social responsiveness (smiling, reaching out) or indiscriminate, inappropriate responsiveness ("overreaction" to stimulation when it occurs). Studies of human infants have indicated that consistent human contact, whether provided by fathers, mothers, or parent-surrogate figures such as nurses or attendants, has been identified as an important variable for preventing the establishment, or at least softening the effects, of a depriving environment.

CULTURAL INFLUENCES ON BEHAVIORAL DEVELOPMENT

The work of anthropologists like Ruth Benedict and Margaret Mead, consisting of studies of culture and cultural differences, has had an impact on the field of child development. As a result of such studies it has become recognized that, among the many variables identified as affecting behavioral development, the culture into which a child is born is one of the more prevailing. A culture may be defined generally as a group of individuals who share a set of values, beliefs, information, and standards of conduct and who transmit these from generation to generation. The experience of being a member of a culture is one common to all children, whether they grow and develop in Cleveland, Ohio, or in a remote village in a South American jungle.

Implications for child development Of special significance to the student of child development is an awareness of the *direct* relationship between children's behavior and the culture of which they are a part. Beliefs about such important behavior-shaping experiences as family life, expression of emotion, use of tools, conduct of sex, organization of time and space, and conduct of social behavior are all components of a child's cultural heritage. Even more specifically, it is the culture that defines the nature of children and prescribes, within the context of that definition, appropriate child-rearing practices.

What people believe about children directly affects the way children are treated and, subsequently, the way they behave. If, for example, a culture defines children as economic assets, children will at an early age be expected to become an active part of the economic enterprise of that culture. In contrast, in a culture in which children are, by definition, to be loved, the period of childhood will be an extended one during which the playful, dependent behaviors of children are encouraged.

Transmission of cultural influences Cultural influences on behavioral development may be transmitted in a variety of ways. Among the most common means is through *direct teaching.* In more primitive societies such teaching may be the responsibility of tribal elders, while more advanced societies provide a body of knowledge from recognized experts to guide the development of children. Another common means of cultural transmission of behavioral guidelines is through *tradition.* Behaviors related to sex roles and sex differences are among those developed on the basis of tradition.

Ritual observances may serve an important function in defining important milestones in behavioral development. In many primitive cultures, for example, it is through prescribed initiation rites that children are made aware of the end of childhood and the subsequent demands of adult behavior codes. Although more advanced societies do not provide definitive rites to guide such behavioral changes, children of such societies may have the benefit of variable behavior-shaping events such as obtaining the right to vote, being licensed to drive, and becoming eligible for employment.

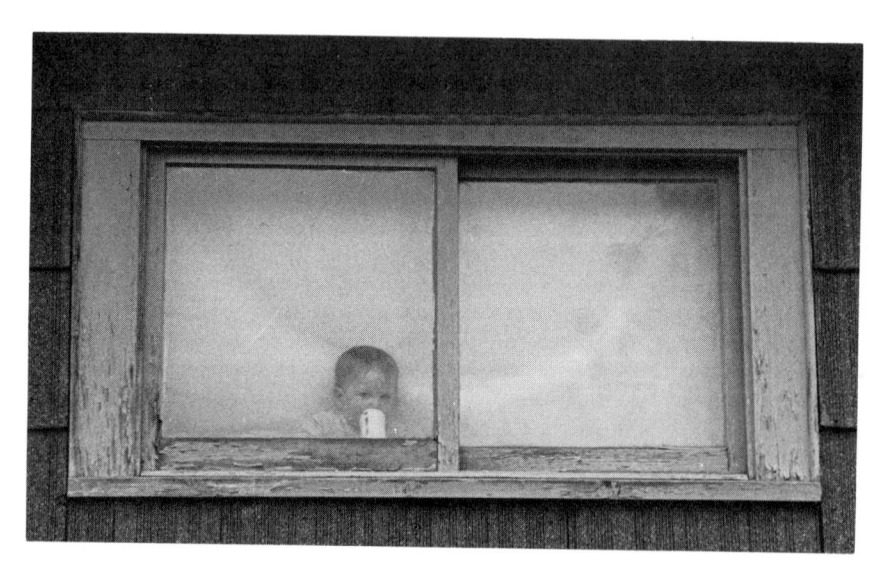

FIGURE 3-2. (*Photo courtesy of Betsy Smith.*)

Cultural influences on behavioral development may also be transmitted to the child through such indirect means as tone of voice, manner and style of movement, or emotional reactions to events. In one culture, for instance, a child may learn that avoidance of eye contact with adults is a sign of respect, while in other cultures such behavior may be indicative of guilt. Reactions to such events as birth, death, weddings, or other such emotionally laden experiences are among those defined by one's culture and can only be interpreted appropriately within the context of the culture.

The social structure of a culture has a decided influence on behavioral development in children. Children reared in cultures in which roles and relations are fixed will develop fewer adaptive behaviors than will children reared in a more fluid structure that encourages such behaviors as initiative and competitiveness.

Changes in social structure in the United States in recent years have been identified as having important implications for behavioral development. The concept of the "shrinking family" is identified as a possible influence on a child's behavior in relationships; the present mobility of families in American society has implications for behavioral development in establishing and maintaining significant relationships; the phenomenon of urbanization and subsequent crowding has been identified as a potentially negative influence on development of behavior; the possible problems and/or benefits confronting the child of the dual-career couple or the single parent continue to be subjects of concern to a variety of professionals in the general area of child welfare.

Cultural variations Although some cultures are more stable than others, cultures in general are subject to some change over time. In many instances such changes may result in the processes of *acculturation* or *assimilation*. Acculturation occurs when individuals from one culture have prolonged contact with members of another culture and interactions produce some changes in one or both of the participating cultures. In the process of assimilation the contact of different cultures results in the complete absorption and integration of the members of one culture into that of the more dominant group.

In addition to processes resulting in cultural revision there exist in more complex societies various cultural subgroups that maintain their own unique sets of standards. Terms such as *subculture, ethnic group,* and *counterculture* are used to describe such groups. A subculture exists within the framework of the majority culture, but its members function according to a set of beliefs and practices based on a departure from general cultural values. Members of the "jet set" in contemporary society are identified as composing a subculture following a more self-oriented philosophy than is characteristic of more general practices.

Ethnic groups are comprised of individuals of a particular racial and cultural origin. In large societies such groups exist within the context of the more dominant culture while maintaining their own unique identity. Neighborhoods such as Chinatown in San Francisco or New York are examples of ethnic group functioning. A more recently experienced phenomenon of culture is that of the development of countercultures, or groups composed of individuals whose value system and practices in some way directly oppose those of the majority culture in which they exist. The "hippie" movement of the 1960s is an example of a counterculture of the United States society.

As is true of any aspect of cultural experience, cultural variability has important implications for behavioral development. A primary consideration is that of the incon-

FIGURE 3-3.

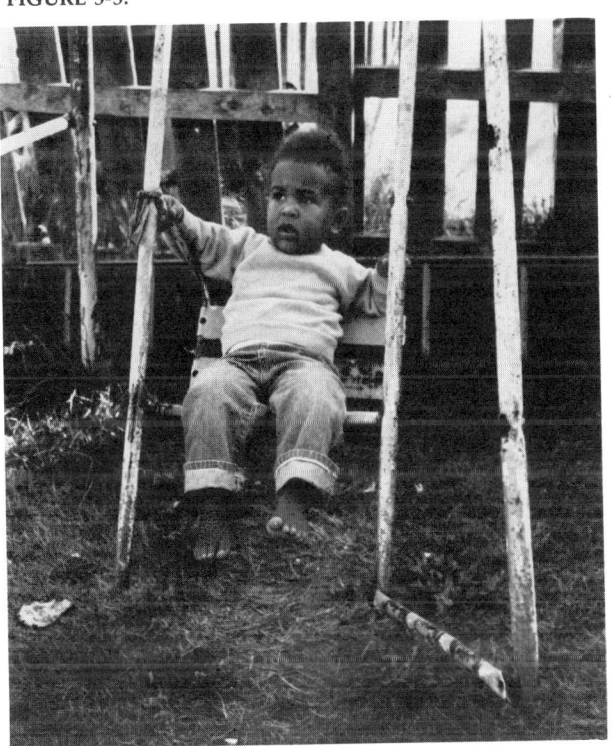

gruities or inconsistencies such experiences may present to children. Both positive and negative behavioral influences can be identified: Positively, such experiences may foster such behaviors as initiative and social adaptability in children; negatively, the confusion the child may experience could lead to a behavioral repertoire based on doubt, contradiction, or conflict.

In summary, what people believe about children (a cultural dictate) affects the way children will be treated and, subsequently, their behavior. Variations within a culture are identified as significant influences on behavior, as they confront growing children with inconsistencies or incongruities in their experiences. The importance of understanding and interpreting behavior in the cultural context in which it is developed is significant for nursing practice.

HEALTH STATUS AND DISEASE

Observations of children at any developmental stage provide evidence that health status and disease are important influences of behavioral development. A general reaction of children is described in the work of Anthony and Koupernik:

> Since the discovery of disease takes place within the normal process of development, the child imperceptibly becomes his illness, but as a result of enhancement of body feeling, the *psyche* and *soma* are not too well integrated, so that, whereas the healthy child *is* his body, the sick child *has* a body that is constantly making its presence felt through pain. It is this suffering appendage that makes him feel acutely different from others. (1972, p. 32)

Physical health as a facilitator of behavioral development It has become a well-recognized fact in the field of child development that healthy behavior in children most readily develops and is demonstrated in conditions of optimum physical health. A healthy, functioning body is a prerequisite for the accomplishment of the age-related developmental tasks children encounter in the process of behavioral development. The physically intact infant, for example, is able to engage in such activities as moving about, thereby experiencing bodily events in relation to normal, or usual, environmental stimuli. These stimuli become associated appropriately with pleasure or discomfort and with many other activities related to behaviors of increasing self-awareness and appropriate social responses. The older child who enjoys good physical health is capable of exploring his world, becoming an accepted part of the increasingly important peer group, and engaging in the many behaviors related to self- and social acceptance.

Illness as a deterrent to behavioral growth Because behavioral development occurs generally within a progressive, sequential framework, it is, as a phenomenon, vulnerable to any interference imposed on that sequence. The occurrence of illness, ranging from a simple cold to the onset of a chronically handicapping condition, poses some threat to the continuing evolution of behavior.

A basic consideration of illness as a negative influence on behavior is referred to above in Anthony and Koupernik's observation that the ill child feels different from others. This is especially true of the older child for whom being with and like others is so important and a necessary condition for positive behavioral development. The infant and younger presocial child will not, of course, experience "feeling different" from others, but illness occurring at these stages causes care givers to treat such children differently, thus exerting an important influence on behavioral development. Illness in the infant, for example, may be so frightening to the parent that she or he fails to provide the infant with the tactile or social stimulation that enhances beginning development of attachment behaviors.

Children's specific reactions to the meaning of and/or manifestations to illness vary to some extent depending on the stage of development of the ill child. There are, however, some reactions with important behavioral implications that appear to occur to some extent across developmental lines. Two such reactions are the development of feelings of guilt and evidence of behavioral regression. (See Chaps. 6 through 10 for further discussion of these reactions.)

Thus, illness is identified as a deterrent to behavioral as well as to physical growth. Physical health as a prerequisite for healthy behavioral development is indicated by the relation of physical abilities to the tasks of behavioral development served in children at all stages of growth.

THE EFFECT OF BEHAVIOR ON HEALTH
AND PHYSICAL DEVELOPMENT

The significance of physical development to various areas of behavioral development has been indicated in many definitive investigations. It has been observed, for example, that certain physical capacities of the child must have been achieved before the behavior of walking can occur. Not as well documented, however, are widespread observations of the effects of behavioral development on the child's health and ability to achieve important physical milestones.

Infancy research In the field of infancy research some evidence has become available that does appear to indicate that development of certain behaviors is prerequisite for physical growth. Early and subsequent reports of the failure-to-thrive syndrome implicate at least a disturbance in the mother-child relationship as a primary etiologic factor. Although early reports tend to identify behavior of parents as the negative valence in the relationship, later studies have reported that the absence from the infant's behavioral repertoire of such social responses as smiling or looking can have an important effect on the care giver's responses and thus on the quality of care the infant receives.

Studies of institutionalized infants have provided dramatic proof of the relation between behavioral development and physical growth. Repeated observations have been made of the phenomenon that occurs when infants are not provided appropriate opportunities for the development of behaviors related to attachment. Such infants may fail to develop physically at the same rate as more stimulated infants. In severe cases, infants have been unable to survive.

The older child The influence of behavior on physical growth beyond the stage of infancy has been noted, although such data are not as readily available. The work of Sigmund Freud provided an important foundation for understanding behavioral experiences characterized by high levels of stress as causative factors in some physical aberrations. The occurrence of such problems, known as psychosomatic illnesses, can well be identified as a behavioral effect on physical development. The child suffering from a physical condition caused by disturbed behavioral development is deprived of many of the activities necessary to foster continued adequate physical development.

Throughout the course of physical development, observations can be made of the correlation between appropriate physical maturity and the behavior engaged in by the child at that stage. Growth and maturity of large muscles and long bones that occur during toddler years is stimulated when the child has achieved mobility. The continued refinement of physical growth and development that occurs in early childhood is fostered by a child's functioning at the appropriate level of behavioral development, which encourages running, jumping, dressing oneself, or learning to manipulate objects. The failure of a child to achieve appropriate levels of behavioral functioning can impair physical growth.

OTHER ENVIRONMENTAL EFFECTS ON BEHAVIORAL DEVELOPMENT

In addition to the effects imposed on behavioral development by such major environmental variables as stimulation, deprivation, culture, nutrition, and health status, other features present in the environment are also recognized as potential influences on or disruptions of this process.

Social class Although somewhat related to the cultural variable, social-class membership has some unique implications for development of behavior. This may be especially true with regard to the effects of lower-class membership, in which the child must learn to cope with the reality of poverty. Various sociological investigations have indicated that conditions of poverty experienced by the developing child increase the possibility of a negative self-image.

Another observation of the effects of poverty is that children reared in such conditions often develop behaviors characteristic of a "now" rather than a future orientation to life. Such children learn, at an early age, to develop necessary survival skills often directed to getting through the day. If, for example, children of lower classes are offered a choice between one candy bar now or three candy bars in a week, their choice is likely to be to take the one candy bar that is available rather than to trust a situation that might never materialize.

Racial minorities Though often related to social-class differences, membership in a racial minority can exert influences on behavioral development that are distinct from those imposed by social-class membership. Development of a unique, positive self-image may be seriously impeded in the experience of a child whose development occurs in a majority environment that defines him primarily in terms of racial difference.

The confusion posed to the child developing a sense of self in situations stressing racial stereotypes rather than individual characteristics has obvious implications for behavioral development. In contemporary United States society efforts at minimizing the negative effects of both social-class and racial differences have begun. Indications are, however, that continued emphasis in this area will be a need for a prolonged period of time.

School The effect of school on behavioral development is often assumed to be a positive one. School does offer such positive experiences as peer interaction, opportunities for development of various skills, and opportunities for expression of self, as well as intellectual stimulation. School experiences can also negatively affect behavioral development. Children with learning problems often may be predisposed to develop negative adaptive behaviors in an effort to cope with the pressures exerted in an achievement-oriented setting such as school.

Mass media Although the actual effect of the various elements of mass media, books, movies, television, remains a point of controversy at the time of this writing, some current observations are relevant in this discussion. It has been observed, for example, that books available to children may have some influence on the development of behaviors characteristic of sexual stereotyping. More recent children's literature makes references to role reversal of such behaviors as housekeeping or going to work, with male and female characters sharing equally in all kinds of tasks and social behaviors.

Television has been implicated as both a potentially positive or negative influence on behavior. The possible negative effect on behavior resulting from constant detailed exposure to violence is a point of continued concern. The negative influence of commercials on the developing child's eating behavior has also been implied. Tele-

FIGURE 3-4. [Child's art (a) and writing (b) courtesy of Marguerite Ryle, R.N., American Red Cross, Harrisburg area chapter, Pennsylvania.]

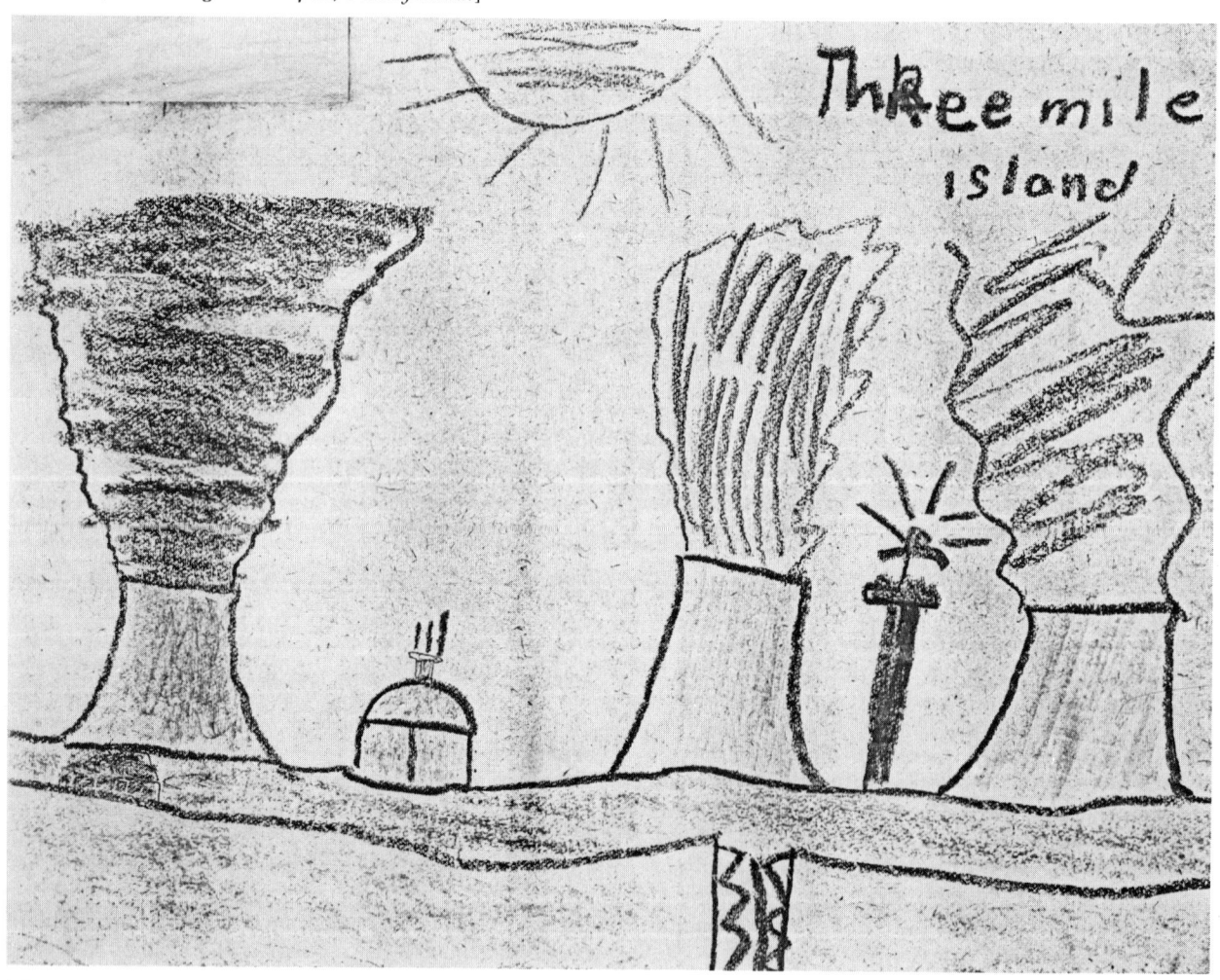

(a)

vision is a sedentary activity and thus could be considered a negative influence on physical development. Positive influences of television include its recognized impact on learning. Another positive effect identified is the role television can play in mitigating effects of social-class differences by exposing children of different socioeconomic strata to similar vocabularies and sources of general information.

Social disruption or disaster A concern for children's reactions to, and the subsequent effects imposed by, a disaster of natural or human origin on behavioral development has been a continuing concern of twentieth-century society. Beginning with the effects of the holocaust of World War II and continuing in the face of political assassinations and national political scandal as well as such natural disasters as fires, floods, and earthquakes, concern for children's behavioral responses to social disruption or disaster has made this a continued focus of investigation.

In a study describing the effects of a natural disaster on behavioral development, Newman (1976) reported significant observations. A major finding in this study was that the stage of development of children at the time of a disaster is an important variable. The majority of negative-response behaviors occurred in children who were under the age of 12 years at the time of the disaster. The negative effects on behavior seen as responses to disaster included development of a modified sense of reality, problems of increased vulnerability to future stress, an alteration in the sense of one's power, and an early awareness of fragmentation and death.

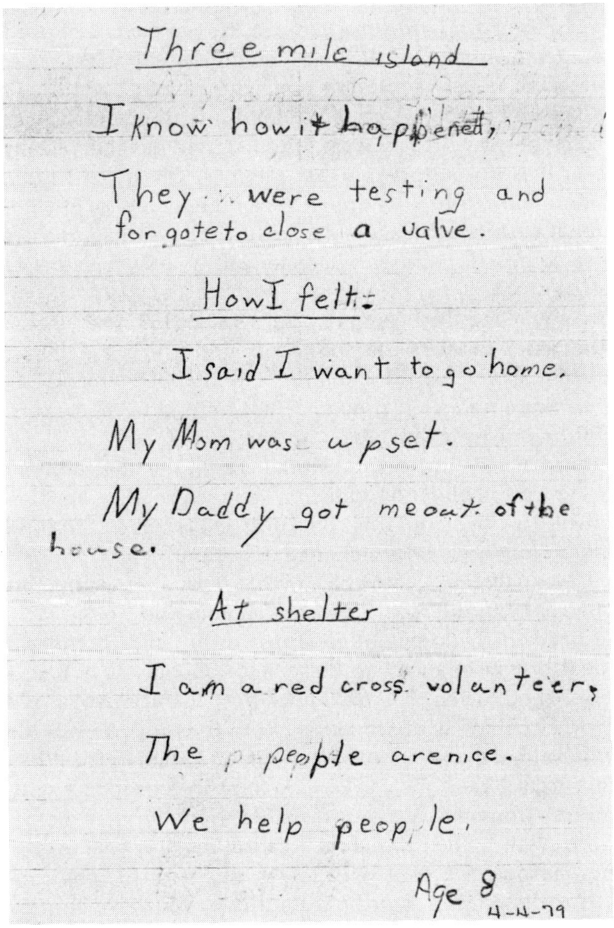

Other studies of reactions to stress indicate that removal from parents, in addition to the child's stage of development, is another important variable influencing the degree to which disaster negatively affects behavior. Still another variable identified is that of the child's ability to talk about the experience. Time required to recover from traumatic experiences is apparently lessened for the child who is encouraged to talk about such experiences.

Although some of these environmental factors remain points of controversy in regard to the quality of their effect on behavioral development, all are aspects of current society whose influences must be recognized.

FIGURE 3-4. (*Continued*)

(b)

Effect of parenting on behavioral development Marion H. Rose

All major theories of child development view parents as playing a major role in the behavioral development of their child, although explanations of how this occurs vary from theory to theory. Various theories explain how parents influence the child's sex-role development, intelligence, moral development, and other aspects of psychosocial development. Most theories see parents as role models for their children with identification an important process by which the child becomes socialized to the norms of a particular culture.

Much of the emphasis in the literature has been on mothering; recently, however, attention has been given to the role of fathers in the child's development (Lamb, 1976; Lynn, 1974). There have also been persistent arguments over time concerning the relative importance of environment versus heredity, nature versus nurture. Currently the reciprocal nature of environment and heredity is being emphasized. Thus parents' influence on a child's behavioral development is generally viewed as being based on interaction between parent and child rather than being a unidirectional influence by a parent on a child.

Yarrow (1968) conceptualizes the human environment as similar to the inanimate environment, that is, the same amount, quality, and intensity of stimulation but in different sensory modalities. However, there are variables distinctive to the human environment. These are the following:

> The affective and affectional characteristics of interaction; the level or depth of relationship with caretakers and other significant persons; the extent of individualized sensitivity to the child; the behavior and personal characteristics of caretaker and peers as identification models; the consistency and predictability of the behavior of caretakers; and the continuity of significant people. (Yarrow, 1968, p. 19)

The impact of the parent on the child is at least partially dependent on characteristics of the child. Yarrow identified several types of organismic variables that would affect the impact of the environment on an individual. These are the following:

- Degree of receptivity or sensitivity to stimuli determined by developmental characteristics
- Response capabilities based on developmental level
- Individualized receptivity, sensitivity, or vulnerability related to basic biological or constitutional factors and cumulative changes in the individual resulting from his unique past history
- Receptivity to stimuli based on immediate past experiences; for example, the level of attentiveness of a hungry infant will differ from that of a satiated one

Thomas, Chess, and Birch (1968) studied temperament and its role in determining development of the child's personality. Temperament reflects the how of behavior rather than the what or why of behavior. They identified nine categories of temperament: activity level, rhythmicity, approach or withdrawal, adaptability, threshold of responsiveness, intensity of reaction, quality of mood, distractibility, and attention span and persistence. Thomas, Chess, and Birch do not view the nine categories listed above as exhaustive but expect that other behavior styles will be identified. They use the term temperament to refer to stylistic characteristics which are evident in early infancy, while the broader term behavioral style includes characteristics or trends which appear in later childhood or adult life.

On the basis of their study, they were able to categorize children as difficult children, easy children, and slow-to-warm-up children. The attributes which characterized difficult children are as follows: irregularity in biological functions, a predominance of negative (withdrawal) responses to new stimuli, slowness in adapting to changes in environment, a high frequency of expression of negative mood, and a predominance of intense reactions. Easy children, on the other hand, were described as children who are highly regular, preponderantly positive in mood, low or mild in the intensity of their reactions, rapidly adaptable, and usually positive in their approaches to new situations. Thomas, Chess, and Birch go on to say: "Indeed, they were children who, not infrequently, contributed to the mother's sense of well-being and to her conviction that she was an effective, skillful, and good parent" (1968, p. 85).

Children who are slow to warm up were characterized temperamentally as children having initial withdrawal reactions to new situations and who adapt slowly. Their moods are characteristically of mild intensity so that their initial negative reaction is quiet. Activity level is usually low. It is not surprising that Thomas, Chess, and Birch found that difficult children have a high incidence of emotional problems by age 4. However, some problems were also found in children characterized as easy or slow to warm up.

As viewed by Thomas and Chess (1977), it is the interaction between the parent and child which is of importance in affecting both child and parental behavior. However, the interaction process is not limited to the parent-child dyad (or triad), for both the parents and child are influenced by and exert an influence on the environment in which they live. In addition, the reciprocal interaction process is not static. It is constantly evolving, as the child and family and society change over time.

In analyzing the nature of the temperament-environment interactive process Thomas and Chess (1977) utilized the concept of "goodness of fit" and the related ideas of consonance and dissonance. Goodness of fit occurs when the child's own capacities, characteristics, and style of behaving are in accord with the properties of the environment and its expectations and demands. When this occurs, the child can be said to be in consonance with the environment; thus optimal development can occur. Conversely, when the child's capacities and characteristics are not in accord with the demands of the environment, dissonance is present, and distorted development and maladaptive functioning occur. Goodness of fit is not an abstraction but is relative to the values and demands of a given culture or socioeconomic group.

Based on the method used in the original research (Thomas, Chess, and Birch, 1968; Thomas, Chess, Birch, Hertzig, and Korn, 1963), several short rating scales or interview protocols have been developed for measuring temperament. Three are mentioned here. Carey (1970, 1972) has developed a short questionnaire for rating temperament in infancy. Thomas and Chess (1977) have developed a separate short questionnaire form for parents and teachers for the 3- to 7-year age period. Graham, Rutter, and George (1973) have developed an interview protocol to rate children on activity level, regularity, approach-withdrawal, malleability, mood, intensity, and fastidiousness.

In summary, parents have an important role in the behavioral development of children; however, the parental impact is mediated by the child's own characteristics and the goodness of fit between parent, child, and the culture in which they live.

Child-development theories
Mary Jane Amundson

For years developmentalists have been concerned with the process underlying growth. The field has been grossly categorized into environmentalists and geneticists, that is, those who feel that development is largely the result of events in the environment versus those who see development as stemming largely from biological maturation. Most developmentalists recognize that the child's growth is a combination of biological and environmental influences interacting within the framework of a specific individual of the species. There is no consensus about the processes underlying child development. It is also evident that there are probably several processes that may differ with each child, depending on the capacities of the child and on the types of learning involved.

During the twentieth century, three theoretical systems about child development have made major inroads into understanding the growth process (Caldwell and Richmond, 1970, p. 5). These are *psychoanalytic theories*, *behavioristic theories*, and *developmental theories*.

The theoretical formulations of psychoanalysis and the body of empirical data collected to test the hypotheses have provided perhaps the most significant and pervasive influence on child-development theories and child-rearing practices in recent decades. By clinically reconstructing the life history of the adult or child through therapeutic efforts, psychoanalysts have developed theoretical formulations concerning the meaning of interaction of the infant or young child with his environment. The Freudian view holds that people are neither active nor passive but always in flux between the two states, always in conflict between their natural instincts and the constraints imposed upon them by society. The nature of these conflicts depends upon the stage of development that a person is in at any one time. To Freud, a child is a reactive organism whose development proceeds through stages. He postulates psychosexual development as being characterized by a maturationally predetermined shift of instinctual energy from one body zone to another. At each stage, the child undergoes a major conflict in either the sexual realm (Freud, 1938) or the social realm (Erikson, 1950). The way each stage is resolved or not resolved determines the individual's ultimate personality development (Papalia and Olds, 1978, p. 34).

John B. Watson exerted the greatest influence in the development of behavioristic (social learning) theories. His concept of an infant was that of an amorphous bit of behavior potential to be shaped by the learning opportunities experienced by the infant. From many experiments, he concluded that most forms of complex behavior were the result of reflexes and simple response systems associated through conditioning. Several other theorists, notably Skinner (1953), Miller and Dollard (1953), and Sears, Macoby, and Levin (1957) have significantly advanced social-learning theory and extended knowledge about the limits of external manipulation and control of infant and child behavior. The infant is seen as reacting, rather than initiating. Behavior theorists see change as quantitative and development as continuous. The focus is on how early experiences affect later behavior. The attempt to understand the effects of experience is accomplished by breaking down complex stimuli and complex behaviors into simpler elements.

Arnold Gesell propounded the developmental (maturational) theory. Gesell's (1956) theory of development is relatively simple yet, in some ways, more global than other more complex theories. The key concept is that of maturation, or growth. It is a theory of intrinsic development, of an infant's maturation proceeding from both the human and the individual nature of the infant. The emphasis is on the growth integrity of the young organism, its inherent potential for healthy development. Implicit in the concept of maturation is self-regulation of growth. Gesell urged recognition of this principle in every aspect of development from the establishment of infant feeding schedules to the acquisition of moral values. Acceptance of the principle calls for a certain considerateness of the child. Developmentalists see infants as active organisms who, by their own actions, set in motion their own development. They initiate acts. Change, both quantitative and qualitative, is seen as an inherent part of life. It is internal rather than external.

Developmental theorists see life experiences, not as the basic cause of development, but as factors that can make it proceed more quickly or more slowly. They often describe development as occurring in a set sequence of qualitatively different stages—as discontinuous. Jean Piaget (1952) explains many aspects of children's thought and behavior by considering them as going through definite stages. Such stage theories have certain characteristic tenets: All individuals go through the same stages in the same order, even though the actual timing will vary from one person to another; each stage builds on the one that went before and constructs the foundation for the one that comes next; and each stage is multifaceted. Kohlberg's (1971) postulations on moral development also fit within this concept.

All theories of child development are concerned with learning, with the interaction of the organism and the environment. They all highlight different facets of development—emotional, intellectual, and behavioral—and utilize different conceptual systems. The major psychoanalytic, behavioral, and developmental theorists will be discussed below. The principles and concepts underlying their views of child development will be outlined.

PSYCHOANALYTIC AND RELATED THEORIES

FREUD AND PSYCHOANALYTIC THEORY

Freud's theory of development is primarily a dynamic, motivational theory of behavior which is concerned with the present conflicts of the individual and how these may be resolved. The theory is essentially interactive rather than developmental, although the conflicts have developed out of the past, whether as a result of constitutional or experiential influences.

Five major types of concepts provide a structure for discussing the basic principles of the theory. These concepts are adaptive, dynamic, economic, structural, and developmental (Starr and Goldstein, 1975, pp. 179–191).

Adaptive Behavior has an overall goal of adaptation. The organization of behavior occurs in such a way as to gratify impulses which refer to instinctual drives associated with sexual and aggressive behavior and feelings.

Dynamic This refers to the energy force behind behavior. The energy source is called *libido* or life force. Its goal is reduction of tension, and it is concentrated on the instinctual drives. Freud acknowledged a wide variety of human motives, or instinctual unconscious drives, but emphasized ego (behaviors necessary for self-preservation), sexuality (behaviors necessary for the survival of the species), and the death instinct (aggression toward self and others).

Economic A limited but constant supply of energy is available for psychic functioning. Freud viewed delay of impulse gratification as necessary for civilization to advance. The ability to channel gratification in creative ways is the highest form of personal expression in Freudian theory.

Structural Freud conceived of mental life in terms of three major structures (hypothetical constructs), *id, ego,* and *superego,* which together are a way of conceptualizing aspects of human functioning (Stone and Church, 1973, pp. 402–404). Developmentally, the baby at birth is considered to be pure id, governed by what Freud called the pleasure principle, the seeking for immediate gratification. The id, conceptualized within the unconscious, consists of instinctual drives, impulsive behavior, and wish fulfillment and is the source of all motive energies. The infant's strivings collide with reality, and the resulting anxieties and frustrations produce a layer of ego (reality principle). The ego orders the relationship between the person and the outside world. Also labeled the conscious, reason, and the will, the ego holds a balance between the strivings for satisfaction of the id, the censures of the superego, and the realities of the world. There is a delay or binding of instinctual energy as the ego utilizes its structuring characteristics. Defense mechanisms are behavioral techniques devised by the ego to reduce anxiety, resolve conflicts, and overcome frustration, any of which occur when unacceptable impulses break into consciousness. Examples of these include the following:

- *Displacement:* The instinctual drive of the individual is diverted from one goal to another, which is usually more socially acceptable.
- *Regression:* An individual who is under stress invokes behavior that was successful at an earlier stage of development.
- *Denial:* A person denies the presence of feelings and impulses that can be assumed to be present.

- *Isolation of affect:* Impulses come into consciousness, but the feeling usually associated with the thought or act is cut off from the individual's awareness.

Finally, in early childhood, as the child assimilates his parents' standards regarding what is good and what is evil, a portion of the ego becomes further differentiated as superego, imparting an ethical-moral, socially responsible dimension to the purely pragmatic reality principle in the search for gratification of the id impulses.

Developmental The classical psychoanalytic theory of Freud posits a theory of psychosexual development to explain personality organization (Lovell, 1969, p. 79). Psychosexual development refers to shifts in the channels or zones of the body through which id gratification is sought and obtained and in the objects which serve as gratifiers. In the first year of life, the child passes through an *oral stage* where, if not severely frustrated in his relationship with a parent figure, he lays the foundation for his capacity to form stable relationships with other persons. Pleasure is obtained in this stage through the lips and mouth, through activities involving sucking, swallowing, and biting. The second year of life is characterized by the *anal stage* of personality development, during which pleasure is obtained through the expulsion and retention of feces and through the exercising of the associated muscular control. Favorable experiences during this period can lead to a creative and productive personality. Between the third and fifth years, the source of pleasure is derived through genital stimulation and functions associated with the genital area. The child becomes jealous of the special relationship between the parents, and at the same time the boy becomes interested in his mother and the girl in her father. The child is now at the *phallic phase* of development. As the Oedipal issue is resolved, the child identifies with his parents, incorporating some of their qualities into his personality. During this phase, the child increasingly develops appropriate roles for his age and sex.

In the Freudian view, there is a *latency period* from about the sixth to the twelfth year. Sexual interests seem to be repressed, and the main source of pleasure comes from the child's interaction with the external world. The child is acquiring basic knowledge and skills to enable him to cope with his environment. Finally in adolescence and adulthood, the individual passes into the *genital phase*, moving away from the dependence upon parents to a greater concern for others. He moves to a position which is characterized by mature sexuality and sexual love for others.

ERIKSON AND PSYCHOSOCIAL THEORY
Erik Erikson's theory of personality development offers vivid descriptions of how each stage of the life cycle is organized around a central theme. His insights and interpretations fit well with several systems' concepts since Erikson considers the multiple interacting factors that influence and are influenced by the developing personality. The theory diverges from the Freudian model in his emphasis on three major areas:

1. Erikson emphasizes the ego, assuming an innate ability of the infant to coordinate activities within an average, predictable environment. He also places stress on continuity of experience involving functioning of the ego beyond the sexual-developmental phases.
2. Erikson introduces a new matrix. The individual is viewed in his relationship with his parents within the context of the family, in relation to a wider social setting, and within the framework of the family's historical-cultural heritage.
3. Erikson viewed his contribution to be that of pointing out the developmental opportunities in the individual which help him to triumph over the psychological hazards of living. His belief is that every personal and social crisis furnishes components that are conducive to growth (Maier, 1969, pp. 16–18).

Erikson emphasizes the crucial, continuous role of the ego throughout the life cycle. He views development as a continuous process with each phase equally a part of the continuum since every phase finds its antecedents in previous phases and its ultimate solution in those subsequent to it. Each successive stage provides the possibility of new solutions for previous questions, while an element of conservatism is always present because every early acquisition lives on in subsequent phases, in some form (Maier, 1968, pp. 28–29). The key concept in Erikson's psychosocial scheme is that of identity. The developing individual pursues his identity throughout the life cycle as it is attained, maintained, lost, and regained through complex feedback processes as the individual interacts with significant others in multiple environments.

The stages are described briefly below (Sutterly and Donnelly, 1973, p. 80).

Stage I—trust versus mistrust—birth to about 1 year
This stage is the foundation for all subsequent personality development. This sense of trust, for the newborn,

requires a feeling of physical comfort and minimal fear or uncertainty. These conditions are highly dependent on the quality of the maternal relationship. Body experiences become the means of the first social experiences and, therefore, provide the basis for a psychological state of trust. The conflict of trust versus mistrust arises at each successive stage of development, which may offer a new chance if needs are not met at earlier periods of development.

Stage II—autonomy versus shame and doubt—2 to 4 years As the infant gains trust in the world around him, he begins to discover that his behavior is his own; he acquires a sense of autonomy. The major theme of this phase is the conflicting pulls in the child—to assert himself and to deny himself the right and capacity to make this assertion, thereby remaining comfortably dependent. The child is engrossed with activities of retaining and releasing perceptions, desires, and manipulative objects; with interpersonal relations; and eventually with bodily products. If parents recognize the young child's need to do what he is capable of doing at his own pace and time, he develops a sense that he is able to control his muscles, his impulses, himself, and his environment.

Stage III—initiative versus guilt—about 4 to 6 years During this period, the child's use of language and locomotion permits him to expand his imagination. He is curious about differences in sizes, in general, and particularly about sexual differences. Play becomes more meaningful since he can now associate with others of his own age. The modality during this period is termed intrusive. Infantile sexual curiosity, genital excitability, and preoccupation with sexual matters are prominent. Because of fantasies, explorations, and acquired autonomy, the child's behavior may be often frustrated by the autonomous behavior of others. As a result, he may incur a deep sense of guilt. He begins automatically to feel guilty for mere thoughts and for deeds which no one has observed. It is at this stage of initiative that conscience becomes established and subsequently forms initiative. If he is made to feel that his actions are bad, a nuisance, silly, he may develop a sense of guilt over self-initiated activities that will persist through life.

Stage IV—industry versus inferiority—approximately 6 to 11 years During this period, the child ventures into the world of school. He is learning to work, to accomplish things, yet there is still the world of play that acts as a harbor. At this time, he develops industry; in other words, he adjusts himself to the inorganic laws of the tool world and develops a sense of competition. This period is a most decisive one from a social aspect since a first sense of division of labor and of equality of opportunity develops at this time. Whether a child develops a sense of industry from his efforts and achievements or develops a sense of inferiority no longer depends solely on parents but on other adults as well. Also, peers are needed for the purpose of maintaining self-esteem and as a measure against which the child can judge his own success and failure. These phases are the foundation with which the child meets the challenge of adolescence, during which time he defines and firms up his sense of identity.

Stage V—identity and repudiation versus identity diffusion—adolescence The ultimate goal of the individual is to acquire a sense of identity, which is constantly lost and regained. Because of the growth spurt and bodily changes, previous trust in the body is shaken. With these changes, there is an upset in the id-ego-superego integration, and the genitals now have physical primacy. There is also a recurrence of the Oedipal theme, which the adolescent has the chance to resolve in the matrix of the peer group and in heterosexual relations. The peer group becomes the essential support and value giver, and family relationships are more transitory. If a young person cannot attain a sense of personal identity, role confusion results, and a negative identity may be preferable to having no identity. Erikson considers that adolescence provides the young person with opportunities to experiment with different identities before making any final decisions.

Stage VI—intimacy and solidarity versus isolation—young adulthood This first phase of adulthood becomes a reality only after the individual has established in himself a sense of identity. By intimacy is meant the sexual and psychological intimacies that two people have in a love relationship and the interpersonal intimacy that he seeks in the form of friendship, combat, leadership, and love. The developmental theme of this phase centers around mutual intimacy in marriage or relationships. Readiness includes the ability and willingness to share mutual trust; to regulate cycles of work, procreation, and recreation for each partner's fullest and most satisfying participation in society; and to prepare a foundation for the healthy development of their potential offspring.

Stage VII—generativity versus self-absorption or stagnation—the middle years The basic theme of this phase is rooted in the interest in establishing and guiding the next generation. Adults may apply this drive to forms of altruistic concern and creativity, which may absorb their kind of parental responsibility. The normative crisis of the middle years is the "crisis of generativity which occurs when a person looks at what he has generated or helped to generate and finds it good or wanting" (Suterly and Donnelly, 1973). Stagnation results when the individual turns inward and becomes self-absorbed and indulges himself only.

Stage VIII—integrity versus despair—old age The basic task of this phase is the acceptance of one's own life cycle. A sense of despair at what might have been is experienced in feeling that time is too short to start another life and to reach this integrity by alternate roads. There may result a fear of death. In contrast, old age can be a time when one can reflect on and enjoy what has been.

BEHAVIORISTIC (SOCIAL LEARNING) THEORIES

SEARS' SOCIAL LEARNING THEORY

Sears founded a theory of social learning and socialization of the child on the basis of psychoanalytic hypotheses and placed the causal explanations and theoretical justifications of these hypotheses within the stimulus-response framework (Maier, 1969, p. 437). Sears focuses upon those aspects of behavior which are overt and can be measured; for Sears, personality development can best be measured through *action* and *social interaction*. He is primarily concerned with evaluating active behavior from this perspective: an emphasis on the learning experience of an individual that results from an action sequence—i.e., the learning effects of the stimulus-response sequence—in which each effect of an action can become the learned cause of future behavior. Action is instigated by a drive that is strong enough to impel the individual to respond to a cue, or stimulus. Initially, all stimuli are associated with primary, or innate, drives such as hunger. The satisfaction or frustration that results from the behavior prompted by these primary drives leads the individual to adopt additional behaviors. During this interactive process, the individual learns new modes of behavior, the satisfactory results of which serve to reinforce the achieving behavior. Constant reinforcement of specific actions, in turn, give rise to new, or learned, drives and to primary-drive equivalents; these are the secondary drives. These secondary drives arise from the social influences on development. Development may be considered a continuous, orderly sequence of conditions which create actions, new motives for actions, and eventual patterns of behavior.

As long as everyday social life proceeds as if developmental phases were a reality, all social learning tends to proceed in comparable patterns. All human functioning must be seen as the result of the interactive effects of all the influences, both constitutional and experiential, that have impinged on the individual. Social behavior depends almost exclusively upon the impact of others, rather than upon any internal developmental processes (Maier, 1969, p. 146). Early training of the infant distinctly implies an expectancy of different levels of readiness. Therefore, social conditions dictate the existence of developmental phases, regardless of whether they are based upon independent fact.

Sears relates each of the following to the three developmental phases which he outlines (Maier, 1969, pp. 155–175):

- Meaning of the particular phase
- Place of primary needs
- Place of secondary motivational systems
- Five major motivational systems in development (dependence, feeding, toileting, sex, and aggression)
- Important processes in development (identification, play, motility, reasoning, and conscience)
- Social factors (parent's own status, sex, ordinal position, class, education, cultural heritage)

Phase I—rudimentary behavior: Native needs and early-infancy learning The first phase connects the biological endowment of the newborn child with the endowment of the social environment. This phase introduces the infant to the environment and provides the foundation for ever-increasing interactions with the environment.

During the early months of a child's life, his environmental experience has not yet directed his learning. An infant's behavior in the first 10 to 16 months of his life involves his attempts to reduce inner tension originating from his inner drives. The way in which these innate needs are met introduces environmental learning experiences. When the infant's behavior tends toward specific goal-directed behavior, each completed action which brings about a reduction in tension is the one which is most likely to be repeated again whenever the tension arises. Successful development is characterized by a decrease in autism and innate need-centered actions and by an increase in dyadic, socially centered behavior. Early child development investigates three essential areas.

1 The conditions for a child's motivational system to be learned

2 The circumstances in which parents and other environmental factors reinforce a child's learning
3 The products or behavioral patterns of a child's learning

Sears' learning theory classifies dependency as a central component of learning. Rewarding reinforcement in all dyadic situations depends upon the child's having consistent contacts with one or more persons. Both child and mother have their repertoire of significant actions which serve to stimulate responses from the other which will be compatible with their own expectancies.

Aggression, on the basis of Sears' early research on the frustration-aggression hypothesis, is a consequence of frustration. Aggression readily becomes an early and vital aspect of learned behavior because frustration occurs from the very moment the infant experiences discomfort or pain and delay in finding relief from the unpleasant experience. Aggression, usually manifested through anger, is primarily a response to this frustration.

Phase II—secondary motivational systems: Family-centered learning Socialization begins to take place during this second phase, when primary needs continue to motivate the child. Aspects of the undisciplined life of the infant become subject to the rigors of parental training. Primary needs are gradually incorporated into repeatedly reinforced social learning or secondary drives. From now on these secondary drives will be the child's main motives to action, unless social environment fails to provide the necessary reinforcement. Social learning depends upon replacing previous learning with newer experiences that are based upon more appropriate satisfaction rather than upon avoiding unpleasant experiences or upon a fear of consequence.

Early-childhood development is essentially anchored in the satisfaction gained from the learned dependency upon the mothering person. As the child grows older, a sensitive mother looks upon excessive emotional dependency as behavior which should be altered. Slowly, the child learns to gratify his dependency drive by performing actions that he previously anticipated and demanded from his mother (imitation). The child discovers a new source of gratification in the very process of self-initiated imitation, which eventually leads from imitation of behavioral sequences to acting like another person. He may behave as if he possesses the psychological properties and skills of another. A nonmotivational system, identification, emerges and becomes a goal response.

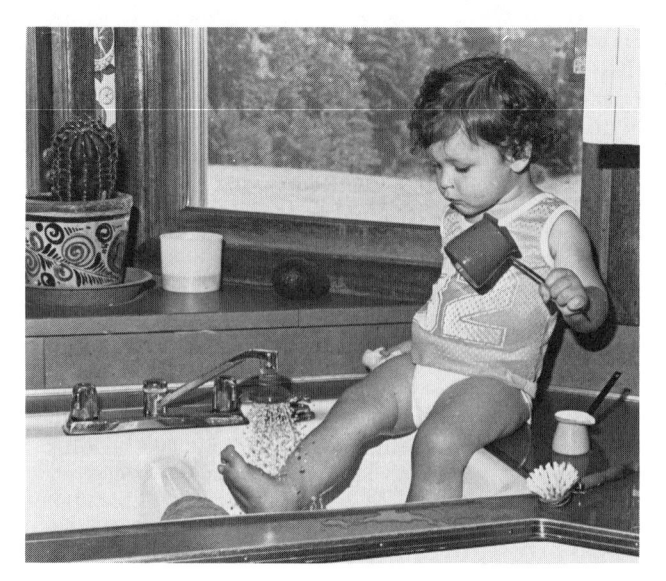

FIGURE 3-5. (*Photo courtesy of Betsy Smith.*)

Phase III—secondary motivational system: Extrafamilial learning By the time the young child is chronologically and developmentally ready for school, he is ready to absorb from a world which lies beyond that of his family. His new and wider environment helps him to achieve social, religious, and eventually political and economic values. All acquisitions of later value judgments are based on his earlier incorporations of his parents' behavior and what he has learned from his parents' teaching.

BIJOU AND BAER'S THEORY
OF SYSTEMATIC ANALYSIS OF DEVELOPMENT
In Bijou and Baer's analysis, development is defined as the progressive changes in the way an organism's behavior interacts with the environment and is limited to the observable, recordable instances of the responses of the developing child and to the specific events which operate on him and thus make up his environment.

The child is conceptualized as an interrelated cluster of responses and stimuli. The environment is conceived as events acting on the child: some specific stimuli and some setting events. The child and his environment interact continuously from fertilization until death. The psychological development of a child, therefore, is made up of progressive changes in the different ways of interacting with the environment. Progressive development is dependent upon opportunities and circumstances in the present and in the past. The circumstances are physical, chemical, organismic, and social. The influences may be analyzed in their physical and functional dimensions.

The theory proceeds by the following chain (Bijou and Baer, 1961, pp. 84–85):

- The developing child is adequately conceptualized as a source of responses, which fall into two functional classes: *respondents,* which are controlled primarily by preceding eliciting stimulation and which are largely insensitive to consequent stimulation, and *operants,* which are controlled primarily by consequent stimulation. The attachment of operant responses to preceding (discriminative) stimuli is dependent upon the stimulus consequence of behavior previously made in the presence of these *discriminative stimuli.* Some responses may share attributes of both respondents and operants.
- Initial understanding of the child's development next requires analysis of the child's environment, which is conceptualized as a source both of *eliciting stimuli,* controlling his respondents, and of *reinforcing stimuli,* which can control his operants.
- Subsequent analysis of the child's development proceeds by listing the ways in which respondents are attached to new eliciting stimuli and detached from old ones, through respondent conditioning and extinction. Similarly, a listing is made of the ways in which operants are strengthened or weakened through various reinforcement contingencies and discriminated to various stimuli which reliably mark occasions on which these contingencies hold. Some respondents are called emotional, and the conditioned eliciting stimuli for them may be provided by people and hence are social. Some of the operants strengthened are manipulatory, and some of their discriminative stimuli consist of the size, distance, weight, and motion of objects; hence, this development is perceptual-motor. Some of the operants are vocal, as are some of the respondents. The discriminative stimuli, reinforcing stimuli, and conditioned eliciting stimuli typically are both objects and the behavior of people. Hence, this development is both cultural and linguistic.
- The processes of the discrimination and generalization of stimuli are applied throughout these sequences of development. Thus, the child's operants and respondents may be attached to classes of eliciting and discriminative stimuli. These classes may have varying breadths, depending upon the variety of conditioning and extinction procedures applied to them. Consequently, the child's manipulatory and verbal behaviors seem to deal in classes; this phenomenon, coupled with the complexity or discriminative stimuli possible in discriminating operants, typically gives the label "intellectual" to such behaviors.
- The equation of discriminative stimuli to secondary reinforcers suggest that many discriminative stimuli will play an important role in strengthening and weakening operant behaviors in the child's future development. Some of these discriminative stimuli consist of the behavior of people (typically parents) and thus give rise to social reinforcers: attention, affection, approval, achievement, pride, status, etc. Again the preceding principles are applied but now to the case of social reinforcement, offered for what are therefore social behaviors under social discriminative stimuli.
- In all these steps, the scheduling of eliciting, discriminative, and reinforcing stimuli, to one another and to responses, is applied. This gives an explanation for characteristic modes of response which distinguish children: typical rates, the use of steady responding or bursts of activity, resistance to extinction, and the likelihood of pausing after reinforcement.

The cultural environment, or, more exactly, the members of the community, starts out with a human infant formed and endowed along species lines, but capable of behavioral training in many directions. From this raw material, the culture proceeds to make, in so far as it can, a product acceptable to itself. It does this by training: by reinforcing the behavior it desires and extinguishing others, by making some natural and social stimuli into discriminative stimuli and ignoring others, by differentiating out this or that specific response or chain of responses, such as manners and attitudes, by conditioning emotional and anxiety reactions to some stimuli and not others. It teaches the individual what he may and may not do, giving him norms and ranges of social behavior that are permissive or prescriptive or prohibitive. It teaches him the language he is to speak; it gives him his standards of beauty and art, of good and bad conduct; it sets before him a picture of the ideal personality that he is to imitate and strive to be. In all this, the fundamental laws of behavior are to be found. (Keller and Schoenfeld, 1950, pp. 365–366)

FRITZ HEIDER AND NAÏVE PSYCHOLOGY

The *naïve theory* of development is concerned with the various concepts that are thought to underlie voluntary action. Several sources of interaction included are personal wants, ulterior reasons, the promptings of sentimental attachment, the inclination to accede to requests, obedience to commands, and moral obligations. Intentional behavior is viewed as stemming from the person himself, as being active rather than passive in its nature. However, naïve psychology also conceptualized the events that impinge on the person and arouse feelings and reactions (Baldwin, 1968, p. 26).

The theory contains a complex set of assumptions and laws that govern much of our understanding of other people. Briefly, these are as follows:

- Nearly all human behavior is cognitively directed, that is, directed toward the attainment of goals which must be cognized before they can become operative. This cognition is seen as a natural process depending merely upon the exposure of the person to the external world.
- Differences in the behavior of different people depend upon differences in motivation, which in turn depend upon differences in dispositional characteristics.
- As well as being motivated by appropriate goal objects, people also respond to external pressure or imposition, which may arouse hostility, gratitude, fear, and other reactions. These feelings and their accompanying behavioral consequences are reasonably predictable. Two other classes of psychological mechanisms, according to commonsense theory, are sentiments and feelings of moral obligation (Baldwin, 1968, pp. 35–36).

Related to development and change, Heider's primary concern is with the naïve theory of social behavior as based on a mixture of these two assumptions:

1. In certain fundamental aspects, *human behavior is innate* and appears without training. These include self-evident actions, e.g., perception, instrumental actions, and emotional reactions.
2. In other important respects, children are not like adults because they are uninformed and untaught. Areas that give meaning to experience, such as information, meanings, and values, are seen as acquired (Baldwin, 1968, p. 36).

Naïve psychology is not a stated theory but a body of beliefs about human behavior. Commonsense beliefs are the ground from which theories of human behavior may grow but are equally the ground in which literary criticism, the historian's understanding of social processes, and the theologian's ideas of the relation of God to people are rooted.

COGNITIVE DEVELOPMENTAL THEORIES

GESELL AND MATURATIONAL THEORY

Arnold Gesell, as a maturational theorist, emphasizes the family as the pivotal center at which the interaction of inner and cultural forces comes to the most significant expression. The household is a cultural workshop for transmitting the social inheritance: a democratic household fosters a way of life which respects the individuality of the growing child. The child as an organism and the environment as a culture are inseparable. Each reacts to the other. The reactions of the child are primary: he must do his own growing. The culture helps him to achieve his developmental potentialities, helps him to learn, but the process of acculturation is limited by the child's natural growth process.

The child's personality is a product of slow and gradual growth. His nervous system matures by stages and natural sequences. All of his abilities, including his moral thoughts, are subject to laws of growth.

Gesell espoused a developmental philosophy of child care that is

. . . sensitive to the relativities of growth and maturity. It takes its point of departure from the child's nature and needs. It acknowledges the profound forces of racial and familial inheritance which determine the growth sequences and the distinctive growth pattern of each individual child. It envisages the problem of acculturation in terms of growth; but this increases rather than relaxes the responsibility of cultural guidance. Developmental guidance at a conscious level demands an active use of intelligence to understand the laws and mechanisms of the growth process. (Gesell and Ilg, 1943, p. 289)

Gesell discusses the dynamics of the growth complex as an overview of total unitary action with the system in dynamic flow. The outstanding features are the following:

- *Day cycle:* Growth is a self-renewing, self-perpetuating, and a self-expanding process which occurs every day.
- *Self-regulatory fluctuations:* The living growth complex during the period of infancy and childhood is in a state of formative instability combined with a progressive movement toward stability. The growing organism oscillates along a spiral course toward maturity.
- *Constitutional individuality:* Each child has a distinct mode of growth which is unique and which is also highly characteristic (Gesell and Ilg, 1943, p. 291).

Gesell emphasized a passionate regard for the individual, which he maintained was crucial to a truly democratic orientation to life. A corollary of this stress on the importance of the individual is the concept of individual differences. Yet, paradoxically, it is here that Gesell seems to have been most generally misinterpreted. This stems from the organization of most of his books in terms of the continued stress on ages and stages of behavioral development throughout childhood and adolescence (Rebelsky and Dorman, 1970, p. 7).

LEWIN AND FIELD THEORY

Kurt Lewin's point of view is called *topological field theory* and is based on his concept of *life space,* which consists of those selected aspects of the environment which stand out for the individual as psychologically meaningful. He viewed the life space as a region marked with *routes* and *barriers*. Routes lead to goal objects with positive and negative *valences,* which indicate attractiveness or repulsion. The person in the field is moved or immobilized by the action of these valences along the pathways that are open to him, representing courses of action. Lewin was less interested in how a life space comes to be constituted as it is than in its structure at the moment of action. He saw the life space becoming progressively more differentiated in the course of development and conceived of regression as a dedifferentiation of the life space. It does not seem incompatible with his views to assume that the life space also undergoes qualitative reorganization and reintegration as development proceeds (Stone and Church, 1973, pp. 404–405).

Lewin's field theory is postulated as a restatement and refinement of naïve theory. A basic concept is life space—which includes the sum of all the facts that determine the person's behavior at a given time. These contemporary facts are directly relevant to the behavior and are divided into two large classes: those that describe the environment and those that describe the person (Baldwin, 1968, pp. 90–124).

The psychological environment is defined in terms of its effect on behavior. All parts of the psychological environment influence the person's behavior, and therefore the environment is a description of the external situation as it affects behavior, which is not physical activity but merely a change in the psychological environment. Behavior is a means for attaining some goal; it is viewed as locomotion in the direction of the goal within some defined space (region). The environment is described in geometrical terms. It is composed of regions which may correspond to varied psychological events, activities of the individual, group memberships, or physical areas. The arrangement of the regions in the psychological environment is called the *cognitive structure*. Lewin postulated the existence of psychological forces in the environment. The movement of the person from one region to another was explained in terms of a force on the person in the first region in the direction of the second region. Any force must have a point of application, a strength, and a direction. A valence represents a force field that is manifested in a particular force on a particular person and may be positive or negative. If there are many different regions with valences, there may be various forces upon the person, some which may be in the same direction and reinforce one another and some which may be in different directions and conflict with one another.

Needs of the person are correlated to forces in the psychological environment. The effect of a need system in a state of tension is that some region in the environment acquires a positive valence. Consequently, there is a force on the person in the direction of that region. Directed action to satisfy this need is one possible consequence, or the need may remain latent until the appropriate goal becomes available.

The basic assumption is that development involves an increase in the number of regions and an increase in the strength of the boundaries of these regions. The aspects of development include the following:

- As the child grows older, he exhibits a greater variety of behavior.
- Behavior becomes increasingly guided by a governing purpose, a main theme.
- The psychological environment of the child expands both in area covered and in time span.
- Growth of the child involves change in the dependence of his activities on one another.
- An increase occurs in realism, which is identified by its psychological properties, not by external reality (Baldwin, 1968, pp. 117–119).

PIAGET AND COGNITIVE DEVELOPMENT

According to Jean Piaget's theory, the major forces which facilitate the developmental process are maturational forces; results of experience and environment; results of explicit and implicit teaching of the child by others in the environment; and the process of equilibration (cognitive development and particularly the development of organized belief systems) (Baldwin, 1968, p. 296).

Unorganized belief systems contain inherent self-contradictions and conflict; force is set up to harmonize the child's ideas one with another and is the process of equilibration.

Piaget (1952), a French biologist, begins from the point of view that as all organisms adapt to their environment, they must possess some form of structure or organization which makes the adaptation possible at all. Thus he views organization and adaptation as the basic invariants of functioning. Adaptation is further subdivided into two closely interwoven components, *assimilation* and *accommodation*.

Assimilation involves changing the elements in the situation, (e.g., experience or food) so that they can be incorporated into the structure of the organism (e.g., intellectual or digestive systems) in order that the individual may adapt to the situation. Accommodation implies modifying the structures of the organism so that the organism can adapt to the situation. Assimilation and accommodation are also regarded as functional invariants. For Piaget, every intellectual act necessitates some intellectual structure, while intellectual functioning is characterized by assimilation and accommodation.

As the baby interacts with his environment, he builds up sequences of actions, or patterns of behavior, called *schemata* which have definite structure. In the postinfancy period, the term schema refers to mental actions and intellectual structures. In assimilation, the child has to absorb new experiences into his existing schemata, whereas in accommodation there is the modification of existing schemata or the buildup of new ones. But once new experience is assimilated; the child's schemata become more complex, and because of this, accommodations of even greater complexity are possible. Changes in the schemata brought about by attempts at accommodation and reorganization brought about independently of external stimulation together ensure schemata of greater complexity and hence intellectual growth.

Piaget has provided much evidence to suggest that there is a fixed sequence of stages in the growth of thought and that thinking at one stage is qualitatively different from that of another (Lovell, 1968, p. 23). The age at which children reach the stages varies because of the educational and cultural backgrounds, the degree of intellectual stimulation they receive, and heredity.

These stages, described in Lovell (1968, pp. 24-33) include the sensorimotor period, the preoperational stage, concrete operational thought, and formal operational thought.

Sensorimotor period In the first 21 months or so of life, the schemata built up need the direct support of information obtained through the senses and through motor action. Each element in the schema comes into being at the exact moment when other aspects of the environment provide the necessary support for it. During the development of sensorimotor intelligence, there is a growth of the more specialized intellectual achievements, e.g., the sensorimotor construction of causality, imitation, objects, play, space, and time. It is during this period that the basic schemata are elaborated for dealing with the environment, as in the case of space when the child adjusts his actions to reach near and distant objects and the case of time when he adjusts his actions to catch a swinging rattle.

Preoperational stage The child moves from the stage of sensorimotor intelligence into what Piaget calls the preoperational stage of thought, when he can differentiate a *signifier* (an image or a word) from a significate (what it is the signifier stands for) and call forth the one to represent the other. The capacity to make this differentiation and to be able to make an act of reference is termed the symbolic function. With the onset of language, the nature of the child's intelligence greatly changes. *Representational thought* can grasp a number of events as a coherent whole, whereas, at the level of sensorimotor intelligence, successive actions and perceptual states are linked one by one. Representational thought provides the child with a less transient and far more flexible model of the outside world and extends the range of thought well outside the present environment, for he is no longer dependent on action and immediate perception for thought.

Between 2 and 4 years of age intellectual development seems to consist largely in the building up of this representational activity and in differentiating image and language, on the one hand, from action and reality, on the other. Between ages 4 and 5½ years, the child is more able to examine and set about a specific task, adapt his intelligence to it, and commence to reason about more difficult everyday problems. Even so, one of the marked characteristics of thought at this stage is its tendency to center on some striking feature of the object about which he is reasoning to the exclusion of other relevant aspects, with the result that the reasoning is distorted. The child is also incapable of seeing a situation from other than a personal point of view. However, around 5½ years of age, the rigid and irreversible intellectual structures begin to become more flexible, and there is a transition to the next stage of thought.

Piaget calls the overall 4- to 7-year-old period one of *intuitive thought*. The term intuition indicates the rather isolated and sporadic actions in the mind which occasionally give a foretaste of later systematized thinking but which do not yet coalesce into an integrated system of thought, as they do when operational thought sets in.

Concrete operational thought At this stage the child's logical thought extends only to objects and events of firsthand reality. The child is able to take into account two contrasting features, e.g., height and width, which could balance and compensate for any distortion brought about by concentrating on one aspect of the situation. At 7 to 8, the schemata which have developed are different in kind from those present at 4 to 5 years of age. The capacity to reason and understand demands a higher-order schema which permits a simultaneous grasp of successive sequences in the mind. The child can now look at his own thinking and monitor it. Also, for any action in his mind, he can now understand that there are other actions that will give the same result. There is now learning with understanding. In Piaget's system, when mental actions have a definite and strong structure, they are termed operations. Thus any action which is an integral part of an organized network of related action is an operation. In Piaget's view, concrete operational thought must possess certain properties, which are *closure, reversibility, associativity,* and *identity.*

Formal operational thought As the child becomes better at organizing and structuring data with the methods of concrete operational thought, he becomes aware that such methods do not lead to a logically exhaustive solution to his problems. The adolescent, due to the maturation of the central nervous system and the continued interaction with the cultural milieu together with the resulting feedback, can now produce more complex operations when faced with certain kinds of data or situations. The adolescent can set up a number of *hypotheses* and establish which are compatible with the evidence in front of him.

Piaget argues that the age of onset of formal thought is relative to the culture pattern, for in some undeveloped societies, adolescents do not appear to attain this level of thought (Lovell, 1969, p. 35). So beyond some minimum ages, perhaps set by neurophysiological factors, the level of an individual's thinking may be a product of the progressive acceleration of individual development under the influence of education and culture.

For Piaget, there are four major influences affecting intellectual growth; these are briefly listed below (Lovell, 1969, p. 38):

1. Biological factors, which probably determine the unfolding of the stages of intellectual growth in a fixed sequence.
2. *Equilibration* (the process of bringing assimilation and accommodation into balanced coordination) or autoregulation factors, which probably lie at the origin of mental operations themselves.
3. General factors resulting from socialization, which arise through exchanges, discussions, agreements, and oppositions in social intercourse between children or between children and adults. Such influences operate to a greater or lesser extent in all cultures, and they are closely linked to the equilibration factor since the general coordination of actions concern the interindividual as well as the intraindividual.
4. Factors related to education and cultural transmission, which differ greatly from one society to another.

Piaget established that intellectual development follows a predictable pattern (Maier, 1969, pp. 141–142):

- All development proceeds in a unitary direction.
- Developmental progressions are in order and can readily be described by criteria marking distinct developmental phases.
- There are distinct organizational differences between childhood and adult behavior in all areas of human functioning.
- All mature aspects of behavior have their beginnings in infant behavior and evolve through all subsequent patterns of development.
- All developmental trends are interrelated and interdependent; developmental maturity means the final and total integration of all the developmental trends.

Piaget's theory is discussed further in "Cognitive Development."

KOHLBERG AND MORAL DEVELOPMENT

Kohlberg's major contribution to the study of human development has been his insight into the development of *moral behavior*. Morality indicates a set of rules for determining one's social actions which have been internalized by the individual. The rules tend to be related to the culture and are internalized because of some inner motivation.

Kohlberg has identified three levels which include a total of six definite and universal stages of development in moral thought (Sutterly and Donnelly, 1973, p. 226). These stages are the products of interactional experience between the child and the world, experience which leads to a restructuring of the child's own organization rather than to the direct imposition of the culture's pattern upon the child. Throughout life the organism receives enormous inputs of information from which he reconstructs his image of the world. In early infancy, the messages he receives are largely undifferentiated sounds, lights, and feelings, but with growth comes consciousness and ability to distinguish people and objects. Growth and the experiences of life bring to the child an expansion in his image of the world of things and human relationships. A child is not born with values but forms them in his relationships with his family and his culture. The value systems of a culture are transmitted in the processes of that culture by the information inputs which the culture generates.

Level I—preconventional—ages 4 to 10 in American middle-class culture Moral value resides in external, quasiphysical happenings, in bad acts, or in quasiphysical needs rather than in persons and standards. The two stages emphasize punishment and obedience orientation and a nonquestioning deference to superior power. Right action consists of that which instrumentally satisfies one's own needs of others.

Level II—conventional—preadolescence Moral value resides in performing good or right rules in maintaining the conventional order and expectancies of others. The two stages focus on orientation to interpersonal relations of mutuality and to approval, affection, and helpfulness. Correct behavior consists of doing one's duty, showing respect for authority, conforming to the fixed rules, and maintaining the given social order for its own sake.

Level III—postconventional—adolescence Moral values reside in conformity by the self to shared or shareable standards, rights, or duties. Within these two stages, orientation is to internal decisions of conscience but without clear rational or universal principles. The growth within this level is toward ethical principles appealing to logic, comprehensiveness, universality, and consistency. Kohlberg concludes that something like the internalization of moral rules depends closely upon the cognitive growth of moral concepts and that conscience develops late. He also states that social class and the extent of participation in peer group activities is related to moral development quite independently of IQ.

SUMMARY

Within the context of a three-dimensional approach (cognitive, affective, and behavioral), each type of theory provides a partial and, consequently, varying answer concerning the child's development. But children, if they are to be guided toward successful and social development, must be viewed in the light of their total development. The focus of the theories is upon developmental readiness and developmental acquisition, both of which are tied to developmental phases. Individual children can be assessed only within the context of their own evolvement, and while developmental theory may help to provide a generalized understanding of the processes of child development, any such theory can be used successfully only when applied to individual children according to the specifics of their own unique situations.

SECTION 2
General Considerations of Behavioral Development

Principles of behavioral development as well as specific, well-known theories have been presented. Further concepts of behavioral development within specific areas of functioning—perceptual, gross motor, fine motor, cognitive, language, self-help, and social—are presented in the following section.

Perceptual development   Veronica A. Binzley

THE NATURE OF PERCEPTION

DEFINITION
Perception refers to the process by which one obtains firsthand information about the environment that enables one to function adaptively. If a person is to survive, which means taking care of the most basic needs and avoiding potential hazards, he must be able to fairly accurately recognize what is "out there" and react appropriately. In lower animals this process is fairly automatic because it is genetically determined and relatively unmodified by experience. All that is necessary is that the lower animal be exposed to the kind of environment for which nature intended it. That is not the case with humans.

As we ascend the phylogenetic scale, perception comes increasingly under the control of cognition, becomes less fixed, and hence becomes more complex. In the human neonate the perceptual system is functional but immature such that only gross selectivity is demonstrable. However, with maturation, experience, and learning, the reflexive perceptual system of the neonate is gradually transformed into the complex information-processing system of the adult, capable of detecting the subtlest sign of emotion in the face of a friend.

CONTENDING THEORIES OF PERCEPTION
Although there is an extensive literature on the topic of perception, actual research in this area did not gather much momentum until the 1950s and 1960s. Prior to that time, most inferences regarding perception and perceptual development were made on the basis of introspection or experiments with adults (Pick and Pick, 1970). Hence the perceptual process, even in the adult, is not well understood. Perception functionally is part of cognition, and as such it historically has been included in the nativism-empiricism controversy concerning the origins of knowledge.

The nativistic position, which is usually associated with the eighteenth-century German philosopher Immanuel Kant (1724-1804), maintains that the ideas of space and things are innate, prototypical, universal, and God given. By ideas, Kant meant principles of ordering that make it possible to understand experience and make incoming sensations meaningful. According to this view, the human infant is born with an adultlike ability to interpret incoming information about the environment.

On the other hand, the empiricists, most notably the British philosopher John Locke (1632-1704), claimed that the neonate's mind is a *tabula rasa*, or blank slate, upon which information is imprinted via the senses. Therefore in the view of the empiricist the world of the neonate is a confusion of insubstantial shadows, sounds, and sensations out of which the infant must laboriously try to make sense. This supposedly is done by gradually building elemental sensations into complex concepts such as color, form, depth, and distance. Today no such simple view of perception is held. Nor are there many psychologists who would dichotomize perception as an exclusively learned or unlearned process, as was done in the past.

PRESENT CONSENSUS
Although there remain areas of disagreement which will be noted where appropriate, the general consensus is that the human begins with certain unlearned, wired-in programs which are reflexive and necessary to start the adaptive process. Disagreement exists, particularly among developmentalists, over the extent and quality of the wired-in programs possessed by the neonate. Some researchers have reported finding amazing abilities in the neonate (Bower, 1977). Notwithstanding this controversy, it is generally agreed that the neonate's basic abilities improve with age. The improvement results from a complex interaction of maturation, experience, and learning which enables the child to develop more efficient ways of detecting and organizing the available information about the environment.

While agreeing that maturation, experience, and learning are all important for the development of perception, theorists disagree about what experiences are important, what is learned, and how it is learned. Eleanor Gibson (1969) has classified the various theories of perceptual learning according to the psychological status of their main concept. According to her classification there are *cognitively oriented, response-oriented,* and *stimulus-oriented* theories.

A cognitively oriented, or judgmental, theory, of which there are several, assumes that as a result of experience with the environment and objects in it, the young child progressively elaborates and organizes his knowledge of the environment. Supposedly this is accomplished by a process of unconscious inference or schema formation. On the other hand, the response-oriented theories assume that perceptual learning occurs as the result of association of motor acts with visual and other sense data. An extreme form of this view maintains that perception develops from and is isomorphic with a motor copy of objects and events. In this theory all depth and form perceptions are dependent upon motor experiences with objects and forms. That is, just looking experience would not be adequate. However, there is very little empirical data to support this view.

Jean Piaget views perception as a subset of cognition which increasingly comes under the active direction of cognition. His theory of perceptual development incorporates aspects of both the cognitive and response theories. According to Piaget, perceptual learning occurs as a result of schema building, which is enhanced by the actual motor exploration of the environment and things in it. Further he assumes that every intellectual act presupposes an interpretation of the environment, thereby making perception the very cornerstone for intellectual development.

The last type of theory, the stimulus-oriented theory, holds that all the necessary information about the environment is contained in the available stimulus and that perceptual development, or learning, is simply a matter of improvement in one's ability to discriminate this information. In this view, which has been most strongly argued by J. J. Gibson (1966), perception is an active, information-seeking process which improves with development as the child learns to detect the properties, patterns, and distinctive features of the environment.

Although various theorists differ as to the exact nature of perceptual development, they do agree that abilities improve with age as a result of a complex interaction of maturation, learning, and experience. That is, ability to make sense of the environment is limited by cognitive ability at the time, but cognition, in turn, is affected by experience with that environment as well as by maturity and integrity of the central nervous system. As cognitive abilities increase, so presumably do perceptual processing abilities. This interaction is graphically depicted in Fig. 3-6.

THE PROCESS OF PERCEPTION

The above are some of the general theories of perception that have been proposed; now the process itself can be discussed in more detail. Perception begins with stimulation from the environment—stimulation in the form of energy such as light, sound, movement, and touch, to name a few. However, the central nervous system is only sensitive to certain aspects of these energy sources. For example, in the area of auditory perception of pitch, the average adult is stimulated informationally only by sound vibrations that fall between 10 and 20,000 hertz (Hz) and is deaf to bases lower than 10 Hz and trebles higher than 20,000 Hz. (More detailed information regarding specific sensory physiology is given later in this section.) It is sufficient here to point out that senses are differentially sensitive to specific aspects of the energy information available in the environment and that the range of this sensitivity is much the same for the neonate as for the young adult. Perceptual development for the most part involves improvement in the ability to discriminate within this range.

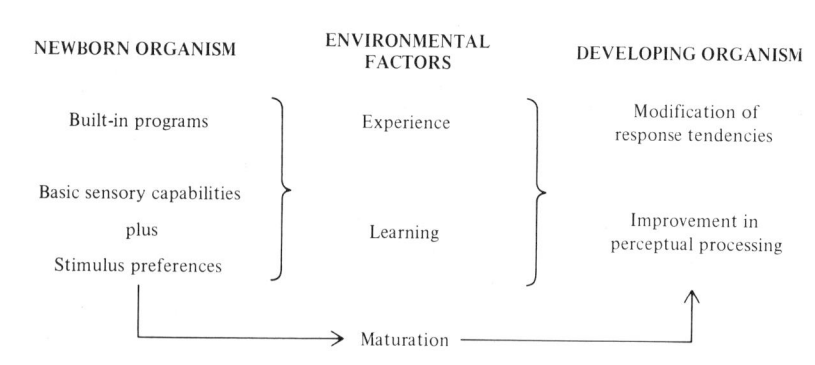

FIGURE 3-6. Model of perceptual development.

Sense organs translate the informational aspect of the physical energy into a form the central nervous system can use. The specific sense organs and the kind of information they transduce are listed below (Forgus, 1966):

- The *exteroceptors,* or distance senses.
  1. Vision, which transduces light energy.
  2. Audition, which transduces sound energy.
- The *proprioceptors,* or near senses.
  1. Cutaneous (tactile) or skin senses, which transduce changes in touch—warm, cold, and pain energy.
  2. Taste, which transduces changes in the chemical composition of liquids stimulating the tongue.
  3. The chemical sense of smell, which transduces gases reaching the nose. Taste and smell are closely related such that the discrimination of different flavors within a specific taste requires the interaction of the senses of taste and smell.
- The *interoceptors,* or deep senses.
  1. Kinesthetic sense, which transduces changes in body position and the motion of the muscles, tendons, and joints
  2. The vestibular (static) sense, which transduces changes in bodily balance.

Sensory perceptual experience can also be analyzed in terms of two basic modes: *autocentric* and *allocentric* (Worden, 1966). Autocentric is the mode in which sensory quality is fused into a bodily feeling (pleasure or displeasure), and there is no representation of the stimulus object. This would include the olfactory, gustatory, and proprioceptive (thermal and pain) senses. The allocentric mode is less directly related to bodily feeling and has intellectual qualities which evoke a representation of the object. This mode includes primarily the visual and auditory but also the tactile.

Once the incoming stimulus energy is transformed into the code of the nervous system, the process of perception starts. At one time it was thought that the sensory systems relayed their coded information to the cortex, where in some mysterious way it was interpreted.

Although it is still not clear exactly what the intervening brain activity is between stimulus input and perceptual response, it has recently become evident that active processing goes on at the subcortical level, indeed in some instances even at the receptor level. This new evidence has come primarily from the work of neurophysiologists using microelectrodes to record the responses of individual cells within the sensory system to various stimuli. Most notable in this area is the pioneering work of Torsten Wiesel and David Hubel of Harvard Medical School on the visual system of the cat. They found neurons in the cat's visual system that functioned like feature detectors: they responded only to certain attributes of the visual world. Some neurons responded only to movement, others to vertical lines or contours. The human visual system may work something like the cat's, in which case the intervening brain activity, although the exact neurophysiological mechanism has not been identified, would consist of filtering out irrelevant information while detecting and elaborating meaningful patterns. Pattern recognition can be accomplished by either a buildup of a schema or a clustering of distinctive features. In either case with development there is progressive elaboration and organization of the available patterns such that the individual becomes more efficient at extracting information from the immediate environment.

The last stage of the perceptual process is the response, or perceptual experience, which is the only evidence that the individual has perceived something in the environment. Often this involves just a verbal report of what one has experienced or, in the case of the preverbal child, simply an observed change in behavior correlated with a stimulus, from which the act of perception is inferred.

Detailed analysis of the perceptual experience itself has shown that it is a complex task which may involve several subtasks. These subtasks can be ordered hierarchically from the simplest to most complex as follows:

- Simple detection of a stimulus
- Discrimination of a figure from its background or of one stimulus from another
- Identification or recognition of a form or pattern
- Manipulation of the identified form, as in problem solving and social perception

Each successive subtask requires the extraction of progressively more information from the stimulus energy. That is, more stimulus information is required to pick a figure out from its background than is needed to simply detect the presence of a stimulus. In addition, studies have shown that detection and discrimination are more heavily determined by sensory factors, while the more complex tasks are increasingly influenced by learning and experience.

The implication of this hierarchy of perceptual subtasks is that it is the order of their occurrence developmentally. That is, the neonate's and young infant's perceptual responses consist primarily of simple detection of a stimulus and the discrimination of two stimuli as being physically different. Later, with the development of cognition, the older infant and toddler recognize a form or pattern as being familiar. This kind of perceptual experience is evident when the child recognizes the parent's face or voice from all other faces and voices in the environment. Lastly the child develops the ability to manipulate identified forms, as in the process of learning to read.

SOME DEVELOPMENTAL TRENDS

Although knowledge of what the developing child can perceive at different ages is limited, certain developmental trends are apparent. First, with learning and development there is a progressive increase in the specificity of discrimination to stimulus information. For example, the young infant will smile as readily at a scrambled face, a picture of two dots, or a cyclops, among other things, as he will to the human face. But with development and experience the smile soon is only elicited by a smiling human face. Additional evidence for this trend comes from the reported reduction of variability in judgment or increase in precision and consistency of discrimination as a function of age.

Secondly, there is what Eleanor Gibson (1969) has labeled as *optimization of attention.* What begins in the young infant as captivelike attention becomes more exploratory and random in nature. The random, exploratory activity then becomes more systematic, selective, and finally exclusive in nature. Thus by school age, the normal child is no longer easily distracted by extraneous stimuli in the environment but can focus his attention to the point of screening out competing and irrelevant stimuli. And lastly, there is progressive economy in the extraction of information from stimulation as the growing child learns to detect the distinctive features of things, to recognize invariants over time (perceptual constancy), and to process larger units of structure. These trends will become apparent as the emerging abilities of the developing child are presented.

Gross motor development Fay F. Russell and Beverly R. Richardson

Upon his entrance into the world, the neonate has few gross motor skills and is thus rendered almost helpless and quite dependent on others around him. Most of his gross motor movements are random, uncoordinated, generalized, nonproductive, and dominated primarily by primitive reflexes arising chiefly from the spine and midbrain. The transformation of this helpless neonate into a motorically independent adolescent depends largely on development and refinement of gross motor skills. Specifically, gross motor development refers to large motor skill development and is demonstrated as the child develops tone, control, and strength for such functions as postural stability, balance, coordination, and other movements involved in these functions.

PRINCIPLES OF GROSS MOTOR DEVELOPMENT

General principles of gross motor development demonstrated in the progressively and sequentially acquired gross motor skills of the infant and child are basic and predictable; however, each child, as a unique individual, develops large motor skills in his own way and at his own pace. These skills emerge largely within the first 2 years of

FIGURE 3-7. *(Photo courtesy of Betsy Smith.)*

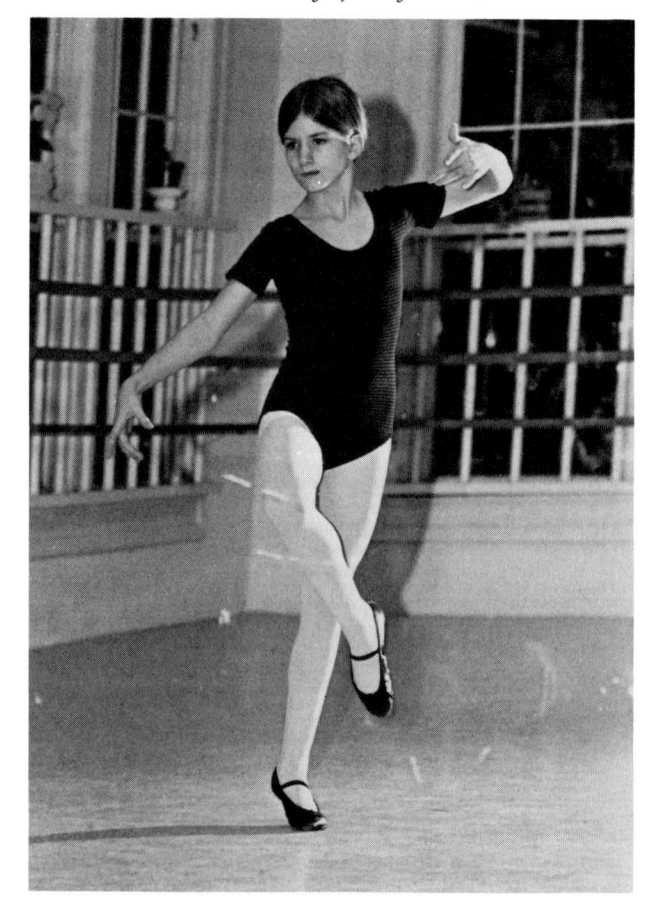

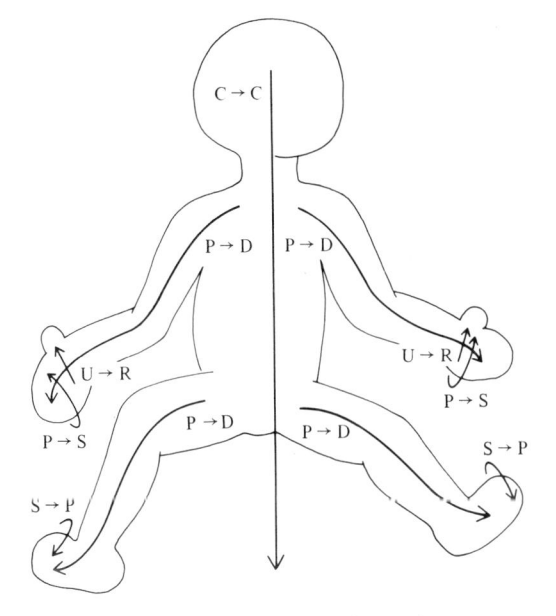

FIGURE 3-8. Anatomical directions of gross motor development. C → C: cephalad to caudad; P → D: proximal to distal; U → R: ulnar to radial; P → S: pronation to supination; S → P: supination to pronation.

life and are only being refined and becoming more functional as the child grows older.

ANATOMICAL DIRECTIONS

Seven basic principles, two relating to differentiation of behavior and five to the anatomical directions of gross motor development, are evident (see Fig. 3-8). The first principle is that the infant progressively exhibits less reflexive and more purposeful, integrated behavior. The second is that the infant goes from a predominately *flexed* to a predominately *extended* posture. Functional adult posture is that of predominate extension. This principle relates to the third in acquisition of motor control.

The third principle is that the infant acquires gross motor skills and muscular control in the *cephalocaudal* direction, that is, from his head in a downward fashion to his feet. This principle is demonstrated functionally as the infant lifts his head before he gets on his elbows or hands, sits before he stands, and crawls before he walks. The fourth principle is that development proceeds in the *proximodistal* direction. This is seen as the infant learns to move and control the joints closest to the central axis of his body before he masters use of the joints farther away, for example, he uses his shoulder joints before his wrists.

The fifth principle is that gross motor development proceeds in a *ventrodorsal* direction, that is, from the front to the back surfaces. For example, the infant uses his anterior trunk muscles to pull to a sitting position before he uses the muscles in his back to sit unsupported. Sixth, motor development occurs from near midline in the anatomical position outward in the *ulnar-to-radial* direction. As this principle is of significance in development of fine motor skills, it is discussed in more detail in that area. Finally, in motor development, especially in regard to posture, the upper extremities develop in a pronation-to-supination pattern and the lower extremities in a supination-to-pronation pattern. This pattern is particularly evident in the fetus and neonate.

Development of gross motor skills is a sequential process whereby each step of development prepares the way for the step to follow. Simple skills occur first with more complex ones emerging as the child's development proceeds. Accompanying this progression from simple to complex is the evolvement of specific and purposeful activity from the generalized and random movements of the neonate.

POTENTIALITY, PROMOTION, AND READINESS

Three factors to consider in development of gross motor abilities are *potentiality*, *promotion*, and *readiness*. Each child's potential for gross motor development is genetically determined and to a lesser extent environmentally influenced. These environmentally influencing factors include opportunity and stimulation for learning skills. Freedom from ill health and handicapping conditions and a supportive, nurturing environment promote acquisition of gross motor skills. Readiness refers here to the child's being equipped physiologically and psychologically for attainment of each skill. Of particular relevance to the degree of physiological readiness for development of gross motor skills is the status of the neuromuscular system.

NEUROMUSCULAR SYSTEM

Of greatest importance in consideration of the neuromuscular system is the degree of maturation as well as integration of the nervous, muscular, and sensory systems. Absence or abnormalities of any of the above will result in alterations in muscle tone, control, and/or strength, producing deficiencies in postural stability, movement, coordination, and balance, with the ultimate result being interference in the acquisition of gross motor skills.

MAJOR GROSS MOTOR MILESTONES

Gross motor development is reflected in the functional skills attained and can be divided into average age-level attainments. These skills represent milestones in the child's development.

Lack of gross motor skills is evident in the neonate, but given an intact, maturing neuromuscular system and a supportive environment, he soon begins acquiring those gross motor skills which will culminate in his evolution from a helpless neonate to an independent adolescent.

Fine motor development Barbara Newcomer McLaughlin and Nancy L. Morgan

Throughout an individual's lifetime, some type of fine motor activity is the major means of reacting to and coping with the environment. Fine motor function is the primary method that humans have of responding to external stimulation. Fine motor ability is often the yardstick for evaluation of a young child's mental functioning.

PRINCIPLES OF FINE MOTOR DEVELOPMENT

The distinction between gross motor activity and fine motor activity is important; the significance of fine motor skills and their proper development lies in the use of these skills for expression of cognitive ability, emotional response, and personal adequacy (Stott, 1974). The fine motor behavior is fundamentally *prehension*—the use of the hands and fingers in the reaching for, grasping, and manipulating objects. Many other abilities are essential to the development of fine motor skills, such as correct posturing, visual accuracy, and neuromuscular coordination; these, however, are not actually within the realm of fine motor skills but are functionally integrated, as are gross motor skills.

ANATOMICAL DIRECTIONS

Fine motor development, as development in general, progresses from flexion posturing to extension posturing, gross movements to fine movements, and proximal control to distal control. Control in the arm is first gained over the shoulder, giving large, gross, whole-arm movements (proximal to distal), and progressing then to finer movements of the elbow and finally to the wrist. Arm movement progresses from a more flexed posture with the hand close to the face to an extension position. Initially, move-

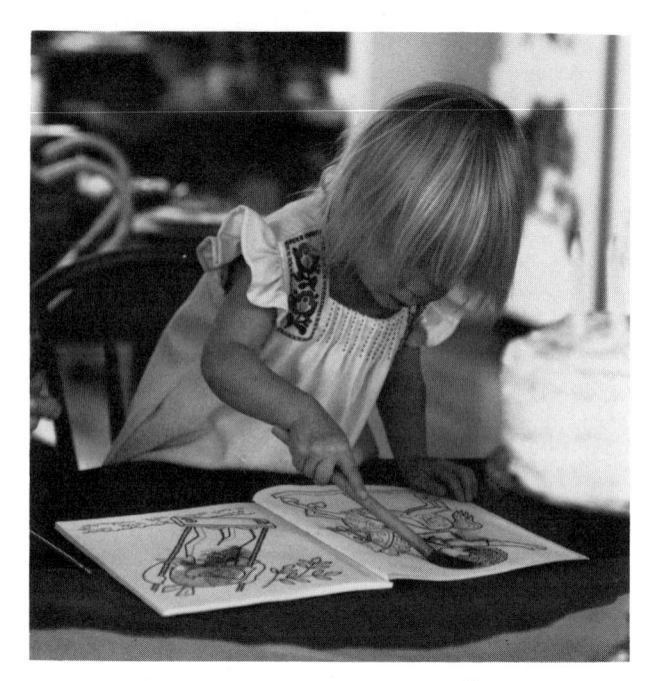

FIGURE 3-9. (*Photo courtesy of Grant C. Allen.*)

ments of the arm are *bilateral* (mirror) and then progress to *unilateral* and finally to a coordinated interaction.

Hand motion involved in prehension progresses from palmar to fingertip (proximal to distal) and ulnar to radial resulting in transformation from an ulnar-palmar to a radial-digital grasp. Prehension also progresses from primarily pronate to more supinate (see Fig. 3-10). Grasp progresses from maximum stretch to adaptation to the object to be grasped as movements develop from gross to finer. Hand release develops from gross, undirected release to fine, directed release.

POTENTIALITY, PROMOTION, AND READINESS

Other factors significant to fine motor development are age-related expectations, the continuum of development, and the refinement of skills. Age-related expectations should be realistic and incorporate the readiness factor basic to all learning and development. Child-development researchers have cataloged the age level for each skill acquired in prehension (fine motor development) as in the other areas of development. There are, however, many individual variations dependent upon maturity level and environmental stimulation. Certainly particular behaviors are characteristic of the neonate, the infant, the toddler, the preschooler, and the school-age child; the development of expected behaviors, however,

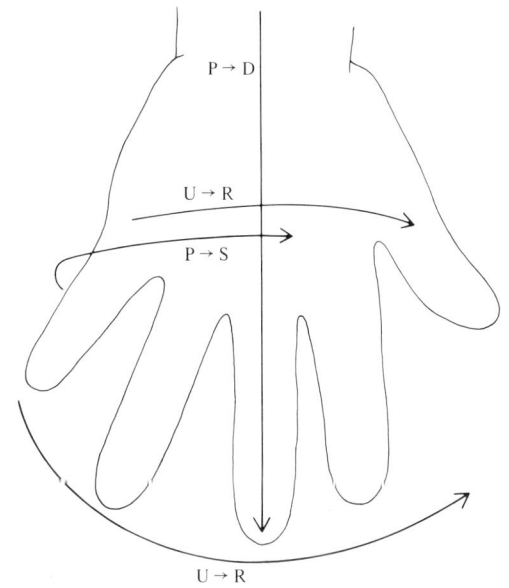

FIGURE 3-10 Anatomical directions of fine motor development. P → D: proximal to distal; U → R: ulnar to radial; P → S: pronation to supination.

is dependent upon other areas of growth and development, especially cognitive processes. Therefore, the correlation of chronological age and specific fine motor skills may not always follow the predicted schedule.

Acquisition of fine motor skills moves along a continuum of development from the neonatal grasp reflex to the complex school-age usage of "tools" in meaningful personal expression. Movement along this progression of fine motor skills is a deliberate, methodical process involving the child's mastery of sequential abilities. At many points along the continuum, moving to the next action requires abandoning more primitive skills. For example, the characteristic open-handedness and beginning of object grasping by the 8- to 16-week-old child means he has ceased the close-handed behavior of the 4- to 6-week-old. The mastery of sequential abilities also means a building relation of achievement, with each step making it possible for the child to move on to the next level of fine motor behavior. For example, the bidextrous approach to objects characteristic of the 20- to 24-week-old child gives rise to the ability, at a slightly older age, of transferring objects from one hand to the other.

Another significant concept in fine motor development is the refinement of skills. As a child moves along the continuum, he not only increases the number of actions he can perform with his hands and fingers, but he also improves his performance of particular behaviors. Much of this process depends upon the basic principle of improvement with practice, but it also involves a progressively higher level of coordination and integration of abilities due to neuromuscular maturation. When the child first holds a crayon, for example, he may do so in an awkward and rather ineffective manner; as he continues to become familiar with the crayon, however, he refines his ability to hold and manipulate it, reaching a level of meaningful involvement.

ENVIRONMENTAL INPUT

Environmental factors play an important role in development of fine motor abilities as well as of cognitive and gross motor abilities. The availability of toys and other objects for manipulation as well as parents' conscious efforts to allow exploration of the environment will greatly influence fine motor development.

Cognitive development Virginia Pidgeon

The development of the human mind from the fitful attentiveness of the neonate to the abstract theorizing of the adolescent is a fascinating process. How does the mind develop? Is human learning the product of increasingly complex stimulus-response sequences and behavioral shaping? Or is it the result of maturational changes in cognitive structures and abilities? Is the learner a passive recipient of information through conditioning or an active agent in the acquisition of knowledge? For insights and answers to these questions three cognitive theories will be explored, with recognition of the bias inherent in this selection.

FUNCTION OF COGNITION

What is the function of cognition or intelligence? The function of cognition, to Jean Piaget, is in adaptation to the environment achieved through the dual processes of accommodation and assimilation. Freud similarly described the ego, with its cognitive functions (reality testing, perception, memory, judgment, and reasoning) as an organ of adaptation. The ego was seen however in the context of other aspects of the personality (id and superego) as an organ of internal as well as external adaptation. Not only does the ego have a reality-testing function (acquisition of knowledge about the environment) but also a mediating function between the demands of the disparate parts of the personality (id and superego) and the demands of external reality. Piaget deals with cognition in isolation from the personality. Freud embeds the ego and its cognitive functions in the context of personality and assigns to the ego the more complex task of achieving an adaptation between internal and external demands. The cognitive theories of Heinz Werner, Jean Piaget, and Jerome Bruner will now be discussed.

WERNER'S THEORY OF COGNITIVE DEVELOPMENT
Cognitive development according to Werner proceeds from undifferentiation to differentiation. The thought of the young child is characterized by *syncretic thinking,* or a tendency to fuse affects, actions, perceptions, and self with objects in the environment. Objects to the young child are not out there, separate and distinct from self and fixed in meaning. Instead objects are permeated with his motor and affective experience of them as well as their sensory qualities. An infant's concept of a bottle may be suck + pleasure + milk + mommy. Objects are conceptualized by the young child in terms of his actions on them as "things of action." A rattle is a "shake and hear noise" and a towel is a "wipe it dry."

Another characteristic of undifferentiated thinking is *physiognomic perception,* or the tendency to perceive the dynamic, rather than the static, qualities of objects. The static details of the object are not perceived by the young child. He responds to the dynamic qualities of the object that speaks out to him of motor and affective experience. A dog is perceived as a thing that barks and bites; a cup lying on its side, as tired; a towel hook, as a cruel thing.

In addition, undifferentiated thinking is also diffuse, or *global.* The young child perceives globs. He may be able to distinguish a cat glob from a dog glob but does not clearly perceive their distinguishing characteristics. He conceives of an object in terms of one or two qualities that are striking and does not clearly perceive the parts of the object and their relation to the whole. Consequently his concept of the object may include only one or two qualities which stand out and take on the character of the whole. Fur and tail may comprise his concept of a cat.

Situations also may be perceived diffusely. Werner (1948) tells of a $4\frac{1}{2}$-year-old boy whose fear of spiders included fear of the spider web and of bits of web that caught onto his clothes. The quality of biting was generalized not only to the spider but to the entire situation. In the doctor's office or hospital the quality of hurting may not simply be associated with the syringe and the needle but may impregnate the whole situation.

Cognitive development not only proceeds from undif-

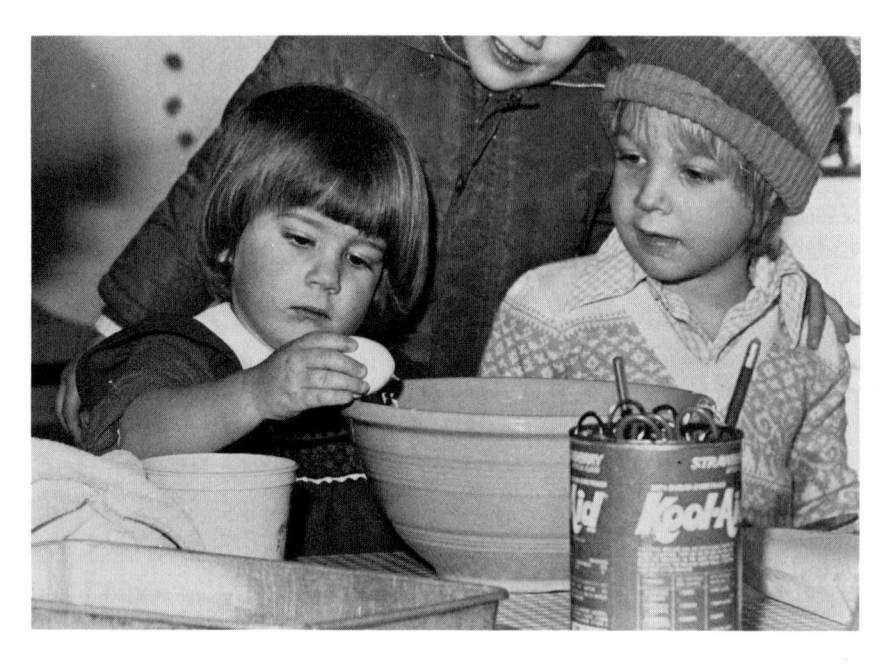

FIGURE 3-11. (*Photo courtesy of Betsy Smith.*)

ferentiation to differentiation but also to *hierarchic organization*. Hierarchic organization is a process by which differentiated parts or elements are organized and subordinated in relation to the whole. Object concepts become centralized as the child recognizes certain essential or central parts or qualities and other parts or qualities that are nonessential or are peripheral. The same child who did not recognize his mother in a hat now recognizes the hat as a nonessential part that does not alter her essential gestalt.

PIAGET'S THEORY OF COGNITIVE DEVELOPMENT

Cognitive development according to Piaget (1954) is characterized by the development and organization of systems of related motor or mental acts in dealing with the environment. The first cognitive structures to develop are a set of motor acts, or *schema*, which the infant uses in interacting with the environment. A schema is a class of similar action sequences, for example, the schema of sucking or the schema of grasping. Each schema includes variations as it is applied to different objects. The sucking schema includes the different forms of sucking inherent in the sucking of different objects like bottles, fingers, and blocks. The cognitive structures that appear later in childhood are a set of mental acts (multiplication, division, ranking, composition of classes) which are used by the child in dealing with the environment.

These sets of mental or motor acts are to Piaget cognitive structures or, actually, the organizational properties of intellectual activity at each age level. They develop and are refined through interaction with the environment. The organizational properties of intelligence change and are discernible as stages in cognitive development.

Cognitive development is a process of adaptation to the environment. It proceeds through the dual processes of assimilation and accommodation (see Fig. 3-12). The child in the process of assimilation generalizes a schema to a new object in the environment. In so doing he incorporates new information about the object and the schema into his meaning system. The infant grasping a ring for the first time learns of its roundness and hollowness and the need to curve his fingers to adapt to its contour. The child in the process of accommodation has assimilated this new information and modifies the schema to accommodate to the newly discovered aspects of reality. The experienced infant now approaches the ring with fingers curved to accommodate to it.

Mental activity involves the assimilation of reality to old schemata and the alteration or accommodation of old schemata to new aspects of reality. Fumbling to unlock an unfamiliar door, one applies the old and familiar schema for unlocking doors. That failing, there follows a trial-and-error period during which one discovers that modification of the old unlocking schema which accommodates to the reality of the unfamiliar door. Cognitive development is characterized by states of equilibrium and disequilibrium in which assimilation and accommodation are alternately in and out of balance. The young infant grasping and mouthing objects is in a state of disequilibrium in which assimilation predominates.

The child in the course of development is continually in the process of seeking a new equilibrium. Confounding the achievement of an equilibrium, or balance between assimilation and accommodation, is the *egocentrism* of the young child. He is egocentric in the sense that he is only aware of his own point of view and is unaware that other points of view exist. Egocentrism favors the dominance of assimilation over accommodation, as the young child is unaware of other points of view and does not question his own. In the middle years the child develops objectivity and becomes aware of his own and others' viewpoints and the inaccuracies of his own thinking. With the development of objectivity, assimilation and accommodation become complementary and balanced.

Cognitive development according to Piaget is characterized by the emergence of qualitatively different cognitive structures (or properties of intelligence) at different

FIGURE 3-12. Assimilation and accommodation.

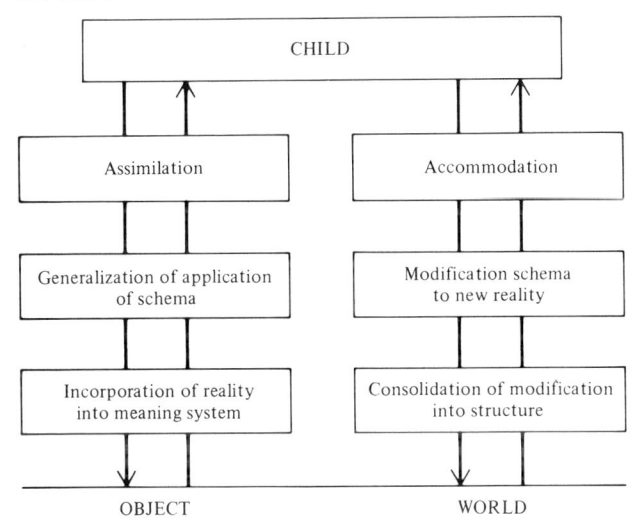

```
                    CHILD
          ↑                    ↑
    Assimilation          Accommodation
          ↑                    ↑
  Generalization of      Modification schema
  application of schema  to new reality
          ↑                    ↑
  Incorporation of reality  Consolidation of modification
  into meaning system       into structure
          ↓                    ↓
        OBJECT              WORLD
```

stages in development. Refer to the previous discussion of Piaget's theory for explanation of these stages.

BRUNER'S THOUGHTS ON COGNITIVE DEVELOPMENT

Cognitive growth according to Bruner (1966) occurs as the result of an internal push and an external pull. The internal push is the will to learn and is similar to competence motivation. It is evident in the young child's impelling curiosity about the world and activity directed toward the achievement of competence. The external pull is stimulation from the environment and culture, a powerful factor in shaping cognitive development. Western culture has developed implementation systems that act as *amplifiers* of people's capacities: amplifiers of motor capacities (the lever and the wheel), amplifiers of sensory capacities (the microscope and radar), and amplifiers of reasoning capacities (language, theories, computers). These amplifiers constitute an external pull and favor the development of an internal organization of motor, perceptual, and reasoning skills that matches their requirements. The culture transmits and selectively stimulates and reinforces in the child those cognitive activities consonant with its requirements.

The child's experience of the world is represented and organized in his mind by three different modes of representation. These modes are *enactive, iconic,* and *symbolic* representation. In the enactive mode the child knows and represents the world in terms of his habitual actions in dealing with it. He knows an object by the usual pattern of action he has mastered in dealing with it. A bed is a lying-down place. In the iconic mode the child represents objects in his mind in pictures, or images, and knows objects by his pictures of them. The young child, seeing an unfamiliar bed, may or may not recognize it depending on whether or not it matches his internal picture of a bed. In the symbolic mode the child represents and describes the object in his mind with words. He may describe the object in terms of its characteristics or his actions upon it, in specific terms (high, hard), or in general terms as one of a class of objects (crib, twin bed).

The purpose of representation is also important. Each mode of representation may be used to facilitate doing or sensing or symbolizing. Symbolic representation, or words, may be used as guides for action, as in recipes or directions. The young child may say "Don't touch my oowie." Words also may be used to describe an object or situation ("It was a big needle." "She stuck me.") or to describe abstract relations between states and processes ("I am sick because my tummy hurts.").

Modes of representation initially operate independently of each other and require integration by the child. When two modes of representation exist parallel to each other, a segment of reality represented in one mode may either match or not match that segment of reality as it is represented in the other mode. A distant light in the night sky may be represented iconically in one's mind as a star. Seeing it move, one senses a mismatch between visual or iconic appearance and the symbolic reality of a star (a fixed or infinitely slowly moving object). Upon further inspection, it proves to be an airplane. When reality, as represented in two systems, does not match, conflict arises. The outcome is either that one system is suppressed or that a correction is made through problem solving. Experience is reorganized and restructured so that reality as represented in different modes is articulated and made congruent.

INFLUENCE OF AFFECT ON COGNITION

The impact of emotion on cognition is not acknowledged by Piaget. Affectivity and cognition are seen by him as complementary processes in which affectivity is the energizer or motivator. Emotions develop but do not intrude upon the cognitive process. Erroneous ideas or distortions in the child's thinking are due to immaturity of his cognitive structures. Freudian theory in contrast explicity points out the effect of strong emotions on thinking. Freud described the deterioration of secondary process thinking (rational, ordered, reasoned thinking) under the impact of strong emotions and the prevalence of primary process thinking (irrational thinking characterized by free association and fantasy) in times of emotional turbulence. In addition Freud described as an ego function the use of defense mechanisms as protection against anxiety. The defense mechanisms (repression, denial, projection) introduce blind spots or distortions of reality into thinking and preclude accurate knowledge of self and the environment. Reduction of anxiety is achieved at the cost of loss of accurate reality perception.

In summary, the function of cognition is adaptation to the environment; cognitive development is characterized by qualitative changes in the properties of intelligence. To the above three theorists the child is an active learner continually engaged in the construction and reconstruction of the reality of his world. They agree that the child brings to this task an increasing capacity to organize, integrate, and articulate his experience in his mind. According to Werner and Piaget the child also brings, in time, a sense of differentiation from the object world that lends him objectivity.

Language development Shirley Joan Lemmon

How children learn to talk is a fascinating and complex developmental process. The dynamics of communication pervade every aspect of human tasks, functions, and interactions. Feelings, ideas, and experiences are conveyed through gesture, motion, body language, and verbal language. Language is a function of communication. Language is a common symbolic communication system with an arbitrary order that allows two or more persons to convey meanings, ideas, feelings, and experiences (Coggins and Carpenter, 1978). It is a phenomenon which begins soon after birth, and although in many ways it continues to develop through life, its essential components are mastered well within the first decade.

Although language has a broad range of variability in the normal population, language also has a predictable sequential development. Language develops horizontally and vertically; there are horizontal lines of complexity of expression and in-depth (vertical) concepts of knowing and understanding symbolic language. These are *expressive* and *receptive* language, respectively.

Before understanding a child's emerging language, one must ask, "What is language?" Language has three overlapping dimensions: *function, form,* and *content.*

THREE LANGUAGE DIMENSIONS

FUNCTION
Function is how language is used. The environmental situation has a strong influence on the function of language. What is the task being performed; what is the surrounding physical environment; what is the topic of conversation; and who are the persons involved? For example, a 3½-year-old child is visiting the zoo with his parents and is interested in gaining information about what is happening. The child has learned to use the question to gain information, which is the function.

FORM (SYNTAX)
Form, or syntax, includes the production of consistent sounds to form words (phonology), rules of grammar, intonation, and stress. The combination of words and parts of words in a child's speech seem to be systematic rather than random and productive rather than merely imitative or rote-learned (McNeil, 1971). The vast majority of syntax has unfolded in children by the age of 5 years.

CONTENT (SEMANTICS)
Content, or semantics, refers to relationships and meanings of words. Syntax is very closely tied to semantics.

INTERACTION OF LANGUAGE DIMENSIONS
The most current research in the field of language acquisition focuses on the interaction and relationship between these three overlapping dimensions of language: function, form (syntax), and content (semantics). At one time emphasis in the study of child language was on the spoken word exclusively, and language development was described as the acquisition of the form of language (Bloom, 1976). At the end of the 1960s, researchers realized that children do not learn form alone; they learn form to represent content. Thus, learning the content of language is as much a part of language development as learning the form of language. Again in the 1970s there was a change in emphasis away from manners of form and content in language toward the goal of the acquisition of language use.

The integration of content, form, and function makes up language competence, or knowledge. One authority states, "Such knowledge can be conceived of as a plan for the behaviors involved in speaking and understanding messages. There is a mutual influence between plan and behaviors. At the same time that the plan directs the behaviors, it is evolving and changing as a result of those behaviors. Children learn language as they use language: both to produce and understand messages" (Bloom and Lahey, 1978, p. 23). A child's communication is constantly shifting and not only relates to what he understands in form, content, and use but is also contingent upon the extent to which the child is motivated to communicate.

Language acquisition or, more specifically, vocabulary growth, phonology, relationship of words (semantics), grammar (syntax), and the function of language are processes learned within a social context. Language also implies that there are aspects of intrapersonal relations between thought and language: linguistic behaviors and nonlinguistic behaviors such as perceptual support and adaptation to the needs of the listener. These interactions between the three forms of language relate to both understanding and speaking receptive and expressive language.

For the purpose of research and assessment, the three dimensions may be considered separately; for the child the three components come together in the process of language learning. The three dimensions have a predictable sequence; however, they do not progress evenly, and the rate at which a child acquires language and how language is used are variable.

VARIABLES AFFECTING LANGUAGE DEVELOPMENT

In considering the developmental process of language acquisition, two important factors should be considered: the rapid growth of language skill and the many variables that influence how the child uses language to communicate to others.

Variables in language acquisition cannot be discussed in detail within this text; however, the following aspects of the child and environment that facilitate language acquisition and communication should be considered:

- Cognitive development: Especially in the first 2 years of life, cognitive development is of major importance to language development. In fact, it is impossible to fully separate the two processes. Researchers in language development are particularly interested in a child's concepts related to object permanence, means-to-end activity (goal-directed activity), and imitation skills.
- Motor development: During the first 2 years of life motor development is especially important for readiness to utilize a symbolic system language. The child who is free from physical constraints of immaturity and his volitional movement will have a rich interaction with the environment. Children need this continuous experience with objects and persons to begin to identify similar as well as unique characteristics of objects and regularities in the world.
- Environmental stimulation: Sensory input and the moment-to-moment experience of the child are very important to language development. The integrity of all sensory modalities and how stimuli are integrated and processed influence language acquisition. Environment is culturally bound and for the young child is largely determined by the parents.
- Parent-child interaction: Parent-child interaction is the fourth critical variable in language acquisition. In the 1970s there was a flourish of research activity and clinical interest in the richness of the dynamics of parent-child interaction. How interaction specifically influences a child's development has not been wholly defined. The research generally investigates infant characteristics; few studies have been done in terms of sequence interaction between parent and child. How different styles of interaction between parent and child influence the child's use of language as a communicative form should be the subject of future study.

The rate of linguist acquisition is probably determined by a combination of level of maturation and environment; the richness of communication and quality of linguistic ability may depend more directly on environmental input, or social content.

An enlarging field of research in language acquisition deals with pragmatics in which language is seen primarily as a social act. Any utterance of the child needs to be interpreted as having two parts: the *proposition* representing the semantic content (meaning) of the sentence and the *performative* or *elocutionary force,* which specifies how the content is to be taken by the listener.

The younger the child and the less complete the form of verbal communication, the closer the listener must attend to other cues within the environment because of the lack of elocutionary force. These cues are intonational patterns of the vocalization and what the child is doing. The closer the child's communication to the adult model, the less the listener has to rely on other situational cues to determine what the child is trying to communicate.

THEORIES AND CONCEPTS OF LANGUAGE ACQUISITION

The impetus to study a child's emerging language was the realization by researchers that children speak their own language (Dale, 1972). In other words, a child's language is not simply a version of adult language. There are two predominant theories of language acquisition. One is that language is universal. The child develops language because he is innately equipped to do so. The environment helps him further structure a task that is built into the biological-neurological mechanism. The other theory is one of stimulus-response mode of language acquisition.

The infant's communication style, especially in relation to cognition, motor development, and social interaction, is a focus of recent research. The toddler presents a rapid change in acquisition of language and communication. There is strong evidence that by $2\frac{1}{2}$ years of age the child understands the rudiments of content, form, and function of language; he has progressed from having about 10 words at 15 months to beginning to use 2- to 3-word phrases with a lexicon (vocabulary) of 275 words by 3 years of age. The 3-year-old uses language to express experience of the here and now and can talk about past events, can anticipate events, can gain new information by asking questions, and can use language to facilitate social interaction.

Children during the preschool years have increased sophistication in the basics of language. They have concepts relating to time, quantity, and qualities of objects, such as size, shape, and use, and they can provide verbal information in relation to their experiences. Vocabulary growth continues to increase to 1500 to 2500 words.

The school-age child is faced with additional academic experiences that will require elaborate use of communication: reading, writing, and expressing ideas that will facilitate his ability to expand knowledge as well as engage in more cooperative social interaction.

Self-help skill development and independent functioning Doris Julian

The acquisition of skills necessary for the care of basic physical needs is a primary task of children as they move toward functioning as independent beings in their environment. An optimal goal of families is to promote those abilities and attitudes which permit all of its members to function adequately within the immediate family and, later, the community. This acculturation process leads the child to an eventual independence from care givers and a productive role within society.

PRINCIPLES OF SELF-HELP SKILL DEVELOPMENT

Self-help skill development in general encompasses the abilities to do the following:

- Feed oneself using appropriate utensils and equipment
- Recognize internal cues for elimination and attend to toileting needs
- Manipulate clothing and fastenings for undressing and dressing and choose clothing appropriate for the activity and weather
- Care for personal grooming (face and hand cleaning and later bathing and the care of hair, teeth, and nails)

Advanced abilities are added as the child's dexterity and discrimination improve. These include the following:

- Care of personal belongings such as toys and clothing
- Care of bedroom or personal space
- Contribution to broader family needs through assisting with household-maintenance chores

FOUNDATIONS FOR OPTIMAL DEVELOPMENT OF SELF-HELP SKILLS

A number of factors contribute to optimal development of self-help skills in the young child. These same factors are operative from infancy through the early adolescent years, at which time the individual assumes increasing initiative for learning new tasks. Self-help skills are most readily learned when these conditions exist:

- An appropriate level of physiological maturation
- A state of cognitive and psychological readiness
- An environment conducive to skill learning

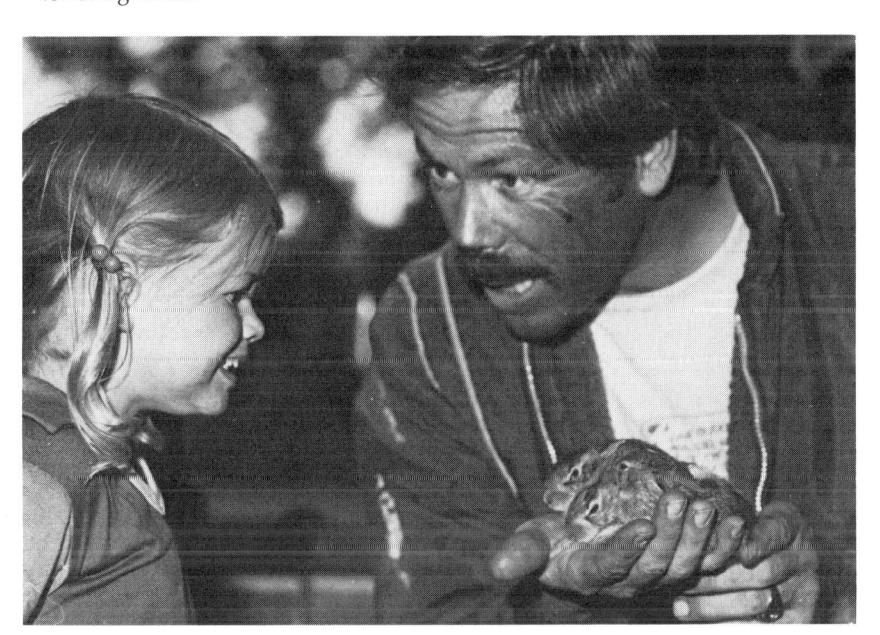

FIGURE 3-13. (*Photo courtesy of Betsy Smith.*)

The first two factors are specific to the child, and the third pertains to the child's total environment of people, objects, and setting.

Physiological maturation Physiological maturation incorporates components of central nervous system maturation with concomitant sensory-motor integration. The relevance of this to self-help skill acquisition can be illustrated by describing sensory-motor prerequisites for a skill achieved early: independent eating.

For independence in eating to occur, the young child must have achieved a level of physiological maturation permitting head, neck, trunk, and upper extremity control. Arm and hand control must be such that the child can manipulate finger foods or eating utensils. In addition, the child must develop sensory integration to permit visual fixation and necessary eye-hand coordination to complete the task. Thus, physiological maturation, viewed as complex central nervous system integration, is a prerequisite to and determines readiness for specific self-help skill acquisition.

Cognitive and psychological readiness Additional aspects of readiness are those of cognitive ability and psychological motivation. Although interrelated, these two factors are not considered synonymous. Certainly, a child's ability to function within a mental or cognitive potential can be influenced by psychological or emotional factors. Such factors can have a negative or positive impact on learning ability. A key element influencing these aspects of readiness is sensitivity of the environment to the individual child's learning potential and emotional needs. The reciprocal impact of the child on the environment (animate and inanimate) is a significant part of this consideration (Escalona, 1968; Lewis, 1971; Thomas, Birch, Chess, Hertzog, and Koru, 1963; Westman, 1973).

Consideration of individual difference in learning ability is important in promoting development of self-care skills. A range of abilities in all attributes assigned to cognition (memory, recall, problem solving, abstract thinking, judgment, and discrimination) are typically found in any sample of children of a specific chronological age.

Communicative abilities parallel cognitive development. In learning rules and classifying and organizing experiences, cognition and communication may demonstrate equivalent growth (Striffler, 1976). A child's level of competence in communication, nonverbal as well as verbal, will therefore be a helpful clue in determining ability to understand and follow through with a task expectation.

Parental attitudes The above discussion is concerned with factors related to the child's development which are considerations in facilitating self-help skill development. Parental perception of individual developmental differences is also a part of this process. Parents bring to their roles of care givers, nurturers, and teachers a wide variety of backgrounds and skills. Appreciation of this diversity is as essential as awareness of individual differences in their children. No single variable can be identified as the most significant attribute of a parent for effective teaching of facilitating self-help skill development. However, parents who have achieved the following goals in relation to their overall role will have a useful framework for assisting the child:

- *A trust in personal capacity to be a parent.* This may be based on previous parenting activities, including sibling or child-care responsibilities or prolonged contact with an individual identified as a positive model for parenting. The significance of role models as a basis for acquiring a frame of reference is described by social-learning theorists Bandura and Walters and others.
- *Recognition of the child as a separate individual in relation to other family members.* This perception permits the parent to view the child, not as a personal extension, but as a quite special and unique individual with distinctive qualities and needs unlike any other family member. Recognition that each child is different from siblings, children in the neighborhood, and youthful relatives is essential in supporting personal differences in abilities and methods of learning new tasks.
- *Recognition of independence as a desirable goal of child rearing.* Parents with attitudes based on their own experiences, needs, and values may have varying goals for achievement of independence by their children. This may range from an expectation of very early assumption of total self-responsibility on the part of the child to a prolonged delay (postteens) in permitting appropriate independence. Although desirable levels of self-responsibility will relate to the individual child's capacities and circumstances, parental facilitation of gradually decreasing dependence can be seen as a desirable goal in child rearing.

FACTORS INFLUENCING DEVELOPMENT OF SELF-HELP SKILLS

CHILD'S ENVIRONMENT

Although parental attitudes are viewed as major factors in promoting self-help skill development, the child's environment makes a significant contribution also. The importance of a setting which provides the child with material to practice skill acquisition cannot be overlooked. Toys or household items can serve as props for exploration, manipulation, and problem solving of the relation of objects to tasks of self-care.

Contact with children the same age or older has proved helpful in demonstrating steps needed in acquiring a skill. If there are no siblings in the home, parents may be alerted to the value of encouraging exchange visits with other children and may find specific skills more readily learned with the help of child models. Well-planned daycare and preschool programs incorporate self-care competencies as part of the daily curriculum and capitalize on peer influence in promoting such skills.

CULTURAL INFLUENCES

Home, school, and day care as learning environments for the child are all influenced by the broader culture of which they are a part. Cultural expectations play a major role in defining the specifics of when and how a self-help skill is introduced (Whiting, 1973). Because of the multiplicity of factors implied in the term culture, consideration must be given to ethnic origin, economic status, and the general heritage of religious and social values as contributors to socialization practice (Spencer, 1964). As depicted in Fig. 3-14, self-care skills as well as other behaviors are an outgrowth of cultural values and socialization practices. Self-care skill abilities, sex-role expectations, relationship styles, and communication patterns all constitute essential components of the foundation needed for independence.

CONTEMPORARY TRENDS

No discussion of general considerations for self-help skill development and ultimate independent functioning would be complete without noting changing trends in child-rearing practices of families in the United States. Today's child may be reared by a variety of care givers in group care as well as home settings. The family may be limited to parents and siblings if other relatives are geographically isolated.

An additional trend is an increase in the number of families with a single parent. A child may be exposed to a variety of models and stimulation, as television, movies, and a large variety of printed material become a part of the child's daily world. As Yarrow notes, "Today's children are reared by more influences and fewer significant persons" (1973, p. 209). An understanding of these multiple influences and contemporary trends is essential in identifying those factors which would most facilitate a child's movement toward independence.

In summary, acquisition of self-help skills is strongly influenced by the child's state of readiness, the parent or care giver's ability to promote optimal independence based on cues provided by the child, and an environment contributing opportunity and support. Age-related considerations are discussed in following chapters.

Social development Susan Blanch Meister

THE BASIS OF SOCIALIZATION

Socialization is a lifelong process—one that is traced along generations, found in cross-cultural study, and personally experienced. It is an underlying theme which runs throughout human development. Its nature, processes, and effects have been most extensively studied in the childhood period of human development.

The basis of socialization lies in *interaction*. Interaction can be considered a process in and of itself. Rosenthal (1969) encouraged conceptualization of the *open system* of interaction. An example of an open system would be a

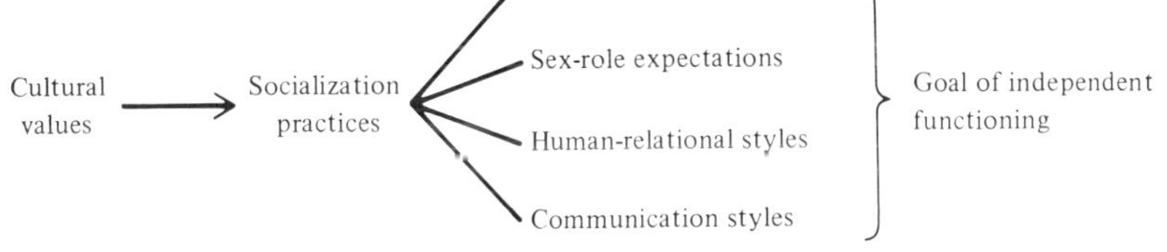

FIGURE 3-14. Relationship of culture to growth of independence. (*Adapted from M. Ramirez, III, and A. Castenoda, Cultural democracy, bicognitive development and education. New York: Academic, 1974, p. 60.*)

situation in which the child relates to the parent, the child's reactions affect the parent, the parent reacts to the child in a new way, and the entire cycle repeats itself, but on a new level (see Fig. 3-15).

It is clear that interaction is a concept which includes the idea of mutual effect. The child may have interactions with parents, siblings, peers, and the inanimate environment. The actual importance or impact of each type of interaction varies throughout childhood. When all four interactions are placed into the mutual-effect cycle, an abstraction of the context of the socialization process of childhood is designed (see Fig. 3-16).

Mary Ainsworth's (1974) approach represents a central school of thought regarding goals of socialization. She adopts the stance that children enter the world with a predisposition to become social adults. In other words, the naturally occurring social experiences of children interact with the tendency to become social, and the result is effective social development.

Within this framework, the goal of socialization becomes very clear. Socialization is not purely a process of transforming an asocial newborn into a social person. Rather, the goal of socialization is to promote the natural tendency toward social development.

This promotion occurs along several lines. The child learns about affective relationships, moral behavior, empathic responses, and gender identity. Socialization promotes development along these lines.

Several concepts are essential components of social development. One such concept is readiness. A child is a complex, total being. Development within each component of that total being affects development in all other components. All components are not bound to a rigid and harmonious rate of development; a child may advance in some areas prior to other areas. Therefore, social development will occur at various rates and in variant patterns in individual children.

Another essential concept is that of sociocultural environment, or milieu. The child lives within an environment and is, therefore, in continual interaction with it (note that in Fig. 3-16 "environment-child" comprises one cell of mutual effect). Sociocultural milieu influences the child's development. On the other hand, the child's level of development will also affect the nature of the sociocultural milieu which a child experiences (Parsons and Bryan, 1978). The environment plays a dual role in social development: It encourages continued development, and it concurrently supports the child's present level of development.

A third concept underlying social development is that of social learning. Through experiences with a broad range of social learning, the child proceeds with a broad scope of social development (note that in Fig. 3-16 "parent-child," "sibling-child," and "peer-child" comprise three cells of mutual effect). It is important to recognize that differences exist between these relationships and that the nature of early affective relationships will be related to the *specific* differences an individual child experiences.

A final note on the goals of socialization concerns the role of the society in which it occurs. Social development will reflect the goals of the greater social environment. When cross-cultural, cross-class and cross-race comparisons are made, differences in both rate and content of social development are found. Note that this variance is a *difference;* deficits in socialization rate and content are validly measured only within a group of children who at least share culture, class, and race membership.

PROCESSES INVOLVED IN SOCIALIZATION

Socialization has been noted to be a process which occurs throughout life. The tremendous impact of socialization is

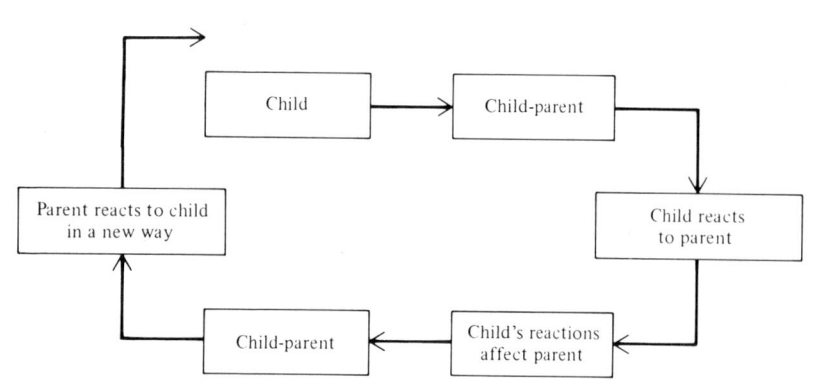

FIGURE 3-15. Open system of interaction. *(After M. K. Rosenthal, The study of infant-environment interaction: Some comments on trends and methodologies. J. Child Psychiat., 1969, 14, 301–317.)*

Parent-child (mutual effect)	Sibling-child (mutual effect)
Peer-child (mutual effect)	Environment-child (mutual effect)

FIGURE 3-16. Context of the socialization process.

generated by the many processes which occur within its boundaries. The contributing processes which are discussed as part of social development are the development of attachment, the emergence of moral internalization and empathy, and the learning of gender identity, or sex role.

ATTACHMENT

Attachment is a social relationship which develops over time. Its emergence can be tracked during the first year of life, but it is important to recognize that attachment behaviors rather than the attachment relationship itself are observed. Attachment behaviors have been defined in many ways. Cohen (1974) defined them as the behaviors which are stimulated by a small number of familiar people and are notably more intense and frequent than other behaviors. Ainsworth (1972) defined attachment behaviors in a broader sense; she constructed them as behaviors which establish a relationship. This relationship is affectional, differential, and discriminating.

Attachment may be viewed as an interactive relationship which includes specific people. Attachment behaviors are used in two ways: to draw specific people into physical proximity and to intensify the relationship. For example, a crying infant draws its parents into close proximity; an infant's smile is highly valued by the parents.

Bowlby (1969) has been a major force in emphasizing the use of attachment behaviors to draw the members of the relationship together. He argued that the defenseless infant requires protection in order to survive and that this protection must be provided by someone other than the infant. Therefore, attachment to an adult would be highly adaptive for the infant. Using attachment behaviors, the infant could draw adult attachment figures closer and thus be nourished and kept warm, dry, and safe. Maintaining proximity to adults meets the early survival needs of an infant.

When individual attachment relationships are examined, great differences are usually seen which have long-range effects upon social development. These differences are presented in following chapters. At this point, attachment is considered as an affective, interactive relationship, and attachment behaviors as powerful, effective mechanisms.

MORAL INTERNALIZATION

Moral standards are not part of the neonate's makeup; they are developed through socialization. Moral development includes a second, crucial element; the standards cannot be simply learned, because if they were learned in the same manner as, say, table manners, they could be easily violated or forgotten. Social control is highly dependent upon the moral actions of society's members. Moral development must include acquisition of an internal motivation to comply with learned moral standards. This internal acquisition is moral internalization.

Hoffman (1970) defined three types of moral internalization. One type is primitive and based upon conditioned fear or anxiety. For example, if a child is repeatedly punished for an act, the child learns to avoid punishment by avoiding the act itself. The child has acquired fear of punishment rather than a motivation to comply with moral standards.

The second type of internalization is based upon the child's relationship with a respected person. The child identifies with this person and learns to believe in that person's standards. The child will comply with these standards, even when the valued person is absent, out of an internalized sense of obligation to the person, not the standards.

The third and most advanced type of internalization requires a developmental ability to judge right and wrong. At this level of development, a child considers the moral standards and accepts them. These standards become part of the self (rather than part of a respected other), and the child acquires the motivation to comply.

In following chapters, this process of internalization will be further discussed. Parental discipline techniques and their effects will also be examined. At this point, moral internalization is defined as a process of socialization which is intimately bound to the child's relationships, experiences, and other developmental capabilities.

EMPATHY

Empathy is a social response experienced by a person who has learned that other people exist (social cognition) and recognizes the feelings of others in a situation (affective learning). When this person experiences a desire to help distressed others, regardless of reward (altruistic motivation), he demonstrates empathic response.

Development of empathy is a particularly clear example of the interdependent nature of child development. Empathy is part of social development, but it requires advances in several other areas of development. One such area is cognitive development. In order to experience and act upon empathy, the child must be capable of thinking about other people. The child must acquire social cognition: the cognitive ability to attend to, receive, and process information about other people (Shantz, 1975).

The development of empathy also requires specific social learning. Affective cues from others serve as a stimulus for empathic or helping behaviors. The child must learn to recognize and interpret these affective cues prior to demonstrating empathic development (Bryan, 1975). The concept of motivation bridges social cognition and response to affective cues. What is it that stimulates a child to help another when neither reward nor recognition are likely? Hoffman (1975) calls this component of empathy "altruistic motivation." His conceptual framework of the development of altruistic motivation is discussed in Sec. 3.

At this point, empathy is considered to be comprised of three elements: social cognition, affective learning, and altruistic motivation. Development of empathy is clearly related to many other developmental processes and is examined in following chapters.

GENDER IDENTITY AND SEX ROLE

Development of gender identity and the corollary process of sex-role socialization are multifaceted concepts. Both involve learning from many sources. Two major sources for such learning are significant others, especially parents, and social systems.

Developmental theorists differ in their descriptions of how and why gender-linked learning occurs. In later sections, discussion will include the role of the parents as "trainers" and sex-type "labelers" (Mussen, 1969). Theories of sex-linked differential treatment of children (Hoffman, 1972) will also be examined.

One aspect of gender identity development is the effect of significant others. The child's unique relationships with mother, father, siblings, and peers contribute to gender identity (Hetherington, 1965; Johnson, 1971; Lamb, 1978b) and will be examined in later chapters. Development of gender identity and sex role are vital components of socialization, and the results of this development will accompany the child throughout the life cycle.

EFFECT OF CHILDREN ON PARENTS

An introduction to social development of children must include recognition of their effect upon their parents.

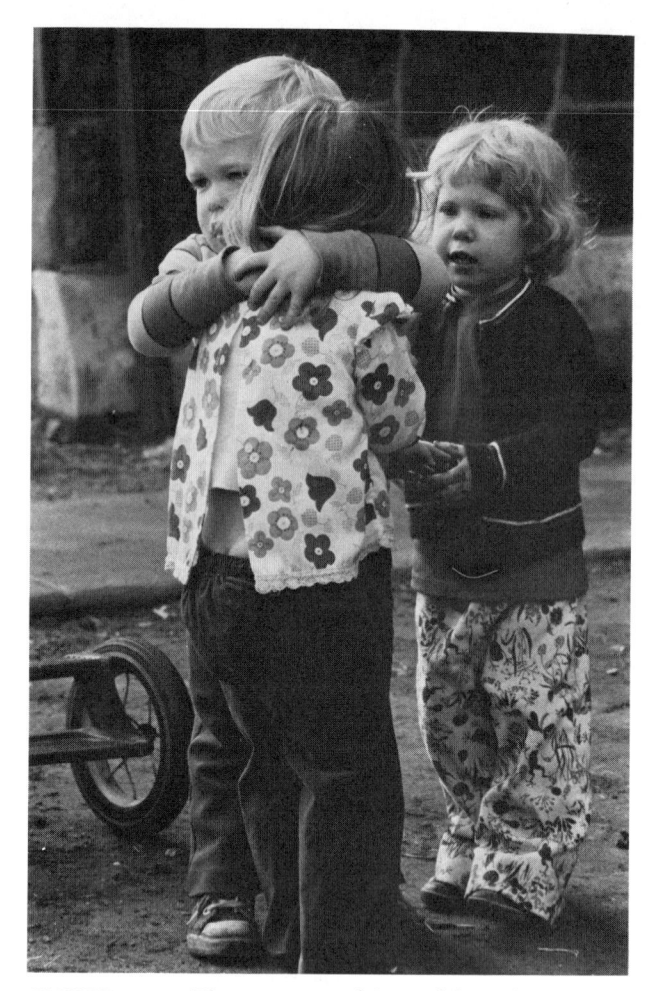

FIGURE 3-17. *(Photo courtesy of Armand Scavo.)*

Children become salient elements in the parents' own contexts of social development. Parents are involved in at least two socialization processes: socialization of their children and continuing their own adult socialization.

It seems likely that these two socialization processes may exist as conflicting or concordant parental experiences. The developmental needs and abilities of children may exist in conflict or concordance with the developmental needs and abilities of their parents. In the case of concordance the child acquires an additional value—one of fostering and supporting the parent's own development. There is a paucity of research in this area; however, this potential effect remains a hypothesis worthy of further study as well as a consideration in the developmental assessment of children.

SIBLING RELATIONSHIPS

Studies of sibling relationships represent a maturation of the older concepts of birth order and ordinal position. These older concepts made an important contribution in terms of definitions. Birth order is simply that: listing siblings in the order of their birth. Birth order becomes ordinal position when the child's gender and age as well as the gender of adjacent siblings are identified (Krout, 1939). In this movement to go beyond simply listing children in order of birth, these early works offer indications of the complexity of factors related to sibling relationships.

A major component of the sibling relationship is ongoing proximity. This is a major component because of sibling care giving. *Proximity* occurs in many cultures (Weisner and Gallimore, 1977). This proximity is characterized by two factors: it occurs within the family, and it involves an element of ongoing responsibility. These characteristics are important in differentiating peer and sibling relationships, relationships founded on very different rules. A child is freer to fight with and reject a peer than to fight with and reject a sibling. The proximity of siblings is colored by its origin in the family in that family membership is nonchanging and a sufficient condition for sibling interaction.

Family structure includes several implications for sibling relationships. The family represents at least three sets of *generational influences* for a child: the parent generation, the intergenerational relationship (parent-child), and the intragenerational relationship (sibling). The influence of siblings is grounded in regular, intimate contact which is long-standing in nature. Intragenerational relationships are most likely to continue through the entire life span. It may be that these early relationships between siblings are responsible for the continuity of family sentiments and solidarity (Irish, 1964).

In fact, siblings form the major portion of the "family peer group." They have the potential to serve as models, confidants, pacesetters, and teachers for each other (Cicirelli, 1977a). This potential is facilitated by the frequency of interaction within the family as well as by the fact that siblings share dominant socializers—parents. The power of the sibling relationship is second only to that of the mother-child relationship (Irish, 1964) and, hence, carries great influence over the life span.

Through ongoing interaction and social learning, the child uses siblings as a means of self-definition (Davis and Northway, 1957). This process within sibling interaction is also affected by other family members. For example, parents are active in defining sibling relations; their responses to each child affect the siblings' responses to each other (Lamb, 1977). Perhaps this parental factor accounts, in part, for the individual nature of children in the same family. Individuation is one of the most interesting aspects of sibling relationships. It implies a specialization of sibling *roles*: each child develops a role which is related to, but not redundant with, roles already in existence in the family (Bossard and Boll, 1955).

Role emphasizes diversity in effects of sibling relations. Roles are highly complex, mutually interactive components of the person. Therefore, roles which are mutually developed between siblings are more likely to be related to an interaction of factors rather than to direct effects. For example, the effectiveness of helping is related to the ordinal positions of the siblings. However, it is not simply a situation of older sibling helping younger sibling being more effective than the converse. The *width* of the age difference is a critical variable related to effectiveness of helping (Cicirelli, 1974). This example points out an interaction effect rather than a direct effect.

As noted, sibling relationships extend across the life span. The elderly person reports expanded kin networks but also reserves a special solidarity with siblings (Cumming and Schneider, 1961). There is evidence of differential response to male versus female siblings during childhood, and the elderly appear to maintain a differentiation in feelings about brothers and sisters (Cicirelli, 1977b).

The effects of sibling relationships are not fully understood; current research is directed at increasing knowledge. At this time it is known that the sibling relationship carries powerful effects, but the nature and outcome of such power is uncertain. For example, there is evidence that a younger sibling in a cross-sex dyad is likely to demonstrate some degree of androgyny (Brim, 1958), but life-span effects of this androgyny are unknown.

Studies of adolescents have demonstrated wide variability in sibling relationships. Adolescents reveal trends in feelings for brothers and sisters, but these trends are weakened in various family sizes (Bowerman and Dobash, 1974). This is an example of another set of unknowns in describing sibling relations: the factors which affect the quality of the relationship itself.

It may be best to summarize sibling relations and their effects in a more general fashion. Siblings share many experiences, including play. Through play, they not only acquire skills but more importantly learn about the establishment and maintenance of social relations. Significant emotional ties are developed, and children learn to receive and offer influence through their relationships with siblings. In short, the sibling relationship is both a mediator and an active force in a child's world (Lewis and Feiring, 1979). Beyond this capsule summary, one must consider the all-important factor of subjectivity. It is the individual child and setting which play a major role in determining the actual effects of sibling relationships.

In summary, socialization has been presented as a life cycle experience. The overall goal of socialization has been identified as promotion of the natural tendency to become social. One significant process of socialization is development of attachment. A second is emergence of moral internalization. A third process is development of empathy, and a fourth is acquisition of gender identity and sex role. Parent-child developmental matches or mismatches are powerful factors within the interactions of social development. Sibling relationships also play a significant role in social development.

SECTION 3
Assessment of Behavioral Development

The above theories and principles of behavioral development, as overall concepts as well as in specific areas of functioning, provide a framework for professional nursing in the field of child development. Application of these principles in assessment of child behavior, an initial step in the nursing process, is presented in the following section.

Behavioral assessment Ruth Hepler

Children's behavior often serves as an important indicator of their reactions to situations or their perceptions of factors within a situation. Behavioral assessment, in conjunction with its correlate, physical assessment, has become a recognized component of the total health care of the developing child. Child health care is often anticipatory guidance offered to prevent development of physical or behavioral disorders. Such guidance is based on an awareness of the child's current level of physical and behavioral functioning acquired through systematic methods of assessment. Basic considerations in the assessment of behavior include an awareness of behavioral "norms," the consideration of all the individuals involved in the assessment process, the appropriateness of the assessment method, and the limitations of behavioral assessment.

IMPLICATIONS OF BEHAVIOR
Behavior may be simply defined as any observable activity, or response of an organism. Human behavior includes such responses as talking, playing, working, crying, laughing, sleeping, and eating. The way a child reacts to a situation is inferred primarily from his behavior. Such abstract conceptualizations of reactions as fear, excitement, and confusion all have related, often culturally defined, behavioral correlates by which they are identified. For instance, young children may be said to demonstrate fear in a situation if they display behaviors such as crying and clinging to mother.

SIGNIFICANCE OF BEHAVIORAL NORMS
Acceptance of the proposition that "normal" behavior assumes characteristic patterns that differ according to developmental stage is basic to the conduct of appropriate, meaningful assessment of children's behavior. Evidence obtained from numerous studies of the process of behavioral development supports a concept of behavioral norms: the presence of average, age-related trends in behavior.

Although behavioral assessment will always be lacking in precision because of the absence of absolute (unvarying) units of behavior, established behavioral norms serve as available, reliable standards against which observed behavior can be measured. An illustration of the use of behavioral norms in assessment is presented in terms of the observation of behavior related to stranger anxiety. One infant reacts to a stranger by crying and clinging to the parent, avoiding contact with the stranger. A second infant reacts by smiling, reaching out for the stranger, and babbling. It can be said that the behavior of the second infant was more positive and sociable. When behavioral norms are consulted, however, it is found that indiscriminate, apparently "accepting" behavior occurring in response to people is characteristic of infants prior to 5 or 6 months of age and that stranger anxiety is characteristic of infants at about 8 months of age.

In terms of this norm, if the infant who demonstrated stranger acceptance is 8 months of age, he may be considered abnormal with respect to this feature of social behavior. If, however, the infant is 3 months of age, his behavior is considered normal. Of course, sociocultural factors must be considered. For example, if the 8-month-old has multiple care givers, his behavior may be interpreted differently. Thus, assessment of behavior is based on observed responses considered in terms of age-related, culturally appropriate norms of behavior. The necessity of continued assessment of behavior over time (longitudinal study) is an important implication of this concept of age-related norms of child behavior.

GENERAL CONSIDERATIONS

ESTABLISHING RAPPORT WITH CHILDREN
The ability to establish with children relationships that have positive effects is necessary for conducting objective-assessment procedures as well as for forming interactive relationships. An awareness of behavioral norms is once again an important consideration.

Recognition of the vulnerability of children's behavior to a number of variables is a basic assumption of the assessment process. Although many variables are beyond the assessor's control, the important variable of the influence resulting from the presence of people, including the person conducting the assessment, can be at least partially controlled. Knowledge of norms of social responsiveness of children is crucial. At almost any stage of development the "too-intrusive" adult can exert significant influence on a child's behavior.

Awareness of a child's unique characteristics, such as language skills and his home environment, facilitates formation of adult-child relationships that are conducive to behavioral assessment. Such awareness enables the assessor to plan and conduct assessment procedures which are more easily tolerated by the child.

RECOGNITION OF PARENTS AND SIGNIFICANT OTHERS

The recognition of parents and significant others in the behavioral assessment of children has implications for the quality of the procedure as well as for the eventual utilization of information which has been collected. In most cases parents represent the constant feature in a child's experience and environment and thus must be included as active participants in the assessment process.

In an ongoing assessment of behavioral development, parents' assistance can be enlisted to observe and document the occurrence of changes in response patterns demonstrated by the child. Utilizing the parent-child relationship is an important means of increasing the quality and reliability of behavioral-assessment procedures. Parents can provide data that are collected consistently over time periods that usually exceed those available to the outside observer.

Another important consideration related to parental involvement in behavioral assessment is that of the responsibility parents must accept for implementing any development-facilitating program based on the results of the assessment. Planned parental involvement in some way throughout the assessment process is a vital factor in the effective behavioral assessment of the growing child.

METHODOLOGICAL CONSIDERATIONS

A basic consideration regarding method of behavioral assessment is defining a purpose for the assessment. Behavior is a dynamic, complex phenomenon that can be observed along many dimensions at almost any time. An efficient approach to assessment of behavior is one based on the assessor's awareness of the most specific, significant behavior to be considered and the persons or circumstances surrounding that behavior.

After the purpose, or focus, of the assessment is identified, choosing an appropriate method is a subsequent concern. The major consideration is whether the method will provide answers to questions raised about the child's behavior. If, for example, questions have been raised about the child's general developmental level, the nurse would select an appropriate, standardized developmental screening test rather than carry out observation of the child in a nonstructured situation.

A related consideration is that of the feasibility of the method. The assessor must address such questions as the following: What is the cost of the method? Is special equipment required? How much time will be involved? Can the method be conducted easily, or are special arrangements required? Am I qualified to administer the test and interpret the results?

LIMITATIONS

A significant characteristic of behavioral assessment is its status as a still somewhat imprecise endeavor susceptible to experimental or observer errors. Physical assessment is guided by definite parameters such as temperature, height, weight, and pulse rate. While the field of developmental psychology provides an ever-increasing data base of phases and features of behavioral development, interpretation of such data is subject to the consideration of numerous intervening variables that can directly or indirectly affect behavioral response.

Another important consideration in behavioral assessment is the necessity for the development of specific examiner skills related to the measurement and interpretation of behavior. Although behavioral assessment can be accomplished to some degree through such means as direct observation and reporting, many of the techniques available for systematic analysis of behavior require specific training and certification of the personnel authorized to use them.

THE PROCESS OF BEHAVIORAL ASSESSMENT

METHODS OF BEHAVIORAL ASSESSMENT

Systematic methods of behavioral assessment range in form from recording observations of behavior in nonstructured situations to general screening procedures to measuring specific areas of functioning, such as intelligence, by means of a highly structured test or measure. Awareness of assessment measures and specific considerations relative to their use are important adjuncts of effective work with children.

Observational techniques A basic and readily available means of assessing behavior is through observation. Observation of behavior can be conducted in a variety of ways ranging from casual to planned. Casual observation, although the term might seem to imply a nonrigorous effort, actually requires a high level of awareness of child development, which enables the observer to be instantly aware of developmental discrepancies. Observations of this sort are best made in the natural setting, such as the child's home or school. Observation can also occur, however, in settings such as the hospital or clinic.

Planned observations require more time and have become an important part of overall developmental assessment. Methods of planned observation include (1) descriptive techniques, such as diaries; (2) sampling techniques, in which selected times or events specify the behaviors observed; and (3) various rating techniques, such as behavioral checklists, which the observer uses to structure observations.

Descriptive observational techniques consist of carefully recording everything the child does. Such observations may be carried out over long periods of time (the diary method) or in relation to a particular section of a child's activity (the specimen method).

Sampling techniques are also used in observational assessment procedures. In event sampling, a particular behavior is specified (e.g., thumb-sucking) and each time the behavior occurs during the observation period a record is made of its occurrence and the circumstances surrounding it. In time-sampling methods, a particular behavior is identified, and observations are made at specified time intervals (e.g., every 10 s). A record is kept of the presence or absence of the behavior every tenth second.

Measures of intensity or severity of a particular behavior are often achieved through the use of observations utilizing rating scales. In this method a behavior is identified, and the possible range of that behavior, from its absence to its most marked presentation, is specified. The assessor then checks the degree of demonstration of that behavior in the child's observed activity.

Although observational methods are among the most widely used assessment techniques, important limitations must be recognized. The use of human perception and judgment in observational methods predisposes such methods to bias and inaccuracy. The danger of seeing what one is "looking for," a particular bias, is an ever-present one. Recording exactly and only what is seen without the use of interpretive language is a basic guideline for the observer. The following examples of recordings of observations illustrate the importance of this consideration:

Example 1
Child pulls chair around playroom. Mother asks child to "leave chair alone." Child continues pulling chair around room. Mother leaves playroom. Child continues pulling chair around.

Example 2
Child pulls chair around playroom. Does not hear mother ask him to "leave chair alone." Child continues pulling chair. Does not hear mother leave room.

Example 1 represents a straightforward recording of the actual behavior observed. In example 2 the observer demonstrates the inclusion of a bias, in this case "deafness," as a contaminant of the observation.

Another inherent problem in observational methods is the effect of the observation process on the behavior of the child being observed. A method of countering this effect in observations is to allow the child time to adjust to the situation, including the presence of the observer, before recording of observations is initiated.

Formal measures of behavior In an effort to overcome, or at least control, some of the problems of observational methods of behavioral assessment, various tests of specific areas of behavioral development have been constructed. Such tests actually sample a child's behavior in a specific area of functioning. Development of a satisfactory test of behavior development must include consideration of many factors; among the most important are the following:

1 Range: A structured test of behavior must include items that span performance possibilities of the behavior. A satisfactory test must include easy items reflecting the slowest, or least developed, appropriate response as well as difficult items that will challenge the most capable child.
2 Standardization: In order for test results to be meaningful the performance of an individual child must be compared with that of a representative sample of peers. Tests accused of "cultural bias" are those in which the allegedly representative peer group has failed to include sufficient cultural variability. Standardization also implies precise methods of test administration that do not vary in any test situation.
3 Reliability: A satisfactory test must produce essentially similar results for different examiners and at different

times of administration. If examiner A obtains the same results as examiner B in an assessment of a child's behavior, the assessment is considered reliable (interobserver reliability). If examiner A obtains the same or similar results on a test administered at two different times, the test is considered reliable (intraobserver reliability).

4 Validity: This feature refers to how well a test measures what it claims to measure. Tests of behavioral development, for example, are considered valid if they include items characteristic of child behavior appropriate to the age of the child being tested.

Formal measures of behavior can be divided into two categories: screening and, more precise, in-depth assessment. "The primary task of screening is to identify children who manifest a high probability of significant developmental deficits. . . . The task for assessment is to identify as specifically as possible the nature and degree of handicap and the domains of residual competence in order that assistive intervention may be mobilized to attempt to overcome the disability" (Friedlander, 1975, pp. 521–522).

A screening tool is utilized with children whose behavioral development is presumed normal. It can be applied rapidly but systematically. It is not intended to be diagnostic but determines only which children are probably within normal limits and those who may be delayed developmentally. A positive screening test indicates a need for, and must be followed by, an in-depth assessment of behavior for the purpose of diagnosis of specific areas and degree of abnormality.

Both behavioral screening and assessment tests are readily available. However, there is often some disagreement as to in which category a particular test may be classified. Examples of both screening and in-depth assessment tests are given which demonstrate observation, manipulation, or questionnaire format and evaluate a broad range or a more circumscribed group of behaviors.

Screening tests *DENVER DEVELOPMENTAL SCREENING TEST* The Denver Developmental Screening Test (DDST) is a tool widely used in screening children aged 1 month to 6 years. Its features include the ease with which it is administered by professionals and paraprofessionals. It also meets criteria for reliability and validity; it requires minimum time to administer and score; and it can serve as a useful basis for health care according to developmental needs.

Specific behaviors are observed or elicited in four areas (sectors) by an examiner: personal-social, fine motor–adaptive, language, and gross motor (see Fig. 3-18). In each of the four sectors, the three items which are immediately to the left of but not touching the age line should be given plus all of the items which intersect the age line. The test is continued until the child fails three items in each sector. If a child fails an item which is to the left of his age line (over 90 percent of children his age pass the item), it is considered a *delay*. One also notes whether the child's age line intersects a passed item or whether all passed items are to the left of his age line.

The test is interpreted based on the presence of delays or lack of intersected passed items. Results will indicate that the child's behavioral development is probably within normal limits, should be retested after a short period of time, or is probably delayed and should be referred for in-depth assessment (see Table 3-1).

TABLE 3-1 Interpretation of the Denver Developmental Screening Test

Interpretation	Test results
Normal	Any condition not listed below
Questionable	(1) Any one sector has two or more delays (*or*) (2) One or more sectors have one delay *and* in the same sector the age line does not intersect an item which is passed
Abnormal	(1) Two or more sectors each have two or more delays (*or*) (2) One sector has two or more delays and one other sector has one delay and in the same sector the age line does not intersect one item that is passed

Source: W. K. Frankenburg, A. D. Goldstein, and B. W. Camp, The revised Denver Developmental Screening Test: Its accuracy as a screening instrument. *J. Pediat.*, 1971, 76(6), 990.

FIGURE 3-18. The Denver Developmental Screening Test Scoring Sheet. (*Denver developmental screening test scoring sheet,* © *1969 by William K. Frankenbug and Josiah B. Dodds. Reprinted by permission.*)

DENVER DEVELOPMENTAL SCREENING TEST

STO.=STOMACH
SIT=SITTING

PERCENT OF CHILDREN PASSING: 25 50 75 90

May pass by report → R | Test Item

Footnote No. → see back of form

Date

Name

Birthdate

Hosp. No.

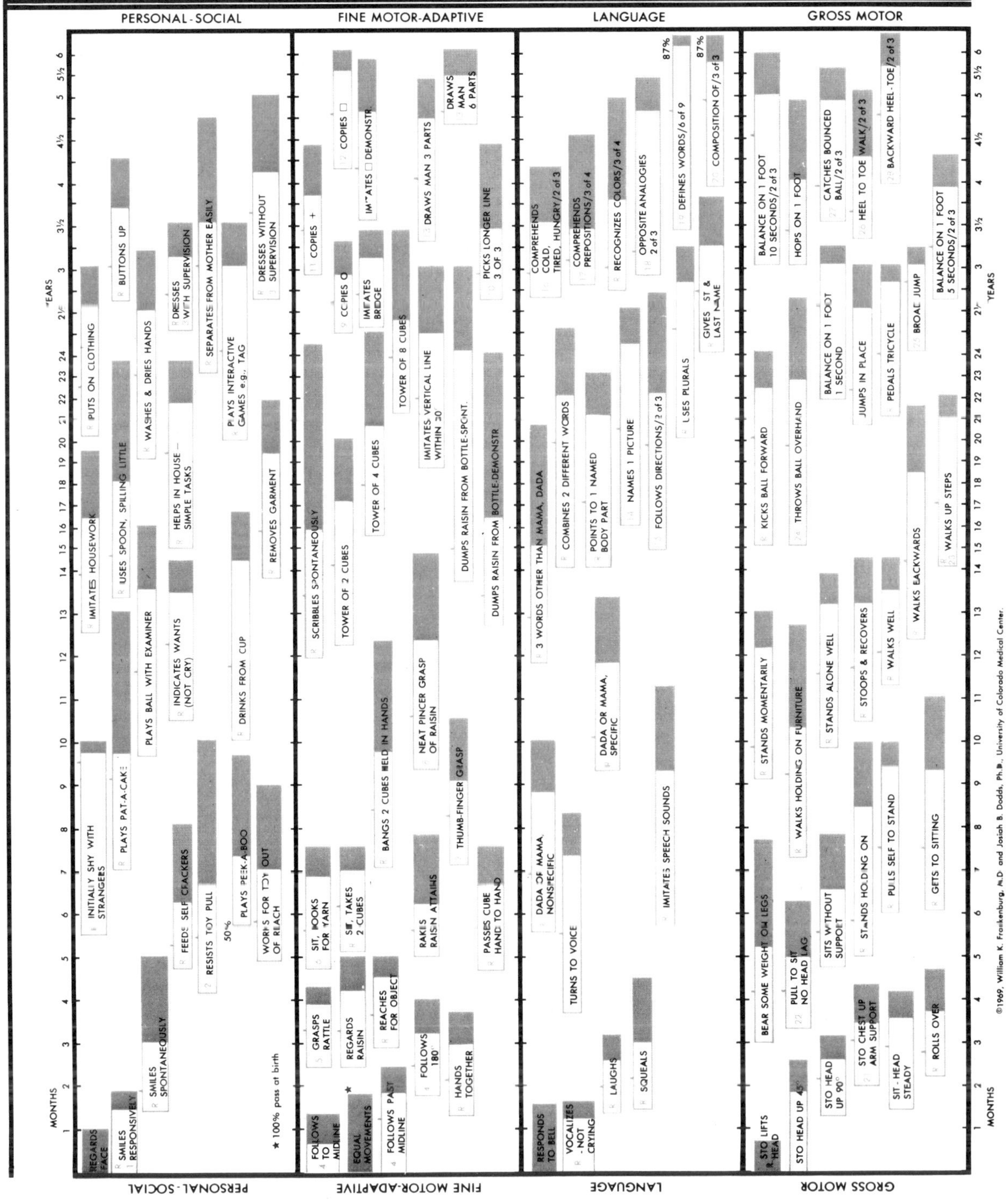

A DEVELOPMENTAL SCREENING INVENTORY A Developmental Screening Inventory is a rapidly applied, condensed version of the Gesell Developmental Schedules. Administered by an examiner, it screens behavioral development of children from 1 to 18 months of age in the areas of adaptive, gross motor, fine motor, language, and personal-social behavior. As with the DDST, the child may pass items by observation or report. These areas are discussed in more detail in the discussion of the full Gesell Developmental Schedules.

A Developmental Screening Inventory supplement is also available for children 21 to 36 months of age.

GUIDE TO NORMAL MILESTONES OF DEVELOPMENT The Guide to Normal Milestones of Development is a wheel device which displays milestones and primitive reflexes expected for children 1, 2, 3, 4, 6, 9, 12, 15, 18, 24, and 36 months. It is used as part of an assessment protocol presented in U. Haynes (1977) (see Fig. 3-19).

Through serial observations of children, primarily in the nursery or at home, the nurse can detect signs of physical, developmental, or neurological abnormality. A child who is suspected of an abnormality in one or more of the areas is referred for in-depth assessment.

MINNESOTA CHILD DEVELOPMENT INVENTORY The Minnesota Child Development Inventory, developed by H. Ireton and E. Thwing (1976), is a paper-and-pencil assessment tool completed by the child's primary care giver, requiring neither formal observations nor directed interview. It is used to evaluate children 1 to 6 years of age. The instrument elicits information regarding past or present behaviors of the child in a forced choice, for example, "Talks or asks about death," "Kicks a ball." The parent answers, "yes" indicating that the behavior has been observed or "no" indicating that it has not been observed.

The test is divided into eight behavioral categories: general development, gross motor behavior, fine motor behavior, expressive language, conceptual comprehension, situation comprehension, self-help, and personal-social. The test includes 320 items covering all categories and age groups.

Results are presented in the form of a developmental profile which depicts the child's level of achievement in each of the eight categories. Analysis of this profile presents an indication of the child's general level of behavioral functioning in terms of accepted norms. The profile also enables the examiner to identify strengths and weaknesses in the child's behavioral development, as indicated by the graphic presentation of data related to each of the eight areas of functioning.

A score which is 20 to 30 percent below age range indi-

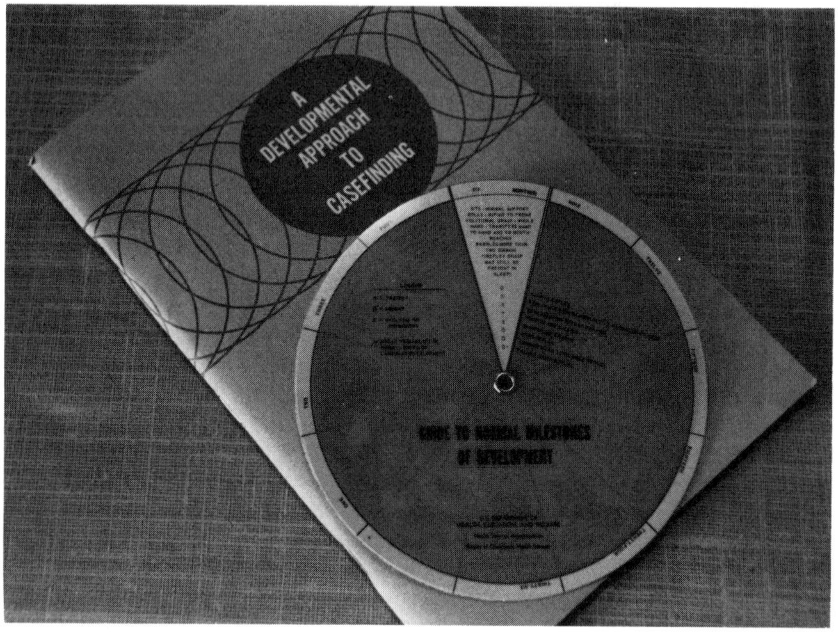

FIGURE 3-19. The wheel device, Guide to Normal Milestones of Development, and accompanying pamphlet, *A Developmental Approach to Casefinding.*

cates a "borderline" level of development in that category. A score 30 percent or more below age range indicates "developmental retardation" in that category. One extreme weakness of this tool is that the age norms are based on suburban white children.

OTHER SCREENING TESTS Two broad but very brief screening tools are the Denver Prescreening Developmental Questionnaire (PDQ) and the Rapid Developmental Screening Checklist.

The PDQ consists of items similar to or the same as those of the DDST. It is completed by the parent with "yes," "no," "child refuses to try," or "child has not had the chance to try." The age-appropriate form is given at well-child appointments with 10 questions per form. It is recommended that the DDST be administered if the child's PDQ indicates a possible delay.

The Rapid Developmental Screening Checklist was compiled by the Committee on Children with Handicaps, of the American Academy of Pediatrics (Frankenburg, 1976). It covers ages 1 month through 5 years. One to four (a mean of two) behavioral items are given in each chronological age. Two examples are: "Can he walk by himself." "Does he say six words." A "yes" or "no" answer is given. Although the checklist was designed to be administered by a professional, the parent could as easily complete the form as most items must be answered by report.

These two brief and simple tests are examples of a possible entry level of developmental screening in a setting or situation where time is critical and thus screening is not carried out. These tests may not determine those children who need developmental assessment, but they can be used to determine which children should have a more thorough developmental screening test.

In-depth assessment tests *GESELL DEVELOPMENTAL SCHEDULES* The Gesell Developmental Schedules, one of the classic behavioral assessment instruments, was developed from a longitudinal study of infant behavior conducted by Arnold Gesell and his associates at the Yale Clinic of Child Development (Knobloch and Pasamanick, 1974). This instrument is utilized in assessing the normal course of behavior in the human infant. Combining the methods of formal observation and parent interview, the instrument measures behavioral development in the following areas:

- Motor behavior: This category includes data relative to both gross body movements and finer motor coordination. Examples of behaviors observed include head balance, standing, reaching, and manipulation of objects.

- Adaptive behavior: Data collected here relate to the behaviors of eye-hand coordination, solution of practical problems, and exploration and manipulation of objects. Examples of specific behaviors observed include reactions to selected stimuli (e.g., the ring of a bell, the presentation of objects) as well as the solving of simple form boards.

- Language behavior: Observations in this area are directed at all forms of communication—verbal and nonverbal—as well as at the child's ability to comprehend language.

- Personal-social behavior: The child's personal reactions to the social culture in which he lives are the bases of observations reported in this category. Types of specific behaviors observed include eating, toileting, playing, and responding to people.

BAYLEY SCALES OF INFANT DEVELOPMENT The Bayley Scales of Infant Development evaluate the development of children from 2 through 30 months. It is a three-part tool consisting of the following scales: mental scale, motor scale, and infant behavior record. All three scales are used with each administration of the test, and three scores are obtained.

The mental scale is designed to assess sensory-perceptual acuities, discriminations, acquisition of object constancy, memory, problem-solving ability, vocalizations, beginning verbal communication, and the bases of abstract thinking. The motor scale is designed to assess gross and fine motor control. The infant behavior record assesses the "nature of the child's social and objective orientations toward his environment as expressed in attitudes, interests, emotions, energy, activity and tendencies to approach or withdraw from stimulation" (Bayley, 1969, p. 4).

Raw scores are converted to be expressed as the child's mental development index (MDI) and psychomotor developmental index (PDI). Both are numerical scores which can be translated to an age equivalent. This is considered a developmental quotient, not an intelligence quotient, and reflects the child's current, not future, performance.

NEONATAL BEHAVIORAL ASSESSMENT SCALE The Neonatal Behavioral Assessment Scale by T. B. Brazelton evaluates 3-day-old infants on 27 behavioral items and 20 elicited responses (primitive reflexes). Each behavior item is scored on a nine-point scale; each reflex is scored on a three-point scale. The state of the infant is observed and taken into consideration on each item, and descriptive comments of the neonate are made.

The best response obtained on each item is recorded. A total score, a development quotient, is not obtained. The author states that its purpose is as a means of scoring interactive behavior to assist in understanding a care giver's response to the neonate. In this respect it is unique among assessment tools. This behavioral assessment tool can also be used to evaluate at-risk neonates in conjunction with a neurological evaluation.

HUMAN FIGURE–DRAWING TESTS The use of figure drawings as indicators of emotional or behavioral functioning is widespread in the assessment of child development. A variety of reliability studies have supported

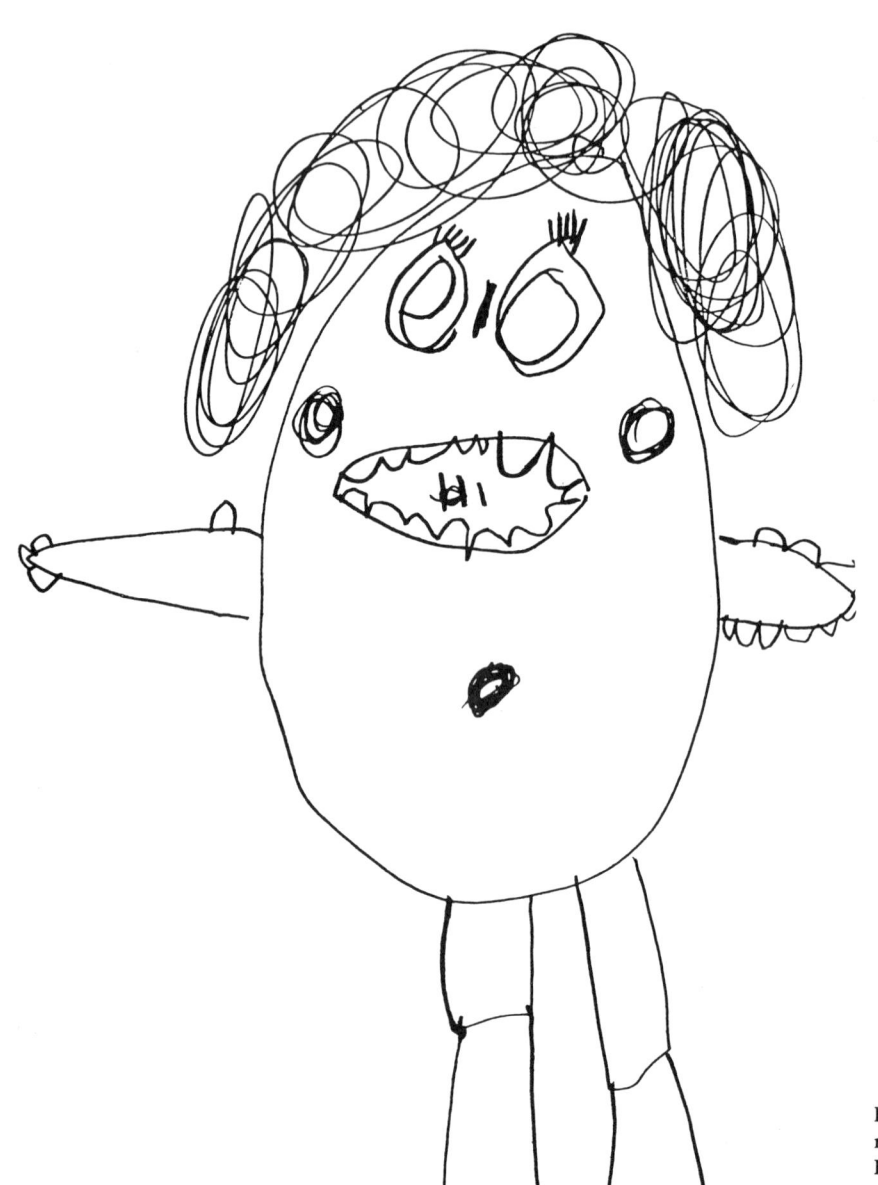

FIGURE 3-20. A child's drawing which received 15 points on the Goodenough-Harris Drawing Test, equivalent to age 6 years, 9 months.

the use of this measure. Such drawings do require clinical interpretation, best provided by professionals trained in their use. Information is available, however, to facilitate understanding of some of the basic features of drawings of the human figure.

The Goodenough-Harris Drawing Test is one example of a human figure–drawing test. It is used for children 3 to 15 years of age to test intelligence as well as personality traits. The child draws a woman, man, and self-portrait. Specific items on the figure are given a score of 1 point. Each point equals 3 months added to a base age of 3 years. Figure 3-20 illustrates a child's drawing which received 15 points, equivalent to 6 years, 9 months. It is debatable whether a test such as the Goodenough-Harris Drawing Test is truly diagnostic and thus considered an assessment tool. It may be more appropriately used as a screening test.

VINELAND SOCIAL MATURITY SCALE The assessment of behaviors related to an individual's ability to meet practical needs and to take responsibility is facilitated by the use of the Vineland Social Maturity Scale. Used on people from 1 year of age to adulthood, the tool is especially appropriate in the behavioral assessment of young children. A directed interview is used to obtain the information regarding the child's behavioral development. In this interview the child's primary care giver is asked to respond to specific questions related to behaviors the child has actually performed in daily living.

Items are developed to elicit information about a child's behavior in the following categories: general self-help behavior, self-help in eating, self-help in dressing, self-direction, occupation, communication, locomotion, and socialization. On the basis of information obtained in the interview a social age and social quotient are derived for the child, which indicate the level of the child's behavioral development as compared with accepted norms.

Other assessment measures In addition to the instruments described above, numerous other measurement tools are available which facilitate behavioral assessment. Another type of measure providing information about development is the general intelligence test (behavioral competence being an aspect of intelligence). Among the intelligence tests most frequently employed in the testing of children are the Stanford-Binet Intelligence Scales and the Wechsler Intelligence Scale for Children—Revised, both of which are largely verbal measures. The Merrill-Palmer Scale of Mental Tests and the Leiter International Performance Scale are representative of nonverbal or performance measures of intelligence.

SUMMARY

Assessment of behavior is an important component of effective health and developmental management of children. Methods of behavior assessment include observation techniques and the use of formal measures of behavioral development. In all methods of assessment important characteristics and limitations of the method must be considered. In addition, the purpose of assessment, nursing intervention, is an important criterion to guide the selection of the assessment procedure.

Bibliography

GENERAL CONSIDERATIONS
OF BEHAVIORAL DEVELOPMENT

Anthony, E. J., and C. Koupernik: *The child in his family: The impact of disease and death.* New York: Wiley, 1973.

Bayley, N.: Comparisons of mental and motor test scores for ages 1 to 15 months by sex, birth order, race, geographical location, and education of parents. *Child Develop.*, 1965, 36, 379–412.

Bowlby, J.: *Attachment.* New York: Basic Books, 1973.

Brown, J., and R. Hepler: Stimulation—A corollary to physical care. *Amer. J. Nurs.*, 1976, 76, 578–581.

Capute, A. J., and R. F. Biehl: Functional developmental evaluation: Prerequisite to habilitation. *Pediat. Clin. N. Amer.*, 1973, 20(1), 3–26.

Developmental psychology today: Del Mar, California: Communication Research Machines, 1971.

Erikson, E. H.: *Childhood and society* (2d ed.). New York: Norton, 1963.

Frankenburg, W. K.: Developmental screening of infants and children. In *Brennemann's practice of pediatrics.* New York: Harper & Row, 1976.

Gerber, M.: The psycho-motor development of African children in the first year and the influence of maternal behavior. *J. Soc. Psychol.*, 1958, 47, 185–195.

Gochman, D. S.: Children's perceptions of vulnerability to illness and accidents. *Public Health Rep.*, 1970, 85, 69.

Henderson, R. W., and J. F. Bergan: *The cultural context of childhood.* Columbus, Ohio: Merrill, 1976.

Hepler, R.: Teachers' sensitivity to children, measured by responses to hypothetical situations and peer observations of teacher-child interactions (Doctoral dissertation, 1977).

Hess, E. H.: Imprinting in birds. *Science*, 1964, 146, 1128–1129.

Jones, M. C.: Psychological correlates of somatic development. *Child Develop.*, 1965, *36*, 899–911.

Kagan, J., and R. Klein: Cross-cultural perspectives on early development. *Amer. Psychol.*, 1973, *28*, 947–961.

Korner, A. F.: The effect of the infant's state, level of arousal, sex, and ontogenetic stage on the caregiver. In M. Lewis and L. A. Rosenblum (Eds.), *Origins of behavior: The effect of the infant on its caregiver.* New York: Wiley, 1974.

Malmquist, C. P.: Depressive phenomenon in children. In B. B. Wolman (Ed.), *Manual of child psychopathology.* New York: McGraw-Hill, 1972.

Monroe, R. L., and R. H. Monroe: *Cross-cultural human development.* Monterey, California: Brooks/Cole, 1975.

Murphy, L. B.: Development in the first year of life: Ego and drive development in relation to the mother-infant tie. In L. J. Stone, H. T. Smith, and L. B. Murphy, *The competent infant.* New York: Basic Books, 1973.

Newman, J.: Children of disaster: Clinical observations at Buffalo Creek. *Amer. J. Psychiat.*, 1976, *133*, 306–312.

Osofsky, J. D., and B. Danzger: Relationship between neonatal characteristics and mother-infant interaction. *Develop. Psychobiol.*, 1974, *10*, 124–130.

Sackett, G.: Some effects of social and sensory deprivation during rearing on behavioral development of monkeys. *Rev. Interamer. Psicol.*, 1967, *1*, 55–80.

Spitz, R. A.: Anaclitic depression. *Psychoanal. Stud. Child*, 1946, *2*, 313–342.

Stone, L. J., and J. Church: *Childhood and adolescence: A psychology of the growing person* (3d ed.). New York: Random House, 1973.

———, H. T. Smith, and L. B. Murphy (Eds.): *The competent infant.* New York: Basic Books, 1973.

White, R. N.: Motivation reconsidered: The concept of competence. *Psychol. Rev.* 1959, *66*, 297–333.

Whiting, B. B. (Ed.): *Six cultures: Studies of child rearing.* New York: Wiley, 1963.

EFFECT OF PARENTING ON BEHAVIORAL DEVELOPMENT

Carey, W.: Measuring infant temperament. *J. Pediat.*, 1972, *81*, 414.

———: A simplified method of measuring infant temperament. *J. Pediat.*, 1970, *77*, 188–194.

Graham, P., M. Rutter, and S. George: Temperamental characteristics as predictors of behavior disorders in children. *Amer. J. Orthopsychiat.*, 1973, *43*, 328–339.

Lamb, M.: *The role of father in child development.* New York: Wiley, 1976.

Lynn, D.: *The father: His role in child development.* Monterey, California: Brooks/Cole, 1974.

Thomas, A., and S. Chess: *Temperament and development.* New York: Brunner/Mazel, 1977.

———, ———, and H. Birch: *Temperament and behavior disorders in childhood.* New York: New York University Press, 1968.

———, ———, ———, M. Hertzig, and S. Korn: *Behavioral individuality in early childhood.* New York: New York University Press, 1963.

Yarrow, L.: Conceptualizing the early environment. In L. Dittmann (Ed.), *Early child care.* New York: Atherton, 1968.

CHILD-DEVELOPMENT THEORIES

Baldwin, A.: *Theories of child development.* New York: Wiley, 1968.

Bijou, S., and D. Baer: *Child development—A systematic and empirical theory.* New York: Appleton-Century-Crofts, 1961.

Caldwell, B. M., and J. B. Richmond: The impact of theories of child development. In F. Rebelsky and L. Dorman (Eds.), *Child development and behavior.* New York: Knopf, 1970.

Erikson, E.: *Childhood and society.* New York: Norton, 1950.

Freud, S.: *Basic writings of S. Freud* (A. A. Brill, Ed.). New York: Random House, 1938.

Gesell, A.: *Youth—The years from 10–16.* New York: Harper, 1956.

———, and F. Ilg: *Infant and child in the culture of today.* New York: Harper, 1943.

Keller, F. S., and W. N. Schoenfeld: *Principles of psychology.* New York: Appleton-Century-Crofts, 1950.

Kohlberg, L., and C. Gilligan: The adolescent as a philosopher: The discovery of the self in a postconventional world. *Daedalus*, Fall 1971.

Lewin, K.: Behavior and development as a function of the total situation. In L. Carmichael (Ed.), *Manual of child psychology.* New York: Wiley, 1954.

Lovell, K.: *An introduction to human development.* Toronto: Macmillan, 1969.

Maier, H. W.: *Three theories of child development.* New York: Harper & Row, 1969.

Miller, N. E., and J. Dollard: *Social learning and imitation.* New Haven: Yale University Press, 1953.

Mussen, P. H., J. J. Conger, and J. Kagan: *Child development and personality.* New York: Harper & Row, 1969.

Papalia, D. E., and S. W. Olds: *Human development.* New York: McGraw-Hill, 1978.

Piaget, J.: *The origins of intelligence in children.* New York: International Universities Press, 1952.

Rebelsky, F., and L. Dorman (Eds.): *Child development and behavior.* New York: Knopf, 1970.

Sears, R. R., E. E. Macoby, and H. Levin: *Patterns of child rearing.* New York: Harper & Row, 1957.

Skinner, B. F.: *Science and human behavior.* New York: Macmillan, 1953.

Starr, B. D., and H. S. Goldstein: *Human development and behavior.* New York: Springer, 1975.

Stone, L. J., and J. Church: *Childhood and adolescence.* New York: Random House, 1973.

Sutterley, D. C., and G. F. Donnelly: *Perspectives in human development.* Philadelphia: Lippincott, 1973.

Watson, J. B.: *Psychological care of infant and child.* London: Allen & Unwin, 1928.

PERCEPTUAL DEVELOPMENT

Bower, T. G. R.: *The perceptual world of the child.* Cambridge: Harvard University Press, 1977.

Brian, W. R.: *Mind, perception and science.* Oxford: Blackwell, 1951.

Forgus, R. H.: *Perception: The basic process in cognitive development.* New York: McGraw-Hill, 1966.

Gibson, E. J.: *Principles of perceptual learning and development.* New York: Appleton-Century-Crofts, 1969.

Gibson, J. J.: *The senses considered as perceptual systems.* Boston: Houghton Mifflin, 1966.

Hubel, D. H.: The visual cortex of the brain. *Scientific American,* November 1963.

Illingworth, R. S.: *The development of the infant and young child.* Baltimore: Williams & Wilkins, 1962.

Pick, H. L., and A. D. Pick: Sensory and perceptual development. In P. H. Mussen (Ed.), *Carmichael's manual of child psychology* (Vol. I). New York: Wiley, 1970.

Worden, F. G.: Attention and auditory electrophysiology In E. Stellar and J. M. Sprague (Eds.), *Progress in physiological psychology.* New York: Academic, 1966.

GROSS MOTOR DEVELOPMENT

Banus, B. S.: *The developmental therapist.* Thorofare, New Jersey: Charles B. Slack, 1971.

Gesell, A., H. M. Halverson, H. Thompson, F. L. Ilg, B. Castner, L. B. Ames, and C. S. Amatruda: *The first five years of life.* New York: Harper, 1940.

———, and F. L. Ilg: *The child from five to ten.* New York: Harper, 1946.

Johnston, R. B., and P. R. Magrab: *Developmental disorders.* Baltimore: University Park Press, 1976.

Knobloch, H., and B. Pasamanick: *Gesell and Amatruda's developmental diagnosis.* New York: Harper & Row, 1974.

FINE MOTOR DEVELOPMENT

Gesell, A., H. M. Halverson, H. Thompson, F. L. Ilg, B. Castner, L. B. Ames, and C. S. Amatruda: *The first five years of life.* New York: Harper, 1940.

———, and F. L. Ilg: *The child from five to ten.* New York: Harper, 1946.

Illingworth, R. S.: *The development of the infant and young child—Normal and abnormal.* Edinburgh, London and New York: Churchill Livingstone, 1975.

Knoblock, H., and B. Pasamanick: *Gesell and Amatruda's developmental diagnosis.* New York: Harper & Row, 1974.

Kopp, C. B.: Fine motor abilities of infants. *Develop. Med. Child Neurol.,* 1974, 16, 629–636.

Porter, L. S.: The impact of physical-physiological activity on infants' growth and development. *Nurs. Res.* 1972, 21, 210–219.

Stott, L. H.: *The psychology of human development.* New York: Holt, 1974.

Touwen, B. C. L.: A study on the development of some motor phenomena in infancy. *Develop. Med. Child Neurol.,* 1971, 13, 435–446.

COGNITIVE DEVELOPMENT

Bruner, J.: *Studies in cognitive growth.* New York: Wiley, 1966.

Piaget, J.: *The construction of reality in the child.* New York: Basic Books, 1954.

Wenar, C.: *Personality development from infancy to adulthood.* Boston: Houghton Mifflin, 1971.

Werner, H.: *Comparative psychology of mental development.* New York: International Universities Press, 1948.

LANGUAGE DEVELOPMENT

Allen, R. R.: *Developing communication competence in children.* Skokie, Illinois: National Text Book, 1976.

Anglen, J.: The extensions of the child's first terms of reference. (Paper presented at the Society for Research in Child Development, 1975.)

Bellugi, U.: Development of language in the normal child. In McLean, Yodeu, and Schiefelbusch (Eds.), *Language intervention with the retarded—Developing strategies.* Baltimore: University Park Press, 1972.

Bloom, L.: An integrative perspective on language development. (Papers and reports on child language development, Department of Linguistics, Stanford University, Stanford, California, 1976.)

———, and M. Lahey: *Language development and language disorders.* New York: Wiley, 1978.

Coggins, T. E., and R. L. Carpenter: Developmental changes in language and communication: What children acquire from eight months to eight years. In M. Cohen and P. Gross (Eds.), *Developmental pin points.* New York: Grune & Stratton, 1978.

Dale, P.: *Language development structure and function.* New York: Dryden Press, 1972.

Greenfield, P.: Who is "dada"? Some aspects of the semantics and phonological development of a child's first words. *Lang. Speech,* 1973, *16,* 34–43.

Katz, J., and J. Fodor: *The structure of language.* Englewood Cliffs, New Jersey: Prentice Hall, 1964.

Kriegsmann, E.: Providing an optimal language environment for the young child. (Unpublished paper, 1978.)

McNeil, D.: The capacity for the ontogenesis of grammar. In D. L. Slobin (Ed.), *The ontogenesis of grammar—A theoretical symposium.* New York and London: Academic, 1971.

Skinner, B. F.: *Verbal behavior.* New York: Appleton-Century-Crofts, 1957.

SELF-HELP SKILL DEVELOPMENT AND INDEPENDENT FUNCTIONING

Connally, K: Learning and the concept of critical periods in infancy. In S. Chess, and A. Thomas (Ed.), *Annual progress in child psychiatry and child development.* New York: Brunner/Mazel, 1973.

Escalona, S. K.: *The roots of individuality: Normal patterns of development in infancy.* Chicago: Aldini, 1968.

Lewis, M.: *Clinical aspects of child development.* Philadelphia: Lea & Febiger, 1971.

———, and L. Rosenblum (Ed.): *The effect of the infant on its caregiver.* New York: Wiley, 1974.

McBride, A. B.: *The growth and development of mothers.* New York: Barnes & Noble, 1973.

Murphy, L. B.: Spontaneous ways of learning in young children. *Children,* Nov/Dec 1967, pp. 211–216.

Ramirez, M., III, and A. Castaneda: *Cultural democracy, bicognitive development and education.* New York: Academic, 1974.

Spencer, K.: The family and child development: A sociocultural viewpoint. In H. C. Stuart, and D. G. Prugh (Eds.), *The healthy child.* Cambridge: Harvard University Press, 1964.

Striffler, N.: Language function: Normal and abnormal development. In R. B. Johnston and P. Magrab (Eds.), *Developmental disorders: Assessment, treatment, education.* Baltimore: University Park Press, 1976.

Thomas, A., H. G. Birch, S. Chess, M. E. Hertzog, and S. Koru: *Behavioral individuality in early childhood.* New York: New York University Press, 1963.

Westman, J. C. (Ed.): *Individual differences in children.* New York: Wiley, 1973.

Whiting, B., and C. Edwards: A cross-cultural analysis of sex differences in the behavior of children aged three through eleven. *J. Soc. Psychol.,* 1973, *91,* 171–188.

Yarrow, M. R.: Research on child rearing as a basis for practice. *Child Wel.,* 1973, *52*(4), 209–219.

SOCIAL DEVELOPMENT

Ainsworth, M. D.: Individual differences in the development of some attachment behaviors. *Merrill-Palmer Quart.,* 1972, *18,* 123–143.

———: Infant mother attachment and social development: "Socialization" as a product of reciprocal responsiveness to signals. In M. P. Richards (Ed.), *The integration of the child into a social world.* Cambridge: Cambridge University Press, 1974.

Bossard, J. H., and E. S. Boll: Personality types in the large family. *Child Devel.,* 1955, *26,* 71–78.

Bowerman, C. E., and R. M. Dobash: Structural variation in intersibling affect. *J. Marriage Family,* 1974, *36,* 48–54.

Bowlby, J.: *Attachment and loss.* New York: Basic Books, 1969.

Brim, O. G.: Family structure and sex role learning by children: A further analysis of Helen Koch's data. *Sociometry,* 1958, *21,* 1–16.

Bryan, J. H.: Children's cooperative and helping behaviors. In E. M. Hetherington (Ed.), *Review of child development research* (Vol. 5). Chicago: University of Chicago Press, 1975.

Cicirelli, V. G.: Family structure and interaction: Sibling effects on socialization. In M. McMillan and S. Henao (Eds.), *Child psychiatry: Treatment and research.* New York: Brunner/Mazel, 1977a.

———: Relationship of siblings to the elderly person's feelings and concerns. *J. Geront.,* 1977b, *32,* 317–322.

———: Relationship of sibling structure and interaction to younger sib's conceptual style. *J. Genet. Psychol.,* 1974, *125,* 37–49.

Cohen, L. J.: The operational definition of human attachment. *Psychol. Bull.,* 1974, *81,* 207–217.

Cumming, E., and D. Schneider: Sibling solidarity: A property of American kinship. *Amer. Anthrop.,* 1961, *63,* 498–507.

Damon, W.: *The social world of the child.* San Francisco: Jossey-Bass, 1977.

Davis, C., and M. Northway: Siblings—Rivalry or relationship. *Bull. Inst. Child Stud.*, 1957, *19*, 10–13.

Hetherington, E. M.: A developmental study of the effects of sex of the dominant parent on sex-role preference, identification and imitation in children. *J. Personality Soc. Psychol.*, 1965, *2*, 188–194.

Hoffman, L. W.: Early childhood experiences and women's achievement motives. *J. Soc. Issues*, 1972, *28*, 129–156.

Hoffman, M.: Developmental synthesis of affect and cognition and its implication for altruistic motivation. *Develop. Psychol.*, 1975, *11*, 607–622.

———: Moral development. In P. H. Mussen (Ed.), *Carmichael's manual of child psychology*. New York: Wiley, 1970.

Irish, D. P.: Sibling interaction: A neglected aspect in family life research. *Soc. Forces*, 1964, *42*, 279–288.

Johnson, M.: Sex role learning in the nuclear family. In G. C. Thompson (Ed.), *Social development and personality.* New York: Wiley, 1971.

Krout, M. H.: Typical behavior patterns in twenty-six ordinal positions. *J. Genet. Psychol.*, 1939, *55*, 3–30.

Lamb, M.: The father's role in the infant's social world. In J. H. Stevens and M. Matew (Eds.), *Mother/child, father/child relationships.* New York: National Association for the Education of Young Children, 1978a.

———: Observational analysis of sibling relationships in infancy. (Paper presented to the International Conference on Infant Studies, 1978b, at Providence, Rhode Island.)

———: A re-examination of the infant social world. *Hum. Develop.*, 1977, *20*, 65–85.

Lewis, M., and C. Feiring: The child's social world. In *Contributions of the child to marital quality and family interactions through the life span.* New York: Academic, 1979.

Mussen, P. H.: Sex-typing and acquisition of sex-role identity. In D. A. Goslin (Ed.), *Handbook of socialization theory and research.* Chicago: Rand McNally, 1969.

Parsons, J., and J. Bryan: Adolescence: Gateway to androgyny. *Occasional Papers Series,* Women's Study Program. Ann Arbor: University of Michigan Press, 1978.

Rosenthal, M. K.: The study of infant-environment interaction: Some comments on trends and methodologies. *J. Child Psychol. Psychiat.*, 1969, *14*, 301–317.

Shantz, C.: The development of social cognition. In E. M. Hetherington (Ed.), *Review of child development research* (Vol. 5). Chicago: University of Chicago Press, 1975.

Weisner, T. S., and R. Gallimore: My brother's keeper: Child and sibling caretaking. *Curr. Anthrop.*, 1977, *18*, 169–190.

BEHAVIORAL ASSESSMENT

Anastasi, A.: *Psychological testing* (4th ed.). New York: Macmillan, 1976.

Bayley, N.: *Bayley scales of infant development manual.* New York: Psychological Corporation, 1969.

Brazelton, T. B.: Neonatal behavioral assessment scale. *Clinics in Developmental Medicine* (No. 50). Philadelphia: Lippincott, 1973.

Erickson, M. L.: *Assessment and management of developmental changes in children.* St. Louis: Mosby, 1976.

Frankenburg, W. K., and J. B. Dodds: The Denver developmental screening test. *J. Pediat.*, 1967, *71*, 181.

———, A. D. Goldstein, and B. W. Camp: The revised Denver developmental screening test: Its accuracy as a screening instrument. *J. Pediat.*, 1971, *79*(6), 988–995.

Friedlander, B. Z.: Notes on language: Screening and assessment of young children. In B. Z. Friedlander, G. M. Sterritt, and G. E. Kirk (Eds.), *Exceptional infant* (Vol. 3): *Assessment and intervention.* New York: Brunner/Mazel, 1975.

Haynes, U.: *A developmental approach to casefinding.* U.S. Department of Health, Education, and Welfare Pamphlet No. (HSA) 77-5210, 1977.

Holt, K. S.: *Developmental paediatrics.* London: Butterworth, 1977.

Ireton, H., and E. Thwing: Appraising the development of a preschool child by means of a standardized report prepared by the mother. *Clin. Pediat.*, 1976, *15*(10), 875–882.

Johnson, O. G., and J. W. Bommarito: *Tests and measurements in child development: A handbook.* San Francisco: Jossey-Bass, 1971.

Kenny, T. J., and R. L. Clemmens: *Behavioral pediatrics and child development.* Baltimore: Williams & Wilkins, 1975.

Knobloch, H., and B. Pasamanick (Eds.): *Gesell and Amatruda's developmental diagnosis* (3d ed.). Hagerstown, Maryland: Harper & Row, 1974.

Marshall, C. L.: Attitudes toward health among children of different races and socioeconomic status. *Pediatrics*, 1970, *46*, 422.

National Center for Health Statistics: *Intellectual maturity of children as measured by the Goodenough-Harris drawing test.* U.S. Public Health Service Pamphlet No. 1000 (Series 11, No. 105), 1970.

Robertson, J.: *Young children in hospital* (2d ed.). London: Tavistock, 1970. (Also New York: Barnes & Noble, 1970.)

Sundberg, N.: *Assessment of persons.* Englewood Cliffs, New Jersey: Prentice-Hall, 1977.

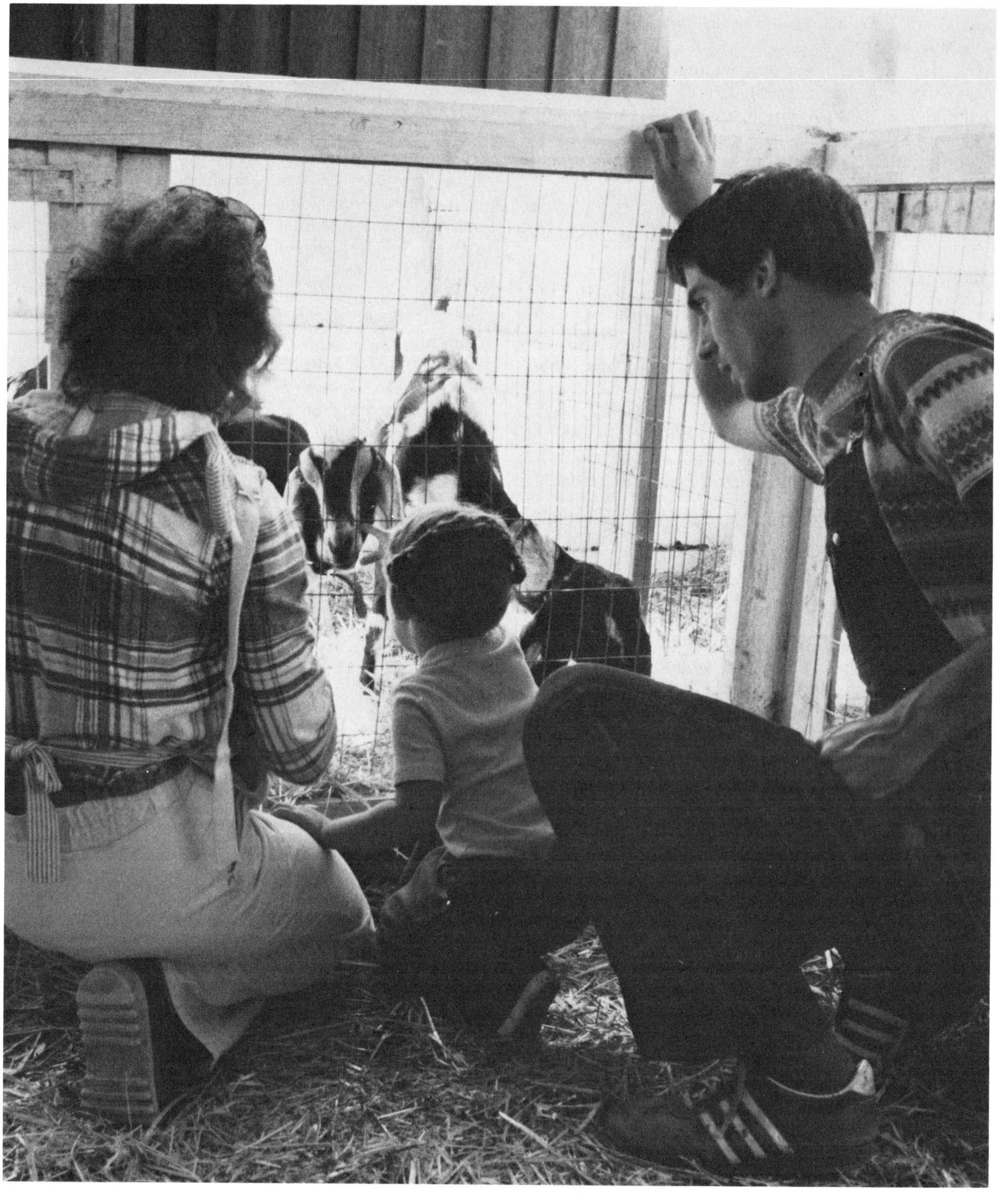

CHAPTER 4
Parenting and the Developing Child

Introduction

Parents are the enablers of child development. As the critical environmental "variable," their impact on the child, physically and behaviorally, is most profound. The child's individuality, capabilities, and limitations cannot be overlooked. However, it is through parents that the child is able to impact the world and achieve developmental tasks.

The parent-child relationship and evaluation of the home environment are discussed in this chapter. Also, an overview of current resources that parents are using to aid and direct them in their parental roles is presented.

The parent-child relationship Marion H. Rose

CONCEPT OF PARENTING

Webster's New Collegiate Dictionary (1956) defines a parent as "One who begets or brings forth offspring; a father or a mother" (p. 610). Today, *parent* is more broadly defined to include adults who are legally responsible for the health and welfare of a child, be they biological parents, adoptive parents, foster parents, or stepparents. People may also assume all or part of the role of a parent even though they are not legally responsible for the child, providing the child also sees this person as a parent. Recently the word parent has been translated into a verb form, *parenting*, to describe what parents do to and for children. Unfortunately the exact meaning of the word is usually left to the reader to define.

Parenting is often discussed in isolation from the social and cultural milieu in which it occurs. Families are often viewed as consisting of mother, father, and child (or children) with little if any attention to the influence of various relatives and friends. Although many nuclear families today do not live in close physical proximity to an extended family, a close communication system often exists via the telephone, letters, or audiotapes. Another aspect which is often overlooked is the development of substitute families and their influence on parenting and child rearing.

In his book titled *Parents in Modern America*, LeMasters (1974) discusses folk beliefs about parenthood. Folklore or folk beliefs are widely held beliefs that are not supported by facts.

These beliefs are as follows (pp. 19–30):

- That child rearing is fun
- That children are sweet and cute
- That children turn out well if they have "good" parents
- That girls are harder to rear than boys
- That today's parents are not as good as those of yesterday
- That child rearing today is easier because of modern medicine, modern appliances, child psychology, and so on
- That children today really appreciate all the advantages their parents are able to give them
- That the hard work of rearing children is justified by the fact that we are going to make a better world
- The sex education myth: That children will not get into trouble if they have been told the facts of life
- There are no bad children—only bad parents
- That two parents are necessary to rear children successfully
- That modern behavioral science has been helpful to parents
- That love is enough to sustain good parental performance
- That all married couples should have children
- That childless married couples are frustrated and unhappy
- That children improve a marriage
- That parents are mature and grown up
- That parents are parents because they wanted to be parents
- That parenthood receives top priority in our society

FIGURE 4-1.

- That American parents can be studied without interviewing the father

These beliefs tend to romanticize the truth; however, the reverse might be true in some cases. (For a complete discussion of these folk beliefs see LeMasters, 1974.)

One way to look at parent-child interaction is through role theory and role analysis. A role is defined as "a task that some person is supposed to perform" (LeMasters, 1974, p. 50). Every role is a position which has a certain status and prestige within the interaction system. For every role there is a complementary role. To be a parent, for example, one must have a child; to be a sister one must have a sibling.

> In a well-organized family, the major roles have been identified, assigned, and performed with some degree of competence. When this does not occur, the family may be said to be disorganized to a certain extent. (LeMasters, 1974, p. 50)

Minor roles (such as cutting the grass) may be ignored or performed indifferently without producing too much difficulty, but major roles (such as caring for young children) require consistent and adequate role performance.

Based on role theory and role analysis, LeMasters (1974, pp. 50-53) identifies 13 features of the parental role which produce problems for some parents:

- The role of a parent in modern America is not well defined. It is often ambiguous and hard to pin down.
- The parental role is not adequately delimited. Parents are expected to succeed where even the professionals fail.
- Modern parents are not well prepared for their roles as fathers and mothers.
- There is a romantic complex about parenthood.
- Modern parents are in the unenviable position of having complete responsibility for their offspring but only partial authority over them. LeMasters' thesis on this point is that parental authority has been eroded gradually over the past several decades without equivalent reduction of parental responsibilities.
- The standards of role performance imposed on modern parents are too high. This arises from the fact that modern fathers and mothers are judged largely by professional practitioners, such as nurses, psychiatrists, and social workers, rather than by their peers, other parents who are "amateurs."
- Parents are victims of inadequate behavioral science. They have been told repeatedly by the psychiatrists, social workers, sociologists, ministers, and others that nothing determines what the child will be like but the influence of the parents.
- Parents do not choose their children, unless they are adoptive parents. Thus, they have responsibility for children whether they find them congenial or not.
- There is no traditional model for modern parents to follow in rearing children. The old model has been riddled by critical studies; yet no adequate new model has developed. Instead, there has been a series of fads and fashions in child rearing based on research of the moment.
- Contrary to what some may think, parenthood as a role does not enjoy the priority one would expect in modern America. The needs of the economic system, in particular, come first, as can be seen in the frequency with which large firms transfer young managers (and, as a result, their families) around the country.
- Other new roles have been assumed by modern parents since World War I which are not always completely compatible with the role of parent.
- The parental role is one of the few important roles in contemporary America from which one cannot honorably withdraw.
- And, last but not least, it is not enough for modern parents to produce children in their own image; the children have to be reared to be not only different from their fathers and mothers but also *better*.

Although most studies presented in the remainder of this chapter are *not* based on role theory, one can see that they often deal with a specific role or role task within the framework of parent-child interaction and often do not attend, or attend minimally, to all other related role relationships and tasks. This is a reminder to the reader that studies of specific aspects of parent-child behaviors and interactions need to be seen as part of a complex interacting system.

PARENTAL-INFANT BONDING OR ATTACHMENT

MOTHER-INFANT ATTACHMENT

Until recently the entire focus of theory and research on parent-infant attachment has been on maternal-infant attachment. Fortunately, paternal-infant attachment is now receiving attention. So far, *how* the attachment occurs and/or is facilitated in the mother-father-infant triad is not known. Rather, *what* happens in the attachment process has been the focus of research. (*Bonding* is beginning to replace the word *attachment* in more current literature; however, in order to be consistent, the word *attachment* will be used in this chapter.)

Bowlby At the third session of the Social Commission of the United Nations held in April 1948, it was decided to study needs of homeless children. Undoubtedly, the study was stimulated, at least in part, by the separation of many children from their parents during World War II. The World Health Organization offered to contribute a study of the mental health aspects of the problem. The result was the famous and somewhat controversial report by John Bowlby (1966), titled *Maternal Care and Mental Health,* published by the World Health Organization (WHO) in 1950.

Bowlby's report is an important and historic document. It points out the fact that current interest in maternal-infant attachment is an outgrowth of concerns about maternal-infant separation and maternal deprivation and their relation to the mental health of children. The document also serves as a base line to judge the progress made in this area since 1950. The emphasis of this report was on the impact of maternal separation and/or deprivation on the mental health of children. In the first chapter Bowlby states the following:

> It is sufficient to say that what is believed to be essential for mental health is that the infant and young child should experience a warm, intimate, and continuous relationship with his mother (or permanent mother substitute) in which both find satisfaction and enjoyment. Given this relationship the emotions of anxiety and guilt, which in excess characterize mental ill health, will develop in a moderate and organized way. When this happens the child's characteristic and contradictory demands, on the one hand for unlimited love from his parents and on the other for revenge upon them when he feels that they do not love him enough, will likewise remain of moderate strength and become amenable to the control of his gradually developing personality. It is this complex, rich, and rewarding relationship with the mother in the early years, varied in countless ways by relations with the father and with siblings, the child psychiatrist and many others now believe to underline the development of character and of mental health. (p. 11)

Bowlby goes on to say:

> The ill effects of deprivation vary with degree. Partial deprivation brings in its train acute anxiety, excessive need for love, powerful feelings of revenge, and, arising from these last, guilt and depression. These emotions and drives are too great for the immature means of control and organization available to the young child (immature physiologically as well as psychologically). The consequent disturbance of psychic organization then leads to a variety of responses often repetitive and accumulative, the end product of which are symptoms of neurosis and instability of character. Complete deprivation has even more far reaching effects on character development and may entirely cripple the capacity to make relationships. (p. 12)

Although Bowlby focused on maternal-infant separation and deprivation in his report, he did recognize the importance of and the need for further study in the area of parent-child relationships.

In discussing the theoretical problems regarding personality development, Bowlby goes on to say the following:

> Ego and superego development are thus inextricably bound up with the child's primary human relationships; only when these are continuous and satisfactory can his ego and superego develop. In dealing here with the embryology of the human mind, one is struck by a similarity with the embryological development of the human body, during the course of which undifferentiated tissues respond to the influence of chemical organizers. If growth is to proceed smoothly, the tissues must be exposed to the influence of the appropriate organizer at certain critical periods. In the same way, if mental development is to proceed smoothly, it would appear to be necessary for the undifferentiated psyche to be exposed during certain critical periods to the influence of the psychic organizer—the mother. For this reason, in considering the disorders to which ego and superego are liable, it is imperative to have regard to the phases of the child's capacity for human relationships. These are many and, naturally, merge into one another. In broad outline, the following are the most important: (a) The phase during which the infant is in the course of establishing a relationship with a clearly identified person—his mother; this is normally achieved by five or six months of age. (b) The phase during which he needs her as an ever present companion; this usually continues until about his third birthday. (c) The phase during which he is becoming able to

maintain a relationship with her in absentia. During the fourth and fifth years such a relationship can only be maintained in favorable circumstances and for a few days or weeks at a time; after seven or eight the relationship can be maintained, though not without strain, for periods of a year or more.

The process whereby he simultaneously develops his own ego and superego and the capacity to maintain relationships in absentia is variously described as a process of identification, internalization, or introjection, since the functions of the ego and superego are incorporated within the self in the patterns set by the parents. (pp. 53–54)

Although Bowlby's theoretical conclusions were subjected to a considerable amount of criticism, his report stimulated a great deal of interest, which led to changes in child-care practices and to further research.

In his original report, Bowlby emphasized the need for further study. Specifically, he encouraged researchers both to study basic processes and to identify and unravel the effects of the many variables operating. He stated that though some variables, such as age and emotional development of the child, length of deprivation, degree of deprivation, and relations with the mother figure before and after deprivation, have been identified as variables, there are undoubtedly other variables still to be identified. He also stated that matters of immediate practical significance on which information was needed were limits of the safety margins during which deprivation can, if absolutely necessary, be permitted and within which damage already done can be repaired.

A summary of some of the controversy and thoughts following the original report is given in another publication called *Deprivation of Maternal Care: A Reassessment of Its Effects*. In this volume, Ainsworth (1966) lists nine controversial questions which were prevalent at the time the book on reassessment was written. These are as follows: (1) the question of definition of maternal deprivation, (2) the question of multiple mothers, (3) the question of variability in the degree of damage following deprivation, (4) the question of specific versus general effects of deprivation, (5) the question of diversity in the nature of the adverse effects of deprivation, (6) the question of permanence of the effects of deprivation, (7) the special question of delinquency, (8) the question of maternal versus environmental deprivation, and (9) other controversial questions such as the place of defective genetic constitution in contributing to the retardation of young children in institutions or to the frequency of undiagnosed organic brain damage in cases of infants manifesting a "hospitalism" syndrome.

Many studies following Bowlby's original report have continued to focus on the effects of maternal-infant separation and/or deprivation. However, other studies have focused on how maternal-infant bonds or attachments are achieved.

Rubin Reve Rubin's study "Attainment of the Maternal Role" was reported in *Nursing Research* in 1967. In this study, the childbearing period was assumed to be a preparatory period for maternal role acquisition. Rubin looked at the "taking-in" process of the role to determine if the role and an orderly sequence of taking-in acts could be specified. She also investigated what models were used by pregnant women and what aspects of the models' behavior are taken in by pregnant women. Both women who were primiparas and women who were multiparas were studied.

In Rubin's study, a high rate of relevant role–taking-in items was elicited. These items increase in the neonatal period and are consistently higher for multiparas than for primiparas. Five distinct operations of taking-in of the maternal role were elicited. Mimicry and role play were found to be early, tentative forms of taking-on the role. Fantasy and a circular process of introjection, projection, and rejection were found to be a later and a more discriminating process of taking-in of the role. Grief work, the fifth operation, was found to be a letting go of former roles incompatible with the new role. Grief work appeared as a catalyst for other role-taking operations.

Identity was the end point or goal in Rubin's investigation in role taking. When subjects had a sense of being in their roles, a sense of comfort about where they had been and where they were going, role achievement could be said to exist. Two major factors designated role achievement. The subject was clearly "I" without reference to a model or to a reflection of self, and the tense was clearly present: "I am"; "I do"; "I like."

There seemed to be an ordering in the sequence of the operations manifested. No one operation of taking-in occurred independently of the other operations. However, more mimicry occurred earlier in the process of taking-in than any other operation. There was a long interval before introjection, projection, and rejection replaced mimicry as a dominant operation. Within this interval, role play occurred, and fantasy became a significant feature.

This progression in dominance of operations could be seen in each long-term subject. The progression was cyclical in nature during the prenatal period, more like incoming and outgoing waves than a straight-line progression. This was true for both primiparas and multiparas.

Selection of models tended to be sex- and situation-specific. All subjects began with their own mothers as models for each phase of maternal role taking. Their own mothers were soon replaced by peers who seemed to be defined as women in contemporary or advanced stages of role acquisition. Women who were primiparas tended to select peer models outside the family. Women who were multiparas tended toward peer models within the family.

Identification with the infant was a concurrent phenomenon of role taking. The operations were precisely the same as those of role taking earlier described. In mimicry, however, the object of the operation, and consequently the model, became the infant, not the anticipated role. The infant was "like someone in appearance and behavior." He was identified by associations within the subject's experiences and memories of other people who were significant to her. There was a mental searching for similarities, for "best-fit"—"Her hands are like her father's";

FIGURE 4-2.

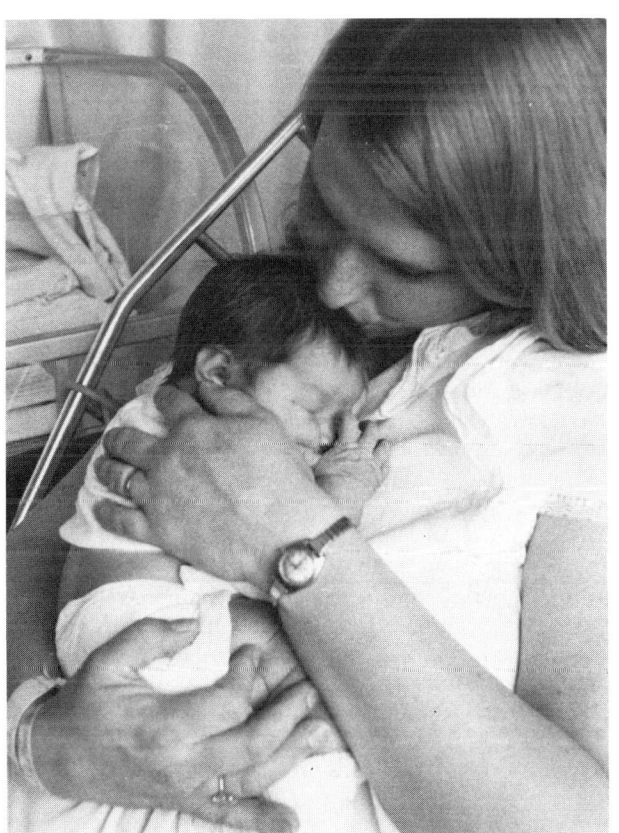

"His head is like my father's." Models for identification of the infant tended to be sought in a narrower family radius by multiparas than by primiparas. All operations involved in role taking were also used in identification with the infant. The extent of role achievement was largely dependent upon the extent of identification with the infant.

Reva Rubin (1963) is also well known for her descriptions of development of maternal touch. She states that a woman who loves impulsively enfolds the person that she loves. Such impulsive action by the new mother in response to her infant is usually not seen in the maternity section of the hospital. Thus Rubin believes that feelings of maternal love are not endowed but are acquired over time and in experiences within the relationship with two people.

Rubin describes the course of development of such a loving relationship as "a definite progression and an orderly sequence in the nature and amount of contact the mother makes with her child" (p. 829). The mother moves from making contact first with only her fingertips, then with her hands, and much later with her whole arms as an extension of her body.

Three factors operate in determining the extent to which she does permit herself to become progressively more intimately involved. These are (1) how she feels about herself in this particular function of her role, (2) how she perceives the infant's reciprocal response to her, and (3) the character of the relationship at any given time.

Reva Rubin comments that the mother's commitment to her infant seems to await some personal evocative response from the infant. This may be a burp or more likely the way he cuddles or, as he becomes older, the way he expresses pleasure at his mother's contacts. She also points out that the mother is very vulnerable at this time to signs of rejection as well as responsiveness from her infant. According to Rubin, the beginning stages of maternal self-involvement begin in the maternity unit. Somewhere between the third and fifth days postpartum the mother has advanced from fingertips to the whole cupped hand to stroke the neonate's head. She may also start using the length of two or three fingers to turn his head. Then she begins to slip her whole hand under his back to turn him. Her arms and shoulders become progressively more relaxed as the distance between her body and that of the neonate becomes shorter.

Rubin sees changing body posture of the mother and the increasingly large body surface involved in contact as indicative of an ongoing relationship in which the mother is becoming involved. At this time she begins to ask realistic questions about the infant's well-being and care and wants to assume more maternal functions than feeding. The mother's body language indicates that psychological work has progressed from the exploratory, information-seeking phase of an intimate relationship to that of involvement.

These stages are seen in women with more than one child as well as in women having their first child. Some women who are multiparas seem to move more rapidly from one phase to the next. However, some of these reported that they moved too fast in assuming that one child was just like another.

Rubin states that mothers who have a very recent experience of appropriate and meaningful bodily touch from a ministering person, for instance during labor, delivery, or the postpartum period, use their own hands more effectively. Conversely, if the mother's most recent experiences of contact in relation to her own body have been of a remote and impersonal nature, she seems to stay longer at this stage in her own activities with her infant.

Klaus and Kennell A number of studies have been reported in the last few years by Marshall Klaus, John Kennell, and their associates (1970; 1971; 1972; 1974; 1976). Many of these studies have focused on development of mothering in women who have premature or sick infants. Their findings tend to support Rubin's earlier findings regarding the use of fingertips followed by later incorporation of the neonate toward the body. However, they found that there was a rapid progression from fingertip to palm and trunk contact within a period of 10 min rather than the several days reported by Rubin. They speculated that the nude state of the infant during the contact period might have stimulated more rapid progression. Furthermore, differences in maternal anesthesia might also have altered the effective state of either the mother or infant. A limp, sleepy, unresponsive infant whose eyes are closed will not provide the same stimulus as an active, wide-awake baby. A more rapid flow of the sequence may be correlated with early hospital discharge.

Mothers of premature infants, studied on their first three contacts (over a period of 1 to 17 days), exhibited an attenuated sequence of the behavior observed in the mother of full-term infants during the first contact. The progression from fingertip to palm contact did not occur over the time span of the first three contacts of mothers of

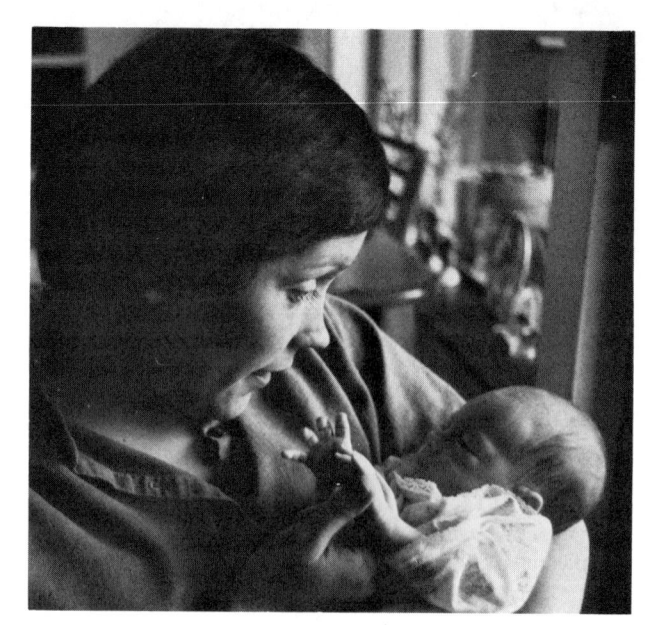

FIGURE 4-3. The *en face* position.

premature infants. Instead, fingertip contact increased in the second and third contact. With the full-term infants, the mother showed a marked increase in the *en face* position within the first 5 min (see Fig. 4-3). Klaus, Kennell, Plumb, and Zuilkke (1970) speculated that early mother-to-infant eye-to-eye contact appears to be a significant interaction during development of maternal affectional ties.

Kennell and Klaus (1971) identify nine steps in maternal attachment: (1) planning the pregnancy, (2) confirming the pregnancy, (3) accepting the pregnancy, (4) fetal movement, (5) accepting the fetus as an individual, (6) birth, (7) seeing the infant, (8) touching the infant, and (9) caretaking. They discuss the multiple variables which may play a role in development of disorders or distortions of maternal behavior, which can range from severe (battered-child syndrome) to mild (undue persistent concerns about minor illness long since completely resolved). Their contention is that separation in the immediate neonatal period may be a major component in these mothering disorders. In support of this hypothesis they cite the high number of premature infants who later return to the hospital with failure to thrive with no organic cause. Studies of failure-to-thrive infants have shown that 15 to 30 percent have no organic disease; 25 to 41 percent of this group were premature. Kennell and Klaus report a study by Solnit and Green on the vulnerable-child syndrome (children whose parents expect them to die prematurely). They note that 44 percent of these children were either born prematurely or were severely ill and separated from the mothers in the immediate neonatal period. Furthermore, they speculate that if adoptions occurred at 1 day of life, behavioral problems of adoptive children, which are far out of proportion to the instances of adoption, would be decreased.

In an attempt to study the importance of the first postpartum days on maternal attachment, Klaus, Jerauld, Kreger, Alpine, Steffa, and Kennell (1972) placed 28 primiparous women in two study groups shortly after delivery of normal, full-term infants. Fourteen mothers, who were the control group, had usual physical contact with their infants, and fourteen mothers in the extended-contact group had 16 h additional contact. Mothers' backgrounds and infants' characteristics were similar in both groups. Maternal behavior was measured 28 to 32 days later during a standardized interview, an examination of the infant, and a filming of the infant being bottle-fed. They found that extended-contact mothers were more reluctant to leave their infants with someone else, usually stood and watched during the examination, showed greater soothing behavior, and engaged in significantly more eye-to-eye contact and fondling.

While previous studies have focused on the process by which the infant becomes attached to his mother, Klaus, Kennell, and associates felt that their observations helped in describing the process in the opposite direction, the attachment behavior of the mother. They suggest that the neonatal period may be a special attachment period for an adult woman—special in the sense that what happens during this time may alter the later behavior of the adult toward a young infant for at least as long as 1 month after delivery. They suggest the use of the term *maternal sensitive period* as a special term to describe this period.

In a follow-up study (Kennell, 1974) of these same mothers when their infants were 1 year of age, the mothers in the two groups also proved to be significantly different in their answers to interview questions and in their behavior during the physical examination of the infants. In discussing these findings, Kennell speculated that possible differences in the control and the extended groups might be due to a few mothers in one or both groups. However, "the ranking of the mothers within each of the two groups showed no significant correlation for the measures at the one month and one year examination (that is, a mother ranking high in a certain activity at one month might be low at one year)" (p. 177).

This finding can be interpreted to mean that while one can predict that *as a group* mothers who have extended contact with their infants in the neonatal period and those who have usual hospital contact will be different, one cannot predict that any one mother's behavior will show consistency over the period of 1 year. Thus, one needs to be careful not to assume that *any* mother who has extended contact with her neonate will show high mothering behavior at 1 year or, conversely, that a mother who has minimal contact with her neonate will have low mothering behavior. In other words, data in this study are reporting consistency in behavior for the two groups but not for individuals within those groups.

Broussard and Hartner Broussard and Hartner (1971) focused on the dissonance between mothers' expectations of an average infant and their perception of their own infants using the Neonatal Perception Inventories (NPI). These inventories measure the mother's perceptions of an average infant and of her own infant. The behavioral items included are crying, spitting, feeding, elimination, sleeping, and predictability. These inventories were completed by 318 primiparas on the first or second postpartum day (time 1) while in the hospital. Of these, 46.5 percent rated their infants as better than average. The perception inventories were administered again when the infants were approximately 1 month of age (time 2). At this time, 61.2 percent of the women rated their infants as better than average.

One hypothesis was that mothers who originally rated their infants as not being better than average at time 1 were experiencing dissonance between their expectations of the average infant and their perception of their infants immediately after delivery. One could further expect that these mothers would attempt to reduce their dissonance. Those who were successful in doing so were expected to have low problem scores at time 2. On the other hand, if mothers were unable to reduce dissonance or if they experienced an increase in dissonance, the problem score would be expected to be high. Since the threshold of parental annoyance varies widely in accordance with parents' emotional orientation to the child, the ultimate decision as to what constitutes a problem for a specific mother varies among mothers. In order to measure problems in infant behavior, a Degree of Bother Inventory was designed. Administered when the infants are 1 month old, this assesses the degree to which mothers were bothered by their infants' behavior in regard to the same six behavioral items on the NPI.

The results of the studies showed that the mother's perception of her infant, as compared with her perception of the average infant, on the first or second postpartum day is not predictive of the child's subsequent development. However, of the 120 children from the original population who were followed to age 4½ years, there was less psychopathology among the children viewed as better than average by their mothers at 1 month of age than among those not viewed as better than average. Of the 85 children from whom a diagnosis was established, 40 percent were judged to have a degree of psychopathology sufficient to require psychiatric intervention.

Broussard and Hartner's research did not determine why mothers rated their infant's behavior as better than or not better than average. They postulated that perhaps the unique personality characteristics of the neonate, or innate genetic characteristics, are detected very early by the mother and that her rating represents a true picture of the child. However, they counterpostulated that the mother's expectations may influence the child's behavior, thus producing a self-fulfilling prophecy. In any case, they suggest that by administering the perception inventories at 1 month of age a significant proportion of children who may experience subsequent developmental and emotional problems can be identified. Broussard and Hartner emphasize the need for long-term research on intervention strategies with the high-risk group for developing primary prevention methods in the mental health area.

Other theorists Recent work of Korner (1967; 1971) has further advanced knowledge of behavioral variables of the neonate. She hypothesizes that an understanding of the earlier stages of development must involve, not only assessment of a mother's mothering, but also the infant's characteristics and what these represent as a stimulus to his care giver. Korner's observations have implications for child rearing in that if infants differ significantly from each other from the start, this suggests there is more than one way to provide good child care.

Brazelton (1961; 1969; 1973) has also made important contributions to the study of individual differences in infants. Much of his research deals with behavioral differences in other cultures and effects of maternal medication on the neonate. In addition, he has developed a neonatal behavioral assessment scale (1973) to be used to score an infant's available responses to the environment and the infant's effect on the environment (see Chap. 3).

FATHER-INFANT ATTACHMENT

Until this point, discussion has centered on mother-infant attachment, and nothing has been presented about the role of the father in the infant's development or about father-infant attachment. This does not mean that father-infant attachment is not important but does reflect the great scarcity of literature in general, and studies in particular, on fathering and on father-infant interaction or attachment.

Parke Recently, however, an exploratory study was done by Parke (1973) at the Fels Research Institute. In the first study, 19 Caucasian couples and their firstborn infants served as subjects. Mothers ranged in age from 19 to 30, while fathers ranged between 20 and 38 years of age. With one exception, the fathers were present during both labor and delivery; one-half of the couples had attended childbirth classes. Two sets of observations were made: (1) mother-father-infant, and (2) mother-infant alone. All observations took place in the mother's hospital room between 6 and 48 h after delivery. For the mother-only sessions, the neonate was placed in the mother's arms prior to commencement of the observations. In the case of the mother-father-infant sessions, the investigator brought the neonate to the mother's room, and the observer asked, "Whom shall I give the baby to?" The neonate was then handed to the parent who indicated a preference to hold the child.

Infant behaviors recorded were cries, vocalizations, moves, mouth movements with or without object, looks at mother, looks at father, and looks around. For both mother and father, behaviors recorded were looks, smiles, vocalizations, holds, kisses, touches, imitations, explorations, feedings, and handing over the neonate to the other parent. In this study Parke found that the father is a very active participant in the family triad. Statistical analysis indicated only one significant difference, and that was that mothers smile more than do fathers. Fathers tended to hold the infant more than mothers; they rocked the neonate more in their arms than did their spouses. On all other measures, the father was just as likely to interact with the neonate as the mother.

In comparing the mother's behavior when the father was or was not present, Parke found that the presence of the father reduced the amount of interaction between mother and neonate. Mother was less likely to hold, change position, rock, touch, or vocalize when father was present. It was also found that both mothers and fathers touched male babies significantly more than female babies. However, this sex difference was not present during the sessions when mother and neonate were alone.

A second and more extensive investigation extended the previous study in two ways. First, observation of father-infant interaction as well as mother-infant and mother-father-infant interactions were included in the second study. Second, the fathers in the original study were well-educated, middle-class fathers, many of whom had attended prenatal classes. In the second study, the sample was drawn from a large, metropolitan general hospital with 51 Caucasian and 31 Negro families of lower socioeconomic status participating. The age range for mothers was 15 to 43 years, while fathers ranged in age from 17 to 47. The infants sampled consisted of 48 girls and 34 boys; 17 boys and 17 girls were firstborn, while the remaining boys and girls were later born. No fathers were present during delivery. All contacts were made in the hospital within the first 48 h. Three types of observations were made: (1) mother-infant, (2) mother-father-infant, and (3) father-infant. The parents were informed that they could either pick up the infant or leave him in his crib.

Again, in this study, Parke found that the father was a very active participant. Statistical analysis revealed that the father is significantly more likely than the mother to hold and visually attend to the infant and to provide physical and auditory stimulation. Only in smiling did the mother outdistance the father. When the father was alone with the infant, he was significantly more likely to touch and rock his infant than was the mother when she was alone with the infant. The presence of the mother had one positive effect: The father smiled more in her presence than alone. When the mother and infant were alone, the mother-infant interaction was much higher than when the father was present. Statistical analysis indicated that the mother is significantly less likely to hold, touch, rock, vocalize, imitate, and feed her neonate when the father is present. However, the mother is more likely to explore the infant and smile at him when the father is present than when she is alone with her neonate. Perhaps the most important comparison involved the mother and father alone with their infant. When they are alone, fathers and mothers differ only slightly in their pattern of interaction; mothers feed the baby more frequently than do fathers.

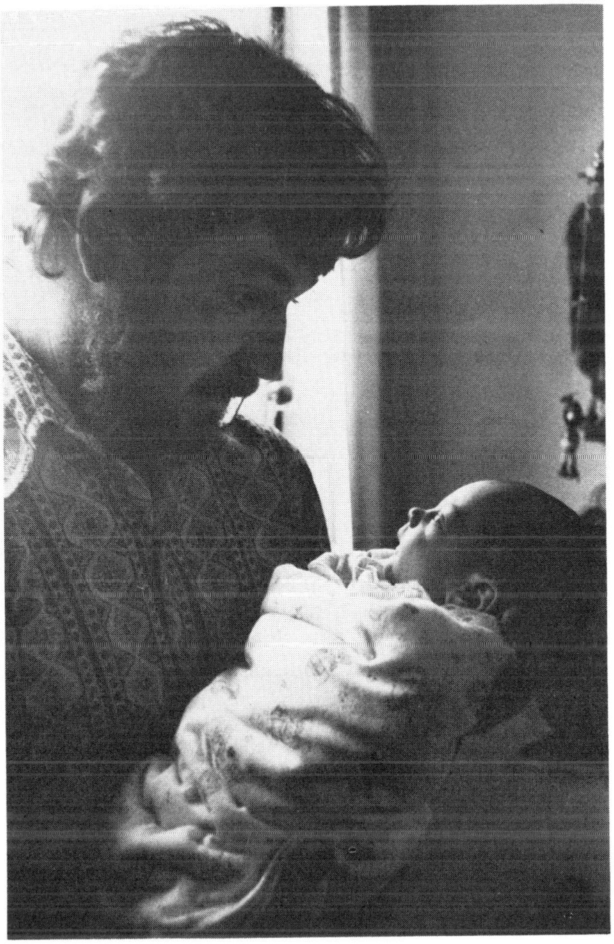

Some sex and ordinal-position differences were noted in the second study. When the mother and father were together, parents tended to hold firstborn infants in their arms but to hold later borns in their laps. Parents were more likely to walk with the firstborn than the later-born infant, particularly if the firstborn was a boy. Parents walked girls equally, regardless of ordinal position. Finally, fathers touched the firstborn more than the later born, while mothers tended to touch later-born infants slightly more than firstborn infants.

The analysis involving the mother alone, compared with the mother in the presence of the father, indicated that mothers rocked firstborn infants more than later born infants and boys more than girls. However, these ordinal-position differences in maternal behavior varied with the presence or absence of the father. When the father was present, the mother rocked firstborn and later-born infants equally. Fathers, regardless of being alone or with the mother, touched firstborn boys more than either later-born boys or girls of either ordinal position. Fathers vocalized more to firstborn boys than to firstborn girls, while they vocalized equally to later-born infants irrespective of sex. In summary, sex and ordinal position of the infant and presence of the spouse are important modifying variables in the early parent-infant interaction.

Greenberg and Morris In a study entitled "Engrossment: The Newborn's Impact upon the Father," Greenberg

FIGURE 4-4. The *en face* position.

and Morris (1974) studied two groups of first fathers: (1) a group of fathers whose first contact with the neonate occurred at the birth (in the delivery room), and (2) a group whose first contact with the neonate occurred after the birth, when shown to them by nursery personnel. Both groups of fathers showed evidence of strong paternal feelings and of involvement with their neonate.

Results of this study suggest that fathers begin developing a bond to their neonate by the first 3 days after the birth and often earlier. Furthermore, there are certain describable characteristics of this bond, which the authors call *engrossment,* which were observed in clinical interviews. The findings suggest that the fathers develop a feeling of preoccupation, absorption, and interest in their neonate. The father is gripped and held by this particular feeling and has a desire to look at, hold, and touch the infant. It is as if he has been "hooked" by something that has transpired in the father-infant relationship. Greenberg and Morris (1974, p. 526) state the following:

> The term engrossment is meant to mean more than involvement. The derivation of the word engross means "to make large." When the father is engrossed in his individual infant, the infant has assumed larger proportions for him. In addition, it is suggested that the father feels bigger, and that he feels an increased sense of self-esteem and worth when he is engrossed in his infant.

SEPARATION

The influence that the family has on child development cannot be argued. The family is particularly important in early childhood, when strong emotional ties are formed and when the child is in a particularly rapid growth period. As noted in preceding sections, special emphasis has been placed on the importance of a close maternal-child relationship. What happens, then, if children are separated from their families, and particularly from their mothers, for brief or extended periods of time?

As presented earlier, Bowlby predicted dire consequences if young children are separated from their mothers. It is sometimes claimed that the normal growth of children is dependent on the mother's full-time occupation in the role of rearing children. A WHO expert committee (World Health Organization, 1951) stated that the use of day nurseries and crèches inevitably caused permanent injury to the emotional health of children. It is no wonder many mothers feel guilty when they work. Margaret Mead (1954) suggested that the campaign on evils of mother-child separation is another attempt by men to shackle women to the home.

Most children experience some separation from their parents during childhood, and presumably most of these children turn out to be quite normal. Thus, it is not strictly a question of whether a child should be separated from his parents but at what age, for how long, and from which parent. Another question is: What other support does a child have when separated from one or both parents?

EFFECTS OF SHORT-TERM SEPARATION

The effects of short-term separation have been studied mostly in children admitted to the hospital. Bowlby and his colleagues, noting the frequency with which children were upset after admission to the hospital, described three phases of disturbance (Bowlby, 1969; Robertson, 1958). First is the period of *protest,* when the child cries and shows acute distress. Next is the phase of *despair,* when the child appears miserable and withdrawn. Finally the stage of *detachment* occurs, when the child seems to lose interest in his parents. When the child returns home, he often ignores his parents initially and then becomes clinging and demanding.

Some investigators have failed to confirm these findings (Davenport and Werry, 1970; Rose, 1972, 1973), but Bowlby's and Robertson's observations have been supported by other studies (Vernon, Foley, Sipowicz, and Schulman, 1965; Yarrow, 1964). However, certain factors need to be considered. Reaction to separation is most noted in children ages 6 months to 4 years, but even at this age it occurs only in some children (Illingworth and Holt, 1955; Prugh, Staub, Sands, Kirschbaum, and Lenihan, 1953; Schaffer and Callender, 1959). Furthermore, children are strongly attached to other family members besides mothers. The importance of this is supported by the finding that children admitted to the hospital with a sibling show less distress than children admitted alone (Heinicke and Westheimer, 1965). Branstetter (1969) showed that the presence of a substitute mother, even though unknown to the child before hospitalization, alleviated the usual responses to hospitalization and separation from mother in 2-year-olds. Finally, it appears that children used to brief, happy separations are less distressed by unhappy separations such as a hospital admission (Stacey, Dearden, Pill, and Robinson, 1970).

In summary, it appears that brief separation has the potential for causing short-term distress and emotional disturbance. However, many factors, such as presence of a sibling or another supportive person, happiness of previous separations, and the child's own ability to cope, determine whether and how much distress actually occurs.

EFFECTS OF LONG-TERM SEPARATION

It has often been claimed that children of working women are likely to become delinquent or develop some form of emotional problem. However, there is considerable evidence that this is not so. In fact, some children of working mothers may be less likely to become delinquent than children whose mothers do not work. In addition, there is no evidence that children suffer from having several mother figures as long as the relationships are stable and that good care is provided. Furthermore, the view that putting children in day nurseries and crèches will lead to psychological damage has not been supported by research (Rutter, 1971). In fact, there is some evidence that with adequate substitute care a mother's working need not be detrimental and can be beneficial to the child's development in terms of positive gains in the developmental quotient (Wallston, 1973).

Working fathers, conversely, have not had to face the role conflict or child rearing decisions of working mothers. Even when both parents work, mothers often also take on total responsibility for child care. However, it is becoming more common today for a working father to assume equal child-care responsibility with the working mother. Also, in more families today the father is the primary, full-time care giver, not employed outside the home.

Poor child care, whether at home with a parent or a baby-sitter or in day-care setting, is undesirable and may lead to disturbed behavior in children. However, studies generally have not looked at the quality of care given children as opposed to the type of care (mother versus father versus baby-sitter versus day care). In addition, the child's individual ability to cope with various types of care has not been studied.

Transient separation As has been discussed in a previous section, brief separations can lead to some short-term distress. Does extended separation lead to long-term psychological disturbance? Some studies have shown that children can be separated from their parents for quite long periods in early childhood with little, if any, ill effects. However, other studies indicate that children separated from their parents in early childhood have a slightly increased risk of later psychological disturbance (Rutter, 1971).

In order to separate differences in these findings, Rutter (1971) and associates undertook a study of families, dividing separation experiences into those involving separation from one parent only and those involving separation from both parents at the same time. Only a few of the findings can be reported here.

They found that children separated from both parents come from more disturbed homes than do children who never experience separation. Many of the children are separated from their families because of a family crisis. Investigating the relation between parent-and-child separation and antisocial behavior in boys, after controlling for the quality of the parental marriage, it was found that the greatest differences in antisocial behavior are associated with quality of the marriage and not with the experience of separation. Furthermore, Rutter reports, "regardless of the parental marriage relationship, separations from one parent only carried no increase in the rate of antisocial disorder" (1971, p. 240). This is true regardless of the age of the child at the time of separation. On the basis of these findings, Rutter suggested that the association between marriage ratings of parents and disturbed behavior in children may be due to discord and disturbance which surrounds separation rather than to separation itself.

To study this, the investigators divided separations from both parents into those due to some event not associated with discord (for example, a child admitted to the hospital) and those in which the separation was due to deviance or discord (for example, breakup due to quarrels or mental illness in one parent).

As indicated by Fig. 4-5, it is the *reason* for separation that matters, not the separation itself. When the children are separated because of physical illness or vacation, the rate of antisocial behavior is low. However, when separation from both parents is due to some type of family discord or deviance, almost one-half the children exhibit antisocial behavior. These findings are true regardless of the age of the child when the separation takes place.

Permanent separations Rutter (1971) and his associates also investigated the effects of permanent separation due to death or divorce on the behavior of children. They concluded that while parental death may play a part in the pathogenesis of some disorders, delinquency is primarily associated with separations which follow parental discord rather than the loss of a parent as such. Rutter also suggests that the disturbances which do occur in children following the death of a parent may be due to a long illness preceding the death, grief of the surviving parent, and economic and social deterioration of the family following the death of the father.

FACTORS IN THE CHILD

Sex and temperment, two factors in the child which might aggravate or ameliorate the adverse influence of family discord, were investigated by Rutter (1971). In regard to sex, the effects of parental discord were found to be much more marked in boys than in girls.

The other factor which Rutter considered was the temperamental makeup of the child. Temperaments of the children were assessed at 4 and 8 years of age, and the influence of temperament was measured against behavioral deviance in school 1 year later. Children who show deviant behavior are more likely to be nonfastidious, lack malleability, and be markedly irregular in their eating and sleeping patterns. These findings are very similar to those reported by Thomas, Chess, and Birch (1968) and indicate that children differ in their capacity to deal with family stress. Rutter (1971, p. 254) summarizes by saying, "It is no new observation that children differ in their responses to stress situations but until recent years surprisingly little attention has been paid to this side of parent-child interaction."

In summary, the literature suggests that while the child's separation from his family may lead to short-term distress, it is not of direct importance as a cause of long-term behavioral disorder. Other factors need to be considered in explaining deviant behavior in children, some of which may be family discord and the sex and temperament of the child. Rutter suggests several possible mechanisms that may explain why and how family discord interacts with a child's temperamental characteristics to produce antisocial behavior. First, both retrospective and prospective studies give evidence that parents of delinquent boys differ from other parents in their approach to the discipline and supervision of children. Second, studies show that children readily imitate other peoples' behavior. Thus, when family discord is present, it may provide the child with a model of aggression, inconsistency, hostility, and antisocial behavior. The third alternative is that the child learns social behavior by having warm, stable relationships with his parents; thus, difficulties in interpersonal relationships are the basis of antisocial conduct.

SINGLE-PARENT FAMILIES OR MULTIPLE-PARENT FAMILIES

Much of what is written about parent-child relationships assumes a two-parent team made up of the biological mother and father. However, many families do not fit this idealistic model. There are many single-parent homes in the United States primarily due to divorce but in other cases due to the death or absence of one parent. In addition, many children have adoptive parents (single or married) or foster parents. Except in the case of death, the fact that a parent is not living in the home does not mean that contact with or responsibility for the children is lost.

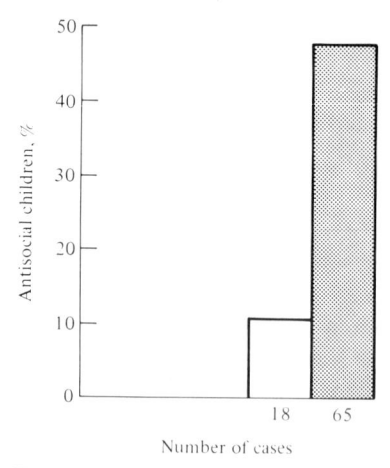

FIGURE 4-5. Reasons for total parent-child separation and antisocial behavior in children. ☐ Separation due to physical illness or holiday; ▨ separation due to family discord or psychiatric illness. (From M. Rutter, Parent-child separation: Psychological effects on their children. *J. Child Psychol. Psychiat.*, 1971, 12, 239. Reprinted by permission.)

SINGLE PARENTS

Mothers Financial stress is one of the major problems in households where the mother is the sole parent. The problem may range from abject poverty to relative deprivation as compared with the income available if married. Lack of money or change in available money can create considerable stress in the parent-child relationship. In most cases the mother is employed outside the home. Particularly with small children there may be difficulties finding appropriate substitute care for the child. With school-age children the hours of school rarely coincide with the mother's working hours, and special arrangements have to be made when school is not in session or a child is ill. While these problems also exist for the working mother who is married, the presence in the home of a father allows more flexibility, since he is able to undertake his share of tasks.

Since only one person is available for the parental role, the mother must assume role responsibilities of mother and father. This often leads to role overload with some roles, of necessity, being slighted.

Fathers Undoubtedly many of the same problems exist for fathers raising their children alone. However, this is mostly speculation since there are few studies about single fathers. Financially the fathers may be more independent; their salaries are likely to be higher than that of single mothers, though single fathers are less likely to receive alimony and child support. The same problems of role overload and role conflict, however, probably will exist.

EXTENDED FAMILIES
There are very little data about the influence of grandparents or other members of the extended family on child rearing. For many parents, grandparents are a supportive resource. They may provide temporary or permanent child care, counseling, and financial help. Other grandparents may be a major source of conflict.

For the adolescent parent, grandparents may be the primary source of help. Often the adolescent parent and the child live with grandparents, at least until the parent finishes high school. How successful this is often depends on the degree to which the adolescents have resolved their own role conflicts with their parents. Not infrequently the grandmother assumes, or tries to assume, the role of mother with the child (particularly if it is her daughter's baby). In some instances this may be agreeable to both persons. In such a situation the parent often assumes the role of older sibling rather than a mother or father role. In many cases, however, major conflicts about role responsibilities arise between parent and grandparent. The dilemma may be further confounded by the adolescent's own ambivalence about being a parent.

Literature on maternal-infant attachment emphasizes the importance of early and consistent bonding to one mother figure. But that is probably not the situation in a large segment of the population. There is some suggestion in the literature that if bonding does not occur, there may be an increase in child abuse in those families. But what if multiple bonding occurs? Farber (1964, p. 457) has asked this question: "Are two parents enough? . . . in almost every human society *more* than two adults are involved in the socialization of the child." Farber goes on to say that in many societies a "third parent," outside the nuclear family, acts as a sort of "social critic" of the child.

ASSESSMENT OF PARENT-CHILD INTERACTION: GENERAL CONSIDERATIONS
Much has been written about the assessment of parent-child behavior—maternal-infant and paternal-infant interaction; however, most of the tools actually measure infant or child behavior or mother (and sometimes father) behavior or ideas and attitudes about the child. A great deal of the research in the area of parent-child relationships is based on the assumption that there is a direct and discernible relation between parents' behavior, attitudes, and personality and child behavior (Mcdinnus, 1967). This assumption does not take into account the multiple variables that influence a child's behavior and development. Nor does it consider parents' and children's mutual influence on each other.

The major tool historically used in psychological studies of parent-child relationships has been the research interview. Questions concerning the validity and reliability of this method have been raised (Yarrow, 1963). Yarrow suggests that the use of direct observation would be of value in answering the unanswered question about parent-child interaction. Directly observing the parent

FIGURE 4-6. (*Photo courtesy of Betsy Smith.*)

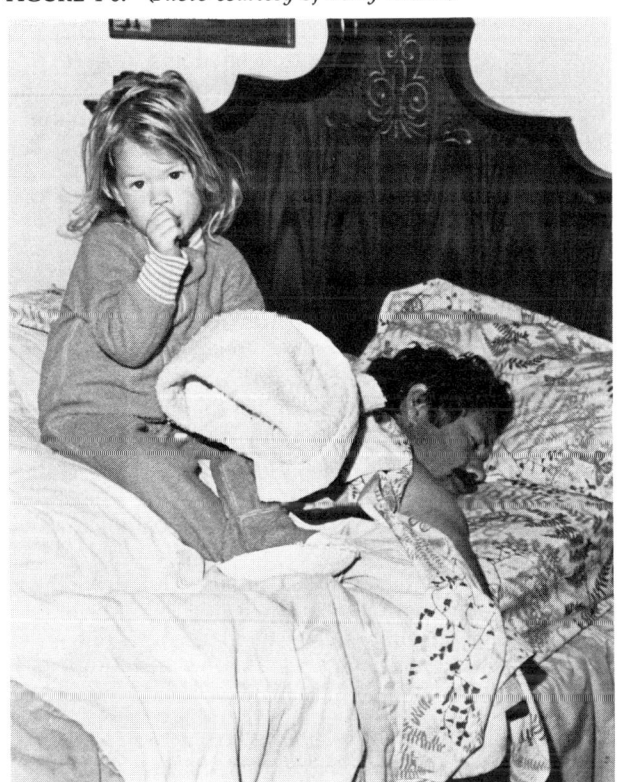

with the child would allow for the study of the context in which particular parental behavior occurs and also the role of the child in eliciting parental behavior. Rubin (1963) made use of this method in her study of maternal touch, as did Klaus and Kennell (1976) in their studies on maternal-infant bonding.

In deciding what type of assessment to use, important questions to be considered are the following: For what purpose is the assessment being made? Is it for research purposes? Are the data collected applicable to the total group only or to individuals within the group? Are the data to be used as a basis for intervention, and if so, when? Now, or in several years? Has intervention based on the assessment tool been studied (or is it being studied) adequately? Have adequate validity and reliability studies been done on the assessment tool?

The tools used to assess parent-child interaction do not necessarily give direction as to the type of intervention strategies most useful to help improve parent-child interactions. In addition, most assessment tools that measure interaction measure a parent interacting with a child, not the interaction between both parents and child. In other words most current tools can be symbolized by

Parent ↔ child

rather than by

Mother ↔ father
       ↘ ↙
       child

or by

Mother ↔ father
  ↕ ╳ ↕
child ↔ child
   ↘ ↙
   child

Many assessment tools in use today document what happens between parents and children and what effect this has on the child's development. Less emphasis has been placed on systematically studying how parent-child interaction can be improved, though some studies are being done in this area (Kogan, 1969). In discussing the possible relation between early intervention with mothers and infants and later emotional problems of children, Rexford (1976) concludes that a number of well-planned and -staffed intervention projects need to be set up before there is proof that early intervention will prevent or ameliorate later emotional problems and mental illness.

The major misuse of an assessment tool comes from using it on populations for which it was not designed or by not following the written protocol on how to use it. Thus, results may be based on incomplete or inappropriate data.

Assessment of the child's environment[1]
Marcene Powell Erickson

A great deal of attention has been focused in recent years on standardizing tools that accurately assess growth and development of children. Less attention has been directed at assessing the animate and inanimate aspects of the child's environment that either foster or impede a child's growth and developmental processes. There is more concern for ways to assess the quality and quantity of social, emotional, and cognitive support that is available in a young child's environment. Although there have been almost no tools available that permit the precise measurement of the child's developmental and learning environment, this trend is changing.

Dr. Bettye M. Caldwell has been doing research for many years to develop hypotheses about the nature of the environment and how it best meets the needs of children. Over the past decade she formulated the view that it is not the social status or family structure that necessarily predicts a child's subsequent cognitive outcomes. She hypothesized that what was most important were various characteristics of the environment that could predict a child's developmental outcomes. This theoretical view stimulated her and her associates to devise a tool by which the subtle aspects of the young child's environment could be measured to determine which specific features were most likely to influence the child's development. They endeavored to create a measure of the home environment that could warn of developmental risk before age 3 years.

Based on clinical observations and observations in the home, an inventory was developed that was intended to tap the environmental characteristics of a child from birth to 3 years of age that might be associated with favorable developmental outcomes for the child. This instrument is called the Home Observation for Measurement of the Environment (birth to three) (see Table 4-1). The inventory

[1] Reproduced with permission from M. P. Erickson, *Assessment and management of developmental changes in children.* St. Louis: Mosby, 1976.

endeavors to measure the following six subscales: (1) the emotional and verbal responsivity of the mother, (2) avoidance of restriction and punishment, (3) organization of the physical and temporal environment, (4) provision of appropriate play materials, (5) maternal involvement with the child, and (6) opportunities for variety in daily stimulation.

Caldwell also developed the Home Observation for Measurement of the Environment (three to six) (see Table 4-2). This inventory is intended to tap the changing environment of the older child between 3 and 6 years of age. This inventory endeavors to measure the following seven subscales: (1) provision of stimulation through equipment, toys, and experiences; (2) stimulation of mature behavior; (3) provision of a stimulating physical and language environment; (4) avoidance of restriction and punishment; (5) pride, affection, and thoughtfulness; (6) masculine stimulation; and (7) independence from parental control.

The Home Observation for Measurement of the Environment (referred to as the HOME), developed by Caldwell and associates over the past 10 years, is one of the first major tools of its kind to focus on the environment.

Because of Caldwell's research, means of providing substantive feedback to parents about the way they regulate their child's environment and how to effect environmental changes that best facilitate their child's growth and development are available. Such feedback can also be used to help parents meet their own needs for assuring their child an appropriate environment at different stages of development.

As an infant or child progresses in his adaptive functioning, there are corresponding needs for the developmental environment to change simultaneously. Parents may experience the need for help in creating and sustaining an environment that is most suitable for their child or may need reassurance that the environment is regularly and consistently providing appropriate input both in terms of timing and frequency that enhances the child's growth and development. Nurses, physicians, and early child educators can respond in more appropriate ways by expanding their roles in terms of developmental assessment and management of infants and children, as well as assessment of the child's developmental environment. By doing so, such professionals can improve their ability to provide counseling and guidance within a preventive framework.

Both inventories (birth to three and three to six) offer a valuable framework for systematically and objectively collecting information about the subtle aspects of a child's environment that can be used for the mutual benefit of both the child and his parents. The HOME may be used to assess not only the home environment but any environment in which the child spends time. It can be administered to the mother or any other primary care giver. (It should be noted that the instruction manual relates only to the birth to three inventory.)

Although extensive standardization data are not available, both inventories measure inanimate and animate

TABLE 4-1 The six subscales and two sample items from each subscale of the inventory, *Home Observation for Measurement of the Environment, Birth to Three*

Subscale	Sample items
1 Emotional and verbal responsivity of mother	1a Mother responds to child's vocalizations with a verbal response. b Mother caresses or kisses child at least once during visit.
2 Avoidance of restriction and punishment	2a Mother does not shout at child during visit. b Mother neither slaps nor spanks child during visit.
3 Organization of physical and temporal environment	3a Child gets out of house at least four times a week. b Child's play environment appears safe and free from hazards.
4 Provision of appropriate play materials	4a Child has push or pull toy. b Mother provides toys or interesting activities for child during interview.
5 Maternal involvement with child	5a Mother "talks" to child while doing her work. b Mother invests "maturing" toys with value via her attention.
6 Opportunities for variety in daily stimulation	6a Father provides some caretaking every day. b Mother reads stories at least three times weekly.

Source: From B. M. Caldwell and R. H. Bradley, Home observation for measurement of the environment, birth to three. By permission.

qualities and quantities and the variation and complexity of the child's environment.

Caldwell (1970) states that the purpose of the HOME is to obtain samples of certain aspects of the quantity and quality of social, emotional, and cognitive support available to a young child within his home.

> The selection of items has been guided by empirical evidence of the importance of certain types of experience for nourishing the behavioral development of the child. Included were such things as the importance of the opportunity to form a basic attachment to a mother or mother substitute; an emotional climate characterized by mutual pleasure, sensitive need gratification, and minimization of restriction and punishment; a physical environment that is both stimulating and responsive, offering a variety of modulated sensory experience; freedom to explore and master the environment; a daily schedule that is orderly and predictable; and an opportunity to assimilate and interpret experience within a consistent cultural milieu. (Caldwell, 1970, p. 1)

Indices of health and nutritional status are not included in the inventory. As Caldwell asserts:

> The development of this Inventory represents a conviction that such a gross structural designation as social class is insensitive to the cumulative transactions that occur daily between the infant and his environment and that an attempt to describe and measure these transactions will not only provide a more accurate description of the learning environment but will in addition help to pin-point areas in which intervention is needed. (Caldwell, 1970, p. 2)

She further states:

> The original intention was that all items should be based on direct observation of the interaction between caretaker (usually the mother) and the child. A large pool of items was generated, all of which required actual observation of mother-child behavior. But a conceptual examination of the items suggested that many important areas of infant experience were unfortunately excluded with this restriction on the type of items. Accordingly, with succeeding versions of the Inventory (the present is the fourth revision), items requiring interview data were added. (Caldwell, 1970, p. 2)

Caldwell (1970) suggests that prior to use, observation, and scoring of the HOME, the observer should be reasonably familiar with the content of each individual item.

The HOME can be of significance in the following ways:

1 Determining the frequency of contacts between adult care givers and children
2 Determining that the child is in an environment that is both stimulating and responsive to his needs
3 Helping determine whether the emotional climate is positive or negative in nature

TABLE 4-2 The eight subscales and one sample item from each subscale of the inventory, *Home Observation for Measurement of the Environment, Preschool* **(Three to Six)**

Subscale	Sample items
1 Stimulation through toys, games, and reading material	1 Toys or game permitting free expression (finger paints, play dough, crayons or paint and paper)
2 Positive social responsiveness	2 Parent encourages child to relate experiences or takes time to listen to him relate experiences.
3 Physical environment: safe, clean, and conducive to development	3 The interior of the apartment is not dark or perceptibly monotonous.
4 Pride, affection, and warmth	4 Parent holds child close 10 to 15 min/day (e.g., during TV, story time, visiting).
5 Stimulation of academic behavior	5 Child is encouraged to learn colors.
6 Modeling and encouragement of social maturity	6 Child can express negative feelings without harsh reprisal.
7 Variety of stimulation	7 Child's artwork is displayed someplace in house (anything that child makes).
8 Physical punishment	8 Mother neither slaps nor spanks child during visit.

Source: From B. M. Caldwell and R. H. Bradley, Home observation for measurement of the environment, preschool (three to six). By permission.

4 Helping determine if there is provision for sensory experiences that are neither understimulating nor overstimulating to the child
5 Helping determine the adequacy of novelty and range of contacts with others
6 Helping identify areas of strengths and weaknesses in a family
7 Planning appropriate guidance for a family
8 Identifying developmental risk before a child is 3 years of age
9 Planning intervention strategies when weaknesses or deficits are observed

One of Caldwell's original goals in developing the HOME was to have information gained from observations available for family guidance. It was her intent to be able to identify areas of strength and weaknesses in a family. She emphasizes that if the care-giving disciplines could profile a family's patterns, then those working with families could determine those areas which were in need of extra efforts by professionals in child health.

The HOME (birth to three) measures 45 items in six major categories. The HOME (three to six) measures 80 items in seven major categories.

GENERAL INSTRUCTIONS FOR THE HOME

The HOME is administered by a person who goes into the home at a time when the child is awake and can be observed in his normal routine for that time of day. The entire procedure in the home generally takes about an hour (Caldwell, 1970).

MAKING ARRANGEMENTS FOR THE VISIT

The visit should never be made without careful advance arrangements; otherwise the mother might be led to think that an attempt is being made to catch her "off guard" (e.g., when her house is not clean or she is not tidy). Caldwell (1970) advises that advance contact may be made either by letter or telephone, making certain that the mother being contacted knows the following: (1) whom the interviewer represents and what kind of information he needs, (2) how much time she should allow for the visit, (3) that it is important for the child to be present and awake, and (4) that the mother will be giving something of value to the interviewer, the group he represents, and to all people who are concerned about how young children grow and develop.

Caldwell suggests that in making the contact the interviewer might wish to use the following speech, with appropriate changes made:

> I am from the Center for Early Development and Education at Kramer School. We are interested in seeing what your child does when he is in his home territory—how he occupies his time, what he likes to play with, whether he plays by himself or with someone else, etc. Because of this we will want to come at a time when he is likely to be awake and going about his usual routine. My visit will last about an hour. I would very much appreciate the opportunity to visit with you. (Caldwell, 1970, p. 20)

It is crucial that the home visit be made at a time when the child is awake (at least for part of the visit). If after an appointment has been carefully arranged the interviewer makes a trip to the home and finds that the child has just gone to sleep, it is probably wise to forgo that visit and make another appointment (preferably for later the same morning or afternoon). This inconvenience to the interviewer is necessary, since scoring on at least one-third the items is predicated on interactions between the mother and child during the visit. However, if the child is asleep when the interviewer arrives but is expected by the mother to awaken any moment, it is all right to go ahead and begin the visit with the mother. The interviewer should save all items that require observation of the

FIGURE 4-7.

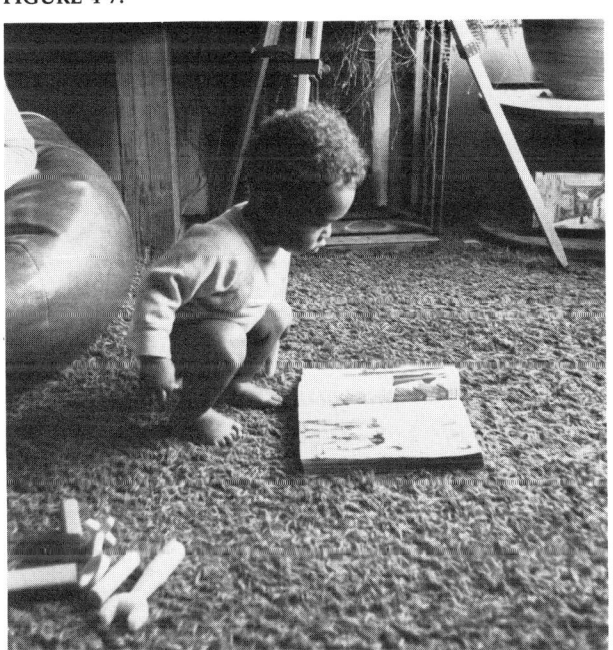

mother and child together and go on to items that rely on the interview (Caldwell, 1970).

THE INTERVIEW

Caldwell does not recommend a standard interview for eliciting the information necessary to score those items which require information that cannot be obtained by observation (e.g., whether the child is taken to the grocery store). She does, however, recommend one standard feature—good interviewers. As defined by Caldwell:

> A good interviewer is a person who can be at ease herself or himself in the situation, can put the mother or caregiver at ease, can easily adjust subsequent questions to answers given by the mother, and can ask questions in such a way as to avoid putting the informant on the defensive and thereby trying to second guess the interviewer as to what is the "right" or "expected" response. (Caldwell, 1970, p. 20)

The interviewer's goal is to be objective and accepting as opposed to approving or disapproving. This is essential if the interviewer is to find out how the mother feels and what she does with the child rather than what she may think you want her to say. It is highly recommended that if at all possible an observer accompany a person already trained in the use of the inventories prior to initiating the interview all alone.

Caldwell suggests an appropriate technique for beginning the interview and for helping the mother to relax. This is to ask her to describe a typical day in the home, using the following statement or something similar:

> You will remember that we are interested in knowing the kinds of things your infant (child) does when he is at home. A good way to get a picture of what his days are like is to have you think of one particular day—like [today]—and tell me everything that happened to him as well as you can remember it. Start with the things that happened when he first woke up. It is usually easy to remember the main events once you get started. (Caldwell, 1970, p. 22)

If the mother cannot get started, help her with questions like "Was he the first one to wake up?" or "Where did he eat his breakfast?"

Caldwell (1970) cautions that the interviewer must be careful not to ask questions in a threatening or seemingly judgmental manner. For example, rather than ask, "Do you ever read stories to your child?" (item 44 on the birth to three HOME), it is preferable to ask, "Do you ever manage to find time to sit down and read to him?" If the mother answers affirmatively, the interviewer can explore further by inquiring, "How often does he like you to do that?"

Almost all the items in sections I and II of both inventories require observation only and must not be based on verbally supplied information.

Caldwell suggests that it is advisable to complete the coding of the HOME before leaving the house. The interviewer must *not* trust his memory. Before the interviewer leaves the home, he should have placed a check in either the Yes or No column for every item.

Caldwell reinforces the concept that ". . . the intent of the assessment procedure is to get a picture of what the child's world is like from his perspective—i.e., from where he lies or sits or stands or moves about and sees, hears, smells, feels, and tastes that world" (Caldwell, 1970, p. 30).

The inventory is attempting to assess the home environment from the perspective of the child, and Caldwell (1970) reminds the interviewer not to think in terms of the respondent's "passing" or "failing" HOME items or the HOME as a whole. Caldwell also discourages conveying that the respondent is passing or failing in his answers.

The interviewer is reminded too that not everything unfolds exactly according to the assessment guide. The interviewer may be observing items in section I and observe or note an important interaction or event in section III of the HOME.

SCORING

Observations that are made and answers that are given by the mother or primary care giver to a semistructural interview administered within the home serve as the basis of scoring.

All items on the HOME receive binary scores—Yes or No—and no attempt is made to rate finer gradations. In clinical use of the instrument, however, interviewers are encouraged to make notes on the form and to jot down their general impressions after each home visit. It is also important to keep in mind the fact that all observation items refer to the contemporary situation, that is, to conditions prevailing at the time of the visit (Caldwell, 1970).

It is suggested that a judgment of "not applicable" be avoided; instead, interpret the item in terms of reasonable limits of the child's age and score accordingly even if a rating of No seems unfair for a baby whose mother does not read to him at 3 months. Each item is to receive a Yes or No.

Caldwell relates that the score for a given home consists of the total number of items marked Yes. In scoring the inventories, special care should be taken to interpret correctly those items in which failure to act in a given way identifies the behavior assumed to be facilitative to development. For example, item 14 on the HOME (birth to three) states, "Mother neither slaps nor spanks child during visit." If neither occurs, then this should be marked in the Yes rather than in the No column. This seemingly awkward procedure is preferable to the even more awkward alternative of having to remember to subtract from the total score those Yes responses that correlate negatively with the total score (Caldwell, 1970).

The HOME yields subscores for each of the subscales and a total score. At the end of each set of items belonging to a given subscale, space is provided for recording the total score for that particular subscale. On the cover sheet, space is provided for transcribing all raw scores for the subscales and then computing the total raw score.

TRAINING

In lieu of formal training by the developers of the instrument, the best procedure is to have people work in pairs on at least a dozen home visits. On the first two visits they should alternate serving as interviewers and score jointly, with each giving reasons for his decisions whenever there is disagreement. Both should consult with each other frequently to clarify scoring for individual items. The next ten interviews should be scored independently, although all scoring differences should be discussed and clarified. If these two persons agree on their coding for 90 percent of the items on each of the last ten inventories administered, then both should be able to administer the inventory individually (Caldwell, 1970). It is reported that raters can quickly be trained to achieve a 90 percent level of agreement.

PREDICTIVE VALUE OF THE HOME

Elardo and associates (1975) designed a study using the HOME with 77 mothers and infants. Their purpose was to explore the inventory's ability to predict later mental test performance. Data were collected on all the infants by using the Mental Development Index (MDI) of the Bayley Scales of Infant Development at 6 and 12 months of age and scores from the Stanford-Binet scale at 36 months. Each infant's home environment was assessed at 6, 12, and 24 months with the HOME.

Results of the study indicate that measures of the home environment when the infant is 6 months old does not correlate highly with the infant's performance on the MDI at 6 or 12 months of age; however, the correlation between measures of the home environment at 6 months of age and Stanford-Binet performance at 3 years of age is extremely significant (Elardo, Bradley, and Caldwell, 1975). The correlation between home environment measured at 12 and 24 months and Stanford-Binet performance is also significant. The investigators found that during the first year of life, the HOME subscales relating to organization of the physical and temporal environment and, to a lesser extent, opportunity for variety in daily stimulation seem most highly related to mental test performance. Elardo and coworkers point out that beginning at 12 months of age, provision of appropriate play materials to and maternal involvement with the child seem to show the strongest relationships to mental test performance.

The data generated from the study showed that the most enriching environments for children in the study sample were those in which a mother or other primary care giver provided an infant with a variety of age-appropriate learning materials and at the same time promoted developmental advances by attending, talking, and positively responding to the child (Elardo et al., 1975).

A major result of this study was to maintain and strengthen the predictive value of the HOME. The inventory was also scrutinized for reliability as the study was carried out.

Because of its predictive aspects, the HOME has major diagnostic and management possibilities for all child-care professionals.

Although the concept and objectives of the inventories have been accepted as valid from the beginning, the tool has undergone many revisions primarily in an attempt to make it applicable to almost any child's environment and usable by a variety of professional observers, with a scale that is valid, reliable, and easy to administer. Throughout the vigorous testing period, the HOME has emerged as one of the best means of assessing the subtler aspects of the quality and quantity of social, emotional, and cognitive support that is available to a young child within his home environment.

IMPLICATIONS OF ENVIRONMENTAL ASSESSMENT FOR THE CHILD

It is universally recognized that optimal development can be achieved when there is emphasis on assessment of the child's environment. Changes in a child's development may depend on both the quality and quantity of kinesthetic, auditory, visual, and other sensory inputs he receives from his environment. A child may be receiving too little or too much change or novelty. His environment may not be organized, predictable, or nurturing, or it may be supportive and sensitive to his needs for consistency, trust, dependability, and organization. It may be introducing change at a rate compatible with the child's pace of assimilating change, or it may be one in which there is not too much pressure to succeed. On the other hand, the environment may be nurturing. It may provide optimal amounts and timing of social, emotional, and cognitive support for the child. There may be sufficient feedback, appropriate kinds of attention for appropriate kinds of behavior, and a consistency in feedback and responsiveness provided by parents that fosters all facets of the child's changing needs.

A child is potentially vulnerable for being at risk in his present and subsequent development if he is not receiving adequate, individualized, and variable sensory inputs of an animate or inanimate nature that direct the way a child processes information. An adequate environment will influence the extent and timing of a child's gains in mastery of himself and his environment and how he progressively makes gains in fine motor, gross motor, personal-social, and language skills. At the same time, if a child is deprived of the ingredients that are necessary for the acquisition of social, emotional, cognitive, personal-adaptive, and motor skills, his parents may not feel adequate about their ability to provide what is best for their child. These same parents may lack adequate support systems themselves. A child whose environment is deficient may correspond to a parent who is also suffering a lack of environmental stimuli.

IMPLICATIONS OF ENVIRONMENTAL ASSESSMENT FOR PARENTS

Just as fulfilling a child's environmental needs are important for a healthy continuum of change, parents, too, need reassurance, support, guidance, and opportunities to discuss their perceptions of providing an environment that meets their child's needs. In addition, a parent's need to know "Am I doing the right things for my child?" must be met.

Parents who are responsive to their child's needs and are attempting to offer substantial input or refrain from too much stimuli deserve acknowledgment of the ways they have elected to create a healthy, appropriate, nurturing environment.

Sometimes parents try too hard, expect too much of themselves, and tend to go to extremes in doing the right thing for their child at exactly the right time. Parents may need support to relax their efforts, to take the pressure off

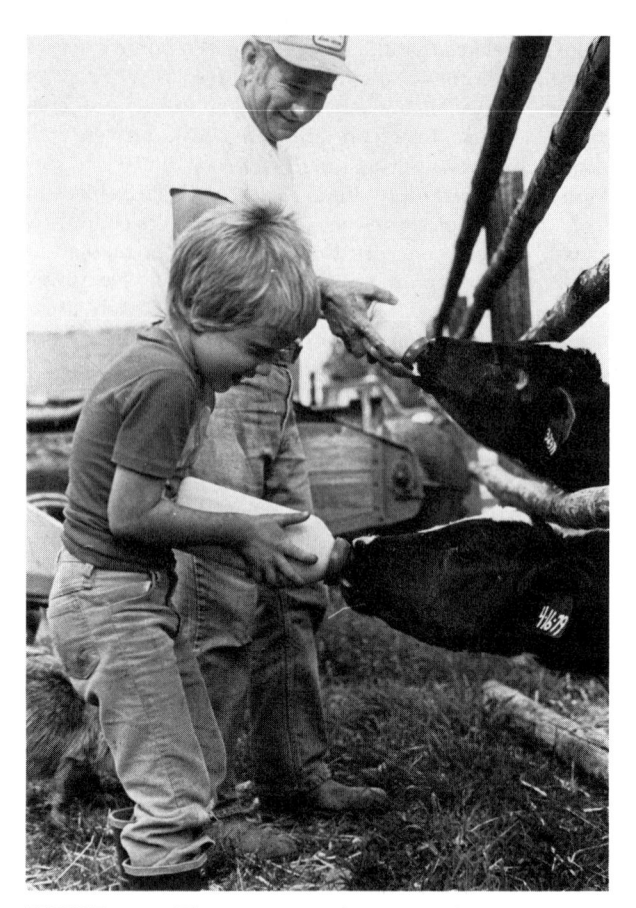

FIGURE 4-8. (*Photo courtesy of Betsy Smith.*)

themselves, and to give themselves credit for the appropriate environment they have created and maintained for their child.

A systematic assessment of the child's environment can be a reference for feedback to parents. This feedback is characterized by giving the parents specific examples of observations that were made about the child's environment. If an environment is found lacking, excessive, or deficient in particular stimuli, the parents can participate in discussing change. Naturally the strengths of the environment are described first. Parents can be queried whether they have any questions or concerns or if they have thought about the way they select toys, provide opportunities for variety, or respond when their child initiates a conversation with them.

The parents' observations of the environment can be a significant point of reference for discussion purposes. They can be asked specifically if their observations concerning activities and interactions and their descriptions of a typical day are congruous with what the assessment guide revealed. Is there anything about the environment that they wish to change? Of all the aspects of the environment they would change, what would their first priority be? How would they begin to initiate change? Do they think this change would be an advantage to the child (or children) or themselves. What disadvantages do they see? Have they thought of ways in which the environment could be altered for the benefit of the child? Have they thought of ways of changing the environment that would make it more positive for themselves or other family members? Is there anything that they would change, for example, to make it easier for them and their child to communicate better in words? Is there any way that parents might make it easier for their child to pay attention, get interested in, or play with a toy in a different way?

HELPING PARENTS SET LIMITS FOR THEIR CHILDREN

Many parents need to know that setting limits for children is an extremely important concern. Most parents need reassurance that all parents at some time are confronted with setting limits and that they may find it easier to achieve their goals by trying something different than what they have tried before. For example, if spanking or yelling does not seem to work, is there another way that parents can get the child to conform to their expectations? It is important to convey to parents that they have tried a variety of methods, some of which seem to be working, whereas others are not as successful for them in achieving the results they desire. At the same time, parents may need to hear that it must be tiresome and even frustrating to keep trying something that does not work. Some parents need to hear from an astute observer and an active listener that maybe they are preferring a change. It is important to check with this perception. Is either of the parents in fact saying, "Yes, I would like to see a change in the way I set limits"? Parents need to realize that changing everything at once is not possible or even desirable. What one single change might the parents consider necessary? After the parents have set a realistic goal and have discussed the ways they would initiate change and evaluate its effectiveness, their ability to solve problems, to make choices, and to make decisions should be acknowledged.

USEFULNESS OF THE HOME FOR TEACHING PARENTS

There is increasing awareness and sensitivity to the need to use the HOME for teaching parents. As a teaching tool, it serves to foster more appropriate interpersonal interactions between parents and children. It can help parents feel more potent and confident about their parental abilities to provide an environment that is most responsive to their child's individual needs, as well as their own. Used properly the inventories can be valuable in reassuring parents about their unique capabilities to determine the child's readiness for new or different stimuli. It can be a helpful guide in selecting appropriate learning experiences that correspond with the child's level of development. Used for the purpose for which it was created, the HOME can focus on both the child's changing needs and the parents' resourcefulness in meeting these on-going needs.

This tool in combination with other developmental assessment tools can serve as a reliable index to assist parents with anticipatory guidance, to prevent problems, to diminish those that are present, to help parents in an educational process of change, to assist them in setting reachable objectives and individualized goals, and to facilitate better communication between parent and child. The results of an environmental assessment can serve as a reference for discussing a mother's or father's concerns, can serve as a framework for giving reinforcement to parents for efforts to promote an environment that responds to their child's needs, and help to differentiate concerns and priorities of change. Most importantly, the HOME offers a reliable framework for determining which parts of the environment merit change. An overall assessment does not necessarily correspond to overall change. Parts of the environment may require special attention to best meet the needs of the child based on his different developmental rates.

CONSIDERATIONS FOR THE OBSERVER

A unique facet of the HOME is that the observer rates the interactions that he sees; he does not make judgments or conclusions about his interactions with a child or mother but rather the interactions that occur between the mother and child.

Like other tools, the HOME relies on beginning interrater reliability. Caldwell suggests that observers work in pairs on the first 12 home visits to increase objectivity of assessment and to decrease subjective interpretations.

One assessment in the home can never be considered sufficient to determine adequacy of the environment. The HOME is best used in combination with selected developmental assessment tools.

If change of the environment is recommended for meeting the needs of the child or parent, it is suggested that the tool be used on a routine basis. The first record would serve as base-line information against which subsequent assessments of the environment could be compared.

By using the inventories on a serial basis, changes in the environment can be observed in a systematic and reliable manner. Parents can be offered valuable feedback on a more objective, concrete basis and can be assisted in seeing the changes they were able to implement. Changes in the child's development can be documented as well.

The nurse, physician, and early-child-care professional could benefit from using objective methods in their continuing observations of the stability of change or lack of it. Subsequent and systematic observations are made possible by the structure of the HOME.

SUMMARY
The HOME gives sensitive indicators of appropriate kinds and amounts of animate-inanimate stimulation an infant or child may need at one time compared with another time. This inventory offers a valid way of observing the structure of the environment and the consistency or inconsistency of stimuli presented to or thrust at a child; it gives a profile of what a day is like within a specific home environment; it presents objective information about who helps or does not help with selected aspects of care giving; it gives a picture of what activities or events a child can predict or expect; and it offers a way of determining both the positive and negative aspects of the environment and how these meet the needs of a child. Most importantly, the HOME inventories are designed to evaluate the environment from the child's point of view.

In their endeavors to meet the challenge of promoting optimal development in young children, child-care professionals have one more instrument that enables them to measure the subtle aspects of a child's environment, which are crucial in the formative period of life. It is clear that Caldwell's research has helped develop reasonably reliable, sensitive, and predictive measures of those aspects of the environment that influence a child's outcome. These measures are based on objectively discriminable animate and inanimate aspects of a child's environment. Studies with HOME have produced significant findings such as the not surprising finding that an optimal environment in the child's first year of life has a dramatic influence on cognitive performance at 3 years of age.

Child-care and development theorists: Resources for parents Jeanene B. Brown

As the nuclear family becomes the dominant family form in society, parents turn to nonfamily members for advice about child rearing. Members of the extended family are often not readily available to young parents. In some cases, young families feel that methods of child rearing used by their parents are no longer relevant to their own needs and life-styles. Authoritarian methods of child rearing may seem inconsistent with the belief in the right to equality of all persons and the importance of each individual.

Advice about child rearing is available to parents from a variety of sources. Many professionals, such as teachers, counselors, psychologists, nurses, physicians, and religious leaders, are sought out by parents for assistance in guiding their children. In addition to these direct, personal contacts, many parents rely on the printed word for guidance. Articles and regular columns appearing in popular magazines discuss many topics of interest to parents. Likewise a variety of books is available to aid parents in raising and educating their children.

This abundance of references may present conflicting or contradictory advice. For inexperienced parents this inconsistency may cause confusion and lower their self-confidence. On the other hand, a parent may decide that the disagreement among these so-called authorities implies that none of the advice is to be completely trusted.

Nurses increasingly are in a position to offer guidance and counseling to parents. Familiarity with current popular child-care and developmental theorists is essential for a variety of reasons. One reason is that many helpful approaches can be derived from the experience and advice offered by these authors. Another is that, before any source is suggested to parents, the counselor must be familiar with the content. Finally, if nurses have an understanding of the different child-care and developmental theorists, they can help parents interpret seemingly conflicting advice based on knowledge of child development. Helpful techniques for rearing children can be individualized, and parents can increase their own skill and confidence in dealing with their children.

BENJAMIN SPOCK
One book which through the years has continued as a favorite among parents is Dr. Spock's *Baby and Child Care*. Since the 1940s, Dr. Spock has continued to revise and update his advice according to the needs of parents. Many of his original views on child rearing have not changed and are as applicable today as they were when they were first written. In fact much of Spock's advice, such as the flexibility and individuality of children and a relaxed, loving approach, has provided a foundation for many subsequent authors.

Baby and Child Care is arranged as a handbook for parents, which can be read from cover to cover or can provide advice on a specific problem. Health, medical, physical, and psychological care of children are discussed; however, Spock does not deal as extensively with parent-child relationships or the psychological aspects of child rearing as do many other authors.

A refreshing aspect of the latest revision of the book is the emphasis on parenting and raising children as individuals rather than focusing so much attention on "mothering" and raising a boy or a girl for a specified role in life. Spock has tried to "eliminate the sexist biases of the sort that help to create and perpetuate discrimination against girls and women" (1976, p. XIX).

He points out that sexual discrimination continues to be a problem today. Many small acts and child-rearing practices in early childhood bring about the subordination of women. Whether conscious or unconscious, the message which is given to many girls and women is that they are inferior to boys and men in many capabilities such as abstract reasoning, executive ability, and emotional control. Likewise men are affected by sexual stereotyping by being taught that they should not show their feelings and that they are supposed to be aggressive, competitive, and tough if they are to be successful. When individuals feel obliged to conform to a conventional sexual stereotype, valuable traits are lost. The hope for liberation for both sexes is expressed so that a more relaxed, whole existence for all is possible.

Spock believes the first 2 to 3 years of life are most important in the formation of the child's personality, and parents are vital in providing continuity of care and in focusing the child's development in a healthy direction. However, he states that "Both parents have an equal right to a career if they want one . . . and an equal obligation to share in the care of their child, with or without the help of others" (p. 37). A positive relationship with the parent of the same sex is more important in giving children a strong sex identity than are the toys they are given, the chores they are assigned, or the clothes they wear.

Spock encourages parents to trust their own common sense and points out the love they give their children is more important than any other aspect of care. He encourages parents to relax and enjoy their children and not to take any one method of child rearing too seriously but rather do what seems best for their child. Spock counsels parents that they should realize they are human; they have needs of their own; they will become cross at their children; they may have doubts and ambivalent feelings about a new baby; and they may not feel the same about each of their children. He assures the parent these feelings are normal and should not cause guilt.

Although Spock says that parents should develop a relaxed attitude toward child rearing and use their own common sense, he deals extensively with the details of ways parents should clothe, feed, and care for their child. This might prove useful to some parents; however, other parents might feel overwhelmed with the multitude of specific instructions for the many different tasks of child rearing. The book does not give parents a general approach for handling situations.

Infant feeding is discussed in several chapters of the book. Dr. Spock recommends feeding the baby on demand but within bounds which are comfortable and convenient for the parents. The discussion of weight gain includes a warning that "fatness in infancy tends to foster fatness for the rest of life" (p. 91).

Mention is made of the values of breast-feeding and the techniques of how to proceed and problems which may develop. However, additional resources should be suggested for the mother who is considering or desires to breast-feed. The mechanics and methods of bottle-feeding are also outlined. However in discussing both methods of feeding, emphasis is placed on the "how to" aspect rather than the parent-child relationship.

Spock's recommendations in certain aspects of nutrition during childhood vary somewhat from other experts in this field. He recommends supplemental vitamins, initiating solid foods at 2 to 4 months, and changing over to fresh milk sometime between 3 and 6 months of age.

Many specific pointers on daily care of a baby are outlined. Spock encourages quiet play with the baby but cautions against too much holding and game playing for fear the child may become dependent on the parents' attentions. He seems very concerned that by 3 months of age a child may become "spoiled." In this respect Spock apparently differs from other authors who are more liberal in encouraging parents to respond to their infant's messages to help develop the sense of trust.

Quick, easy-to-use references to common problems of infancy as well as childhood illnesses are provided in the book. Pointers are given helping parents know what treatments they can institute and when they need professional help.

Baby and Child Care discusses aspects of child development and care through adolescence, giving specific advice for a variety of situations. In discussing toilet training, Dr. T. Berry Brazelton's (1969) philosophy that "children should become trained of their own free will" is suggested with specific suggestions given on ways this can best be accomplished.

Anticipatory guidance and counseling is given on common problems for the preschooler, the school-aged child, and the adolescent. The advice is specific and encourages parents to understand the child's developmental stage but to be firm and consistent in their dealings with the child.

BOSTON CHILDREN'S MEDICAL CENTER AND RICHARD I. FEINBLOOM

Another book, much newer to the area of child care than Spock's book, is the *Child Health Encyclopedia* (Feinbloom, 1975). An example of the several encyclopedia-type source books, this book is written for parents to use as a reference regarding the health of their child. (Many health professionals, nurses included, will also find the book a useful reference in caring for children.) The editor states that the focus of the book is on the physical, rather than the psychological, health of the child and encourages the reader to consult other references for additional information in this latter area. The book does concentrate mainly upon physical health problems; however, the authors expertly incorporate the psychosocial aspects of these problems. It also gives considerable attention to health maintenance and anticipatory guidance such as toilet training, dental care, common feeding issues, accident prevention, preparation for school, television viewing, and stimulation.

The book is divided into three sections. The first section is in essay form and provides general discussions regarding health care for children. Dr. Feinbloom discusses the right of all children to "comprehensive health care," including both curative and preventive services. He encourages expansion of the nurse's role while cautioning that the family should be the major focus in a well-thought-out health care plan which would keep the numbers of health workers involved with any particular family small.

This comprehensive, first-line, first-contact type of care is termed *primary care*, which is distinguished from secondary or consultative care and tertiary or third-level care. Dr. Feinbloom feels that most deficiencies in health services are in primary care. He points out the great advances of secondary and tertiary levels of care, while such advances have not been made in primary health care. He feels that medical specialization has contributed to fragmentation of care in a variety of ways. In spite of these deficiencies, a promise for a brighter future for primary care is seen with involvement by lay groups and a shift in attitudes about health and illness. More education and a better understanding of life processes are seen as positive forces.

Greater human fulfillment and medical economy are viewed as products of accurate information and psychological preparation, which can decrease dependence on health professionals, drugs, and hospitals.

A chapter concerning the diet of infants and children includes many of the most recent findings and suggestions in the field of nutrition. The chapter includes a discussion of obesity and infant feeding as well as guidelines for feeding infants and children.

Dr. T. Berry Brazelton discusses complaints with an emotional component and gives suggestions for ways parents might deal with these. In addition, the book includes discussions of the sick child at home and in the hospital, focusing on ways parents can help their children during times of illness.

A second section of the book discusses safety. Included in this section are chapters on accident prevention; first aid; poisoning; and bicycle, minibike, and car safety. At the front of the book is an index for quick reference listing pages that discuss specific emergencies.

The third section of the book is a compilation of diseases and conditions of childhood. Since this section is intended to be used as the need for information arises, it is arranged alphabetically with cross-referencing of many items. Overall, the *Child Health Encyclopedia* serves to help parents become better consumers of health care on behalf of their children.

Other books dealing with child rearing focus on child health in a more psychological, rather than physical, sense. Although varying somewhat in their interpretations and recommendations, several authors present approaches which stem from similar philosophies.

RUDOLF DREIKURS

Children the Challenge, by Rudolf Dreikurs (1964), considers child discipline and is based on an Adlerian philosophy. Dreikurs discusses the dilemma many parents face over whether they should embrace a strict or permissive approach to discipline. He feels that this may arise from confusion about the application of democratic principles. The social atmosphere has changed from the autocratic relationship of the superior-inferior to the democratic relationship of equals. However, he feels that we have frequently mistaken license for freedom and anarchy for democracy. Dreikurs advocates abandoning autocratic methods of forcing children into compliance for newer principles of child rearing based on principles of freedom and responsibility which stimulate and encourage voluntary compliance to maintain order.

Dreikurs maintains that all behavior is goal-directed. Although the child is not aware of the motive behind his behavior, the desire to belong is his basic goal, while the method he devises for attaining this basic goal becomes his immediate goal. Factors in both the child's inner and outer environments influence his personality.

Parents are advised that encouragement is the single most important aspect of child raising. Encouragement gives the child a sense of self-respect and accomplishment. Lack of encouragement is the basic cause of misbehavior. Dreikurs states that "a misbehaving child is a discouraged child" (p. 36).

A clear distinction is to be made between the deed and the doer. Parents are advised to avoid indicating that the child is a failure if he makes a mistake or fails to accomplish a certain goal. A failure is said to indicate only a lack of skill and does not affect the value of the person.

Punishment and reward are said to belong in an autocratic social system with the "authority" having a dominant position of meting out rewards or punishments. Since democracy implies equality, stimulating the child so that he has a desire to conform to the demands of order is a preferable approach.

When children misbehave, one method parents can use instead of punishment and reward is allowing the child to experience the natural and logical consequences of his action. These consequences should not be turned into punishment but rather convey to the child that he has the power to take care of his problems.

Dreikurs gives parents guidelines for relating to their children with examples of successes and failures in applying these guidelines. Among these guidelines, parents are advised to be firm without dominating, to show respect for their child, to induce respect for order and for the rights of others, and to eliminate criticism and minimize mistakes.

In addition parents are advised to maintain a routine; to avoid giving undue attention to their children; not to become involved in a struggle for power; and when there is a disturbance, to withdraw from the conflict. Substituting action for words and giving a matter full attention until the requirement has been met are effective ways to influence change in a child's behavior.

Throughout the book communication is encouraged between parent and child by talking *with* each other instead of *to* each other. In all, the book discusses 34 principles of child raising, explaining ways parents can influence their child's behavior in a democratic manner.

HAIM G. GINOTT

In the book *Between Parent and Child,* Haim Ginott (1965) also focuses on communication between parents and children. He states that communication with children is based on respect and skill. Messages should preserve the child's and parent's self-respect, and statements of understanding should precede statements of advice and instruction.

Dreikurs advised parents to separate the deed from the doer. Ginott further explains that only conduct, not feelings, can be condemned or commended. Ginott holds that all feelings are legitimate, including the positive, the negative, and the ambivalent. Strong feelings cannot be banished; however, a sympathetic and understanding listener can diminish their intensity.

During conversations, parents are advised to respond to the relationship implied by the child rather than to the event. Likewise, when a child tells of an event, responding to the feelings around it, rather than to the event itself, is sometimes more helpful. Finally, rather than agree or disagree with a child's statement about himself, parents should convey an understanding of his feelings. In these ways children can be helped to know what they are feeling by the parent serving as a mirror to the child's emotions.

Praise, if used, should deal only with the child's efforts and accomplishments, not with character and personality. Constructive criticism should only point out what has to be done without remarking on the personality of the child. Children's self-concepts are formed by the way parents respond to their actions and feelings.

Several patterns of relating to children are considered to be self-defeating. These include treats, bribes, promises, sarcasm, sermons on lying and stealing, and the rude teaching of politeness. Ginott gives examples of ways parents can respond to misbehavior with more effective methods.

Dreikurs proposes stimulating and encouraging voluntary compliance to maintain order. Likewise, Ginott states that responsibility cannot be imposed; it can only grow from within. He states, "Values cannot be taught directly. They are absorbed, and become part of the child only through his identification with, and emulation of, persons who gain his love and respect" (p. 81). Allowing children a voice and, when indicated, a choice in matters that affect them fosters responsibility.

Parents are encouraged to listen attentively to their child to convey that his ideas are valued and respected. They should consciously avoid words and comments that create hate and resentment. When conflicts do arise, parents should state their own feelings and thoughts without attacking their child's personality.

The cornerstone of Ginott's approach to discipline is distinguishing between feelings and acts. Children are allowed to speak about what they feel, but undesirable acts are limited and directed. There is a need for a clear definition of acceptable and unacceptable conduct. The guideline for stating a limit is that the child knows what constitutes unacceptable conduct and what substitutes will be accepted. For example, "Dishes are not for throwing; pillows are for throwing" (p. 116). Application of these principles is provided through specific advice for dealing with daily situations.

Some helpful guidelines are given to help parents understand and deal with the sexual education of their children. However, the sexist biases which Spock tried to eliminate in the 1975 revision of his book are still very evident in this 1965 book by Ginott.

Instead of focusing upon parenting, Ginott makes a clear distinction between mothering and fathering. He states that mothers represent love and sympathy while fathers personify discipline and morality. Ginott's Freudian background becomes most apparent regarding his views of sexual role and social function. He advocates not demanding the same standard of conduct from both sexes. Rather he would allow boys to be more boisterous because they have more energy and will need to be more assertive later in life. Girls, he says, should be complimented on their appearance but must not be allowed to engage in rough play. Ginott feels that the majority of women are destined to be wives and mothers and that life will be easier if most men and women do not engage in competition and rivalry. By advocating these child-rearing practices Ginott reinforces practices of sexual discrimination.

FITZHUGH DODSON

While Dreikurs and Ginott deal primarily with discipline, Fitzhugh Dodson applies many of these same principles to parenting in general. In his book *How to Parent* (1970), Dodson deals with many of the situations parents face in the first 5 years of their child's life. He tells parents they are the most important teachers their child will ever have. Although specific advice and recommendations are given, parents are advised to follow their own feelings and apply what works best in their own situations.

Dreikurs and Ginott advise parents to focus on their child's actions rather than their child's feelings when disciplining. Likewise Dodson tries to advise parents about what they should *do*, not what they should *feel*, since parents as people have feelings which cannot be controlled at will. Dodson advises new parents that feelings of inadequacy, panic, and resentment are normal and that confidence grows with experience.

Emphasis in this book is placed upon the first 5 years of the child's life, since it is felt that these are the most important, formative years. Dodson feels that a child's basic personality structure is formed by the time he is 6 years old. These first 5 years are vital to emotional as well as intellectual development.

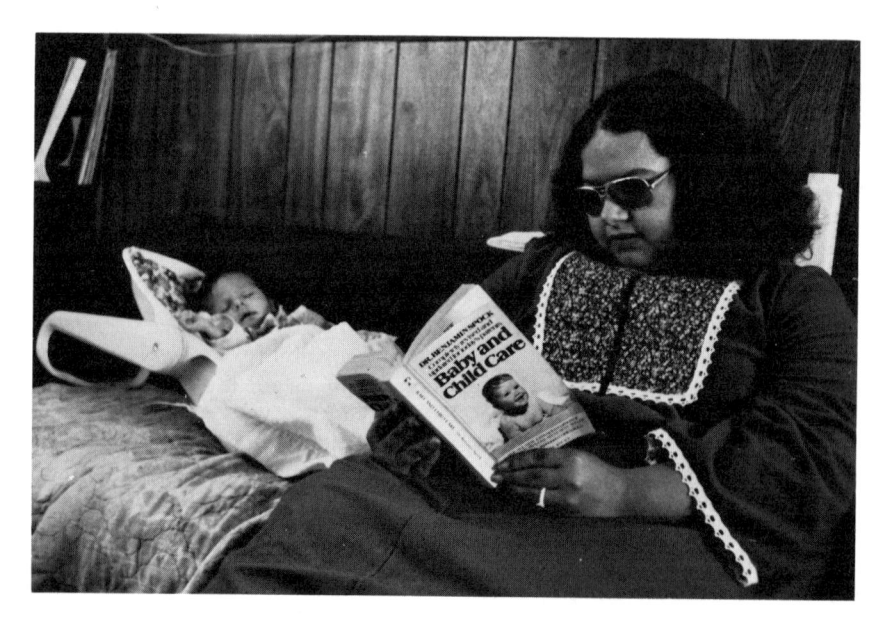

FIGURE 4-9.

The child's self-concept is held to be the single most important factor in forming this basic personality structure. The book traces the way self-concept begins in infancy and develops through the first 5 years of life. Dodson incorporates the stages of personality development outlined by Erikson and shows parents how they can help develop a strong and healthy self-concept in their child.

A child's self-concept begins during infancy, when he is developing his basic outlook on life. "He is developing either a basic sense of trust and happiness about life, or one of distrust and unhappiness" (p. 41). Dodson gives specific advice to parents regarding this period. He feels that there is no one method of feeding which is physically or psychologically best for infants. However, whether breast- or bottle-feeding, the parent should hold and cuddle the infant. Feeding an infant when he is hungry is seen as the most important thing a parent can do to help an infant develop a basic trust in himself and his world. Parents are encouraged to cuddle, rock, sing to, and play with their child. Instead of spoiling their child, they are letting him know he is loved.

By providing adequate intellectual stimulation the parent helps the child bring his world into focus. Although a child may have a maximum potential intelligence, the degree to which he achieves this maximum will depend greatly on how much sensory and intellectual stimulation he receives in the first year of life.

In toddlerhood, when the child learns to walk, the learning task is to actively explore his environment with the opportunity to learn self-confidence. This forms the phase of the child's self-concept when he learns either self-confidence or self-doubt. The child explores his physical environment, including his own body.

> If he is allowed to play and explore freely in such a stimulating environment, he will acquire feelings of confidence about himself. . . . But if he meets a constant stream of "no-no's," he will develop feelings of self-doubt which will be devastating to his initiative and drive as an adult. (p. 97)

First adolescence is the term used to describe the period of disequilibrium which occurs at approximately 2 years of age. This is seen as a transition stage between infancy and childhood and as necessary for the child's development to proceed. Although the negativism and rebelliousness of this age cause parents difficult moments, Dodson points out that it is actually a positive stage. The child is learning self-identity versus social conformity. Negative self-identity is said to be part of the struggle for positive self-identity. During this time rules and limits should be flexible. Limits should be reasonable and consistent. Children should be allowed to express negative as well as positive feelings. A feedback technique similar to the one proposed by Ginott mirrors the child's feelings and shows him that the parent knows how he feels.

The next stage of development, the preschool stage, runs roughly from the child's third to sixth birthday. The child faces many developmental tasks in this stage. The way he deals with these tasks will determine his self-concept and personality structure. Dodson says the preschooler passes into and out of periods of equilibrium. At age 3 he displays a spirit of cooperation and a desire for approval; 4 years is marked by disequilibrium, insecurity, and incoordination, while 5 tends to be reliable, stable, and well adjusted.

Dodson defines discipline as training and points out that it is not synonymous with punishment. The ultimate goal of this training is to produce an adult who has learned self-regulation. Techniques of behavior modification through reinforcement are thought to be helpful in disciplining the child and should be understood and utilized by parents. However, Dodson points out that methods of child training which strengthen the self-concept of the child are unique to humans and must be included in the parents' approach to discipline. Teaching methods which a parent can use to help strengthen the child's self-concept are outlined with examples of applications of these methods. Although there are some minor differences in their approaches, Dodson supports most of the principles outlined by Ginott.

Although Dodson discusses parenting, he generally uses this term synonymously with mothering and mentions fathers only in passing. Emphasizing the roles of both mothers and fathers in parenting would give an added dimension to the book.

While discussing children and violence, Dodson also displays some sexist biases. For instance he advocates teaching male children to grow up to become aggressive adults and warns against molding a boy to be like a passive little girl. His words on violence would have had just as much and possibly more validity had he focused more on human traits, rather than male and female ones.

THOMAS GORDON

Parent Effectiveness Training, by Thomas Gordon (1975), is similar to those books previously reviewed in that it deals with skills parents need to be more effective in raising their children. Like the others, this book gives specific skills to help keep lines of communication open and strengthen the parent-child relationship. The method encourages children to accept responsibility for finding their own solutions to their own problems. Parents are not expected to know all the answers. However, instead of giving advice and recommendations for specific problem areas, Dr. Gordon teaches skills and methods of interaction which can be applied to many situations. His method is not age-specific. In fact, *Parent Effectiveness Training* (PET) is "based on a theory of human relationships that is applicable to any and all relationships between people, not only to the parent-child relationship" (p. XII).

Gordon portrays parents as persons who have feelings of both acceptance and nonacceptance toward their children. The degree of acceptance a parent has toward a child is partly a function of the kind of person that parent is and also the kind of person the child is. This degree of acceptance does not remain stationary but is influenced by many factors such as the state of mind of the parent and the immediate situation.

Gordon differs with some of the authors previously reviewed in that he does not feel that parents necessarily need to be consistent or present a united front to their children. He knows that parents are human and that to pretend consistency or total agreement would be unrealistic. He states that false acceptances will be perceived by children. The mixed message of acceptance and nonacceptance puts the child in a bind which can be more harmful to the child's psychological health than realizing that a parent does not accept him all of the time. In addition, Gordon does not feel that it is possible to accept the child but not his behavior. He feels the child is the behaving child, and the two cannot be separated by either the parent or the child himself.

PET is a method of communication. An essential component is the language of acceptance. When one person can feel and communicate genuine acceptance, that person has the capacity to help the other. Acceptance of the other fosters growth, development, constructive changes, problem solving, and actualization to the fullest potential. Gordon points out that acceptance must be demonstrated. A parent can nonverbally communicate acceptance by not intervening in a child's activities. Passive listening or saying nothing also communicates acceptance. Verbally communicating acceptance is also necessary. However, Gordon points out that most parents verbally communicate with their children with messages which carry more than one meaning. They may cause the child to stop talking, make him feel guilty or inadequate, reduce his self-esteem, produce defensiveness, trigger resentment, or make him feel unaccepted.

PET suggests some alternative responses. One of these is the "door opener" or "invitation to say more." This is a response that does not communicate any of the listener's own ideas or judgments or feelings but invites the child to share his own. The person is encouraged to start or to continue talking. Another way of responding to people's messages is termed *active listening.* In active listening the receiver of the message tries to understand what the sender is feeling. Active listeners then put their understanding into their own words and verify this with the sender. The feedback should include only what the receiver feels the sender's message meant.

Another principle of PET is one of problem ownership. There are times in every human relationship when one person "owns a problem," or some of that person's needs are not being met with her or his behavior. At other times one person's needs are being met by the behavior, but that behavior is interfering with a second person's needs. Consequently that second person owns the problem. In the parent-child relationship the child may own the problem, or the parent may own the problem.

Active listening by the parent is most appropriate when the child owns the problem but often inappropriate when the parent owns the problem. Entirely different skills in communication are needed when the child causes the parent a problem.

Parents often send children a "solution message" when the child causes a problem for the parent. They do not wait for the child to initiate considerate behavior; instead they tell him what he must, should, or ought to do. At other times parents send a "put-down message" communicating blame, judgment, ridicule, criticism, or shame. Both the solution message and the put-down message are "you"-oriented.

PET suggests an alternative message, an "I message," in which a parent simply tells a child how some unacceptable behavior is making the parent feel. It is felt that I messages are more effective in influencing a child to modify behavior that is unacceptable to the parent as well as healthier to the parent-child relationship.

There are other times in family relationships when problems are not owned solely by the child or solely by the parent. The needs of both parent and child are at stake. In this situation it is said that the relationship owns the problem, and thus a conflict has occurred. The way conflicts are resolved is thought to be the most critical factor in parent-child relationships.

Often conflict resolution is solved by one of two "win-lose" approaches; either the parent or the child wins, and the other must lose. However, Gordon states, "It is paradoxical but true that parents lose influence by using power and will have more influence on their children by giving up their power or refusing to use it" (p. 192). He proposes an alternative "no-lose" method of resolving conflicts with which nobody loses. Both parent and child win because the solution must be acceptable to both. With this method parent and child participate in a joint search for some solution. When a final decision is made, no selling of the other is required since both have accepted the solution. Also no power is required to force compliance because neither is resisting the decision.

Gordon feels that parents need only to learn this single method for resolving conflicts. There are no best solutions, only solutions which are right for a particular parent-child relationship at a particular time.

LEE SALK

While Gordon proposes communication and problem-solving methods which parent and children could use in their interactions with each other, Dr. Lee Salk takes a different approach. Salk, in *What Every Child Would Like His Parents to Know* (1972), structures his book in a series of questions and answers. He takes a much more directive approach, giving advice about selected problems rather than teaching problem solving. Salk's approach to most issues is from a psychoanalytic background.

In discussing the newborn infant, Salk points to the importance of bonding between the mother and newborn infant. He also encourages early stimulation as a way to give the infant an increased capacity for learning. Parents are advised not to let infants cry since during the first 9 or 10 months of an infant's life he develops a lifetime sense of trust or distrust in people based upon his experiences with having his needs satisfied.

Salk feels that parents are the best persons to care for their children. He encourages fathers to be involved in the care of the child. Other persons can care for children if they are carefully selected by the parents; however, long separations are not encouraged. Mothers are encouraged not to work, especially during the first 9 or 10 months of her baby's life if at all possible. If the mother does work, she is encouraged to arrange her schedule so that she and her child are not separated for prolonged periods.

Weaning and toilet training are discussed in terms of oral and anal stages of development. Salk gives much advice about what not to do in these instances.

Discipline is defined as rules, regulations, and expectations that regulate a child's conduct. It is seen as establishing an organized world with organized limitations which make things predictable. Unlike some of the previous authors, Salk sees parents in positions of power. They should consistently apply the rules and regulations they have established. Because their love and affection are so valued by the child, parents are capable of using them to correct unacceptable behavior. Love and affection can be withheld as a form of discipline. Parents are advised to be consistent and to set limits for their children.

In discussing sex education, Salk advises parents to be well informed about sex and reproduction and to begin their child's education at an early age. When a child begins to ask questions, the parent is advised to answer honestly, directly, and with information the child can understand. In general, young children have questions about reproduction, while the child approaching puberty has questions about the feelings of sex. Sexual experiences, such as masturbation and sexual exploration among children, are seen as natural, and parents are advised to deemphasize their importance. Parents are cautioned against allowing a child to interfere with the intimacy of the husband-wife relationship.

Relating to others outside the immediate family can increase a child's skill in social interaction. Salk discusses many factors involved in relationships with grandparents, relatives, and others. Also discussed in the book are a child's emotional reactions to doctors, medicine, and illness, and suggestions are given to help children deal with these experiences.

Suggestions are given concerning relationships among siblings; areas included are the arrival of a new sibling, twins, ordinal position of children, and the adopted child.

Salk advises parents to educate their child from the time of birth onward. He encourages sensory stimulation and a variety of environmental experiences. He feels that children are ready for school around age 3, and play groups before this time may be helpful for the child but are primarily helpful and valuable in freeing the mother. Different problems which children may encounter in school are discussed.

Salk sees disobedience as a natural part of children's development. Once the parent sets expected standards of behavior, the child will challenge them. This is seen as positive in that the child is finding the "structure and meaning to life." Total obedience may indicate too-harsh discipline, while constant misbehaving indicates lack of internal mechanisms of control. Again in this area Salk gives much advice to parents about what they should and should not do with their children, but he does not tell how parents might carry out this advice.

It is interesting to note the parallel between his approach toward parents and the recommendations he gives parents in dealing with their children. Much of the advice is helpful but is given in terms of relationships of power and authority. Salk is the expert authority giving advice to the parent; likewise the parent is in the position of power and authority and is advised to guide and direct the child. In neither relationship are participants seen as equal. Set answers are given rather than encouraging participants to find their own solutions.

BURTON L. WHITE

The First Three Years of Life, written by Burton White (1975), deals exclusively with the early years indicated by the title. This book delves into these first years in much greater detail than any of the other books reviewed. Dr. White is convinced that the first 3 years of life deserve the most attention because these years form the foundations of all later development. The book deals in the broad sense with the education of children. Sensorimotor developments are discussed because of their importance in the young child's behavior. However, the primary focus of the book is the comprehensive discussion of educational goals, since this is the area in which parental intervention is most influential.

Through his research, White has concluded that "the informal education that families provide for their children makes more of an impact on a child's total educational development than the formal educational system" (p. 4). If the family, early on, has not done its job well, the professional is limited in the degree to which he or she can help the child.

White contends that most American families do a reasonably good job of assisting the education and development of their children through the first 6 to 8 months. However, few families manage their child's education and development during the next 8 to 36 months as well as they could.

White divides the first 36 months into seven phases. He devotes a chapter to each phase and includes in the chapters general remarks about the phase, the general behavior characteristics of the phase, a child's apparent interests at that age, the educational developments of the phase, recommended child-rearing practices for the phase (also practices which are not recommended), materials which are recommended for that phase (and sometimes materials not recommended), and finally behaviors that signal the onset of the next phase.

Phases I to IV, or the first 8 months of the baby's life, are seen by White as the most problem-free for parents in terms of the development and education of their child. Nature is thought to play a major role in the child's development during this period. The goals parents are given to work toward during these months are giving the infant a feeling of being loved and cared for, helping him develop specific skills, and encouraging his interests in the outside world by stimulating his curiosity.

When the child reaches 8 months of age, the parent is said to assume a more significant role in the child's education and development. Three ways of describing the educational goals for the period of 8 months through 3 years are described. One way deals with the child's major interest patterns. The three major interests (aside from physiological ones) are the primary caretaker, exploration of the world as a whole, and mastering newly emerging motor abilities. A second way of discussing educational goals is in terms of the emerging competencies which are of special importance. A third way is to focus upon the four key goals of language development, the development of curiosity, social development, and nurturing the roots of intelligence.

Beginning with phase V, from 8 to 14 months of age, the primary caretaker assumes three major functions. The primary caretaker is the designer of the child's world and daily experiences. Safety and playthings take on new importance. The primary caretaker is in a role of consultant to provide assistance and advice to the child. White points out that if mothers have full-time jobs, they do not have a chance to assist during the times they are gone. Mothers are advised to stay home at least part of the day. The primary caretaker also has the role of authority and is the source of discipline and the setter of limits.

Phase VI is the period from 14 to 24 months. During this phase White recommends a balance across all three major directions of the child's interest: the primary caretaker, exploring the world, and mastering the use of his body. Goals for phase VI are also considered in terms of the four fundamental educational processes as well as the special abilities of the child. Coping with negativism, language development, the emergence of thinking ability, the development of curiosity, and social development as well as nurturing the roots of intelligence are all discussed as goals for this period.

Phase VII is from 24 to 36 months. The four educational goals of language development, development of curiosity, social development, and nurturing the roots of intelligence continue throughout the child's third year of life. Also the three major interests, listed above, continue to prevail. Fostering the dimensions of the child's competence is a major focus of this phase.

White recommends spacing children at least 3 years apart so that the parent can give each child the special help he needs during these important first years. He feels that no job is more important than raising a child in the first 3 years of life and sees this job as providing a deep satisfaction. White is confident that the average family, given some help and guidance, has the resources for effective child rearing.

STELLA CHESS

While White focuses on the similarities of the development of children, other authors focus on children's individual differences. Stella Chess, Alexander Thomas, and Herbert Birch, in their book *Your Child Is a Person* (1965), emphasize the individuality of children. These authors agree with other authors that parents can have an important influence on their child's development. However, they feel that personality characteristics are a result of the continuous interaction between individual temperamental styles and life experiences. Books previously reviewed emphasize the influence of the child's parents and his early environment in personality development. Chess, Thomas, and Birch present an alternative approach to child care based on a longitudinal research study which suggests that the developing personality is shaped by the constant interplay of temperament and environment.

The book focuses on the age period from infancy to first grade. However, the research study has followed children through adolescence, and the authors, in other publications, deal with a broader age range. The book is not meant to be a manual of child care; instead the authors discuss some principles of interrelationship important to psychological development.

Your Child Is a Person is said to be a psychological approach to parenthood without guilt. The authors point out that most parent-education experts identify mistakes parents make, including even the most innocent-appearing acts, and imply that parents are totally responsible for the psychological as well as physical health of their child.

In addition, psychoanalytic theory has increased the burden of responsibility and guilt for parents, especially mothers. If something goes wrong in the child's development, the mother is usually seen as the cause. If something she has consciously done cannot be identified, then her unconscious is suspected.

The authors question the validity of parents' reports of their children's development as the main source of data for psychoanalytic theory. They cite studies which document the inaccuracy of mothers' memories and show that memories edit the child-care methods used to conform to the popular method of the day. Doubt is cast on the theory that the quality of the mother's care is the sole determining influence in the child's development. These authors do not minimize the mother's importance but show that there is no proof that her influence is the decisive factor. They feel that the picture is much more complex. The problem may be, not the parent's, but the parent's and the child's and result from the pattern of interaction between the two.

They write, "Events in themselves can have no developmental meaning. Only if the child has characteristics which lead him to respond to an event in a given way can its influence on development be understood. Consequently, the environment is first filtered by the child's own characteristics" (p. 21). The child is not only said to screen his environment but also to influence it. Just as the parent and environment influence the child, so the child also influences the parent and the environment.

The longitudinal study carried out by the authors was designed to directly study the traits of infants rather than to rely only on parental reports. The study systematically analyzed individuality in behavior from infancy onward. The term *temperament* is used to describe the "how" of behavior. Whether initial temperament was persistent or varied as the child grew up was studied. In addition, the authors tried to characterize the interactive processes between temperament and environment as these processes affected development.

Nine headings to classify individual characteristics of children's behavior were identified. These included activity level, regularity, approach or withdrawal as a characteristic response to a new situation, adaptability to change in routine, level of sensory threshold, positive or negative mood, intensity of response, distractibility, and persistence and attention span.

The child's usual pattern of functioning in these nine categories is called his temperament. Certain characteristics clustered into general types of temperament. A category called *easy children* was described by attributes of positiveness in mood, regularity of body function, low or moderate intensity of reaction, adaptability, and positiveness in a new situation. Another category of children was termed *slow to warm up*. These children typically showed a low activity level, tendency to withdraw on first exposure to new stimuli, slow adaptability, and a somewhat negative mood. They responded to situations with a low intensity of reaction. A third category, termed *difficult children*, showed irregularity in body functions, intensity in reactions, withdrawal in the face of new stimuli, slow adaptations to changes in the environment, and negative moods. The highly active child and the persistent, non-distractible child were also described. The interaction between parent, child, and environment for children with these different temperamental characteristics would vary greatly.

From this conceptual framework, Chess and her colleagues discuss common problems parents encounter as their child grows and develops. Sleep, feeding, toilet training, discipline, sex, play, siblings, and education are all discussed in terms of individuality of children. Ways parents might identify and interact with their individual child are explained. Special advice for parents of the difficult child, "late bloomer," and the handicapped child is given. These authors also say that the working mother is "not guilty." They feel that the fact that a woman works need not interfere with her children's development. The quality of the parent-child relationship is much more important than the amount of time involved.

This book does not replace other child-care manuals. However, it does present important additional information concerning the personality development of the child. (See Chap. 3 for discussion of Thomas's and Chess's professional writing.)

T. BERRY BRAZELTON

T. Berry Brazelton's work also focuses upon individual differences in children. Two of the books Brazelton has written are *Infants and Mothers* (1969) and *Toddlers and Parents* (1974).

Infants and Mothers presents a perspective of the first 12 months of life. Brazelton states that the obvious fact that normal babies are not all alike has been overlooked in the literature for new parents. By describing the developmental paths of three different infants, Brazelton shows the very different ways they affect their environment. These differences are apparent from the moment of birth and influence the reactions of parents to their child. It is believed the neonate affects his environment as much as it influences him. Brazelton does not feel that parents should feel guilty when they find themselves in conflict with their infant.

Brazelton states that parents can enjoy and find rewarding the relationship with their infant when they recognize the individual strengths. He finds most of the literature for new parents full of advice but says it does not support individual reactions and intuition. Mothers are told that there is no one right answer and that they must find their own way with their own infants.

Brazelton demonstrates this advice by developing composite descriptions of three infants and following the development of these infants through their first year. He points out the individual strengths and weaknesses of each child and the manner in which the child influences the reactions of his parents and environment. At the same time he includes ways in which parents and the environment affect the child's responses and development.

The three different kinds of infants described are a quiet one, an active one, and an intermediate or "average" one, all expressing variations of the "normal" infant. Interspersed among the descriptions of the three infants are discussions about physical and psychological aspects of child development. Many of Brazelton's research findings on individual differences among neonates and infants are presented to parents in an interesting style. The importance of stimulation to the development and growth of the infant is stressed. The way infants are able to selectively repress stimuli is also discussed.

The book expertly combines useful information and support for the parent in an easy-to-read form. If the parent has a specific question, he or she can refer to the index at the back.

Toddlers and Parents discusses the years 1 to 3. The same focus on particular strengths and marked individuality of each child is apparent. Brazelton states that no parent ever feels the same about two children since each child elicits a different set of responses. "Because of the strengths and a resilient individuality, a child can absorb a great many mistakes on his parents' part" (1974, p. X).

The years from 1 to 3 are seen as turbulent ones. The child has the job of resolving the struggle between being controlled by outsiders and learning controls for himself. The parent is advised to support and encourage self-expression but also to show the way to its mastery when self-expression gets out of control. Parents are also encouraged to take the opportunity to influence their child's development during this time as these are the last years that parents will play such an important role.

CONCLUSION

There are a variety of approaches to management of child development and of child-rearing practices. Although individual recommendations and advice may differ, general trends can be found. Parents can be encouraged to read several different sources and then helped to apply this advice to their own individual children. The most helpful advice will probably be repeated by many authors. Parents can also better select advice which is appropriate for them if they are aware of the different theoretical frameworks and philosophies from which advice stems. There is no one correct method or theory of child rearing. Parents and children together must find the answers which are correct for them.

Bibliography

THE PARENT-CHILD RELATIONSHIP

Ainsworth, M. D.: The effects of maternal deprivation: A review of findings and controversy in the context of research strategy. In *Deprivation of maternal care*. New York: Schocken, 1966.

Bowlby, J.: *Attachment and loss* (Vol. 1). *Attachment*. New York: Basic Books, 1969.

———: *Maternal care and mental health*. New York: Schocken, 1966.

Branstetter, E.: The young child's response to hospitalization—Separation or lack of mothering care? In M. Batey (Ed.), *Communicating nursing research: Problem identification and the research design*. Boulder, Colorado: Western Interstate Commission for Higher Education, 1969.

Brazelton, T. B.: *Neonatal behavioral assessment scale*. Philadelphia: Lippincott, 1973.

———: Psychophysiologic reactions to the neonate, I, The value of the observation of the neonate. *J. Pediat.*, 1961, 58, 508–512.

———, and G. A. Collier: Infant development in the Zinncantico Indians of southern Mexico. *Pediatrics*, 1969, 44, 274.

Broussard, E., and M. Hartner: Further considerations regarding maternal perception of the first born. In J. Hellmuth (Ed.), *Exception infant: Studies in abnormalities*. New York: Brunner/Mazel, 1971.

Davenport, H. T., and J. S. Werry: The effect of general anesthesia, surgery and hospitalization upon the behavior of children. *Amer. J. Orthopsychiat.*, 1970, 40, 806–824.

Farber, B.: *Family organization and interaction*. San Francisco: Chandler, 1964.

Greenberg, M., and N. Morris: Engrossment: The newborn's impact upon the father. *Amer. J. Orthopsychiat.*, 1974, 44(4), 520–530.

Heinicke, C. M., and I. J. Westheimer: *Brief separations*. London: Longmans, 1965.

Illingworth, R. S., and K. S. Holt: Children in hospital: Some observations on their reactions with special reference to daily visiting. *Lancet*, 1955, 2, 1257–1262.

Kennell, J.: Maternal behavior one year after early and extended postpartum contact. *Develop. Med. Child Neurol.*, 1974, 16(2), 172–179.

———, and M. M. Klaus: Care of the mother of the high risk infant. *Clin. Obstet. Gynec.*, 1971, 14, 926.

Klaus, M., R. Jerauld, N. Kreger, W. Alpine, M. Steffa, and J. Kennell: Maternal attachment: Importance of the first postpartum days. *New Engl. J. Med.*, 1972, 286(9), 460–463.

———, and J. Kennell: *Maternal-infant bonding*. St. Louis: Mosby, 1976.

———, ———, N. Plumb, and S. Zuilkke: Human maternal behavior at the first contact with her young. *Pediatrics*, 1970, 46(2), 181–192.

Kogan, K., H. Wimberger, and R. A. Bobbitt: Analysis of mother-child interaction in young mental retardates. *Child Develop.*, 1969, 40, 799–812.

Korner, A. F.: Early stimulation and maternal care as related to infant capabilities and individual differences. *Early Child Care Develop.*, 1973, 2, 307–327.

———: Individual differences at birth: Implications for early experience and later development. *Amer. J. Orthopsychiat.*, 1971, 41, 608–619.

———, and R. Grobstein: Individual differences at birth: Implications for the mother-infant relationship and later development. *J. Amer. Acad. Child Psychiat.*, 1967, 6, 676–690.

LeMasters, E. E.: *Parents in modern America*. Homewood, Illinois: Dorsey, 1974.

Mead, M.: Some theoretical considerations of the problem of mother-child separation. *Amer. J. Orthopsychiat.*, 1954, 24, 471–483.

Medinnus, G. R. (Ed.): *Readings in the psychology of parent-child relations*. New York: Wiley, 1967.

Parke, R. D.: Family interaction in the newborn period: Some findings, some observations, and some unresolved issues. (Unpublished paper presented at the Biennial Meeting of the International Society for the Study of Behavioral Development, Ann Arbor, Michigan, 1973.)

Prugh, D. G., E. M. Staub, H. H. Sands, R. M. Kirschbaum, and E. A. Lenihan: A study of the emotional reactions of children and families to hospitalization and illness. *Amer. J. Orthopsychiat.*, 1953, 23, 70–106.

Rexford, E. N.: Forward. In L. W. Sander, L. Shapiro, and T. Shapiro (Eds.), *Infant psychiatry*. New Haven, Connecticut: Yale University Press, 1976.

Robertson, J.: *Young children in hospitals*. New York: Basic Books, 1958.

Rose, M. H.: Ann copes with open heart surgery. In E. Anderson, B. Bergersen, M. Duffey, M. Lohr, and M. Rose (Eds.), *Current concepts in clinical nursing* (Vol. IV). St. Louis: Mosby, 1973.

———: The effects of hospitalization on the coping behaviors of children. In M. Batey (Ed.), *Communicating nursing research: The many sources of nursing knowledge.* Boulder, Colorado: Western Interstate Commission for Higher Education, 1972.

Rubin, R.: Attainment of the maternal role: Part I—Processes. *Nurs. Res.*, 1967a, *3*, 237–245.

———: Attainment of the maternal role: Part II—Models and referents. *Nurs. Res.*, 1967b, *4*, 342–346.

———: Maternal touch. *Nurs. Outlook*, 1963, 828–831.

Rutter, M.: Parent-child separation: Psychological effects on their children. *J. Child Psychol. Psychiat.*, 1971, *12*, 233–260.

Schaffer, H. R., and W. M. Callender: Psychological effects of hospitalization in infancy. *Pediatrics*, 1959, *24*, 528–539.

Stacey, M., R. Dearden, R. Pill, and D. Robinson: *Hospitals, children and their families: The report of a pilot study.* London: Routledge, 1970.

Thomas, A., S. Chess, and H. Birch: *Temperament and behavior disorders in children.* New York: New York University Press, 1968.

Vernon, D. T. A., J. Foley, R. Sipowicz, and J. L. Schulman: *The psychological responses of children to hospitalization and illness.* Springfield, Illinois: Charles C Thomas, 1965.

Wallston, B.: The effects of maternal employment on children. *J. Child Psychol. Psychiat.*, 1973, *14*, 81–95.

Webster's New Collegiate Dictionary. Springfield, Massachusetts: Merriam, 1956.

World Health Organization Expert Committee on Mental Health: Report on the second session, 1951. *World Health Organization Monograph,* Technical Report Series No. 31. Geneva, 1951.

Yarrow, L.: Separation from parents during early childhood. In M. C. Hoffman and L. W. Hoffman (Eds.), *Review of child development research* (Vol. I). New York: Russell Sage, 1964.

Yarrow, M. R.: Problems of methods in parent-child research. *Child Develop.*, 1963, *34*, 215–226.

ASSESSMENT OF THE CHILD'S ENVIRONMENT

Caldwell, B. M.: *Instruction manual inventory for infants (Home observation for measurement of the environment).* Little Rock, Arkansas: Infant Development and Education Center, 1970.

Elardo, R., R. Bradley, and B. M. Caldwell: The relationship of infant's home environments to mental test performance from six to thirty-six months: A longitudinal analysis. *Child Develop.*, 1975, *46,* 71–76.

CHILD-CARE AND DEVELOPMENT THEORISTS: RESOURCES FOR PARENTS

Brazelton, T. B.: *Infants and mothers.* New York: Dell, 1969.

———: *Toddlers and parents.* New York: Dell, 1974.

Chess, S., A. Thomas, and H. G. Birch: *Your child is a person.* New York: Viking, 1965.

Dodson, F.: *How to parent.* New York: New American, 1970.

Dreikurs, R.: *Children the challenge.* New York: Hawthorn, 1964.

Feinbloom, R. I. (Ed.): *Child health encyclopedia.* New York: Dell, 1975.

Ginott, H. G.: *Between parent and child.* New York: Avon, 1965.

Gordon, T.: *Parent effectiveness training.* New York: New American, 1975.

Salk, L.: *What every child would like his parents to know.* New York: Warner, 1972.

Spock, B.: *Baby and child care.* New York: Pocket Books, 1976.

White, B. L.: *The first three years of life.* New York: Avon, 1975.

PART TWO

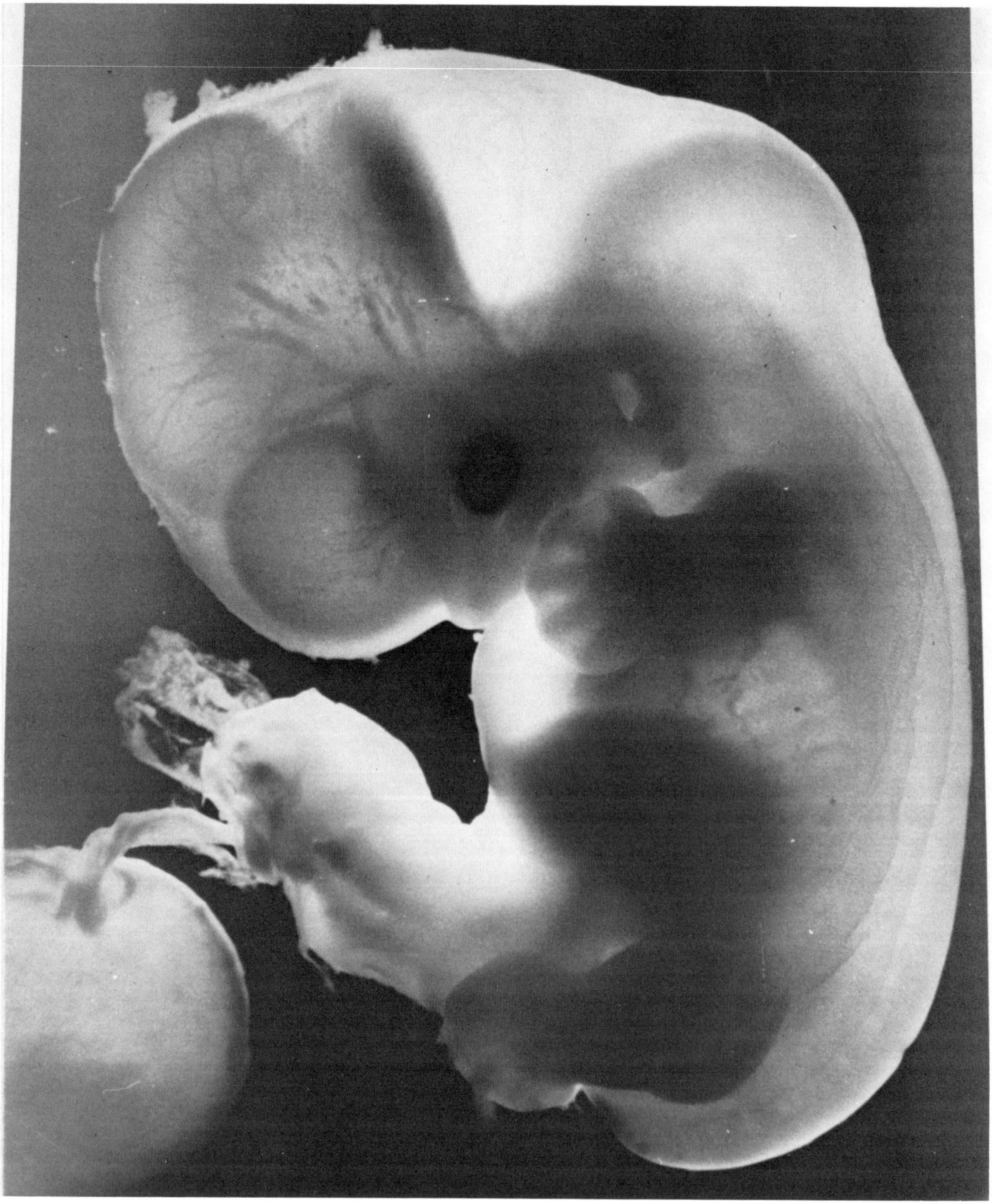

CHAPTER 5
The Embryo and Fetus: Conception to Birth

Introduction

The forgotten era of child development is the very beginning, and yet the vast percentage of physical development occurs during the first 266 days of life! The child in utero is also covertly practicing behaviors which will later be observed directly. The importance of this critical beginning stage to normal development of the child and to eventual status of the adult is now recognized.

The earliest weeks of life are most decisive to normal development. Formation of gametes; implantation; and early, rapid differentiation are high-risk events. This embryonic period is one of organogenesis; major body systems are formed, and some initiate function.

The fetal period is one of elaboration and growth. Relative to body size, the rate of growth will never be more rapid. The fetus also exhibits reflexive behavior as well as some behaviors which will be necessary for extrauterine life. As monitoring capabilities improve, the level of complexity of fetal life is appreciated more.

Prenatal development is not free from environmental influences. The moment the week-old embryo begins implantation in the endometrium (and perhaps before), the environment impacts development. Although initiated and directed by genetic activity, the maternal and surrounding environments determine the perfection of morphogenesis and the dimensions of growth. Environmental insults can result in abnormal morphology and compromised growth and health.

The nursing profession provides health care to those children who are physically impaired; the profession is also active in prevention of deterrents to maximal development. It is to these ends that this knowledge of prenatal period is applied.

FIGURE 5-1.

SECTION 1
Development of the Embryo: The Period of Organogenesis

Conception through establishment of body form   Mary Tudor

GAMETOGENESIS AND FERTILIZATION

Conception, the moment of fertilization, when oocyte and sperm unite, is generally considered the point at which new life begins—the start of human development. The genome of the resulting *zygote,* the one-cell product of conception, directs this development and is the combined genotypes of the two parental gametes. *Gametogenesis,* the process by which gametes are formed in the parents, is prerequisite to conception and normal development.

Gametogenesis in the female, oogenesis, and male, spermatogenesis, although differing in some aspects, share five basic steps:

- Formation and segregation of primordial germ cells prenatally.
- Repeated mitotic divisions of primordial germ cells resulting in a large number of available cells for reproduction.
- Generalized growth of germ cells signaling the end of mitotic stage and beginning of final maturation.
- Meiotic cell division, a two-step process resulting in transformation of diploid germ cells into haploid gametes. (The female primordial germ cell completes meiosis to prophase by the end of gestation.) Without this critical step, chromosomal number would double with each succeeding generation.
- Structural and functional change in preparation for the role in fertilization including release, transport, and energy requirements.

As described in other sections (see "Reproductive System," Chaps. 2, 6, and 10, and "Development of the Reproductive System," Chap. 5), gametogenesis begins in prenatal life with development and segregation of the primordial germ cells in the fetal testis and ovary. However, final maturation of sperm and ovum do not occur until after puberty; this discussion covers ongoing production after puberty.

OOGENESIS

Oogenesis begins, as noted above, prenatally and is completed in the mature ovary. All primordial germ cells, *oogonia,* are present in fetal life. Their development proceeds through the primary oocyte stage when they are arrested at meiotic prophase by the end of gestation: 38 weeks conceptual age. After puberty, with each 28-day reproductive cycle, a primary oocyte will complete prophase and mature through ovulation. (More than one primary oocyte may mature to the point of ovulation but will become atretic. Multiple ovulation may occur, however, which would result in a fraternal multiple pregnancy.)

Each primary oocyte has a full chromosomal complement of 46XX. The primary oocyte, still within the ovary, is surrounded by follicular cells; the entire structure is the *primary follicle* (see Fig. 5-2). As the primary follicle matures, it increases in size, and a thick membrane, the *zona pellucida,* forms around the oocyte. At this stage, it is designated the *growing follicle.* The follicular cells multiply and secrete a fluid, liquor folliculi, producing a fluid-filled space, the *follicular antrum.* The primary oocyte is suspended in the fluid and then displaced to the border of this antrum, where it is surrounded by follicular cells, the *cumulus oophorus.* The structure is now designated the *vesicular follicle.*

At this time, the primary oocyte completes the first meiotic division, which was arrested at prophase prenatally. The result is the *secondary oocyte* with a haploid chromosomal complement of 23X and the inconsequential first polar body (oocyte with no supporting cytoplasm), which soon degenerates. Unlike most cell lines which equally share cytoplasm in the process of division, the oocyte receives the bulk and the polar body, virtually none. The cytoplasm serves a critical function in nutritional support before placental circulation is established. The mature *graafian follicle* is larger and has a large antrum (see Fig. 5-2).

The follicle moves toward the ovarian surface as hormonal changes cause the oocyte and surrounding cumulus oophorus to detach from the follicle wall. A vesicle forms on the ovarian wall which ruptures, ejecting the secondary oocyte into the abdominal cavity. The secondary oocyte is surrounded by the zona pellucida and remaining follicular cells (cumulus oophorus), the *corona radiata*.

The secondary oocyte begins a second meiotic division at about the time of ovulation. This division, however, is arrested at metaphase and will not be completed unless fertilization occurs. Thus, the unfertilized oocyte does not complete gametogenesis. The mature oocyte is a large cell due to the relatively large amount of cytoplasm, needed during the first 3 days after fertilization.

The secondary oocyte remains in the abdominal cavity, probably adherent to the ovarian surface (Speroff, Glass, and Kase, 1978, p. 314), only briefly before it is carried into the ampulla of the oviduct. The sweeping movements of its fimbria covered by ciliated epithelium pull the oocyte into the tubal lumen, where fertilization may occur. If not fertilized, the oocyte degenerates within 12 to 24 h (Shettles, 1970; Speroff et al., 1978).

Concurrently, in the ovary, the wall of the now-empty follicle collapses and develops into the *corpus luteum*, a glandlike structure which secretes both progesterone and, to a lesser degree, estrogen. If fertilization does not occur, the corpus luteum will degenerate, usually within 10 to 12 days. If fertilization does occur, the corpus luteum is maintained, enlarges, and continues hormonal secretion for the first 10 to 12 weeks of gestation (see Fig. 5-3).

Reproductive cycle Maturation of the primary follicle as well as proliferation and secretion of the uterine endometrium are under hormonal control (see Fig. 5-4). The gonadotropins, follicle-stimulating hormone (FSH), and luteinizing hormone (LH) are released from the anterior lobe of the hypophysis under the stimulus of the hypothalamus. FSH and LH cause follicle maturation, ovulation, and initial development of the corpus luteum. The growing follicle in turn produces estrogen, and the corpus luteum produces progesterone and estrogen. The steroids, estrogen and progesterone, cause proliferation of the endometrium in preparation for implantation of the fertilized oocyte.

The reproductive cycle can be described in terms of ovarian and uterine events that occur approximately every 28 days and are hormonally synchronized to maximize potential for successful implantation. In terms

FIGURE 5-2. Schematic diagram of the ovary showing maturation of the ovarian follicle, ovulation, and corpus luteum formation and retrogression. Follow clockwise starting at the primary follicle. (*Adapted from C. E. Corliss, Patten's human embryology. New York: McGraw-Hill, 1976, p. 15.*)

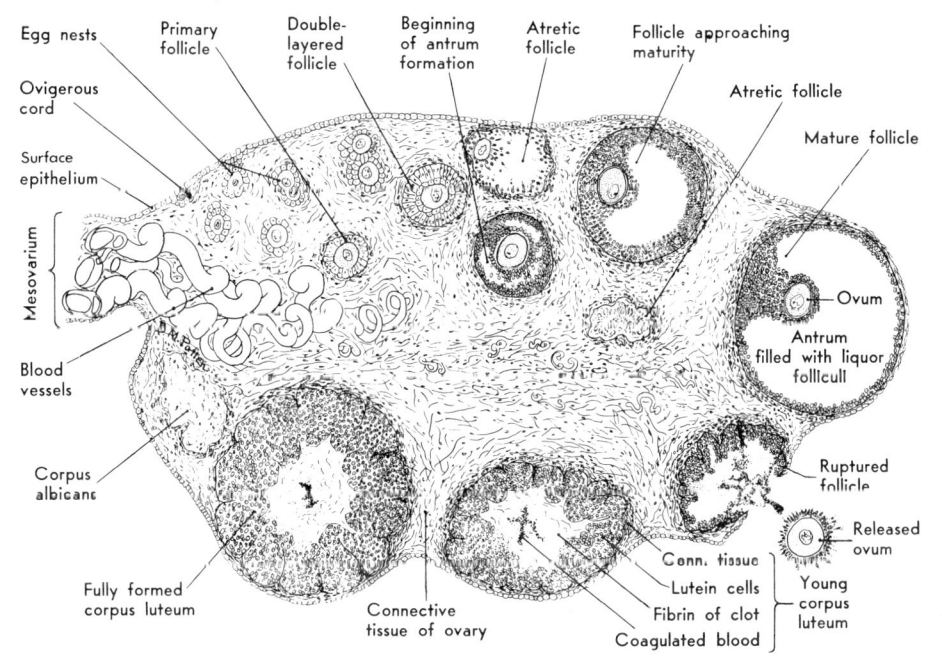

of ovarian events, day 1 through day 13 is considered the follicular or preovulatory phase (follicular development); day 14 is defined as the ovulatory phase or midcycle; and day 15 through day 28 is the luteal or postovulatory phase, when luteinization of the ruptured follicle occurs.

The uterine events may be described in three phases: the menstrual phase, days 1 through 5; the proliferative phase, days 6 through 14; and the secretory phase, days 15 through 28 (see Fig. 5-4). During the proliferative phase (corresponding to the follicular phase of the ovary) the endometrium thickens in response to estrogen produced by the maturing follicle. The secretory phase (corresponding to the luteal phase of the ovary) produces further endometrial proliferation and increased glandular secretion of a glycogen-rich substance due to progesterone secretion by the corpus luteum. If fertilization does not occur, the corpus luteum degeneration and decreasing level of both estrogen and progesterone result in ischemia of the endometrium. The reproductive cycle then begins again with the menstrual phase and sloughing of the ischemic endometrium.

SPERMATOGENESIS

Spermatogenesis occurs in the seminiferous tubules of the mature, descended testis. In the male fetus, as in the female, primordial germ cells are formed during embryogenesis. Unlike the female, initial stages of germ cell maturation do not occur prenatally. Some of the germ cells of the male fetus will differentiate into *spermatogonia* at puberty, but many will degenerate during postnatal development. Unlike oogenesis, spermatogenesis is a continual process; sperm at every level of maturation can be found in the seminiferous tubules at any one time (see Fig. 5-5).

Spermatogenesis begins with several mitotic divisions of spermatogonia. Each spermatogonium will give rise to both primary spermatocytes and replacement spermatogonia. Because cell size does not double prior to division as with most cells, the resulting primary spermatocytes are smaller. Unlike oocyte formation, what cytoplasm exists is divided equally. A primary spermatocyte has a diploid (46XY) complement. The first meiotic division then occurs, resulting in two secondary spermatocytes which are smaller and haploid, having a chromosomal complement of 23X or 23Y (see Fig. 5-5).

The secondary spermatocytes rapidly divide again, resulting in four smaller haploid spermatids. The sper-

FIGURE 5-3. The ordinary (nonpregnant) reproductive cycle followed by a reproductive cycle in which fertilization occurs followed by implantation and placentation. The corpus luteum does not regress but becomes the corpus luteum of pregnancy. (From C. E. Corliss, *Patten's human embryology.* New York: McGraw-Hill, 1976, p. 27. Reprinted with permission of the publisher.)

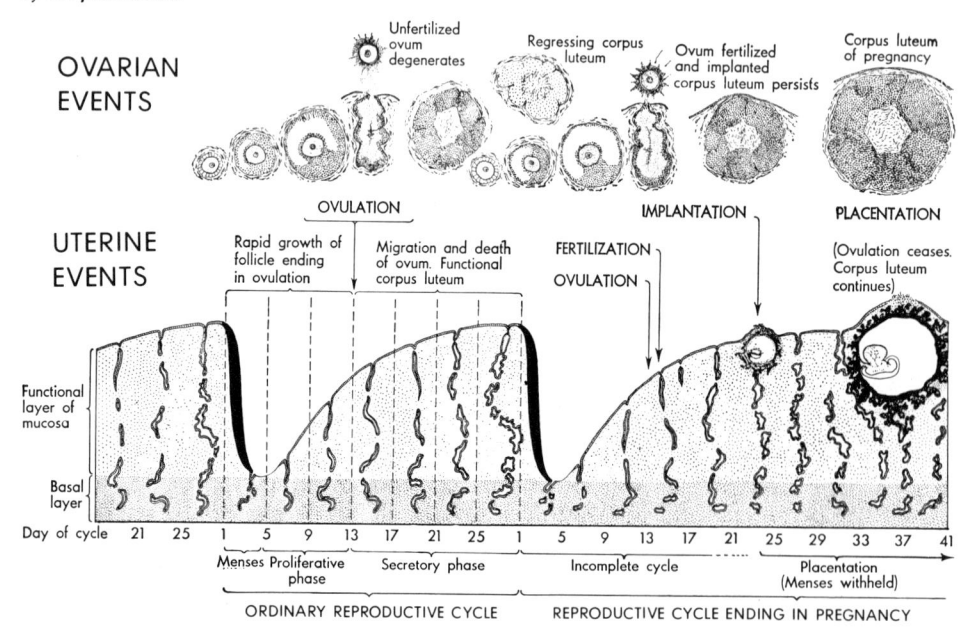

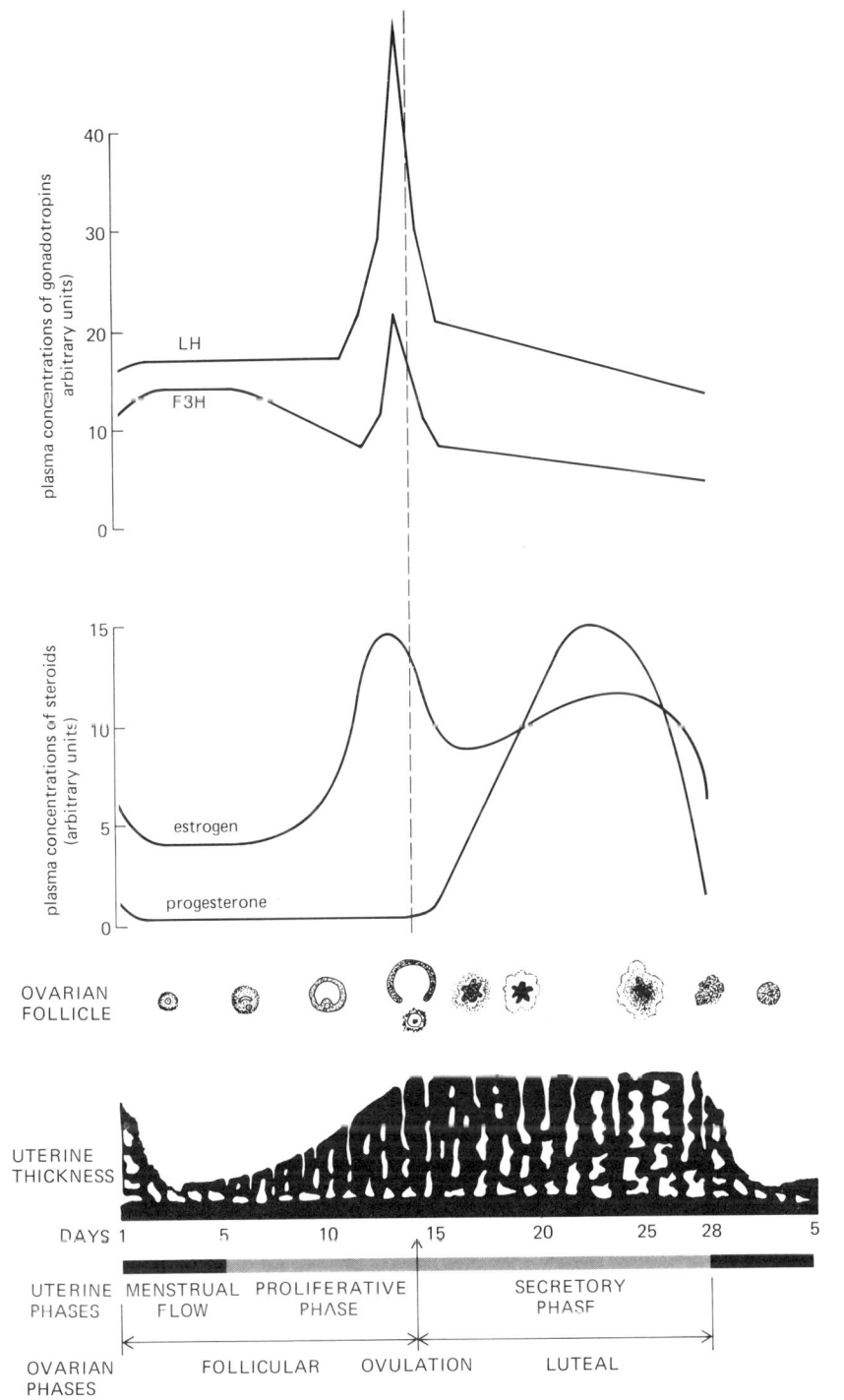

FIGURE 5-4. Summary of plasma hormone concentrations, ovarian and uterine events of the female reproductive cycle. (From D. Luciano, A. Vander, and J. Sherman, Human function and structure. New York: McGraw-Hill, 1978, p. 633. Reprinted by permission of the publisher.)

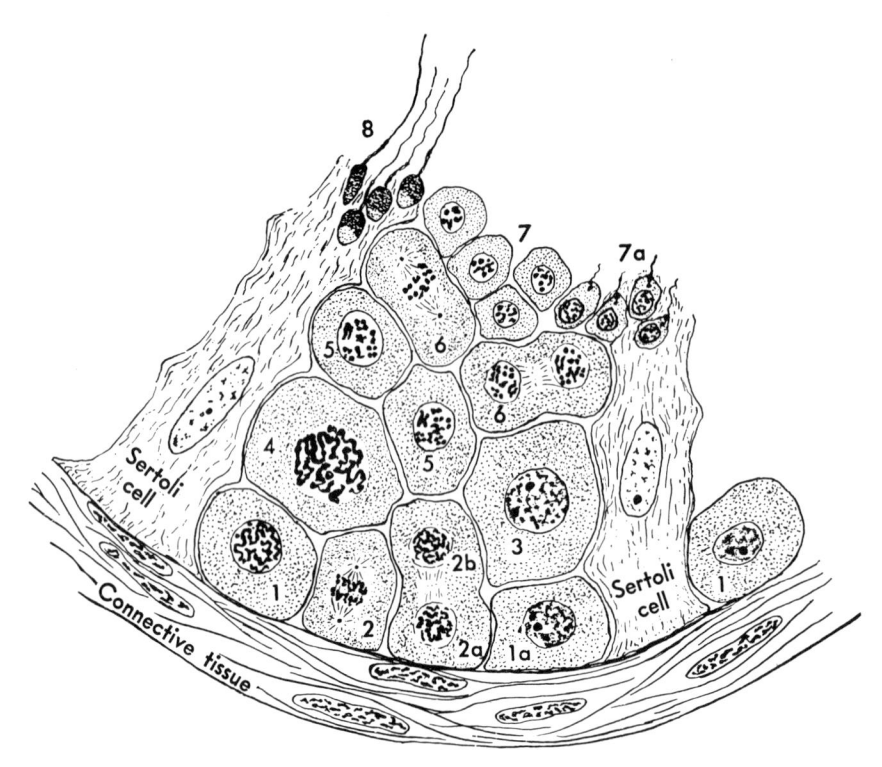

FIGURE 5-5. Semischematic representation of the wall of an active seminiferous tubule. Sequence of events in spermatogenesis is indicated by numbers. A spermatogonium (1) undergoes mitosis (2), producing two daughter cells (2a,2b). One (2a) may remain peripherally located as a new spermatogonium, eventually occupying position 1a. The other daughter cell (2b) may grow into a primary spermatocyte (3), being moved nearer the lumen of the tubule. When fully grown, the primary spermatocyte will go into mitosis again (4) and produce two secondary spermatocytes (5,5). Each secondary spermatocyte at once divides again (6,6), producing spermatids (7). The spermatids become embedded in the tip of a Sertoli cell (7a), there becoming morphologically mature sperm (8). When mature, they are detached into the lumen of the seminiferous tubule.

matids become embedded in the Sertoli cells and through a final differentiation process of spermiogenesis are transformed into sperm. Cell size is diminished, and structure is modified for motility and penetration of the oocyte. However, maturation is not complete until sperm are exposed to storage in the epididymis, where they acquire motility and fertilizing capacity. The entire process of spermatogenesis takes a total of approximately 70 days (Speroff et al., 1978, p. 365) in contrast to oogenesis, which is completed over a number of years.

The mature sperm is composed of four basic parts: head, neck, middle piece, and tail. At the tip of the head is the acrosome, important for penetration of the oocyte. The head contains the nucleus with the chromosomal material. The middle piece contains the mitochondrial helix, source of energy for motility, which is achieved by lashing movements of the tail. When mature, the sperm move into the lumen of the seminiferous tubule and are stored in the epididymis and ductus deferens. During ejaculation, sperm are mixed with fluid from the seminal, prostate, and bulbourethral glands (stimulating motility), and the semen then passes through the urethra.

FERTILIZATION

During sexual intercourse, the male ejaculates approximately 3 to 5 mL of semen, which contains 200 to 300 million sperm, into the vagina of the female, near the cervix. [A sperm count of 20 million has been suggested as the minimum for conception to be possible (Speroff et al., 1978, p. 364).] In order for fertilization to occur, sperm must travel through the cervical os and uterine cavity to the ampulla of the oviduct. Movement of the sperm is a combination of intrinsic motility as well as muscular contractions of the uterus and uterine tubes. It is estimated to take only 5 min for the sperm to travel from the cervix to the ampulla; however, less than 200 sperm arrive at the vicinity of the oocyte (Speroff et al., 1978, p. 313).

Although some sperm are viable for 3 to 4 days after ejaculation, the ability to fertilize probably lasts only 24 to 48 h. In order to fertilize the oocyte, the sperm must undergo a process of capacitation (exposure to the female reproductive tract environment) after ejaculation. This process, taking several hours, is thought to result in instability of the sperm plasma membrane, facilitating penetration of the oocyte by the sperm. Once the sperm reaches the oocyte, fertilization is completed in approximately 24 h (Moore, 1977).

A single sperm penetrates the corona radiata and zona pellucida by motility and acrosomal enzyme action. The sperm then passes into the cytoplasm of the oocyte leaving its plasma membrane fused to that of the oocyte. The tail of the sperm degenerates, and the head forms the male pronucleus—the paternal chromosomal material—either 23X or 23Y. In response to penetration, the oocyte becomes impenetrable to other sperm, the zonal reaction. The oocyte finally matures, a process begun decades before during embryogenesis, as the second meiotic division is completed. The second polar body is extruded and soon degenerates (see Fig. 5-6).

The female pronucleus and the male pronucleus fuse into a single cell, the zygote, and at that moment of conception form a new individual with a full set of chromosomes, either female (46XX) or male (46XY). The maternal and paternal chromosomes mingle within the single nucleus to make up the genotype of the offspring and begin to direct the development of the child.

If the reproductive cycle is regular, ovulation can be determined by noting a biphasic pattern in basal body temperature. An increase in temperature above 46.6°C (taken upon awakening and before activity) occurs about 2 days after ovulation and is maintained for the duration of the cycle due to thermogenic effects of progesterone. Sexual intercourse every other day 4 days prior to and 3 days after ovulation will maximize potential for conception.

CONCEPTION TO BIRTH: GENERAL CONCEPTS

The prenatal period represents the most significant period in physiological development in terms of degree of morphogenesis, "the progressive attainment of bodily forms and structures" (Berrill and Karp, 1976, p. 219), as well as increase in size and the rapidity of this change. Although Aristotle is considered the "founder of embryology" (Moore, 1977, p. 8), it was not until the twentieth century that the greatest strides were made in human genetics and embryology. Major advances are recorded with astonishing regularity including the recent birth of an apparently normal child after fertilization and early development in vitro and successful implantation in the uterus of her mother 2½ days later at the eight-cell stage (Steptoe and Edwards, 1978).

Over a period of approximately 266 days, the one-cell zygote, its genome determined by the genetic contribution of ovum and sperm, becomes a human infant and emerges from the uterine environment. "Genetics tells us of developmental potentialities and experimental embryology analyzes mechanisms involved in their fulfillment" (Corliss, 1976, p. 140).

Clinically, the prenatal period is divided into trimesters: three periods, each 3 calendar months long. In embryology, prenatal development is divided into three periods:

- The early period: conception through 14 days
- The embryonic period: 15 through 60 to 62 days (weeks 2 through 8)
- The fetal period: 60 through 266 days (weeks 9 through 38)

In addition to age of the conceptus, prenatal development can be further described and calibrated by anthropometric measurements or by the stage of development, determined from external and internal characteristics: morphological change (see Table 5-1). These descriptions are essential to discussion of embryological development as well as to clinical application of this knowledge.

AGE

In calculating the age of an embryo or fetus, conceptual age or menstrual age may be used. Conceptual age (ca) is the actual age of the developing human, beginning at the moment of conception. Using conceptual age, the actual length of gestation is 266 days, 38 weeks, or 8.75 calendar (9.5 lunar) months. Because of the difficulty in determining the moment of conception, in clinical practice gestational age is calculated from the onset of the last menstrual period (LMP) giving menstrual age (ma). Using *Nagele's rule,* date of birth is estimated:

$$\text{LMP} + 7 \text{ days} - 3 \text{ months} + 1 \text{ year} = \text{expected date of birth}$$

As conception would not occur until about 2 weeks after the last menstrual period, menstrual age is conceptual age plus 14 (±2) days. Using menstrual age, the date of birth is calculated to be at 280 days or 40 weeks or 9.25 calendar (10 lunar) months.

A woman's recall of menstrual history may be inaccurate, ovulation may not occur at 14 ± 2 days after the last menstrual period, and implantation (6 to 10 days after conception) may cause spotting and be mistaken for menstruation. Uterine size, fetal heart tones, and movement are also used clinically to estimate gestational age, in order of accuracy.

References giving gestational age should note whether menstrual or conceptual age is used. Often, however, this is not done. Generally, embryologists use ca and practitioners use ma. In the following sections, ca is used; in addition, ma will be noted as well when clinical application is discussed.

Early period: conception through day 14 The initial period of development begins with fertilization, which results in the one-cell zygote. Through mitosis, the zygote evolves into an embryonic structure with two primary cell layers. This 14-day period comprises *Carnegie stages* 1 through 6 (see below, "Stages"). Anthropometric measurements are not appropriate as the conceptus is minute.

Embryonic period: days 15 through 60 to 62 (second through eighth weeks) The embryonic period is often referred to as the *period of organogenesis;* growth by hyperplasia, differentiation, and specialization are key features of this period. During these 6 weeks, the three primary germ layers evolve, and the embryo changes from disk- to cylinder-shaped and then to human form with all systems present and functioning to some degree. The remainder of the Carnegie stages, 7 through 23, comprise the embryonic period. Crown-rump length in millimeters is the anthropometric measurement most commonly utilized.

Fetal period: days 60 to 62 through 266 (ninth through thirty-eighth weeks) The fetal period is one of elaboration and growth. The final stages of differentiation are completed during this time; however, the primary task is growth. Hypertrophic cellular growth begins at 25 weeks ca. Fetal weight, length, and body circumferences are noted in monitoring growth. Increase in size is dramatic, and physiological preparations for extrauterine life are completed during the fetal period. The fetus becomes more extended and flexible; a variety of spontaneous and reflexive movements are seen which contribute to, as well as reflect, normal development.

STAGES

In embryology, the first 8 weeks are divided into 23 stages of development based on morphological change, the Car-

TABLE 5-1 Prenatal developmental timetable drawn to represent actual length of gestation and notable events

		Conception ↓			FHT (dopler) ↓	Fetal movement noted (quickening) ↓	Extrauterine viability 20% ↓ / 97% ↓		Birth ↓
Developmental period		Early	Embryonic	Fetal					
Highlight of period		Implantation	Organogenesis	Elaboration and growth					
		Stages	Stages	Anthropometric measurements: C-R or C-H length and weight					
Morphogenesis/growth		1–6	7–23	30 mm C-R / 1 g	90 mm C-R / 51 g	140 mm C-R / 220 g	190 mm C-R / 480 g	37 cm C-H / 990 g	45 cm C-H / 1460 g	50 cm C-H / 3250 g
				Week 8	Week 12	Week 16	Week 20	Week 25	Week 32	Week 38
Conceptual age	days weeks	1–14 1–2	15 → 56 3 → 8	57 → 266 9 → 38					
Menstrual age	days weeks	1–28 1–4	29–70 5–10	71–280 11–40					
		↑ LMP	1st trimester ↑ 1st MP missed	↑ 2d MP missed	2d trimester		3d trimester		

negie stages (Streeter, 1942). The degree of morphogenesis is used as a reliable, systematic method to calibrate development. Each stage is 1 to 5 days in length and includes a significant morphological change. The fetal period, weeks 9 through 38, does not have a comparable staging.

ANTHROPOMETRIC MEASUREMENT

Development of the embryo and fetus is also described in increments of length, weight, and other measurements. Anthropometric measurements historically have been obtained directly from aborted embryos and fetuses; consequently, they must be viewed as such, possibly varying from normal intrauterine size. More recently, ultrasonography has been used to obtain measurements with the fetus in utero from 3 weeks ca. Anthropometric measurements give information on growth as well as gestational age in the embryonic and fetal periods.

Greatest length, crown-rump length, and crown-heel length are used to evaluate growth and to estimate developmental level. Foot length is also used as a measurement of growth; however, the possibility of error is greater due to the smaller dimension.

Weight is a relatively simple measurement to obtain directly and is less prone to error in technique. It can also be extrapolated from linear measurements obtained by ultrasound. Head circumference as well as diameter are used in assessment of fetal development. Chest and abdominal circumference are also used to mark fetal growth.

ANATOMICAL DIRECTIONS

In the embryo, as in the adult, *ventral* refers to the anterior aspect or front of the body and limbs (in the anatomical position); *dorsal* refers to the posterior aspect or back of the body and limbs. *Proximal* and *distal* are used as in the adult. *Cranial* or *cephalic* refers to the head portion; *caudal* refers to the tail end. *Rostral* is also used in describing embryonic anatomical position and refers to the nose of the embryo. This is necessary due to the cephalic flexure early in development which results in a C-shaped body.

EVALUATION OF FETAL STATUS

Evaluation, visualization, and measurement of the fetus is currently possible by amniocentesis, radiography, ultrasonography, amniography or fetography, and fetoscopy.

Amniocentesis Prenatal diagnosis of genetic (including metabolic) disorders, chromosomal abnormalities, and some structural disorders as well as determination of lecithin and sphingomyelin levels to evaluate fetal lung maturity and delta OD to determine status of Rh sensitization are possible by amniocentesis. Transabdominal amniocentesis is possible from the twelfth week ca (14 ma) and should be performed as soon after that time as possible (except to determine lecithin/sphingomyelin ratio, which is done near term).

The placenta is localized by ultrasound, and fetal heart tones are monitored. The abdominal wall, uterine wall, and amnion are punctured, and 10 to 15 mL of amniotic fluid is withdrawn. Fetal cells, which are sloughed into the amniotic fluid, are cultured and studied by karyotyping or other analysis. Metabolites and other substances in the amniotic fluid can also be studied. Tests performed depend on the concern: the purpose of the amniocentesis. The risk appears low; spontaneous abortion, fetal death in utero, and stillbirths were reported in 3.5 percent of patients undergoing amniocentesis compared with 3.2 percent in the control group (National Institute, 1976).

Ultrasonography Ultrasonography uses short pulses of high-frequency, low-intensity sound which are transmitted through the maternal abdomen. As a sound pulse (wave) crosses the interface of different tissues, a partial reflection of the wave occurs. The remainder of the ultrasonic pulse continues to the next tissue junction, and the same reflection occurs. The gestation sac (embryo and surrounding membranes) can be visualized from 3 weeks ca (Campbell, 1976).

The reflection (echo) of the pulse or sound waves can be displayed in several ways. An A scan gives a display of vertical spikes on a horizontal time base. This is most often used to determine distance between two tissue structures as well as for recording fetal heart and respiratory rates. B scan displays a two-dimensional picture of deflected sound waves as the transducer travels over the maternal abdomen. B scan is used to display several tissue interfaces at one time.

By combining A and B scans, the most precise measurements are obtained (Campbell, 1976). A scan converter displays the full range of sound waves in shades of gray (gray scale), according to the strength of the wave, as television. Detailed, life-sized images of the fetus are possible, which can be transferred to paper and measured directly. Real-time ultrasonography has been introduced more recently and has been used to evaluate fetal movement.

Many studies have been done to detect any harmful effects of repeated ultrasound on the developing embryo

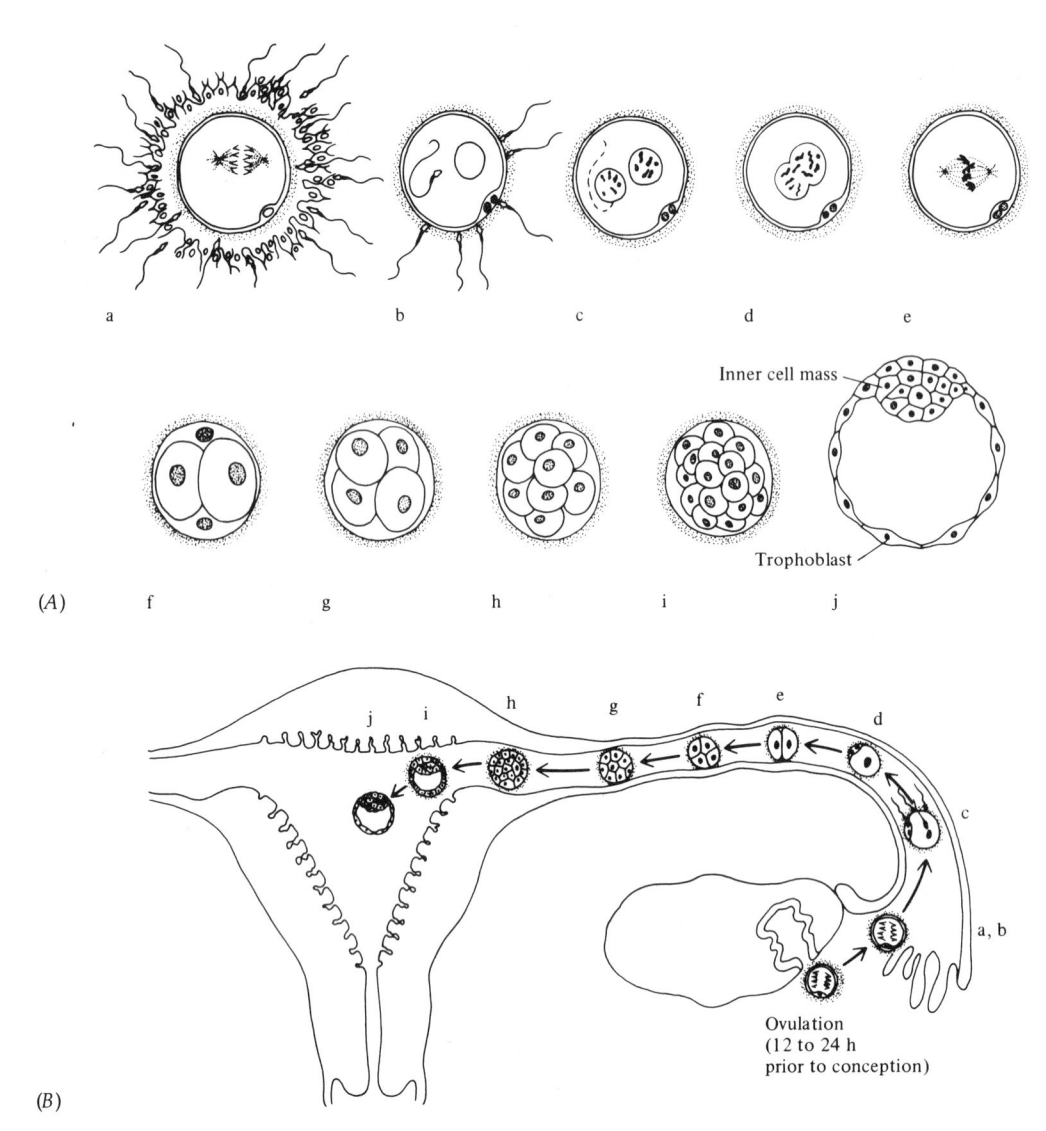

FIGURE 5-6. (A) Fertilization, cleavage, and blastocyst formation, days 1 through 5. (a) Sperm penetrating corona radiata and zona pellucida; second meiotic division of oocyte begins. (b) Penetration is complete, and the zonal reaction prohibits penetration by other sperm. (c) The female and male pronuclei are formed. (d) The zygote is formed as the pronuclei fuse. (e) The first mitotic division begins, starting cleavage. (f) Two-cell stage. (g) Four-cell stage. (h) Eight-cell stage. (i) Sixteen-cell stage, morula. (j) Blastocyst. (B) Passage through the uterine tube into the uterine cavity; the blastocyst is now ready for implantation on the posterior uterine wall. [Adapted from K. L. Moore, The developing human (2d ed.). Philadelphia: Saunders, 1977, pp. 26; 31. Used with permission of the publisher.]

and fetus; none have been found. Ultrasonography is preferred over radiography prior to term due to hazards of serial radiation. Both x-ray and ultrasound at term can detect malformation, multiple pregnancy, and other complications. Cephalopelvic disproportion is not detected by ultrasound; it is detected by radiography.

Amniography and fetography In amniography, a water-soluble contrast medium is injected into the amniotic fluid by amniocentesis. A radiograph then allows visualization of the fetus. Fetography utilizes an oil-soluble medium which has an affinity for vernix caseosa. Thus a more defined picture of fetal extremities and surface anomalies is possible.

Fetoscopy Fetoscopy allows direct visualization and blood sampling of the fetus by a fiberoptic endoscope inserted into the uterus. This technique is with significant risk and is not widely available.

ESTABLISHMENT OF BODY FORM

THE EARLY PERIOD: WEEKS 1 AND 2

Week 1 (period of cleavage) During the first week of life, the conceptus undergoes significant change in form as well as location in the maternal reproductive system. The single-cell zygote, still within the outer one-third of the oviduct, begins rapid mitotic division, each daughter cell termed a *blastomere*. As these divisions, or *cleavages,* occur, the zygote moves through the oviduct (see Fig. 5-6). On the third day, the zygote has reached the 16-cell (16-blastomere) stage, the *morula,* and has passed into the uterine cavity.

On days 4 and 5, the morula is transformed into the *blastocyst,* composed of an inner fluid-filled cavity and two cell masses, the *inner cell mass* and *trophoblast.* These cell masses represent initial differentiation—the process that will eventually transform the single-cell zygote into the human adult with a multitude of cell types.

The inner cell mass, the *embryoblast,* is the future embryo, and the outer cell mass, the trophoblast, will give rise to the *syncytiotrophoblast,* the future fetal portion of the placenta. On day 6, the blastocyst (previously free-floating in the uterus) begins implantation in the endometrial lining (see Fig. 5-6). The section of the trophoblast overlying the inner cell mass is thought to be "sticky," and thus implantation occurs with the inner cell mass next to the endometrium. Implantation may occur in any part of the uterus; however, the posterior wall is the most common site.

Week 2 (period of the bilaminar embryo) During the second week, implantation is completed as the early embryo disappears beneath the endometrium, placental circulation begins, and the inner cell mass differentiates further into the bilaminar embryonic disk. Implantation occurs as a result of the syncytiotrophoblast invading the endometrial epithelium causing the blastocyst to be completely buried. The invasive syncytiotrophoblast establishes primitive placental circulation by day 12.

The embryonic disk now consists of two layers (*bilaminar*): the epiblast, future ectoderm and mesoderm; and the endoderm. The embryonic disk lies between the amniotic cavity and the primitive yolk sac (see Fig. 5-7).

By day 14, one end of the embryonic disk shows a thickening of the endodermal cells, the *prochordal plate.* This is the future cephalad region and is a critical marker for organization of the embryo. The amnion and yolk sac are surrounded by the *extraembryonic coelom* (chorionic cavity), a fluid-filled cavity formed by the chorion with a connecting body stalk attaching the amnion to the chorion at the caudal end, opposite the prochordal plate (see Fig. 5-7).

Multiple pregnancy Twinning occurs once in every 85 to 90 pregnancies (Moore, 1977). The incidence is higher in Negroes than Caucasians (Arey, 1965). Two mature oocytes fertilized by different sperms will result in dizygotic twins, which account for two-thirds of all cases of twins. Monozygotic twins originate from one oocyte and one sperm. At about 7 days' gestation, however, the inner cell mass divides, eventually giving rise to two embryos which will have a shared placenta. Earlier separation, at the morula stage, may occur, in which case the identical embryos will have separate placentas.

THE EMBRYONIC PERIOD

The embryological period, the period of organogenesis, is one of differentiation and specialization with less dramatic change in actual size. During this period, the embryo develops from a relatively simple bilaminar disk to a clearly human form with all internal structures and organ systems present but immature. All future body structures will differentiate from one of these three chemically and positionally different germ layers of the *trilaminar* embryo: endoderm, ectoderm, and mesoderm.

Week 3 (period of the trilaminar embryo) The third week of life is significant in the transformation of the

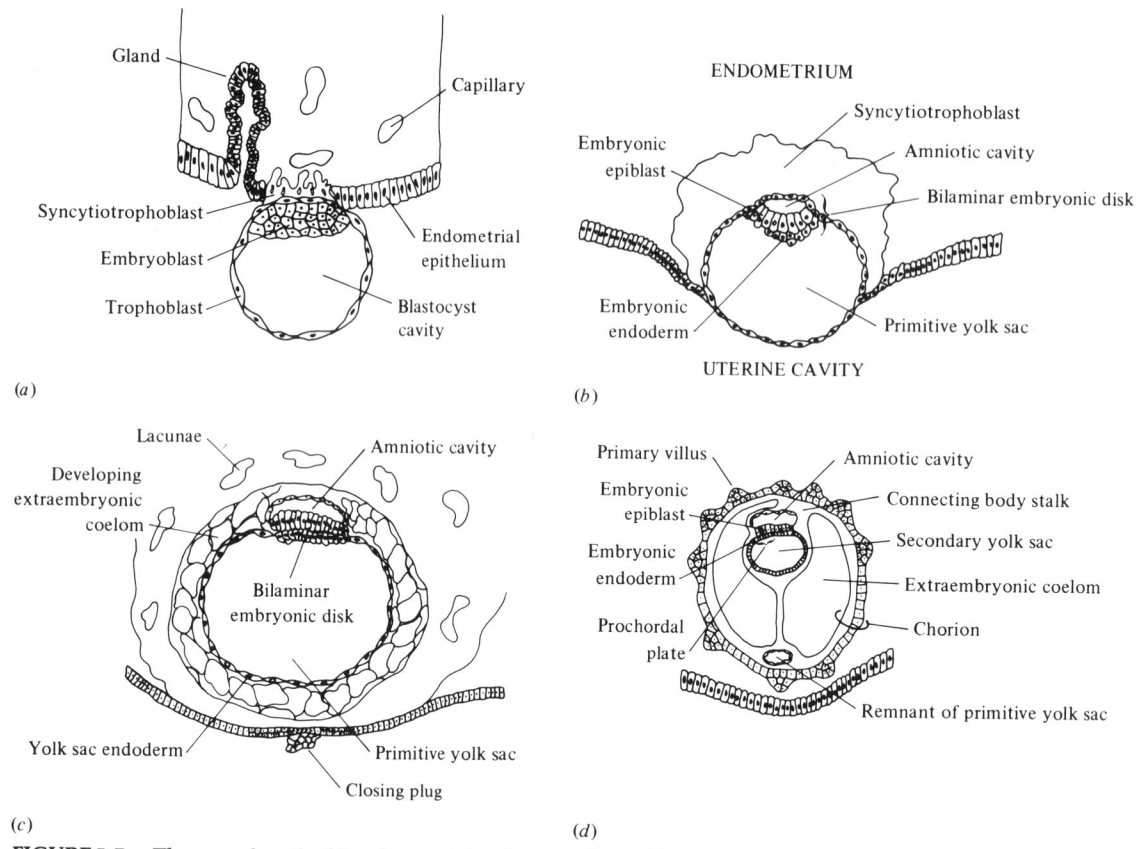

FIGURE 5-7. The second week of development: implementation and formation of the bilaminar embryo (sagittal section). (a) Sixth to seventh day: beginning implantation. (b) Day 7½. (c) Day 12. (d) Day 14. [a adapted from many sources; b and c adapted from C. E. Corliss, *Patten's human embryology.* New York: McGraw-Hill, 1976, pp. 38–39; d adapted from K. L. Moore, *The developing human* (2d ed.). Philadelphia: Sanders, 1977, p. 38.]

bilaminar embryonic disk to the trilaminar embryonic disk with the development of mesoderm. Cellular differentiation is further evidenced by development of the notochord, the neural tube, somites, and a primitive cardiovascular system. In addition, the primitive placental circulation becomes more complex and substantial to provide the needed oxygen and nutrients of the rapidly developing embryo.

A dorsal view of the 15-day-old embryo shows the midline *primitive streak* beginning at the caudal end on the dorsal side and defining the longitudinal axis of the embryo. From the primitive streak, the primitive groove and primitive pit appear, which initiate and organize development of the trilaminar embryo (see Fig. 5-8).

At 16 days, embryonic mesoderm migrates peripherally from the primitive streak between the epiblast, now the embryonic ectoderm, and the endoderm. Mesenchymal cells, which will form embryonic connective tissue, evolve from mesoderm (see Fig. 5-8).

The notochordal canal develops within the process, and the once-circular trilaminar embryo elongates with notochordal process growth. Simultaneously, the embryonic ectoderm gives rise to the neural groove and the notochord, the beginning development of the nervous system.

The embryonic mesoderm continues to proliferate and differentiate. At about 20 days, cube-shaped somites, which will differentiate into *sclerotome* (axial skeleton)

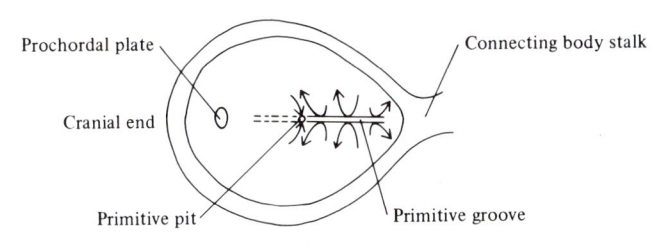

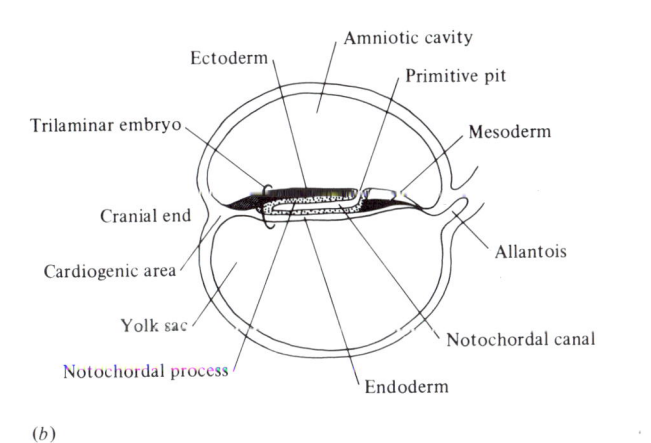

FIGURE 5-8. Days 16 to 18. (*a*) Dorsal view of embryo. Arrows indicate cell migration to form the mesodermal layer. (*b*) Sagittal section showing trilaminar embryo. (*a* adapted from C. E. Corliss, 1976, p. 41, and K. L. Moore, 1977, p. 49; *b* adapted from K. L. Moore, 1977, p. 50.)

and *myotome* (skeletal muscles), begin to develop in pairs in a cephalocaudal direction (see Fig. 5-9). Two pairs develop during the third week. One portion of each somite, designated *dermatome*, has been thought to give rise to the dermal layer of the integument. This is now in question.

The *intraembryonic coelom*, a horseshoe-shaped space within the mesoderm, develops, dividing the mesoderm into two layers, the *somatic layer* and the *splanchnic layer*. The intraembryonic coelom will eventually give rise to the *peritoneal, pericardial,* and *pleural cavities*.

The primitive cardiovascular system is composed of a pair of heart tubes which develop in the cardiogenic area of the endoderm and a simple vascular system formed in

FIGURE 5-9. Day 20. (*a*) Dorsal view showing beginning somite formation. (*b*) Transverse section of trilaminar embryo. (*Adapted from K. L. Moore, 1977, p. 52.*)

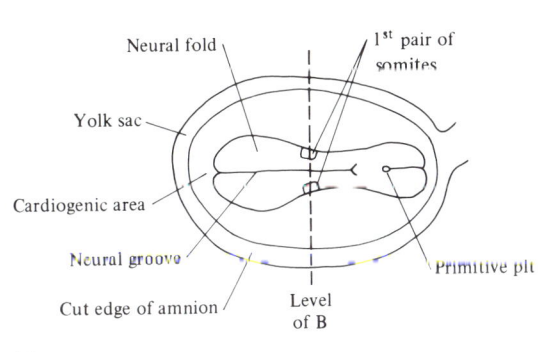

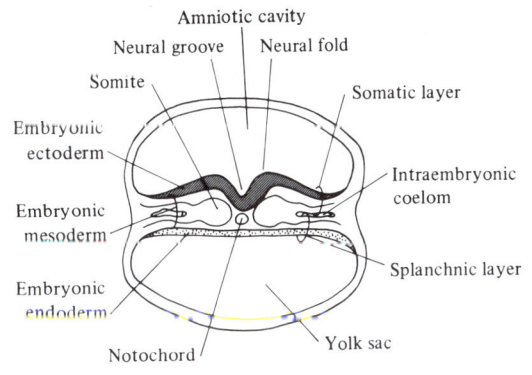

the yolk sac. The heart tubes and vascular plexus interconnect and also extend through the connecting body stalk to the villi of the developing placenta. By the beginning of the fourth week, this primitive cardiovascular system is functional with circulation of embryonic blood. This blood is formed in the yolk sac and allantois; blood formation does not begin within the embryo proper until week 5 (Moore, 1977).

Week 4 During the fourth week, many of the processes begun during week 3 are completed. The major change is in overall form of the embryo. The neural folds continue to fuse, forming the neural tube, closing first cephalically and 2 days later caudally. Neural crest cells remain outside the tube. The neural tube will develop into the brain and spinal cord and its lumen into the ventricles and spinal canal. The neural crest cells give rise to the sensory cells of the peripheral nervous system and melanocytes of the integument. By the end of the fourth week, the three major segments of the brain can be identified, and the number of somites has increased to 29 pairs (see Fig. 5-10).

During the fourth week, the embryo folds in two planes: longitudinally and transversely. The longitudinal fold occurs with flexion of the embryo, first at the cephalic end and later at the caudal end (see Fig. 5-11a and b). The cephalic flexion results from growth and folding of the primitive brain. As the future head folds, the primitive

FIGURE 5-10. (a) and (b) Dorsal views of embryos during the fourth week showing somite formation and neural tube closure: (a) 7-somite stage, 21 to 22 days. (b) 10-somite stage, 22 to 23 days. (c) and (d) Lateral views: (c) embryo with 19 somites, 24 to 25 days; neural tube is nearly closed. (d) embryo with 27 somites, about 26 days. [Adapted from L. B. Arey, Developmental anatomy (7th ed.). Philadelphia: Saunders, 1965, p. 96 and K. L. Moore, 1977, p. 68.]

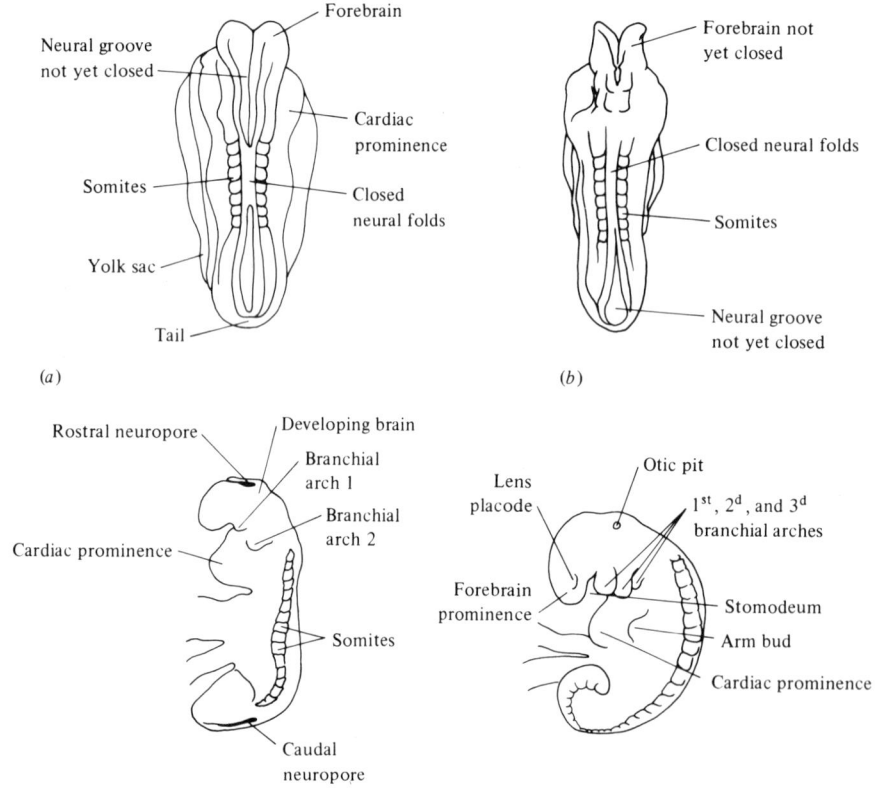

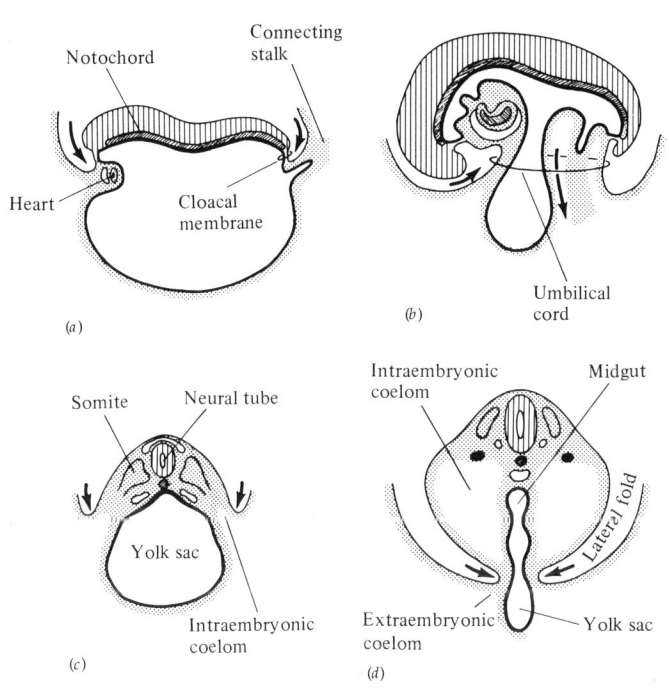

FIGURE 5-11. (a) and (b) Longitudinal fold during the fourth week: (a) 24 days. (b) 28 days. (c) and (d) Transverse fold during the fourth week: (c) 22 days. (d) 26 days. (*From K. L. Moore, 1977, p. 60.*)

heart swings under from the cardiogenic area to the ventral surface of the embryo. The caudal end then folds ventrally and amnion, yolk sac, and connecting body stalk form the more constricted umbilical cord.

Simultaneously, transverse folding results in the embryo changing from disk- to cylinder-shaped. The lateral edges of the disk move ventrically and fuse, incorporating the intraembryonic coelom, which will eventually give rise to body cavities. The yolk sac is constricted with the midgut, the primitive digestive system, remaining within the embryo and connected by a stalk to the remaining yolk sac (see Fig. 5-11c and d).

The heart tubes fuse into a single tube, and on day 22 peristaltic-type myogenic contraction begins, initially as an "ebb and flow" (Moore, 1977, p. 262) and by 28 days in a unilateral pattern.

As the brain rapidly grows and develops and flexion increases, paired prominences in the ventrolateral area of the cephalic flexion are formed. These *branchial arches*, separated by branchial grooves, form in a cephalocaudal direction. By the twenty-eighth day, all six pairs are present, the fifth and sixth in rudimentary form. The branchial arches will give rise to structures of the lower face and neck.

At the end of the fourth week, the increasing complexity of the brain is indicated by external evidence of development of the sensory system. The *otic pit*, indicating the future inner ear, and the pair of *lens placodes*, future lenses, appear on the lateral aspects of the head region. The primitive mouth, *stomodeum*, becomes patent, and two *nasal placodes* develop in the ventral portion of the head region.

The human form is approximated even more as arm buds and leg buds appear as small, blunt swellings. By the end of the fourth week, the embryo is approximately 4 to 5 mm crown-rump length.

Week 5 By the beginning of the fifth week the embryo is fully C-shaped with the facial region in contact with the heart prominence (see Fig. 5-12a). The brain, sensory end organs, and face continue to dominate the morphological change. The primitive eyes, ears, nose, and mouth continue to develop as well as change in relative placement. The brain, however, shows the greatest increase in size as well as morphological complexity.

The heart continues to develop, and left and right lung buds, future lung and bronchi, appear. The (permanent) kidney also develops during the fifth week of gestation (see Fig. 5-12b). Somite formation is completed, a total of about 44 pairs including the tail bud. The arm buds begin to lengthen and become paddle-shaped. The embryo doubles in length during the fifth week to approximately 8 mm crown-rump length.

Week 6 During the sixth week, the head increases significantly in size and the arm and leg buds continue to develop, becoming finlike, with the leg buds less developed than the arms in cephalocaudal pattern. The embryo becomes less flexed with growth, the head lifting from the heart prominence (see Fig. 5-13). Cartilage formation begins as well as formation of tooth buds.

The gastrointestinal system and other visceral organs are well developed by this stage; the stomach, liver, spleen, and pancreas are recognizable. The liver as well as heart prominences are visible on the external surface. The primitive small intestine and part of the colon begin to herniate into the umbilical cord; this accommodates growth, not possible within the small pelvic girdle and thorax. The tail bud begins to disappear during the sixth week. By 42 days, crown-rump length is approximately 14 mm.

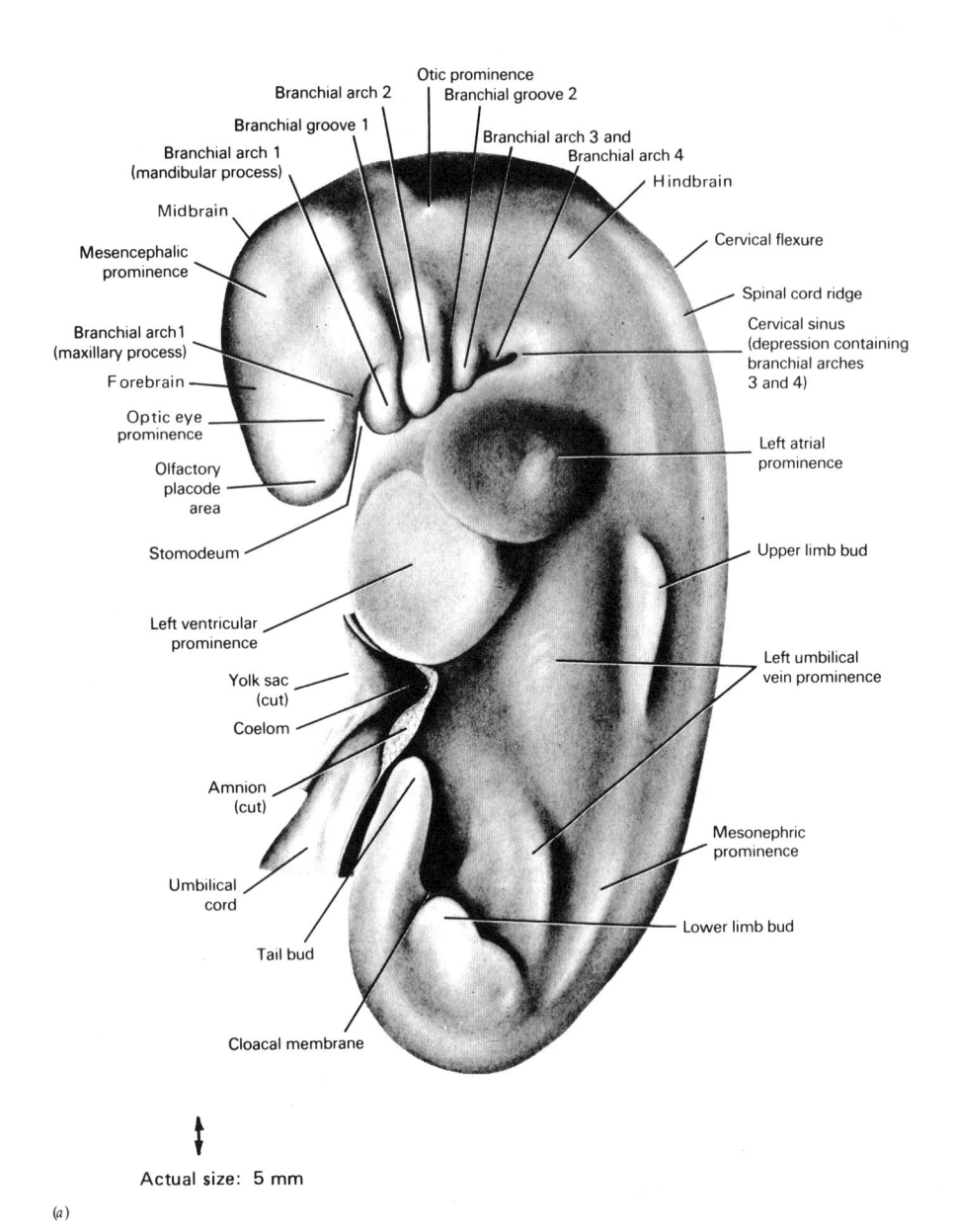

FIGURE 5-12. (a) Embryo at the beginning of the fifth week, lateral view. Actual crown-rump length of 5 mm is shown. (b) Sagittal section of the embryo in the fifth week showing development of internal organ systems. (a modified from R. F. Gasser, Atlas of human embryos. New York: Harper & Row, 1975, p. 49; b from C. E. Corliss, 1976, p. 62. Used with permission of the publisher.)

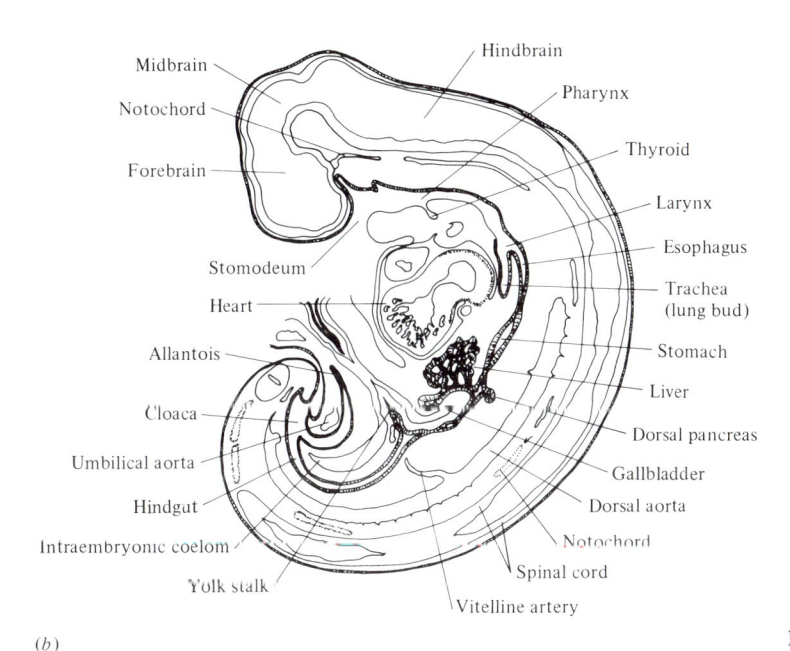

[Figure 5-12 (b): labeled diagram of embryo showing Midbrain, Hindbrain, Pharynx, Notochord, Thyroid, Forebrain, Larynx, Esophagus, Stomodeum, Trachea (lung bud), Heart, Stomach, Allantois, Liver, Cloaca, Dorsal pancreas, Umbilical aorta, Gallbladder, Hindgut, Dorsal aorta, Intraembryonic coelom, Notochord, Yolk stalk, Spinal cord, Vitelline artery]

FIGURE 5-12 (*Continued*)

Week 7 The external form of the embryo continues to appear more human as the facial components develop and migrate medially, the limbs and lower body lengthen, and the neck and trunk straighten (see Fig. 5-14). The limb buds assume a more ventral position with palms and soles facing medially. The upper limb buds develop form with the forearm and hand evident. Likewise, the lower limb bud segments develop. Digit formation also begins. The tail bud has almost disappeared.

Although determined at the moment of conception, the sex of the embryo is not evident physiologically until the gonads begin to differ morphologically at 7 weeks. Externally, however, sex cannot be differentiated at this stage. The embryo has reached approximately 20 mm by the end of the seventh week. During the eighth week, the embryo will increase 10 mm in length.

Week 8 By the final week of the embryological period, the human has developed from one cell to an embryo approximately 30 mm in length, weighing 1 g, with all basic components formed (see Fig. 5-15). The embryo becomes even less flexed with rapid development of the lower body during this week. The head remains relatively large, making up one-half of total body length. The face is recognizable as childlike, and the head is rounded with less frontal prominence. The eyelids will soon fuse. The arms and legs have rotated to their proper position with palms and soles facing caudally; elbows and knees are distinct, and digits are obvious. The tail bud has disappeared and the anal opening becomes patent; the kidneys begin to function. The sex of the embryo becomes externally evident.

DEVELOPMENT OF THE PLACENTA AND FETAL MEMBRANES

The *placenta*, responsible for respiration, nutrition, excretion, endocrine secretion, and immunology, is obviously critical for fetal survival and growth. Normal and adequate development and function of the placenta as well as coordinated interaction between fetus, placenta, and mother are a means for realizing the potential of the fertilized ovum. The placenta is a major determinant of fetal size and, along with other maternal factors, is probably more important than genetic factors in determining fetal growth and size at birth (Cheek, Graystone, and Niall, 1977; McKeown, Marshall, and Record, 1976).

The mature placenta consists of four major parts: *villi*, *placental membrane*, *intervillous spaces*, and *decidua basalis*

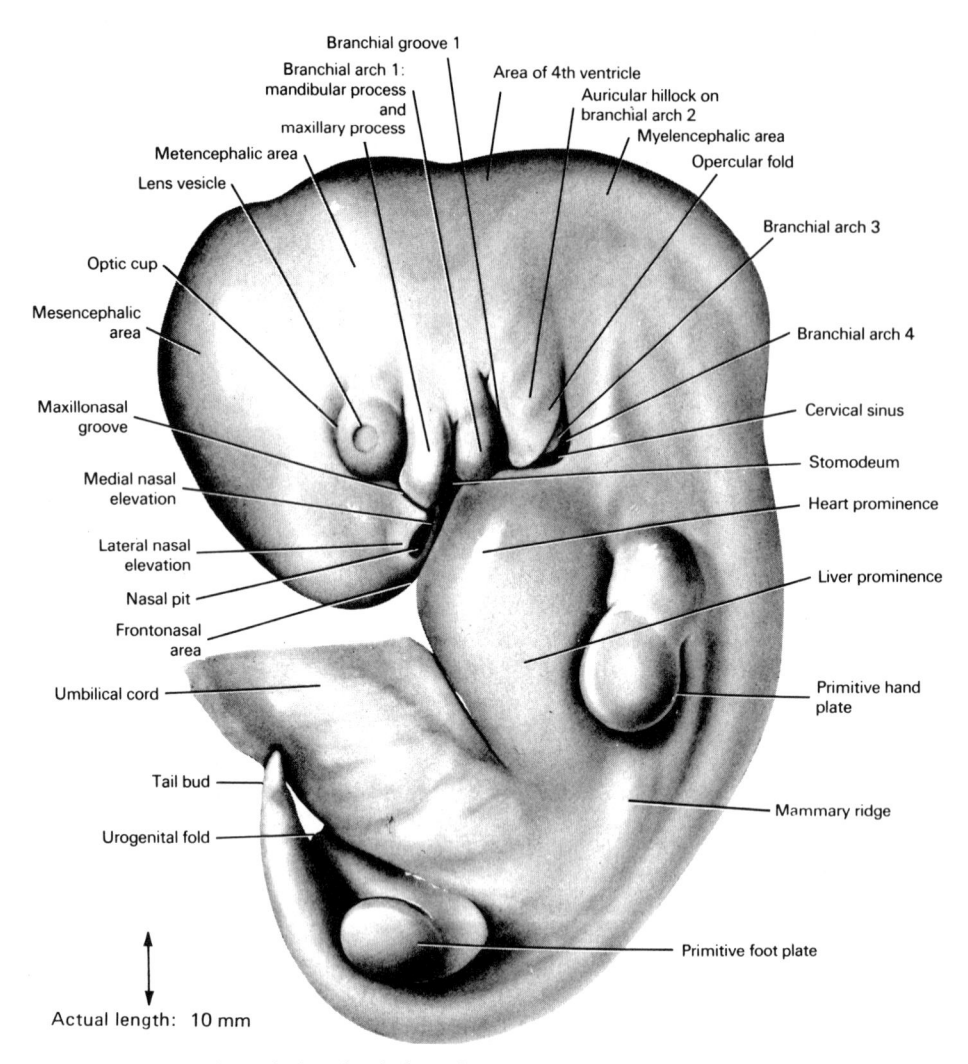

FIGURE 5-13. Embryo during the sixth week, 38 to 40 days. Actual crown-rump length of 10 mm is shown. (*Modified from R. F. Gasser, 1975, p. 105.*)

(superficial part). The *umbilical cord*, originating as the body stalk, connects fetus and placenta, acting as the lifeline for the critical exchange. It contains three vessels: two arteries and one vein which, opposite to corresponding systemic vessels, carry unoxygenated and oxygenated blood, respectively. It also allows fetal movement and birth of the infant without cessation of placental-fetal exchange.

As noted in the early development of the embryo, the trophoblast gives rise to the fetal portion of the placenta. This differentiated portion of the trophoblast, syncytiotrophoblast, begins invasion of the endometrium by the sixth day (see Fig. 5-8). The functional layer of the uterine endometrium, the decidua, contributes the maternal portion of the placenta.

Implantation Implantation occurs most often on the posterior wall of the uterus. Implantation in the lower

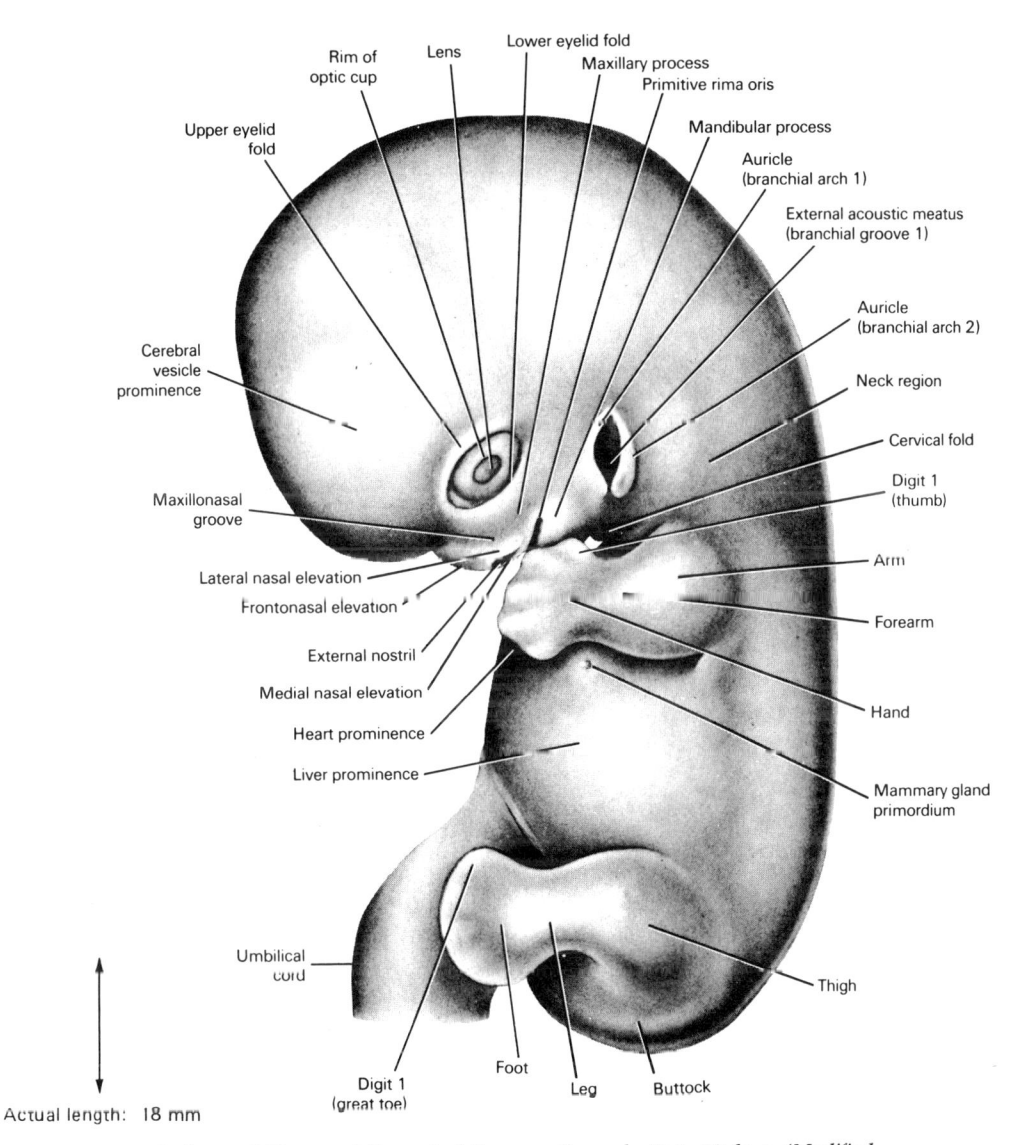

FIGURE 5-14. Embryo of 18 mm, at the end of the seventh week, 48 to 49 days. (*Modified from R. F. Gasser, 1975, p. 165.*)

portions of the uterus, more common in higher parity, can cause complications during pregnancy and birth and may result in spontaneous abortion. Abnormal fetal growth can result, probably due to bleeding secondary to partial placenta previa. One study reported term fetal head size of below the 10th percentile in 25 percent of cases of uncomplicated placenta previa (Adamsons, 1978). Ultrasound techniques have facilitated localization of the placenta for amniocentesis as well as diagnosis of abnormal implantation.

Early embryo-maternal exchange by diffusion begins at 10 to 12 days when *lacunas,* spaces within the syncytiotrophoblast, fill with endometrial blood and glandular secretions. A network of lacunas evolves and will eventually

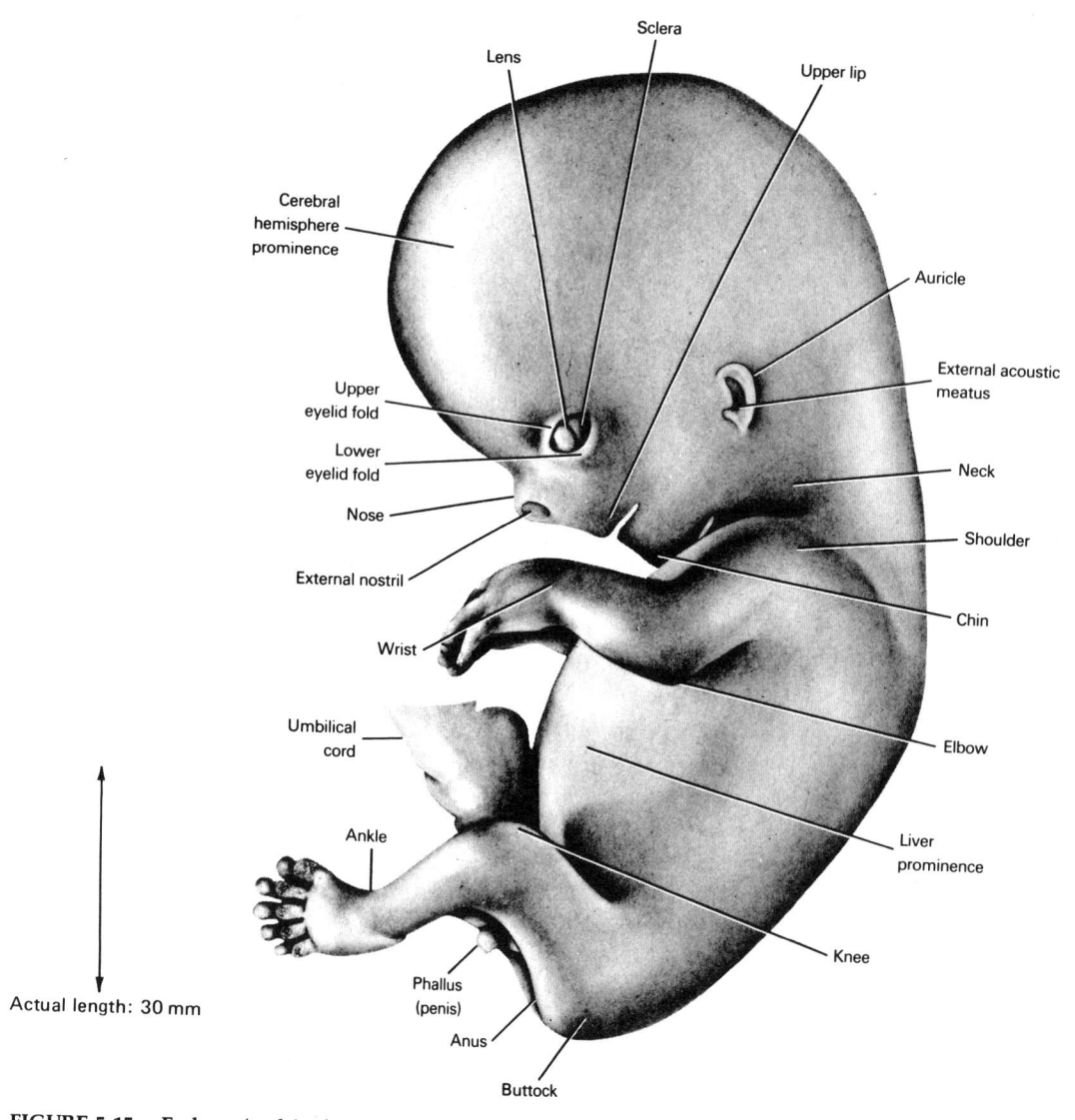

FIGURE 5-15. Embryo (male) of 8 weeks, 30 mm crown-rump length. (*From R. F. Gasser, 1975, p. 243.*)

form the intervillous spaces of the mature placenta. By about 10 days the blastocyst is completely embedded in the endometrium (see Fig. 5-7).

At about 13 days, the chorion, underlying the trophoblast (*cytotrophoblast*), begins to form the primary (primitive) villi which invade the intervillous spaces of the syncytiotrophoblast (see Fig. 5-16a). Although initially formed over the entire chorionic sac, all villi, except those in communication with the decidua basalis, degenerate. Thus, there is a smooth portion and a villous portion of the chorion.

By 15 to 20 days, vessels form within the villi, and by 21 days embryonic blood circulates through the vessels of the villi, embryonic heart, and yolk sac vessels. Nutrients and wastes are exchanged, and thus by the beginning of the fourth week basic placental function is established. At this stage the placenta takes up about one-fifteenth of the uterine interior. It will continue to grow in synchrony with fetal growth.

Placental structure The growing embryo, surrounded by the amnion and chorion, bulges the overlying decidual layer of the endometrium and by 4 weeks has expanded into the uterine cavity (see Fig. 5-16b). The decidua overlying the embryo is the *decidua capsularis*. The *decidua basalis* is the portion of the endometrium underlying the chorionic villi, and it will form the maternal portion of the placenta. The remainder of the decidua lining the uterus is the *decidua parietalis*.

When the chorionic villi invade the decidua basalis, they segregate in groups of two or more to form a *cotyledon*. Thus, a cotyledon consists of two or more villi with a surrounding hollow space, previously the lacunas, the intervillous space. The term placenta has 15 to 30 cotyledons containing approximately 100 villi (Shanklin, 1978). Between the cotyledons are wedge-shaped sections of decidua basalis, placental *septa*. The continuous basal layer of the placenta opposite the decidua basalis, not separated by septa, is the *chorionic plate*. Chorionic villi secured to the decidua basalis are anchoring villi. The placental membrane (barrier) is actually the membrane of the chorionic villi, thus entirely of fetal origin.

Upon inspection of the placenta after birth, the fetal and maternal sides are readily distinguished. The umbilical cord inserts on the smooth, shiny fetal surface; both cord and placenta are covered by the amniochorionic membrane, which extends to and beyond the placental margin. The maternal side has a cobblestone appearance—cotyledons with the dividing septa—which is covered by a thin layer of the decidua basalis.

Placental function Circulation of blood through the placenta allows exchange of nutrient substances for and waste products from fetal metabolism (see Fig. 5-17). Ma-

FIGURE 5-16. Implantation, placenta formation, and fate of the fetal membranes. (*a*) Early implantation. (*b*) The embryo and overlying decidua capsularis expand into the uterine cavity. (*c*) The amnion approaches and fuses with the chorion. (*d*) The uterine cavity is nearly obliterated; the decidua capsularis is degenerating. (Adapted from C. E. Corliss, 1976, p. 76 and K. L. Moore, 1977, p. 97.)

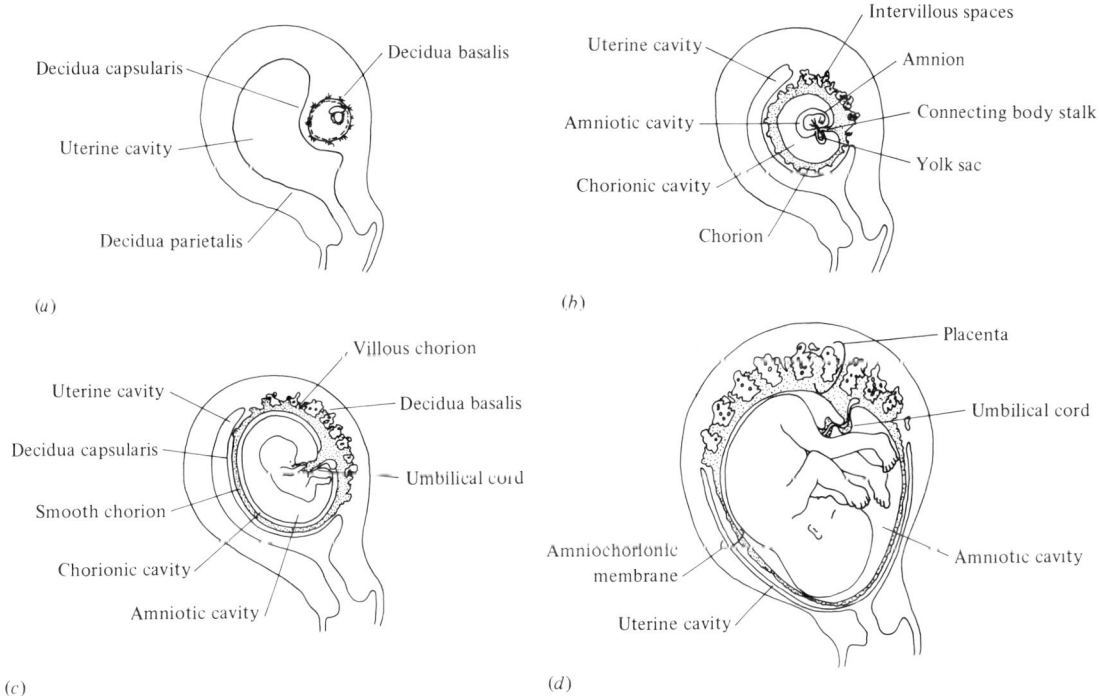

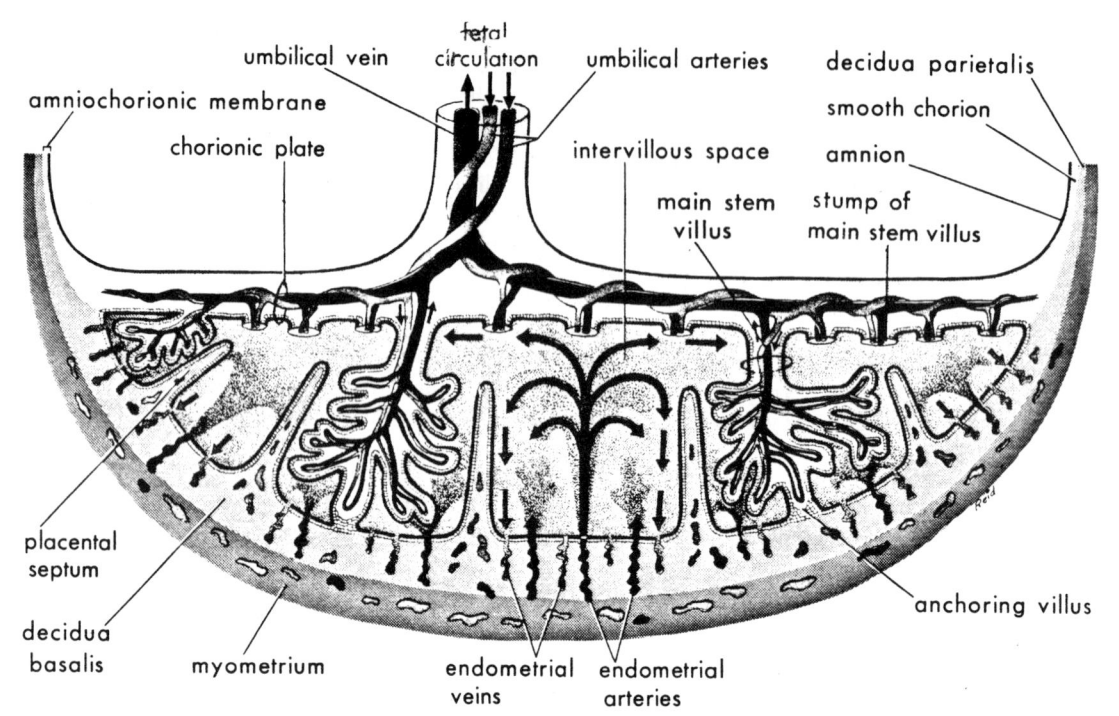

FIGURE 5-17. Schematic drawing of a section through a mature placenta showing fetal-placental circulation and maternal-placental circulation. Maternal blood enters the intervillous spaces through the endometrial arteries in spurts. Exchange occurs as maternal blood bathes the villi. The maternal blood leaves the intervillous spaces through the endometrial veins. Unoxygenated fetal blood enters the placenta through the two umbilical arteries, is oxygenated and receives nutrients in the villi, and returns to the fetus through the umbilical vein. (*From K. L. Moore, 1977, p. 102.*)

ternal blood flows with pulsatile force through endometrial arteries into the intervillous spaces, where it bathes the chorionic villi. Nutrients, oxygen, and other substances cross the placental membrane of the villi and enter the fetal capillaries. Carbon dioxide and other waste products leave fetal circulation through movement in the opposite direction. The nutrient- and oxygen-rich fetal blood continues through the umbilical vein to the fetus. The two fetal arteries return blood from the fetus to the placenta (see Prenatal Circulation, in "Development of the Cardiovascular System"). Under normal conditions, fetal and maternal blood do not intermingle. However, nucleated fetal cells have been detected in maternal blood samples as early as 13 weeks ca. Cell-sorting techniques are now possible (when the fetus is male) by detection of Y-chromatin–positive cells or by immunogenetic techniques detecting antigens of paternal origin (assumed to be carried on the Y chromosome). *How* as well as *how early* fetal cells enter the maternal circulatory system is uncertain. This technique is promising in the future as a noninvasive prenatal screening technique for chromosomal abnormalities (Herzenberg, Bianchi, Schröder, Cann, and Iverson, 1979). Maternal blood leaves the intervillous spaces through endometrial veins.

The endocrine and immunologic functions of the placenta are discussed elsewhere. Transport of nutrients, O_2, CO_2, and other waste products occurs across the placental membrane by simple and facilitated diffusion, active transport, and pinocytosis. The placental membrane was once thought of as a protective barrier, but it is now recognized that most substances, including harmful ones, will cross the placental membrane into fetal circulation and may even be sequestered (Corliss, 1976; Dancis and Schneider, 1978).

Gases, water, and solutes of low molecular weight are exchanged rapidly by simple diffusion. Diffusion capacity of the placenta increases proportionately with fetal growth and placental surface area (Cheek, 1977). Nutrients vary in method of exchange. Glucose is transferred to the fetus by diffusion. Glucose was long considered the primary source of metabolic fuel; this is now being investigated (Adam and Felig, 1978; Dancis and Schneider, 1978). Amino acids are now believed to also contribute significantly to fetal nutrition; they are received from the mother by active transport, and the fetus then synthesizes the necessary proteins. Large molecules, viruses, and gamma globulins cross the membrane by pinocytosis. (Gamma-G globulin, or IgG, is one protein received from the mother.) The placental transport of lipids is unclear. It is thought that maternal lipids do contribute to part of the fetus's adipose tissue (Dancis and Schneider, 1978). Fatty acids are transferred in small amounts (Metcoff, 1978). Less is known about vitamins; it is thought that fat-soluble vitamins cross the placental membrane by simple diffusion and water-soluble vitamins by active transport (Dancis and Schneider, 1978).

Electrolytes are exchanged by either diffusion or active transport, depending primarily on whether the ions are univalent or divalent. Hormonal transport is also variable; although protein hormones do not cross the placental membrane in appreciable amounts, steroids are rapidly transported. Waste products, bilirubin, urea, uric acid, and creatinine are removed from fetal circulation by movement in the opposite direction to maternal circulation.

The placenta itself requires significant O_2 and other nutrients for metabolism, energy required for transport, and endocrine secretion. Under conditions of nutritional deprivation, placental nutritional needs are met first, before fetal, and can result in diminished fetal growth (Cheek, 1977). The placenta may even remain a living and active organ up to 2 months after fetal death.

Placental growth Placental growth is influenced by the two placental hormones: *chorionic gonadotropin* and *placental lactogen*. These hormones also have been theorized to play a part in blocking the response of maternal lymphocytes to the fetus preventing rejection of this "allograft" (see "Development of the Endocrine System"). Placental growth stops or is greatly diminished at 34 to 35 weeks' gestation (Shanklin, 1978).

Placenta and cord sizes as well as morphology often give clues to pathophysiology of some small-for-gestational-age (SGA) and other infants. The placentas of SGA infants are much smaller than average. They may be proportionate or smaller relative to fetal weight, probably reflecting varying etiology (Ounsted and Ounsted, 1973). Placental infarction also diminishes maternal-fetal exchange and is associated with SGA neonates. Chronic maternal hypertension has been reported to be correlated with a small placenta with mean villous surface area less than 60 percent of normal (Adamsons, 1978). Cords small in diameter, some with vascular anomalies, are also associated with intrauterine growth retardation (Ounsted and Ounsted, 1973). A two-vessel cord (one artery and one vein) warrants further inspection for other physical anomalies, particularly of the gastrointestinal, cardiovascular, and urogenital systems (Ainsworth and Davies, 1969).

Fetal membranes As the amniotic sac surrounding the embryo increases in size faster than the chorionic sac which surrounds both, the two membranes, amnion and chorion, fuse to become the *amniochorionic membrane*. This membrane overlies the cervical os and acts as a protective cushion for the fetal head during labor. It ruptures before or during birth, releasing the amniotic fluid (see Fig. 5-16c).

By 22 weeks, the fetal sac has enlarged to fill the uterine cavity. The decidua capsularis, still covering the fetus and amniochorionic membrane, comes in contact and fuses with the decidua parietalis on the opposite uterine wall. The uterine cavity is then obliterated (see Fig. 5-16d).

The amount of amniotic fluid increases during pregnancy from 30 mL at 10 weeks to between 500 and 2000 mL at term. There is disagreement regarding the primary sources of amniotic fluid; however, it appears that there are both fetal and maternal contributions (Corliss, 1976; Moore, 1977). Before the fifteenth week, the epithelium of the amniotic sac is probably the primary source (FitzGerald, 1978).

The organic constituents of amniotic fluid are albumin; enzymes; carbohydrates and organic acids; lipids; non-protein nitrogen; vitamins A, B, and C; hormones; and pigments (Thompson, 1978). The amniotic fluid supplies about 40 cal/day to the growing fetus through gastrointestinal system absorption (Liley, 1972). It is thought that perhaps 18 percent of the protein utilized by the fetus is provided through swallowing amniotic fluid albumin (Thompson, 1976).

The water in amniotic fluid is completely exchanged every 3 h by diffusion (Rugh, 1975). The amniotic fluid also circulates within the amniotic cavity as the fetus swallows, absorbs, and excretes it beginning early in gestation. A reduced amount of amniotic fluid, oligohydramnios, can represent placental insufficiency or renal abnormality or agenesis, reflecting reduced fetal output. Increased amount of amniotic fluid, polyhydramnios, is associated with a central nervous system (CNS) deficit resulting in reduced fetal swallowing behavior, congenital atresia of the gastrointestinal system, diabetes, Rh disease, and other abnormalities (Moore, 1977; Smith, 1976). Normally, amniotic fluid is clear and colorless. Stained amniotic fluid, from meconium, bile pigment, or red blood cells, is an indication of fetal distress or other complications.

The yolk sac, which aids in transfer of nutrients until placental circulation is established, is eventually incorporated in part as gut lining. The yolk sac is the initial site of blood formation and embryonic circulation. The primordial germ cells first appear in the membrane of the yolk sac. There is some evidence that yolk sac can sequester teratogens (Stevens, 1980). The allantois also is an early site of blood formation and contributes vessels to the body stalk which eventually become the umbilical arteries and vein.

Establishment of Organ Systems

Development of the face   Mary Tudor

Development of the face, nasal and oral cavities, and neck region results from an interlocking of two regions of the embryo: the *frontonasal prominence* and the *branchial apparatus* (see Fig. 5-18).

The frontonasal prominence overlies the developing forebrain, the enlarged head end of the neural tube. It will eventually form the major portion of the upper midportion of the face: the forehead, all but the most lateral aspects of the nose, the philtrum of the upper lip, and the primary palate and related gingivae and teeth.

Four paired components make up the branchial apparatus: branchial arches, branchial grooves, pharyngeal pouches, and branchial membranes (closing plates). The branchial arches are paired prominences on the ventrolateral aspects of the head region with branchial grooves separating one pair from the next. Six arches are formed in a cephalocaudal direction; however, only the first four are of great significance. The fourth and sixth arches will be considered together; the fifth is insignificant.

The first branchial arch, the mandibular, is in two sections: the *maxillary process* and the *mandibular process*. The mandibular will contribute primarily to formation of the lower face. The second, or *hyoid*, arch and third arch will form major portions of the neck (see Fig. 5-18). The fourth and sixth arches will contribute more caudal sections of the neck.

The *stomodeum* (primitive mouth), which becomes patent at about 24 days, is bounded by the frontonasal prominence and first branchial arch. It opens into the primitive pharynx, which in turn narrows to join the esophagus. The endodermal *pharyngeal pouches* develop in the lateral walls of the pharynx between the branchial arches and opposite the external branchial grooves. The pharyngeal pouches give rise to the middle ear and inner ear, eustachian tube, palatine tonsils, parathyroid glands, and thymus.

By the time the 4-week-old trilaminar embryo undergoes ventral flexion, the head portion is underlying more enlarged neural tube section: the future brain. During the fifth to eighth weeks, the forebrain especially continues to develop and enlarge in all dimensions: frontal, parietal, and occipital. This enlargement not only changes head size and contour but, as it occurs more rapidly than facial growth, the relation of facial structures to the head also changes markedly.

Although facial development is noted by change in external appearance, orderly and timely migration of underlying mesenchymal cells is critical to normal facial development and midline fusion.

During the fifth week, the frontonasal prominence enlarges and broadens, reflecting the growth of the underlying intermediate forebrain. The paired lens placodes, induced by the optic evaginations, and the nasal placodes are visible on the frontonasal prominence. The otic pits are visible on the lateral aspects of the head during the fourth week. They sink below the surface (between branchial arches 1 and 2, which are enlarging), becoming otocysts, during week 5. As the forebrain enlarges laterally, it begins to cause the primitive eyes and nose to assume more forward-directed (medial) positions. The eyes enlarge, and the nasal placodes become patent nasal pits, which are surrounded by the lateral and medial nasal prominences.

The paired maxillary processes of the first branchial arch develop toward the midline as they fuse with the frontonasal prominence along the nasolacrimal grooves. In response to this midline migration, the nasal promi-

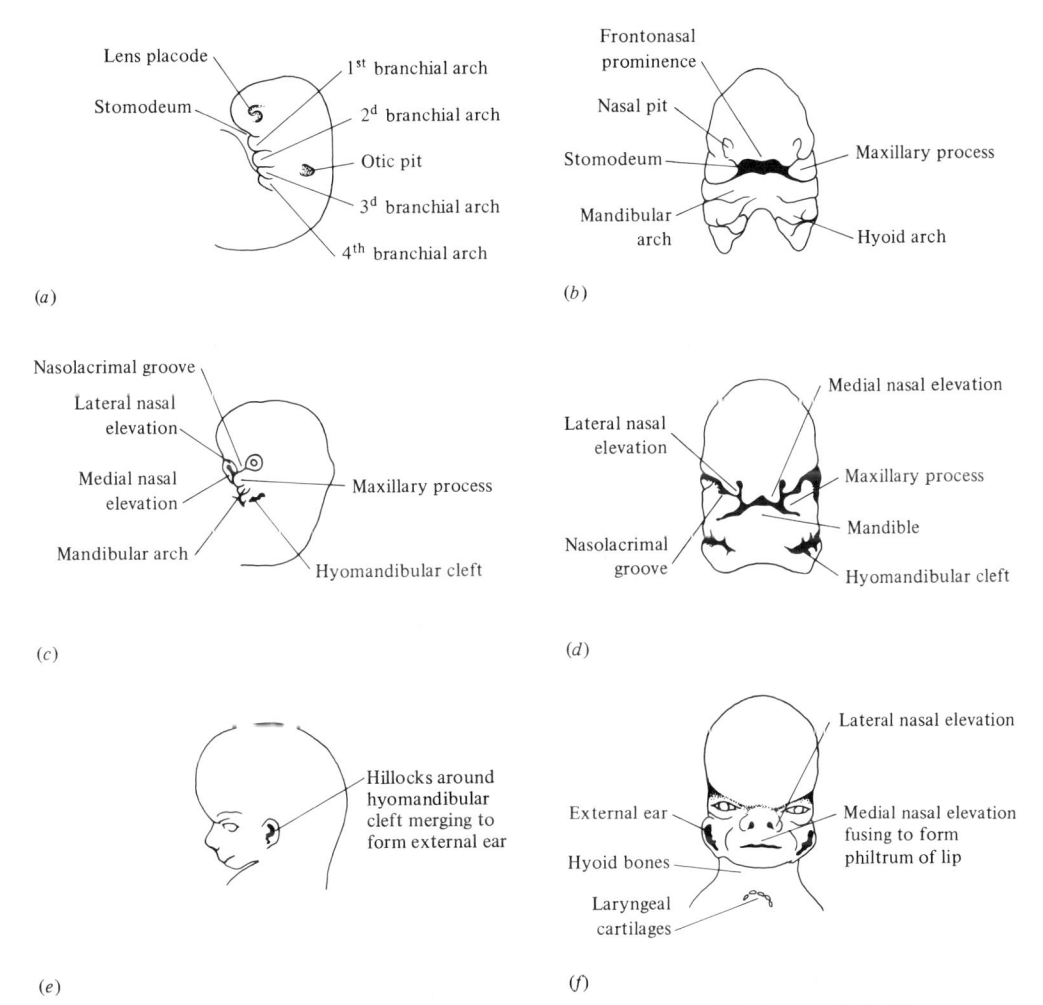

DEVELOPMENT OF THE EMBRYO: **223**
THE PERIOD OF ORGANOGENESIS

FIGURE 5-18. The developing face. (a) Four branchial arches are visible (28 ± 1 day). (b) The stomodeum is prominent. The nose and eyes become more visible and begin forward migration (33 ± 1 day). (c) The nose is evident with medial and lateral elevations (42 ± 1 day). (d) Further medial orientation of eyes and ears is noted with increasing forebrain area. The hyomandibular cleft has formed from the first branchial groove and will become the external ear (42 ± 1 day). (e) The eye is more fully developed. The external ear is moving to its final position, and the growth of the mandible and maxilla give the embryonic face a human appearance by 8 weeks. The brain grows rapidly during this period, making up a greater percentage of the total cranial area (56 ± 1 day). (f) Forward orientation is achieved by 8 weeks although the eyes remain hyperteloric, nose and mouth prominent, and ears low-set (56 ± 1 day). (From C. E. Corliss, 1976, pp. 258; 262.)

nences are further caused to converge. The mandibular processes, fused during the fourth week, continue to develop somewhat later than the upper face. Between the mandibular process and the hyoid branchial arch, the external auditory meatus and auricle also begin elaboration from the distal end of the first branchial groove. The first and second branchial arch derivatives are innervated by the trigeminal (V) and facial (VII) nerves respectively.

By the end of the fifth week, all facial features are readily apparent and directed more medially. The face is smaller relative to the head, however, and the profile remains flat. During weeks 6 and 7, the facial features continue to move toward their final position. The eyes, continuing to enlarge, are directed to a forward-looking position. Eyelids begin to develop, fuse by 10 weeks, and reopen late in fetal life. The medial nasal prominences approach and fuse in the midline, and internally the nasal septum is formed. The maxillary prominences come to the midline, fusing with the narrow portion of intervening frontonasal prominence. The external ears, originally in the site of the future neck, move cephalically and dorsally to the side of the head at eye level as a result of cerebral growth.

The developing oral structures and mandibular prominence cause the mouth and lower jaw to develop forward. By the seventh week, the nasal and oral cavities are in communication. The midline primary palate, of frontonasal prominence origin, and the bilateral secondary palate, derived from the maxillary prominences, begin development in the sixth week. Fusion occurs sometime during the ninth or tenth weeks.

The third, fourth, and sixth branchial arches recede, giving the neck region a smooth external appearance. The hyoid bone, thyroid, cricoid cartilages, and pharyngeal and laryngeal muscles, as well as other structures of the neck, are derived from the third, fourth, and sixth branchial arches. Innervation of the third branchial arch derivatives is by the glossopharyngeal (IV) nerve and of the fourth and sixth arches, by the vagus (V) nerve. Internally, the four pharyngeal pouches are developing into their respective derivatives during the same stage (see "Development of the Gastrointestinal System").

At the end of the seventh week, the head begins to extend, lifting the face away from the receding heart prominence. The 8-week-old embryo's face is directed more forward than caudally, is more proportionate to the rest of the head, and in profile is less flat due to development of the nose, mouth, and mandible.

Although the major portion of facial development is achieved during embryonic life, subtle changes occur during the fetal period and childhood until the final adult facial form is achieved. The deep indentation of the nasal bridge is lost during the early fetal period; the lower jaw continues to grow out; and during the late fetal period deposition of subcutaneous fat is evident in the face, especially with formation of the sucking pads of the cheeks. Thus, the face of the neonate is more rounded and cherublike than that of the 8-week-old embryo.

TOOTH FORMATION

Teeth develop from ectoderm (enamel) and mesenchyme (remaining tissue) in three stages: *bud, cap,* and *bell* (see Fig. 5-19). Teeth form and calcify in approximately the same order as emergence into the oral cavity beginning with the anterior mandibular teeth followed by the anterior maxillary teeth.

BUD STAGE
During the sixth week ca, dental laminas form along the primitive jaws. Tooth buds of the deciduous teeth begin to form from each lamina at 7 weeks ca.

CAP STAGE
The cap stage begins at 8 weeks ca as the bud is invaginated with tissue destined to become the future pulp and dentin.

BELL STAGE
The bell stage begins about 10 weeks ca. Formation of enamel and dentin, calcification of the tooth, begins at the cusp and proceeds toward the root. The root forms later than the crown. Ossification of the fetal jaws and alveolar development secure the root in this bony tissue. The permanent teeth, which have deciduous predecessors, appear as buds at 10 weeks beneath the deciduous teeth. Permanent molars with no deciduous predecessors form directly from the dental laminas.

All teeth, deciduous and permanent, form through initial stages during the fetal period except for the second and third permanent molars. These buds form after birth. A tooth is not completely formed and calcified until the root is completed. Thus, even the deciduous incisors are not completely developed prenatally. Complete root formation results in complete eruption. For example, the lower central incisors, which emerge at about 6 months, are completely calcified when they reach the occlusal level.

Certain agents, such as tetracycline, which permanently discolor enamel will have an effect during fetal development through the first several years of childhood as deciduous and permanent tooth enamel is forming.

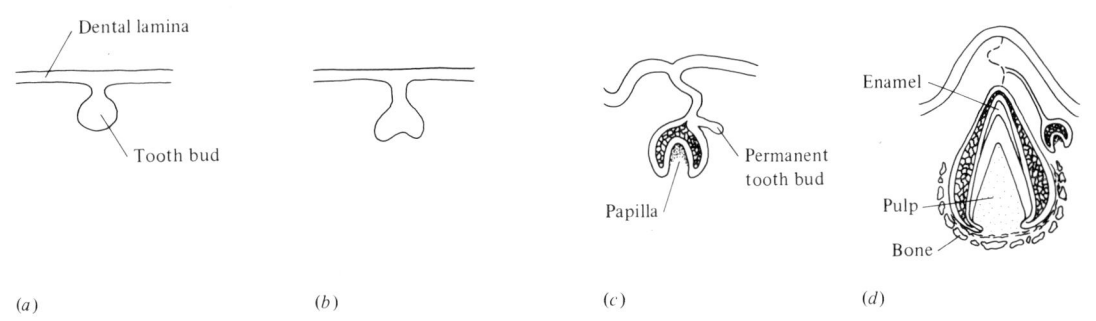

FIGURE 5-19. Prenatal tooth development. (*a*) Bud stage, 7 weeks; (*b*) cap stage, 8 weeks; (*c*) bell stage, 10 weeks; (*d*) 28 weeks. (*Modified from K. L. Moore, 1977, p. 381.*)

Development of the central nervous system Mary D. Guthrie

EARLY DEVELOPMENT

As the primitive embryo becomes disk- or saucer-shaped, the primitive streak appears in the caudal quadrant (see Fig. 5-8a). It is a thickened area of rapid cell growth brought about by both multiplication of ectodermal cells in that area and migration of cells from other areas into that one. The primitive streak rapidly extends in length. It grows rostrally and becomes quite precocious in cell growth; these multiplying and migrating cells push other nonneural cells deeper into the growing body region. The rostral end of the streak extends and is well established before that of the slower-growing caudal end.

The rostral end of the embryonic head can be identified as the neurocranial and visceral portions. The visceral portions are slower growing and form the primitive branchial arch complex, facial structures, and termination of the respiratory and digestive tracts (see "Development of the Face"). The neurocranial portion forms the brain, retina of the eyes, olfactory system, and internal ears. These structures soon become quite conspicuous because their rate of growth is faster than that of the visceral portions. This predominance is never lost throughout fetal development and infancy.

After the primitive streak and notochord are clearly defined at approximately 3 weeks ca, the notochord induces further growth and thickening of the streak. The well-thickened streak, the *neural plate*, displays differential growth in two dimensions. The lateral edges grow faster than the middle, thus forming two elevated longitudinal ridges between which is an indented or depressed area, the neural groove (see Fig. 5-21). There is also differential growth in the rostrocaudal axis; the rostral area, which foreshadows the brain, grows faster and larger than the caudal area, which is to become the spinal cord. At this stage the orientation of the embryo can be established by gross observation.

As the lateral ridges of the neural groove continue to grow more rapidly than the center portion, there are also microscopic changes in the cells. The apical portions of the cells become narrower, while the basilar portions remain wide. By this mechanism, the lateral ridges that have grown dorsally are induced to bend toward the midline and touch. The fusion of the two ridges results in formation of the neural tube, which is a characteristic beginning of all mammalian CNS. The closure of the tube does not take place uniformly along its length. It fuses first in the region of the hindbrain, and fusion is extended toward both the caudal and rostral ends. This closure starts during the third week of fetal life ca and is completed at the end of the fourth week ca. The CNS does not have its own vascular system until the eighth week.

There is additional ectoderm that also takes part in the formation of the nervous system. This neural crest ectoderm is lateral to the ectoderm forming the neural plate (see Fig. 5-21). During the time the neural groove is formed, the neural crests each draw nearer the midline until they become a single midline structure. As the neural tube is formed, it sinks below the surface and becomes a separate tissue. The neural crest ectoderm and the undifferentiated superficial ectoderm fuse and make a continuous layer of ectoderm.

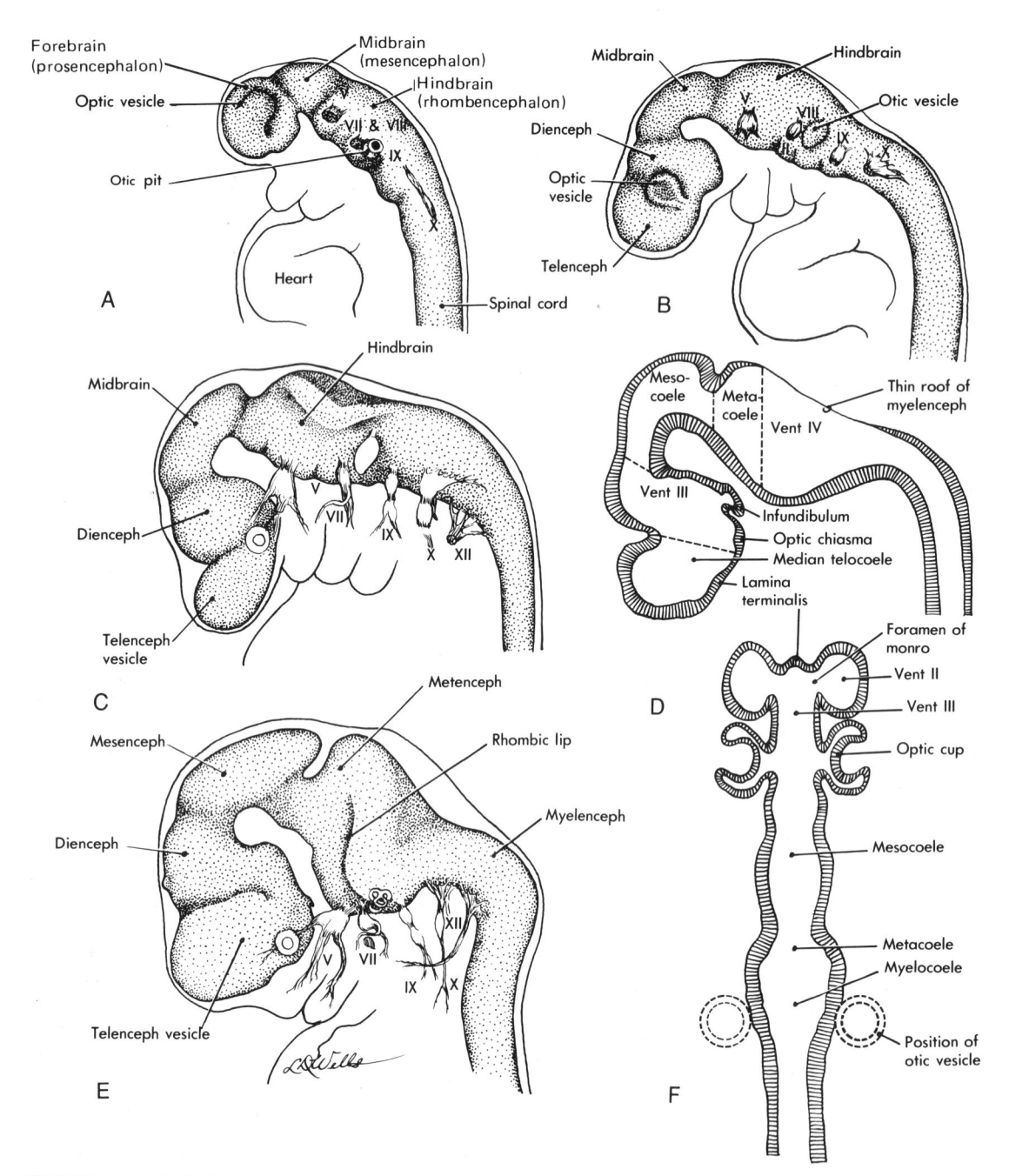

FIGURE 5-20. Early development of the brain and cranial nerves (approximate ages). (*a*) 24 days; (*b*) 28 days; (*c*) 36 days; (*d*) sagittal section; (*e*) 49 days, cranial nerves are indicated by the appropriate Roman numerals; (*f*) schematic frontal plan of the brain as it would appear if the flexures had been straightened before cutting. (*From C. E. Corliss, 1976, p. 61.*)

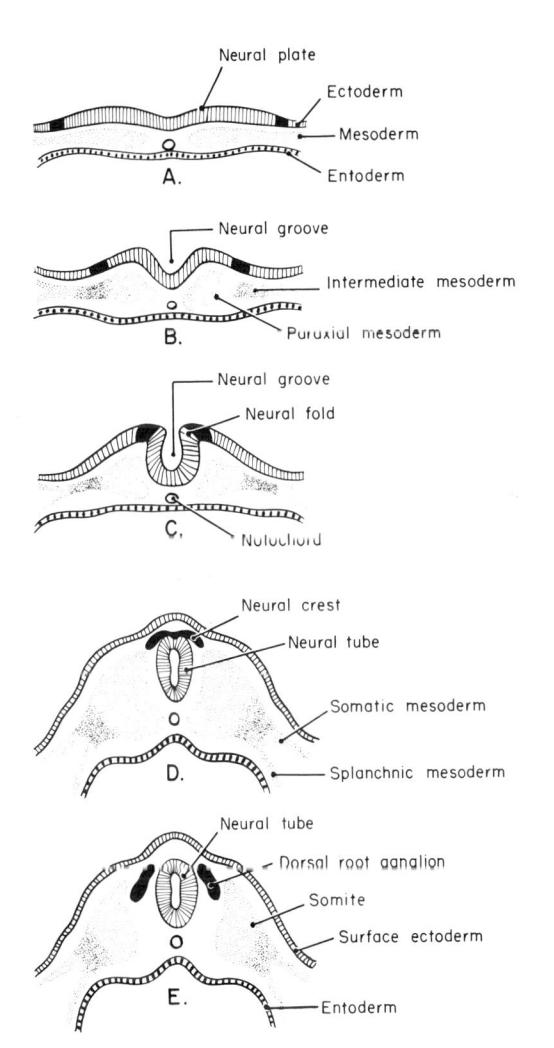

FIGURE 5-21. Diagrams of transverse sections of embryos at different ages showing development of the spinal cord. (a) Neural plate stage; (b) early neural groove stage; (c) late neural groove stage; (d) early neural tube and neural crest stage; (e) neural tube and dorsal root ganglion stage. (From M. B. Carpenter, Human neuroanatomy. Baltimore: Williams & Wilkins, 1976, p. 51. Reprinted by permission of the publisher.)

Shortly thereafter the cells of the neural crest material divide and migrate to positions dorsolateral, on either side of the neural tube. In this position a mass of cells is in a longitudinal dimension in the angle between the neural tube and superficial ectoderm. The cells within these masses migrate and become aggregated in paired clusters at segmental levels. These clusters of cells form the primordium of the dorsal root ganglion cells of the spinal nerves and the sensory ganglia of those cranial nerves having sensory modalities. The neural crest primordium also contributes indirectly to the sympathetic ganglia and cells of the adrenal medulla. This versatile tissue also forms progenitor cells for non-CNS structures such as pia and arachnoid meninges, most of the skull, integumental pigment cells, neurolemma (sheath of Schwann cells), tooth buds, and mesoderm of the branchial arches.

BRAIN MORPHOGENESIS

During the fourth week ca the walls of the neural tube in the rostral region undergo very rapid and very uneven growth while growth in some portions of the neural tube lags. This differential growth, by the end of the fourth week, results in three bulges, or enlargements, called the three *primary vesicles*. The most rostral is the forebrain, or *prosencephalon*, from which the optic vesicles sprout and start to grow during the fourth week. The second and third vesicles are called *midbrain*, or *mesencephalon*, and *hindbrain*, or *rhombencephalon*, respectively (see Fig. 5-20b).

By the end of the fifth week ca, this short-lived three-vesicle stage has become the five-vesicle brain that grows into the adult brain. The prosencephalon divides into the *telencephalon*, which forms the cerebral hemispheres, and the *diencephalon*, from which the optic vesicles form and which forms the thalamus, infundibulum, and epiphysis (see Fig. 5-20c).

TELENCEPHALON

At no place in the CNS is differential growth more marked than in the prosencephalon. The cerebral hemispheres expand in lateral, rostral, and caudal directions. At the end of the eleventh or twelfth week ca they have covered the diencephalon, and at the time of birth they cover the diencephalon and mesencephalon. The bony cavity of the skull develops concurrently with cerebral hemisphere development, and in addition to the other directions of growth this enclosure causes a downward and forward growth of the hemispheres that thus forms the temporal lobes. In addition, the continued overgrowth of the cerebrum within a closed cavity causes it to wrinkle, or form the gyri and sulci that are seen in the adult brain. Phylogenetically, the cerebral cortex is the newest part of the brain.

The *corpus striatum*, composed of the *lentiform nucleus* and the *caudate nucleus*, form in the ventral part of the lateral walls of the telencephalon during the fifth to sixth week ca. By the end of the twelfth week the lentiform nucleus may clearly be seen to have divided into the *putamen* and the *globus pallidus*. The relation of these nuclei to the cerebral cortex is not well understood. It is difficult to separate these structures from the surrounding cortex in experimental animals, and most knowledge of humans comes from pathology discovered during autopsy. At one time these nuclei were considered to have functions antagonistic to the cerebral cortex. Now it is believed that the two centers work together and that the corpus striatum dampens, coordinates, and modifies voluntary movement of the cerebral cortex.

The olfactory system is first seen as a bulb continuous with the telencephalic vesicle at the end of the sixth week. These three structures, the olfactory system, the corpus striatum, and the cerebral cortex, give the features of the adult telencephalon.

The *commissural* system of axons of the telencephalon is of interest in that it is through these systems that one side of the brain communicates with the other. The corpus callosum is the largest and most conspicuous set of fibers and is in evidence during the third prenatal month. The *anterior commissure* and the *hippocampal commissure* are much smaller, are concerned with olfactory information, and appear much earlier than the corpus callosum. The posterior commissure is very small in humans. The association fiber system allows for communication from one gyrus of the cerebral cortex to another gyrus. Projection fibers are those that transmit information to and from the cortex and brainstem.

DIENCEPHALON

Relatively speaking, the diencephalon is much slower in growth. It is not until the third month that the infundibulum and the thalamic mass can be identified. The distal end of the infundibular stalk extends to form the *pars nervosa*, or posterior pituitary, between the eighth and twelfth weeks of fetal life. The exact function of the epiphysis, or pineal gland, in the human is unknown and the subject of much current investigation; it can be identifiable at 6 weeks ca. The thalamus is a sensory relay station for modalities whose information is sent to the cerebral cortex and efferent centers.

MESENCEPHALON

The mesencephalon becomes one of the five secondary vesicles by virtue of the fact that it does not divide. It is the slowest-growing part of the brain. The lumen of the middle vesicle forms the aqueduct of Sylvius and remains the smallest part of the ventricular system. Dorsal to the aqueduct is the tectum, or roof of the mesencephalon. This tectum forms the corpora quadrigemina, which do not appear until late in embryonic life. The inferior and superior colliculi, or corpora quadrigemina, handle auditory and visual modalities respectively; it stands to reason that these centers would not need to fully develop until the fetus comes nearer to having an independent life. Ventral to the aqueduct is the tegmentum, or floor of the mesencephalon. This is largely made up of fiber tracts that ascend and descend the brainstem.

RHOMBENCEPHALON

The rhombencephalon, the hindbrain, divides into the *metencephalon* and the *myelencephalon*. With this division the brain makes a sharp ventral bend at the level of cranial nerve V. Rostral to this bend is the metencephalon. From the forward area develops three functional sections of the metencephalon, namely, the *pons,* composed of ascending and descending fiber pathways between the more rostral brain and the myelencephalon; the *pontine branchii*, composed of fiber tracts to and from the cerebellum; and the cerebellum itself, which develops bilaterally on the dorsal plate of the metencephalon and then fuses to form a single midline structure. The cerebellum controls and modifies posture and movements of the body. It is a phylogenetically primitive part of the brain.

The myelencephalon lies to the caudal extent of the cervical or cranial nerve V flexure and is henceforth known as the medulla. It is continuous with the spinal cord. At the time the CNS is still a neural tube, it is easy to identify the thickened lateral walls as lateral plates and the thinner roof and floor plates. The lumen of the tube is slitlike in some places; but in the myelencephalon the roof plate thins out, and the dorsal part of the lateral walls move apart to form the fourth ventricle of the medulla. The *sulcus limitans* is an indentation on the internal part of the lateral plate that demarks the areas of sensory functions in the dorsal portion and motor functions in the ventral portion. This same topography is preserved in the spinal cord. The medulla is noteworthy as the seat of nuclei for cranial nerves having to do with vital functions of the body. The term *nuclei of the central nervous system* does not mean nuclei within cells, but rather it is a designation of an aggregate of cells having a common origin and common function.

Microscopically, neurons are developing by the seventeenth week. Glial cell development follows this and continues through the second year of postnatal life.

SPINAL CORD

The spinal cord develops at the same time as the brain but on a much simpler and more generalized plan. The walls of the original neural tube display three different laminas of cells. They are the ventricular ependymal cells, the intermediate or mantle cells, and the marginal cells. The ventral and dorsal columns of gray matter of the cord are derived from the mantle cells. In contrast to the outer cells, or gray matter, and internal fibers, or white matter, of the brain, the spinal cord has inner cells and outer fibers. The posterior cellular mass contains entering sensory fibers and internuncial cells, while the anterior cellular mass contains motor, or efferent, cells. The afferent, or sensory, cell bodies are in the dorsal root ganglia. Axons of both the sensory cells and the motor cells unite at each level to make the peripheral nerve of that segment. It is in these sensory and motor roots of the peripheral nerve that the earliest *myelinization* takes place. This is about the fourth and fifth months. Other nerves display myelin as they become functional in the embryo.

Some of the cranial nerves are like the peripheral nerves in that they are mixed motor and sensory with the sensory cell body in ganglia outside the CNS and derived from neural crest cells. Other cranial nerves are purely sensory or motor. An additional difference is that the strict segmentation of the peripheral nerves is not maintained by the cranial nerve in the developed brain.

The autonomic nervous system is made up of the antagonistic sympathetic and parasympathetic nervous system. These functionally and anatomically overlapping systems give double innervation to all the chest and abdominal viscera and glands of the body. Both the sympathetic and parasympathetic systems are two-neuron effector systems with the first neuron being within the CNS. The sympathetic bodies are in the intermediate column of the spinal cord at the thoracic and lumbar level, whereas those of the parasympathetic are in the brain and sacral areas of the spinal cord. These nerves develop concurrently with the viscera they innervate, but they are not myelinated until late in fetal life.

THE VENTRICULAR SYSTEM

Just as the walls of the straight, primitive neural tube develop differentially to form the adult brain, the hollow part of the tube develops differentially to form the ventricles of the adult brain.

The ventricles of the telencephalon form equally to either side of the midline. They are not designated by numbers but simply called the *lateral ventricles*. First bulges are formed, the body of the ventricles. They then extend forward into the frontal lobes and become the *anterior horns*. The *posterior horns* grow backward and down into the occipital lobes. As the temporal lobes develop, the lower anterior parts of the ventricular bodies follow to make the rounded inferior horns. Each lateral ventricle is roughly C-shaped with the inferior limb more laterally situated than the superior limb, and from the body of the C the inferior horn projects backward (see Fig. 5-22). It is at the upper part of the superior limb that each lateral ventricle communicates with the third ventricle through a narrow space, the *foramen of Monro*.

The third ventricle, whose roof is the corpus callosum and floor is just above the infundibulum and optic chiasma, is narrow and slit-shaped due to the bulging medial walls of the thalami. The third ventricle opens caudally into the very narrow *aqueduct of Sylvius*, or the ventricle of the mesencephalon.

At the level of the metencephalon and myelencephalon the lumen forms the fourth ventricle. At the rostral portion of the fourth ventricle are two lateral openings, the *foramens of Luschka*, and a single midline opening, the *foramen of Magendie*. The caudal aspect of the ventricle narrows and is continuous with the central canal of the spinal cord, which is quite small in diameter but extends the length of the cord. Even though this canal remains patent throughout life, it does not participate in circulation of cerebrospinal fluid.

CEREBROSPINAL FLUID

There may be some seepage of cerebrospinal fluid from the walls of the ventricles, but most of it is formed by the specialized *choroid plexus*. The choroid plexus evolves from an area of ependymal cells in the roof of the lateral, third, and fourth ventricles and grows down into the ventricular spaces as highly vascularized, tufted tissues. The cerebrospinal fluid from the lateral ventricles circulates through the patent ventricular system and is increased in volume by the choroid plexus of the third and fourth ventricles. It escapes through the foramens of the fourth ventricle. Outside the ventricular system, it fills the space between the brain and the arachnoid membrane. Due to the pressure gradient caused by the formation of new fluid, that cerebrospinal fluid in the subarachnoid space circulates around the CNS, both the brain and spinal cord.

The dura mater, the thick outer meninges, folds at given areas around the brain to form venous sinuses. In addition to collecting venous blood from the brain, these sinuses also collect cerebrospinal fluid via *arachnoid villi*. Each villus is a protrusion of arachnoid tissue into a dural sinus which provides a passageway for cerebrospinal fluid to be returned to the bloodstream.

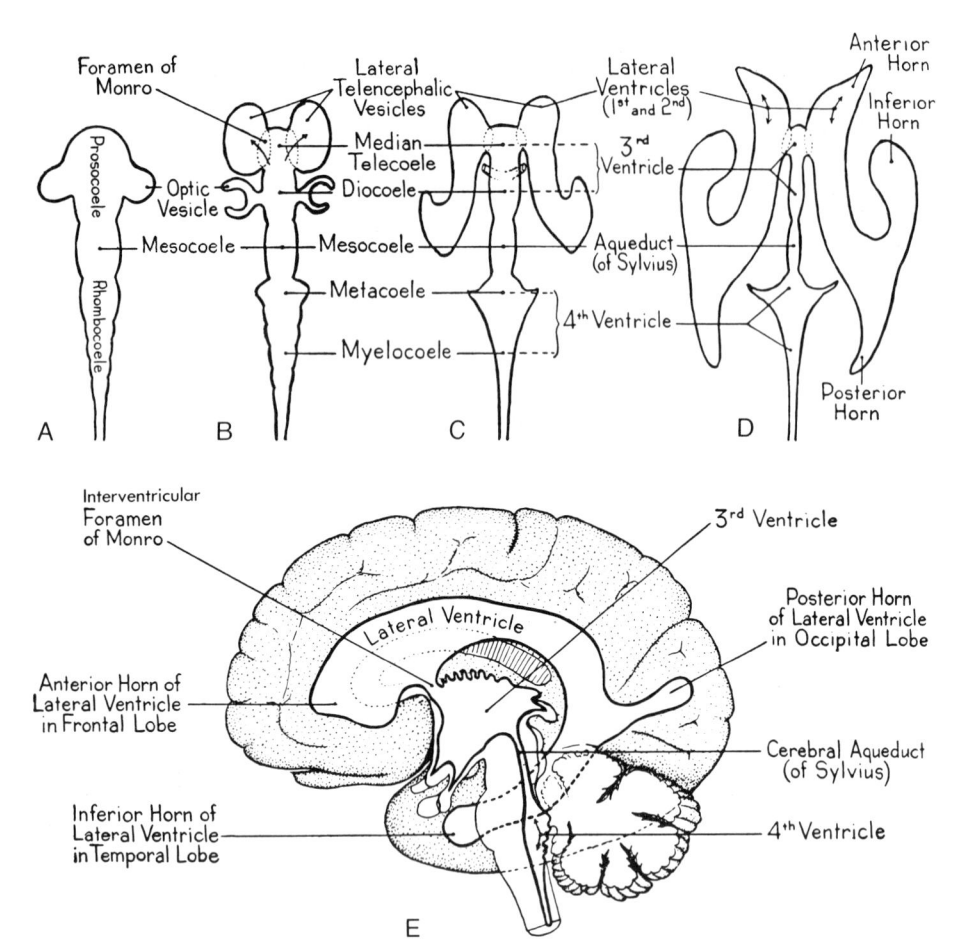

FIGURE 5-22. Schematic diagrams showing the development of cerebral ventricles from the cavities of the embryonic brain. (*a*) Primitive three-vesicle stage; (*b*) early five-vesicle stage; (*c*) expansion of lateral telencephalic vesicles; (*d*) final arrangement (schematic) as viewed from above; (*e*) final arrangement as viewed from the side. Contours of the brain are indicated for orientation. (*From C. E. Corliss, 1976, p. 218.*)

Development of the sensory system
Anna M. Tichy

Development of sense organs begins early in prenatal life in unison with the CNS.

VISUAL SYSTEM

Development of the eye involves a complex but orderly sequence of developmental interaction of tissue components which assemble so that size, configuration, orientation, and relative position are optimal for function. The eye and related structures are often referred to as a displaced CNS tract. Development of the eye from mesoderm and from surface and neural ectoderm can be identified in embryos at the eight-somite stage, about 22 days.

A pair of minute invaginations in the neural fold at the cranial end of the embryo, the beginnings of the optic sulci, or grooves, are the first indications of ocular development. The optic vesicles evaginate to form two double-walled *optic cups,* which project from the sides of the diencephalon (see Fig. 5-20). Lateral growth of these vesicles is accompanied by expansion of their distal segments and constriction of connections with the forebrain to form the *optic stalks* (see Fig. 5-23).

The retina develops from the double-walled optic cup. The inner layer of the cup becomes the sensory neural layer of the retina, and the outer layer forms the pigmented retina. At 8 weeks the neuroepithelium of the retina shows three strata; in a fetus of 6 months, all the layers of the adult retina can be identified, including the photoreceptive rods and cones.

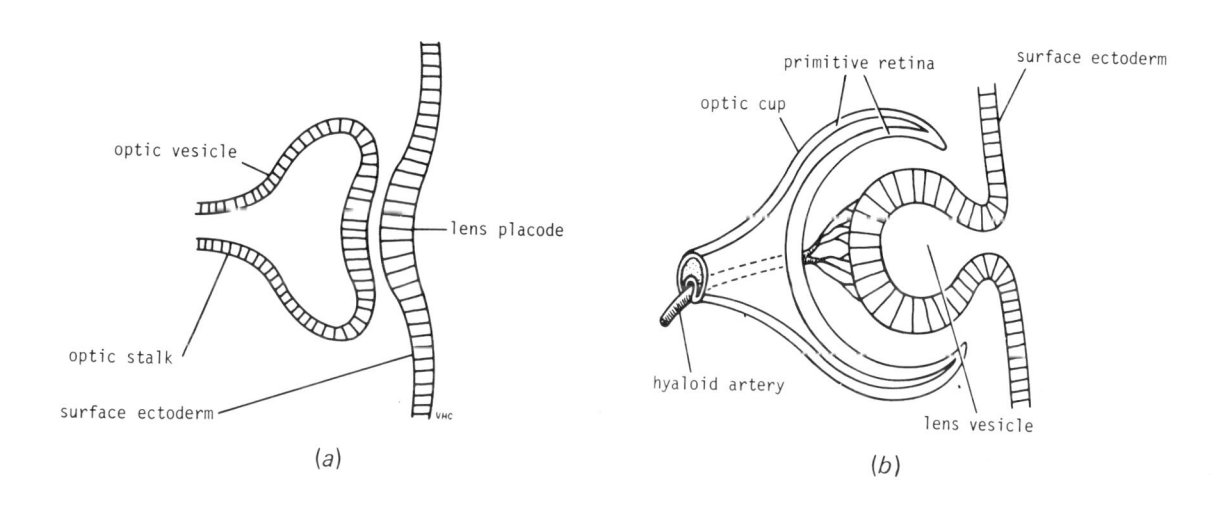

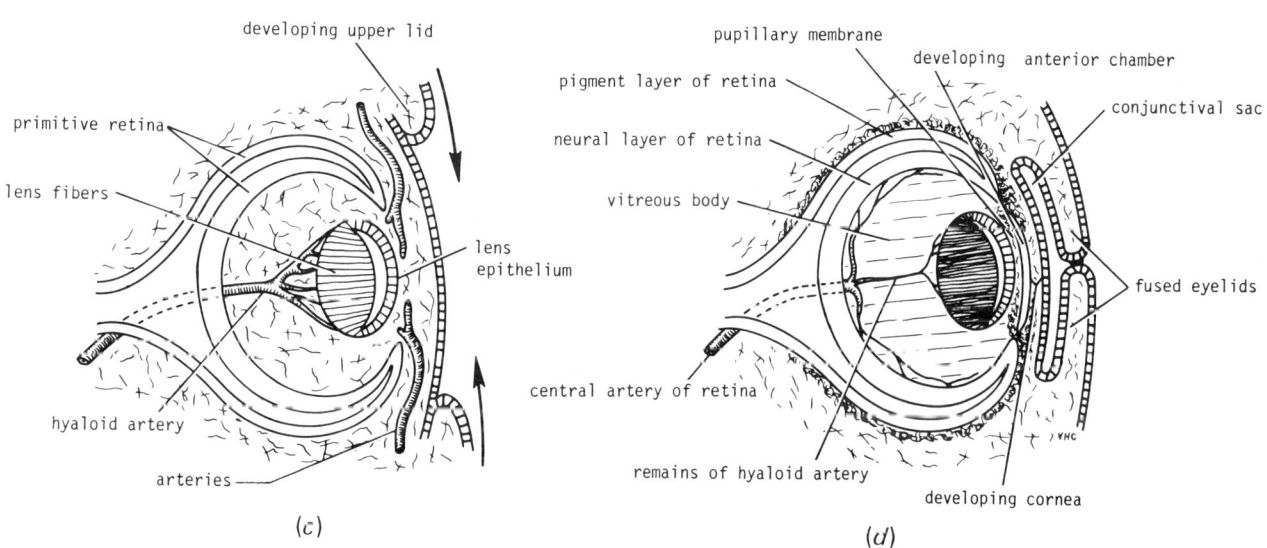

FIGURE 5-23. Development of the eye. (*a*) Optic vesicle and overlying lens placode from surface ectoderm; (*b*) invagination of optic vesicle to form optic cup and the depression of the lens placode to form the lens vesicle; (*c*) and (*d*) development of the eye including lens formation and fusion of the eyelids. [*From R. S. Snell, Clinical embryology for medical students* (2d ed.). *Boston: Little, Brown, 1975, pp. 306; 325. Reprinted by permission of the publisher.*]

Development of the macula lutea begins in the third month but proceeds slowly. At birth, the retina is fully developed except for the central foveal region.

The space separating the double wall of the optic cups gives rise to a cleft communicating with the cerebral vesicle through the optic stalk. By the seventh week nerve fibers that arise from ganglion cells converge to an area where the optic stalk emerges from the cup and continue growing toward the brain; the optic stalk becomes the *optic nerve*. The process of myelinization of the optic nerve begins in the twenty-fourth week of fetal life and has reached the optic disk by 38 weeks.

The *lens placodes* form as a result of thickening of a small area of surface ectoderm overlying the optic vesicle. By a process of invagination of the lens placode, the *lens vesicles* form. These are subsequently cut off from the surface ectoderm and form the lens. Though the lens is an avascular structure during its development, blood vessels do spread over its surface. This vascular tunic flourishes during the time of rapid lens growth; however, it degenerates about the fifth month leaving behind the central retinal artery, which will ultimately provide the vascular supply for the inner retinal layers.

The *vitreous body* forms within the optic cup partly from mesenchyme and partly from neural ectoderm. The accessory coats, sclera and cornea, as well as the aqueous chamber and associated eye organs, begin to develop about the seventh week of prenatal life and are complete at the time of birth.

AUDITORY SYSTEM

The inner ear is the first structure of the auditory apparatus to develop, reaching adult configuration early in the third month of gestation (see Fig. 5-24). Early in the fourth week an *auditory placode,* a thickened area of surface ectoderm, appears on each side of the hindbrain. Invagination of the surface of the placode forms the auditory pit. The edges of the pit approximate and fuse to form the *auditory vesicle.* These derivations of the auditory placode constitute the membranous labyrinth.

The auditory vesicle is constricted into an upper vestibular complex and a ventral cochlear portion. During the sixth week of embryonic life, the vestibular part of the auditory vesicle gives rise to the semicircular canals. The cochlear portion of the auditory vesicle is divided into a superior portion, the saccule, and an inferior segment which rapidly elongates and becomes curved to form the cochlea. By the ninth week, each cochlea achieves its final form of two and one-half turns. The organ of Corti differentiates from the cochlear portion.

The differentiation between the organ of equilibrium and the organ of hearing takes place during the first and second months of intrauterine life. The mesenchyme surrounding the developing membranous labyrinth differentiates into a cartilaginous capsule, the beginning of the bony labyrinth. The cartilage surrounding the membranous labyrinth is replaced by bone in the fifth month. The cochlea undergoes a number of changes to differentiate into the highly receptive spiral organ of Corti. The middle and inner ear approximate during development to form a functional unit.

The first pharyngeal pouch, or tympanic recess, forms the eustachian tube, while the blind outer pouch becomes the tympanic cavity. It is surrounded by connective tissue in which the bones of the middle ear—incus, stapes, and malleus—develop from mesenchyme of the first and second branchial arches. The tympanic cavity expands in the final months of intrauterine life so that the ossicles are eventually suspended in the middle ear chamber. This process extends into postnatal life.

OLFACTORY SYSTEM

During the fourth week of gestation the first indication of an olfactory organ appears as paired oval areas of thickened ectoderm, the olfactory placodes, on each ventrolateral surface of the head. The placodes are transformed into olfactory pits, which are surrounded by the medial nasal process, the lateral nasal process, and the maxillary process (see Fig. 5-18d). With fusion of the nasal processes, the olfactory pits deepen and form blind sacs. The opening into each of the sacs is the external naris.

By the seventh week, an epithelial plate at the distal end of the olfactory sac ruptures providing a route of internal communication for each nostril to the pharynx. From the second to the sixth months of fetal life, epithelial plugs occlude the external nares. The medial nasal processes fuse to form the bridge and upper nose as well as the nasal septum and philtrum. Simultaneous developmental processes include formation of the palate, which will separate the nasal and oral cavities.

By the seventh week, the olfactory bulb and the anterior olfactory nucleus begin to develop. The olfactory bulb differentiates simultaneously from the temporal lobe; subsequently the optic tract develops from the stalk of the olfactory bulb. The lining of the upper part of the nasal passages differentiates into sensory elements. Olfactory perception, though not well established, is present by the eighth month of gestation.

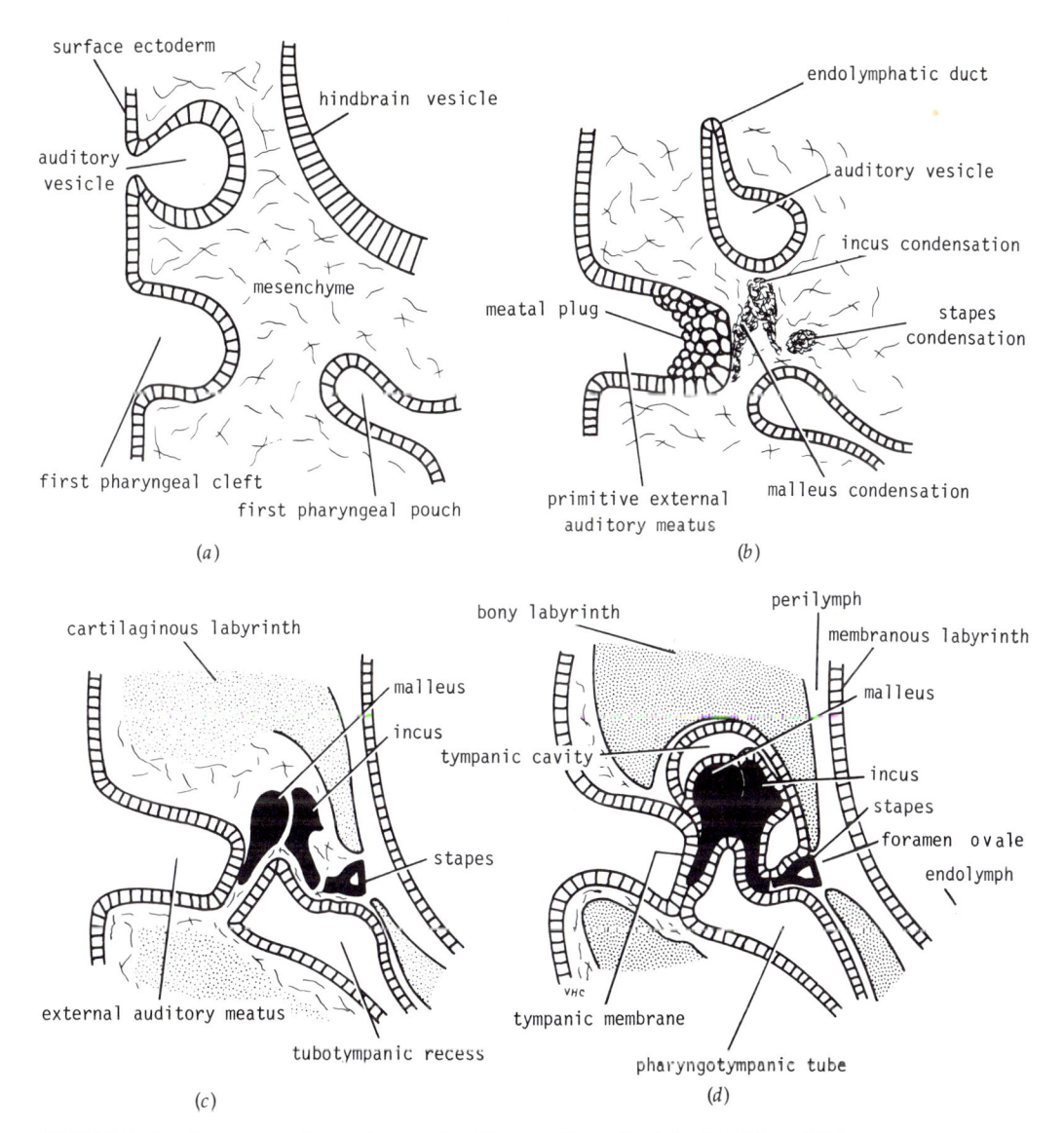

FIGURE 5-24. Four stages in development of the ear. (*From R. S. Snell, 1975, p. 331.*)

GUSTATORY SYSTEM

Taste buds appear in the third month of gestation, at about the same time that the fetus begins to swallow. Local thickenings of the lingual epithelium, the forerunners of taste buds, may be identified as early as the eighth week of prenatal life. The basal cells of the thickened areas lengthen and extend toward the surface of the epithelium. By the fourth month nerve fibers enter the clearly defined cell clusters and branch about the periphery of the taste cells. These nerves exert an organizing effect on developing taste buds. The integrity of the taste bud depends on its innervation.

Between the fifth and seventh fetal months taste buds are numerous and widely scattered in the mouth, but in late gestation and after birth many taste buds degenerate.

TACTILE SYSTEM

From an evolutionary standpoint, the skin is the oldest sensitive tissue of the body. The fibrous dermis layer houses nerve terminations which give rise to cutaneous sensations. With the proliferation of epidermal ridges, the dermis projects upward into the epidermis in the form of columnar papillae, which contain either capillary loops or sensory nerve endings. From a functional standpoint, the sensory nerve endings seem highly developed at this time. Light tactile stimulation of the upper lip or nose of the fetus induces flexion of the neck or total body movement away from the source of the stimulus (see "Prenatal Behavior").

The simplest sensory receptors, free nerve terminations, are recognizable in the latter part of the third month of prenatal life, while tactile disks appear about 1 month later. Differentiation of tactile corpuscles, which begins during the fourth month of gestation, is not complete until 1 year after birth. Knowledge concerning prenatal development of specialized sensory receptors, such as Krause's end bulbs (cold), Ruffini's end organs (warmth), and genital corpuscles, is lacking. Receptors of the sensations of deep pressure, or proprioception, complete differentiation at 8 months. The organs which provide information about muscle tension and the relative positions of body parts, or kinesthesia, have their origin in the third month of fetal life.

Development of the musculoskeletal system Sherrilyn Passo

The components of the musculoskeletal system, including cartilage, bone, muscle, ligaments, and tendons, differentiate from mesenchymal tissue, which in turn is derived from mesoderm and neural crest. During the fourth week of embryonic life, mesoderm around the notochord condenses into *somites*, which are further differentiated into sclerotome, myotome, and dermatome. Sclerotome is destined to become the vertebrae and ribs; myotome, the skeletal muscle; and dermatome, the skin (although this last component is under question). (See "Development of the Integumentary System.")

The precursors of the long bones in the embryonic limb buds pass through a cartilage phase before bone is formed by endochondral ossification; the flat bones, such as the skull, develop directly from mesenchymal tissue by intramembranous ossification. The vertebrae and ribs arise from the mesenchymal tissue of the sclerotome, the medial wall of each mesodermal somite. Resorption of tissue in the primary ossification center of the bone results in formation of the medullary cavity.

Joints are derived from the primitive joint plate, which appears between bone precursors in the mesenchyme of the limb bud. Ligaments arise from the mesenchyme around the joint and develop into fibrous bands that interconnect bones. The skeletal muscles of the limbs appear soon after the mesenchymal skeleton in the form of condensations of mesenchyme. Muscle contractions begin at the end of the eighth week ca, when the motor nerves have reached the muscle fibers.

THE SKELETON

The axial skeleton, which provides a center of support for the appendicular skeleton, evolves from mesenchyme from the serially arranged pairs of mesodermal somites (see Fig. 5-14). During the fourth week, the medial wall of each somite breaks down into a mass of diffuse cells designated a *sclerotome*, which migrates toward the notochord and surrounds it. The sclerotomes are destined to become the vertebrae and ribs. A recombination of sclerotomic masses takes place to produce the primordia of the vertebrae. Mesenchymal tissue condenses into an intervertebral disk within each somite. Remnants of the notochord become incorporated in the central portion of the intervertebral disks, the nucleus pulposi. Centers of cartilage formation in the vertebrae begin to appear in the seventh week ca. At 9 weeks, ossification begins. Not until well into the third month do the vertebral arches unite and enclose the spinal cord.

The ribs originate from the costal processes, which grow out from the primitive vertebral mass (see Fig. 5-25). Only in the thoracic region do they become long bars, following the curvature of the chest wall. In the seventh week, the mesenchymal rib tissue transforms into cartilage; by the ninth week, ossification begins, and cartilage is transformed into bone. From the cervical, lumbar, sacral, and coccygeal vertebrae, the ribs fuse or are modified so that they appear to be parts of the vertebrae themselves. The sternum first appears around 6 weeks as a pair of longitudinal bands of mesenchyme. The cartilaginous ribs attach to these bands, after which the bands fuse in a cephalocaudal direction. Ossification of the sternum begins toward the end of the fifth month.

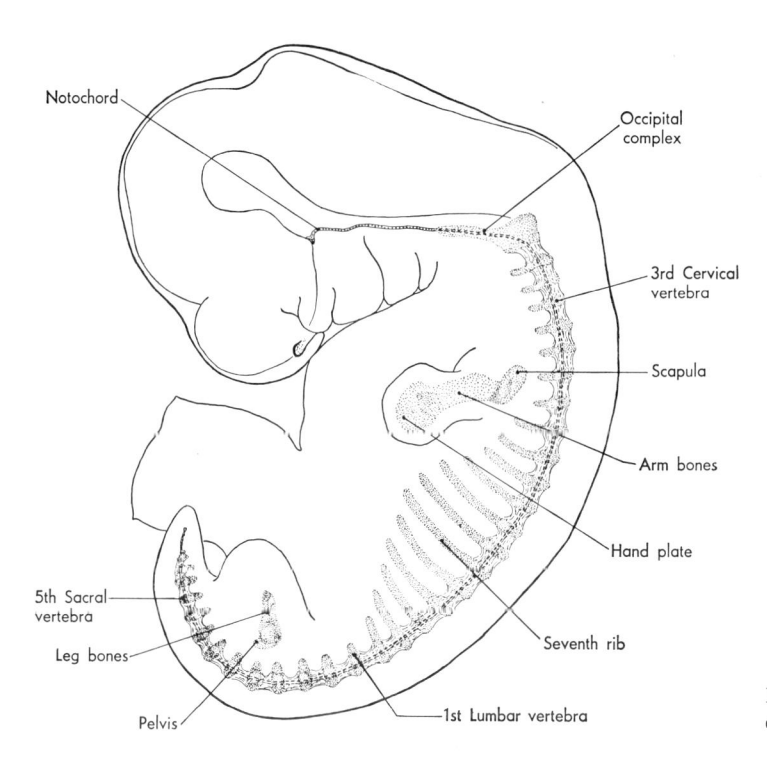

FIGURE 5-25. Precartilage primordia in a 9-mm embryo. (*From C. E. Corliss, 1976, p. 175.*)

The skull is another major part of the axial skeleton (see "Development of the Face"). The earliest indication of skull formation (the basicranium) is a mass of dense mesenchyme of mesodermal origin which, during the fifth and sixth weeks, envelops the cranial end of the notochord. Cartilage formation begins in the basal part of the skull during the seventh week ca. By the middle of the third month, ossification ensues in this area.

Skull bone growth is determined by the growth of the brain, sense organs, and other visceral organs. Thus, abnormal brain growth will be reflected in skull formation. The union of bones of the skull is still incomplete by the time of birth.

Paired limb buds appear late in the fourth week ca (see Fig. 5-11b). In the embryo of 5 weeks, mesenchyme has condensed into definite masses both within the limb buds and at the sites of the future pectoral and pelvic girdles. Each mesenchymal mass is the precursor of a bone (see Fig. 5-26). At 7 weeks, the cartilage model of the bone is formed from the mesenchymal model. In the eighth week, the largest cartilage models begin their transformation into bone as ossification begins.

The first site of ossification is the primary ossification center in the diaphysis, or shaft, of the bone. As in other areas of development, differentiation in the limbs proceeds in a proximodistal direction. Also, ossification proceeds in a cephalocaudal direction, as the arms develop somewhat in advance of the legs; at birth the upper limb is longer. Ossification is incomplete at birth, and some elements of the appendicular skeleton are still wholly cartilaginous.

MARROW

The marrow cavity is formed by the processes of tubulation and resorption, after ossification has already begun. In the flat bones resorption of the center part of the bones results in formation of a medullary cavity. By the sixth prenatal month in the femur and later in other long bones, the process of tubulation occurs. Bone is resorbed at the site of the primary ossification center to form the medullary cavity of the long bone. During the later part of the gestational period, the bone marrow begins to function in production of blood cells.

JOINT

The primitive joint plate, an articular disk of mesenchyme, appears at the site of a future synovial joint in the mesenchyme of the limb bud. Dense tissue, similar to the perichondrium of the cartilage model, surrounds the primitive joint plate and later becomes the joint capsule. By the tenth week, spaces filled with tissue fluid appear in the primitive joint plate and gradually join into a single joint cavity filled with fluid. The outer layer of the joint capsule differentiates into fibrous tissue, while the inner layer forms the synovial membrane.

At birth the synovial joint appears as two opposing surfaces covered by articular cartilage and joined by an encircling band of fibrous tissue. The joint cavity is held in place by ligaments and muscles. The synovial membrane lines the joint cavity except over surfaces of articular cartilage. Synovial fluid lubricates and nourishes the articulation. Full development of a synovial joint, such as the hip joint, does not occur until adulthood.

Ligaments arise from the mesenchyme in regions where joints are developing. These tissues develop into fibrous bands that interconnect bones and allow movement and proper alignment.

MUSCLES

The three types of muscles, skeletal, smooth, and cardiac, differentiate from the myoblast, which originates from myotome segments of the somites (see Fig. 5-27). Muscle development can be considered on two levels: histogenesis, or development of myoblast into muscle fibers, and morphogenesis, the formation of muscles from organization of muscle fibers.

Skeletal muscle fibers of the head, neck, and trunk originate from a thickening of the myotome plate during the fifth week. During histogenesis, cells in the plate differentiate into myoblasts, or muscle-forming cells, which arrange themselves parallel with the long axis of the body and become skeletal muscle fibers. Limb muscles, flexors and extensors, do not develop wholly from myotome migration, but mesenchyme in the limb buds is "seeded" by muscle cells which migrate from the myotome.

Between the sixth to eighth weeks, muscles are capable of movement. Proliferation of new muscle fibers occurs prenatally and for a short time postnatally. After that time, enlargement of a muscle occurs as a result of hypertrophy, increase in diameter and length of individual fibers, rather than hyperplasia.

The spinal nerve corresponding to each somite makes

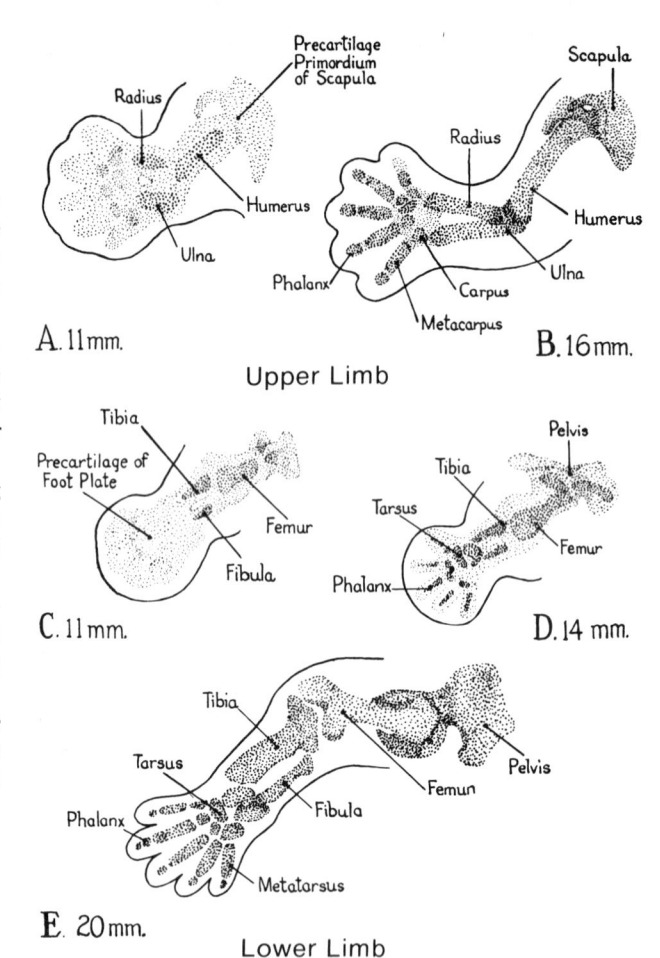

FIGURE 5-26. Early stages in the development of the skeleton of the limbs. The conceptual ages represented are A—40 days, B—46 days, C—40 days, D—44 days, and E—50 days. The fine stippling in the drawings of the younger stages indicates precartilage concentrations of mesenchyme; the more sharply circumscribed and coarser stippling of older stages represents cartilage. (*From C. E. Corliss, 1976, p. 178.*)

contact with the myotome and dermatome at an early stage. At the end of the second month, when the motor nerves reach the muscle fibers, the long muscles of the trunk and neck begin to contract spontaneously. Later, arm and then leg movements are added. By 3 months, the fetus has developed some postural reflexes and shows reaction to skin stimulation (see "Prenatal Behavior"). By the fourth prenatal month, a flattened terminal network differentiates from the spinal nerves. This network enters the skeletal muscle fiber and rests on the motor end plate of the muscle.

The relation of segmental spinal nerve to myotome is

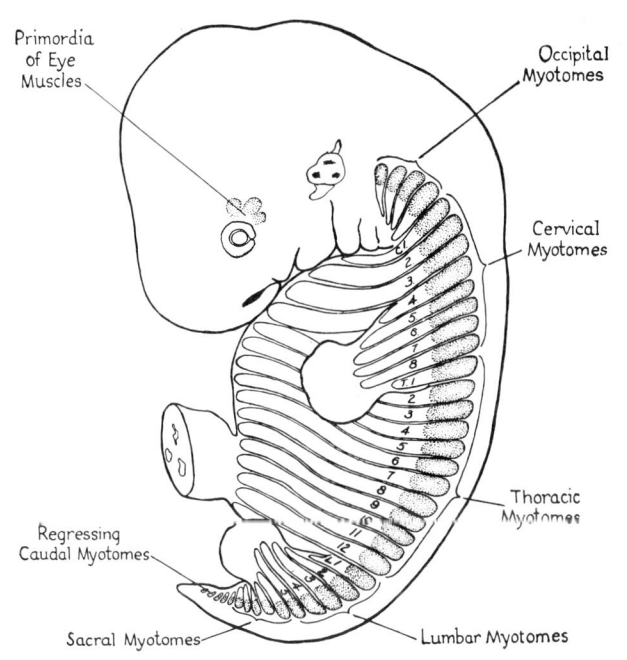

FIGURE 5-27. Schematic diagram showing the myotome region of the somites which give rise to most of the skeletal muscles. The stippled areas show the approximate size of the mesodermic somites when they are first established. The unstippled areas outlined opposite each somite suggest the territory into which the segmental nerves extend. (*From C. E. Corliss, 1976, p. 191.*)

retained throughout life. This is illustrated when myotomes fuse to form a muscle; that muscle remains innervated by several spinal nerves. If myotomes split into several muscles, all these muscles are innervated by the original spinal nerve.

Connective tissue is differentiated from local mesenchyme and binds individual muscle fibers together or encloses an entire muscle. Tendons are fibrous cords that arise independently of muscles and attach muscles to bones.

Movement of the fetus appears to be important for proper muscle and joint development; its role in central and peripheral nervous system development, if any, is unknown.

Development of the cardiovascular system LaNelle E. Geddes

Cells in a multicellular organism, like those of unicellular creatures, exchange nutrients and waste products with their immediate environment. In the case of unicellular organisms the general external and the immediate cellular environments are one and the same; however, for multicellular organisms, the cellular environment is interstitial fluid and very different from the general external environment of the body as a whole. Since individual cells are far removed from direct access to environmental oxygen and ingested nutrients, requirements for cellular metabolism must be delivered by a circulatory system. Likewise, waste products must be continuously removed from the cellular surroundings to distant specialized excretory organs.

During the first few days following fertilization, the embryo is small enough for each cell to be in intimate communication with and have direct access to its external environment. However, the rapidly proliferating cell mass soon outgrows this simple relation. When the embryo reaches a size that is too large for exchange of adequate nutrients, oxygen, and waste products by physicochemical means such as diffusion, osmosis, and bulk flow, development of a circulatory system becomes mandatory. A circulatory system begins to appear about the twentieth day, when the embryo has reached a length of approximately 1.5 mm.

While not the first to actually appear in the embryo, the cardiovascular system is the earliest *functional* system to develop. This fact is not surprising when the functional simplicity of the cardiovascular system is considered. The cardiovascular system is, after all, little more than a system of conduits containing an inherently rhythmic, pulsating portion to move the contents contained within it. Inherent rhythmicity is a very primitive cellular characteristic present in even the simplest organisms. A functional cardiovascular system requires only structural integrity and has no elaborate dependence on enzyme systems, hormonal construction, or intricate organization, such as the digestive, endocrine, and nervous systems. Therefore, the relative simplicity of the emerging cardiovascular system permits it to reach a functional stage ahead of more intricate body systems. Emphasis on functional simplicity does not mean that cardiogenesis is either relatively insignificant or functionally unimpaired by embryological misadventure. Congenital heart defects are consequence of embryological mistakes during cardiovascular development.

The heart, blood vessels, and red blood cells originally develop from the inner mesodermal layer of the yolk sac. Cellular clusters, or "blood islands," develop, and the cells then move away from each other to form a lumen.

Those cells that move to the periphery increase in number and coalesce to form the walls of the primitive vessels. The cells remaining more central develop into early erythrocytes. Vessel development is dynamic and keeps pace with the increased tissue mass of the developing embryo. New vessels appear and grow in size, while others may regress.

In early development a bilateral plexus of vessels coalesce into a primitive vascular system. The vessels increase in diameter and length to keep pace with the perfusion demands of a growing embryo. Later, the heart and major vessels will develop from this primitive plexus. About the twenty-first day a contractile cardiac tube can be identified. This simple heart exhibits all the properties of automaticity, conduction, and contractility that will be refined to a higher degree as it develops. Compared with that of the more mature fetus and the neonate, the heart of the embryo is large compared with the body in which it is confined. But it must be appreciated that the embryonic (and fetal) heart must perfuse extraembryonic tissue, including the developing placenta.

DEVELOPMENT OF THE HEART

The heart develops from a confluence of vessels in the cardiogenic area at the cephalad end of the embryo. Pulsations develop in a portion of the vessels and cause blood to ebb and flow. Valves for imparting a unidirectional blood flow have not yet developed at this stage (see Fig. 5-29). The pulsating cardiac tube later develops into the contracting atria and ventricles. At first, the pericardium and the cardiac tube lie next to each other. The pericardium begins to envelop the endocardial tube as the developing heart invaginates into what is to become the pericardial sac. About 3 days have elapsed between the start of vasculogenesis and the appearance of a pulsating cardiac tube.

Cardiac growth exceeds that of the surrounding pericardium, and the heart is forced to fold on itself much as a tall person must stoop upon entering a child's playhouse. This cardiac folding occurs in an orderly fashion (see Fig. 5-28). What had formerly been the inferior end of the cardiac tube is forced upward. Later, additional folding forces the developing tube into an S shape. Torsion and twisting occur as the cardiac tube folds within the pericardium.

As the primitive atria and ventricles enlarge and twist on each other, vessels located below the cardiac tube are pulled up behind the developing ventricles and come to lie above them. Because of the extensive reorientation of cardiac structures with relation to one another that occurs at this stage of embryological development, certain congenital abnormalities, such as ventricular inversion with or without transposition of the great vessels, can be traced to this point in embryogenesis.

FIGURE 5-28. Early development of the embryonic heart. The arrows indicate blood flow. [*From L. L. Langley et al., Dynamic anatomy and physiology (4th ed.). New York: McGraw-Hill, 1974, p. 399.*]

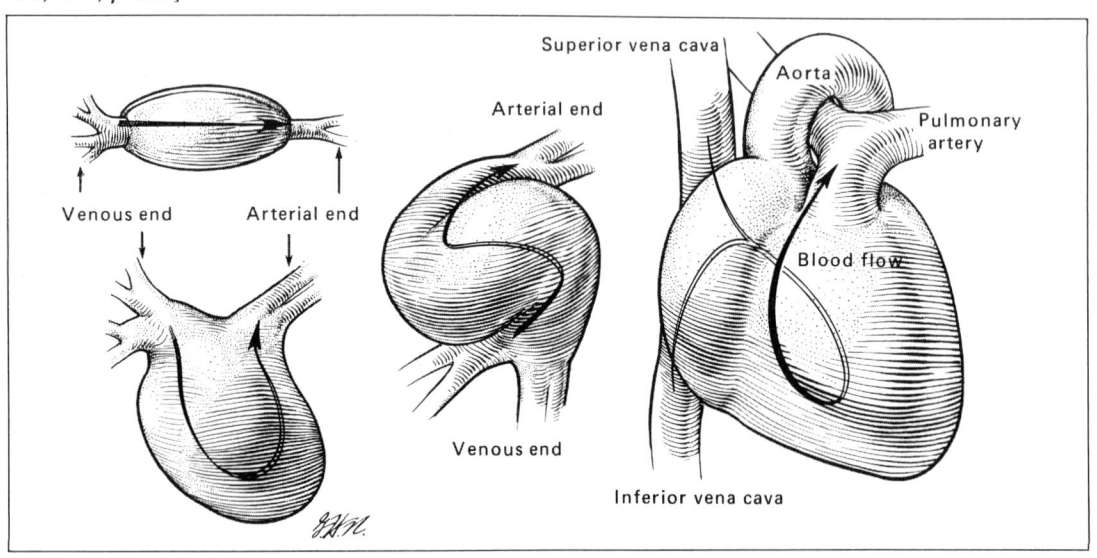

A four-chambered heart develops from the straight cardiac tube between the fourth and eighth weeks of gestation (see Fig. 5-29a, b, and c). This partitioning begins as the endocardial cushions develop in the dorsal and ventral walls of the tube near the atrial and ventricular junction, the *atrioventricular canal*. The endocardial cushions grow toward each other and fuse, dividing the atrioventricular canal into the left and right atrioventricular canals.

The *septum primum*, a crescent-shaped membrane, appears on the dorsocranial wall of the primitive atrium and grows (ventrocaudally) toward the endocardial cushions to divide the atrium. The area between the downward-migrating septum primum and the endocardial cushions is the *foramen primum*. As the foramen primum closes, the *foramen secundum* forms in the upper central portion of the septum, maintaining communication between the two atrial chambers.

A second sheet of tissue, the *septum secundum*, develops just to the right of the septum primum. The septum secundum also has an opening, the *foramen ovale*. The foramen ovale is not in line with the foramen secundum but lies below it and behind the inferior portion of the septum primum that acts as a flap valve over the foramen ovale. Blood flows from the right atrium to the left through the foramen ovale but is prevented from moving in the opposite direction by action of the flap valve (see Fig. 5-29c and d). In the fetus, right atrial pressure exceeds left atrial pressure; therefore, blood is forced from right to left through the foramen ovale.

The interventricular septum develops from the floor of the primitive ventricle near the apex and grows toward the endocardial cushion in the atrioventricular canal. The muscular septum does not extend all the way to the endocardial cushion, and an interventricular opening persists for a time. This interventricular communication is later closed by tissue extending downward from the endocardial cushion. This upper part of the ventricular septum is called the *membranous septum* to differentiate it from the lower muscular portion.

Septation also proceeds in the *truncus arteriosus*, the outflow tract from the heart, dividing this structure into the pulmonary trunk and the aorta. Spiraling continues to occur, with the result that in the fully developed heart the aortic root lies to the right of the pulmonary trunk despite the fact that the pulmonary artery emerges from the right ventricle and the aorta from the left. A lifelong reminder of embryological twisting of the truncus arteriosus is provided by the fact that the auscultatory area for the aortic valve is to the *right* of the sternum while that for the pulmonary valve is located to the *left*.

PRENATAL CIRCULATION

Intra- and extracardiac shunts, considered problematic in the young child or adult, are both normal and necessary during fetal life. There are several features of fetal circulation that disappear after birth. These features include an umbilical vein and the umbilical arteries, a patent foramen ovale, a ductus venosus, and a ductus arteriosus (see Fig. 5-30). Each of these fetal circulatory features subserves a function that is neither necessary nor beneficial to the child postnatally but is important to the unique fetal circulation. Before detailing the function served in the fetus by each of these four features, the differences between fetal and extrauterine circumstances are examined.

Since the fetal pulmonary system is not involved in gas exchange, there is little rationale for directing large amounts of blood through the lungs. To accommodate this fetal reality, much of the blood is shunted away from the pulmonary vascular beds and moved directly from the right side of the heart to the systemic circulation. The placenta not only acts as fetal "lungs," it also acts as an entry and exit port for materials that will later be handled by the liver of the young infant.

Oxygenated blood delivered from the placenta to the inferior vena cava via the umbilical vein and the ductus venosus is directed through the foramen ovale from the right atrium to the left atrium and bypasses the right ventricle and the pulmonary vasculature. It is only in fetal life that inferior vena caval blood is highly oxygenated. Directing this blood through the foramen ovale results in delivery of oxygenated blood to the left side of the heart for perfusion of the rest of the fetal body.

The two umbilical arteries are branches of the iliac arteries and communicate with the placenta. The hemoglobin saturation of blood within the umbilical arteries, as compared with that in the umbilical vein, is somewhat analogous to the situation in the pulmonary artery and veins of the adult, as both pulmonary and umbilical veins carry blood that is more highly oxygenated than their associated arteries. This similarity assumes its proper perspective when it is realized that the gas-exchange organ of the fetus is the placenta.

The ductus venosus is a branch of the umbilical vein and serves to divert a significant quantity of oxygenated

240 THE EMBRYO AND FETUS: CONCEPTION TO BIRTH

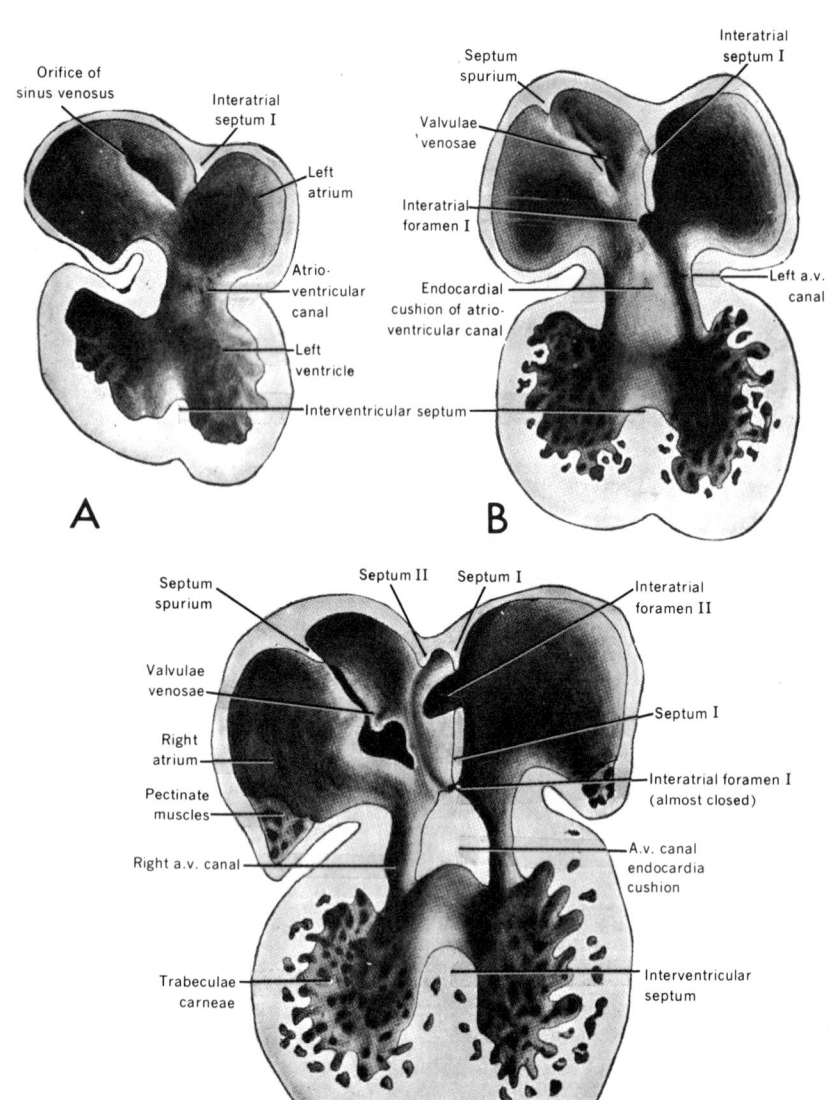

FIGURE 5-29. (a), (b), and (c) Early stages of cardiac septation in the developing embryo. Septum I is also called the septum primum and septum II is the septum secundum. Interatrial foramens I and II refer to foramens primum and secundum respectively. (d) and (e) Later septation in the fetal heart. Trabeculations and valve structures, including the papillary muscles and chordae tendinae, are clearly identifiable at this stage. The arrows in the lower half of the figure indicate the direction of blood flow in the right atrium and through the foramen ovale. [*From Hurst et al., The heart (4th ed.). New York: McGraw-Hill, 1978. Reprinted by permission of the publisher.*]

blood from the liver and deliver it directly to the inferior vena cava. Although functional, the fetal liver is aided by maternal activities, and not all the blood need be directed through fetal hepatic tissue. Therefore, the ductus venosus serves as an umbilical vein to the inferior vena cava shunt.

As noted above, much of the blood delivered to the right heart is shunted across the foramen ovale and bypasses the lungs. However, some blood, especially that returning to the heart through the superior vena cava from the cephalad parts of the body, is directed into the right ventricle and thence into the pulmonary artery.

FIGURE 5-29 (Continued)

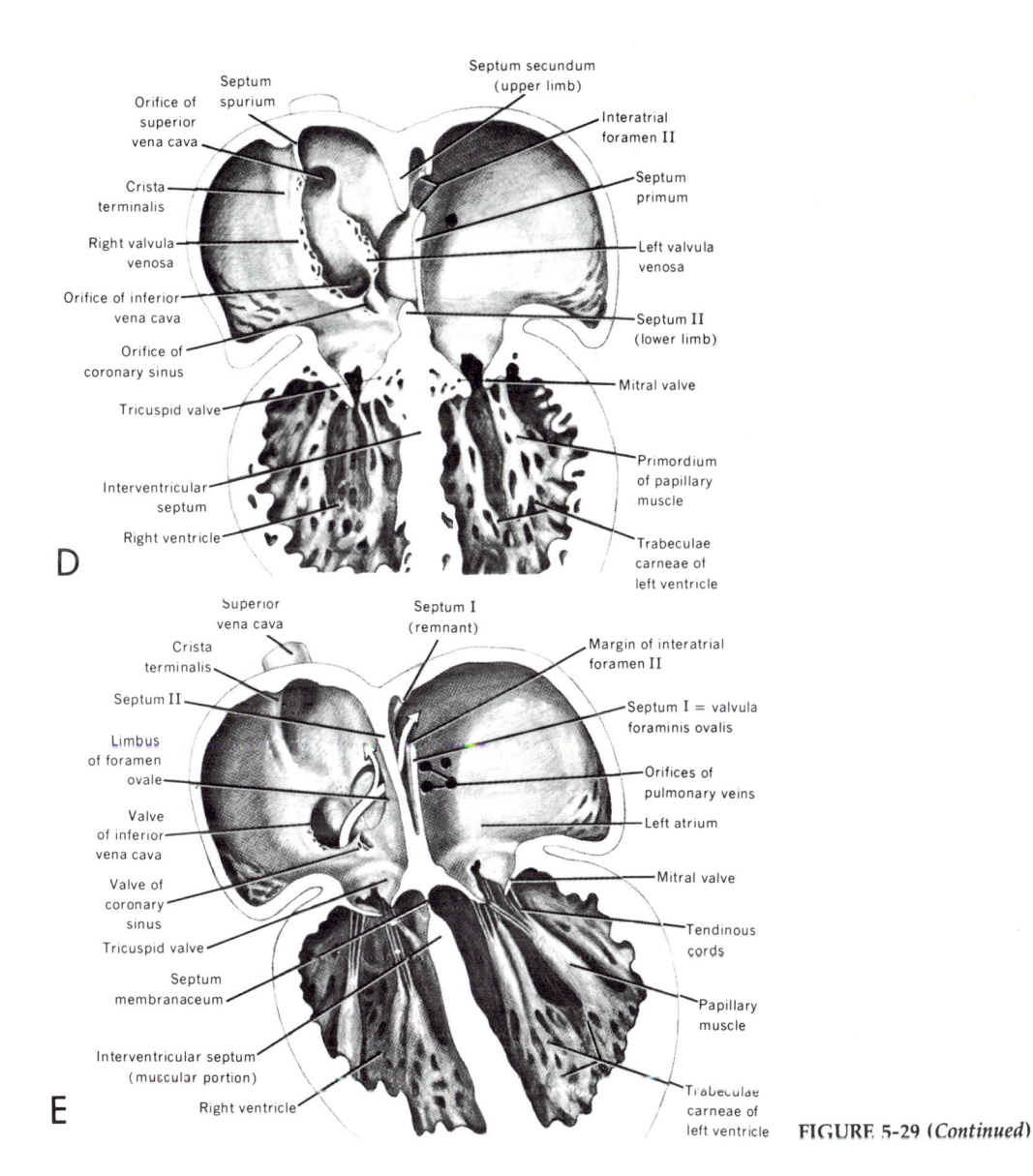

Pulmonary vascular resistance in the fetus is high due to the uninflated state of the lungs, and systemic vascular resistance is low due to the large placental bed. This situation is reversed in extrauterine life because after birth pulmonary vascular resistance decreases and systemic resistance increases. Right atrial pressure is higher than left atrial pressure in the fetus, and this pressure gradient directs blood from right to left through the foramen ovale. From the left atrium, blood enters the left ventricle and is then delivered, through the aorta, to the systemic circulation.

Blood directed from the right atrium into the right ventricle is moved into the pulmonary artery. The fetal circulation contains a patent communication, the ductus ar-

242 THE EMBRYO AND FETUS: CONCEPTION TO BIRTH

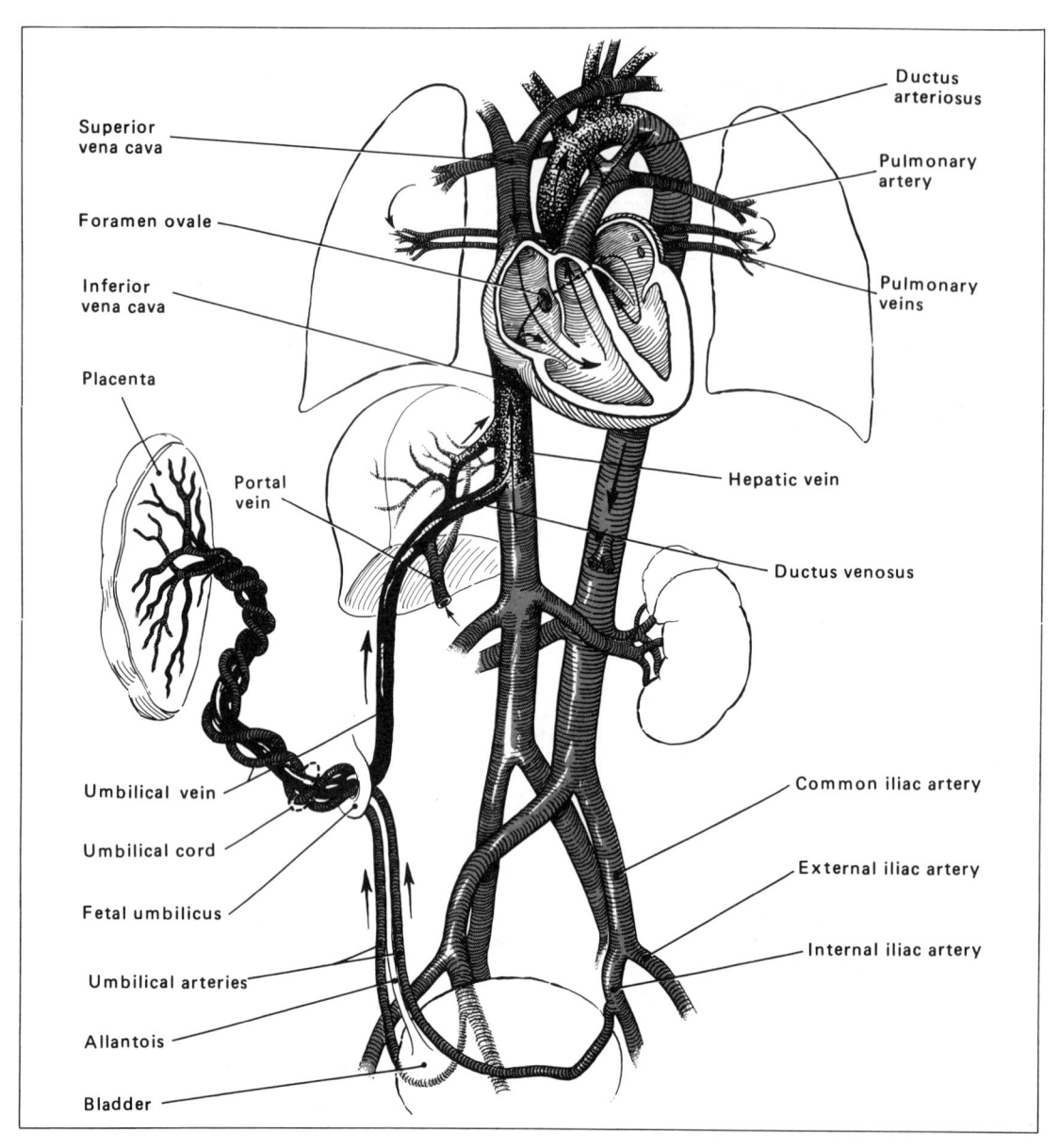

FIGURE 5-30. Fetal circulation. The arrows indicate the direction of blood flow. (*From L. L. Langley et al., 1974, p. 783.*)

teriosus, between the pulmonary artery and the aorta. Since pulmonary artery vascular resistance (and pressure) is higher than aortic resistance (and pressure) during the fetal period, much of the blood entering the pulmonary artery from the right ventricle flows through the ductus arteriosus from the pulmonary artery into the aorta and bypasses the lungs. Although some variations do exist, the ductus arteriosus generally enters the aorta below the aortic arch and the origins of the major vessels (the brachiocephalic or innominate, left common carotid, and left subclavian arteries) serving the upper part of the body.

Fetal circulation provides shunts that result in an economy of pressure gradients and favor directing blood to functioning and developing organs and diverting it from tissues whose function in utero is shared, or even assumed, by placental exchange. Although fetal circulation reflects most of the perfusion patterns appropriate to extrauterine existence, it also has features that are appropriate only to a dependent existence and actually counterproductive to independent life.

ERYTHROPOIESIS

Erythropoiesis (blood formation) in the fetus is shared by several tissues and organs. Erythropoiesis in bone marrow does not begin until approximately the fourth to fifth month of fetal life. Prior to this time, blood cells are formed in the yolk sac, liver, spleen, and endothelial cells of the fetus. Not only are the anatomical sites of red cell production in the fetus and mature individual different, but the relative amounts of hemoglobin variants also differ. Hemoglobin is a tetrameral molecule composed of four heme groups, each of which is attached to a globin chain. Each heme group contains a single ferrous (Fe^{2+}) ion. Differences between the types of hemoglobin reside in the amino acid sequence of the globin chains. Adult hemoglobin (HbA) has two alpha chains and two beta chains, whereas fetal hemoglobin (HbF) has two alpha chains and two gamma chains. At birth about 75 to 90 percent of the hemoglobin is HbF, but by several months of age is has been largely replaced by HbA.

Fetal hemoglobin has a functional difference from adult hemoglobin: It is more highly saturated with oxygen at a given partial pressure of oxygen (P_{O_2}) than adult hemoglobin. Despite the molecular differences in the two types of hemoglobin, the greater oxygen affinity displayed by HbF does not appear to be due to its structure. The P_{O_2} of blood in the umbilical vein is about 30 to 40 mmHg. At this P_{O_2}, HbA is about 70 percent saturated, while HbF is about 80 percent saturated. Thus, the greater affinity of fetal blood for oxygen enables greater quantities to be carried to the fetus from the placental vessels than would be possible in blood with HbA.

Furthermore, the P_{O_2} of fetal tissues is only about 15 mmHg, while it is about 40 mmHg in the adult. The extremely low tissue oxygen pressure of the fetus encourages release of oxygen from HbF. The characteristics of HbF represent an important fetal adaptation to life in an environment of low P_{O_2}. A testament to the value of HbF is the fact that even in the adult the body does not lose the capability for producing it. Faced with conditions of increased destruction of erythrocytes, such as sickle cell anemia, or reduced erythropoietic capability, such as aplastic anemia, the body may again produce HbF.

In addition to production of HbF, the fetus has other ways of coping with the low P_{O_2} of its immediate cellular environment. First, the hemoglobin concentration of the fetus's blood is about 50 percent greater than that of the mother. This increased hemoglobin concentration increases the number of oxygen carriers per unit volume. Second, the effects of pH on hemoglobin transport of oxygen work in the fetus's favor. The effect of pH on oxygen saturation of hemoglobin is the *Bohr effect*. The Bohr effect describes the phenomenon that the higher the pH the more saturated hemoglobin is, with oxygen at a given P_{O_2}. Conversely, the lower the pH, the lower the hemoglobin saturation. The Bohr effect enhances fetal availability of oxygen in the following way: Fetal blood entering placental vessels has a higher P_{CO_2} and, hence, a lower pH than the maternal blood it contacts. Therefore, CO_2 from fetal blood diffuses into the maternal circulation. The exit of CO_2 from fetal blood raises its pH and oxygen affinity at the same time that CO_2 from the fetus entering maternal blood lowers its pH and decreases the affinity of maternal hemoglobin for oxygen. The oxygen thus released from the "acid" maternal blood is picked up and bound by the "alkaline" fetal blood.

The combination of fetal hemoglobin with its increased affinity for oxygen, the elevated hemoglobin concentration in the normal fetus, and the Bohr effect serve to increase the oxygen availability to fetal tissues. Maximization of oxygen-carrying capability along with the anatomical shunts for delivering blood to the most demanding regions of the body of the fetus enable the fetus to survive and thrive in an environment that imposes its share of physiological limitations.

Development of the respiratory system
Virginia J. Neelon

While the primary function of the mature lung is gas exchange, the tasks of the prenatal lung are as follows:

- Organization of growth
- Surfactant synthesis
- Establishment of respiration at birth

ORGANIZATION OF GROWTH
Lung development begins around the twenty-fourth day of embryonic life and continues throughout the period of body growth. The epithelium and glands of the trachea and bronchi and the pulmonary lining epithelium are of endodermal origin. The connective tissue, cartilage, and smooth muscle, however, are of mesenchymal origin (Moore, 1977).

Prenatal development of the lung (see Fig. 5-31) is divided into three periods: the glandular phase, fourth to seventeenth weeks; canalicular phase, seventeenth to twenty-fourth weeks; and terminal sac phase, twenty-fourth week to term. The alveolar period predominates after birth (Fraser and Paré, 1977; Reid, 1967; Strang, 1977b).

GLANDULAR PHASE
The lung is a sac of epithelium derived from the gut as an outpouching around the twenty-fourth day after fertilization. The trachea and esophagus have this common origin which predisposes them to one of the more frequent congenital lung anomalies: tracheoesophageal fistula. Within a few days from the appearance of the first lung bud, two primary branches appear to form the major bronchi. The development of the bronchial tree is completed by the sixteenth week ca (see Fig. 5-31). During this period the lung's appearance resembles a glandular organ. The epithelial cells are columnar in structure and contain a glycogen-filled cytoplasm. The high concentration of glycogen is characteristic of immature epithelial cells. In later development the cells become cuboidal.

CANALICULAR PHASE
The canalicular phase signifies ductlike development and signals the emergence of early respiratory bronchioles. During this period the epithelial cells become differentiated, producing several types of cells whose functions are crucial to the respiratory and nonrespiratory functions of the lung.

Type I alveolar cells appear for the first time. They are characterized by marked thinning and stretching of the cytoplasmic space and represent the major epithelial surface for gas diffusion. Goblet cells and the cells of the bronchial glands, involved in mucus secretion, are present in the lung from the thirteenth week. Secretion by globlet cells is influenced by direct stimulation, such as that produced by inhaled particles, while secretion from the gland cells is influenced more by neurogenic mechanisms (Scarpelli, 1975).

Like type I cells, type II epithelial cells also come from the glycogen-filled, primitive lining cells. These cells have characteristic inclusion bodies, which are considered the storage sites for the essential components of the surfactant system. These inclusions in type II cells first appear during the canalicular stage (twenty-fourth week) and increase in number throughout gestation.

Ciliated cells are present in bronchial branches by the thirteenth week. At term they are found in all conducting airways and extend into the terminal bronchioles (Murray, 1976). The action of the cilia propels the mucous blanket forward to be expelled. Secretion by the bronchial cells is also a main (but not the only) source of amniotic fluid and provides important diagnostic information about fetal development. A deficiency in amniotic-fluid volume results in decreased lung liquids and retarded lung growth.

TERMINAL SAC PHASE AND ALVEOLARIZATION
From the twenty-fourth week, lung development is characterized by the appearance of terminal air sacs, which later give origin to primitive alveolar sacules. True alveoli are not seen until a few weeks prior to birth (Hallman and Gluck, 1977). Alveolar development increases most rapidly during the first neonatal months and continues at a slower rate to 15 years of age. Proliferation of the capillary network close to the developing airways occurs between the twenty-sixth and the twenty-eighth weeks. Extrauterine life is possible at this time and even earlier with modern methods for caring for the premature. However, these infants are at a high risk because of the immaturity of their lung surface and the limited area for gas exchange. (Avery and Fletcher, 1974; Kendig and Chernich, 1977).

Obviously both fetal and maternal factors can stress and limit lung development. Any congenital defect of the fetus which might limit space within the thoracic cavity could affect growth of the respiratory system. Defects in the diaphragm or protrusion of abdominal parts into the chest causes diminished lung size. A deficiency in

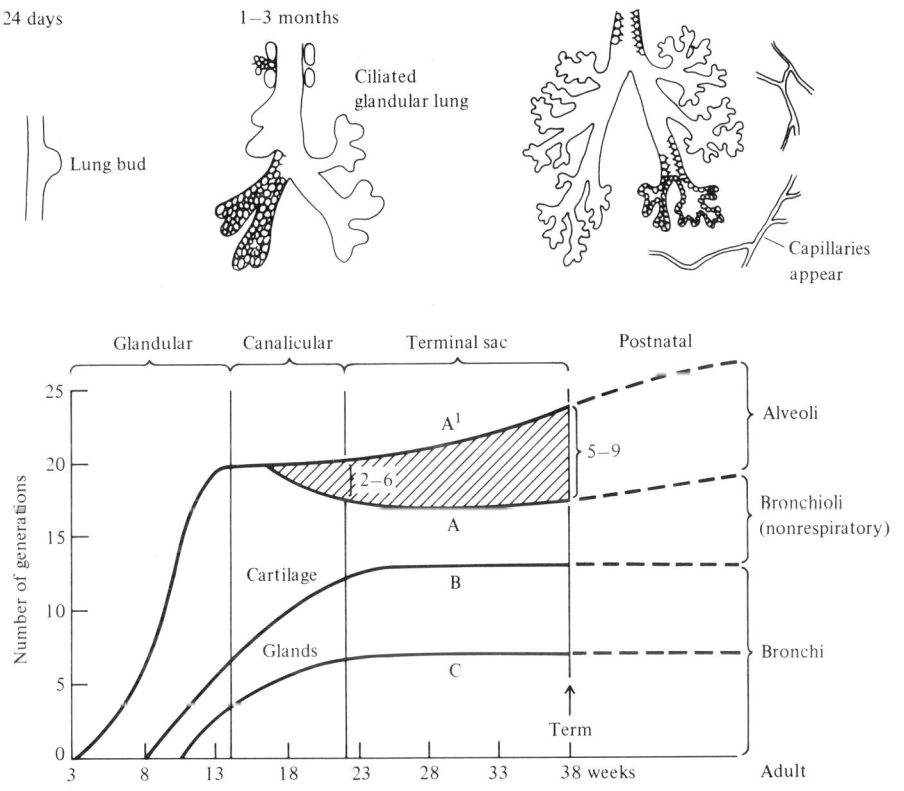

FIGURE 5-31. Organization of prenatal growth of the respiratory system. The glandular, canalicular, and terminal sac phases are represented as well as postnatal development. Line A represents the number of bronchial generations and A¹ the respiratory bronchioles and alveolar ducts. Line B is the extension of cartilage along the bronchial tree, and C is the extension of mucus glands. Conceptual age in weeks is given. (*Adapted from U. Bucher and L. Reid, Thorax, 1961, 16, 207.*)

amniotic-fluid volume results in decreased lung liquids and retarded lung growth. Finally, lung maturation can be accelerated by elevated hormone levels of both glucocorticoids and thyroxine.

LUNG MATURATION AND FUNCTION

SURFACTANT SYNTHESIS

The susceptibility of newborn infants to respiratory distress depends considerably on the stage of lung maturation at the time of delivery and, in particular, on the biochemical maturation of the surfactant system. Surfactant is a surface-tension–lowering material present at the air–liquid interface of the alveolus. It contributes to airway stability by preventing collapse of alveoli at low lung volumes through lowering surface tension during expiration. It also acts as an antiedema factor, inhibiting the leakage of fluid from the pulmonary circulation (Hallman and Gluck, 1977).

Surfactant is composed primarily of phospholipids, the most abundant being lecithin. It is synthesized and released from the type II alveolar cell and can be detected in lung tissue as early as 23 weeks' gestation. Its release to the lung surface occurs later, about 30 to 32 weeks' gestation, and it can be detected in the amniotic fluid at about this time (Strang, 1977b).

The importance of surfactant in respiratory distress syndrome (RDS) was demonstrated in 1959 (Avery and Mead) when infants with RDS (also known as *hyaline membrane disease*) were shown to be unable to synthesize sufficient surfactant for alveolar stability. Subsequent work has shown that fetal surfactant synthesis appears according to a developmental timetable, and at birth critical amounts are released to create the alveolar air-liquid interface. The presence of surfactant is a prerequisite for normal postnatal pulmonary function. Not only must it be present in adequate amounts, but its synthesis by type II cells must be sufficient to offset surfactant breakdown.

EVALUATION OF LUNG MATURITY

Because of the continuity between fetal lung fluids and amniotic fluid, the nature of the phospholipids in the amniotic fluid can be correlated with the functional maturity of the fetus, specifically the maturity of the lung (Gluck, 1974).

The concentrations of the phospholipids sphingomyelin (S) and lecithin (L) in the amniotic fluid are relatively constant during the first 7 to 8 months of a normal pregnancy; the S concentration is slightly more than that of L. At about 28 weeks, L increases sharply and continues to increase until birth. Using the ratio of L to S (to control for variation in the volume of amniotic fluid), a remarkable correlation has been shown between L/S ratios greater than 2 and the absence of neonatal RDS. With lower L/S ratios, the occurrence of RDS increases significantly. Figure 5-32 demonstrates the characteristic changes in L/S ratio in amniotic fluid during a normal pregnancy. The L/S ratio is less than 1 until about 32 weeks' gestation. By 35 weeks the L/S ratio is 2, and by term the ratio is 4 to 6. Postmature infants have ratios of 6 or greater.

High-risk pregnancies have a variable effect on fetal lung maturation, and maternal disease may accelerate or retard functional development. Early maturation, that is an L/S ratio greater than 2 prior to 33 weeks' gestation, is seen in chronic placental bleeding, some types of diabetes, sickle disease, and some narcotic addiction. These occurrences suggest that intrauterine stress may stimulate the synthesis of surfactant.

The control of fetal lung maturity appears to involve the pituitary-adrenal axis in the fetus. Corticosteroids accelerate lung maturation and have been given to women in premature labor to promote surfactant production. However, other organs could also be affected by this treatment, so that the overall effects may not be wholly beneficial to the fetus (Hallman and Gluck, 1977).

FETAL GAS EXCHANGE

In the fetus the gas-exchange system is the umbilical-placental circulation. The umbilical vein contains the highest concentration of oxygen, which is only about 30 mmHg, and feeds into the low-resistance, high-flow systemic circulation via the inferior vena cava. Despite this low oxygen tension, fetal blood is able to carry sufficient oxygen to meet the needs of the developing fetus for two reasons. First, fetal hemoglobin is able to bind more oxygen at any P_{O_2} below 100 mmHg than can adult hemoglo-

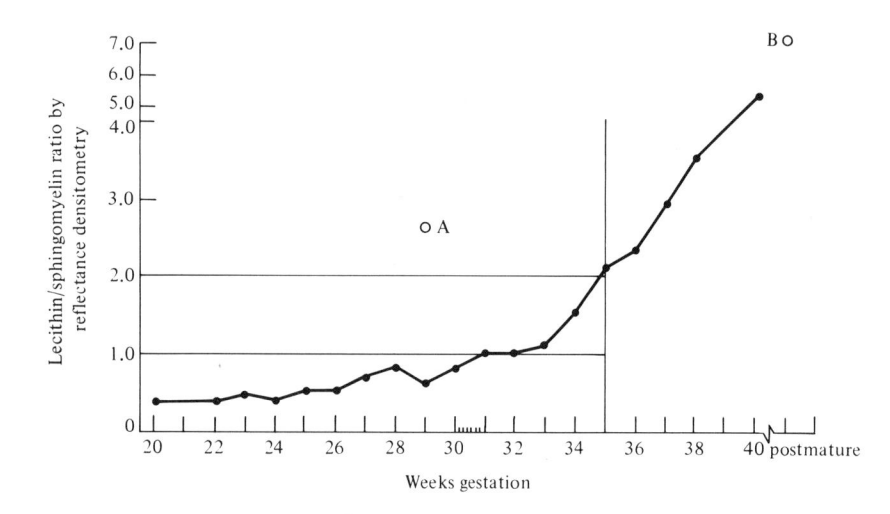

FIGURE 5-32. Curve showing progression of L/S ratios during gestation in normal pregnancy. Note: Menstrual age is given. (A) Acceleration of maturation found in chronic abruptio placentae, diabetes, or heroin or morphine addiction. (B) An L/S value greater than 7 found in postmaturity. (*From L. Gluck, The interpretation and significance of the lecithin/sphingomyelin ratios in amniotic fluid. Amer. J. Obstet. Gynec., 1974, 120, 142. Reprinted by permission of the publisher.*)

bin. Secondly, fetal blood has a higher concentration of hemoglobin, resulting therefore in a greater oxygen-carrying capacity even though the hemoglobin is not fully saturated (see "Development of the Cardiovascular System").

FETAL RESPIRATION

Rapid, shallow respiratory movements occur in the human fetus as early as 9 weeks ca. These respiratory movements probably do not involve a significant exchange of fluid between the lung and amniotic space but may aid in the development of neuromuscular organization required for effective air exchange at birth.

The existence of episodic breathing movements and their association with the rapid eye movement (REM) sleep state suggest early organization of the respiratory centers in the CNS and point to the likelihood of a behavioral-neural, rather than a metabolic, stimulus for fetal respiration. As a consequence, a dramatic change in control of respiration must occur at birth, at which time sensitivity to metabolic and chemical factors becomes the major regulatory stimulus for breathing (Strang, 1977b).

Development of the gastrointestinal system
Anna M. Tichy and Dianne Chong

During the fourth week of gestation the primitive gut forms and later divides into the foregut, midgut, and hindgut. Most of the digestive epithelium and glands are derived from endoderm. The cranial and caudal epithelium arises from ectoderm. Splanchnic mesoderm is the source of the muscular and fibrous components as well as the peritoneum.

ORAL STRUCTURES

Early in development, the embryonic gut is a blind tube with neither oral nor cloacal openings. Two surface depressions appear, cephalically the stomodeum and caudally the *proctodeum*. The stomodeal ectoderm comes into contact with the endoderm of the foregut to form the oral membrane. In the fourth week this membrane ruptures as the stomodeum and foregut merge. The original stomodeal depression is deepened by growth of surrounding structures and forms the oral cavity (see Fig. 5-18; see also "Development of the Face"). At approximately 4 weeks the tongue appears as fusion of two lateral swellings, and a medial swelling occurs.

At approximately the seventh week, salivary gland primordia grow from the wall of the mouth into the underlying mesenchyme. The parotid is derived from the ectoderm, while the endoderm gives rise to the submandibular and sublingual glands.

The major portion of the palate develops from two shelf-like projections extending from the maxillary processes of the upper jaw to the midplane of the oral cavity. During the ninth week fusion occurs, first between the two halves of the palate and then between the palate and nasal septum. Simultaneously, the appearance of bone in the anterior part forms hard palate while in the posterior part no bone appears leaving the soft palate (see Fig. 5-33).

The gastrointestinal tract develops from the endodermal germ layer, which is at first open via the yolk stalk to the yolk sac, and also from mesodermal elements around the yolk sac. The endoderm becomes the epithelial lining, while the mesoderm becomes the thick supporting wall. As with other developing systems, specialization begins sooner in the cranial aspects of the digestive tube than in the caudal portion. The mucosal lining grows faster than the outer wall and thus forms folds which later allow distension of the gut by food and also provide a secretory and absorptive surface.

The endodermal cavity is divided into an intraembryonic section, the primitive gut, and two extraembryonic sections, the yolk sac and the allantois. The primitive gut is divided into three sections: the foregut, midgut, and hindgut.

FOREGUT

From the foregut are derived the pharynx and its derivatives, the esophagus, stomach, duodenum to the common bile duct, pancreas, and biliary apparatus of the liver.

ESOPHAGUS

The esophagus develops from the narrow part of the foregut that extends from the respiratory diverticulum to the stomach. It elongates rapidly at the same time of descent of the heart and lungs; final relative length is reached by the seventh week.

STOMACH

At about the fourth week the stomach appears as a fusiform dilatation of the foregut. A ventral and dorsal mesentery attach it to the body walls. The convex, greater curvature of the stomach is formed by highly active

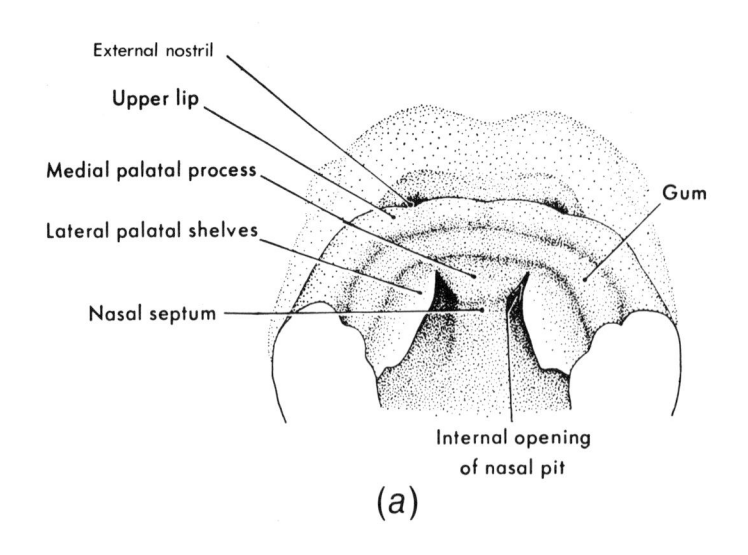

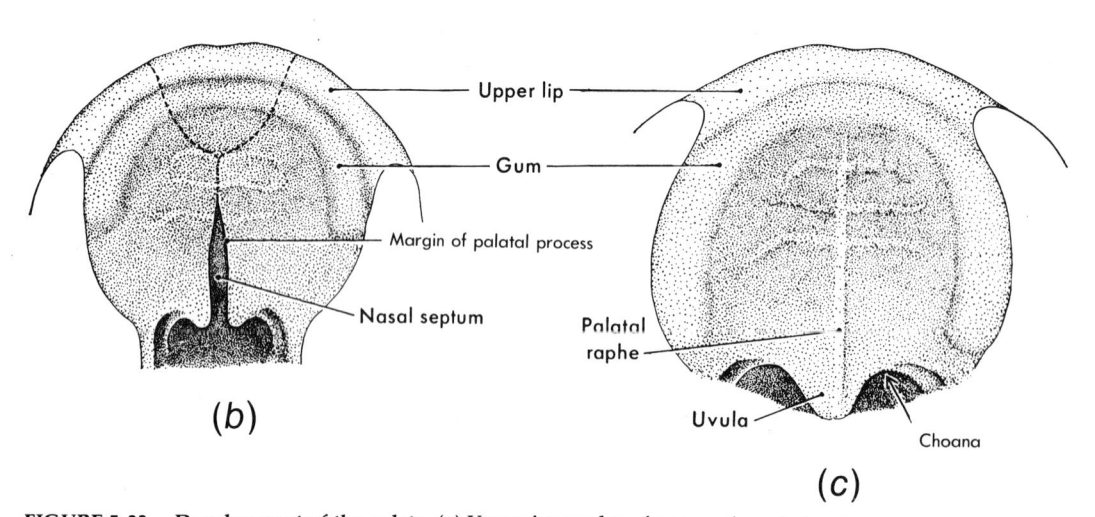

FIGURE 5-33. Development of the palate. (a) Upper jaw and roof as seen from below in an embryo just over 6 weeks ca; (b) the ninth week; (c) late in gestation. (From C. E. Corliss, 1976, p. 266.)

growth along the dorsal border. The fundus is a dilatation of the upper end of the stomach.

By 6 weeks' gestation, the shape of the stomach is similar to the adult shape, but its definitive position is not yet attained. During this time of active growth the stomach rotates causing the left surface to become anterior and the right to become posterior. The ventral and dorsal mesenteries now form the omenta of the stomach. The lesser sac, or omental bursa, is a peritoneal pouch located behind and inferior to the stomach. The cephalic and caudal ends of the stomach, originally in the midline, rotate so that the caudal (pyloric) portion is to the right and rostral and the cephalic (cardiac) portion is to the left. Finally, the stomach assumes a relatively more caudal position migrating from the level of the heart at 4 weeks to the abdominal cavity by 8 weeks.

Sucking and swallowing activities in the human fetus have been identified as early as 12 weeks' gestation, the same time period during which the taste buds appear in the tongue epithelium. Digestion and absorption of the glucose and amino acids contained in the amniotic fluid have been demonstrated. In the full-term fetus, swallowed amniotic fluid provides a daily allotment of 540 mL of fluid and 0.24 to 0.30 g of protein per kilogram of body weight. This comprises a significant component of fetal nutrition; growth retardation is common among fetuses who are unable to swallow as a result of neurological problems or gastrointestinal obstruction. The daily amniotic fluid intake of 540 mL is equivalent to an intake of 4 to 8 L/day of fluid by an adult when computed on the basis of relative body surface area.

DUODENUM

The duodenum is formed from the most caudal part of the foregut and the most cephalic part of the midgut. The duodenum forms a loop that rotates with rotation of the stomach. The caudal portion of the duodenum adheres to the posterior abdominal wall.

HEPATOBILIARY SYSTEM

In the middle of the third week the liver appears as a bud of endodermal cells at the caudal end of the foregut. The liver diverticulum forms only the secretory tubules and duct system. The hepatocytes, forming the glandular tissue, are mesodermal in origin. Although the right and left lobes of the liver are initially the same size, the right becomes much larger. The left lobe later develops into two lobes.

During the sixth week hematopoiesis begins, giving the liver a reddish color. The relatively large size of the liver is mainly due to this hematopoietic activity; the liver weighs about 10 percent of total fetal weight by 9 weeks. Active differentiation of blood cells takes place from the second to seventh months. At birth only small foci are found, however. A latent regenerative ability is retained throughout life.

The second bud of the liver diverticulum is a small caudal portion. This expands to form the gallbladder, and its stalk becomes the cystic duct. These are both solid structures until the seventh week, at which time a lumen is established. The stalk that connects the hepatic and cystic ducts to the duodenum becomes the common bile duct. Beginning from the 13- to 16-week period bile pigment is formed giving the meconium a dark-green color.

MIDGUT

The midgut gives rise to the caudal end of the duodenum, the rest of the small intestine, the cecum and appendix, the ascending colon, and the proximal part of the transverse colon. The midgut initially communicates widely with the yolk sac, but this communication is reduced to the yolk stalk. Elongation of the midgut is more rapid than elongation of the embryo's body. Because of this discrepancy in growth rate, a series of intestinal movements occur in three stages.

Herniation, the first stage, occurs in the sixth week. The elongating midgut forms a ventral umbilical loop which projects out of the abdominal cavity into the umbilical cord. Due to the massive size of the kidneys and the liver, the abdomen cannot accommodate the rapidly growing midgut.

The second stage is the return of the midgut into the abdomen, which occurs during the tenth week. The cause for this return to the abdomen is not certain, but it is thought that the decrease in the relative size of the liver and mesonephric kidney and the increase in the size of the abdominal cavity are important.

HINDGUT

Derivatives of the hindgut are the distal part of the transverse colon, descending colon, sigmoid colon, rectum, upper part of the anal canal, and part of the urogenital system. The hindgut extends from the midgut to the cloacal membrane, which is composed of endoderm of the cloaca and ectoderm of the anal pit. The cloaca receives the allantois ventrally and the mesonephric ducts laterally.

The urorectal septum descends caudally to divide the cloaca into the primitive urogenital sinus anteriorly and the anorectal canal posteriorly (see Fig. 5-39). The upper two-thirds of the anal canal is derived from the hindgut, while the remaining one-third is from the anal pit. The anal pit is formed by mesenchymal proliferation, which elevates the surface ectoderm. Rupturing of the anal membrane at the end of the eighth week establishes the anal canal. The caudal part of the digestive system now communicates with the amniotic cavity, and morphogenesis of the gastrointestinal system is essentially complete.

Development of the endocrine system
Norma J. Briggs

Endocrine tissue is derived from all three embryonic layers. Once differentiation of these germ layers has begun, endocrine tissue begins to emerge.

HYPOTHALAMUS
In the embryonic nervous system the diencephalon gives rise to several structures, one of which is the hypothalamus. The cavity of the diencephalon becomes the third ventricle with the walls and the floor of the diencephalon forming the thalamus and the hypothalamus. The hypothalamus is composed of clusters of cells, called *nuclei*, which produce substances that regulate secretion of hormones from the *adenohypophysis*. These substances are releasing factors, both stimulating and inhibiting, which effect the release of adenohypophyseal hormones. The role of such factors in the developing fetus has not yet been determined.

NEUROHYPOPHYSIS
An outpouching of the diencephalon, the infundibular process, gives rise to the neurohypophysis, which produces two hormones: oxytocin and antidiuretic hormone (ADH). In the adult, oxytocin produces uterine contractions, and ADH influences water balance. While these two hormones have been isolated from fetal pituitaries, their function during fetal development has not been ascertained.

There is some speculation that fetal oxytocin blood levels, which become higher than maternal blood levels near the end of pregnancy, may influence the delivery of the fetus. Women with diabetes insipidus or who have had their pituitary removed surgically have given birth without incident, thus lending support to this speculation.

ADENOHYPOPHYSIS
The adenohypophysis is made up of an anterior and an intermediate lobe. Its formation begins with an evagination of epidermal ectoderm (Rathke's pocket), which separates from the oral cavity and migrates inward, where it ultimately lies next to the infundibular process of the diencephalon.

The adenohypophysis produces between 8 and 10 hormones. The number of hormones depends upon which classification system is used. Each hormone is thought to be produced by a specific cell type; thus the cellular structure of the gland is complex. Differentiation of the cell types begins at about 8 weeks' gestation and is completed by the tenth week.

Somatotropin (STH), or growth hormone, can be found in small amounts in fetal pituitaries by the ninth week of gestation. There then follows a continuing increase in stored STH levels in the pituitaries as well as an increase in blood-level concentration. Despite the availability and abundance of STH, there are no indications that it is necessary for the normal growth of the fetus.

Only two hormones produced by the adenohypophysis seem to have a major influence on the fetus: *adrenocorticotropic hormone* (ACTH) and *thyrotropin* (TSH). ACTH has been detected by the tenth week of gestation. After approximately the twentieth week of gestation, ACTH has been shown to be essential for normal adrenal gland development. TSH has been detected at 11 weeks' gestation in the blood serum. The effects of TSH on fetal development are based on the evidence that if for some reason thyroid function does not develop, the lack of fetal thyroxine feedback results in increased TSH secretion and the development of goiters in the fetus.

ADRENAL CORTEX
The *adrenal cortex*, of mesodermal origin, is derived from a proliferation of coelomic epithelium in the angle between the dorsal mesentery and the urogenital ridge. Proliferation of the cortical cells begins at about 28 days and by 34 days is seen as a discrete mass of cells.

At 5 to 6 weeks' gestation, the adrenal gland is composed of immature cells surrounded by a chin fibrotic capsule. The division of these cortical cells into the outer and inner (fetal) zones occurs sometime after the sixth week. The outer zone has mainly a proliferative activity, while the inner zone shows intracellular changes suggesting steroidogenic activity. The outer-zone cells do not begin to demonstrate functional activity until after midgestation.

Natural and synthetic glucocorticoids can cross the placental barrier. Infants of mothers receiving glucocorticoid administration are at high risk.

ADRENAL MEDULLA
Neural crest cells migrate to form a sympathetic primordium, which lies posterior to the dorsal aorta. It is a recognizable structure by the fourth week of gestation. At about 6 weeks of age, primitive cells (sympathogones) from the sympathetic primordia migrate into the adrenal cortex. The early fetal medulla contains sympathogones and pheochromoblasts, the latter being sympathogones which have undergone further differentiation. The pheochromoblasts mature into pheochromocytes at about

9 to 10 weeks. A positive chromaffin reaction can be seen about the twelfth week and indicates that epinephrine secretion is occurring.

THYROID

The thyroid develops in the fetus as an evagination of the endoderm in the midline of the pharynx. The distal end of the thyroid diverticulum proliferates and becomes a bilobed structure. The thyroid reaches its final location, and the thyroglossal duct atrophies by the seventh week of gestation. The fetal thyroid can accumulate iodide by the tenth week, and triiodothyronine (T_3) and thyroxine (T_4) production is evident by the twelfth week. Fetal thyroid hormones influence the development of bones, teeth, and the CNS, particularly the cerebellum.

Maternal thyroxine can cross the placental barrier, but the quantity is usually not sufficient to prevent brain damage to a fetus in which the thyroid fails to develop or lacks the necessary enzymes to produce fetal thyroxine. Iodides and antithyroid drugs also cross the placental barrier and can produce goiters in the fetus.

The C cells of the thyroid which store and secrete calcitonin are of neuroectodermal origin. This ultimobranchial tissue is derived from the last pharyngeal pouch. At about the sixth week of gestation this tissue is associated with the thyroid. However, not until the twelfth week of gestation are the C cells seen as actually a part of the thyroid gland. The C cells mature about the seventeenth week of gestation. The function of calcitonin in the human fetus is not known at the present time.

PARATHYROIDS

Parathyroid tissue is derived from the third and fourth pharyngeal pouches and differentiates into solid nodules about the fifth week of gestation. They lose their connection to the pharyngeal wall by the sixth week. The tissue from the third pharyngeal pouches migrates with the thymus and becomes the inferior parathyroid glands. The tissue from the fourth pharyngeal pouches attaches to and migrates with the thyroid and becomes the superior parathyroid glands. When parathyroid hormone (PTH) is first secreted in the fetus is unknown. Grown in culture with bone, the parathyroids from a fetus of 12 weeks' gestation demonstrate biologic activity, suggesting that they are functional glands in the fetus.

THYMUS

The ventral portions of the third pharyngeal pouches, with some ectodermal cells of the branchial grooves, give rise to the thymus gland. As the primordia of the thymus gland migrate, they pull the inferior parathyroid glands with them. In its definitive position in the upper thorax, the thymus gland develops as a true lymphoid tissue and by the third month of gestation contains a well-developed lymphocyte population.

The role of the thymus in the human fetus is unknown. In rodents, the thymus has been shown to effect the stem cells of the bone marrow, conferring on them the potential for reacting to antigens. Thus, the thymus does not produce antibodies but facilitates the development of T lymphocytes. There is still some question as to whether the thymus secretes a single hormone, thymosin, or several factors which effect lymphoid structure and function. The influence of other hormones on the thymus can be determined by looking at thymic weight, which is easily observed. Gonadal and adrenocortical hormones have been found to reduce thymic weight, while growth and thyroid hormones increase thymic weight.

PINEAL

The pineal gland (epiphysis) develops from the caudal portion of the roof plate of the diencephalon. The gland begins as an epithelial thickening which then proceeds to evaginate by the seventh week of gestation. The pineal is innervated by the sympathetic nervous system and thought to be indirectly influenced by environmental lighting. There is very little known about the fetal pineal gland. Almost all research on the role of the pineal gland in the adult has been directed toward showing a relation between the pineal and reproductive function.

PANCREAS

A dorsal and ventral outgrowth of the gut fuse at about 7 weeks in the human fetus to form the pancreas. The pancreas is both an exocrine and an endocrine gland. At about the third month of gestation both the acinar cells and the islets of Langerhans have differentiated, and insulin can be measured in the fetal blood. Little or no insulin crosses the placental barrier. Experimentally it has been shown that an increase in blood glucose in a pregnant woman will increase the fetal blood glucose, but the insulin level in the fetus does not increase. This raises the question as to what, then, are the fetal mechanisms of control of insulin secretion. The presence of many alpha cells in the pancreas suggests glucagon may have some control of fetal glucose levels.

PLACENTA

The human placenta forms three protein hormones: human chorionic gonadotropin (HCG), placental lactogen

(HPL), and placental thyrotropin. Only HCG and HPL have been well characterized.

HCG has been detected as early as the seventh day of fetal gestation, and its presence is the basis of one diagnostic test of pregnancy. Maternal blood and urine levels rise during the first trimester and then decline to low levels for the latter part of the pregnancy. HCG enhances production of progesterone by the corpus luteum and may exert an influence on the developing fetal gonads.

HPL appears to have both growth-promoting and lactogenic properties. Maternal blood levels of the hormone increase throughout the pregnancy and disappear rapidly postpartum. The human placenta is also involved in the production of two steroid hormones: progesterone and estrogen.

The endocrine and reproductive systems are closely linked embryologically and functionally. These factors are discussed in "Development of the Reproductive System."

Development of the reproductive system Nancy Reame

PRIMITIVE REPRODUCTIVE TRACT

Although each human being is genetically programmed from the time of conception to develop into either a male or female (sex determination), there is a period during early embryonic life when the individual is bipotential, having neither male nor female characteristics but the capacity to develop either. The bipotential structures that will eventually develop into male or female reproductive organs (sex differentiation) include a pair of indifferent gonads populated with primordial germ cells, two pairs of gonadal ducts (Wolffian and Müllerian), a urogenital sinus, a genital tubercle, and a pair of genital swellings (see Fig. 5-34).

These structures first appear at the fourth and fifth weeks of gestation, although the primordial germ cells are recognizable as early as day 24. Female embryos experience a longer period of asexuality. In both sexes, the indifferent gonads are the first to undergo differentiation, and the external genital structures are the last. It is therefore not possible to determine the sex of the fetus by outward appearance until about the twelfth week of development.

Several events are taking place in the primitive reproductive system of the 5- to 6-week embryo.

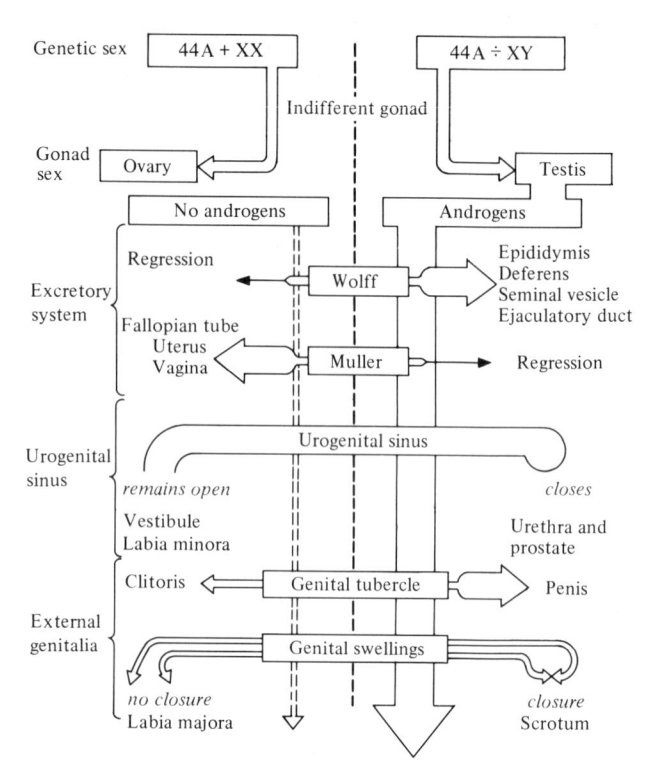

FIGURE 5-34. Developmental fate of the reproductive organs of the indifferent gonad and its hormonal regulation. [From H. Tuchmann-Duplessis and P. Haegel, Illustrated human embryology (Vol. 2): Organogenesis. New York: Springer-Verlag, 1974, p. 100. Reprinted by permission of the publisher.]

ORIGIN AND MIGRATION OF GERM CELLS

Although the gonads are the sites of gametogenesis, the germinal tissue from which future gametes arise does not originate here. Three weeks after conception, even before a gonadal structure is present, primordial germ cells are found in the epithelium of the yolk sac near the developing allantois. By the time the embryo has developed 25 somites (approximately 30 days ca), the majority of germ cells have migrated through the connective tissue of the hindgut, into the region of the developing kidney (mesonephros), and then finally to the adjacent genital ridge, the site of development of the primitive gonads (see Fig. 5-35).

POPULATION OF THE PRIMITIVE GONAD

The gonads appear in pairs on each side of the 4-week-old embryo as small bulges on the surface of the primitive kidney. These genital ridges consist mainly of a proliferating coelomic epithelium overlying a mesenchymal cell

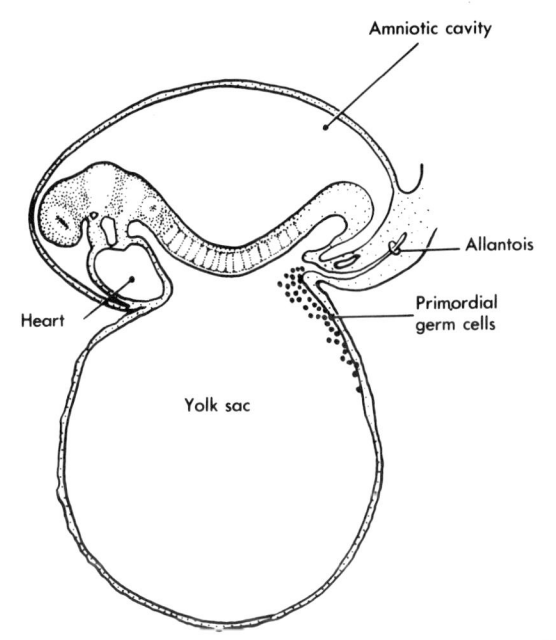

FIGURE 5-35. Origin and migration of the primordial germ cells. Germ cells, first observed in the yolk sac endoderm at day 24, migrate across the hindgut to reach the genital ridges. (*From C. E. Corliss, Patten's human embryology. New York: McGraw-Hill, 1976, p. 11. Reprinted by permission of the publisher.*)

mass (embryonic mesoderm) which has been recently colonized with primordial germ cells. By way of migrating germ cells, the primitive kidney may also contribute cells to the developing gonad and may be essential for its sexual differentiation. Animal experiments have shown that gonads fail to differentiate in vitro unless cultured together with mesonephric tissue.

Although the gonad at this stage is bipotential, its anatomical regions are unipotential: the cortex can only develop as an ovary and the medulla as a testis. The genetic constitution of the germ cells determines the site of gonad colonization and therefore the gonadal sex. If the germ cell sex is female, cells will remain in the periphery (cortex) of the genital ridge; if male, germ cells will continue to migrate into the mesenchyme (medulla). This mesenchymal tissue is regarded as the common origin of the hormone-producing cells of both the ovary (follicle cells) and the testis (Leydig cells).

DETERMINATION OF GONADAL SEX

Development of the medulla of the bipotential gonad into a testis is dependent upon the presence of a Y chromosome. (For a discussion of genetic sex determination, see Chap. 2.) In female embryos, normal differentiation of the primordial germ cells appears to require two X chromosomes, the only cell type in the female that does. In an individual with XO genotype (Turner's syndrome), germ cells undergo degeneration, resulting in a sterile gonad. In addition to being sterile, an individual with Turner's syndrome fails to develop all the female sex characteristics. This is due to the fact that female germ cells induce follicle cell development, which is responsible for ovarian hormone production. In the male, the number of primordial germ cells in no way influences the endocrine activity of the testis. Germ cell sex therefore controls both the fertility and endocrine activity of the ovary, but the testis can continue to secrete testosterone even if the germ cells are totally absent.

DEVELOPMENT OF THE INDIFFERENT GONADAL DUCTS

Until the seventh week of development, the genital tracts of both male and female embryos consist of two Wolffian ducts and two Müllerian ducts (see Fig. 5-36). The initial development of these structures is unrelated to the sex of the zygote, whereas the later phases of differentiation are controlled by the type of fetal gonad. The mesonephric ducts (Wolffian) are the common outlet of the mesonephric tubules of the early renal system. The paramesonephric ducts (Müllerian) develop along the posterior abdominal wall of the embryo. The sex of the embryo determines which set of ducts will proliferate and which will regress; the Wolffian ducts differentiate in the male (25 to 30 days), and the Müllerian ducts develop in the female (44 to 48 days).

DIFFERENTIATION OF THE TESTIS

During the seventh week of development, the germ cells which have migrated to the medullary portion of the gonad are enclosed by the Sertoli cells to become seminiferous cords. Shortly after the seminiferous cords are organized, mitotic division in the male germ cells, now called *gonocytes,* is suppressed. During fetal life, the gonocytes may differentiate into spermatogonia after having migrated to the basement membrane of the seminiferous cord.

Embryonic testes become fetal testes when Leydig cells develop in the interstitium at about the eighth week. The number of fetal Leydig cells gradually increases to a maximum by the third month of fetal life. By the fourth

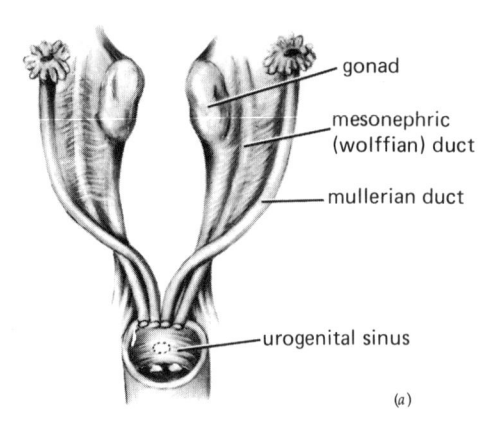

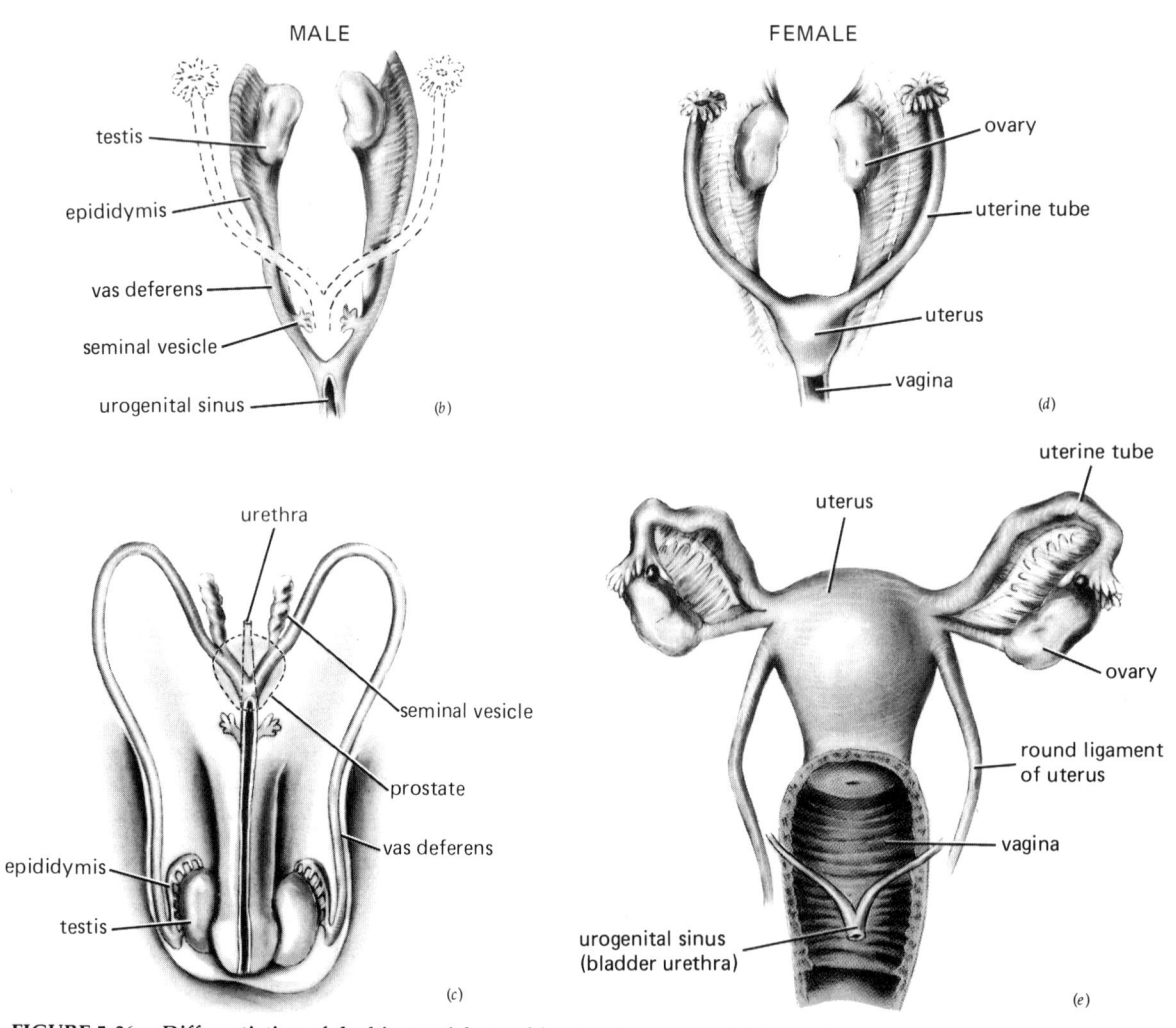

FIGURE 5-36. Differentiation of the bipotential gonad into testis or ovary. (*a*) The primordial germ cells have colonized the peripheral region of the indifferent gonad. (*b,c*) Male germ cells migrate into the central mass of gonadal tissue. The periphery becomes free of cells forming a connective tissue layer. (*d,e*) Female germ cells are surrounded by migrating gonadal cells to form primary follicles. (*From S. Ohno, Sex chromosomes and sex-linked genes. Spinger-Verlag, 1967, p. 163. Reprinted by permission of the publisher.*)

month, Leydig cells begin to decrease and generally have disappeared by the first month of postnatal life. Leydig cells are probably the source of *androstenedione* and testosterone, the androgens responsible for the promotion of further sexual differentiation in the male fetus. During intrauterine life Leydig cells do not influence the differentiation of the Sertoli cells or spermatogonia.

Although all the components of the testis essential for mature reproductive function are present from early embryonic life, their location in the abdomen is deleterious to testicular function. For normal spermatogenesis to take place, the testis must be relocated in a cooler environment. (The mean temperature difference between the abdomen and scrotum is 2.2°C.) During differentiation the embryonic and fetal testis descend to the scrotum. This descent is possible because the testis is attached to a caudal ligament (gubernaculum testis) which terminates in the labioscrotal swelling.

Transabdominal migration of the testis to the inguinal ring occurs during the third month due to the development of the trunk and the abdomen. Usually during the eighth month the testes migrate through the inguinal canal and into the scrotal sac. At birth the inguinal canal is closed in most cases.

DIFFERENTIATION OF THE OVARY

Development of the gonads occurs about 5 days later in females than in males. If the genetic constitution of the germ cells is XX, they will colonize the gonadal cortex rather than migrating to the medullary region. Within the cortex, female germ cells are transformed into oogonia. The number of potential eggs increases greatly in a short length of time, from about 1700 cells during migration to 600,000 during the second month to almost 7 million at the fifth month. After a series of mitotic divisions, the oogonia become transformed into oocytes when they enter upon the prophase stage of the first of two meiotic divisions. The arrest of the meiotic division at this prolonged "resting phase" seems to require the envelopment of the oocytes by a single layer of follicle cells forming the primordial follicle. Primordial follicles are first visible in the embryonic ovary at about 18 weeks and exist in clusters. During later fetal life, a basement membrane is formed, and each follicle becomes completely surrounded by connective tissue, becoming a primary follicle.

Once oocytes have reached the diplotene stages of prophase I, they are incapable of increasing their numbers and can only be lost by atresia or ovulation. During the last 12 weeks of fetal life, the population of viable germ cells declines rapidly to about 500,000 in each ovary at the time of birth. Although germ cells are found in fetal ovaries in all stages of mitosis and meiosis, by the time of birth the ovaries contain only oocytes that have reached the diplotene stage of meiosis. In contrast to the fetal testis, the ovary during fetal life is essentially nonfunctional in terms of secretory activity and does not appear necessary for the differentiation of female organs and genitalia.

DIFFERENTIATION OF THE DUCTAL SYSTEM AND EXTERNAL GENITALIA

HORMONAL REGULATION

The delivery of gametes from the gonads to the site of fertilization requires the formation of the appropriate excretory system. This sex-specific process begins only after the gonads have differentiated so that a long neutral phase exists before further development of the accessory organs.

It appears that differentiation of the secondary sex organs is dependent upon the absence or presence of hormones produced by the early fetal testis. If the testes are removed at a critical period in embryonic life, female differentiation of internal and external organs will occur. Removal of fetal ovaries has no effect on the development of female structures. It is believed that androgens control the masculinization of the external genitalia and maintenance of the Wolffian ducts, thus producing a phenotypic male, while an anti-Müllerian factor causes the regression of the Müllerian ducts. The fetal Sertoli cells of the primitive seminiferous tubules appear to be the source of the factor that causes the Müllerian ducts to regress. If both hormones are absent, differentiation into female sex organs occurs. If only one of the hormones is present, male developmental anomalies result.

The fetal testis exerts its greatest effect on the structures closest to it. The inhibition of oviducts and uterus and the stimulation of epididymis and vas deferens are local events. Laboratory studies have shown that a piece of testis, when grafted onto a fetal rabbit ovary, produces male development only on the one side and fails to affect the other side of the reproductive tract. The masculinization of the external genitalia however is produced by circulating androgens, as in the case of congenital adrenal hyperplasia in female infants or a pregnant woman having received androgenic hormones.

In females, the stimuli necessary for the regression of the Wolffian ducts or the organization of the Müllerian ducts into oviducts, uterus, and vagina are not yet known, although estrogen accelerates the development of the organs of the Müllerian system.

MALE DEVELOPMENT

Providing that both androgens and anti-Müllerian factors are elaborated from the fetal testis, the Wolffian ducts will proliferate and the Müllerian ducts degenerate. Structures which arise from the Wolffian duct system include the epididymis, vas deferens, ejaculatory ducts, and seminal vesicles. Wolffian duct differentiation occurs at a time when fetal testosterone and maternal HCG are at maximal levels (60 to 70 days), suggesting that maternal hormones may be responsible for the initial stimulation of the fetal testis and its effect on sexual differentiation.

The segment of the Wolffian duct opposite the testis forms the epididymis. Below the testis, the Wolffian duct becomes the vas deferens. Just before it joins the urogenital sinus, each duct swells, forming a seminal vesicle. Below the seminal vesicle, the vas deferens is known as the ejaculatory duct. The prostate arises from the urogenital sinus.

During the third month, the phallus continues to elongate and the urethral folds come together to cover the urethral groove and from the penile urethral canal. If development is normal, its orifice will develop on the tip of the glans penis. The genital swellings fuse to form the scrotum, thereby obliterating the potential vagina. A line of closure (raphe) is evident extending along the midline of the scrotum and ventral side of the penis (see Fig. 5-37).

FEMALE DEVELOPMENT

The Müllerian ducts differentiate into oviducts, uterus, and cervix and also contribute to the vagina. The upper portions of the paired Müllerian ducts will remain as two separate tubes forming the oviducts. The septum dividing the two lumen of the midportion will eventually degenerate to form a single uterine cavity, although the uterus passes through a bicornuate stage during development. The myometrium of the uterus forms in the eighth month from the surrounding mesenchyme of the Müllerian system. The body and neck of the uterus become separated by an internal os in the seventh month of development.

The lower ends of the Müllerian system reach the urogenital sinus and fuse with its epithelium to form the vaginal plate, which gradually enlarges and forms a lumen. A defect in the growth, differentiation, or fusion of the Müllerian system can result in paired or malformed structures at any level.

ORIGIN OF THE EXTERNAL GENITAL ORGANS

Development of secondary genital structures is the last phase of sex differentiation to be completed. During the sixth week, a genital tubercle arises (as a swelling below the umbilical cord) and elongates in both sexes to form the phallus with a glans at its end. In the seventh week, urethral folds, a urethral groove, and genital swellings appear. The urogenital sinus, derived from the cloacal membrane, forms the connection from the internal organs to the body surface. These structures remain bipotential until about the third month of prenatal life, which marks the end of the undifferentiated stage.

The difference between the development of the male and female external genitalia depends on the degree of development of the phallus and the extent of obliteration of the urethral groove. In females, the phallus does not enlarge, and the genital folds and labial swellings do not fuse. Instead the rims of the urethral groove form labia minora, and the labioscrotal swellings form labia majora. The phallus bends toward the anus and forms the clitoris. The urogenital sinus elongates, separating the urethral and vaginal orifices. Formation of the female external genitalia is less complex than genitalia formation in the male and more closely resembles the anatomy of the indifferent embryo.

Development of the urinary system
Ida M. Martinson and Nancy V. Rude

STRUCTURE, POSITION, AND SIZE

In contrast to other organ systems which develop in a relatively direct and continuous manner from initial rudimentary organs, the human kidney develops through the differentiation of three cellularly different types of excretory units, or nephrons. Only the last of these three continues to develop throughout fetal and later life to become the mature kidney.

During the middle of the third week of gestation, the first pair of excretory units, the *pronephros,* begin to differentiate from the segmented portion of the intermediate mesoderm on each side of the neural tube, lateral to the seventh somite (see Fig. 5-38). The pronephros is not functional as an excretory organ in the human embryo, and by the end of the fifth week in utero it has degenerated but induces formation of the Wolffian ducts. The ducts extend from the level of the seventh somite to the cloaca, which is the terminal portion of the hindgut before it has differentiated into the rectum, bladder, and rudimentary genital organs.

At the most caudal portion of the pronephros, the second pair of rudimentary excretory organs, the *mesoneph-*

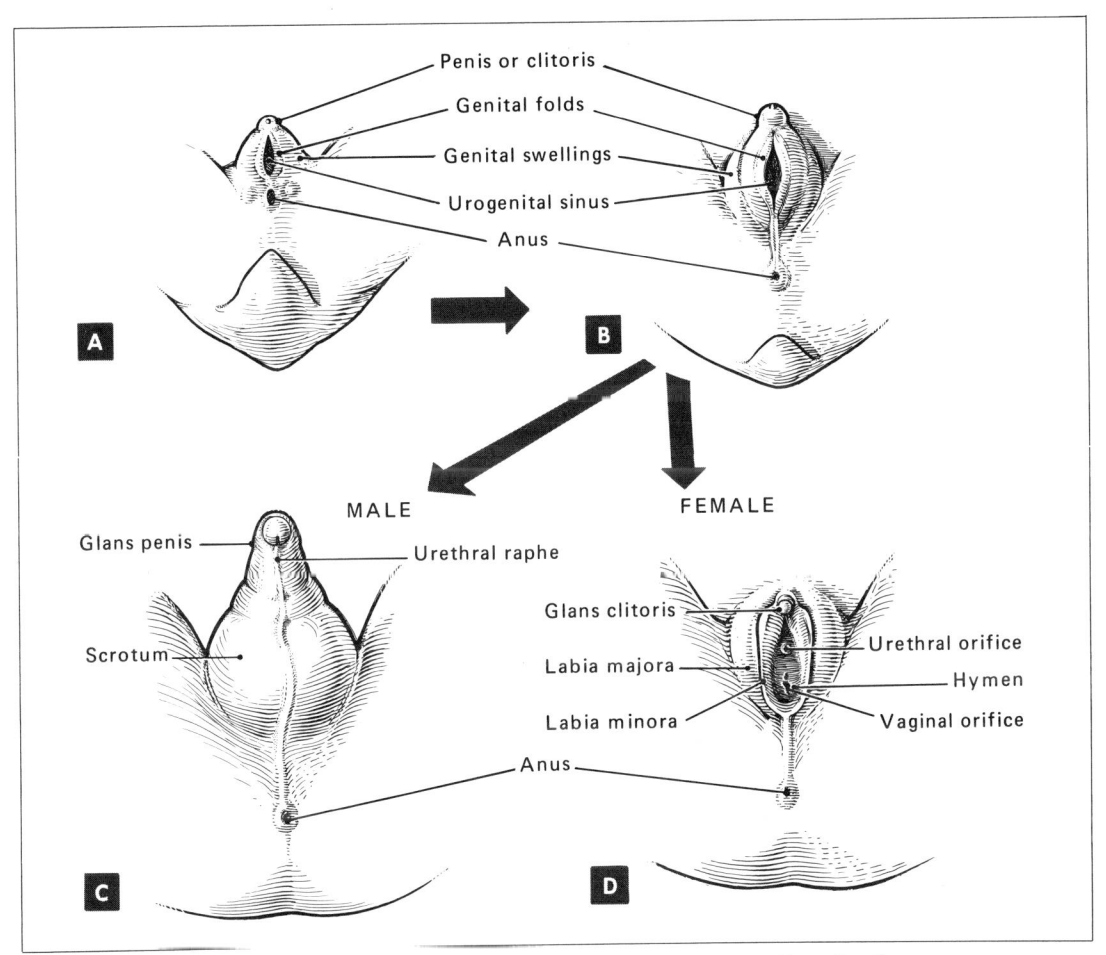

FIGURE 5-37. Embryonic development of external genitalia. (*a,b*) Early undifferentiated stages; (*c,d*) differentiation into male and female genitalia.

ros, begin to develop on the twenty-fourth or twenty-fifth day of gestation from the unsegmented portion of the intermediate mesoderm, also known as the *nephrogenic cord*. Thus, while the most cranial portions of the pronephros are degenerating, the ampulla, or growing tip of the Wolffian duct, which is growing caudally toward the cloaca, seems to provide a chemical stimulus initiating the differentiation and development of *mesonephric vesicles*.

Each small hollow vesicle is formed from a group of cells which segregate medial to the Wolffian ducts. Each vesicle becomes elongated to form an S-shaped tubule, the lateral portion connecting with the Wolffian duct and the most medial portion forming a capsule similar to Bowman's capsule in the permanent kidney. This capsule is indented by branches of a capillary which stems from one of the small arteries diverging from the aorta. This capsule and capillary, a glomerulus, along with its S-shaped tubule, make up the nephron of the mesonephros, which is similar in function and morphology to a nephron of the permanent kidney but lacking Henle's loop. About 40 pairs of these mesonephric nephrons are

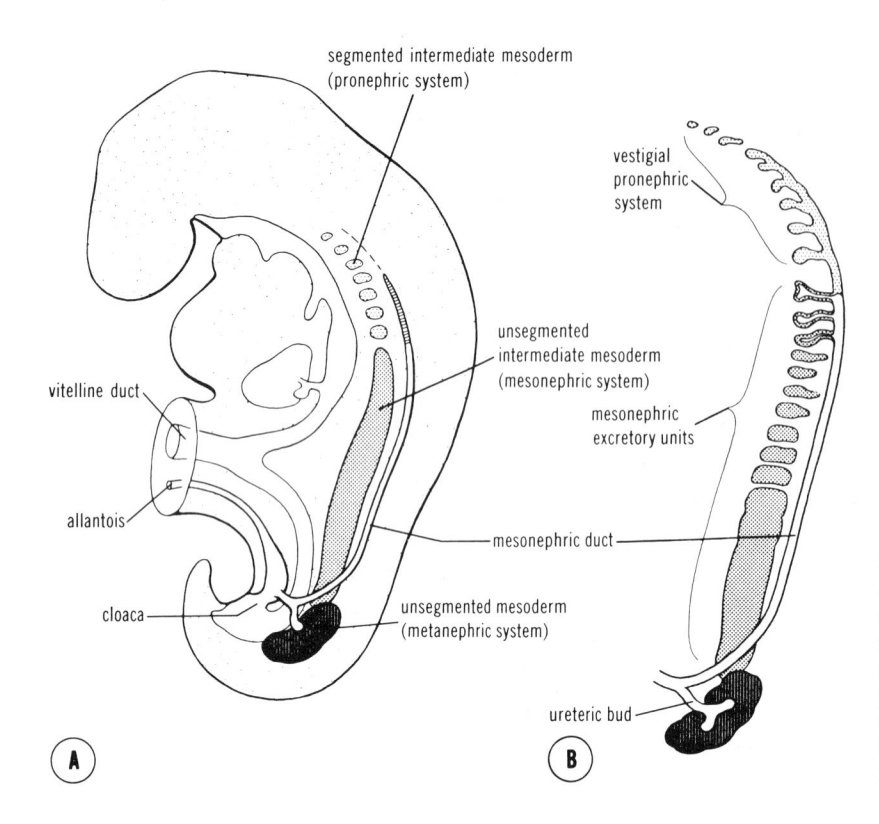

FIGURE 5-38. (a) Schematic diagram showing the relation of intermediate mesoderm of the pronephric, mesonephric, and metanephric systems. (b) Schematic representation of the excretory tubules of the pronephric and mesonephric systems at 5 weeks ca. (From J. Langman, Medical embryology. Baltimore: Williams & Wilkins, 1969, p. 162.)

formed, but only 30 are present at one time since the most cranial nephrons degenerate as the most caudal nephrons are developing.

It is believed that the glomeruli and tubules of the mesonephros begin to function as soon as they are fully differentiated, during the eighth week. The urine excreted by the mesonephric kidney enters the cloaca via the Wolffian ducts and from there is discharged into the amniotic cavity. The mesonephric kidney remains functional throughout the early development of the third and final pair of excretory organs, which will become the permanent kidneys.

The *metanephros*, or permanent kidney, begins development at about the fifth week of gestation. The metanephros appears first as an outbudding of the Wolffian duct near its entrance to the cloaca and penetrates the caudal portion of the metanephric mass of mesoderm. The ureteric bud grows cranially, lateral and parallel to the Wolffian duct, to form the primitive ureter and enlarging at its tip to form the renal pelvis and the treelike branching system of collecting ducts of the permanent kidney. Like the ampulla of the Wolffian duct, the growing end of the collecting duct releases a mucoprotein, which seems to be responsible for the differentiation of nephrons from the metanephric mesoderm. The developing glomeruli become fixed in position as the glomerular arteriole and capillaries develop and become attached to them. The arterioles which enter the glomeruli are extensions of the arcuate arteries, which receive their blood supply from the aorta. The adult pattern of blood supply to the kidney can be recognized by the end of the second month of gestation.

Initially the metanephric kidney is located in the lower lumbar and sacral regions of the fetus, caudal to the bifurcation of the aorta. As the kidney enlarges, it begins to ascend. During the seventh week the kidneys begin to slide forward over the ridges formed by the umbilical arteries and by the ninth week lie above the arterial fork. During their ascent the kidneys rotate about 90° so that the convex borders initially facing dorsally come to lie laterally. Newer blood vessels are continuously being formed at higher and higher levels while the older lower vessels degenerate. This migration of the kidney is thought to be due in part to the diminution of the curvature of the body and in part to the growth of the body caudal to the kidneys as well as to the continuous cranial growth of the ureteric bud.

The permanent kidney begins excretory function after the sixth week of gestation, but the primitive ureter is not functionally open to the urogenital sinus until the ninth week of gestation. Urine formed by the permanent kidney prior to the ninth week of gestation enters the cloaca through the Wolffian duct and is discharged into the amniotic cavity. After about the sixth week of gestation a septum, known as the *urorectal septum*, begins to form in the cloaca, separating the urogenital sinus from the anorectal canal. At about the time when the urorectal septum is completed, the cloacal membrane breaks down forming separate openings to the outside for the urogenital sinus and rectal canal.

The primitive urogenital sinus can be distinguished as having three separate portions. The most cranial portion is known as the allantois. Initially this portion is a narrow canal containing a lumen. Later the lumen shrinks and is obliterated, becoming a thick fibrous cord known as the *urachus* connecting the bladder to the umbilicus. Immediately caudal to the allantois is the largest portion of the primitive urogenital sinus, the urinary bladder. Below the urinary bladder lies the third portion of the urogenital sinus, the phallic portion. The development of this part greatly differs between the two sexes. In the male the phallic part differentiates into the prostatic and membranous urethra and the penile urethra. In the female the phallic part differentiates into the urethra and vestibule (see Fig. 5-39).

When the permanent kidney begins to function, the mesonephric kidney begins to degenerate, leaving only the Wolffian ducts after the third month of gestation. Initially the Wolffian ducts are the only openings into the urogenital sinus. With the growth of the ureteric bud, separate ducts, *ureters*, form and open independently into the bladder. In male fetuses the Wolffian ducts then continue development to become the epididymis and the vas deferens, while in the female they remain only rudimentary structures.

The growth process which segregates all nephrons to the cortex or outer portion of the kidney and the collecting ducts to the medulla or inner portion of the kidney has not been completely defined, but it has been observed that the radial branching of the ureteric bud can account for the formation of the papillary ducts, into which each nephron drains. By the end of the fifth month of gestation, all the nephrons have been arranged toward the periphery of the kidney with the most developed nephrons located more centrally. The boundaries between the cortex and the medulla are well defined, even though only about one-third of the total number of nephrons have been formed. Cortical growth is greatest from this time until birth, with many new nephrons being formed until a mean total of 1.2 million nephrons per kidney are present at birth. Formation of new nephrons normally ceases at birth; most nephrons are fully differentiated and functional after 36 weeks' gestation. The weight of the fetal kidney at the end of the fifth month of gestation is about 3 g, while at birth the kidney normally weighs 20 to 40 g.

FIGURE 5-39. Diagram showing partitioning of the cloaca by the urorectal septum and position of the urinary bladder, ureter, and mesonephric duct. (*Modified from K. L. Moore, 1977, p. 209.*)

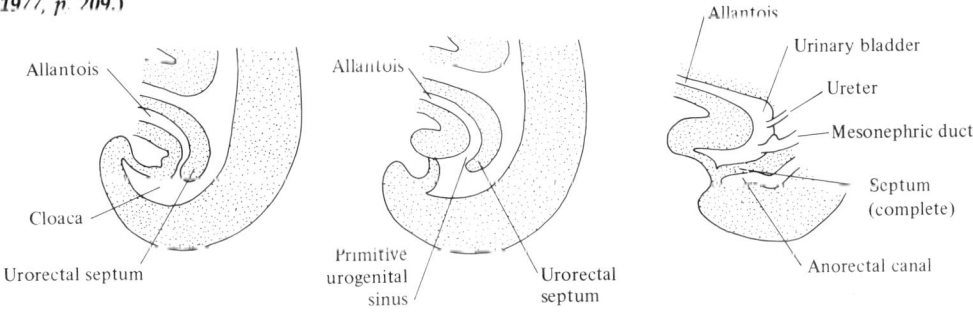

FUNCTION OF THE URINARY SYSTEM

As stated above, the pronephric kidney never functions as an excretory organ in the human embryo. The mesonephric kidney, on the other hand, does function as an excretory organ. Urine elaborated by the mesonephric kidney is a glucose- or protein-free fluid which seems to be simply an ultrafiltrate of fetal serum since its urea and other solute concentrations are the same as fetal plasma.

It has been shown that the metanephric kidney begins to elaborate what can be considered a "true" urine after about the eleventh week of gestation (Gersh, 1937; Keen and Hewer, 1924). This is considered true urine in the sense that it is not simply an ultrafiltrate of plasma but is slightly acidic, free of glucose and protein, contains lower concentrations of sodium and chloride ions than fetal plasma, has a higher concentration of urea and creatinine than fetal plasma, and is hypotonic. The fact that fetal urine is hypotonic to fetal plasma is a good indication that the loops of Henle are functioning properly in removing sodium ions from the plasma filtrate while not allowing water to leave the fluid in the nephrogenic tubule to as great an extent. On the basis of morphological criteria it is thought that the loop of Henle could function in a manner similar to that of the adult after the thirteenth week of gestation (Gersh, 1937). At this early age, then, an osmolar gradient is being established in the fetal kidney with increasing osmolarity of the corticomedullary junction to the tip of the papilla.

Renin synthesized in the kidney and released into the blood combines with other plasma enzymes to form angiotensin II, which is perhaps the most powerful circulating vasoconstrictor in humans. Circulating angiotensin II levels in the fetus increase continuously throughout gestation and are partially responsible for concurrent increases in arterial blood pressure. Fetal circulating angiotensin II levels are greater than maternal levels for some time before birth.

Circulating angiotensin II is also responsible for the stimulation of aldosterone secretion from the adrenal cortex. Circulating aldosterone levels increase throughout gestation until just before birth, when fetal circulating aldosterone levels are two to four times that of the maternal blood. Aldosterone in turn stimulates the reabsorption of sodium. Increasing levels of aldosterone increase the ability of the kidney to reabsorb sodium.

Tubular reabsorption of glucose is believed to begin taking place by the time urine is produced. Glucose is actively transported out of the tubular system of fetal nephrons in a manner similar to the adult mechanism (Alexander and Nixon, 1963). About 60 percent of the filtered sodium is reabsorbed by the fetal nephrons at 12 weeks' gestation, increasing to 90 percent just before birth.

The fetus is in a constant state of mild metabolic acidosis, and the manner in which the fetus regulates blood pH is not known at this time. Secretion of excess hydrogen ions by the fetal kidney is not vital to survival since fetal acid-base balance is controlled via the placenta by the maternal lungs and kidneys. The mild acidosis seen in the fetus may in part be due to low levels of circulating bicarbonate ion in the fetal plasma. It has been shown that the fetus excretes bicarbonate ion to maintain a lower circulating concentration than the adult (Pitts et al., 1949; Tuvad et al., 1954). The reason for this difference has not as yet been accounted for.

In general, the fetal kidney is not the most important excretory organ in utero. Placental membranes are freely permeable to water, urea, and electrolytes, so that fetal and maternal blood are in equilibrium with regard to most metabolites. Fetuses without kidneys will survive until birth, but since the most important function of the kidney in utero seems to be its contribution to the amniotic fluid, these fetuses will have little amniotic fluid.

Development of the integumentary system Mary Tudor

The two-layered integumentary system evolves from two primary germ layers. The epidermis is of ectodermal origin; the underlying dermis, of mesodermal origin, specifically from mesenchyme.

EPIDERMIS

The embryo is initially covered with a single layer of cuboidal ectodermal tissue resulting in the translucent appearance. By the end of the fourth prenatal month, however, the four epithelial layers are present. The basal layer is the germinating layer, responsible for continued growth of the epidermis.

The outermost horny layer of dead cells causes the fetal skin to lose its earlier transparency. These cells also compose a percentage of the vernix caseosa as they are sloughed.

The epidermal ridge patterns (those on the tips of the fingers are used for fingerprinting) on palms, fingers, soles, and toes result from ridging of the germinative layer induced by underlying dermal ridges. Ridge patterns are established by the seventeenth week ca and evident externally by the sixth fetal month. Ridge patterns develop secondary to surface contours, which are genetically determined (Smith, 1976). Abnormal hand or foot morphology gives abnormal ridge patterns or unusual frequency of patterns. Dermal ridge patterns, then, are examined in evaluation for possible genetic disorder.

DERMIS

The dermis evolves from nearby (lateral) mesoderm (mesenchyme); collagenous fibers are present by the third fetal month and elastic fibers by the sixth. It was originally believed that cells from the dermatomes, a portion of the somites, migrated laterally to form the dermal layer. It is now thought that this portion of the somites makes a minimal contribution (Arey, 1965). Subcutaneous fat is deposited beneath the dermal layer primarily during the last trimester.

PIGMENTATION

Dendritic cells, of neural crest origin, migrate through the dermis and eventually become *melanocytes* at the dermis-epidermis junction. Formation of melanin is inefficient before birth. Although dark-skinned fetuses do have more pigmentation than white-skinned ones, they are much lighter at birth than the parents. Pigment formation increases markedly after birth, however, in response to sunlight.

GLANDS

Sebaceous and *sudoriferous* (apocrine and eccrine) glands are of ectodermal origin. Most sebaceous glands form as a budding of a hair follicle. These glands begin to produce sebum prenatally which, along with sloughed primordial epidermal cells and *lanugo* hairs, forms vernix caseosa, the pastelike substance covering the neonate's skin. Sebaceous gland activity diminishes significantly after birth; "cradle cap" is the result of continued high activity of sebaceous glands of the scalp.

Sudoriferous, or sweat, glands evolve as a downgrowth from the epithelium beginning in the fourth month. The glands are believed capable of functioning by the seventh month but most likely to a negligible degree until after birth.

NAILS

Also of ectodermal origin, nails begin development about the tenth week ca. The nails reach the ends of the fingers and toes about 34 and 36 weeks ca respectively.

HAIR

Hair follicles originate from the germinating layer of the epidermis but grow down into the dermal layer. The papillae and capillaries are of mesodermal origin. Epithelial cells of the germinal matrix become keratinized and are pushed outward as hair growth.

Early hair, lanugo, is visible by about the twentieth week, initially on the upper lip and eyebrows and later on the head and body. This lanugo is shed soon after birth and replaced by coarser hair. Hair patterning on the scalp reflects growth and shape of the underlying CNS. Like dermal ridge patterns, it may give clues to abnormal morphogenesis.

Dysmorphology Mary Tudor

Dysmorphology is the study of aberrant development of form. During the first 12 weeks of prenatal development the risk for abnormal morphogenesis and resulting congenital malformations, many of which are incompatible with prenatal or postnatal life, are great. A congenital malformation may be major or minor, external or internal, singular or one of several, and compatible or incompatible with life. In addition to anatomical abnormality, defects at the cellular and intracellular levels also occur (such as Hirschsprung's disease or phenylketonuria). Any part of the body may be affected. Etiology of a congenital abnormality may be a genetic or chromosomal abnormality, environmental insult, or interaction of both. Mechanical forces of uterine constraint can also cause malformation (Smith, 1979). In approximately 60 percent of cases of human malformation, exact etiology is not known.

The worst birth defect, it has been stated, is to never have been conceived at all due to abnormal gametes. It is estimated that 15 to 25 percent of all conceptuses are spontaneously aborted (Lauritsen, 1976). An estimated 6 to 7 percent of all live-born infants have congenital defects, half of which are detected at birth (National Foundation, 1979). Severe congenital abnormalities account for 15 to 20 percent of perinatal deaths (Claireaux, 1973) and are the leading cause of death in the first year of life in the United States (Apgar and Stickle, 1968).

Single minor malformations are not uncommon; 14 percent of normal neonates have one minor anomaly. However, three or more minor malformations indicate that a major problem may exist. Ninety percent of all neonates with three or more minor malformations are found to have either a primary anomaly which initiated the others (collectively termed a *malformation complex*) or a malformation syndrome (Smith, 1976a).

Structural defects result from incomplete morphogenesis; Smith (1976b, p. 415) describes incomplete morphogenesis as resulting from one of the following:

- Agenesis, or lack of development
- Hypoplasia
- Incomplete separation
- Incomplete closure
- Incomplete migration of mesoderm
- Incomplete rotation
- Incomplete resolution of early form
- Persistence of earlier location

The earlier in development abnormal morphogenesis occurs, the more devastating the results. Survival of the embryo is unlikely if the error in morphogenesis occurs prior to 23 days (Smith, 1976b).

GENETIC BASIS

Abnormal chromosome number or structure, a mutant (abnormal) gene, and polygenic inheritance are responsible for a significant percentage of congenital malformations, or defects, at the cellular or intracellular levels. In all cases, the effect is potentially present from conception; abnormal biochemical activity from abnormal gene expression is the assumed mechanism.

Chromosomal abnormalities, such as an extra chromosome (trisomy), translocation, or deletion which involves multiple genes, result in multiple malformations. When a specific pattern of malformation is recognized, it is designated a *malformation syndrome*. For example, Down's syndrome is recognizable clinically by the particular pattern of malformations associated with this disorder.

It is estimated that 3 percent of all conceptuses, 55 to 60 percent of spontaneous abortions, and 0.5 percent of all neonates have chromosomal abnormalities (Boué, Boué, Lazar, and Gueguen, 1973; Lauritsen, 1976; Smith, 1976b). Thus, the majority of fetuses with chromosomal abnormalities are spontaneously aborted or do not survive birth or neonatal life.

An abnormal autosomal dominant or X-linked gene or homogeneity for an abnormal autosomal recessive gene causes abnormal morphogenesis following the laws of Mendelian inheritance. The defect may be expressed in early morphogenesis or later in childhood or adulthood.

Most common, single malformations in otherwise normal persons are thought to be polygenic: the combined effects of many genes. These malformations, including clubfoot, cleft palate, pyloric stenosis, and neural tube defects, make up a major portion, 47 percent, of infants born with congenital anomalies. These malformations are "predominantly the consequence of minor differences at many gene loci, none of which may be held responsible for the abnormality" (Smith, 1970, p. 316).

ENVIRONMENTAL BASIS

Abnormal morphogenesis may be the result of harmful environmental agents, *teratogens*, acting on the embryo either as a mutagenic agent (causing mutation of genes) or by direct influence. A teratogenic agent is "one that produces, during embryonic or fetal development, a major or minor deviation from normal morphology or function in the offspring" (Shepard and Lemire, 1976, p. 3). Teratogens can be classified into five categories:

- Infectious agents (viruses)
- Drugs
- Radiation
- Substance abuse (e.g., alcohol)
- Chemicals (e.g., organic mercury)

Unlike genetically induced defects, environmental agents may affect the developing human at varying times during gestation with potentially variable results. Timing is critical in determining outcome; the earlier in development the environmental insult occurs, the more severe and generalized the abnormality (see Fig. 5-40).

Early development, conception to about 14 days' gestation, has been considered "safe" in terms of malformation from teratogenic agents. At this early stage of rapid development teratogenic agents are more likely to cause disorganization and destruction of the conceptus, to cause complete regeneration, or to prevent implantation. The embryo is highly sensitive to teratogens; the fetus is less affected morphologically; however, growth and/or function may be adversely affected. As with a genetic abnormality, the conceptus may continue to term or be aborted, depending on the severity of the malformation as well as the timing of the insult.

The fetus tends to outgrow the uterine cavity late in gestation and not uncommonly is molded by uterine constraint prior to birth. The resulting deformations, often called *positional* or *postural deformities*, predominantly affect the craniofacies and limbs. The prognosis for most such deformations is usually excellent, though postnatal positioning and/or constraint may sometimes be merited, as in dislocation of the hip (Smith, 1979).

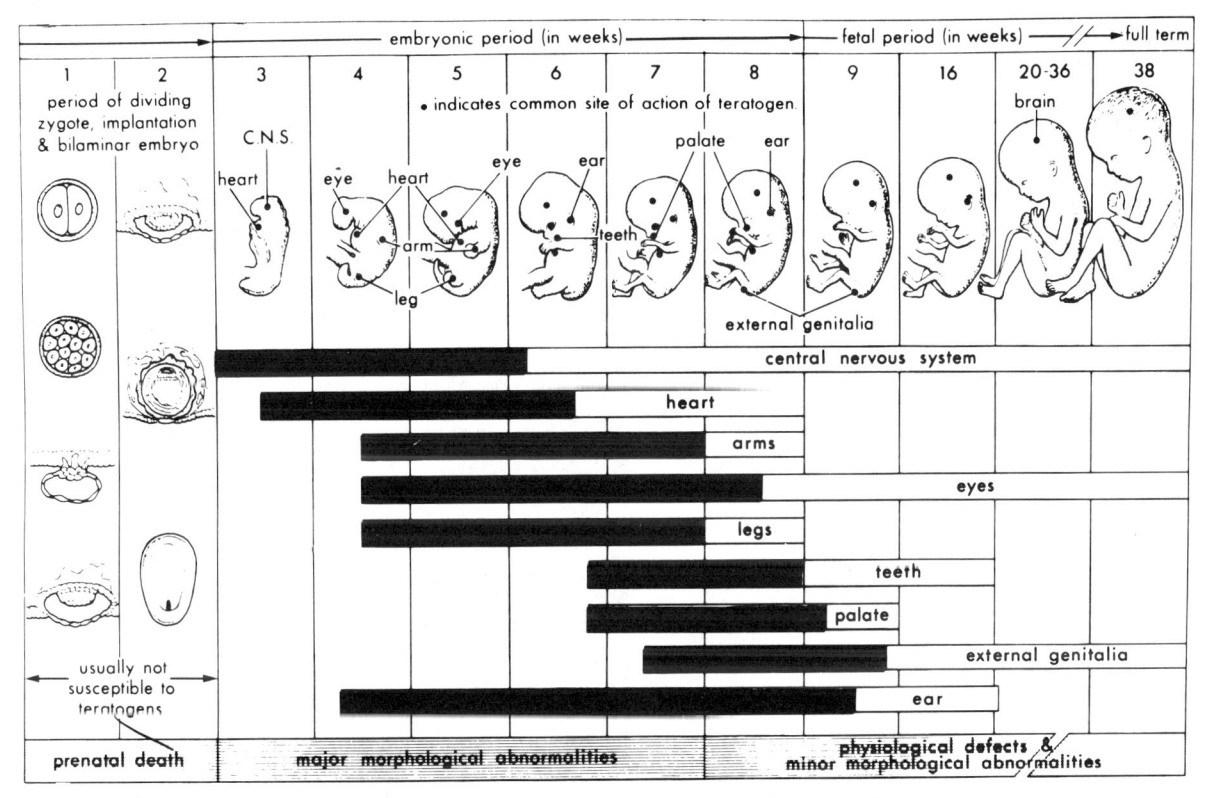

FIGURE 5-40. Schematic drawing of sensitive or critical periods in prenatal development. Dark shading of the bars denotes highly sensitive periods; light shading indicates periods that are less sensitive to teratogens. (*From K. L. Moore, 1977, p. 136.*)

BEHAVIORAL TERATOLOGY

In an attempt to determine more subtle effects of teratogenic agents, the field of behavioral teratology emerged. In the absence of gross morphological abnormalities, the existence of behavioral defects determined by postnatal assessment is used as an indication of teratogenic effects on the CNS. "The discovery of behavioral effects in the absence of morphological alteration of the CNS implies that behavioral testing is a sensitive technique for the detection of adverse consequences of prenatal environmental stresses" (Butcher, 1976).

Great Britain and Japan require animal tests of behavioral toxicology as part of routine drug-toxicity screening procedures. In the United States such animal testing is recommended but not required by state or federal law (Grant, 1976). As interest and data regarding fetal behavior have increased, in utero studies of CNS integrity and possible prenatal behavioral deficits have begun. Thus behavioral toxicology may soon involve prenatal study.

A process as rapid and complex as development during the first 38 weeks of life cannot be expected to be free from inherent failures and external insults. The risks are substantial; the journey from conception to birth is not completed by many. Birth is the momentous end to life's most perilous and extraordinary season.

SECTION 2
The Fetal Period: The Period of Elaboration and Growth

Fetal development Mary Tudor

The fetal period is one of final differentiation and elaboration of the basic form and organ systems and their function achieved in the embryonic period. Although the organ systems are all basically functional by the end of the embryonic period, extrauterine viability is not possible due to immaturity of the systems, especially the nervous and respiratory systems. Increased organ maturation during the fetal period allows tenuous viability outside the uterine environment by 26 weeks' conceptual age (ca).

However, the fetal period is primarily one marked by incremental linear growth and beginning motor, sensory, and other functioning preparatory for and necessary in extrauterine life.

At the end of the embryonic period, the human typically is 30 mm long, crown to rump, and weighs 1 g. Size at birth depends on rate of growth and length of gestation, both of which can be affected by multiple factors including fetal, maternal, placental, and environmental factors. Differentiation of the nervous, sensory, and musculoskeletal systems during embryogenesis makes fetal movement possible. This movement and sensory response become more refined during fetal life.

MORPHOLOGICAL CHANGES
Morphological change is much less striking during the fetal period as primary morphogenesis has been completed. However, there are more subtle changes in external features and general appearance aside from increase in size. A synopsis of these changes with reference to size is given below by conceptual age.

9 TO 12 WEEKS
The fetus's head remains disproportionately large, making up one-half of total body length. The fetal body straightens, and the hands no longer cover the face but drop more to shoulder level. The arms have nearly reached their relative length, and fingernails have appeared; however, the pelvis is small, and the legs remain short and thin. The arms have fully rotated 90° laterally so that they point dorsally. The legs have also rotated 90°, but medially so that the knees point more ventrally than laterally.

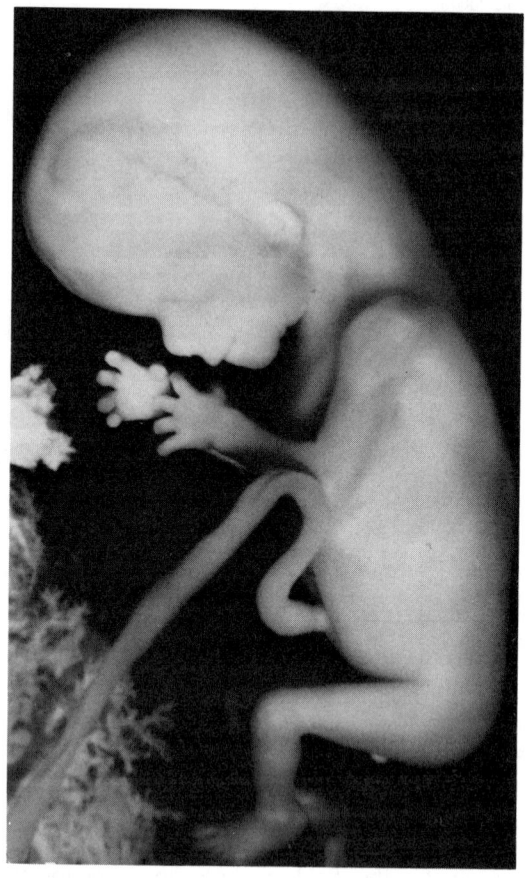

FIGURE 5-41. An 11-week fetus. (*From K. L. Moore, 1977, p. 85.*)

Facial development proceeds, especially in the lower face and mandible. The eyelids fuse, and the eyes remain widely spaced (hyperteloric). The external ears are still below eye level and are relatively small. The neck becomes clearly defined during this period and is less flexed and more mobile. This feature strikingly enhances the more childlike development of the face.

During the tenth week the intestines are accommodated into the enlarging abdomen. The external genitalia can be differentiated by careful inspection. Fetal movement begins early in the fetal period, possible because of neuromuscular development. These movements are not felt by the mother, however.

13 TO 16 WEEKS

The period of major risk for spontaneous abortion is over, and the fetus is no longer at risk for *major* malformation; however, insults after the twelfth week can result in minor malformations or, more likely, growth disturbances. The second trimester is just beginning, but fetal growth has accelerated quickly. This is a period of extremely rapid growth. From the twelfth week until term, the fetus will increase in mass 100 times (Metcoff, 1978).

Amniocentesis is now possible; there is about 200 mL of amniotic fluid present. The trunk and legs continue to lengthen considerably making up a larger portion, two-thirds, of total body length. The skin is beginning to become less translucent. The neck becomes even more defined, the ears stand out from the head close to their relative position. The lower jaw continues to grow out.

Between 8 and 16 weeks ca, the length has almost tripled, and weight has increased 25 times.

17 TO 20 Weeks

Neonatal proportions are reached during this period due to increased trunk and leg length. The head now makes up one-quarter of total body length. The legs reach their final (neonatal) relative length, and toenails are present. Lanugo is evident, and vernix caseosa, sloughed ectodermal cells, accumulate on the fetus's skin. Eyelashes and head hair appear. Subcutaneous (brown) fat is beginning to form in the posterior neck region.

21 TO 25 WEEKS

The fetus during these 5 weeks completes the major tasks of organ maturation, approaching extrauterine viability. As growth continues, fat deposition gives a plumper appearance. The skin is much less translucent and head, face, and body hair is substantial.

26 TO 32 WEEKS

During this last trimester, only "finishing touches" are achieved in outward appearance, but substantial growth continues for the first half of this period, especially in subcutaneous fat deposition. Rate of head growth diminishes in the thirty-second week, but peak body growth velocity occurs between 30 and 34 weeks ca at 200 to 225 g/week.

Tenuous viability is now possible, however, with significant risk of mortality and morbidity. The body is more proportioned with a plumper appearance due to the increasing proportion of body fat. The eyelids are no longer fused. The testes are descending through the inguinal canal. The fetus begins to experience uterine constraint on free body movement and subsequently assumes a more flexed posture with reduced full-body movements.

33 TO 38 WEEKS

As maternal and placental limits are approached, growth rate slows and becomes variable between fetuses. Fetal sex, pariety, and other factors significantly influence growth during this period and thus size at birth. Placental growth essentially stops at about 35 weeks. Changes of extrauterine viability increase with each succeeding week as the fetus increases in size and strength. Movement diminishes greatly the last 2 weeks, and the fetus assumes final position for birth.

BODY COMPOSITION

Change in body composition in prenatal development is significant, reflecting the absolute increase in cell number. Fetal composition also tells a great deal about nutritional needs for this normal growth.

Fetal body composition and nutrient stores are greatly influenced (late in gestation) by maternal nutrition (Apte and Iyengar, 1972). As expected, there is a decrease in percentage of water and an increase in percentage of protein and fat, the greatest increase occurring between 34

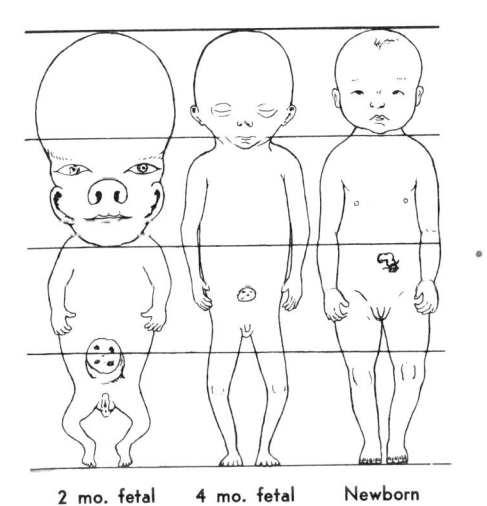

FIGURE 5-42. Change in body proportion during fetal development.

and 36 weeks ca (Ziegler, O'Donnell, Nelson, and Fomon, 1976). During the fetal period the percentage of extracellular water decreases, and intracellular water increases.

FETAL VITAL SIGNS

FETAL HEART RATE

Cardiac contractions, which began about the twenty-second day of life, can be heard by the twelfth to fourteenth week ca (14 to 16 ma) using electronic equipment. With a fetal stethoscope, heart tones are audible by about 4 weeks later. Base-line fetal heart rate (FHR) is normally 120 to 160 beats per minute (bpm) at term. A change in FHR is frequently associated with fetal movement and uterine contraction. As gestation progresses, the heart rate decreases and beat-to-beat variability increases indicating increasing influence of the fetal autonomic nervous system, especially the vagal component (Rochard, 1976).

Monitoring FHR near term has long been used as an evaluation of fetal well-being. However, tachycardia and bradycardia are not 100 percent reliable indications of fetal distress; a normal rate may be maintained until death (Rochard, 1976). The fetus must then be evaluated on other parameters of cardiac response.

The oxytocin challange test (OCT), or stress test, is used to evaluate fetal-placental status. The response of FHR to oxytocin-induced uterine contractions is evaluated. More recently, nonstressed monitoring of FHR has been introduced (Lee, 1975; 1976). In this procedure, FHR and fetal movement as well as uterine contractions (spontaneous) are monitored for 20 to 30 min. (No medications are administered.)

A normal, uncompromised fetus shows the following:

- A stable heart rate of 120 to 160 bpm
- Beat-to-beat variability of 10 to 25 bpm
- FHR acceleration with fetal movement: a reactive pattern

A compromised fetus shows the following:

- A stable heart rate of 120 to 160 bpm
- Decreasing or loss of beat-to-beat variability (less than 6 bpm)
- Absence of FHR accelerations with fetal movement: a nonreactive pattern
- Late FHR decelerations with uterine contractions

RESPIRATORY MOVEMENT

Contrary to past theory, respiratory movement is a normally occurring behavior prenatally and not an indication of fetal distress (Duenhoelter and Prichard, 1977; Manning, 1977; Mantell, 1976; Timor-Tritsch, Dlerker, Zader, and Hertz, 1978). "It is biologically essential to have the structures that make later adaptive responses ready at a period somewhat prior to the time when such reactions must work" (Carmichael, 1970, p. 449). Respiratory movements move amniotic fluid through the lungs and possibly aid in lung development.

Respiratory movement has been detected as early as 9 weeks ca (11 ma) but is highly irregular at this early stage. The fetal pattern is established by 12 weeks ca. After about 34 weeks ca, a respiratory movement rate of 40 to 70 movements per minute is observed, averaging 60 per minute. Fetal respiratory movements are normally discontinuous; movements are continuous for up to 10 min with periods of apnea, usually no longer than 45 s, between. Thus, respiratory movements in a normal fetus are probably present 50 to 90 percent of the time (Dawes and Robinson, 1976; Manning, 1977).

Two different patterns of common respiration movement have been described. The patterns vary in rate, regularity, amplitude, and whether they are accompanied by general fetal movements. The primary pattern is rapid, shallow, and irregular. The relatively uncommon pattern is slow with deeper, gasplike movements. The characteristics of fetal respiratory movements appear to have high intraindividual stability (Marsal, Gennser, and Kullander, 1978).

Fetal respiratory movement is primarily diaphragmatic with indrawing of the thorax due to airway resistance in the fluid-filled lungs. Movements are controlled by the medullary respiratory centers; higher central nervous system (CNS) integrity is not essential as respiratory movements have been observed in anencephalic fetuses. Thus, the pattern is similar to the term neonate with a condition giving airway resistance (Duenhoelter and Pritchard, 1977; Manning, 1977). Blood-gas values also do not directly influence respiratory movements in the uncompromised fetus.

There is a *diurnal rhythm* in incidence of fetal respiratory movements apparently due to variations in the sleep-wake state of the fetus. Respiratory movements have been found to be present about 50 percent of the time around dawn and rise to 90 percent of the time in late evening (Dawes and Robinson, 1976). The primary respiratory pattern is absent when the fetus is awake and in quiet sleep; breathing movements occur primarily during rapid eye movement (REM) sleep, the fetal state 70 percent of the time. (Dawes and Robinson, 1976; Wilds, 1978). Fetal position seems to be correlated with respiration pattern prior to birth; cephalic presentation is correlated with normal respiratory pattern.

Like FHR, fetal respiratory movements are affected by amniocentesis; the procedure produces a significant reduction in respiratory movement (Manning, 1977). Fetal distress (hypoxia) is accompanied by decreased respiratory movements. It is proposed that observations of fetal respiratory movements can predict the fetus that will be in distress during labor and birth (Dawes and Robinson, 1976). In one study, 84 percent of patients with fetal breathing movements occurring less than 50 percent of the time had fetal distress secondary to uteroplacental insufficiency. However, only 1 percent developed fetal distress when respiratory movements were present 60 to 90 percent of the time (Manning, 1977).

TEMPERATURE

Fetal temperature is 0.5 to 1.0°C higher than maternal core temperature. If maternal temperature rises, fetal temperature (and heart rate) rises as well.

FETAL MOVEMENT

Fetal movement can also be considered a vital sign as noted above. Actual number of daily movements is variable between fetuses; thus each fetus determines his normal values. Fetal heart rate response to fetal movement is the more critical variable and indication of well-being. (Fetal movement is discussed in more detail in following sections.)

FETAL GROWTH

Embryonic growth is primarily dependent on inherent (genetically determined) factors, or growth potential; fetal growth, however, is dependent on maternal characteristics, or transplacental growth support, and other extrafetal factors (Cook, 1977). The hyperplasia of embryonic development continues during the fetal period. Hypertrophic growth begins midgestation, about 25 weeks ca, and continues postnatally (Cook, 1977; McCance and Widdowson, 1978)

Embryonic and fetal growth in height and weight follow a sigmoid curve. After the smaller gains of the first 2 weeks, linear growth occurs, which then slows after 32 to 34 weeks ca (34 to 36 ma). Size and degree of maturation are not synonymous. Rate of growth determines size at birth; length of gestation determines level of maturity at birth. Fetal growth rate and length of gestation are not related. Growth rate is familial; length of gestation is not. (Ounsted and Ounsted, 1973).

Clinically, fetal growth continues to be monitored under normal conditions by maternal weight gain and fundal height. Special laboratory procedures and ultrasonic study may be utilized in cases where there is real concern about growth or morphology. Research continues to establish fetal growth parameters. It has been recommended, however, that each specific population have its own fetal growth chart, particularly for the last trimester, due to variations caused by maternal-environmental factors (Ounsted and Ounsted, 1973). (Note: As the fetal growth charts illustrated use ma, so, in this section, will ma be noted first with ca in parentheses.)

Brenner et al. (1976, p. 555) give three reasons for accurate data regarding fetal growth in the clinical setting:

- To identify the effects of pathologic pregnancies on fetal size
- To aid in the evaluation of diagnostic measurements of fetal growth
- To identify potentially abnormal children in the antepartum or immediately postpartum periods

FUNDAL HEIGHT

Fundal height is evaluated during the course of gestation. The *MacDonald rule* states that from about the twelfth week height in inches of the fundus above the top of the symphysis pubis will be eight-sevenths of the duration, in weeks, of the pregnancy. The rule is most accurate between 16 and 36 weeks ma (14 and 34 weeks ca) (Romney, Gray, Little, Merrill, Quilligen, and Stander, 1975).

Low fundal height may mean decreased fetal growth, reduced amniotic-fluid volume, inaccurate dates, or abnormal fetal lie. The reverse is also true, with the added possibility of multiple births. Further studies are warranted when height of the fundus is abnormal by 3 cm for estimated gestational age.

FETAL WEIGHT

Total maternal weight gain during pregnancy in nonpoverty, industrialized countries is 10 to 12 kg (22 to 26 lb): 1 kg in the first trimester, 3 kg in the second, and 6 kg in the third. In the second trimester, 50 percent of the weight gain is fetus, placenta, and amniotic fluid. In the third trimester these account for 90 percent of the weight gain (Metcoff, 1978, p. 418). Although maternal weight gain is related to fetal birth weight, maternal weight gain is not an accurate reflection of fetal weight because of impinging variables.

Fetal weight in utero is important in clinical manage-

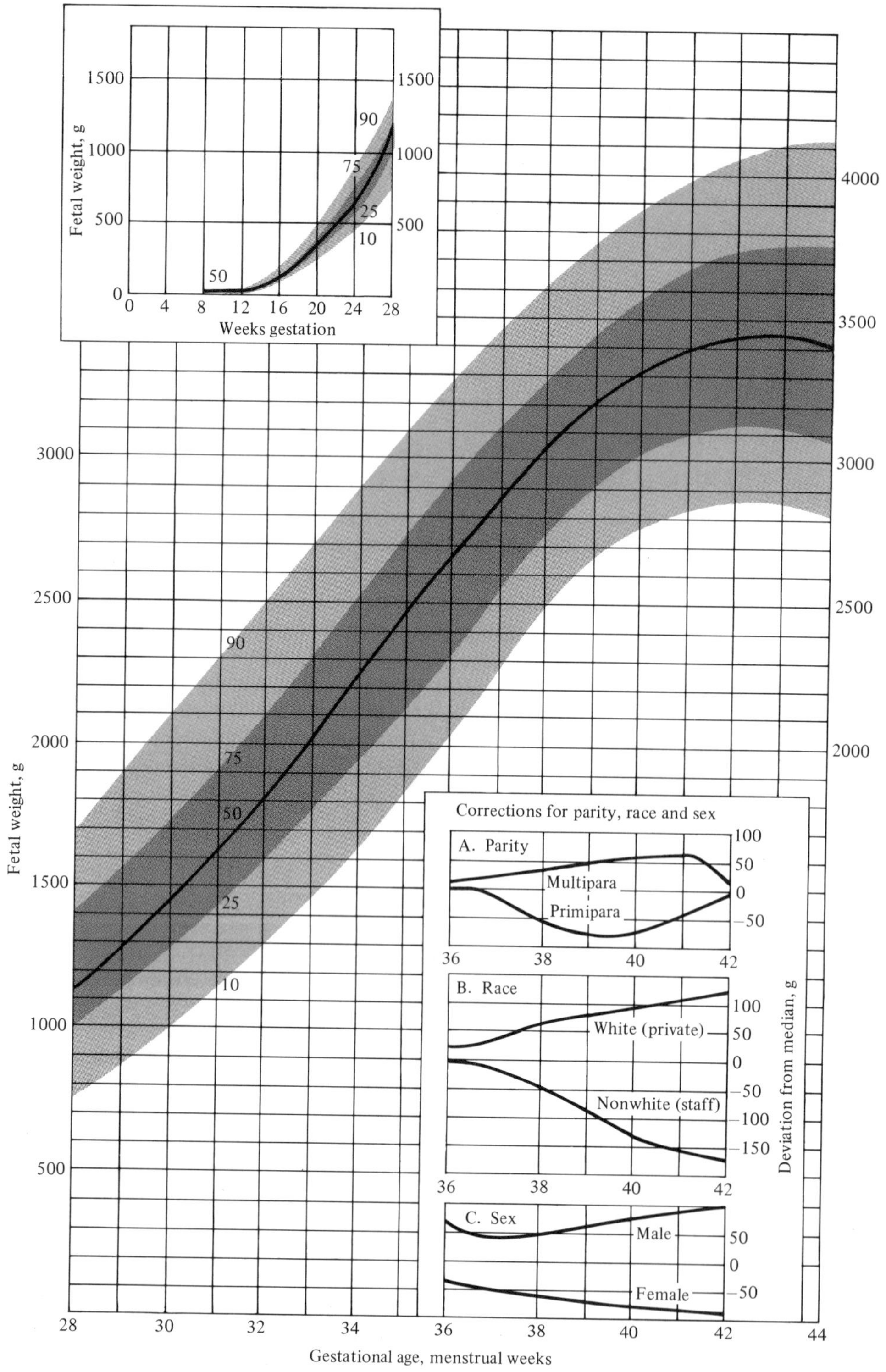

Fetal weight, g
Weeks gestation
50
75
90
25
10
Fetal weight, g
Gestational age, menstrual weeks
90
75
50
25
10
Corrections for parity, race and sex
A. Parity
Multipara
Primipara
B. Race
White (private)
Nonwhite (staff)
C. Sex
Male
Female
Deviation from median, g

ment to evaluate growth and to determine fetal age. Thus, studies of intrauterine fetal weight extrapolated from data obtained by ultrasound have been carried out. Fetal weight is estimated by correlation to a linear measurement: length, head, or trunk circumference.

Fetal weight is the dimension of growth most susceptible to extrafetal influences, most affected by maternal and environmental variables. Thus, normal growth curves of weight must eliminate those fetuses exposed to factors known to cause abnormal weight. As noted above, it has been suggested that fetal growth curves be developed for the specific population under study. This is especially important in weight curves (Ounsted and Ounsted, 1973). Also, of all fetal measurements, weight is least indicative of development or gestational age (Southgate, 1978).

One widely used growth curve for fetuses prematurely born at 24 to 42 weeks ma (22 to 40 ca) is that by Lubchenco, Hansman, and Boyd (1963) (see Fig. 6-12). The data were collected from Caucasian fetuses only with 30 percent of Spanish, Mexican, and Indian extraction. The socioeconomic statuses of the parents were indigent or part-pay. Also, the altitude of residence of this Colorado population is high: over 5000 ft. All of these factors can affect fetal growth. As a result, the findings may be applicable only to other fetuses who fall within these same parameters.

More recently, Brenner, Edelman, and Hendricks (1976) have collected data that they propose give better representation of fetal growth in the United States. The larger sample was made up of voluntarily aborted fetuses and live-born infants from a racially mixed group (50 percent white, 49 percent black, 1 percent other nonwhite) at lower elevation. (*Note:* Menstrual age is used.)

During the 8 weeks of early and embryonic development, total weight gain is approximately 1 g (see Fig. 5-43). However, weight increases rapidly from then to term. Actual fetal weight gain is most rapid, showing a linear pattern, between the twelfth and thirty-sixth weeks of gestation ma (10 to 34 ca); this period is actually the first growth spurt in human development. From 36 weeks to term fetal growth rate slows. Thus, weight for gestation overall shows a sigmoid curve.

Although actual fetal weight gain is significant throughout the fetal period, velocity of weight gain, stated in grams of increase per week, varies significantly during this period (see Fig. 5-44). Peak velocity of weight gain occurs between 32 and 36 weeks ma (30 and 34 ca) when the fetus gains 200 to 225 g/week (Metcoff, 1978). The fetus doubles in weight between 31 weeks ma and term (Brenner et al., 1976). After 36 weeks ma (34 ca), velocity drops rapidly. "Physiological utero-placental insufficiency is proposed as the causal factor for this drop" (Campbell, 1976, p. 273).

While fetal weight is relatively consistent among fetuses throughout most of pregnancy, variations in fetal weight have been demonstrated to occur after 30 to 34 weeks ma (38 to 32 ca) (Brenner et al., 1976; McKeown et al., 1976; Metcoff, 1978; Ounsted and Ounsted, 1973). Brenner et al. offer a system to correct the median fetal weight for maternal parity, fetal sex, and maternal race and/or socioeconomic status (SES).

FETAL LENGTH

Fetal length is less affected than weight by extrafetal factors; thus less variation is seen among fetuses. Length is a better reflection of fetal development, rather than merely increase in size. Although the relative increase in length in the early and embryonic periods is tremendous, from microscopic to 30 mm, the major increase in length, as in weight, is during the fetal period.

Crown-rump length Crown-rump length is the standard measurement for the embryonic period; it is also used during the early fetal period but is often replaced by C-H length at 22 to 26 weeks ma (20 to 24 ca), when the legs reach their final (neonatal) relative proportion (Moore, 1977).

Significant increase in C-R length began in the embryonic period at 6 weeks ma (4 ca). Early C-R growth is exponential until 10 to 12 weeks ma (8 to 10 ca) and then becomes linear (Berger, Edelman, and Kerenyi, 1975; Brenner et al., 1976; Campbell, 1974; Cook, 1977; Golbus and Berry, 1977; Southgate, 1978). The rate of growth be-

FIGURE 5-43. Fetal weight gain from 8 to 44 weeks ma. The 50th (median), 10th, 25th, and 90th percentiles of fetal weight in grams are graphed. [*From W. E. Brenner, D. A. Edelman, and C. H. Hendricks, A standard of fetal growth for the United States of America. Amer. J. Obstet. Gynec., 1976, 126(5), 559.* © *The C. V. Mosby Company. Reprinted by permission of the publisher.*]

tween the sixth and fourteenth weeks ma (4 and 12 ca) is quite predictable at 10 mm/week and is recommended as the measurement (by ultrasound) to determine fetal age at that stage. It is then replaced by a biparietal diameter (Campbell, 1974; Cook, 1977).

Crown-heel length Crown-heel length is a standard measurement for clinical studies, using preterm and full-term infants. Because leg length is a significant proportion of total body length, C-H length is probably a more significant measurement at later gestational ages.

A growth curve for C-H length from 24 to 42 weeks ma (22 to 40 ca), as well as weight, weight/length ratio, and occipital-frontal circumference (OFC), reported by Lubchenco, Hansman, and Boyd from Colorado is widely used. Again, these data represent fetuses from Caucasian, low-SES mothers at a high altitude. Fetal length, as weight, is reported to be diminished by increased altitude (Ounsted and Ounsted, 1973), and SES has a significant if somewhat unclear effect on total fetal growth.

Usher and McLean report C-H length for Canadian fetuses, also Caucasian, from "widely varying socioeconomic backgrounds and national origins" (1969, p. 902) at sea level (see Fig. 5-45). Mean values tend to be similar to those of Lubchenco, Hansman, and Boyd until 36 weeks ma gestation, when the Canadian fetuses are larger. At 40 weeks, there is a difference of 2 cm, which, according to Usher and McLean's data, represents a difference of 3 weeks gestational age (the mean for 37 weeks ma). In addition, the spread between the 10th and 90th percentiles is greater for the Denver sample: there is greater variation from the median.

HEAD MEASUREMENTS

Head size is a reflection of brain growth and is thus critical in evaluating normal fetal development as well as gestational age. Rapid head growth occurs from 14 to 30 weeks ma (12 to 28 ca) and slows from 30 to 34 weeks ma until term. Head growth is least and last affected by malnutrition and other insults, the "brain-sparing" phenomenon. As with height and weight, there is less interfetal variation in early and midgestation, with variability seen during the last 5 to 6 weeks (Adamsons, 1978). In normal growth OFC and BDP bear a linear relation to length and trunk circumference, and thus relative measurements give information beyond either independent head or length measurements (Southgate, 1978).

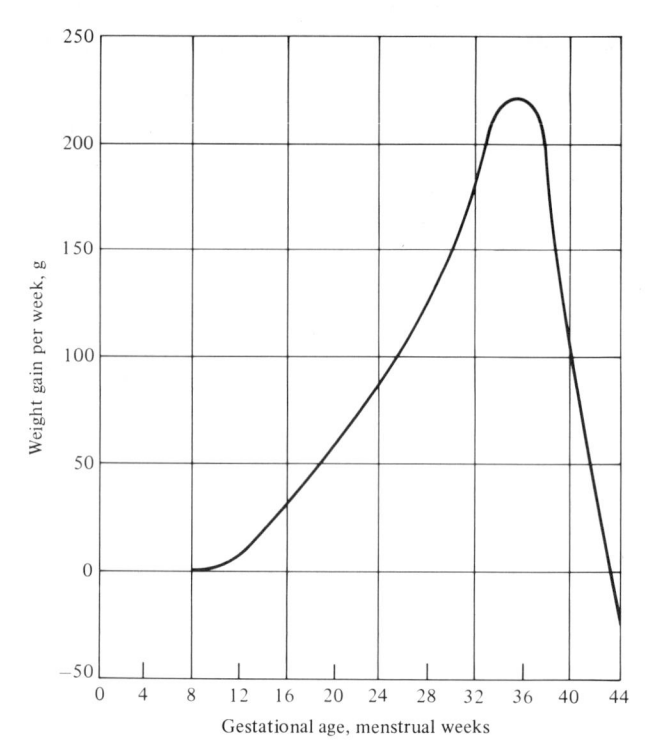

FIGURE 5-44. Velocity graph showing weekly fetal weight gain throughout pregnancy. (*From W. E. Brenner et al., 1976.*)

Occipital-frontal circumference Occipital-frontal circumference is, as postnatally, the maximum value of horizontal circumference across the frontal and occipital areas of the skull. Lubchenco, Hansman, and Boyd (1966) provide a growth curve obtained from live births for 26 to 42 weeks ma (24 to 40 ca). This sample was the same as that for weight and length curves. A difference of 1 cm is noted between Lubchenco, Hansman, and Boyd's mean OFC and that of Usher and McLean after 35 weeks ma, again a 3-week difference in gestational age.

Rapid linear growth in OFC (11.5 mm/week) occurs from 14 to 30 weeks ma. Growth slows at 30 to 36 weeks ma (28 to 34 ca) to 7.2 mm per week (Campbell, 1971).

Biparietal diameter Biparietal diameter, the distance between the two parietal protuberances, has become an invaluable and accurate measurement obtained by ultrasound to evaluate fetal age and intrauterine growth and to detect suspected cephalopelvic disproportion (CPA) requiring cesarean section.

As with other fetal measurements, diameters obtained earlier in gestation are more accurate than those obtained

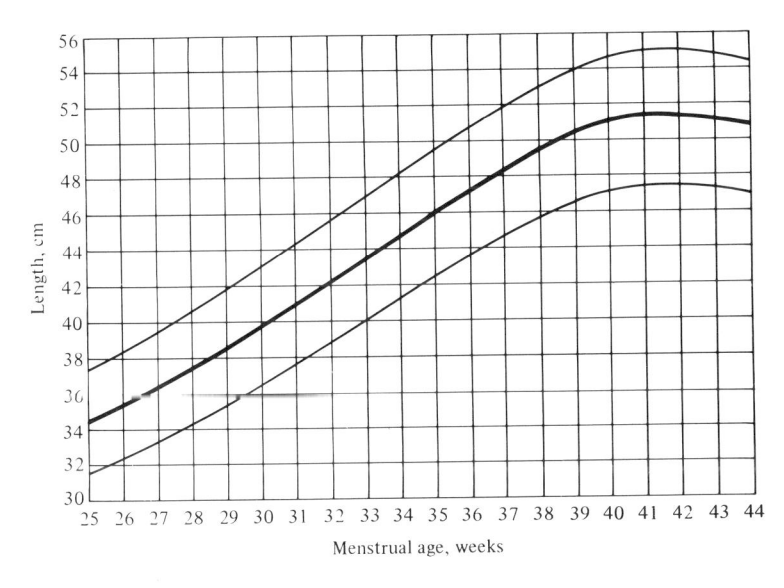

FIGURE 5-45. Smoothed curve values for the mean ± 2 standard deviations of C-H length from 25 to 44 weeks ma (23 to 40 weeks ca) obtained from direct measurement. [*From R. Usher and F. McLean, Intrauterine growth of live-born Caucasian infants at sea level: Standards obtained from measurements in 7 dimensions of infants born between 25 and 44 weeks of gestation. J. Pediat., 1969, 74(6), 901–910.* © *The C. V. Mosby Company. Reprinted by permission of the publisher.*]

later. Biparietal diameters show the same curve as OFC growth: The curve is linear between 14 and 30 weeks ma (12 and 28 ca) (see Fig. 5-46). Between the twelfth and twentieth weeks ma (10 and 18 ca) BPD is so consistent between fetuses that a single measurement is a good assessment of age (Adamsons, 1978; Campbell, 1971).

"The biparietal diameter in the normally growing fetus appears to correlate better with fetal age than any other morphometric or biochemical indicator" (Adamsons, 1978, p. 613). After 20 weeks ma, BPD is more variable, although some recommend its use up to 30 weeks ma (Cook, 1977).

Between the fourteenth and thirtieth weeks ma (12 and 28 ca), BPD increases by about 3.3 mm per week. The rate decreases to about 2 mm/week between 30 and 36 weeks ma and to 1.2 mm/week in the last 4 weeks (Campbell, 1971). This continued rapid growth of the CNS makes it more vulnerable than other body systems during the fetal period. Although fetal age may be determined by one measurement, assessment of head growth is best obtained by a series of measurements (Campbell, 1971).

TRUNK MEASUREMENT

Trunk measurements, chest or abdominal, are also an indication of growth. A relation between trunk and length measurements and trunk and head measurements has been established. Also, a relation between trunk and fetal weight has been established. All measurements are obtained by ultrasound.

The relation between abdominal and head measurements (Jordaan and Dunn, 1978) and chest and head measurements (Cook, 1977) as well as thorax to length measurements can give indications of intrauterine growth retardation. Abdominal circumference (AC) is smaller than OFC before 36 weeks ma. At 36 weeks, AC and OFC are equal, and by term AC is greater than OFC.

Discrepancy from average ratio of chest circumference (CC) or AC to BPD or OFC can identify intrauterine growth retardation where head size (neural growth) has not been affected. Small BPD or OFC with normal chest size may indicate a CNS abnormality. In small-for-gestational-age (SGA) infants, head-to-chest ratio can also indicate duration of slowed growth. Normal head-to-chest ratio in SGA fetuses indicates early onset of growth retardation or chronic growth retardation. With an increased head-to-chest ratio, growth retardation is believed to have started in the third trimester (Wladimiroff, Bloemsma, and Wallenburg, 1978).

FACTORS INFLUENCING FETAL GROWTH

It has long been recognized that early fetal growth proceeds at a relatively unencumbered, consistent, linear pattern until the latter part of gestation. After 32 to 36 weeks ma (30 to 34 ca), variation in growth becomes evident, and final size at birth is a result of the interaction of several factors. These factors can be divided into two categories: fetal and maternal-placental.

FETAL FACTORS

Early growth is genetically directed; rate of hyperplasia, or mitotic cell division, is under polygenic determination (Smith, 1977). (Genetic control of basic growth and differentiation is discussed in Chap. 3.) Fetal growth is considered relatively independent of the fetal CNS and pituitary gland as anencephalic fetuses continue to grow in utero (Cheek, 1977; Cook, 1977). Late fetal growth is, however, influenced by fetal gender and race.

Gender Males grow faster than females during the last trimester, and after approximately 26 weeks ma males are larger. At birth, males are approximately 0.5 to 1 cm longer, 40 to 150 g heavier, and have an OFC approximately 0.5 cm larger than females. One theory regarding this difference in fetal growth rate is that, simply, males are genetically larger. This is true of adults; however, whether this genotype is expressed prenatally is still questioned.

Race Mean size at birth as well as rate of maturation varies significantly between population groups (Ounsted and Ounsted, 1973; Smith, 1977). A percentage of these differences between races is the consequence of multiple gene differences. However, other factors which affect growth (nutrition, health care, and others) are often difficult to separate from race.

Prior to about 34 weeks' gestation, no significant differences in size have been found between racial groups (controlling for other factors). After 34 to 36 weeks ma (32 to 34 ca), several studies have reported size differences. Mean size of term Negro fetuses has been found to be smaller than term Caucasian fetuses (Brenner, et al., 1976; Garn and Bailey, 1978; Smith, 1977). Also, Negro fetuses have a shorter gestation. One study reports twice the prevalence of "preterm" births of Negro fetuses (Garn and Bailey, 1978). As noted, it is difficult to separate racial and socioeconomic factors. The general assumption, however, is that there is variation and to different degrees between different population groups. "It seems unlikely that these differences are explicable in terms of social class, birth-

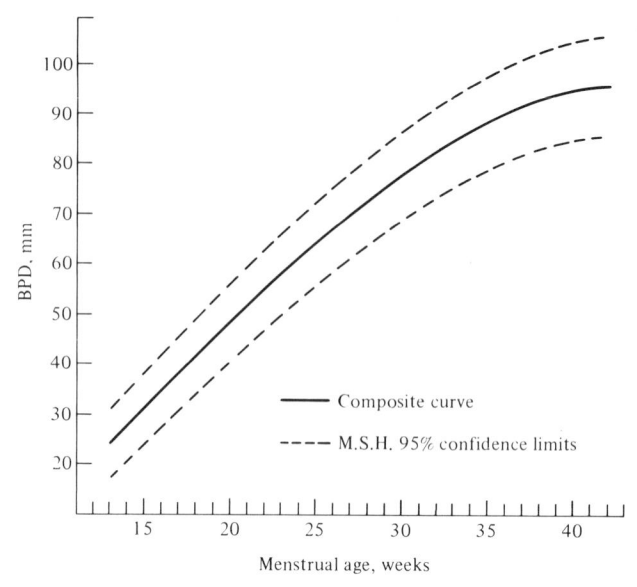

FIGURE 5-46. Biparietal diameter obtained by ultrasound plotted against menstrual age. [From S. N. Weimer, M. J. Flynn, A. W. Kennedy, and F. Bonk, A composite curve of ultrasonic biparietal diameters for estimating gestational age. Radiology, 1977, 122(3), 781–786. Reproduced by permission of the authors and The Radiological Society of North America, Inc.]

rank, maternal height and weight or duration of pregnancy" (Ounsted and Ounsted, 1973, p. 2).

The actual polygenic differences may be compounded or disguised by socioeconomic and other influences; thus, the exact difference may not be evident (Alvear and Brooke, 1978). Again, it has been suggested that fetal growth curves be developed for the specific population in question, which would reflect genetic as well as nongenetic influences.

MATERNAL FACTORS

Although genetic factors are in control of embryonic and early fetal development and have some influence on size at term, later fetal growth is most significantly influenced by maternal factors. In comparison with maternal influences, genotype has a relatively minor impact. In addition to or as a result of these factors, it is postulated that a fixed, maternal influence or constraint operates in every woman and will be expressed with every fetus she conceives (Ounsted and Ounsted, 1973). Only after birth does the fetus return to his own genetically determined growth velocity to achieve his own growth curve.

"Considering the complexities of the relation between maternal variables and fetal growth, a single maternal variable seems unlikely to provide a satisfactory predictor for birth size" (Metcoff, 1978, p. 451).

Maternal size Maternal size is possibly the most significant influence on fetal size near term in normal pregnancies. Height, prepregnancy weight, and weight gain during pregnancy have an effect on fetal size at term. The paternal influence is slight, and birth size is not midparental, supporting the theory that genotype is a minor factor in size at birth (Cheek, 1977; Metcoff, 1978; Ounsted and Ounsted, 1973; Smith, 1977).

In attempting to determine the more significant variable, weight or height, it has been suggested that height is less significant after one corrects for weight. No firm conclusion has been reached; thus, height, weight for height, and weight gain during pregnancy presently are all considered important variables. Larger women will have larger infants; smaller women will have smaller infants.

Uteroplacental factors Uteroplacental factors play a major role in late fetal growth. Uterine constraint of expanding fetal size has been thought to play a role in slowing fetal growth at 32 to 36 weeks ma (30 to 34 ca). This physical limitation, other than as related to maternal height, has more recently been theorized to play a minor role, if any, under normal circumstances (McKeown et al., 1976; Ounsted and Ounsted, 1973).

Placental and umbilical cord limitations may be more important. Placental growth essentially stops at 35 weeks' gestation ma; thus, the rate of nutrients and O_2 exchange levels. The umbilical cord is also proposed to have an upper limit in rate of blood flow, and as the fetal demands increase, the limit may be met.

Uteroplacental vascular insufficiency is a potent cause of fetal growth retardation. An abnormally small or infarcted placenta, abnormally small umbilical cord, preeclampsia, toxemia, chronic renal disease, or placenta previa can result in chronic hypoxia and reduced fetal growth (Campbell, 1976).

Multiple pregnancy results in significantly diminished fetal size. Uterine constraint is considered one factor involved in reduced growth as well as premature delivery. This theory has been questioned (McKeown et al., 1976; Ounsted and Ounsted, 1973). It is proposed that placental size is one factor: a fetus of multiple birth has a smaller placenta. This does not explain the size difference entirely, however, as a twin is smaller than a singleton with the same-sized placenta. The second factor proposed to contribute significantly is increased number of placentas supplied by the maternal uterine artery. "Since rate of blood flow is dependent on pressure, it follows that the greater the number of placentae, the lower is the rate of flow and the less rapid is fetal growth" (McKeown et al., 1976, p. 176).

Parity Parity has a significant effect on fetal size. The firstborn is generally smaller than subsequent children. Size difference is especially striking between the first and second pregnancy. Many have proposed a relaxed or enlarged uterus or improved uterine circulation. Some have found slightly less difference after correcting for women becoming heavier over time. However, because maternal factors are most important in term size and these factors or constraints are seen as basically constant, siblings are generally of similar size, except for the first. Thus, in evaluating for intrauterine growth retardation, one should compare with siblings to account for familial trends (Campbell, 1976; Ounsted and Ounsted, 1973).

Maternal age After correcting for weight gain and increased parity, there does not seem to be an increasing age-related effect on fetal growth (McKeown et al., 1976; Ounsted and Ounsted, 1973). Young mothers, below 17 years, however, do have increased morbidity: a prematurity-rate increase of 7 to 17 percent has been reported. In addition, increased weight gain, toxemia, anemia, prolonged labor, and precipitous labor are more common (Stevenson, 1977).

Nutrition Nutrition of the mother has a significant influence on fetal growth in the last trimester. It was noted in reports of famine conditions that undernutrition did not have an affect on fetal growth during the first two trimesters. The type of food lacking was once thought to be the most significant factor; however, it is now believed to be basic energy need: caloric level of the diet (Metcoff, 1978). Poor spacing of pregnancies may deplete maternal stores and result in less-than-adequate fetal growth.

Birth weight and body composition are most significantly affected by nutrition. Mean term birth weight of fetuses in developing countries is smaller than that in the United States, probably due to nutritional factors and less birth control use as well as to some racial differences. Some theorize that the quality of the mother's prenatal nutrition, affecting her growth as a fetus, is an important variable in size of her infants (Campbell, 1976; Metcoff, 1978).

Maternal health Maternal health and habits that are detrimental to health are important factors in fetal growth. Maternal health influences fetal growth as well as neonatal well-being. The specific effect depends on the actual disease, abnormality, or agent as well as on duration, timing, and treatment.

Hematologic, cardiovascular, and metabolic problems; disability or chronic ill health; and infectious disease all result in varied effects on fetal growth. Diabetes mellitus results in increased fetal weight, primarily tissue hyperplasia stimulated by hyperglycemia and hyperinsulinism. Severe hypertension and toxemia result in reduced rate of cellular hypertrophy. Infectious disease also results in decreased growth from decreased mitotic rate; thus, more of an effect is seen in the embryonic period. There is a positive correlation between prenatal health care and fetal growth, no doubt reflecting multiple variables.

"The single unquestionable effect on the fetus associated with maternal cigarette smoking is growth retardation" (Stevenson, 1977, p. 116) (see Fig. 5-47). Decreased fetal growth, resulting in smaller term weight, and increased rate of prematurity are the major effects of cigarette smoking. There appears to be a direct correlation between reduction in birth weight and number of cigarettes smoked daily. Research gives conflicting indications of exact etiology. Carbon dioxide, smoke or nicotine toxicity, and mild hypoxia have all been proposed. Smaller weight, increased fibrosis, and intimal damage in the uterine artery have been reported in placentas of smoking mothers (Asmussen, 1977). At this time, no long-term effects on postnatal growth have been documented. However, this possibility or other long-term effects, especially on the CNS, as well as possible increased spontaneous abortion rate have not been eliminated.

Significant, chronic alcohol consumption causes pre- and postnatal growth retardation as well as abnormal morphogenesis and developmental disability. Unlike poor nutrition and cigarette smoking, a decrease is seen in head circumference, perhaps even more than weight (Mulvihill, 1976). As in certain genetic disorders, the small size is considered congenital hypoplasia, and catch-up growth does not occur postnatally (Smith, 1977).

Narcotic addiction results in growth retardation which, as with cigarette smoking, appears to be reversed after birth (Stevenson, 1977).

Environment Altitude has a significant effect on fetal growth both in weight and, to a lesser degree, in length. Chronic, low-grade maternal hypoxia is the proposed factor limiting growth. Increased altitude also results in increased placental size (Campbell, 1976; Ounsted and Ounsted, 1973).

Maternal socioeconomic status When fetal growth is assessed in terms of SES, significant differences are noted between higher and lower SES (see Fig. 5-47). However because of the multiple variables defining SES, it is not a meaningful category. Maternal size, nutrition, and health all interact under the various SES labels.

Smith (1977) notes that mothers of low SES have smaller infants but that they themselves are smaller than parents of higher SES. Health status and habits that decrease health vary with SES. One study reports highest incidence of low birth weight in the lowest of four SES groups because of low weight gain, cigarette smoking, drug use, and no prenatal care (Miller, Hassanein, Chin, and Hensleigh, 1976). Medical complications were not distributed in this way.

GROWTH DEFICIENCY

Infants born with growth deficiency placing them below the 10th percentile on an intrauterine growth chart are designated small for gestational age SGA (see Chap. 6). Smith terms this congenital hypoplasia either *primary prenatal onset growth deficiency* or *secondary prenatal growth deficiency* (Smith, 1977, p. 66). Primary growth deficiency is that with a genetic basis. Secondary growth deficiency is secondary to an exogenous cause, primarily the above-listed maternal factors.

In secondary growth deficiency, weight is affected more than length, and head size is least affected except where growth deficiency is secondary to infection. Catch-up growth does not occur with primary growth deficiency. In cases of secondary growth deficiency, catch-up growth can occur and, if it does, will occur during the first 6 months. However, depending on etiology as well as severity, consistently small size may result (Smith, 1977; Toth, 1978).

Prenatal behavior Mary Tudor

INTRODUCTION

Although the embryo is considered a relatively inert being, the fetus is, by contrast, active and responsive. Fetal mobility occurs early; however, the mother's perception of fetal movement, quickening, does not occur until 16 to

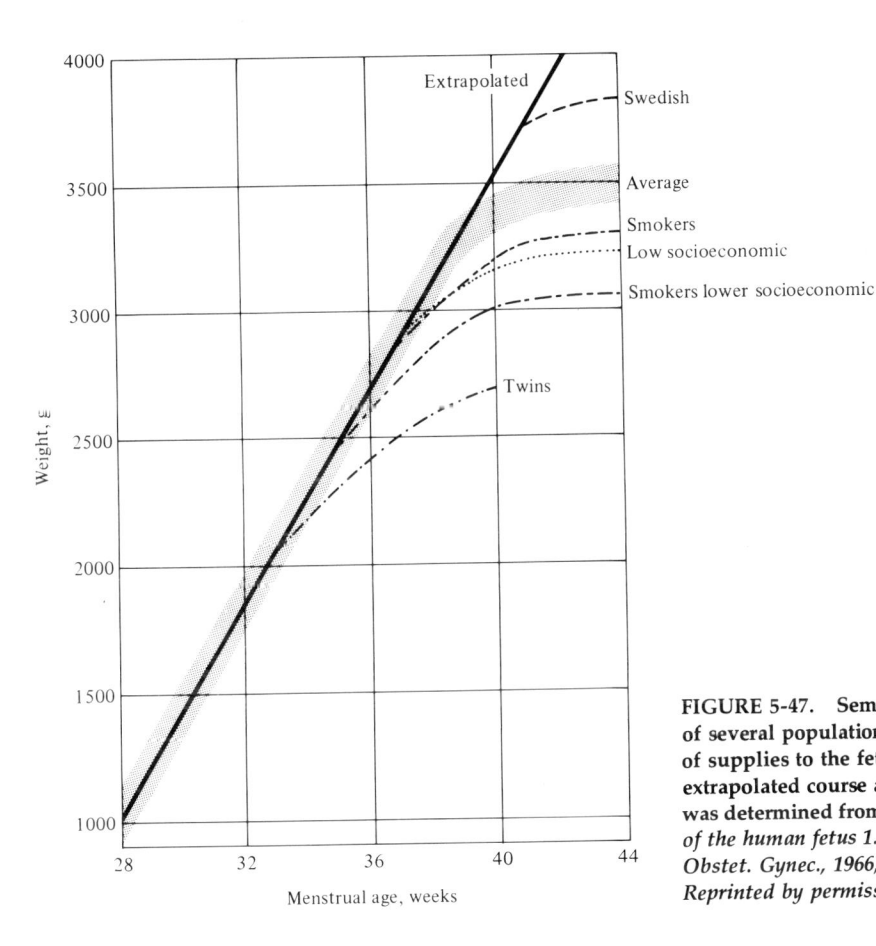

FIGURE 5-47. Semidiagrammatic presentation of fetal growth of several populations. Depending on the time when limitation of supplies to the fetus begins, curves depart from the straight, extrapolated course at different times in gestation. Fetal growth was determined from birth weight. (From P. Grunewald, Growth of the human fetus 1. Normal growth and its variations. Amer. J. Obstet. Gynec., 1966, 94, 112–119. © The C. V. Mosby Company. Reprinted by permission of the publisher.)

20 weeks ca (18 to 22 ma) in the primigravida and 14 to 16 weeks ca (16 to 18 ma) in the multigravida. The uterus, as all internal organs, is insensitive to tactile stimulation; thus, movement is not felt until it is strong enough to stretch the abdominal wall.

When systematic study of human fetal behavior began, data were collected by direct observation or crude tracings of the maternal abdominal wall. More extensive studies conducted in the 1940s and 1950s observed form and pattern of behavior from fetuses expelled from the uterus. Because placental circulation was not intact, the steadily diminishing oxygen supply and accumulating metabolites had a confounding effect. In addition, it is not known what percentage of the fetuses might have been abnormal.

More recently, in situ studies have again assumed importance through the use of ultrasonic and electromagnetic monitoring to observe spontaneous fetal movement in addition to recording heart rate and respiratory movements. Much of the current research is stimulated by the need for diagnosis of high-risk pregnancy. Animal studies have composed and continue to compose a large percentage of research in prenatal behavior.

Prenatal behavior, as defined in this text, refers to movement of all or part of the fetus as well as sensory perception (which may or may not result in movement). The underlying physiological mechanisms (electrical, neurochemical, and hormonal) are discussed in the section on neurogenesis, "Development of the Central Nervous System."

Various descriptive categories of fetal behavior have been proposed. Preyer, who first studied prenatal development of behavior, described six categories of movement: passive (due to uterine contraction), irritative, reflexive, impulsive, instinctive, and ideational (Hamburger, 1971). More recently, fetal behavior has been divided into autonomous, or spontaneous, activity and reflexive activity, in response to sensory stimulation. The question of which occurs first has been debated extensively. In the human, however, it appears that, due to precocious sensory system development, the two capabilities emerge simultaneously (Gottlieb, 1976). In the following discussion, prenatal behavior will be presented in two categories: (1) sensory perception and reflexive activity and (2) early and late movement. The inseparable relationship, however, is acknowledged.

The study of prenatal behavior is, of course, tied to the study of neurogenesis. Organogenesis must precede behavior. "At any particular stage of embryonic development, there can be no doubt that structure does determine function" (Gottlieb, 1976, p. 216). Prenatal behavior results from development of the central and peripheral nervous systems as well as the sensory end organs and musculoskeletal system. Movement is possible immediately upon completion of the first neural connection. A basic tenet of prenatal behavior is that "the state of differentiation of the nervous system at a given stage of development delimits the behavioral capacities of the embryo at that stage" (Hamburger, 1971, p. 46).

Another major question of study of early prenatal behavior has been whether behavior goes from undifferentiated total patterns to individual reflexes or builds from integration of individual reflexes. Neither of these hypotheses has been generally accepted as a single principle to explain early prenatal behavior (Gottlieb, 1976).

Carmichael offers the following view of the evolution of more complex behavior: "Every reaction studied such as grasping, sucking, sneezing, show two phases in development. The first is in a response directly related to the maturation of local and specific morphological structures. The second phase is that of an adaptive action and is due to maturation of appropriate brain centers" (1970, p. 508). Thus function is considered to develop in three stages: the myogenic, neuromotor, and reflex (Reinold, 1976).

An important question as yet unanswered is whether prenatal behavior in turn affects morphogenesis, particularly neurogenesis, and/or subsequent prenatal (and postnatal) behavior. Although this is still unanswered, in the human it is considered possible as both the sensory and motor systems "become functional while they are still anatomically, physiologically, and behaviorally immature" (Gottlieb, 1976, p. 232).

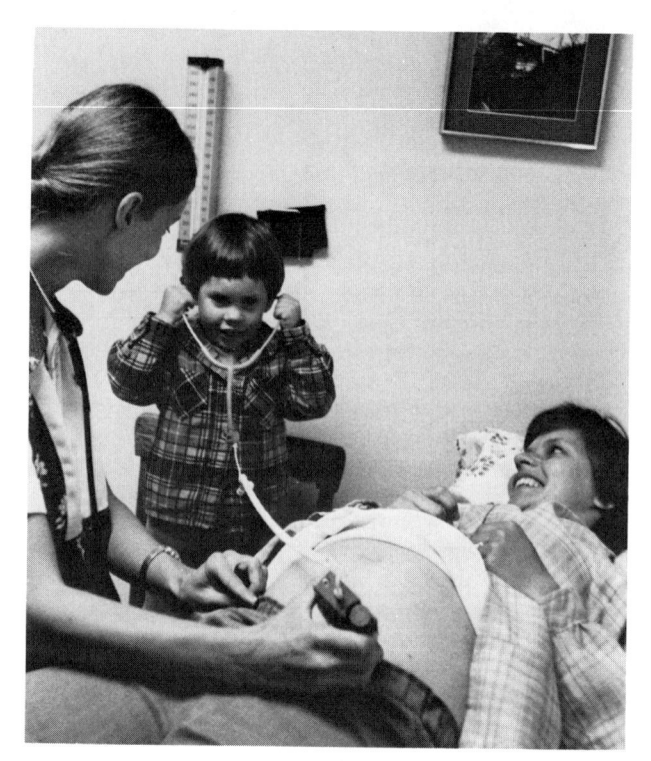

FIGURE 5-48.

Three possible ways in which prenatal behavior (function) has been hypothesized to influence development (embryonic and fetal) are described by Gottlieb:

- Determinative or inductive: channeling of development
- Facilitative: influencing rate of development
- Maintenance: maintaining integrity of prior development

Hamburger has proposed four ways that sensory input might influence motility:

- As a patterning or structuring device (considered doubtful)
- By influencing tone
- By facilitating behavior
- By releasing activity

Movement is known to have some significant effects, primarily on musculoskeletal development, discussed below. For the most part, however, these questions remain unanswered.

It can be generally stated that prenatal behavior, as other areas of development, proceeds in refinement from irregular to more sustained movement, from general to more specialized movements, and from simple patterns to more complex, coordinated, and integrated patterns. More complex movement patterns as well as sensitivity to sensory stimulation proceed (very roughly and inexactly) in a cephalocaudal and proximodistal pattern reflecting development of the CNS.

The area of prenatal learning is an exciting and yet relatively unexplored field. Using fetal response to auditory stimulation, fetal habituation (Sontag and Newbery, 1940) and conditioning (Spelt, 1948) have been demonstrated, although the evidence is somewhat weak. With ever-increasing refinement of techniques of intrauterine observation, data regarding learning in utero will no doubt emerge. Fetal movement patterns signal fetal well-being and are even proposed as developmental milestones in utero (Birnholz, Stevens, and Faria, 1978; Sandovsky and Polishuk, 1977; Timor-Tritsch, Zador, Hertz, and Rosen, 1976).

SLEEP-WAKE PATTERNS

As in the neonate, fetal behavior is influenced by fetal state. Fetal electroencephalogram (EEG) studies demonstrate cyclical activity corresponding with motor and respiratory behavior. Four fetal states have been described: awake, drowsy wakefulness from which the fetus can be aroused by impinging stimuli, REM sleep, and quiet sleep (Duenhoelter and Pritchard, 1977; Liley, 1972). The prominent state is REM sleep, probably present in short duration for 70 percent of the time (Dawes and Robinson, 1976). A diurnal pattern, as discussed above, is established in fetal life.

HEART RATE AND RESPIRATORY MOVEMENTS

As noted previously, fetal movement is closely associated with acceleration of FHR. Simultaneous increased FHR and movement within the normal range is considered a normal response. "The nearly synchronous onset of fetal movement and the observed acceleration suggests a coordinated control of both these functions. Presumably this control resides in the brain" (Timor-Tritsch, 1978, p. 278). Slight, brief movements may not be associated with FHR acceleration. There is thought to be some loss of beat-to-beat variability during fetal sleep states (Rochard, 1976), a consideration important in FHR monitoring.

Fetal respiratory movements appear to be correlated with sleep-wake patterns more than with movement. The most common respiratory pattern occurs just before or just after generalized fetal movement.

SENSORY DEVELOPMENT AND REFLEXIVE BEHAVIOR

Reflexive behavior of mobility results from stimulation of the sensory system. It is proposed to be more specialized than spontaneous behavior from the onset as it is mediated by specific sensory receptors. "Reflexogenic responses are contingent upon the closure of the respective reflex circuits" (Hamburger, 1971, p. 46). Sensory stimulation may precipitate mass or localized movements depending on the stimulus and timing as well as the age of the fetus. Stimulation may be maternal (uterine), environmental, or self-induced. All sensory systems, tactile (cutaneous), proprioceptive, vestibular, olfactory, taste, auditory, and visual, are functional or capable of function during the prenatal period.

TACTILE

Tactile sensitivity develops early, in the late embryonic period. Tactile sensitivity occurs first on the face and moves caudally toward the genital-anal area and distally to the hands and feet. By 16 weeks ca only the top and back of the head are insensitive. Fetal movement is the most obvious response to tactile stimulation. Initially, local stimulation results in a local response due to immaturity of the CNS. Total pattern reflexes emerge and are observed until 8 weeks ca, when again a local but specialized and adaptive response begins to emerge. Flexion is the predominating total response early; later, extension may also occur. Limb movements are passive initially, secondary to head and trunk movement. Later, independent, reflexive limb response is seen emerging in a proximodistal pattern.

It should be noted that the above behavior was observed secondary to direct tactile stimulation by a probe, and there is little evidence that any of these movements occur naturally in utero due to lack of the same stimulus. However, it has not been proved that they do not occur (Humphrey, 1970).

Palmar grasp, as a localized reflex, is elicited at 8 to 9 weeks ca with incomplete finger flexion and no thumb participation following the ulnar-to-radial pattern in development of grasp (see Fig. 5-49). By about 16 to 17 weeks ca a more complete grasp is seen with thumb involvement, and by 25 weeks ca the fetus can almost support his own weight by the palmar grasp. In the fetus 12

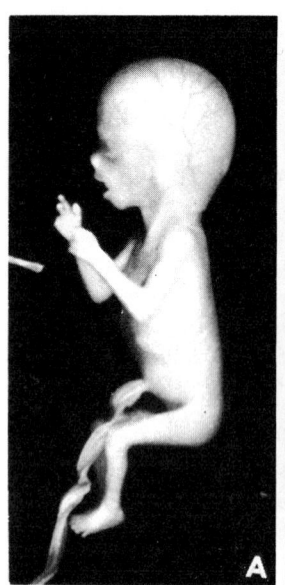

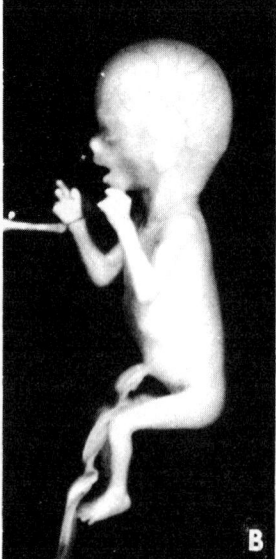

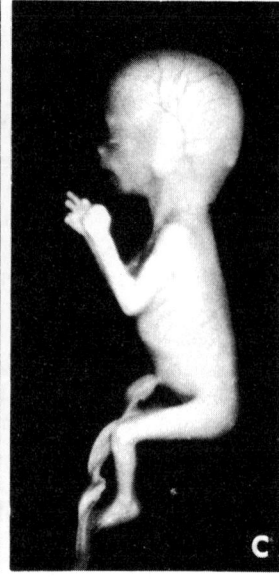

FIGURE 5-49. Finger flexion following stimulation of the palm of a fetus of 12 weeks ca. Mouth opening and tongue elevation and protrusion are also seen. (*From T. Humphrey, The development of human fetal activity and its relation to postnatal behavior. Advances Child Develop. Behav. 1970, 5, 23. Reprinted by permission of Academic Press.*)

weeks and older, palmar stimulation may be accompanied by oral movement. The soles are sensitive to tactile stimulation by 9 weeks ca, and *plantar flexion* is seen. A week later total limb flexion as well as the *Babinski reflex* can be elicited. More complex behaviors follow.

Very early in the ninth week ca perioral stimulation elicits active mouth opening followed by passive closing, a primitive rooting reflex. The 11-week fetus exhibits local facial reflexes, squint and scowl, to tactile stimulation in the eyebrow area. This may be an early blink reflex; however, the fetal eyelids are fused.

Swallowing has been demonstrated in 12-week-old fetuses; tongue retraction and protrusion are elicited at 12 weeks in response to palmar stimulation. By 13 to 14 weeks ca, more refined behavior preparatory to sucking is seen when the lips and tongue are stimulated: the mouth opens, the tongue elevates and forms a longitudinal groove, and the lower jaw lifts, causing mouth closure (see Fig. 5-50). Pursing of the lips occurs at 20 weeks and true sucking at 22 weeks (Humphrey, 1970). The gag reflex can be elicited by 17 weeks. Hiccups are not uncommon after sucking and swallowing behavior emerges.

Self-stimulation (tactile) no doubt does occur early. The hands of the embryo lie aside the mouth until the early fetal period, about 10 weeks. Thus, self-stimulation of the perioral region is likely, and the thumb has been observed inside the mouth as early as 12 weeks ca.

Stimulation of the surface of the intact amnion was demonstrated many years ago to elicit generalized fetal movement (Fitzgerald and Windle, 1942). More recently, FHR monitoring during amniocentesis demonstrated heart-rate acceleration with insertion of the needle into the amniotic sac. This acceleration is interpreted to be indicative of fetal well-being (Ron, Yaffe, and Sodovsky, 1976). Violent movement and protective responses have been observed in fetuses pricked with a needle during amniocentesis (Birnholz et al., 1978; Liley, 1972).

TEMPERATURE

Although the fetus does not normally experience significant variations in temperature, it is known that he responds to thermal stimulation before birth with increased heart rate as well as increased motor activity (Liley, 1972; Reinold, 1976). Thermal sensitivity has been demonstrated in infants born prematurely at 26 weeks ca.

PROPRIOCEPTION

Proprioceptors are functional early in fetal development in muscles, tendons, and possibly joints. Earliest muscle response is the result of direct stimulation of the muscle

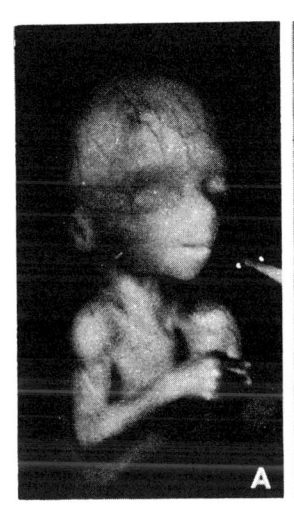

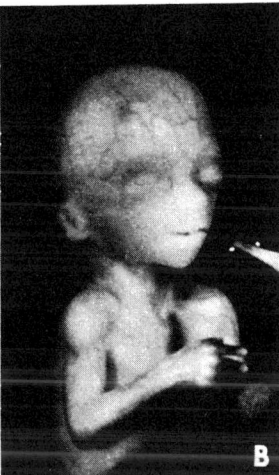

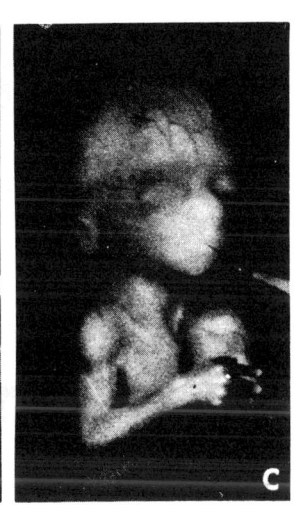

FIGURE 5-50. Lip and tongue reflex activity of a fetus of 13.5 weeks ca. (*From T. Humphrey, 1970.*)

(Reinold, 1976). As it is difficult to avoid tactile stimulation when applying proprioceptive stimulation, the response may involve both. It is known that by 10 to 12 weeks ca stretch reflex responses are seen in the limbs and mouth and influence overall posture of the fetus from that time to term. Self-stimulation (proprioceptive) is involved in spontaneous movement as well. Because of the fluid amniotic environment and relative lack of uterine constraint and gravitational forces until late pregnancy, lesser amounts of proprioceptive stimuli impinge on the young fetus.

VESTIBULAR

Fetal response to vestibular stimulation is less well documented, although it is thought to occur shortly after tactile, possibly in the 8- to 9-week-old fetus (Humphrey, 1970). The vestibular system is well developed at birth. The early reaction to vestibular stimulation is of total pattern response, interpreted as the emerging Moro reflex (Humphrey, 1970).

By the fifth to sixth fetal month, the bony labyrinth is full adult size and assumed to be functional. Increased fetal motor movement has been reported, especially kicking behavior, after 18 weeks' gestation ca when the fetus is in a nonaxial position (Elliott and Elliott, 1964). Evidence has been presented that suggests that assuming vertex or breech position depends on labyrinthine-activated kicking. The dominance of vertex over breech position is thought to occur either because of the interaction of body density and specific gravity of amniotic fluid (Elliott and Elliott, 1964) or because of uterine shape (Liley, 1972).

AUDITORY

When the fetal inner ear is fully differentiated, the potential for hearing exists. Presence of fetal hearing has been established after 20 weeks ca by monitoring FHR in response to 80-dB sound (pure tone, 500 to 1000 Hz) at the abdominal wall. Fetal heart rate increased by 15 bpm (Grimwade, Walker, Bartlett, Gordon, and Wood, 1971). It was determined that the fetus was reacting directly, not secondary to response of the mother.

The fluid environment of the uterus results in higher sound pressure levels. The fetal ear is fluid-filled, thus the sound is fluid-borne rather than airborne resulting in some loss of sound in certain frequencies. The intrauterine noise level has been measured at 72 to 85 dB from maternal voice and cardiovascular and intestinal sounds. Thus, there is some disagreement as to whether the fetus can hear environmental sounds or whether most of these sounds are masked. However, it is generally accepted that after 25 weeks the fetus will startle to a loud sudden noise. Also, many believe the neonate quiets when held against an adult's chest because of the familiarity of the heart sounds he hears.

VISUAL

Bright light next to the maternal abdomen has been shown to cause increased FHR and movement in some fetuses (Sadovsky, 1977; Smyth, 1965). Some natural light may be transmitted through the abdominal wall late in pregnancy. However, it is questionable whether it is of great enough intensity to be a source of stimulation. The fetus is able to see light and dark, especially after 26 weeks ca when the eyelids are no longer fused. Pupillary reflex is present at about 28 to 32 weeks (Carmichael, 1973). It is unlikely, however, that the fetus is significantly visually stimulated or actually sees surrounding structures (Liley, 1972).

TASTE AND OLFACTORY

Rate of fetal swallowing has been used as an indication of fetal taste. Studies have shown a decreased rate of swallowing following injection of a foul-tasting substance into the amniotic fluid and an increase in swallowing after injection of a sweet-tasting substance (Liley, 1972).

True sucking, although weak, is possible at 22 weeks ca, and soon the fetus is able to locate and suck his thumbs, fingers, and toes. Some have a callus already formed at the time of birth.

EARLY FETAL MOVEMENT

MOBILITY

During the first and second trimesters, free movements are possible because of the fluid environment. The fetus may be able to move in ways that will be impossible late in gestation and as a neonate; he has little uterine restraint or limitation on his movement. Ultrasound study (real-time scanning) has been utilized early in gestation, long before the mother perceives movements, and has revealed the fetus's true capabilities in utero.

Early spontaneous-appearing movements, at 6 to 8 weeks ca, may actually be reflexive, elicited by passive uterine movement (Reinold, 1976). Sudden movement, possibly a twitch, causes the buoyant embryo, at rest on the bottom of the amniotic cavity, to float upward and then drift to the bottom again. This may be repeated as soon as the embryo touches the amnion (Reinold, 1976). A second type of early fetal movement is a slow movement of one body part which does not result in total position change. These autonomous movements occur at 8 to 10 weeks ca.

Combined repetitive movements were observed by ultrasound to emerge at approximately 10 to 14 weeks ca. "Locomotive movements" of arms and legs were observed at about 14 weeks ca and hand-to-face and other more complex activity at 22 to 24 weeks ca. Movements initially are jerky but become smooth and more sustained.

LATE FETAL MOVEMENT

As noted above, by 22 weeks more complex behavior patterns and mobility are possible; however, the fetus will soon become somewhat more restricted in the uterine cavity. Maternal movement and change of position cause fetal movement as the fetus attempts to adjust to postural change (Liley, 1972). The fetus will also withdraw from external pressure stimulation. He changes position by propelling himself by his feet and legs. He changes sides by a longitudinal, spiral roll utilizing righting responses possible in the fluid environment.

Spontaneous musculoskeletal activity in utero has been reported subjectively by pregnant women and also by ultrasound and electromagnetic devices. As recorded by the mothers, spontaneous fetal movements (during the sixteenth week of gestation ca and after) increase with the age of the fetus and vary between fetuses. One study of 91 pregnant women reported daily fetal movements ranging from 4 to 1440! All 91 neonates were viable (Sadovsky, 1977). Some fetuses exhibited a constant number of daily movements; some were more variable. However, an individual pattern of rhythm emerged over longer observation.

When fetal movements were simultaneously recorded, electromagnetically and subjectively by the mothers, it was found that the mothers perceived 81 percent of the movements recorded (Sadovsky, 1977). Four basic movements have been described in fetuses 24 weeks ca to term based on duration and pattern (Timor-Tritsch, 1976):

- Rolling movement: "A sustained and rolling movement which seemed to be associated with the entire fetal body in motion" (pp. 72–73). The mean duration was 14 s.
- Simple movement: ". . . relatively short and easily palpable; it felt as though it originated from a fetal extremity" (p. 73). The abdominal wall was visibly displaced. The mean duration was 3 s.
- High-frequency movement: "Short, easily palpable and sometimes readily seen movements of the fetus" (pp. 73–74). Mothers interpreted these movements as kicks which could not be easily localized.
- Respiratory movement

Rolling, simple, and high-frequency movements are felt throughout most of later pregnancy as the fetus turns and moves. When assuming the final presentation 1 to 2 weeks prior to birth, however, rolling movements no longer occur, and the limb movements diminish.

PRESENTATION

After about 36 weeks ca, the fetal movements are significantly reduced as position for birth is taken. Labyrinthine function and the shape of the fetal body have each been postulated to determine fetal presentation. According to the latter theory, the longitudinal shape of the flexed fetal body stimulates a longitudinal lie with the smaller end of the fetus in the smaller, cervical end of the uterus. If the fetus flexes his knees, he will present vertex, the smaller end being the head. If the knees remain extended so that the feet are by the head, breech birth is more likely (Liley, 1972).

Breech presentation is significantly more frequent in preterm births than at term, when it occurs in 3 to 5 percent of births (Adamsons, 1978; Scheer and Nubar, 1976). Thus, cephalic presentation is more likely with longer gestation (see Fig. 5-51). Breech position is also more common in fetuses with hypotonia. Location of the placenta is proposed as a major factor in determining position of the fetal head (occiput presentation) at birth (Liley, 1972).

FIGURE 5-51. Relative frequencies of types of presentation. [From K. Scheer and J. Nubar, Variation of fetal presentation with gestational age. Amer. J. Obstet. Gynec., 1976, 125(2), 269. © The C. V. Mosby Company. Reprinted by permission of the publisher.]

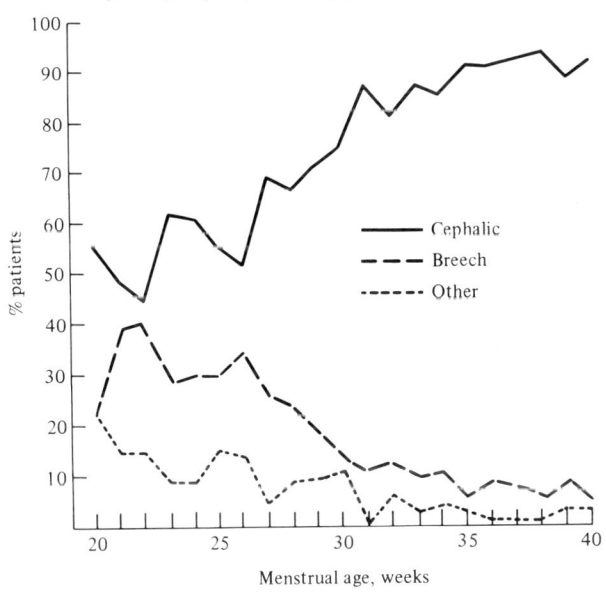

ROLE OF FETAL BEHAVIOR

Spontaneous musculoskeletal activity is known to have some effect on development of the fetus. Normal joint development appears to depend on movement of extremities. Muscle strength is enhanced by intrauterine activity. Positional deformities, caused by one fetal part pressing against another, are less likely to occur with increased movement and position change.

Fetal movements also hold promise as a method of prenatal diagnosis of abnormality or distress. Earliest movements that cause excursion of the embryo within the amniotic sac are proposed for evaluation of the embryo's well-being. The rate of occurrence of movement and duration of periods of immobility are counted during ultrasonic scanning (Reinold, 1976).

Another study describes the "movements alarm system" (MAS) indicating severe fetal distress (Sadovsky, 1978). The MAS is a decrease up to cessation of fetal movements which indicates chronic anoxia and "impending intrauterine fetal death" (p. 51). The MAS is stated to warrant immediate delivery. Furthermore, it is reported that the MAS can be observed when fetal heart tones are still audible and less diagnostic.

The same authors report that sudden, vigorous movements indicate acute fetal anoxia (asphyxia) and are followed immediately with cessation of movement indicating fetal death. The etiology is believed to be cord compression (Sadovsky, 1978).

For the general population, daily fetal movement rate (DFMR) is suggested as a method to monitor fetal well-being, especially in high-risk pregnancies. It is suggested that the woman seek medical treatment "whenever fetal movements are reduced to several a day (four or less) or have ceased altogether" (Sadovsky, 1977, p. 51). Daily records of movement were found to be more reliable than urinary estriol or FHR monitoring in predicting impending fetal death.

SUMMARY

The fetus was once considered a simple creature, charged only with the tasks of gaining in size and randomly moving about. Observation of growth and behavior was traditionally begun at birth or later. Now technology has invaded the fetus's private space, and the science of human development has begun to document the remarkable course of embryonic and fetal development at a much more rapid pace.

The promise of being able to closely link the period of

organogenesis, the first 8 weeks of life, and the emergence of behavior and human function prenatally may reveal some long-sought-after links in human development. In addition, careful observations of fetal growth, movement, and vital signs give data on well-being and readiness for extrauterine life.

Labor and birth Margot Edwards

The onset of labor occurs when a set of hormonal, circulatory, and neurological factors combine to break the balance between maternal progesterone and prostaglandins; it is possible that the process is triggered by signals given from the fetal-placental system (Barden, 1975). When structures designed to maintain intrauterine life are no longer needed, common signs signify the onset of labor. The cervical mucous plug ("show") may be expelled; contractions increasing in frequency and intensity but not always in regularity begin; the amniotic sac ruptures in about 20 percent of pregnancies.

Three classical stages with a recently added fourth define the course of labor:

- First stage of effacement and dilatation of the cervix
- Second stage of birth of the fetus
- Third stage of separation and expulsion of the placenta
- Fourth stage of recovery and parent-infant bonding

LABOR

The Friedman curve, the rate of cervical dilation plotted against the passage of time, is standard for evaluating the normal duration of labor (Friedman, 1973) (see Fig. 5-52). First stage is subdivided into a latent (prodromal or inactive) phase (early labor), lasting 8½ h in women who are nulliparas and 5 h in women who are multiparas. This is followed by an active phase of initial acceleration followed by deceleration or transition lasting 5 h in nulliparas and 2 h in multiparas. Friedman sets the upper limit of second stage as 1 h in nulliparas and 15 min in multiparas and sets that of third stage as less than ½ h.

The labor process consists of three Ps: *powers* or forces of uterine contraction, which is 25 to 55 mmHg in all directions; *passenger* or fetus, his lie, attitude, presentation, and position; and *passage* or resistance of the maternal pelvis, cervix, and pelvic floor. Optimally, the fetal lie is longitudinal, the attitude is one of flexion, the presentation is vertex, and the position is left occiput anterior (LOA) Head flexion is preceded in nulliparas by descent (engagement) prior to onset, and this attitude offers the most favorable diameter of the leading part during labor. The well-flexed head fits into the cervix to exert a dilating effect.

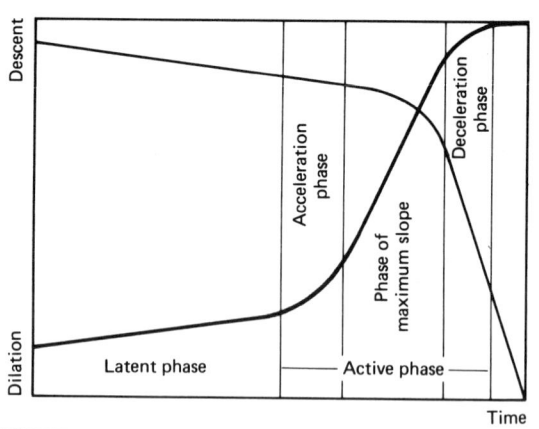

FIGURE 5-52. The Friedman curve of normal labor, a graphic display of the normal patterns of cervical dilation (heavy line) and descent (light line) showing the characteristic phases of the first stage of labor. [From E. Friedman, Normal labor curve. Clin. Obstet. Gynec., 1973, 16(1), 176. © Harper & Row, Publishers, Inc. Reprinted by permission of the publishers.]

One consideration in evaluating efficacy of uterine contractions is the role of maternal abdominal muscles, which should be passive throughout first stage to allow the normal rise of the uterus during contraction. When the uterus rises to its maximum height during contraction, the fetal head faces the cervix, and dilation proceeds normally. If the abdominal muscles are tensed during contraction, the uterus cannot rise properly, and the fetal head faces the uterine wall. These and other influences related to fear, pain, and tension may alter the normal sequence of the first stage.

Throughout the first and second stages, the fetus descends into the pelvis. The liquid cushion provided by the membranes filled with amniotic fluid allows pressure received at any point on the fetus to be equally distributed to prevent excessive disalignment of the fetal skull bones. In normal labor under optimal conditions, uterine contractile pressure produces no change in blood flow to the fetal brain.

FETAL RESPONSE TO LABOR

Continuous electronic monitoring can be used to record FHR: beat-to-beat variability and pressure of the uterine contraction. A normal FHR is 120 to 160 bpm. Three variations in FHR pattern during labor have been identified: type I, type II, and type III dips or decelerations.

The type I dip, or *early deceleration curve,* shows an FHR that gradually slopes downward before the uterine contraction begins and recovers as it ends. The degree of slope forms a uniform pattern that conforms to the shape of the uterine contraction. Early deceleration in normal labor is an indication of head compression.

The type II dip, or *late deceleration,* is a more ominous sign of possible fetal distress. The FHR slows near the peak of contraction and falls to its lowest point after the contraction ends. It has been associated with base-line tachycardia, an increase in FHR between contractions; the FHR can fall as low as 60 bpm as compared with early deceleration, which seldom falls below 100 bpm. Type II dips also have a uniform shape that conforms to the shape of the uterine contraction.

The type III dip, or *variable deceleration,* shows a pattern that may begin at any time during the contraction cycle and that is characterized by steep rises and falls lasting seconds or minutes. The slope of the FHR is not uniform with the uterine contraction as in type I or II. Variable deceleration is caused by cord compression, among other factors, and most often is seen in the supine position or with recumbency over time.

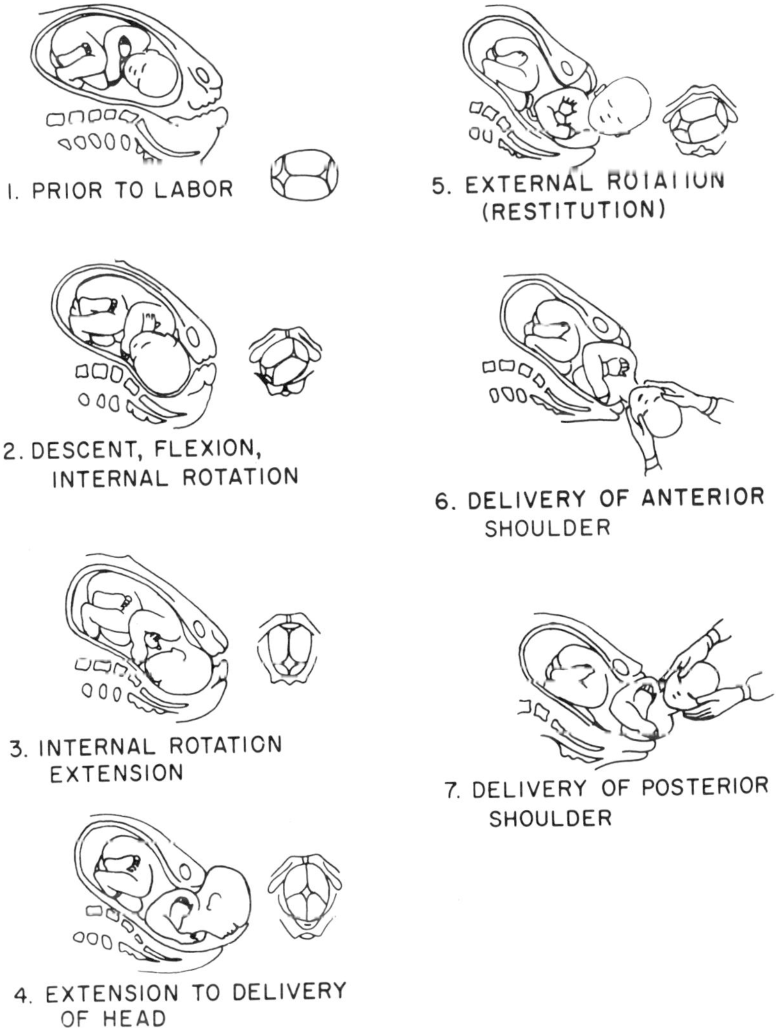

1. PRIOR TO LABOR

2. DESCENT, FLEXION, INTERNAL ROTATION

3. INTERNAL ROTATION EXTENSION

4. EXTENSION TO DELIVERY OF HEAD

5. EXTERNAL ROTATION (RESTITUTION)

6. DELIVERY OF ANTERIOR SHOULDER

7. DELIVERY OF POSTERIOR SHOULDER

FIGURE 5-53. Mechanism of labor for cephalic presentation. *(From S. L. Romney, et al., Obstetrics and gynecology: The health care of women. New York: McGraw-Hill, 1975, p. 661. Reprinted by permission of the publisher.)*

Internal fetal monitoring is precise in reflecting accurate FHR but efficacy of the fetal monitor as a primary method of surveillance during labor is limited by its range of interpretation and the question of whether or not cesarean section is indicated by deceleration patterns. Goodlin and Haesslein (1977) analyzed and quantified the beat-to-beat variability on monitor graphs and compared them with fetal blood-gas readings in a retrospective survey. They found that 60 to 80 percent of the time distress patterns (decelerations) are found in normal fetuses. Haverkamp, Thompson, McFee, and Cetrulo (1976) compared the effectiveness of continuous fetal monitoring with nurse auscultation of fetal heart tones in a double-blind, controlled study of high-risk mothers in Denver. They showed that there is no difference in fetal outcome except for a marked increase in cesarean section in the monitored group.

BIRTH OF THE FETUS

When descent results in the flexed fetal head (occiput) reaching the pelvic floor, it rotates along the side of the pelvis, travels under the symphysis pubis to the crown, and extends as the sinciput, face, and chin sweep the perineum. The fetal head extends, and restitution occurs when the occiput turns to the left and the head rights itself with the shoulders. The anterior shoulder is resisted by the pelvic floor and rotates when the head rotates externally; it escapes under the symphysis pubis, and the posterior shoulder follows. Expulsion of the fetal body occurs by lateral flexion. Thus the cardinal movements of labor are engagement, flexion, internal rotation, extension, restitution and external rotation, and expulsion (see Fig. 5-53).

THE FOURTH STAGE: PARENT-CHILD CONTACT

The routine separation of parents and neonate after second stage is declining as a birth practice and contact occurs during the third or fourth stages in family-centered hospitals. The Division on Maternal and Child Health Nursing Practice of the American Nurses' Association has released *Statement on Parental-Infant Attachment* which defines optimum care and lists the rights of childbearing families.

Bibliography

CONCEPTION THROUGH ESTABLISHMENT OF BODY FORM

Adam, J. A. J., and P. Felig: Carbohydrate, fat, and amino acid metabolism in the pregnant woman and fetus. In F. Falkner and J. M. Tanner (Eds.), *Human growth 1, Principles and prenatal growth.* New York: Plenum 1978.

Adamsons, K.: Fetal growth: Obstetric implications. In F. Falkner and J. M. Tanner (Eds.), *Human growth 1, Principles and prenatal growth.* New York: Plenum, 1978.

Ainsworth, P., and P. A. Davies: The single umbilical artery: A five-year survey. *Develop. Med. Child Neurol.,* 1969, 11, 297.

American Academy of Pediatrics Committee on the Fetus and Newborn: Nomenclature for duration of gestation, birth weight and intrauterine growth. *Pediatrics,* 1967, 39(6), 935–939.

Arey, L. B.: *Developmental anatomy* (7th ed.). Philadelphia: Saunders, 1965.

Berrill, N. J., and G. Karp: *Development.* New York: McGraw-Hill, 1976.

Campbell, S.: Fetal growth. In R. W. Beard and P. W. Nathanielsz (Eds.), *Fetal physiology and medicine.* London: Saunders, 1976.

Cheek, D. B., J. E. Graystone, and M. Niall: Factors controlling fetal growth. *Clin. Obstet. Gynec.,* 1977, 20(4), 925–942.

Corliss, C. E.: *Patten's human embryology; Elements of clinical development.* New York: McGraw-Hill, 1976.

Dancis, J., and H. Schneider: Physiology of the placenta. In F. Falkner and J. M. Tanner (Eds.), *Human growth 1, Principles and prenatal growth.* New York: Plenum, 1978.

Fitzgerald, J. D., and W. F. Windle: Some observations on early human fetal movements. *J. Comp. Neurol.,* 1942, 76, 159–167.

FitzGerald, M. J. T.: *Human embryology, A regional approach.* Hagerstown, Maryland: Harper & Row, 1978.

Gasser, R. F.: *Atlas of human embryos.* Hagerstown, Maryland: Harper & Row, 1975.

Herzenberg, L. A., D. W. Bianchi, J. Schröder, H. M. Cann, and G. M. Iverson: Fetal cells in the blood of pregnant women: Detection and enrichment by fluorescence-activated cell sorting. *Proc. Nat. Acad. Sci. U.S.A.,* 1979, 76(3), 1453–1455.

Langman, J.: *Medical embryology.* Baltimore: Williams & Wilkins, 1969.

Liley, A. W.: The foetus as a personality. *Aust. New Zeal. J. Psychiat.,* 1972, 6, 99–105.

Mastroianni, L.: Fertility disorders. In S. L. Romney, M. J. Gray, A. B. Little, J. A. Merrill, E. J. Quilligan, and R.

Stander (Eds.), *Gynecology and obstetrics, The health care of women*. New York: McGraw-Hill, 1975.

McKeown, T., T. Marshall, and R. G. Record: Influences on fetal growth. *J. Reprod. Fertil.*, 1976, 47, 167–181.

Metcoff, J.: Association of fetal growth with maternal nutrition. In F. Falkner and J. M. Tanner (Eds.), *Human growth 1, Principles and prenatal growth*. New York: Plenum, 1978.

Moore, K. L.: *The developing human* (2d ed.). Philadelphia: Saunders, 1977.

National Institute of Child Health and Human Development National Registry for Amniocentesis Study Group: Midtrimester amniocentesis for prenatal diagnosis: Safety and accuracy. *J.A.M.A.*, 1976, 236, 1471–1476.

O'Rahilly, R.: *Developmental states in human embryos*. Washington, D. C.: Carnegie Institution of Washington, 1973.

Ounsted, M., and C. Ounsted: On fetal growth rate; Its variations and their consequences. *Clinics in Developmental Medicine No. 46*. London: Spastics International, 1973.

Rawlings, E. E., and B. A. Moore: The accuracy of methods of calculating the expected date of delivery for use in the diagnosis of postmaturity. *Amer. J. Obstet. Gynecol.*, 1970, 106(5), 676–679.

Reynolds, S. R. M.: Mechanisms of placentofetal blood flow. *Obstet. Gynec.*, 1978, 51(2), 245–249.

Rugh, R.: Conception and fetal growth. In E. J. Dickason and M. O. Schult (Eds.), *Maternal and infant care*. New York: McGraw-Hill, 1975.

Scheidt, P. C., F. Stanley, and D. Bryla: One-year follow-up of infants exposed to ultrasound in utero. *Amer. J. Obstet. Gynec.*, 1978, 131(7), 743–748.

Shanklin, D. R.: Anatomy of the placenta. In F. Falkner and J. M. Tanner (Eds.), *Human growth 1, Principles and prenatal growth*. New York: Plenum, 1978.

Shettles, L. B.: Fertilization and early development from the inner cell mass. In E. E. Philipp, J. Barnes, and M. Newton (Eds.), *Scientific foundations of obstetrics and gynecology*. London: Heinemann, 1970.

Smith, D. W.: *Recognizable patterns of human malformation: Genetic, embryologic, and clinical aspects* (2d ed.). Philadelphia: Saunders, 1976.

Southgate, D. A. T.: Fetal measurements. In F. Falkner and J. M. Tanner (Eds.), *Human growth 1, Principles and prenatal growth*. New York: Plenum, 1978.

Speroff, L., R. H. Glass, and N. G. Kase: *Clinical gynecologic endocrinology and infertility* (2d ed.). Baltimore: Williams & Wilkins, 1978.

Stephens, T. D.: (Personal communication, 1980).

Steptoe, P. C., and R. G. Edwards: Birth after the reimplantation of a human embryo. *Lancet*, 1978, 2(8085), 336.

Streeter, G. L.: Developmental horizons in human embryos. *Contrib. Embryol. Carnegie Inst.*, 1942, 30, 211.

———: Weight, sitting height, head size, foot length, and menstrual age of the human embryo. *Contrib. Embryol.*, 1920, 11, 143.

Thompson, J. N.: Prenatal detection of heritable metabolic disorders. *Pediat. Ann.*, 1978, 7(6), 25–36.

———: Amniotic fluid protein: A nutritional function. *Nutr. Rev.*, 1976, 34(11), 341–343.

DEVELOPMENT OF THE FACE

Corliss, C. E.: *Patten's human embryology; Elements of clinical development*, New York: McGraw-Hill, 1976.

Langman, J.: *Medical embryology*. Baltimore: Williams & Wilkins, 1969.

Moore, K. L.: *The developing human* (2d ed.). Philadelphia: Saunders, 1977.

DEVELOPMENT OF THE CENTRAL NERVOUS SYSTEM

Blinkov, S. M., and I. I. Glezer: *The human brain in figures and tables*. New York: Plenum, 1968.

Carpenter, M. B.: *Human neuroanatomy*. Baltimore: Williams & Wilkins, 1976.

Cass, R. G., and A. Globus: Spine stems on tectal interneurons in jewel fish are shortened by social stimulation. *Science*, 1978, 200, 787–789.

Corliss, C. E.: *Patten's human embryology; Elements of clinical development*. New York: McGraw-Hill, 1976.

Gessell, A. L.: *Infant development—The embryology of early human behavior*. Westport, Connecticut: Greenwood, 1972.

Hughes, A. F. W.: *Aspects of neural ontogeny*. London: Academic, 1968.

Jacobson, M. A.: *Developmental neurobiology*. New York: Plenum, 1978.

Parnavelas, J. G.: Influence of stimulation of cortical development. *Brain Res.*, 1978, 48, 247–259.

Sarrat, H. B., and M. G. Netsky: *Evolution of the nervous system*. New York: Oxford University Press, 1974.

DEVELOPMENT OF THE SENSORY SYSTEM

Arey, L. B.: *Developmental anatomy* (7th ed.). Philadelphia: Saunders, 1965.

Moore, K. L.: *The developing human* (2d ed.). Philadelphia: Saunders, 1977.

Newell, F. W., and J. T. Ernest: *Ophthalmology: Principles and concepts* (3d ed.). St. Louis: Mosby, 1974.

Snell, R. S.: *Clinical embryology for medical students* (2d ed.). Boston: Little, Brown, 1975.

DEVELOPMENT OF THE MUSCULOSKELETAL SYSTEM

Arey, L. B.: *Developmental anatomy* (7th ed.). Philadelphia: Saunders, 1974.

Haines, R., and A. Mohiuddin: *Handbook of human embryology* (5th ed.). London: Churchill Livingstone, 1970.

Passo, S.: The musculoskeletal system. In G. Scipien, M. Barnard, M. Chard, J. Howe, and P. Phillips (Eds.), *Comprehensive pediatric nursing* (2d ed.). New York: McGraw-Hill, 1979

DEVELOPMENT OF THE CARDIOVASCULAR SYSTEM

DeHaan, R. L.: Embryology of the heart. In J. W. Hurst and R. B. Logue (Eds.), *The heart, arteries, and veins* (3d ed.). New York: McGraw-Hill, 1974.

Erslev, A. J., and T. G. Gabuzda: Pathophysiology of hematologic disorders. In W. A. Sodeman, Jr., and W. A. Sodeman (Eds.), *Pathologic physiology* (5th ed.). Philadelphia: Saunders, 1974.

Moore, K. L.: *The developing human* (2d ed.). Philadelphia: Saunders, 1977.

Netter, F. H.: Embryology. In F. H. Netter (Ed.), *The Ciba collection of medical illustrations, Heart* (Vol. 5). Summit, New Jersey: Ciba Pharmaceutical, 1969.

Sacksteder, S.: Embryology and fetal circulation. *Amer. J. Nurs.*, 1978, *78*(2), 262–264.

DEVELOPMENT OF THE RESPIRATORY SYSTEM

Avery, M. E., and B. D. Fletcher: *The Lung and its disorders in the newborn infant*. Philadelphia: Saunders, 1974.

———, and J. Mead: Surface properties in relation to atelectasis and hyaline membrane disease. *Amer. J. Dis. Child.*, 1959, *97*, 517.

Fraser, R., and J. Paré: *Organ physiology* (2d ed.). Philadelphia: Saunders, 1977.

Gluck, L., M. V. Kulovich, and associates: Diagnosis of respiratory distress syndrome by amniocentesis. *Amer. J. Obstet. Gynec.*, 1971, *109*, 440.

———: The interpretation and significance of the lecithin/sphingomyelin ratios in amniotic fluid. *Amer. J. Obstet. Gynec.*, 1974, *120*, 142.

Hallman, M., and L. Gluck: Development of the fetal lung. *J. Perinat. Med.*, 1977, *5*, 3.

Kendig, E. L., Jr., and Y. Chernich: *Disorders of the respiratory tract in children* (3d ed.). Philadelphia: Saunders, 1977.

Moore, K. L.: *The developing human*. Philadelphia: Saunders, 1977.

Murray, J. F.: *The normal lung*. Philadelphia: Saunders, 1976.

Reid, L.: The embryology of the lung. In *Ciba Foundation Symposium Development of the Lung*. Boston: Little, Brown, 1967.

Scarpelli, E.: *Pulmonary physiology of the fetus, newborn, and child*. Philadelphia: Lea & Febiger, 1975.

Strang, L. B.: Growth and development of the lung. Fetal and postnatal. *Ann. Rev. Physiol.*, 1977a, *39*, 253–276.

———: *Neonatal respiration*. Oxford: Blackwell Scientific, 1977b.

DEVELOPMENT OF THE GASTROINTESTINAL SYSTEM

Auricchio, S., A. Rubino, and G. Nurset: Intestinal glycosidase activities in the human embryo, fetus and newborn. *Pediatrics*, 1965, *35*, 944.

Corliss, C. E.: *Patten's human embryology*. New York: McGraw-Hill, 1976.

Langman, J.: *Medical embryology*. Baltimore: Williams & Wilkins, 1963.

Moore, K. L.: *The developing human*. Philadelphia: Saunders, 1977.

Snell, R. S.: *Clinical embryology for medical students*. Boston: Little, Brown, 1975.

Timiras, P. S.: *Physiology and aging*. New York: Macmillan, 1972.

DEVELOPMENT OF THE ENDOCRINE SYSTEM

Balinsky, B. I.: *An introduction to embryology* (3d ed.). Philadelphia: Saunders, 1970.

Moore, K. L.: *The developing human* (2d ed.). Philadelphia: Saunders, 1977.

Villee, D. B.: *Human endocrinology, A developmental approach*. Philadelphia: Saunders, 1975.

DEVELOPMENT OF THE REPRODUCTIVE SYSTEM

Austin, C. R., and R. V. Short: *Germ cells and fertilization*. Cambridge: Harvard University Press, 1972.

Federman, D. D.: Genetic control of sexual differences. *Progr. Med. Genet.*, 1973, *9*, 123.

Ferguson-Smith, M. A. E., M. E. Boyd, J. G. Ferguson-

Smith, A. F. Prichurd, M. Ysuf, and B. Gary: Isochromosome for the long arm of Y chromosome in patients with Turner syndrome and sex chromosome mosaicism. *J. Med. Genet.*, 1969, 6, 422.

Jost, A., B. Vigier, J. Prepin, and J. P. Perchelle: Studies on sex differentiation in mammals. *Recent Progr. Hormone Res.*, 1973, 29, 1.

Tuchmann-Duplessis, H., and P. Haegel: *Illustrated human embryology* (Vol. 2): *Organogenesis*. New York: Springer-Verlag, 1974.

DEVELOPMENT OF THE URINARY SYSTEM

Alexander, D. P., and D. A. Nixon: Reabsorption of glucose, fructose and megoinositol by foetal and post-natal sheep kidney. *J. Physiol.* (London), 1963, 167, 480.

Gersh, I.: The correlation of structure and function in developing mesonephros and metanephros. *Contrib. Embryol.*, 1937, 26, 35.

Goss, R. J.: Adaptive mechanisms of growth control. In F. Falkner and J. M. Tanner (Eds.), *Human growth 1, Principles and prenatal growth*. New York: Plenum, 1978.

Keen, M. F. L., and E. E. Hewer: Glandular activity in the human fetus. *Lancet*, 1924, 2, 111.

McCrory, W. W.: *Developmental nephrology*. Cambridge: Harvard University Press, 1972.

Moore, K. L.: *The developing human* (2d ed.). Philadelphia: Saunders, 1977.

Pitts, R. F., et al.: The renal regulation of acid-base balance in man. III. The reabsorption and excretion of bicarbonate. *J. Clin. Invest.*, 1949, 28, 35.

Tudvad, F. H., et al.: Renal response of premature infants to administration of bicarbonate and potassium. *Pediatrics*, 1954, 13, 4.

DEVELOPMENT OF THE INTEGUMENTARY SYSTEM

Arey, L. B.: *Developmental anatomy* (7th ed.). Philadelphia: Saunders, 1965.

Corliss, C. E.: *Patten's human embryology; Elements of clinical development*. New York: McGraw-Hill, 1976.

Moore, K. L.: *The developing human* (2d ed.). Philadelphia: Saunders, 1977.

Smith, D. W.: *Recognizable patterns of human malformation: Genetic, embryologic and clinical aspects* (2d ed.). Philadelphia: Saunders, 1976.

DYSMORPHOLOGY

Apgar, V., and G. Stickle: Birth defects: Their significance as a public health problem. *J.A.M.A.*, 1968, 204, 79–82.

Boué, J., A. Boué, P. Lazar, and S. Gueguen: Outcome of pregnancies following a spontaneous abortion with chromosomal anomalies. *Amer. J. Obstet. Gynec.*, 1973, 116, 806.

Butcher, R. E.: Behavioral testing as a method for assessing risk. *Environ. Health Perspect.*, 1976, 18, 75–78.

Claireaux, A. E.: Fetal abnormalities as cause of perinatal death. *Proc. Roy. Soc. Med.*, 1973, 66, 1119–1120.

Grant, L. D.: Research strategies for behavioral teratology studies. *Environ. Health Perspect.*, 1976, 18, 85–94.

Kimmel, C. A.: Behavioral teratology: Overview. *Environ. Health Perspect.*, 1976, 18, 73.

Lauritsen, J. G.: Aetiology of spontaneous abortion. *Acta Obstet. Gynec. Scand.*, 1976, 52, 1–29. (Supplement)

National Foundation—March of Dimes: *Birth defects*. New York: National Foundation—March of Dimes, 1979.

Shepard, T. J., and R. J. Lemire: The causes, mechanisms and prevention of congenital defects. *Univ. Washington Med.*, 1976, 3(4), 3–10.

Smith, D. W.: Dysmorphology: Clinical patterns of human malformation. *Univ. Washington Med.*, 1976a, 3(1), 11–17.

———: *Recognizable patterns of human malformation: Genetic, embryologic and clinical aspects* (2d ed.). Philadelphia: Saunders, 1976b.

———: (Personal communication, 1979.)

———: Growth and its disorders. *Major problems in clinical pediatrics* (Vol. 15). Philadelphia: Saunders, 1977.

———, and J. M. Aase: Polygenic inheritance of certain common malformations. *J. Pediat.*, 1970, 76(5), 653–659.

Weiss, B., and J. M. Spyker: Behavioral implications of prenatal and early postnatal exposure to chemical pollutants. *Pediatrics*, 1974, 53(5), 851–859.

FETAL DEVELOPMENT

Adamsons, K.: Fetal growth: Obstetric implications. In F. Falkner and J. M. Tanner (Eds.), *Human growth 1, Principles and prenatal growth*. New York: Plenum, 1978.

Alvear, J., and O. G. Brooke: Fetal growth in different racial groups. *Arch. Dis. Child.*, 1978, 53(1), 27–32.

Apte, S. V., and L. Iyengar: Composition of the human foetus. *Brit. J. Nutr.*, 1972, 27(2), 305–312.

Asmussen, I.: Ultrastructure of the human placenta at term: Observations on placentas from newborn children of smoking and nonsmoking mothers. *Acta Obstet. Gynec. Scand.*, 1977, 56, 119–126.

Barrada, M. I., L. E. Edwards, and E. Y. Hakenson: Antepartum fetal testing II. The acceleration/constant ratio: A nonstress test. *Amer. J. Obstet. Gynec.*, 1979, 134, 538–543.

Beard, R. W., and P. W. Nathanielsz (Eds.): *Fetal physiology and medicine.* London: Saunders, 1976.

Berger, G. S., D. A. Edelman, and T. D. Kerenyi: Fetal crown-rump length and biparietal diameter in the second trimester of pregnancy. *Amer. J. Obstet. Gynec.,* 1975, *122*(1), 9–12.

Bergsjo, P., T. Bakke, and T. Bjerkedal: Growth of the fetal skull with special reference to weight-for-dates of the newborn child. *Acta Obstet. Gynec. Scand.,* 1976, *55*(1), 53–57.

Brenner, W. E., D. A. Edelman, and C. H. Hendricks: A standard of fetal growth for the United States of America. *Amer. J. Obstet. Gynec.,* 1976, *126*(5), 555–564.

Campbell, S.: The assessment of fetal development by diagnostic ultrasound. *Clin. Perinat.,* 1974, *1*(2), 507–525.

———: Fetal growth. In R. W. Beard and P. W. Nathanillsz (Eds.), *Fetal physiology and medicine.* London: Saunders, 1976.

———: Growth of the fetal biparietal diameter during normal pregnancy. *J. Obstet. Gynaec. Brit. Comm.,* 1971, *78*, 513–519.

Carmichael, L.: Onset and early development of behavior. In P. H. Mussen (Ed.), *Carmichael's manual of child psychology* (Vol. I). New York: Wiley, 1970.

Cheek, D. B.: Factors controlling fetal growth. *Clin. Obstet. Gynec.,* 1977, *20*(4), 925–942.

Cook, L. N.: Intrauterine and extrauterine recognition and management of deviant fetal growth. *Pediat. Clin. N. Amer.,* 1977, *24*(3), 431–454.

Dawes, G. S., and J. S. Robinson: Rhythmic phenomena in prenatal life. *Progr. Brain Res.,* 1976, *45*, 383–389.

Duenhoelter, J. H., and J. A. Pritchard: Fetal respiration. *Amer. J. Obstet. Gynecol.,* 1977, *129*(3), 326–338.

Falkner, F.: Implications for growth in human twins. In F. Falkner and J. M. Tannar (Eds.), *Human growth 2, Postnatal growth.* New York: Plenum, 1978.

Garn, S. M., and S. M. Bailey: The genetics of maturational processes. In F. Falkner and J. M. Tanner (Eds.), *Human growth 1, Principles and prenatal growth.* New York: Plenum, 1978.

Golbus, M. S., and L. C. Berry: Human fetal development between 90 and 170 days postmenses. *Teratology,* 1977, *15*(1), 103–108.

Grunewald, P.: Growth of the human fetus 1, Normal growth and its variation. *Amer. J. Obstet. Gynec.,* 1966, *94,* 1112–1119.

Holsclaw, D. S., and A. L. Topham: The effects of smoking on fetal, neonatal, and childhood development. *Pediat. Ann.,* 1978, *7*(3), 201–222.

Jakobovits, A., N. Westlaker, L. Iffy, M. Wingater, H. Caterihi, R. Chatterton, and M. Lavenhar: Early intrauterine development: II. The rate of growth in black and Central American populations between 10 and 20 weeks' gestation. *Pediatrics,* 1976, *58,* 833–841.

Jordaan, H. V., and E. J. Dunn: A new method of evaluating fetal growth. *Obstet. Gynec.,* 1978, *51*(6), 659–665.

Kearney, K., N. Vigheron, P. Frischman, and J. Johnson: Fetal weight estimation by ultrasonic measurement of abdominal circumference. *Obstet. Gynec.* 1978, *51*(2), 156–162.

Lee, C. Y., P. C. Facog, B. Logrand: Fetal activity acceleration determination for the evaluation of fetal reserve. *J. Obstet. Gynec.* 1976, *48*(1), 19–26.

———, C. D. Panfilo, and J. M. O'Lane: A study of fetal heart rate patterns. *J. Obstet. Gynec.* 1975, *45*(2), 142–146.

Lubchenco, C. Hansman, and E. Boyd: Intrauterine growth in length and head circumference as estimated from live births at gestational ages from 26 to 42 weeks. *Pediatrics,* 1966, *37*(3), 403–409.

Manning, F. A.: Fetal breathing movements as a reflection of fetal status. *Postgrad. Med.,* 1977, *61*(4), 116–122.

Mantell, C. D.: Breathing movements in the human fetus. *Amer. J. Obstet. Gynec.,* 1976, *125*(4), 550–553.

Marsal, K., G. Gennser, and S. Kullander: Intrauterine breathing movements and fetal presentation. *Obstet. Gynec.,* 1978, *51*(2), 163–165.

McCance, R. A., and E. M. Widdowson: Glimpses of comparative growth and development. In F. Falkner and J. M. Tanner (Eds.), *Human growth 1, Principles and prenatal growth.* New York: Plenum, 1978.

McKeown, T., T. Marshall, and R. G. Record: Influences on fetal growth. *J. Reprod. Fertil.,* 1976, *47,* 167–181.

Metcoff, J.: Association of fetal growth with maternal nutrition. In F. Falkner and J. M. Tanner (Eds.), *Human growth 1, Principles and prenatal growth.* New York: Plenum, 1978.

Miller, H. C., K. Hassanein, T. Chin, and P. Hensleigh: Socioeconomic factors in relation to fetal growth in white infants. *J. Pediat.* 1976, *89*(4), 638–643.

Moore, K. L.: *The developing human* (2d ed.). Philadelphia: Saunders, 1977.

Mulvihill, J. J.: Fetal alcohol syndrome: Seven new cases. *Amer. J. Obstet. Gynec.,* 1976, *125,* 937–941.

Ounsted, M., and C. Ounsted: On fetal growth rate; Its variations and their consequences. *Clinics in Developmental Medicine No. 46.* London: Heinemann, 1973.

Pirani, B. B. K., and I. MacGillivray: Smoking during pregnancy, Its effect on maternal metabolism and fetoplacental function. *Obstet. Gynec.*, 1978, *52* (3), 257–263.

Rochard, F.: Nonstressed fetal heart rate monitoring in the antepartum period. *Amer. J. Obstet. Gynec.*, 1976, *126* (6), 699–706.

Romney, S. L., M. J. Gray, A. B. Little, J. A. Merrill, E. J. Quilligan, and R. Stander: *Gynecology and obstetrics, The health care of women.* New York: McGraw-Hill, 1975.

Smith, D. W.: *Growth and its disorders, Major problems in clinical pediatrics* (Vol. 15). Philadelphia: Saunders, 1977.

Southgate, D. A. T.: Fetal measurements. In F. Falkner and J. M. Tanner (Eds.), *Human growth 1, Principles and prenatal growth.* New York: Plenum, 1978.

Stevenson, R. E.: *The fetus and newlyborn infant: Influences of the prenatal environment* (2d ed.). St. Louis: Mosby, 1977.

Timor-Tritsch, I. E., L. J. Dierker, I. Zador, and R. H. Hertz: Fetal movements associated with fetal heart rate accelerations and decelerations. *Amer. J. Obstet. Gynec.*, 1978, *131* (3), 276–280.

Toth, P.: Physical growth of children born small for gestational age. *Acta Paediat. Acad. Sci. Hung.*, 1978, *19* (2), 99–104.

Usher, R., and F. McLean: Intrauterine growth of liveborn Caucasian infants at sea level: Standards obtained from measurements in 7 dimensions of infants born between 25 and 44 weeks of gestation. *J. Pediat.*, 1969, *74* (6), 901–910.

Wiener, S. N., M. J. Flynn, A. W. Kennedy, and F. Bonk: A composite curve of ultrasonic biparietal diameters for estimating gestational age. *Radiology*, 1977, *122* (3), 781–786.

Wilds, P. L.: Observations of intrauterine fetal breathing movements, A review. *Amer. J. Obstet. Gynec.*, 1978, *131* (3), 315–338.

Wilson, R. S.: Twins: Measures of birth size at different gestational ages. *Ann. Hum. Biol.*, 1974, *1*, 175–188.

Wladimiroff, J. W., C. A. Bloemsma, and H. C. S. Wallenburg: Ultrasonic assessment of fetal head and body sizes in relation to normal and retarded fetal growth. *Amer. J. Obstet. Gynec.*, 1978, *131* (8), 857–864.

Ziegler, E. E., A. M. O'Donnell, S. E. Nelson, and S. J. Fomon: Body composition of the reference fetus. *Growth*, 1976, *40*, 329–341.

PRENATAL BEHAVIOR

Adamsons, K.: Fetal growth: Obstetric implications. In F. Falkner and J. M. Tanner (Eds.), *Human growth 1, Principles and prenatal growth.* New York: Plenum, 1978.

Birnholz, J. C., J. C. Stephens, and M. Faria: Fetal movement patterns: A possible means of defining neurological developmental milestones in utero. *Amer. J. Roentgen.*, 1978, *130*, 537–540.

Boddy, K., and J. S. Robinson: External method for detection of fetal breathing in utero. *Lancet*, 1971, *2* (7736), 1231–1233.

Carmichael, L.: Onset and early development of behavior. In P. H. Mussen (Ed.), *Carmichael's manual of child psychology* (Vol. I). New York: Wiley, 1970.

———: William Preyer and the prenatal development of behavior. *Perspect. Biol. Med.*, 1973, *16* (3), 411–417.

Davis, M. E., and E. L. Potter: Intrauterine respiration of the human fetus. *J. A. M. A.*, 1946, *131* (5), 1194–1201.

Dawes, G. S., and J. S. Robinson: Rhythmic phenomena in prenatal life. *Progr. Brain Res.*, 1976, *45*, 383–389.

Duenhoelter, J. H., and J. A. Pritchard: Fetal respiration. *Amer. J. Obstet. Gynec.*, 1977, *129* (3), 326–338.

Elliott, G. B., and K. A. Elliott: Some pathological, radiological and clinical implications of the precocious development of the human ear. *Laryngoscope*, 1964, *74* (8), 1160–1171.

Fitzgerald, J. D., and W. F. Windle: Some observations on early human fetal movements. *J. Comp. Neurol.*, 1942, *76*, 159–167.

Fox, H. E.: Fetal breathing movements and ultrasound. *Amer. J. Dis. Child.*, 1976, *130*, 126–129.

———, J. Inglis, and M. Steinbrecher: Fetal breathing movements in uncomplicated pregnancies I. Relationship to gestational age. *Amer. J. Obstet. Gynec.*, 1979, *134*, 544–546.

Gottlieb, G.: Conceptions of prenatal development: Behavior embryology. *Psychol. Rev.*, 1976, *83* (3), 215–234.

Grimwade, J. D., D. W. Walker, M. Bartlett, S. Gordon, and C. Wood: Human fetal heart rate change and movement in response to sound and vibration. *Amer. J. Obstet. Gynec.*, 1971, *109* (1), 86–90.

Hamburger, V.: Development of embryonic motility. In E. Tobach, L. Aronson, E. Shaw (Eds.), *The biopsychology of development.* New York: Academic, 1971.

Humphrey, T.: The development of human fetal activity and its relations to postnatal behavior. *Advances Child Develop. Behav.*, 1970, *5*, 1–57.

Kasatkin, N. I.: First conditioned reflexes and the beginning of the learning process in the human infant. *Advances Psychobiol.*, 1972, *1*, 213–257.

Lewis, P., and P. Boylan: Fetal breathing: A review. *Amer. J. Obstet. Gynec.*, 1979, *134*, 587–597.

Liley, A. W.: The foetus as a personality. *Aust. New Zeal. J. Psychiat.*, 1972, *6*, 99–105.

Mistretta, C. M., and R. M. Bradley: Taste and swallowing in utero. *Brit. Med. Bull.*, 1975, *31*(1), 80–84.

Reinold, R.: Ultrasonics in early pregnancy: Diagnostic scanning and fetal motor activity. *Contrib. Gynec. Obstet.*, 1976, *1*, 1–148.

Rochard, F.: Nonstressed fetal heart rate monitoring in the antenatal period. *Amer. J. Obstet. Gynec.*, 1976, *126*(6), 699–706.

Ron, M., H. Yaffe, and E. Sadovsky: Fetal heart rate response to amniocentesis in cases of decreased fetal movements. *Obstet. Gynec.*, 1976, *48*, 456–462.

Sadovsky, E.: Timing of delivery in high risk pregnancy by monitoring of fetal movements. *J. Perinat. Med.*, 1978, *6*(3), 160–164.

———, and W. Z. Polishuk: Fetal movements in utero: Nature, assessment, prognostic value, timing of delivery. *Obstet. Gynec.*, 1977, *50*(1), 49–55.

Scheer, K., and J. Nubar: Variation of fetal presentation with gestational age. *Amer. J. Obstet. Gynec.*, 1976, *125*(2), 269–270.

Smyth, C. N. L.: Experimental methods for testing the integrity of the foetus and neonate. *J. Obstet. Gynaec. Brit. Comm.*, 1965, *72*, 920.

Sontag, L. W., and H. Newberry: Normal variations of fetal heart rate during pregnancy. *Amer. J. Obstet. Gynec.*, 1940, *40*, 449–452.

Spelt, D. K.: The conditioning of the human fetus in utero. *J. Exp. Psychol.*, 1948, *38*, 338–346.

Timor-Tritsch, I. E.: Fetal movements associated with fetal heart rate accelerations and decelerations. *Amer. J. Obstet. Gynec.*, 1978, *131*(3), 276–280.

———, I. Zador, R. H. Hertz, and M. G. Rosen: Classification of human fetal movement. *Amer. J. Obstet. Gynec.*, 1976 *126*(1), 70–77.

Walker, D., J. Grimwade, and C. Wood: Intrauterine noise: A component of the fetal environment. *Amer. J. Obstet. Gynec.*, 1971, *109*(1), 91–95.

LABOR AND BIRTH

American Nurses' Association: *Statement on parental-infant attachment.* Kansas City, Missouri: American Nurses' Association, Division on Maternal and Child Health Nursing Practice, 1979.

Barden, T.: *Perinatal care.* New York: McGraw-Hill, 1975.

Clark, A. L., and D. D. Affonso: *Childbearing: A nursing perspective.* Philadelphia: Davis, 1976.

Friedman, E.: Normal labor curve. *Clin. Obstet. Gynec.*, 1973, *16*(1), 176–183.

Gassner, C., and W. J. Ledger: The relationship of hospital-acquired maternal infection to invasive intrapartum monitoring techniques. *Amer. J. Obstet. Gynec.*, 1976, *126*(1), 33–37.

Goodlin, R., and H. C. Haesslein: When is it fetal distress? *Amer. J. Obstet. Gynec.*, 1977, *128*(4), 440–445.

Haverkamp, A., H. E. Thompson, J. G. McFee, and C. Cetrulo: The evaluation of continuous fetal heart rate monitoring in high risk pregnancy. *Amer. J. Obstet. Gynec.*, 1976, *125*(3), 310–320.

Martell, M., J. M. Belizan, F. Nieto, and R. Schwarcz: Blood acid-base at birth in neonates from labors with early and late rupture of the membranes. *J. Pediat.*, 1976, *89*(6), 963–967.

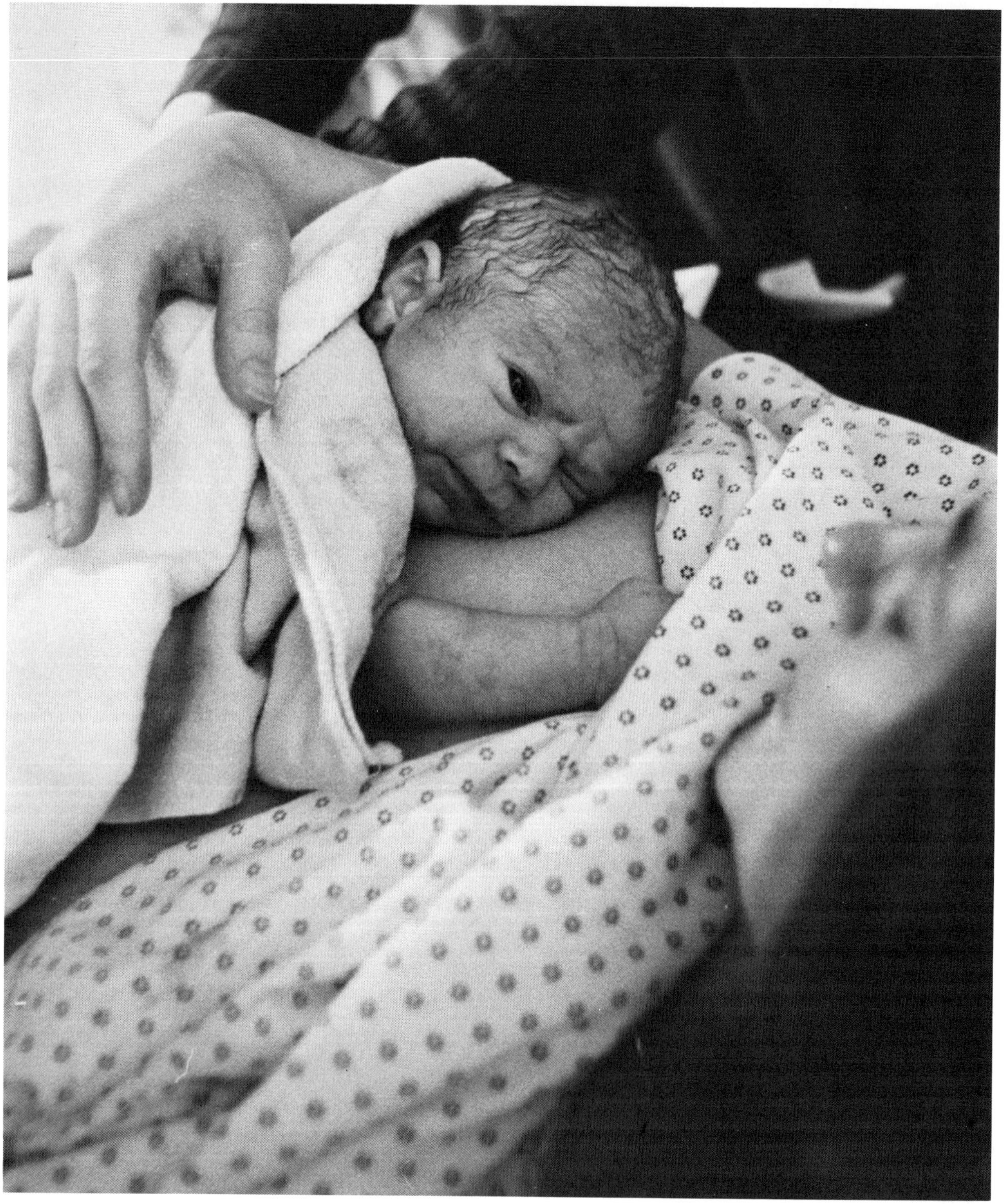

CHAPTER 6
The Neonate: Birth to 1 Month

Introduction

Birth is not a beginning for the child; the neonate—newly born—was the fetus just moments before. The neonate is on a continuum which started at conception. Only to those in his environment (except his parents!) does he "suddenly appear."

The environmental surroundings impinging on the neonate are abruptly changed, and he must instantly cope and gradually adapt. The prenatal environment was life supporting; the postnatal environment demands independence in physiological function. The neonate is morphologically and maturationally prepared to meet this challenge. All body systems are functional, although most to an immature degree. The physical task now is not formation but growth and maturation.

In the first few days of extrauterine life, gaining physiological stability and recovering from birth takes precedence. During the following first weeks, the neonate spends most of the time asleep. When awake, the neonate nurses in order to grow, the second priority. Having slowed near term, rate of growth soon accelerates rapidly. Gains in head circumference, length, and weight are significant during the first month.

The neonate alternates between sleep and wakeful periods, pausing only briefly in the latter. During his wakeful times, the neonate demonstrates notable behavior and response to the environment; when quiet and alert, the neonate will attend to his parent's face and voice. These periods are brief, however, and more often the child resembles an unopened bud at this age. Nevertheless, the neonate shows individuality in his "time clock" of states of sleep and wakefulness as well as his reactions to hunger, discomfort, and comforting.

The neonatal period lasts 1 month. Toward the end of that month it can be seen that the neonate is "waking up" and beginning to stay awake for longer periods. The neonatal period is a time of transition and stabilization, a time of readying for the task of development that lies ahead, and a time of acquaintance with family, those who will assist in the journey.

FIGURE 6-1.

SECTION 1

Physical Development

Physical status and development of the neonate   Jean A. Foster

EFFECTS OF BIRTH

At the moment of birth, the neonate undergoes the most profound physical and physiological changes of his life. He emerges from a warm, relatively quiet, aquatic womb into the colder, noisy extrauterine environment; the contrast of womb to world is dramatic. The neonate's dependent, symbiotic existence is forever relinquished, and he alone must manage all the complicated processes of living.

Physiologically, numerous alterations must occur for the neonate to survive. Some changes, such as expansion of his lungs and the drop in pulmonary vascular resistance, occur almost immediately after birth. Others, such as closure of the ductus arteriosus, may take several hours to days. A measure of the neonate's adaptation to extrauterine life (as well as a prediction of his survival potential) may be made in the first and fifth minutes of his life utilizing the *Apgar Newborn Scoring System*. This scale, developed by Dr. Virginia Apgar, is used in most delivery rooms to evaluate the five critical signs of heart rate, respiratory rate, muscle tone, reflex irritability, and color. As illustrated in Table 6-1, a score of 0 to 2 is assigned to each sign, depending upon the degree to which it is present or absent. A total score of 8 to 10 at 1 or 5 min of age demonstrates that the neonate is making a successful transition from intrauterine to extrauterine life. A score of 2 or less at 1 min or less than 5 at 5 min indicates that the neonate requires resuscitation to support life (Avery 1975).

The effects of labor and birth upon the neonate may be reflected in the Apgar score. If the mother has been recently sedated, for example, the infant may exhibit depressed respirations. A long and difficult labor may produce an exhausted infant with little reflex irritability.

Depending upon the type of birth, other effects may include edema of the presenting part (*caput succedaneum*), abnormal shaping (molding) of the head, and bruises and/or forceps marks. These will disappear in a few days to weeks of life and generally require no intervention.

TABLE 6-1   Apgar newborn scoring system

Sign	0	1	2
Heart rate	Not detectable†	Below 100	Above 100
Respiratory rate	Absent	Slow, irregular	Good (crying)
Muscle tone	Flaccid	Some flexion of extremities	Active motion
Reflex irritability	No response	Grimace	Vigorous cry
Color*	Pale†	Blue†	Pink†

* If the natural skin color of the child is not white, alternative tests for color are applied, such as color of mucous membranes of mouth and conjunctiva and color of lips, palms, hands, and soles of feet.

Source: Used by permission of Dr. Virginia Apgar, with recent modifications indicated by a dagger.

DEVELOPMENTAL APPROACH TO PHYSICAL ASSESSMENT

A special approach must be utilized in the physical assessment of the neonate which is based on developmental stage. The cephalocaudal sequence is disadvantageous with the neonate because observation and auscultation of cardiopulmonary function occur in the middle of the process. The neonate may be either irritable or exhausted by midpoint, causing the assessment of cardiopulmonary status to be inaccurate.

It is preferable, therefore, to begin the physical exam of the neonate by observation of his respiratory status, followed by auscultation of heart and lung sounds. The nurse may then choose to return to the head and move downward, as in a typical physical exam. Whichever approach is chosen, it should be followed consistently with each neonate, thus ensuring completeness of assessment.

Five behavioral states of a normal neonate have been

identified (Prechtl, 1974) (see Sec. 2) and must be considered during physical assessment. General observation of the neonate as well as the previously described assessment of cardiopulmonary status can best be accomplished while the infant is in a quiet sleep (state 1). Quiet alert (state 3) is best for most of the physical exam, and particularly for the neurological assessment. In this state, the neonate's eyes are open; he is alert and attentive and best able to respond. To bring a sleeping or crying neonate to this state, hold him upright with one hand under his head and one hand under his bottom, and gently rock him up and down. This technique is especially helpful before a funduscopic exam.

Symmetry of movement of the neonate's extremities may be observed while he is in state 4, active alert. And finally, facial symmetry and vigorousness of cry will be evident while the neonate is in state 5, crying. The nurse must be fully aware of all responses that require demonstration and then watch for these responses throughout the exam. Feeling for the palate with the index finger may also elicit a sucking reflex; holding the neonate to palpate vertebrae may also demonstrate horizontal positioning. Another reason to combine physical and neurological assessments is to shorten the exam period. A complete physical followed by a lengthy neurological assessment can lead to unreliable results from an irritable or exhausted baby.

The environment in which the neonate is examined is critical; temperature, noise, and lighting will affect his physical well-being and influence his ability to respond. The neonate's anatomy and physiology predispose him to a greater-than-normal rate of heat loss. His surface-to-volume ratio is very large, providing a greater surface area for loss to take place. Also, his subcutaneous fat layer is inadequate and affords little insulatory protection. And finally, due to his rapid respiratory rate, large amounts of heat are lost through evaporation on the lung surfaces.

The neonate's physiological response to heat loss is to produce heat through increased metabolic activity of visceral organs and brown fat. Since increased metabolism requires increased oxygen consumption, the neonate may become compromised if the period of cold stress is severe or prolonged. To prevent these consequences, physical assessment of the neonate should always occur in a warmed environment.

A noisy environment is not conducive to observation of the neonate. Repeated startling of the neonate causes him to become irritable and to cry, thus making the exam difficult or impossible to complete. The neonate, being photophobic, will tightly close his eyes in bright lighting. Thus, he is more likely to move into a quiet, alert, attentive state if the lighting is dim and indirect.

GENERAL APPEARANCE

At birth, the healthy neonate is ruddy red and covered with *vernix caseosa,* a white cheesy material. The vernix need not be removed; it will be absorbed by the neonate's skin in the first 24 h of life, providing beneficial lubrication. *Acrocyanosis* (cyanosis of hands and feet) due to sluggish peripheral circulation and *cutis marmorate* (mottling in response to cold) may also be noted.

During the first month of life, the Caucasian neonate's skin color will diminish from bright pink to a pale-pink color. The Negro neonate will be very light brown at birth, and his color will darken noticeably during the first month of life. (Genitalia are usually darker at birth and may indicate the eventual color of the child's skin.)

The neonate's head is large in relation to his body and accounts for approximately one-quarter of his total length. Often the head will appear elongated in the first few days due to molding during birth; it generally resumes its normal shape in 2 to 3 days. The neonate's chest is cylindrical and approximately the same circumferential size as, to 2 cm smaller than, the head. Rapid, irregular respirations are observed to be abdominal rather than thoracic.

The neonate assumes a "fetal" posture, the position he had in utero. His head and back are fully flexed. With hands held in fists, he holds his arms close to his chest. His hips are also flexed, and his knees are drawn up on his chest, with feet dorsiflexed. During the first month of life, the neonate frequently resumes this position when sleeping, cold, or stressed.

NORMAL GROWTH PARAMETERS

Soon after birth, measurements are taken of the neonate's weight, height, and head and chest circumferences. These parameters reflect the growth of the fetus in utero, influenced by a variety of factors, both maternal and fetal (see Chap. 5). Variability in size exists between neonates of different races as well as between sexes. Thus, these factors must be taken into account before conclusions are drawn from the growth charts. Whereas eventual size of the child is determined by genetic predilection combined with environmental factors, size at birth is determined primarily by maternal factors. Mature size cannot be predicted from initial measurements. However, shortly after birth, the neonate's growth parameters, freed from maternal constraints, begin to reflect his genotype.

THE NEONATE: BIRTH TO 1 MONTH

WEIGHT

The average weight of a female neonate is 3250 g (7 lb 2 oz) with males averaging 50 g (2 oz) larger than females. Variability is greatest in this parameter; the range for 90 percent of all neonates is 2400 g (5 lb 4 oz) to 4100 g (9 lb). During the first few days of life, most neonates lose 5 to 10 percent of their body weight due to passage of meconium and urine as well as to delay in feedings. This weight is usually regained by 10 days of age. Throughout the first month of life, the neonate gains at a rate of 150 to 180 g (5 to 6 oz) per week.

Composition of body weight in neonates is different from that of older infants. Water constitutes 75 percent of body weight in neonates, compared with only 56 percent in the 1-year-old infant. Conversely, the neonate's weight is made up of only 11 percent fat, while the 1-year-old infant has 23 percent (Fomon, 1966).

LENGTH

Less variable than weight, length for 90 percent of all neonates ranges from 44 to 53 cm ($17\frac{1}{2}$ to 21 in). Average length is 49 to 50 cm ($19\frac{1}{2}$ in), with males about 0.5 cm longer than females. By 1 month, the average neonate's length has increased 4 cm (2 in).

HEAD AND CHEST CIRCUMFERENCES

Occipital-frontal circumference (OFC) is the least variable parameter and is little influenced by nutritional, social, racial, and other factors (Nellhaus, 1968). In 90 percent of all neonates, the range is 32 to 37 cm ($12\frac{1}{2}$ to $14\frac{1}{2}$ in), with an average of 34.5 cm ($13\frac{1}{2}$ in). The OFC of males is on an average 0.5 cm ($\frac{1}{4}$ in) larger than females. Chest circumference is usually equal to or slightly less than OFC. By 1 month, both circumferences are 3 cm (1 in) larger.

NORMAL VITAL SIGNS

At birth and throughout the first month of life, the neonate's heart rate ranges from 120 to 160 bpm, and may be irregular. His respiratory rate may also be irregular at 40 to 60 breaths per minute. While he sleeps, the neonate may exhibit periodic breathing: several rapid respirations followed by a 5- to 10-s period of nonbreathing. No change in heart rate or color is associated with this harmless breathing pattern, thus differentiating it from apnea.

The neonate should be maintained at an axillary (skin) temperature of 36 to 37°C (96.8 to 98.6°F). Core temperature (as measured by rectal thermometer) changes only when the neonate's thermoregulatory mechanisms have been exhausted and thus is a very late sign of cold stress.

LABORATORY VALUES

Several laboratory values are commonly determined in the neonatal period to evaluate physiologic status. Hematocrit, sampled via heel stick, is relatively high in the neonate, ranging from 53 to 68 percent. This value is, of course, dependent upon the position of the neonate in relation to the placenta before the umbilical cord is clamped as well as the amount of time before the cord is clamped. Observable signs of high hematocrit in the neonate include acrocyanosis, cool hands and feet, and sluggish blood flow from heel sticks. By 1 month of age, the hematocrit falls to 35 to 45 percent.

Bilirubin levels in the neonate may also be higher than those of older children and adults. Due to the immaturity of the neonate's liver as well as hemolysis from bruising or cephalohematoma, neonates often demonstrate physiological jaundice during the first 2 to 3 days of life. The bilirubin level generally begins to drop after 5 to 7 days and reaches a normal childhood level by 1 month of age.

COMMON PHYSICAL VARIATIONS

Each neonate is an individual and is born with physiological differences that are neither normal nor abnormal but acceptable variants.

Epstein's pearls, found in the mouth of the neonate, are epithelial cysts which appear as white nodules. They are completely without significance and are usually sloughed unnoticed in the first few postnatal weeks.

Milia, which appear as white dots across the bridge of the nose and the chin, are tiny sebaceous retention cysts. These cysts disappear spontaneously after 1 to 2 weeks. *Erythema toxicum,* or newborn rash, appears most commonly on the abdomen and perineum during the first 24 h. The rash is characterized by tiny, raised, yellowish wheals surrounded by areas of redness. Although the lesions may appear and disappear over 1 to 2 weeks' time, treatment is unnecessary.

Cephalohematoma is subperiosteal hemorrhage of the cranial bones. Although it appears similar to caput succedaneum, cephalohematoma may be distinguished by its later onset (several hours after birth) and its conformation to suture lines. While the obvious swelling disappears by 6 weeks, x-ray evidence of calcification may persist for years. Additionally, cephalohematoma may be accompanied by linear skull fracture. *Subconjunctival hemorrhage,* a broken conjunctival capillary as a result of birth, occurs quite frequently and is of no clinical significance. The red "halo" effect around the iris usually disappears in 1 to 2 weeks.

Stork's beak marks are light pink splotches frequently seen on the eyelids and the back of the neck. They tend to fade when the neonate is quiet and become darker when he cries. Usually, these benign hemangiomas lighten and disappear over time. *Mongolian spots*, most frequently observed in Oriental and Negro babies, are large dark-blue or purple spots located over the lumbosacral area. Also benign, they usually disappear by 4 years.

The emphasis in nursing care today is on health and development promotion as well as prevention of illness. An adequate data base is a primary requirement for these interventions, and physical assessment is essential to that data base.

Maturation and growth deviation in the neonate Holly E. Miner

ESTIMATION OF GESTATIONAL AGE

Estimation of gestational age is of primary importance to consideration of the neonate being evaluated. Only after this information has been obtained is it possible to interpret additional information which is based on this finding. Gestational age is determined prenatally in several ways (see Chap. 5). Gestational age can also be determined by clinical examination of the infant. To date, two major areas of clinical examination have been researched: neurological assessment and external characteristics as they relate to gestational age.

In 1970, Dubowitz, Dubowitz, and Goldberg developed a method of determining gestational age which encompassed both physical and neurological characteristics. Their scoring system is the most accurate for determining gestational age. It requires an examination at birth for external criteria with an examination after 24 h of the infant's neurological system. The scales available to assess gestational age include observation of physical signs, as described in Table 6-2, and neurological signs, as shown in Fig. 6-2 and Table 6-3.

Neurological signs include resting posture (see Fig. 6-3) and recoil of extremities. Hypotonia is present until 30 weeks' gestation. Flexion of the thighs and hips occurs at 34 weeks ma, followed by arm flexion at 35 weeks. At 36 to 38 weeks the resting posture includes total flexion. After 2 weeks more, at any point of flexion there is sufficient muscle strength to produce recoil.

Examination of muscle tone includes measurement of

TABLE 6-2 Scoring system for external criteria

External sign	Score*				
	0	1	2	3	4
Edema	Obvious edema of hands and feet; pitting over tibia	No obvious edema of hands and feet; pitting over tibia	No edema		
Skin texture	Very thin, gelatinous	Thin and smooth	Smooth; medium thickness; rash or superficial peeling	Slight thickening; superficial cracking and peeling especially of hands and feet	Thick and parchment-like; superficial or deep cracking
Skin color	Dark red	Uniformly pink	Pale pink; variable over body	Pale; only pink over ears, lips, palms, or soles	
Skin opacity (trunk)	Numerous veins and venules clearly seen, especially over abdomen	Veins and tributaries seen	A few large vessels clearly seen over abdomen	A few large vessels seen indistinctly over abdomen	No blood vessels seen
Lanugo (over back)	No lanugo	Abundant; long and thick over lower part of back	Hair thinning, especially over lower back	Small amount of lanugo and bald areas	At least half of back devoid of lanugo

* If score differs on two sides, take the mean.

TABLE 6-2 Scoring system for external criteria (*Continued*)

External sign	0	1	2	3	4
Plantar creases	No skin creases	Faint red marks over anterior half of sole	Definite red marks over > anterior half; indentations over < anterior third	Indentations over > anterior third	Definite deep indentations over > anterior third
Nipple formation	Nipple barely visible; no areola	Nipple well defined; areola smooth and flat, diameter < 0.75 cm	Areola stippled, edge not raised, diameter < 0.75 cm	Areola stippled, edge raised, diameter > 0.75 cm	
Breast size	No breast tissue palpable	Breast tissue on one or both sides, < 0.5 cm diameter	Breast tissue both sides; one or both 0.5–1.0 cm	Breast tissue both sides; one or both > 1 cm	
Ear form	Pinna flat and shapeless, little or no incurving of edge	Incurving of part of edge of pinna	Partial incurving of whole of upper pinna	Well-defined incurving of whole of upper pinna	
Ear firmness	Pinna soft, easily folded, no recoil	Pinna soft, easily folded, slow recoil	Cartilage to edge of pinna, but soft in places, ready recoil	Pinna firm, cartilage to edge, instant recoil	
Genitals:					
Male	Neither testis in scrotum	At least one testis high in scrotum	At least one testis right down		
Female (with hips half abducted)	Labia majora widely separated, labia minora protruding	Labia majora almost cover labia minora	Labia majora completely cover labia minora		

Source: From L. Dubowitz, V. Dubowitz, and C. Goldberg, Clinical assessment of gestational age in the newborn infant. *J. Pediat.*, 1970, 77(1). As adapted from Farr and associates, *Developmental medicine and child neurology.* St. Louis: Mosby, 1966. Reprinted by permission of the C. V. Mosby Company.

extremity tone, trunk tone, and overall body tone. The *heel-to-ear* test and the *scarf sign* determine extremity tone by the resistance offered to passive movement (see Figs. 6-4 and 6-5). Measurement of trunk tone includes neck flexors, head lag, neck extensors, body extensors, and increasing motor control as gestation progresses (see Fig. 6-6). Overall body tone is measured in the vertical and horizontal positions (see Fig. 6-7).

Tests of flexion angle include measurement of the popliteal angle (see Fig. 6-4) and ankle and wrist angles (see Figs. 6-8 and 6-9). The popliteal angle is indirectly related to muscle tone in the lower extremities; the greater the tone, the smaller the angle. Measuring the ankle and wrist angles will also aid in determining the degree of maturation.

Most common to neonatal assessment is the presence of

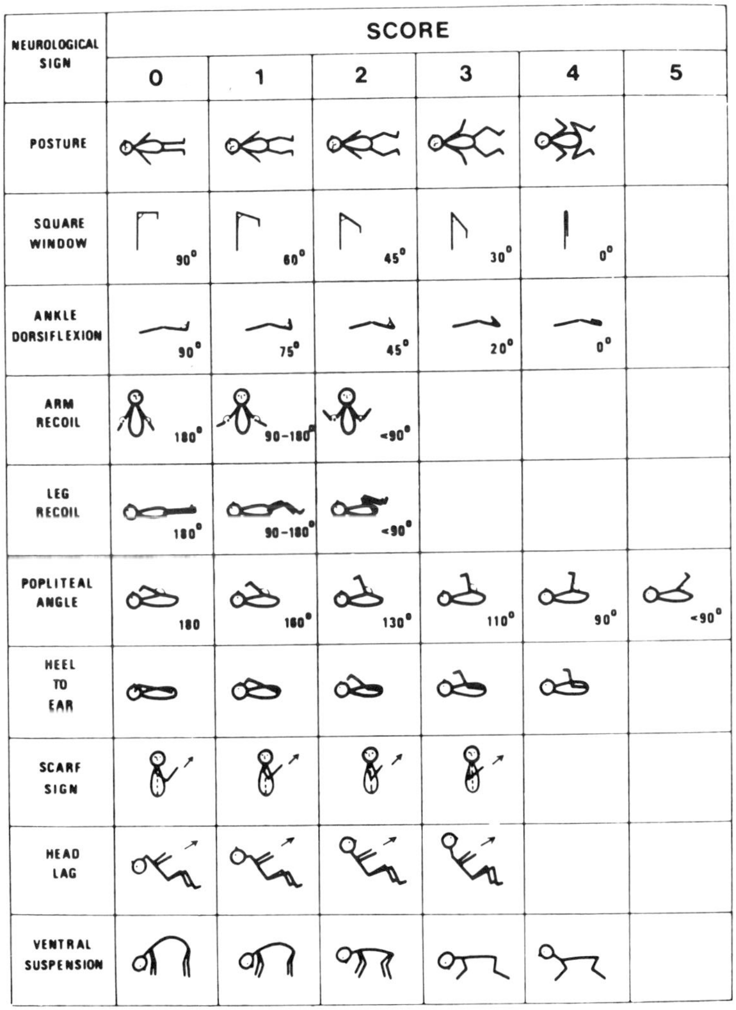

FIGURE 6-2. Scoring system for neurologic criteria; see notes on techniques. [*From L. Dubowitz, V. Dubowitz, and C. Goldberg, Clinical assessment of gestational age in the newborn infant. J. Pediat., 1970, 77(1), 1–10. Reprinted by permission of The C. V. Mosby Company, St. Louis.*]

reflexes. The reflexes of the preterm infant are absent or weaker, slower, more random or uncoordinated, may have a long latency period, and are not elicited consistently. Gestational age is determined by total score (see Fig. 6-10).

Once gestational age has been assessed, it is possible to determine whether the infant is premature, small for gestational age, full term, or postmature depending upon the relation of gestational age to weight, length, and head circumference. Values are plotted on intrauterine growth charts. The Colorado Intrauterine Growth Chart is widely used (see Fig. 6-11). Other growth standards are available, including growth curves from Portland, Oregon, and Baltimore, Maryland. The Colorado curves are widely accepted as they encompass a broader representation of racial groups. However, as discussed in Chap. 5, high altitude (as in Colorado) affects intrauterine growth.

THE PREMATURE INFANT

A universally accepted definition of the premature infant is one who has a gestational age of less than 37 weeks menstrual age yet whose weight surpasses the 10th percentile for gestational age on the Colorado Intrauterine Growth Chart (Korones, 1972).

Most frequently, the premature infant is born intact for its relative gestational age. Problems most commonly encountered with these infants relate to their functioning gestational age and are the result of a faulty maternal physiological system. The more common of these problems are multiple pregnancy, placenta previa, incompetent cervix, and iatrogenic delivery.

The premature infant has been categorized into three degrees of prematurity. (Using menstrual age, the full-term infant is born at 40 weeks gestation.) The borderline

TABLE 6-3 Some notes on techniques of assessment of neurologic criteria

Posture	Observed with infant quiet and in supine position. Score 0: arms and legs extended; 1: beginning of flexion of hips and knees, arms extended; 2: stronger flexion of legs, arms extended; 3: arms slightly flexed, legs flexed and abducted; 4: full flexion of arms and legs.
Square window	The hand is flexed on the forearm between the thumb and index finger of the examiner. Enough pressure is applied to get as full a flexion as possible, and the angle between the hypothenar eminence and the ventral aspect of the forearm is measured and graded. (Care is taken not to rotate the infant's wrist while doing this maneuver.)
Ankle dorsiflexion	The foot is dorsiflexed onto the anterior aspect of the leg, with the examiner's thumb on the sole of the foot and other fingers behind the leg. Enough pressure is applied to get as full flexion as possible, and the angle between the dorsum of the foot and the anterior aspect of the leg is measured.
Arm recoil	With the infant in the supine position the forearms are first flexed for 5 s, then fully extended by pulling on the hands, and then released. The sign is fully positive if the arms return briskly to full flexion (score 2). If the arms return to incomplete flexion or the response is sluggish, it is graded as score 1. If they remain extended or are only followed by random movements, the score is 0.
Leg recoil	With the infant supine, the hips and knees are fully flexed for 5 s, then extended by traction on the feet, and released. A maximal response is one of full flexion of the hips and knees (score 2). A partial flexion scores 1, and minimal or no movement scores 0.
Popliteal angle	With the infant supine and his pelvis flat on the examining couch, the thigh is held in the knee-chest position by the examiner's left index finger and thumb supporting the knee. The leg is then extended by gentle pressure from the examiner's right index finger behind the ankle, and the popliteal angle is measured.
Heel to ear maneuver	With the baby supine, draw the baby's foot as near to the head as it will go without forcing it. Observe the distance between the foot and the head as well as the degree of extension at the knee. Note that the knee is left free and may draw down alongside the abdomen.
Scarf sign	With the baby supine, take the infant's hand and try to put it around the neck and as far posteriorly as possible around the opposite shoulder. Assist this maneuver by lifting the elbow across the body. See how far the elbow will go across. Score 0: elbow reaches opposite axillary line; 1: elbow between midline and opposite axillary line; 2: elbow reaches midline; 3: elbow will not reach midline.
Head lag	With the baby lying supine, grasp the hands (or the arms if a very small infant) and pull him slowly toward the sitting position. Observe the position of the head in relation to the trunk, and grade accordingly. In a small infant the head may initially be supported by one hand. Score 0: complete lag; 1: partial head control; 2: able to maintain head in line with body; 3: brings head anterior to body.
Ventral suspension	The infant is suspended in the prone position, with examiner's hand under the infant's chest (one hand in a small infant, two in a large infant). Observe the degree of extension of the back and the amount of flexion of the arms and legs. Also note the relation of the head to the trunk.
	If score differs on the two sides, take the mean.

Source: From L. Dubowitz, V. Dubowitz, and C. Goldberg, Clinical assessment of gestational age in the newborn infant. *J. Pediat.,* 1970, *77*(1), 5. Reprinted by permission of The C. V. Mosby Company.

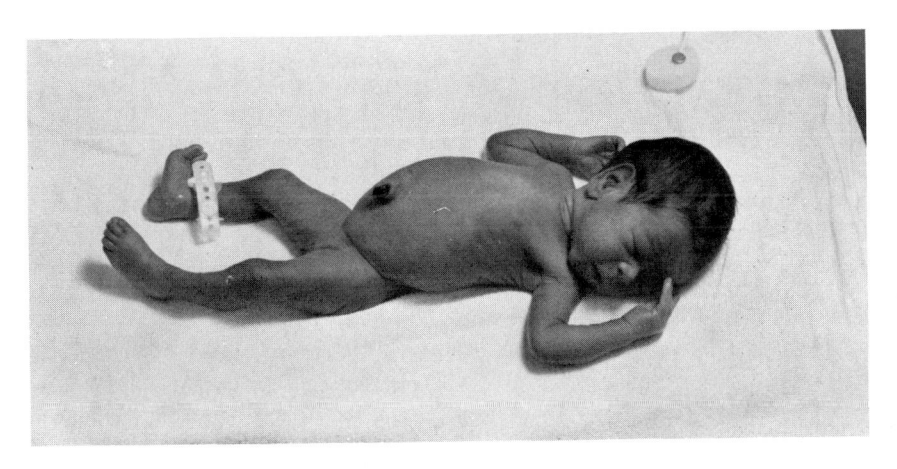

FIGURE 6-3. The resting posture of the premature infant is characterized by only partial flexion in the arms or legs. The term neonate exhibits flexion in all extremities. [*From R. Sullivan, J. Foster, and R. L. Schreiner, Determining a newborn's gestational age. MCN 4(1): 38-45, 1979. Reprinted by permission.*]

premature infant is that one born from the thirty-seventh through the thirty-eighth weeks of gestation ma; the moderately premature infant, 31 to 36 weeks' gestation; and the severe, or extreme, premature infant, 24 to 30 weeks' gestation. Although physical findings are related to gestational age, it is important to note that these factors represent a continuum. There is an inverse relation to gestational age: The greater the gestational age, the fewer problems found in the infant.

FIGURE 6-4. Heel-to-ear test is done with the neonate supine. The neonate's foot is brought as close to the ear as possible without forcing it. The distance between foot and ear as well as the popliteal angle (degree of extension at the knee) is noted. The premature infant exhibits little resistance and more extension of the knee than the full-term neonate. (*From Sullivan et al., 1979. Reprinted by permission.*)

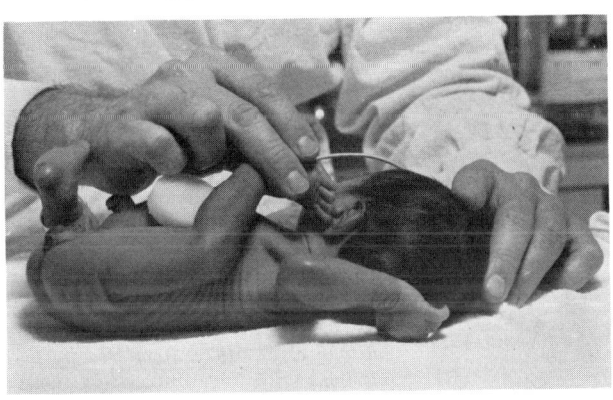

THE SMALL-FOR-GESTATIONAL-AGE INFANT

The small-for-gestational-age (SGA) infant is referred to by several phrases which describe his condition. These include dysmature, fetal malnutrition syndrome, chronic fetal distress, and intrauterine growth retardation.

The SGA infant is one who, by definition, falls below the 10th percentile on the Colorado Intrauterine Growth Chart for his gestational age. The SGA infant can also be defined as one who falls two standard deviations below the mean for any given week of gestation. Births of SGA infants are the result of many factors. Among these are vascular insufficiencies, toxemia, hypertension, renal disease, collagen disease, multiple pregnancy, high altitude, nutritional status, excessive smoking, and economic conditions (Bard, 1970) (see Chap. 5). Approximately 1.5 to 2 percent of neonates are determined to be SGA.

The cause of intrauterine growth retardation is either fetal or placental. "Fetal causes may be genetic, chromosomal, infection (rubella, cytomegalic inclusion disease), twinning, anencephaly, single umbilical artery, drugs, and radiation. Placental causes stem from faulty implantation, malformation and metabolism" (Miner, 1978). The problem, however, is that these reasons fail to explain the SGA infant that is free of abnormalities.

Fetal malnutrition does not appear to be a major factor in the development of the SGA infant until the third trimester. In the first and second trimesters, the umbilical cord is able to supply more than what is demanded by the fetus even in the presence of moderate nutritional deprivation. Clinical studies indicate that even in the event of acute shortage of food, the human female is more prone to

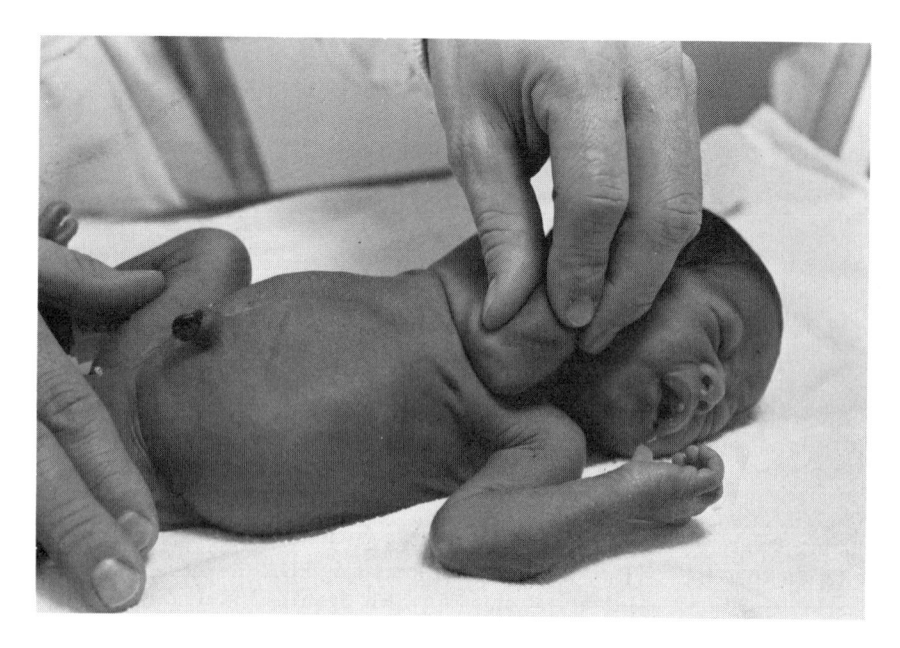

FIGURE 6-5. In elicitation of the scarf sign, the neonate is placed supine and his arm is brought across his chest as far as possible without forcing. In the premature, the elbow reaches near or across the midline as shown. In the full-term neonate, the elbow will not reach the midline. (*From Sullivan et al., 1979. Reprinted by permission.*)

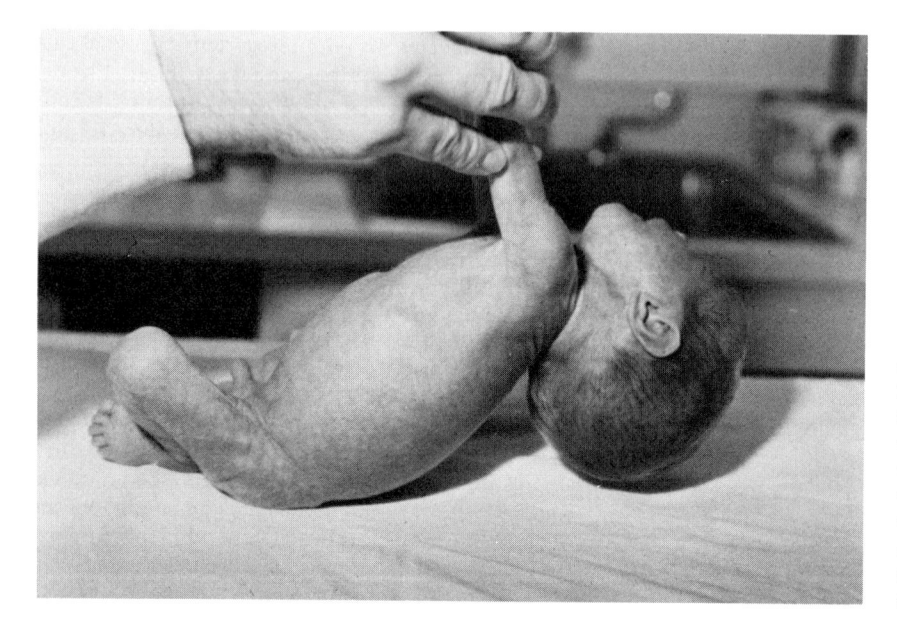

FIGURE 6-6. Head lag (neck flexors and extensors) is tested in pulling the infant to sitting and holding him upright. When pulled to sit, the premature evidences little or no neck flexion and the head falls back as shown. When held upright, the premature's head falls forward and he is unable to use neck extensors to lift his head upright. (*From Sullivan et al., 1979. Reprinted by permission.*)

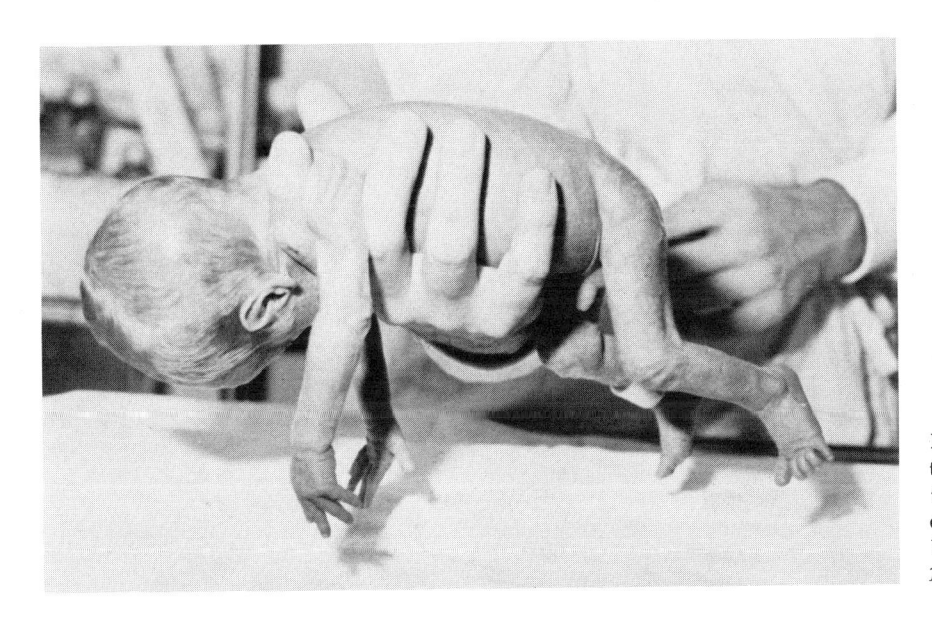

FIGURE 6-7. The premature's low tone is evidenced as he is held in ventral suspension. There is little flexion of the arms and legs and little head and back extension. (*From Sullivan et al., 1979. Reprinted by permission.*)

FIGURE 6-8. In evaluation of ankle dorsiflexion, the foot is pressed onto the anterior aspect of the leg, obtaining as much flexion as possible. The angle between the dorsum of the foot and the anterior aspect of the leg is measured. (*a*) In the premature neonate there will be an angle of 45 to 90°. (*b*) In the full-term neonate the ankle will flex until the foot touches the leg. (*From Sullivan et al., 1979. Reprinted by permission.*)

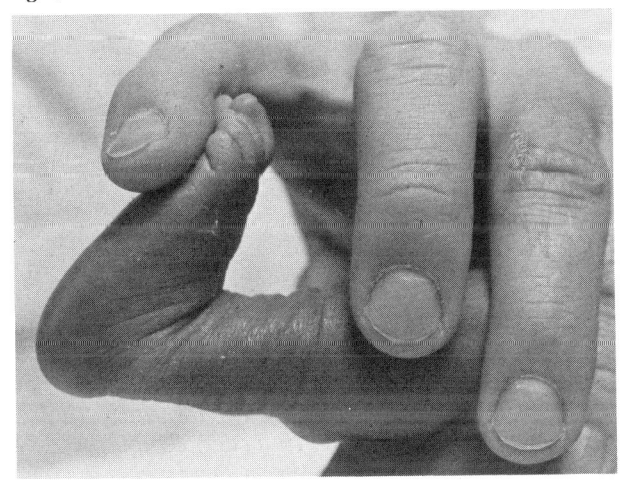

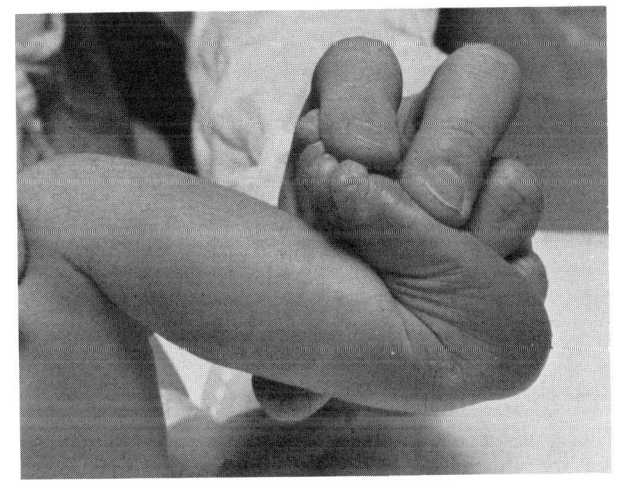

(*a*)   (*b*)

FIGURE 6-9. Wrist flexion, or "square window," is evaluated by flexing the wrist as much as possible and measuring the angle between the hypothenar eminence and the ventral aspect of the forearm. (*a*) The premature will exhibit a 45 to 90° angle. (*b*) It is possible to completely flex the full-term neonate's wrist. (*Sullivan et al., 1979. Reprinted by permission.*)

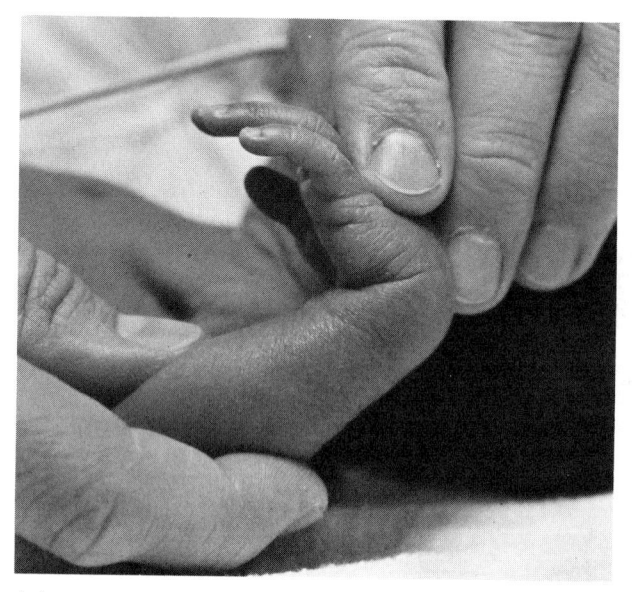

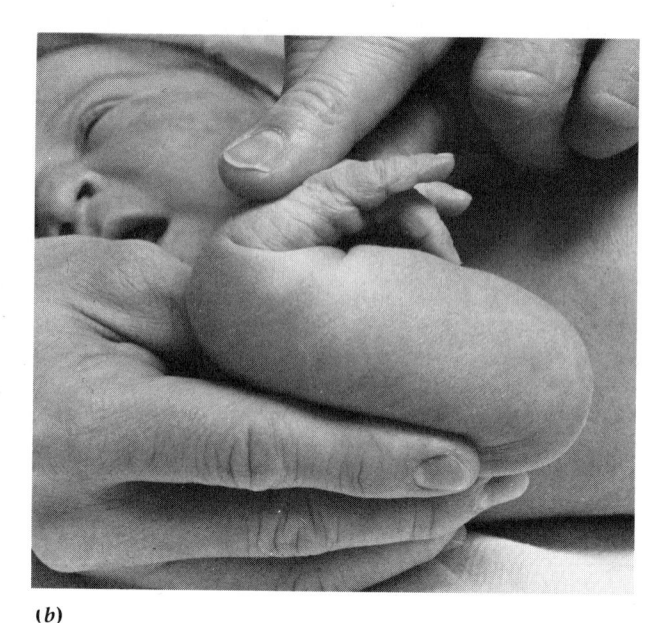

increased frequency of early abortion and failure to conceive than to a decrease in the overall birth weight of the fetus (Drillien, 1970).

THE POSTMATURE INFANT

The postmature, or postterm, infant is that neonate of more than 42 weeks' gestation ma. A majority of the neonates thought to be postmature are often younger, the result of a miscalculation in conception dates. Those infants which are truly postmature have physical signs which include oligohydramnios, meconium-stained amniotic fluid, loss of fetal subcutaneous fat, long fingernails, "golden" vernix, and meconium staining of membranes and cord. Postmature infants are quite active shortly after birth and display developmental skills appropriate to their gestational age.

THE LARGE-FOR-GESTATIONAL-AGE INFANT

The large-for-gestational-age (LGA) infant is defined as that infant who is on or above the 90th percentile on the Colorado Intrauterine Growth Chart in relation to his gestational age. Most often the etiology of the LGA infant is unknown, except in the case of the diabetic mother.

The infants of diabetic mothers are LGA approximately one-third of the time. These infants are large when the mother's blood-glucose level is not strictly controlled. Recent studies have shown that if the mother's blood-glucose level is controlled below 120 mg/mL, these infants are no longer oversized at birth. The infant of the diabetic mother is fat rather than edematous (Avery, 1975). The LGA infant is anxious to suck and eager to eat. However, patterns of feeding will depend on the monitored situation of the glucose levels of the neonate, which will fluctuate significantly.

Development of Organ Systems

The majority of the development of body systems is accomplished prior to birth in order that the neonate can be physically self-sufficient. However, significant adaptations do take place on the system level at the time of birth.

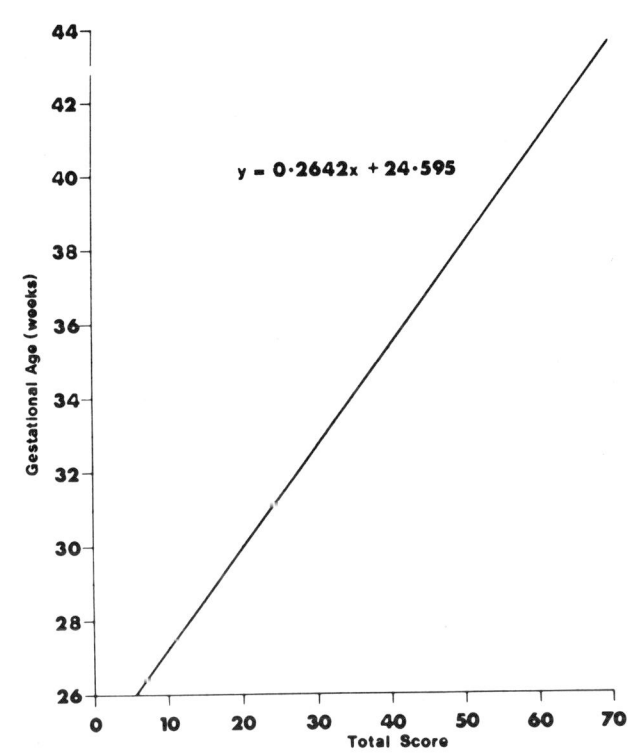

FIGURE 6-10. Graph for reading gestational age from total score of Dubowitz assessment. The score from Fig. 6-2 and Table 6-3 are added. A line is then drawn from the horizontal axis at the score to intersect the diagonal line. Then, from the intersecting point, a line to the perpendicular axis will give age in weeks. [From L. Dubowitz, V. Dubowitz, and C. Goldberg, Clinical assessment of gestational age in the newborn infant. J. Pediat., 1970, 77(1), 10. Reprinted by permission of The C. V. Mosby Company.]

The central nervous and sensory systems, the most precocious in morphogenesis, are remarkably functional in the neonate. Growth and final maturation and, of course, functional elaboration will occur over the years of childhood. However, major physiological development occurred prenatally.

In contrast, the cardiovascular, respiratory, and endocrine systems must make immediate transformations in order to sustain life. Other systems mature and grow over the neonatal period at relatively the same rate as prenatally. The status and development of these body systems will now be discussed.

Nervous system Mary D. Guthrie

It is believed that all the neurons of the central nervous system (CNS) are present at birth; however, it is thought that there is additional development of glial, or supporting, cells after birth. The neonate brain has far fewer glial cells than does the adult brain.

In addition, there is growth and development of the dendritic processes of neurons after birth. This has been shown in a variety of experiments using mammals and lower vertebrates, in which the visual environment is either enriched or deprived. There is also continued myelination of peripheral nerve axons as the muscular system becomes more functional.

Sensory system Anna M. Tichy

The neonate's limited capacity to respond specifically and selectively to stimuli may be due to the sensory input not being picked up by the sensory receptor, incomplete myelination and function of the cortical pathways and the cortex, and inadequate interpretation or processing of afferent information. Any or all of these factors may be involved in the neonate's generalized behavioral response to an environmental or internal stimulus.

VISUAL SYSTEM

Evaluation of the neonate's eyes is difficult because the eyelids are normally tightly closed due to photophobia. The pupil, iris, sclera, and extraocular movements can be evaluated in dim light by holding the infant upright and turning him slowly. The eyes of the neonate are not structurally or physiologically fully developed, nor do they possess the functional capacities of the mature eye. Pupillary reactivity to light is present but sluggish. Inequality of pupil size is not uncommon; however, it may be indicative of pathology if it persists or is associated with other ocular or CNS findings.

The globe is elongated, or *hyperopic*, and will continue to grow in diameter. At birth, the lens has attained two-thirds of its final diameter and its full thickness. New lens fibers develop throughout life though the diameter of the lens increases very little in adult years.

Maturity of the peripheral area of the retina is demonstrated by directionally appropriate eye movements to peripheral stimuli. The macula, however, is poorly developed and will not be fully developed until about 12 months of age. The peripheral retina is sensitive to spatial location, movement, and gross shape or forms, whereas the fovea is critical for form discrimination and identifica-

306 THE NEONATE: BIRTH TO 1 MONTH

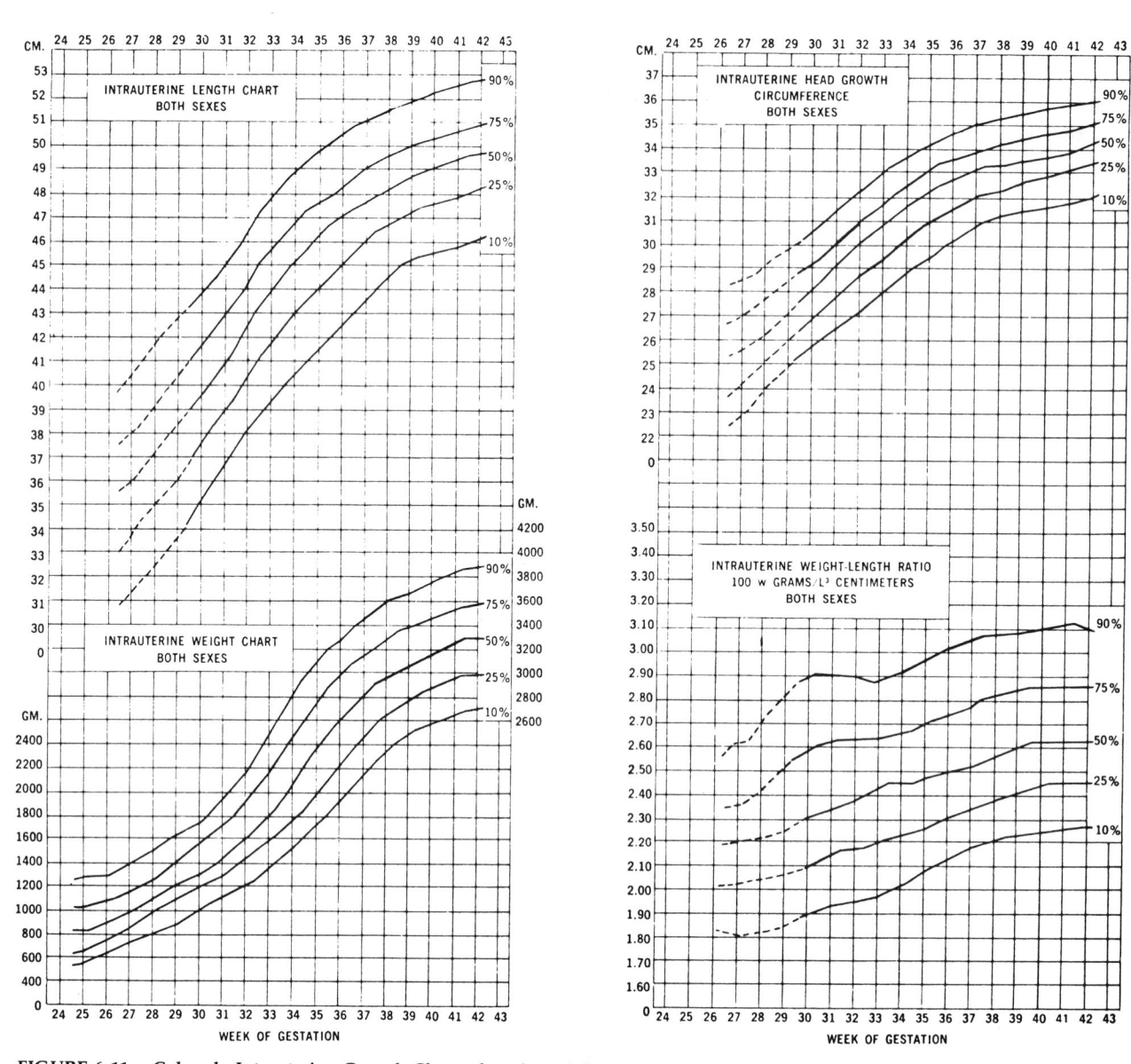

FIGURE 6-11. Colorado Intrauterine Growth Charts: length, weight, occipital-frontal circumference, and weight/length ratio. [From L. O. Lubchenco, C. Hansman, and E. Boyd, Intrauterine growth in length and head circumference as estimated from live births at gestational ages from 26 to 42 weeks. Pediatrics, 1966, 37(3), 403–408. Reprinted by permission of the American Academy of Pediatrics.]

tion. Data on visual acuity in the neonate are conflicting, ranging from 20/150 to 20/400. Visual assessment, visual acuity, and light perception in the neonate are based on the presence of visual reflexes: opticokinetic nystagmus induced by a rotating drum; direct and consensual pupillary constriction in response to light; and blinking when an object is moved quickly toward the eyes or in response to a bright light.

Small scleral, subconjunctival, and retinal hemorrhages are not uncommon in the neonate. Tears are not present before 1 month of age; the lacrimal duct normally opens several weeks after birth. The peripheral fundus in the neonate is not highly pigmented. The optic disk is normally paler; the foveal light reflection is absent; and the peripheral vessels are not well developed.

At birth extraocular movements are not coordinated; thus gaze is primarily monocular, occasionally binocular. Turning the neonate causes the eyes to gaze in the direction of rotation. Cessation of movement is followed by a few nystagmoid movements and a gaze in the opposite direction. The doll's eye test is useful in diagnosing weakness in the lateral rectus muscle and paresis of the abducens nerve. To perform the doll's eye test, the neonate is held supine, and his head is turned to the side. The eyes remain stationary as the head is turned (in the first 10 days of life). At birth, the setting-sun sign, in which the eyes gaze downward with sclera visible above the iris, may be seen for brief periods in a small number of neonates. The corneal reflex is present at birth.

AUDITORY SYSTEM

Examination of the ear structure is included in assessment of the neonate's auditory status. The level and angle of the external ear is noted. The middle ear cavity is nearly filled with a gelatinous tissue which hinders the movement of the eardrum and ossicles, and the external auditory meatus is not completely free of accumulated vernix caseosa. As a result, auditory function in the early neonatal period is imperfect. The vernix is progressively resorbed during the first week of life.

Because of the accumulated debris, visualization of the tympanic membrane is not possible in the first 3 days of life. However, examination of the ear is useful in establishing the patency of the external auditory canal.

OLFACTORY SYSTEM

The apparatus for olfaction is readied during gestation, but it is doubtful if adequate chemical stimuli are ever present in the absence of air currents in the nasal passages. In both the premature infant and full-term neonate, evidence of olfactory function has been obtained.

GUSTATORY SYSTEM

At birth, taste buds are principally located on the tongue and palate, although they may also be found on the epiglottis, pharynx, and lips. Postnatal taste is not highly developed, but sweet, acid, sour, and bitter substances evoke a response. The location of taste buds on the pharynx, just before swallowing becomes an involuntary act, may serve a protective function. The neonate accepts sweetened fluids and resists acid, bitter, or sour ones.

TACTILE SYSTEM

The neonate's sense of touch is well developed; it seems to be most acute on the lips, tongue, ears, and forehead. Studies have shown that neonates are more responsive to tactile stimuli on the right than on the left side of the perioral region. The neonate, by a general discomfort reaction, has demonstrated sensitivity to cutaneous pressure, temperature change, and pain.

In summary, the sensory system of the neonate, with the exception of the visual apparatus, is morphologically mature. Functional limitations are due more to the immaturity of the cortex and cortical pathways.

Musculoskeletal system Sherrilyn Passo

Much of the development of the musculoskeletal system occurs during the 9 months of prenatal life. However, at birth, the skeleton is incompletely ossified (see Fig. 6-12). In the hands and feet only the shafts of the phalanges, the metacarpals, and the metatarsals have enough ossification to appear on an x-ray. Some elements, like the carpals in the wrist, are wholly cartilaginous. In many neonates, a secondary center of ossification (in addition to the primary center in the shaft of the bone) has appeared in the epiphyses at the lower end of the femur and the upper end of the tibia. Because there is a wide variability in time of appearance of the epiphyseal centers, estimation of fetal age, based on the number of centers present at birth, is not generally reliable.

Rapid growth of the skeleton and the muscles proceeds after birth. The cranial vault increases in size rapidly, although union of cranial components is still incomplete. This allows for overriding of cranial bones and molding of the head to the birth canal (see Fig. 6-13). The anterior fontanel in the neonate is 2 to 3 cm wide and 3 to 4 cm long. The posterior fontanel is fingertip-sized or smaller in

97 percent of full-term neonates (Popich and Smith, 1972). The face and base of the skull develop at a slower rate, and the mandible is characteristically small. The pelvic cavity is small and funnel-shaped as a result of the more upright position of the sacrum and ilea. Only the thoracic and pelvic curves are present in the spine at birth, giving the neonate a spinal curve shaped like a C rather than the double-curved S of later life.

At birth, the lower limbs are shorter than the upper limbs, and the bones of the pelvis are less advanced than those of the shoulder girdle, demonstrating the cephalocaudal developmental pattern. The acetabulums are relatively shallow compared with their appearance later in infancy. Both adequate nutrition and intermittent stress from normal muscle activity are important for adequate growth and development of musculoskeletal components.

Muscle mass accounts for about 25 percent of total body weight at birth, compared with 45 percent in young adults. The skeletal musculature continues to grow by hyperplasia, although formation of new muscle fibers begin to slow by 1 month of age (Malina, 1978). In the term infant, the individual muscle fibers are still small, but they become more closely packed as they increase in number.

Cardiovascular system LaNelle E. Geddes

Persons of all ages encounter situations in interaction with their environment (internal as well as external) that require adaptation to new circumstances; however, few stresses are more abrupt, of greater magnitude, or more demanding of adaptation than those experienced at the time of birth. The sudden metamorphosis from a dependent being in a protected existence to a physiologically independent individual in a demanding environment requires adjustment of the greatest proportions.

While in utero, the fetus has many body functions either completely assumed or at least partially assisted by maternal mechanisms. Birth, however, suddenly thrusts the neonate "on his own." From one moment to the next, the neonate must transfer obligation for exchange of respiratory gases from the placenta to his lungs, a transition that requires profound changes in both pulmonary and cardiovascular systems.

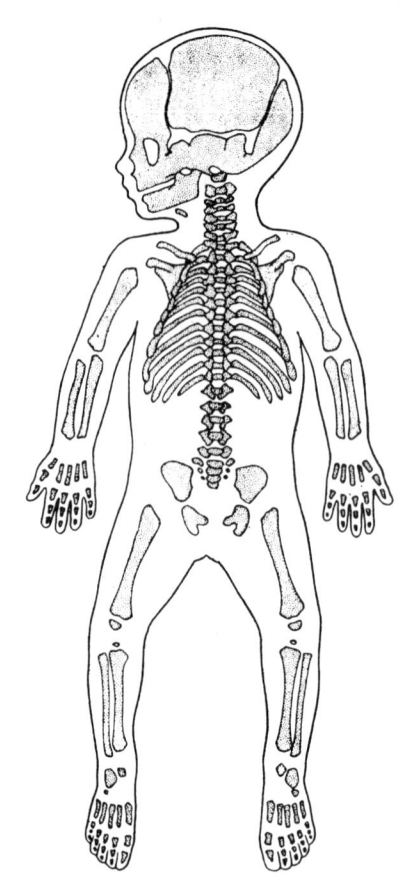

FIGURE 6-12. Ossification of the skeleton of the neonate. Note the absence of ossification centers in the wrist, the separate centers for the components of the hip girdle, and the lack of secondary centers for the long bones (except the distal end of the femur and proximal end of the tibia). [From D. Sinclair, *Growth after birth* (3d ed.). London: Oxford University Press, p. 71. Reprinted by permission of the publisher.]

CIRCULATORY CHANGES AT BIRTH

Two major changes imposed on the cardiovascular system are decreased pulmonary vascular resistance and interruption of the placental circulation. Both subserve redirection of blood flow through the neonate's lungs. In fetal circulation, vascular resistance is greater in pulmonary than in systemic vessels. As a result, blood is directed away from pulmonary vessels and into the systemic vasculature, a scheme facilitated by fetal vascular shunts, such as the foramen ovale and the ductus arteriosus. After the neonate takes his first breath, pulmonary vascular resistance decreases, and pulmonary blood flow increases.

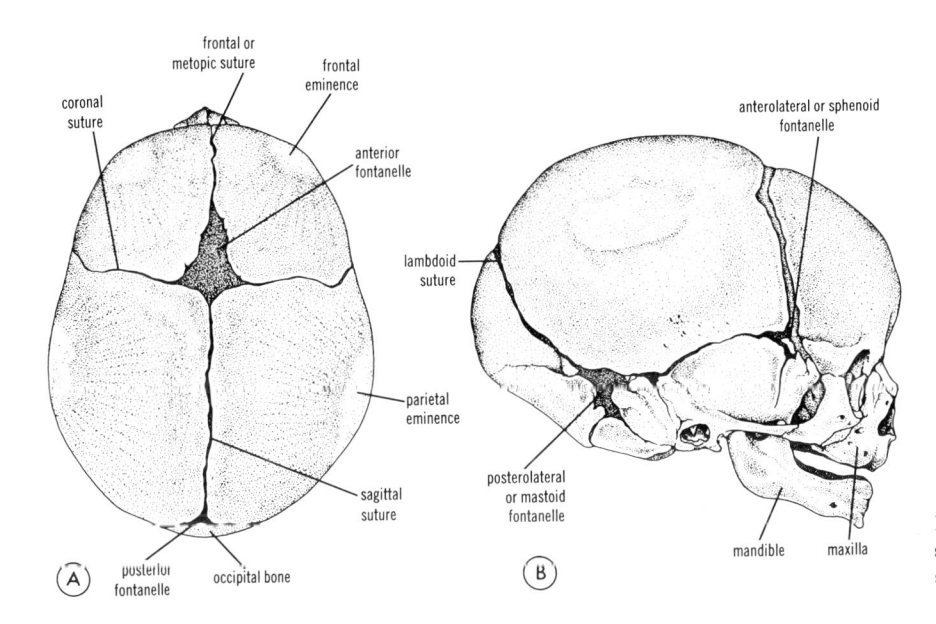

FIGURE 6-13. Skull of the neonate seen from (a) above and (b) the right side.

Separation of the neonate from low-resistance placental circulation increases systemic vascular resistance and decreases right-to-left blood flow through the ductus arteriosus.

The increased oxygen tension of blood flowing in the neonatal pulmonary circulation promotes pulmonary vascular dilation. Thus, venous return to the left atrium through the pulmonary veins increases. At the same time, venous return to the right atrium decreases as the placental circulation that had previously supplied a large quantity of blood is interrupted. As a result of increased venous return to the left atrium and decreased return to the right atrium, left atrial pressure rises above that in the right atrium and forces the flap valve over the foramen ovale into the closed position.

Furthermore, as pulmonary vascular resistance falls and systemic pressure rises, direction of flow through the ductus arteriosus reverses. In the fetus the ductus arteriosus directed blood from the high-resistance (and nonfunctional) pulmonary vessels to the aorta. Elevation of aortic pressure and decrease of pulmonary pressure reverse the direction of flow, and blood passes from the aorta into the pulmonary artery through the ductus arteriosus.

Functional demands on the left and right ventricles, dictated by the relative pressures against which they contract and the relative volumes of blood they pump, are reflected by cardiac anatomy. In the fetus, the right ventricle faces a greater vascular resistance (outflow impedance) than the left. Also, it delivers a slightly greater flow than the left. As a result, the ventricular mass of the fetal right ventricle is approximately equal to that of the left. After birth, pulmonary vascular resistance decreases to about one-half of the prenatal value, while that of the systemic circulation doubles. This transition requires an increase in left ventricular myocardial mass and allows a decrease in right ventricular thickness (see Fig. 6-14).

This changeover from right ventricular dominance in the fetus and neonate to left ventricular dominance characteristic of the older child and adult is reflected by the electrocardiographic patterns. In the neonate, the right precordial leads are characterized by an Rs pattern that undergoes a transition to an rS pattern typical of the older individual. The mean QRS vector also shifts from right to left as left ventricular dominance emerges. In the frontal plane, the QRS vector moves from about $+130°$ shortly after birth to $+90°$ at about 2 months of age to the adult normal reading of $+60°$ by 1 year.

As noted in "Development of the Cardiovascular System" in Chap. 5, four anatomical cardiovascular features—the foramen ovale, the ductus venosus, the umbilical vessels, and the ductus arteriosus—are functional in fetal but not in postnatal life (see Fig. 6-15). The involution of these structures, appropriate to fetal but not to extrauterine existence, is brought about by several influences. As explained above, the foramen ovale ceases to shunt blood from the right to the left atrium primarily as a result of rising left atrial and falling right atrial pressures. In the neonate, closure of this orifice has occurred by several hours postnatally. While in normal conditions it is functionally occluded, the foramen ovale is not sealed shut and can accommodate right-to-left shunting under some circumstances, such as crying, that effectively increase right atrial pressure and decrease left atrial pressure. Crying is accompanied by marked increase in pulmonary vascular resistance. This situation decreases right ventricular outflow and increases right ventricular pressure. Increased right ventricular pressure is reflected back to the right atrium, raising its pressure. Since pulmonary vascular resistance is increased, pulmonary flow and venous return to the left atrium are reduced, and, in turn, left atrial pressure declines. The combination of increased right atrial pressure and decreased left atrial pressure then exists, and flow through the foramen ovale can be reestablished. Since flow is right to left, poorly oxygenated blood is delivered to the left heart, and the systemic circulation and the infant may become cyanotic.

The ductus venosus, which shunted blood from the umbilical and portal veins to the inferior vena cava, bypassing a large part of the hepatic circulation, also appears to close shortly after birth. Closure of this vessel forces blood from the portal vein through the liver, and perfusion of the hepatic vessels increases. The left lobe of the liver is considerably larger in the fetus than in the neonate, but its size decreases after birth. The relatively larger size of the left lobe in the fetus is suggested to reflect a preferential delivery of oxygenated blood to this part of the liver by the patent ductus venosus; however, after birth and closure of the shunt, the left lobe decreases in size relative to the right lobe. Closure of the ductus venosus is primarily attributed to mechanical factors, such as interruption of flow in the umbilical vein. The occluded ductus venosus is identified as the *ligamentum venosum* (see Fig. 6-15).

CORD CLAMPING AND PLACENTAL TRANSFUSION

Closure of the umbilical vessels has been attributed to a decrease in temperature, exposure to elevated oxygen tensions, vasoactive substances, and a combination of

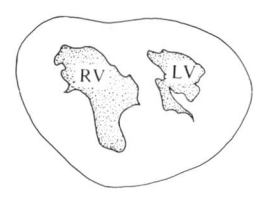

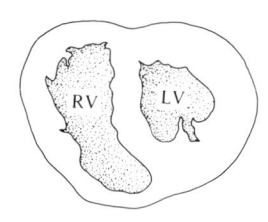

FIGURE 6-14. Relative sizes of the right and left ventricles in the fetus and the older child. During fetal life the thickness of the walls of the two ventricles is approximately equal; however, in the older individual the wall thickness of the left ventricle is greater than that of the right ventricle.

these factors; however, the precise mechanism is not known. The common obstetrical practice of clamping the umbilical cord and occluding the vessels in this manner preempts the physiological closure mechanisms. Early occlusion of the umbilical vessels has implications beyond interruption of vascular paths no longer appropriate to the circumstances.

The umbilical and placental vessels contain about 100 mL of blood that could be transferred to the neonate. When the neonate is elevated above the introitus immediately after birth and the cord is clamped within seconds of delivery, little, if any, of the placental blood is transfused into the infant. Arguments both for and against any benefits of the placental transfusion have been offered. When the total volume of available blood is transfused, the neonate's blood volume is increased by about 25 percent. A transfusion of this magnitude over a matter of just a few minutes corresponds to a transfusion of about 1200 to 1300 mL of blood into an adult in the same amount of time. Needless to say, the transfused infants exhibit signs of vascular distension.

Vascular distension resulting from the placental transfusion is evidenced by an increase in the radiographic cardiac silhouette and by increased pressure in both the pulmonary and systemic vascular beds. Cardiac auscultation reveals cardiac murmurs in transfused infants more often than in those not receiving transfusion. These murmurs are explained by a greater flow through the patent ductus arteriosus. The electrocardiogram (ECG) also suggests transient distension of the cardiac chambers and myocardial strain.

Most of the transfused blood is apparently accommodated by the pulmonary vessels. Transfused neonates have a higher respiratory rate and a lower functional residual capacity than nontransfused infants. The higher respiratory rate is attributed to decreased pulmonary compliance due to increased blood volume in pulmonary vessels. The lower functional residual capacity may also

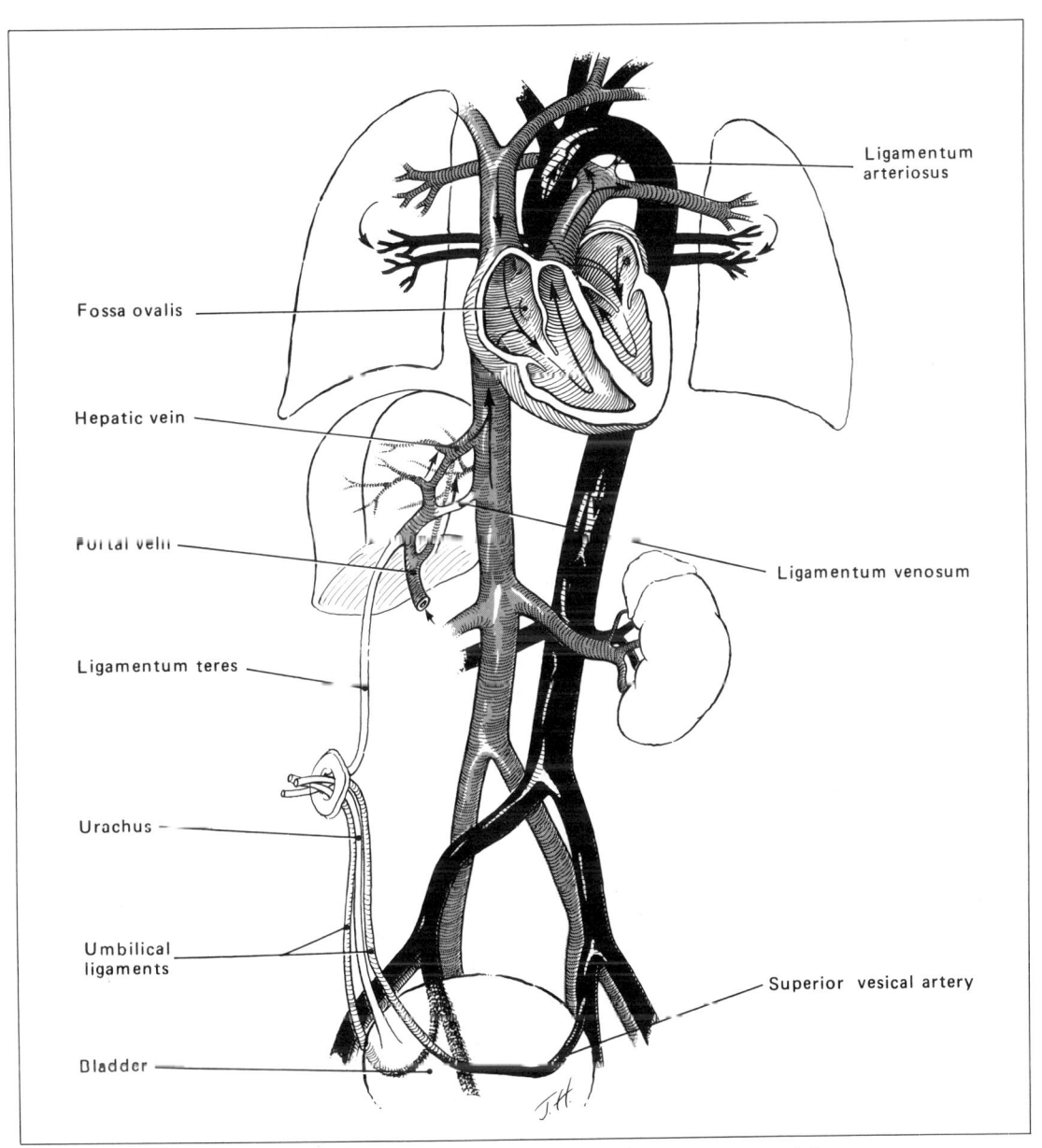

FIGURE 6-15. Circulation after birth. The umbilical vessels, the ductus venosus, and the ductus arteriosus are occluded and present as ligaments. Normally, the foramen ovale also closes. [From L. L. Langley, I. R. Telford, and J. B. Christiansen, Dynamic anatomy and physiology (4th ed.) New York: McGraw-Hill, 1974, v. 785, by permission.]

reflect altered ventilatory mechanics imposed by pulmonary vascular distension. Somewhat unexpectedly, blood gases measured in the transfused neonate suggest a less efficient gas exchange (lowered Po_2 and elevated Pco_2) for the first few hours after birth.

Renal perfusion appears to be higher in transfused than in nontransfused neonates on the basis of increased glomerular filtration rate and urine production. Placental transfusion also increases the hematocrit level.

Several benefits have been argued for late clamping of the cord (after pulsations cease, or later than about 3 min). These include an increased iron supply contributed by the transfused red blood cells. Although blood from placental transfusion initially reaches and affects pulmonary circulation, it does so at a time when right-to-left shunts, such as the foramen ovale and ductus arteriosus, are open. The presence of these shunts allows the directing of some of the increased volume from the right atrium to the left atrium and from the pulmonary artery to the aorta. The increased blood volume may also aid in "opening up" circulations, such as the pulmonary, hepatic, and renal beds, that were relatively occluded in the fetus.

DUCTUS ARTERIOSUS

Closure of the ductus arteriosus appears to be mediated mainly by the increasing oxygen tension of the neonate's blood. Vasoconstrictor substances, such as bradykinin and acetylcholine, may support closure, but they do not appear to be as influential as increased oxygen. The ductus arteriosus is a highly muscular vessel with relatively thick walls and a small lumen. Oxygen sensitivity of ductal smooth muscle appears to parallel gestational age, an observation that is supported by a higher incidence of patent ductus arteriosus in premature than in term infants.

Obliteration of the ductal lumen occurs in two stages. The first stage begins the first $\frac{1}{2}$ h after birth and continues for up to 12 h. Blood flow through the vessel is maintained during this phase, and while it is usually from the aorta to the pulmonary artery (left to right), it may proceed in the opposite direction (right to left). Flow may occasionally be bidirectional and directed from left to right for part of the cardiac cycle and in the opposite direction during the other part of the cycle.

The second phase, in which the intimal layer proliferates and the muscular layer atrophies, lasts from the age of about 12 h to 10 days. The ductus is usually completely closed in several weeks, although it may remain open as long as a year before spontaneously closing. The vestigial *ligamentum arteriosus* (see Fig. 6-15) remains after ductal closure.

Circulatory changes that occur shortly after birth include closure of the umbilical vessels, foramen ovale, ductus venosus, and ductus arteriosus and opening of vascular beds in the lungs, liver, and kidneys. The circulatory modifications are accompanied by a change from right to left ventricular dominance in the heart. Coupled with major changes in the pulmonary system and relatively less profound changes in other organ systems, the neonate progresses from a physiologically parasitic existence to a functionally independent one.

Respiratory system Virginia J. Neelon

THE LUNG AT BIRTH

The establishment of independent respiratory activity capable of effective gas exchange requires complex and extensive internal adjustments within the neonate. Paramount among these adjustments are the removal of lung liquids, alteration of the flow and resistance of the fetal circulatory system, and establishment of a ventilation pattern responsive to metabolic-chemical control.

The fetus is accustomed to a low-oxygen environment. With the onset of labor, the fetus is subjected to a traumatic upheaval of internal state as a consequence of the contractions of the uterus and passage through the birth canal. He enters the world hypoxic, lungs filled with liquid, and with a circulation that is mostly shunted away from the lungs.

LUNG LIQUID ABSORPTION

Inflation of the lung and removal of lung liquids must necessarily occur together. The volume of liquid in the lung, about 30 mL/kg, must be replaced with an equal volume of gas. Although this would seem a difficult task to place on a neonate, the work required to inflate a totally collapsed lung would be far greater than that required to inflate a lung already expanded by a liquid volume. Some of the liquid is removed through the gravitational and mechanical forces of birth, but more than one-half remains to be absorbed; in cesarean delivery almost all of it must be absorbed.

Three distinct factors contribute to the rapid absorption of the remaining lung liquid. First and foremost, the formation or secretion of liquids into the respiratory spaces stops. Secondly, the epithelial lining of the lung becomes much more permeable, permitting the rapid uptake of liquids from the alveoli. Finally, with inflation of the lungs, hydrostatic pressure of the interstitial space falls, encouraging the flow of fluids from the alveolar atrium into the tissue spaces. The fluid is then either removed through the lymphatics or resorbed by the pulmonary capillary network (Strang, 1977). Removal of the liquid across the lung epithelium is an advantage in itself since this process facilitates coating of the respiratory-air surface with the all-important components of the surfactant system.

CIRCULATORY ADAPTATION AND GAS EXCHANGE

In the fetus the gas-exchange system is the umbilical-placental circulation. The potential postnatal gas-exchange system is the pulmonary circulation, which during fetal existence is a high-resistance, low-flow system. Most of the placental flow is directed away from the lungs, shunted to the systemic circulation through the foramen ovale across the atrium and via the ductus arteriosus into the aorta. Thus, with birth, significant circulatory adjustments are critical to establishing effective pulmonary gas exchange (see "Cardiovascular System"). Table 6-4 shows the extreme changes which occur in arterial blood gases and pH over the first 24 h following birth.

The neonate is in a transitional circulatory state during the first hours after birth. The onset of respiration triggers a sequence of arterial pressure changes and circulatory shifts. The crucial circulatory adaptation is the rapid fall of pulmonary vascular resistance initiating a ten- to fifteenfold increase in pulmonary capillary flow and establishing alveolar-capillary gas exchange (Scarpelli, 1975). Left atrial pressure now exceeds that of the right atrium, and flow through the foramen ovale stops. The flow through the ductus arteriosus is at first reversed due to the increased systemic arterial pressure and then diminishes as the increased arterial oxygen tension stimulates closure

TABLE 6-4 Comparisons of partial pressures of gases and pH before and after birth and in the adult

	Fetal umbilical vein	At birth	1 h	24 h	Adult
Po$_2$, mmHg	30	20	60	90	100
Pco$_2$, mmHg	42	58	40	40	40
pH	7.3	7.2	7.3	7.4	7.4

Source: Data adapted from L. B. Strang, *Neonatal respiration.* Oxford: Blackwell Scientific, 1977; from M. H. Klaus and A. Fanaroff, *Care of the high-risk neonate*. Philadelphia: Saunders, 1973; and from A. C. Guyton, *Textbook of medical physiology* (5th ed.). Philadelphia: Saunders, 1976.

of the ductus itself. This transitional process occurs at different rates, but by 24 h after birth the adult pattern of flow is functionally established.

This complex adaptation is dependent on immediate and adequate respiratory function, however. Any disease or stress leading to hypoxia and pulmonary arterial hypertension may result in a persistent fetal circulatory pattern with right-to-left shunting and cyanosis.

THE FIRST BREATH

A variety of factors work together to initiate respiration in the neonate. Included are mechanical factors involved in the process of labor and multiple tactile, temperature, and metabolic changes (hypoxia and acidosis) which trigger sensory stimulation to the respiratory control centers in the medulla.

The chest of the infant is compressed during vaginal delivery, and with the appearance of the head, fluid frequently gushes from the nose and mouth. As the upper thorax is delivered, the chest expands causing a passive inspiratory movement which draws air into the lungs. Although, as a result of these mechanical factors, passage through the birth canal facilitates the onset of breathing, infants born after cesarean delivery nevertheless have a similar onset of respiratory activity (Strang, 1977).

The normal infant breathes immediately, taking several big inspirations interspersed with periods of breath holding and loud cries. The effort required for the first breath is significant and reflects as much the work of moving the lung liquid through the air passages as it does expansion of the airspaces.

The critical event in stabilizing ventilatory function and preventing airway collapse is the establishment of an adequate functional residual capacity (FRC). An adequate FRC allows effective respiration with the least amount of work and acts as a buffer to prevent extreme variations of blood gases (Auld, 1975). Although the first breath does well in inflating the lung, a stable state of aeration is not reached for several hours following birth. Big breaths (sighs) and crying may be important to forming an adequate and stable FRC.

VENTILATORY FUNCTION

The values of ventilation and the mechanics of breathing in normal neonates and in the normal adult are similar when expressed by unit weight, volume, or surface area. The neonate has a higher breathing frequency than the adult. This difference reflects the infant's need to establish a rate which requires the least total energy expenditure. The work of overcoming elastic forces (compliance) and surface tension is greatest at the extremes of lung volumes. The most efficient breathing frequency avoids extremes in either inflation or deflation and for the neonate occurs at a frequency of about 40 breaths per minute. Slow, deep respiratory patterns would require far more work given the highly collapsible (compliant) chest wall and the less compliant lung of the neonate. Lung compliance increases in the normal neonate during the first days after birth and rapidly approaches the value for the adult lung.

CONTROL OF RESPIRATION

There are two major systems for the control of respiration: a *neural system,* which coordinates the depth, frequency, and rhythmic pattern of breathing, and a chemical, or *neurohumoral,* system which regulates alveolar ventilation to maintain normal blood gas tensions. The primary center in the control of breathing is the medulla followed by neural innervation to the pons. Spontaneous respiration originates from the medulla, and transection below this level eliminates respiratory movements. Neurons in the pons exert their influence primarily by regulating medullary rhythmic respiration (Murray, 1976). Almost all afferent nerve fibers go from the lung to the CNS via the vagus nerve, and these innervations contribute significantly to the breathing pattern and reflex activity present in the newborn period (Murray, 1976).

There are two reflexes which, although not fully understood, appear important to regulation of respirations during the newborn period, particularly for the preterm infant. The *Hering-Breuer reflex* involves vagal impulses from receptors in the lung which inhibit inspiration as the lung distends. This reflex is active in the first few days after birth and may persist longer in the premature infant. It appears to help maintain lung volume by increasing breathing frequency; in an infant with an immature respiratory center, this neural stretch response may be critical to maintaining normal rhythmic breathing (Strang, 1977). The reflex is not necessary to normal inspiration in the adult.

A second reflex seen in the neonate is the *Head's paradoxical reflex,* or "inspiratory gasp." This is almost the reverse of the Hering-Breuer reflex; rather than inhibiting inspiration, it initiates a quickly increased inspiration, or gasp. The Head's reflex may be important in the initial process of regulating inspiratory volume.

The predominant respiratory regulatory system in the adult is the chemical, or neurohumoral, system: response to changes in blood gases through central and peripheral chemoreceptors located in the medulla and the great arterial vessels (carotid and aortic bodies). The neonate adapts rapidly to neurohumoral regulation after birth, but the preterm infant is frequently less able to respond to blood gas alterations such as hypoxia or hypercapnia.

THE NORMAL NEONATE

At birth the normal infant breathes at once, and within a few hours his lungs are free of liquids and his arterial oxygen has reached normal neonatal values of about 80 mmHg. His regulation of respirations reflects the shift from fetal neural control to one responsive primarily to metabolic factors involving blood gas levels and pH. His respiratory activity is also increasingly sensitive to behavioral influences such as emotional distress (Strang, 1977).

The neonate is an obligatory nose breather, and any nasal obstruction can cause respiratory distress. Cyanosis and respiratory difficulty which appear to be relieved by crying are frequently dramatic clues to nasal obstruction in the neonate.

Two major postnatal factors influence respiratory adaptation: compliance of the lung and chest wall and oxygen tensions of the inspired air and arterial blood. The neonate breathes primarily with his diaphragm at frequencies between 30 and 40 breaths per minute at rest. Because of the instability of his chest wall (high compliance) and his relatively "stiff" lung (low compliance), the neonate is vulnerable to airway collapse. This precarious state resolves rapidly during the first week of life as the lung becomes more elastic, facilitating a more stable ventilatory exchange. Similarly, during the next months the chest develops a more fixed, bony cage, and muscle growth is significant. These changes, along with an adequate surfactant system, are responsible for stabilizing respiratory volume and preventing airway collapse.

THE PRETERM INFANT

PHYSIOLOGICAL LIMITATIONS

Preterm infants have different problems, depending on both the degree and the cause of prematurity. The single most life-threatening problem for these infants is development of respiratory distress arising from the immaturity of their lungs.

Respiratory distress is rare in infants who are born by normal delivery after 36 weeks ma and who have no other high-risk problems. Infants born prior to this time are at increasing risk, depending on their gestational age, because of incomplete development of the lung and other systems important to effective respiratory function. The premature infant struggles with his first breath because of poor chest wall musculature and precarious neural control. The risk of alveolar collapse is ever present because of the underdeveloped chest wall and limited ability to synthesize surfactant. The frequent deep-sighing respiration observed in premature infants may reflect the infant's attempt to maintain an adequate lung volume and stimulate surfactant release into respiratory airways.

The premature infant appears to tolerate lower levels of arterial oxygen, and values below the normal newborn range may persist for days without apparent distress. The maintenance of these low values might possibly protect maturing organs, such as the retina, which are vulnerable to higher oxygen concentrations at preterm stages.

BREATHING PATTERNS

The breathing pattern of the premature infant is frequently irregular and periodic. Even the normal neonate does not sustain even breathing at all times. The more immature the infant, the more frequent and lengthy are the irregular patterns characterized by episodes of apnea interspersed with periods of respirations of irregular depth and frequency.

Recurrent apnea is uncommon after the thirty-sixth week ma and may not be present in some infants born before this time. The mechanism causing these spells is not clear. There seems to be some relation to hypoxia, and oxygenation of the infant reduces their occurrence. Diminished sensitivity of chemoreceptors to blood gas levels or depressed central respiratory centers are thought to contribute to this problem.

Apnea at birth is usually due to intrapartum asphyxia and depression of the respiratory centers. In contrast, recurrent apnea of prematurity is probably due more to immaturity of the respiratory control centers and persistent dependence on reflex neural stimuli to maintain breathing. As the infant matures, the link between breathing and metabolism develops and dominates, maintaining normal respiration during both waking and sleep states.

EARLY GROWTH PATTERNS OF THE
RESPIRATORY SYSTEM

Growth of the lung is limited somewhat by size of the chest wall during the first 3 months. After that time the thorax enlarges faster than the lung. The respiratory unit in the neonatal lung is not typically a true alveolus but is an immature ductlike structure. Following birth there is a rapid period of alveolarization with enlargement of the existing respiratory units as well as an increase in the number of units.

Although the lung surface per unit weight is about the same for the infant and the adult, the infant has a smaller reserve surface area because of his higher resting metabolic needs. In times of stress, illness, or increased metabolic demand, this limited reserve may not be sufficient to meet respiratory needs.

CONTINUED GROWTH

Lung growth and development of more alveoli will continue as the child grows, although the major morphological changes took place prenatally. There is disagreement regarding the exact age that alveolar development is completed with estimates from the first few years to 15 years of age (Brasel and Gruen, 1978). There may be a correlation between number of alveoli and height, although this has not been established (Brasel and Gruen, 1978).

The nonalveolated airways grow in relation to body growth; thus, the lungs double in weight by 6 months, and triple by 1 year (Gross, 1978). There is also a growth spurt in the lungs corresponding with the pubertal growth spurt. The upper airways descend with growth to a lower position relative to other upper body structures. Respiratory rate decreases, and pulmonary-function values increase as the child grows. As the respiratory system must respond to needs of the body, which are related to size, it is not surprising that lung growth and function parallel body growth.

Gastrointestinal system Anna M. Tichy and Dianne Chong

During the neonatal period, the infant adapts to the extrauterine challenge of ingestion, digestion, and absorption of sufficient nutrients for growth and maintenance of health. Excretion of gastrointestinal waste products, under normal circumstances, is initiated following delivery. The normal full-term infant is capable of digesting and assimilating the nutrients in breast milk and infant formula although significant differences in absorption, secretion, and motility exist between neonate and adult. The alimentary tract of the neonate is physiologically immature, even though it was functional in fetal life.

ORAL STRUCTURES

MOUTH

The anatomical structure of the oral cavity of the neonate and young infant differs from that of the adult. The oral cavity, including the posterior soft palate, is relatively longer, and the opening from the mouth to the pharynx is smaller. Adipose tissue in the space between the buccinator and masseter muscles of the cheeks, the sucking fat pads, equalizes pressure and prevents drawing in of muscle and cheek during sucking. The neonate's lips are well adapted for forming an airtight seal around a nipple.

TONGUE

The tongue of the neonate appears relatively large in proportion to the size of the oral cavity. The frenulum varies considerably in length; it may attach near the tip or midway on the tongue's undersurface, and the consistency may range anywhere from a fragile filamentous membrane to a thick fibrous cord. If the length or consistency of the frenulum prevents protrusion of the tongue beyond the gums, the infant may experience difficulty in sucking and later encounter speech difficulties if not corrected. This, however, is rare.

PALATE

The hard palate at birth is shallow and U-shaped, unlike the typical V shape of the adult bony palate. The hard palate of the neonate is slightly arched, whereas it is deeply arched both transversely and anteroposteriorly in the adult. The series of five or six irregular transverse folds that assist the neonate in holding the nipple during sucking are obliterated before adulthood.

SALIVARY GLANDS

Cellular maturation of the salivary glands is incomplete until the third postnatal month of life or later. Salivation in the neonate is sparse; however, the amount of saliva is adequate to maintain moisture of oral mucous membranes. Salivary amylase, the starch-digesting enzyme, is present only in small quantities in the first 3 months of life.

FOREGUT

PHARYNX

At birth the pharnyx is approximately one-third the adult length. It has a nasal part which gradually curves downward to connect with the oral part without a definite demarcation point. The anatomic arrangement of the posterior pharynx is such that an upward and backward movement of the posterior tongue against the soft palate effectively prevents milk from entering the trachea and forces the contents of the pharynx into the esophagus. The simultaneous closure of the epiglottis prevents entry into the larynx, while muscles of the soft palate obstruct passage of milk into the nasal cavity.

The laryngeal opening into the pharynx is located just below the opening of the oral cavity into the pharynx. This anatomical characteristic limits phonetic ability so that the human infant could not produce articulate speech even if the necessary CNS connections were intact. The laryngeal opening into the pharynx must be situated at a lower level than that in the neonate so that the column of air emitted from the larynx traverses a long expanse of the pharynx before it enters the oral cavity.

TONSILS

The palatine tonsils are present in the neonate but are situated higher in the tonsillar fossa than are the older child's. Lymphoid tissue has been identified in the palatine tonsils during the sixth month of gestation; however, lymphoid nodules are not present until birth or shortly thereafter.

SUCKING AND SWALLOWING

In the full-term neonate the ability to suck and swallow in the first few days of life is relatively inefficient even though swallowing occurs in utero. The coordination of sucking, swallowing, and breathing is usually effective in neonates whose weight exceeds 1500 g or whose gestational age is 32 weeks ma or more. The initial feeding experiences are characterized by three to four short, consecutive sucks preceded or followed by swallowing activity. By 48 h of life these immature sucking efforts are replaced by more efficient groupings of 10 to 30 sucks and intermittent swallows (Gryboski, 1977).

The mechanisms of sucking and swallowing have been studied in neonates by measuring pressures in the oral cavity and by cineradiographic techniques in which nipples are coated with radiopaque dyes. Milk flow is accomplished by grasping the nipple between the tongue and hard palate and creating negative intraoral pressure by alternating compression and relaxation of the tongue against the nipple and hard palate. The volumes of milk obtained are identical whether the nipple is breast or artificial. Sucking and swallowing activities of the neonate are influenced by many factors including the level of neuromuscular maturity, the type of milk, and whether medication was given to the mother during the birth process. Both bite and gag reflexes are active within the first few days of life.

In neonates whose weight exceeds 1500 g, a unique reflex breathing-feeding pattern has been identified, which persists for 6 to 8 months. The swallowing procedure is coordinated so that continuous, simultaneous sucking and breathing activities take place for periods of 5 to 10 min. Simultaneous sucking and breathing is possible because the airway is open during the sucking process and the oral cavity is separated from the pharynx by the posterior portion of the tongue, which is elevated when the infant initiates each suck. Upon swallowing, contraction of the pharyngeal muscles is accompanied by relaxation of the esophageal sphincter. The bolus of milk, acting as a piston, pushes air present in the posterior pharynx into the stomach. Small amounts of air swallowed in this way cause little if any distress. In fact, absence of air in the gastrointestinal tract of the neonate is abnormal and has diagnostic significance in instances of obstruction. However, larger quantities of air in the stomach, which may result from inadequate nipple flow or crying, cause distress.

ESOPHAGUS

Motility studies in the first few days of life have shown that esophageal peristalsis is frequently nonpropagative with numerous simultaneous contractions and an extremely rapid rate of peristaltic activity. After the first week esophageal peristalsis becomes more effective.

In the first postnatal month, there is low tone in the gastroesophageal sphincter. As a result, the phase of sphincter relaxation following swallowing is prolonged with subsequent regurgitation of small amounts of milk. Tone increases rapidly after the first week in mature neonates, and esophageal sphincter pressures are equal to adult levels by 3 to 6 weeks of life (Gryboski, Thayer, and Spiro, 1963).

ABDOMEN AND PERITONEAL CAVITY

At birth the abdominal anteroposterior and transverse diameters, when compared with the adult, are greater in comparison with total body length. As a result of the small size of the pelvic portion of the body cavity at birth, pelvic viscera occupy a higher position than they do in the adult. The ovaries, uterus, and bladder are located in the neonate's abdominal cavity. The only segment of the gastrointestinal tract that is situated wholly in the pelvic cavity is the rectum.

At birth, the liver edge is readily palpable 1 to 2 cm below the right costal margin but is not usually sharply demarcated. Unlike the adult, the spleen may be palpable 1 cm below the left costal margin, and the lower half of each kidney may be palpable at the level of the umbilicus halfway between the midline and the side. When distended, the urinary bladder may lie as high as the level of the umbilicus. Abdominal reflexes, commonly found in older children and adults, are absent in the neonate.

STOMACH

The neonate's stomach is aptly suited to a liquid diet. Both the shape and capacity of the stomach change with age. At birth and during the first 2 years of life the stomach has a round configuration. Its position in the neonate is transverse in relation to the spinal column. The stomach holds approximately 20 mL at birth, 80 mL after 2 weeks, and 100 mL at the end of the first month (Timiras, 1972). (The adult's average stomach capacity is 1000 to 1500 mL.) However, the maximum capacity of the stomach varies widely due to such factors as size of the infant, degree of stomach distension, and quantity of air swallowed.

MOTILITY

At birth, the musculature of the stomach is only moderately developed. As with the gastroesophageal sphincter, the musculature of the pyloric canal sphincter is also poorly developed. At birth, gastric contractions consist of nonperistaltic movements; true peristalsis is absent during the first few days of life. The basis for this is not known; however, factors theorized to be partially responsible are a thin muscular wall and delayed maturation of various intestinal receptors.

Though the range is extremely broad, the majority of values of neonatal gastric emptying fall between 5 and 8 h. Gastric emptying time in the neonate is longer than in any other period of the life cycle. Since true peristalsis of the stomach does not occur until 2 to 4 days after birth, stomach emptying prior to that time is the result of a combination of tonus (generalized gastric contractions) and simple hydrostatic pressure of the milk bolus. Gastric emptying, though erratic at birth, is under similar regulatory mechanisms that operate in the adult.

Formulas which contain large quantities of saturated fatty acids delay gastric emptying. Entry of fat into the duodenum results in the elaboration of a hormone, enterogastrone, that inhibits gastric motility. Cow's milk is retained in the stomach longer than human milk. Hypertonic formulas, large milk curds, larger-volume feedings, colder formula, or solid food prolong gastric emptying, whereas breast milk and isotonic formulas or those with a highly denatured protein or carbohydrate content accelerate early emptying (Davidson, 1973).

Infants fed in the upright, prone, or right lateral position experience the most rapid rate of gastric emptying, whereas the supine position retards emptying. Nursing the infant in a prone or upright position results in a smaller amount of swallowed air passing into the small intestine and lessening of the gastroesophageal reflux, which is attributed to poor gastroesophageal sphincter tone.

Milk leaves the stomach before feeding is completed; the pylorus opens about 90 s after formula reaches the cardia of the stomach. In general, the smaller the stomach, the shorter the interval between feedings. Hunger contractions have been recorded in neonates 2 to 4 h after feeding. Since these hunger contractions occur when the stomach is not yet empty, they do not cause waking or crying in the neonate. They may be attributed to the physiological immaturity of the gastrointestinal tract.

The inefficient, immature peristaltic waves may occur in the reverse direction. This phenomenon, together with the small stomach size and incompetence of the gastroesophageal sphincter, may be responsible for the frequent regurgitation characteristic of the neonate.

SECRETION

The nearly neutral pH of gastric contents immediately after birth is attributed to the presence of swallowed alkaline amniotic fluids. Within a few hours a strongly acid secretion is noted which implies secretory adequacy of the parietal cells. In studies of gastric acidity in a series of neonates with fractional fasting gastric analyses, it was found that the most striking increase in gastric acidity occurs in the first 8 h of life (Ahn and Kim, 1963). The significance of the initial lack of gastric acidity is that the antiseptic effect of the gastric contents is not available to protect the neonate from ingestion of infectious agents (Ebers, Smith, and Gibbs, 1956). In the premature infant, output of gastric acid is well below the level of the full-term neonate (Ames, 1960). The ability to secrete hydrochloric acid may be persistently impaired in low-birth-weight infants or in malnourished infants of higher weights for a number of weeks.

In the full-term neonate, values of gastric acidity, which achieve maximal levels between 4 and 10 days, gradually decrease over the next 10 to 30 days. It is postulated that the initial high level of gastric acidity in full-term neonates and the gradual decline during the subsequent days reflect hormone stimulation in utero from either the placenta or the mother. A direct relationship exists between gastric acidity and parietal cell mass. In neonates parietal cell mass is two to three times as great as in the adult (Polacek and Ellison, 1966). This finding also may explain the hypersecretion of gastric acid that occurs early in the neonatal period.

In addition to secreting hydrochloric acid, gastrin, and mucus, the secretory mucosa of the term neonate's stomach is able to secrete pepsinogen and intrinsic factor. Available data suggest that pepsin secretion parallels acid secretion in the neonate (Rodbro, Krasilnikoff, and Bitsch, 1967). At birth peptic activity is proportional to the neonate's level of maturity and is three- to fourfold greater in average-weight full-term infants than in premature infants weighing 1000 g. The effect of these variations on digestion is not clear.

By the second week of life, the concentration of intrinsic factor in gastric juice approximates that of normal adults (Agunod, Yamaguchi, Lopez, Luhby, and Glass, 1969). However, if the output of intrinsic factor in 2-week-old infants is calculated in terms of body weight, it is approximately two times less than the adult value. Despite this low level in the neonatal period, the average infant has a sufficient output for adequate absorption of vitamin B_{12}.

Some literature reports the presence of an enzyme *rennin* in the neonate's stomach. Rennin coagulates milk casein at pH values between 6.0 and 6.5. Though this enzyme has been identified in the neonatal calf, its presence in the human infant has not been established.

HEPATOBILIARY SYSTEM

The liver at birth is large; it constitutes 4 percent of the body weight and occupies two-fifths of the abdominal cavity. The superior border is in contact with the diaphragm, and the inferior border may extend as low as 1 cm above the iliac crest. As a result of its attachment to the diaphragm, the liver moves with respiration. In the neonate the left lobe composes more than one-third of the total liver mass.

Though the liver appears structurally mature, it is physiologically immature. In the early postnatal period it evolves from a major site of blood cell formation to perform a myriad of functions including digestion, metabolism, and detoxification. The neonatal liver is deficient in glucuronyl transferase, the enzyme that catalyzes the transfer of glucuronic acid from uridine diphosphate glucuronic acid to bilirubin to form bilirubin glucuronide. Only the conjugated water-soluble form of bilirubin is excreted. The glucuronyl transferase enzyme approaches adequate levels by 5 to 14 days of life in full-term neonates. Hepatic immaturity is pronounced in the premature infant, who is usually more jaundiced than the full-term infant. In normal neonates, accumulation of unconjugated bilirubin does not reach levels that are toxic to the CNS. Physiological jaundice, which occurs in 50 percent of the full-term neonates and 80 percent of the premature infants, becomes visible in the third or fourth day of life. It disappears within a week in the full-term neonate and persists for several weeks in the premature.

In addition to the glucuronyl transferase deficiency, the hepatocyte is also deficient in the intracellular Y protein which is responsible for transport of bilirubin for conjugation within the liver cell. Hyperbilirubinemia is further intensified by an increased intestinal absorption of bilirubin secondary to deficient bacterial degradation in the neonate's intestine.

The bile acid pool in the neonate is approximately one-half of the adult value when compared on the basis of body surface area. The values in the premature infant are even lower. Two factors which have been identified as contributing to bile acid deficiency include diminished concentrating capacity of the gallbladder and rapid gastric emptying. Bile acid deficiency in the premature infant leads to malabsorption of fat-soluble vitamins. Despite deficiency of bile acids the neonate adequately handles the high percentage of fats in human milk. A lipase found in human milk, activated by bile salts, is believed responsible for this ability.

A number of coagulation factors, II, VII, IX, and X, which are synthesized by the liver under the influence of vitamin K, are decreased for 2 to 3 days postbirth. Thereafter the values rise slowly but do not approach adult values for about 1 year. The neonate, with a sterile intestinal tract, lacks the vitamin K necessary for hepatic prothrombin formation. As bacterial flora become established, vitamin K synthesis is augmented.

The liver of the neonate is less efficient than it is in adulthood in deamination of amino acids, ketone body formation, and gluconeogenesis. The low blood-glucose values characteristic of the neonatal period may be due to diminished gluconeogenesis from protein. Conversion of fructose and galactose to glucose is also decreased in the neonate. Also, the liver is limited in its capacity to store vitamins; therefore, the neonate is dependent on a daily exogenous supply.

PANCREAS

At birth the subdivisions of the pancreas are typical of the adult, but the head makes up a greater percentage of the organ. The endocrine islets of Langerhans number about 120,000 in the neonate compared with 800,000 islets in the adult.

The humoral stimulatory mechanisms (secretin and pancreozymin) for regulation of pancreatic secretion are present in the neonate. Volume and secretory rates correlate with the neonate's size (Tyson, 1969).

Pancreatic secretion of digestive enzymes appears to be sufficient for the neonate's diet. The amylase content of pancreatic fluid in the neonate is less than that in the adult (Searcy, Berk, Hayashi, and Ackerman, 1967) but increases gradually with age. The capacity to hydrolyze starch is incomplete in the neonate.

Pancreatic lipase activity in neonates is low or normal; however, hydrolysis of triglycerides is incomplete in both full-term and premature infants. Trypsin activity is lower than the other proteolytic enzymes at birth (Lieberman, 1966). The activity is less in the premature than full-term infant and is not stimulated by food entering the duodenum.

MIDGUT

SMALL INTESTINE

The entire intestinal tract wall is relatively thin at birth due to lack of development of the musculature. The duodenum lacks circular folds throughout its length; the jejunum and ileum are strikingly similar and also lack circular folds. Villi are located throughout the small intestine, as is the process of epithelial cell regeneration.

Motility Transit time through the small intestine in the neonate is extremely variable, averaging 3 to 6 h. Peristalsis in the duodenum consists of wave forms similar to the adult, though the motor activity is much less. Radiologic studies have disclosed the presence of an irregular intestinal lumen, segmentation, and collection of the meal in large masses. This may be partially attributed to a poorly developed local mechanism in the small intestine at birth.

Digestion Although initiated in the mouth by salivary amylase, the primary site of carbohydrate hydrolysis is the small intestine. At birth, amylase activity of duodenal fluid is low; however, it gradually increases with age.

At birth, maltase and sucrase activity exceed lactase activity. However, the lactase activity in full-term neonates is two to four times greater than that found in older infants. In contrast, premature infants are relatively deficient in intestinal lactase activity.

Hydrolysis of triglycerides is initiated in the stomach of the neonate by gastric lipase. However, the bulk of fat digestion takes place in the small intestine in the presence of pancreatic lipase and bile salts. Lipase activity is low, and bile salt concentration of the full-term neonate is inadequate for micellar formation. Thus, absorption of long-chain unsaturated fatty acids and cholesterol is poor.

In general, protein digestion in the neonate does not differ appreciably from the digestive capabilities of older infants or adults. However, gastric hydrolysis of proteins is unimportant in the neonatal period; the major proteolytic activity occurs in the small intestine. Enterokinase, necessary for conversion of trypsinogen to trypsin, is present at birth. Intestinal mucosal peptidase activity is well developed and remains highly active in the postnatal period.

Absorption Many of the transport mechanisms essential for absorption are less efficient in the early postnatal period. The capacity of the small intestine to absorb monosaccharides is present at birth. Active-transport processes for glucose and galactose require energy which is dependent, in the mature intestinal tract, upon adequate oxygenation. The neonate is capable of tolerating anoxia for longer periods than the adult; thus, it is possible that the energy sources for transport in the young infant may differ. The anaerobic-transport capacity is lost soon after birth. Approximately 98 percent of the ingested starch, a complex carbohydrate, is absorbed in the neonate.

Fat absorption is quantitatively deficient in the neonatal period. Ease of absorption is determined by the chemical constitution of the fat. Short-chain fats and those with unsaturated linkages are absorbed readily. Neonates absorb 85 to 90 percent of the fat in human milk. Fat in cow's milk is not as well absorbed. Animal fat is not assimilated to the same extent as vegetable oils, which contain more unsaturated fatty acids. Infants under 1 year of age absorb approximately 80 percent of the fat ingested; adult fat absorption is equal to 95 percent of an ingested fat load. In contrast, the premature infant's ability to handle a fat load is even more limited; absorption of an unsaturated fatty acid fat diet may vary from 20 to 90 percent of the intake.

Transport mechanisms required for active absorption of amino acids, which occurs in the upper small intestine, are at adult levels in the neonate. The anaerobic active-transport mechanism for amino acids is functional during the first 2 days of life. When present in high concentrations, amino acids may be absorbed by simple diffusion. Limited evidence suggests that polypeptides may be absorbed as such and hydrolyzed within the mucosal cells by peptidases.

The gut of the neonate is also permeable to some intact proteins; the macromolecules are absorbed by pinocytosis, which is more pronounced during the neonatal period. Increased intestinal permeability to protein macromolecules has implications for potential absorption of endotoxins, proteolytic and hydrolytic enzymes, and ingested antigens. Furthermore, the absorbed protein may escape intracellular proteolysis secondary to immature lysosomal function with intact protein molecules transported into the circulation (Walker, 1975). Absorption of macromolecules from the gut at a time when local immune mechanisms are lacking may result in clinical disease states. The neonate may develop a sensitivity to ingested food antigens or bacterial breakdown products which could result in health problems, such as allergy, in later life. Breast-feeding for the first 3 months of life creates a passive immune state within the intestine and minimizes absorption of foreign proteins in antigenic amounts.

Mechanisms and sites for fluid absorption in the neonate have not been shown to differ markedly from the mature gastrointestinal tract. However, the role of the gut in regulating fluid and electrolyte balance is crucial because of the inefficiency of the immature renal system. In health, the alimentary tract of the neonate maintains fluid and electrolyte balance remarkably well. The response to stress is often an acceleration of the passage of food through the gastrointestinal tract resulting in deficient fluid absorption and dehydration.

HINDGUT

LARGE INTESTINE

Certain common characteristics of the ascending, transverse, descending, and sigmoid colons of the neonate differ from those of the adult. As a result of poorly developed musculature, intestinal walls are thin. The rectum and anal canal are relatively longer at birth, and the rectum is also characterized by a very thin muscular wall. The musculature of the anal sphincter is well developed.

Physiologically the large intestine of the neonate is similar to that of the adult. Fluid- and electrolyte-absorptive capacities of the colon are well established, and fluid absorption in the infant is proportionately greater than that in the adult. Segmentation and coordinated propulsive motor activity is characteristic of colonic motility of the neonate. The *gastrocolic reflex*, usually initiated with feeding, results in mass movement of colonic contents into the terminal rectum. The small capacity of the neonatal rectum results in a more frequent passage of small-volume stools that have a larger fluid content.

At birth the intestinal tract is filled with meconium, a

dark, brownish green, viscid material. Meconium is the residue of amniotic fluid, bile, and embryonic intestinal secretion. The normal neonate passes the first meconium stool within 48 h of birth. The initial meconium discharge is sterile, but within hours a bacterial flora is established.

Meconium stools are generally passed four to six times a day for 2 or 3 days. Transitional stools, which are thin, sour-smelling, and brown to green in color, are passed from the fourth to seventh day. The changing character of the stool is due to the type of milk ingested and the nature of the intestinal flora. Stools of the breast-fed infant are pasty to loose, pale to yellow or green, and homogeneous. In formula-fed infants, the stools are firm, pale in color, and have an unpleasant odor. The number of stools per day varies considerably; the breast-fed infant averages two to four, whereas the formula-fed infant has fewer, usually one to three per day. In the first weeks of extrauterine life the average daily weight of the stool is 30 to 45 g.

ROLE IN IMMUNOLOGY

Within 24 h of birth the neonate's intestinal tract is rapidly colonized by bacterial entry through the mouth and anus. The stomach and duodenum generally do not harbor aerobic organisms, which are present in increasing numbers in the rest of the gastrointestinal tract. The intestinal flora is affected by diet and competitive interactions with other organisms. A well-balanced intestinal flora is important as a defense against pathogens and in synthesis of B vitamins, folic acid, biotin, and vitamin K.

The predominant immunoglobulin (Ig) produced by the intestine is IgA. Small concentrations of IgG and IgE are also present in the gut. IgA has a vital role in control of bacterial proliferation within the gut. This defense mechanism is important protection against potential dangers of invasion of the mucosal barrier (Walker, 1976).

Endocrine system Norma J. Briggs

Endocrine tissue development begins early in fetal life; however, some of these endocrine tissues may or may not be used by the fetus prior to birth. The neonate, who can no longer depend on maternal support, must now activate all his endocrine tissues. Thus, until the neonate's endocrine tissues are functioning in a normal way, he is at risk.

ADRENAL CORTEX

During the first 2 weeks of the neonate's life, the fetal zone of the adrenal cortex, which composes 80 percent of the adrenal cortex, undergoes rapid degeneration. As the fetal zone degenerates, the adult adrenal cortex increases in size and becomes more prolific in secretion of steroid hormones.

Structural and functional maturity of the adult adrenal cortex is reached during the first month of life. With increasing amounts of steroid hormones being synthesized and secreted into the circulatory system, any metabolic problem will become evident in a relatively short period of time.

THYROID

It has been shown that a surge of thyrotropin (TSH) from the adenohypophysis occurs within 30 min following birth. This surge of TSH produces a hyperfunction of the thyroid, which lasts for approximately 2 days. This brief episode of hyperfunction seems to activate the thyroid system. The structural and functional maturity of the thyroid system is normally present in the neonate.

Neonates with an intact thyroid system who were born of mothers with hyperthyroidism may suffer from a transient hyperthyroidism. The length of the transient hyperthyroidism will be influenced by the severity of the maternal hyperthyroidism and the homeostatic regulatory ability of the neonate's thyroid system.

PANCREAS

The fetal pancreas does secrete insulin and glucagon. Functional maturation of the pancreas is seen in terms of regulatory mechanisms. Glucose concentration as the stimulus for insulin release in the neonate is not well developed, and when this adult regulatory mechanism does develop is not known.

Neonates of diabetic mothers have been in all likelihood exposed to hyperglycemic episodes during fetal life. These episodes appear to bring about an early functional maturation of the pancreas and its ability to secrete insulin. This early maturation is based on the neonate's ability to handle glucose and a proneness to hypoglycemia in the early days of postnatal life.

GLUCOSE BALANCE

Carbohydrate metabolism is influenced by many hormones. Growth hormone, glucocorticoids, epinephrine, insulin, and glucagon all help to regulate glucose levels. In the neonate, the activities of respiration, temperature regulation, and muscle activity utilize glucose and rapidly deplete the glycogen stored in the heart, liver, and muscles during fetal life. If the metabolic rate of the neonate is increased by acidosis, hypoxia, or a cold stressor, there is an increased demand on glucose and glycogen stores. Hypoglycemia may occur in the neonate if glycogen stores are below normal; if there is excessive insulin available; or if cortisol, epinephrine, and glucagon are insufficient to aid in carbohydrate metabolism.

TEMPERATURE BALANCE

Maintenance of body temperature in the neonate is under the hormonal influences of glucagon, epinephrine, and thyroxine. In response to a cold stressor, there is an increase in metabolic rate, which increases heat production. Activation of glycogen phosphorylase, which is involved in the breakdown of stored glycogen, can be achieved either by epinephrine or glucagon. The conversion of stored glycogen to glucose provides a source of energy to maintain the metabolic rate necessary to maintain body temperature.

Brown adipose tissue in the neonate is the main site of thermogenesis. Under the influence of catecholamines, brown adipose tissue produces heat by oxidizing fatty acids. The effect of the catecholamines is transient, while a more sustained heat production is dependent upon thyroid function.

WATER BALANCE

Water balance in the neonate is precarious. In addition to the functional immaturity of the kidneys, there may be hormonal influences to explain why the neonate's kidneys do not concentrate urine well. A function of antidiuretic hormone (ADH) is to help concentrate urine. Two possible hormonal mechanisms are an insufficient amount of ADH being released from the neurohypophysis or ADH being produced by the neurohypophysis in sufficient amounts but the target-cell receptors not being fully functional in the immature kidneys.

ELECTROLYTE BALANCE

While a wide range of electrolyte intakes is tolerated by the neonate, a matter of concern is sodium chloride intake. The neonate seems predisposed to salt retention when the salt intake is above normal. Aldosterone is the hormone associated with sodium retention by the kidneys. It may be that the control mechanism initiating aldosterone release is faulty in early neonatal life.

MINERAL BALANCE

Hypocalcemia developing between the fifth and tenth days of life is usually related to diet and is called *neonatal tetany*. Infants unable to excrete large amounts of phosphorus contained in their formulas due to immature parathyroids or kidneys may have low calcium levels.

Other mechanisms involved in causing hypocalcemia need to be explored, for breast-fed infants also have been found to develop hypocalcemia. Parathyroid hormone (PTH) plays a role in maintaining serum calcium levels. Thus, it is possible that high levels of PTH in the maternal blood (hyperparathyroidism) may lead to in utero suppression of the fetal parathyroids. In the neonate, there would then be a period of time required for the parathyroids to become active and adjust to the change in environment. Mothers of breast-fed hypocalcemic infants should be investigated for the possibility of hyperparathyroidism.

Reproductive system Nancy Reame

PHYSICAL ASSESSMENT OF REPRODUCTIVE ORGANS AT BIRTH

Unlike other organ systems at birth the reproductive system of the neonate does not undergo a dramatic adjustment or change in function. In fact, reproductive organs may even regress somewhat in size, especially in female neonates, as the influence of the maternal hormones subsides after delivery. However, the physical appearance of the genitals at birth is commonly used as a criterion for assessment of gestational age, especially when the date of conception is in doubt.

In the normal full-term neonate, areolar and breast tissue are present and 4 to 7 cm in diameter. Because of high levels of maternal estrogens and prolactin in placental circulation at the end of pregnancy, both male and female neonates may exhibit breast enlargement and even secrete a milklike substance. This swelling subsides shortly after birth once the hormonal stimulation is removed.

MALE NEONATE

The genitalia of male neonates vary in size, but the weight of the testis in the neonate is about 1 g, and its volume less than 1 mL. Scrotal edema may be present at birth due to the delivery process but generally subsides during the first week of life. In a full-term neonate the scrotum will hang loosely and have extensive rugae and pigmentation. In most cases, the testes will have descended into the scrotal sac. Occasionally descent is delayed until shortly after birth especially in premature infants.

The cremasteric reflex is not well developed at birth. In the older infant, this reflex, elicited by stroking the inner aspect of the thigh, will cause ipsilateral testes to ascend into the inguinal canal. If the passage traversed by the testis during descent into the scrotal sac is not eliminated by atrophy, intestinal loops may be forced by abdominal pressure into this space, causing an inguinal hernia.

Internally, the testis of the neonate is somewhat different from that of the fetus. The interstitial cells, which are the Leydig cell precursors and have been multiplying during fetal life, diminish rapidly in the early postnatal period, not becoming prevalent again until near puberty. There is little change in either the growth or differentiation of the primitive seminiferous tubules until the time of puberty.

In the neonate the testis is composed of solid cords containing two cell types—the immature interstitial cells (Sertoli-like cells) and the primitive germ cells, or gonocytes. These gonocytes may undergo a series of changes leading to the development of early forms of spermatogonia. Many primordial germ cells, however, degenerate during postnatal development without differentiating into spermatogonia. The primitive type A spermatogonia (stem cells) appear in the testis as early as 2 months after birth, although they have no function or even a route for elimination since the tubular lumen does not develop until later in childhood (see Chap. 10).

The penis in the normal, full-term male will be about 4 cm in length with a urethral opening at the tip rather than on the dorsal or ventral side (hypospadias). The external meatus of the penis is covered by the prepuce, or foreskin. A degree of narrowing of the foreskin (phimosis) is normal, and thus it is *not* retractable for the first 4 to 6 months. Smegma, a whitish, opaque secretion, may collect around the glans penis. It is still a common practice in the United States to remove the foreskin by circumcision during the early neonatal period to facilitate cleansing of the glans and reduce the risk of infection. Since the foreskin plays no role in the reproductive process, this surgical procedure has no effect on future reproductive function. Research has been done to try to determine whether the incidence of cancer of the penis and cancer of the cervix in the sexual partner is reduced when circumcision has been performed in early infancy. Opponents of this procedure feel that the circumcised penis is more prone to ulceration and possible meatal stenosis.

Erection of the penis is possible even in neonates, as it is essentially a vascular phenomenon and dependent only on the integrity of the blood and nerve supply to the penis. The vascular spaces between the corpus cavernosum and the corpus spongiosum fill up with blood (tumescence) following either physical or psychological stimuli. Ejaculation is not possible until after the onset of puberty, when semen production is initiated.

FEMALE NEONATE

In the female, the reproductive tract at birth and for a short time after shows evidence of stimulation by the maternal hormones. Usually by the end of the first month of life the neonatal organs revert to an atrophic state which is characterized by a slow growth rate until the onset of puberty. At birth the external genitalia lie in a more exposed position than in the adult due to the underdeveloped state of the labia majora and the smaller amount of subcutaneous fat. In malnourished and premature infants, the clitoris and urethra are even more exposed. The clitoris of the neonate has almost approached its adult size so that it appears prominent in relation to the other external genitalia. The size and anatomy of the clitoris varies widely among neonates but, if exceptionally large, may be evidence of ambiguous sex differentiation. Fusion of the glans to the prepuce is a common finding which may become attenuated at puberty.

The hymen, a membranous diaphragm with a central opening, surrounds the outlet of the vagina; it has no known physiological function. It varies greatly in anatomical structure and may appear as a single, irregular opening, a longitudinal slit, or multiple perforations. Under the influence of maternal estrogens it is fairly thick at birth but becomes thin and flat once the hormonal effects regress. Sometimes an extra piece of tissue, a hymenal tag, will protrude from the floor of the vagina at birth but usually sloughs after 2 or 3 weeks.

Between birth and the third postnatal week the length of the uterus declines from 35 mm to about 24 mm and undergoes essentially no significant growth until age 9 or 10 years. During infancy, the length of the cervix accounts for about two-thirds of the entire uterus compared with about one-third in the adult. The uterine endometrium of the fetus may be so stimulated by the placental estrogens that a pseudomenstruation may occur in the neonate as evidenced by a white, mucoid, vaginal discharge tinged with blood, which disappears after 1 or 2 days.

Although the ovaries at birth weigh less than 0.5 g, they

contain about 2 million germ cells; one-half of these are in the form of developing primordial follicles, and the other one-half are in various stages of degeneration (atresia). This elimination process of large numbers of germ cells continues from about midfetal life to the menopausal years in the adult. By the time of birth, many oocytes will be "arrested" in the diplotene stage of meiosis and will remain so until just before the time of ovulation, which may occur up to 30 years after the onset of puberty. Although considered a resting phase, the oocytes undergo a high degree of metabolic and synthetic activity during this prolonged meiotic stage. Growth of the ovary is not nearly as influenced by maternal hormones as the uterus and vagina and is minimal during the postnatal period. However, when compared with testicular development, the ovary grows twice as fast during the first 3 years of life (Faiman and Winter, 1971).

REPRODUCTIVE ENDOCRINOLOGY OF THE NEONATAL PERIOD

The fetal pituitary gland has been shown to secrete low, but detectable, levels of luteinizing hormone (LH) and follicle-stimulating hormone (FSH) as early as 10 to 14 weeks' gestation (Kaplan, Grumbach, and Shepard, 1969). These hormones show sex differences in terms of secretory patterns during gestation, but under the influence of high levels of placental steroids at term, gonadotropins are suppressed in both males and females. At birth, the pituitary gland of the neonate becomes freed of feedback inhibition by maternal hormones and discharges a postnatal surge of LH and FSH.

In boys, gonadotropin levels are elevated for the first 4 months of life and then subside to prepubertal concentrations. The testis of the neonate responds to this hormonal stimulation by secreting large amounts of testosterone, up to 40 times the normal prepubertal levels. In the female neonate, dramatic surges of gonadotropins, especially FSH, also occur, which subside gradually during the first year. Both FSH and LH concentrations are significantly higher in the blood of females during infancy. Unlike the male gonad's response, estrogen secretion from the ovary is minimal during infancy and does not respond to the neonatal surge of gonadotropins.

The physiologic significance of these endocrine changes is not yet clear, but it appears that some aspects of hypothalamic-pituitary regulation of the reproductive system are functional at a very early stage of development. It has been shown that the pituitary gland of a 5-week-old infant is capable of responding in a postpubertal fashion to the administration of gonadotropin-releasing hormone (GnRH) (Root, Smith, Dhariwal, and McCann, 1969).

Urinary system Ida M. Martinson and Nancy V. Rude

STRUCTURE, POSITION, SIZE

Anatomic changes in the urinary system after birth are generally considered to be minimal. No new nephrons are believed to be formed after birth except in the premature infant. The main developmental changes of the kidney are the further maturation of the individual nephrons. Since intrauterine development of the kidney is from the cortex outward, the more mature nephrons are those toward the center of the kidney, and the least developed are those toward the periphery. When such heterogeneity of maturational development is noted, the major differences appear in the collecting ducts and loop of Henle, respectively. Greatest development, therefore, occurs in these sections. Equality of maturation among the successive levels within the kidney is believed to be reached by 12 to 14 months of age.

Heterogeneity of nephron development is also noted among nephrons of the same cortical level. The greatest heterogeneity that has been noted is the variation in the length of the proximal tubule. A difference of elevenfold has been noted. While the glomeruli also show variations, they are generally much more uniform. This heterogeneity is reduced to only a twofold difference by adulthood.

At birth, high columnar epithelium surrounds the neonatal renal glomerulus. Thus the visceral layer of the glomerular capsule is thicker than that in the adult. Shortly after birth this covering begins to thin out, first in isolated regions and then the entire glomerulus. This structural change is believed to affect the change noted in glomerular filtration rate (GFR) after birth. The infant kidney is demarcated on the surface, lobulated, at birth. Lobulation usually disappears by early childhood.

As noted in Chap. 5, the lumen of the allantois obliterates and toughens, becoming the urachus. Postnatally the urachus lengthens as the fundus of the bladder descends and becomes known as the median umbilical ligament.

Positional changes of the kidney are minimal with perhaps a slight movement more cephalad and settling deep into the subperitoneal fat and connective tissue on the inner side of the dorsal body wall. The upper portion of the adult kidney lies at the level of the twelfth thoracic vertebra.

One of the more visible changes in the kidney from birth to adulthood is the change in size. The kidney at birth is approximately 4.5 cm in length, 2.0 to 2.5 cm in width, and 1 cm thick. The kidney increases in size until the adult proportions are reached—approximately 11.5 cm in length, 4 to 7.5 cm in width, and 2.5 cm thick—an increase of 2 to $2\frac{1}{2}$ times.

RENAL FUNCTION

The ability of the neonate's kidney to concentrate urine is often considered when comparing the function of the neonatal kidney with that of the more mature kidney. It is important to remember, when comparing concentrating ability, that urea is the solute most responsible for determining urine solute concentration, and dietary protein intake is an important determinant of urea excretion. Both adults and neonates increase urine concentration with increases in dietary protein consumption. It has been shown that infants on high-protein diets may increase their mean maximum urine concentration to 1000 mosmol/L, which is above the mean concentration found for children up to puberty (Edelmann, Barnett, and Troupkou, 1960).

The mechanism by which the neonatal kidney conserves or excretes water is identical to that of the normal mature kidney except for a few special factors present only during the perinatal period. It has been postulated that the neonatal secretion of ADH is not great enough to allow concentration of urine to mature levels and also that the immature kidney is not as responsive to circulating ADH as the mature kidney in increasing the permeability of the distal convoluted tubule and collecting duct to water (Heller, 1951). The normal mean value for urine concentration is 515 mosmol/L from 2 years through the rest of childhood.

Perhaps the most important factor causing differences between neonatal and mature renal function is difference in GFR. The GFR is partially determined by the permeability of the epithelial portion of the glomerulus. Glomerular permeability increases with age, and increasing glomerular permeability correlates well with increasing GFR (Arturson, Growth, and Grottee, 1971; Robillard, 1954). GFR is also dependent in part upon renal blood flow, which increases dramatically at birth as blood flow is rerouted from the placenta to the other fetal organs, notably the lungs and kidneys. These changes in renal blood flow are primarily responsible for a doubling of GFR during the first 2 weeks after birth (Guignard, Torrado, DaCunna, and Gautier, 1975).

Angiotensin II levels, while greater than maternal levels before birth, increase dramatically during and after normal parturition (Mott, 1975). This increase is partially responsible for increased arterial blood pressure and perhaps for accompanying increases in GFR at birth. Considering that adult glomeruli are about four times more permeable than those of infants and that the capillary surface area available for filtration in the glomeruli is increased five times from birth to adulthood, GFR should undergo a twentyfold increase from birth to maturity, which agrees well with empirical observation (Guignard et al., 1975).

Another factor influencing the changes in renal function with age is the anatomic and cellular immaturity of the tubular portions of the kidney during the neonatal period. Since the hypertonicity, or osmolar gradient, established in the medullary interstitium is directly related to the length of the loops of Henle, it can be assumed that as the loops of Henle grow in length during and after the perinatal period, the osmolar gradient across the medullary interstitium will increase, allowing increases in the urine-concentrating ability of the kidney. Recent studies have provided support for this assumption.

Sodium excretion in the neonate has not been shown to differ from adult values if differences in GFR are taken into account. Ninety percent of the sodium ions are reabsorbed by the neonatal nephron. The dramatic increase in circulating angiotensin II at birth accounts for the concurrent increase in aldosterone. Aldosterone in turn increases the reabsorption of sodium. This mechanism is believed to be responsible for the large percentage of sodium reabsorption seen at birth.

If allowances are made for differences between adult and neonatal GFR, there is no significant difference between their respective abilities to excrete hydrogen ion. Yet it has been shown that infants excrete bicarbonate ions to maintain a lower circulating concentration than the adult (Pitts, Ayer, and Schiess, 1949; Tudvad, McNamara, and Barnett, 1954). As stated above, the reason for this difference has not as yet been accounted for.

The neonatal kidney is able to excrete phosphate in amounts equal to the adult but only if infant plasma-phosphate levels are very high. Differences in GFR seem to be the main factor responsible for relatively low phosphate excretion (McCrory, 1952). It seems probable that inorganic phosphate is retained because of increased growth requirements.

The most important changes functionally beyond the neonatal period are in GFR. It appears that this functional ability increases rapidly up to 2 years of age and then begins to slow down, finally reaching the adult level after puberty. Renal blood flow also increases in a similar manner to GFR.

Bladder size and capacity vary among children. In each child, bladder capacity increases with age through adolescence. Thus, an older child can retain a higher volume of urine which, along with increased neurological maturation, progressively increases the length of time between voiding.

In summary, while the kidneys certainly are functional at birth, differences in composition of the urine as well as structure of the kidneys exist between the neonatal kidney and adult kidney. Great differences in maturational level between the nephrons exist, but in general homogeneity among the nephrons is accomplished early in life. Glomerular filtration rate appears to be the single most important function that undergoes dramatic changes early in life and continues to increase through puberty. Many of the differences noted between the neonatal kidney's capabilities and adult kidney's capabilities are accounted for through maturation of this function.

Development of body concept and concepts of illness and wellness
Judith Anne Ritchie

BODY CONCEPT, CONTENT, AND FUNCTION

The differentiation between self and the outer world becomes one of the foremost tasks to be accomplished in formulation of body image. The ongoing process of integration of sensory impression and perceptions leading to a body concept begins in the embryologic period (Freytag, 1961; Kolb, 1975). Throughout fetal life and the neonatal period the child learns about the body and formulates the initial image of its parts and boundaries through vestibular and kinesthetic stimulation (Greenacre, 1958; Kolb, 1975).

The major mode of input of information about the body is tactile. As the neonate is stroked, patted, and cuddled, he receives messages from the body surface. Increasing body motion through rocking and carrying provides the neonate with proprioceptive messages about his body mass and position in space. The neurological reception of these messages is possible at this age because the kinesthetic and tactile sensory paths are the first to complete myelinization (Langworthy, 1975).

As the child develops, body openings have greater import in the body concept than other body parts (Schilder, 1964). The beginning area of prominence is the oral zone, and initially the child's world is said to consist of the "face-hand-breast cluster" (Benfeld, 1929). The mouth becomes a primary area of stimulation by the nipple of the breast or bottle and by the neonate's hand. It is the separation from the nipple that first establishes the differentiation between the mouth and the outer world. The neonate's concept of his body appears limited to surface impressions, beginning awareness of postural changes, and awareness of the oral zone as a source of satisfaction.

WELLNESS, ILLNESS, AND HOSPITALIZATION

When the neonate is well, has his needs satisfied, and is rested, his behavior may be quiet awake (alert) or active awake (Wolff, 1973b). However, during periods of illness or experiences of unpleasant procedures, the behavioral responses are vastly different. These responses tend to be global and to gain in specificity only as the child develops.

PAIN AND RESTRAINT

The exact age prenatally at which the child begins to perceive pain is unknown, but it is clear that the normal full-term neonate responds to painful stimuli from the time of delivery (Swafford and Allan, 1968). The consistent response to pinprick in the neonate is movement of the upper and lower limbs accompanied by crying, grimacing, or both (Rich, Marshall, and Valpe, 1974). Crying during minor surgical procedures is said to be susceptible to elimination by distraction (Poznanski, 1976), but frequently crying persists until the neonate can be comforted at the end of the procedure only by soothing measures such as provision of warmth and cuddling.

It may be difficult to determine whether the neonate's vigorous protest is precipitated by pain or restraint. Protest may begin, for example, as soon as the foot is grasped for access to the heel in order to obtain a blood sample. It may be that this response is due to the cutaneous stimulation rather than the restraint alone (Poznanski, 1976).

Very ill neonates and those whose arms and legs are restrained almost continuously tend to lie very quietly with little evidence of interest in their environment. They seem to have no energy for expression of pain or protest. The effects of such restraint of mobility in the neonate are insufficiently studied. However, children who were restrained for a period of time as ill neonates have been observed to resume the restrained posture when they are feeling insecure, unhappy, or sick (Oremland and Oremland, 1973).

ORAL DEPRIVATION

The necessity of elimination of oral feedings for seriously ill neonates prevents normal satisfaction of nutritive and nonnutritive sucking needs. The ill neonate frequently engages in an individual pattern of rhythmic nonnutritive sucking. This behavior disappears if the neonate is kept from purposeful sucking for prolonged periods. When oral feedings become feasible, the infant often must learn sucking behavior. Occasionally the process of learning is difficult.

SENSORY STIMULATION

The hospitalized, ill neonate, particularly if cared for in an intensive-care nursery, is subjected to multiple sources of sensory stimulation. He receives tactile stimuli from handling, surgical incisions, and various intrusive probes or procedures; auditory stimuli from monitors, other infants, unit personnel, and visitors; and visual stimuli which are often distorted by oxygen hoods or Plexiglas incubators. Visual stimuli may be absent because of eye patches. Often normal sensory stimuli, such as that provided by gentle stroking, patting, clothing, and cuddling, the parents' talking and singing to the neonate, and the normal patterns of lightness and darkness, are absent. The neonate may, in reality, be experiencing almost total sensory isolation because the multiple inputs are continuous and lack variation. Both normal and ill neonates have been observed to habituate to stimuli (Bridger, 1973; Oremland and Oremland, 1973). For example, very young, premature infants exhibit considerable purposeless limb movements despite all the continuous stimuli.

Introduction of an intermittent auditory stimulus is effective in decreasing these movements (Wolff, 1973a).

DISRUPTION OF BONDING

Hospitalization of the neonate is said to be likely to disrupt the process of bonding both for the child and the family. Klaus and Kennell (1976) suggest that increased exposure of the neonate to the mother during the first 3 days of postnatal life positively affects maternal behavior over a period of 2 years and the child's IQ and language behavior over a period of 5 years. They express concern that interruption of this sensitive period, due to illness, for example, may cause serious disruption in the parenting process.

During the first few days after birth the neonate's priority task is stabilization of body function. Not only is the neonate now independent of maternal support, but he is subject to all manner of new, fatiguing environmental assault.

These same environmental stimuli, however, will coax the neonate to respond and to adapt. And, although he sleeps the majority of the time this first month, the neonate exhibits notable behavior and emerging skills. Neonatal behavioral development is discussed by area in the following section.

SECTION 2
Behavioral Development

The neonate: Awakening Mary Tudor

Behavior of the neonate has become a focus of professional attention for both researchers and clinicians. Pursuit of the "answer" to the nature-versus-nurture question and early identification of deviation are two motivating forces. In the past, the neonate's inabilities were noted, but abilities were obscured or overlooked.

Because of changing obstetrical practice, the neonate can now be observed exhibiting behaviors previously thought beyond his capabilities. In addition, increasing information regarding prenatal behavior has been a clue to potential in the neonatal period. Parents as well as professionals are affected by the neonate's behavior, and thus infant care giving as well as assessment and intervention have been impacted.

It cannot be denied, however, that the child is born basically helpless, with limited capabilities. Behaviorally, he remains in the germinal stage; eventual adaptive functioning will evolve from differentiation and elaboration of basic abilities present at birth.

BEHAVIORAL STATE

In all areas of neonatal behavior one must take into consideration behavioral state. Investigation of the neonate has resulted in recognition of behavioral state as a critical variable and determining factor for behavior exhibited by the neonate. P. H. Wolff was the first to describe states of the neonate. He outlined seven descriptive categories of behavior which are regular sleep, irregular sleep, periodic sleep, drowsiness, alert inactivity, waking activity, and crying (1959; 1966).

H. Prechtl also studied these "prolonged and characteristic epochs of stable behavior" (1974, p. 185) and redefined five states or "vectors," based on the presence or absence of a specific collection of behavioral criteria. These are presented in Table 6-5 and Figs. 6-16 through 6-19.

Other researchers continue to identify a stage between 2 and 3, drowsiness, which can also be considered a transitional state.

The behavioral states were initially considered part of a continuum, different levels of one variable: arousal. However, based on clinical testing as well as EEG tracings, Prechtl defines states as "distinct conditions, each having its specific properties and reflecting a particular mode of nervous function" (Prechtl, 1974, p. 207). Thus, behavioral state is thought to be more than a descriptive behavior classification; states may represent "distinct modes of brain activity" (Prechtl, 1974, p. 186).

State is a critical consideration in infant behavior in three ways. First, during assessment, the neonate will respond to stimuli differently in different states. Prechtl offers this fact as support of the mutual exclusivity of states. In this sense, state is a variable to be respected and controlled. Thus, in assessment of neonatal response to stimuli, certain responses are elicited (or observations made) in certain states.

Second, observations of spontaneous (nonelicited) state changes over time, a "state profile" (Prechtl, 1974) give data on neurological status of the neonate. These quantitative descriptions "give an important insight into the organization and regulation of neonatal behavior" (Prechtl, 1974, p. 201).

In the first few hours after birth, most neonates demonstrate a significant alert period. After that, the neonate's state profile shows rapid and large fluctuations in the first 2 to 3 days after birth. The profile is different from that seen prenatally or at 3 days of age and older. This apparently reflects response to the birth process and adaptation to extrauterine conditions (Brazelton, 1973; Prechtl, 1974). Thus, observations of state changes over time are recommended after the third day of postnatal life, when stabilization should occur.

In the quiet-alert state, state 3, the neonate will visually scan the environment and be more receptive of and responsive to external stimuli. It is the optimal time for reciprocal parent-child interaction; however, this state is, on the average, the shortest in duration (Prechtl, 1974). The infant is awake but motorically active in state 4; he kicks, waves, turns his head, and squirms. These generalized motor movements interfere with prolonged attention, but this stage is also an enjoyable time for the parent observing the neonate.

During the transitional time between awake and sleep states, when the neonate exhibits drowsy behavior, he is not very responsive to outside stimuli; even food or play attempts to rouse him generally are unsuccessful. Quiet

TABLE 6-5 Behavioral states of the neonate

State	Behavioral correlates
1 Quiet (NREM) sleep	Eyes closed; no rapid eye movements Regular respiration No movement except for occasional startles and rhythmic mouthing
2 Active (REM) sleep	Eyes closed; rapid eye movements More rapid, irregular respiration No gross movement; small movements of face and limbs
3 Quiet awake	Eyes open; scanning or rapid eye movements No gross movement
4 Active awake	Eyes open; rapid eye movements Variable gross movements of head, limbs, trunk
5 Fussing or crying	Eyes open or closed Crying; variable gross movements
6 Indeterminate	Transitional; drowsiness

and active sleep, states 1 and 2, are discussed in "Sleep," p. 330.

A third important aspect of behavioral state is the impact on parents and the implications for care giving. Parents' understanding of behavioral states can aid in timing feeding, responding to vocalizations or startles, and other parenting behavior and can result in a more rewarding parent-infant interaction. Also, parents' awareness of their infant's particular state profile can enable them to better understand their child's temperament and read his cues.

FOUNDATIONS OF BEHAVIOR

Two other predominant themes in neonatal study are areas of behavior which are foundations of the soon-differentiating areas of perceptual, motor, cognitive, language, and social behavior. These foundations for future development are primitive reflex functioning and behaviors representing higher cortical functioning.

REFLEXIVE FUNCTIONING

The neonate's predominately flexion posture and primitive reflexes have been evaluated and described by many. Evaluation of reflex function is used as early neurological assessment, primarily of lower brain centers. It is partly because of these reflexes that the neonate's behavior has been described as stereotyped and stable. In actuality reflexive behavior is affected by state. Some reflexes, such as the palmar grasp and rooting, cannot be elicited in state 1. During states 4 and 5, the deep-tendon reflexes cannot be elicited (Prechtl, 1977). Primitive reflex functioning as foundation to motor skill development is dis-

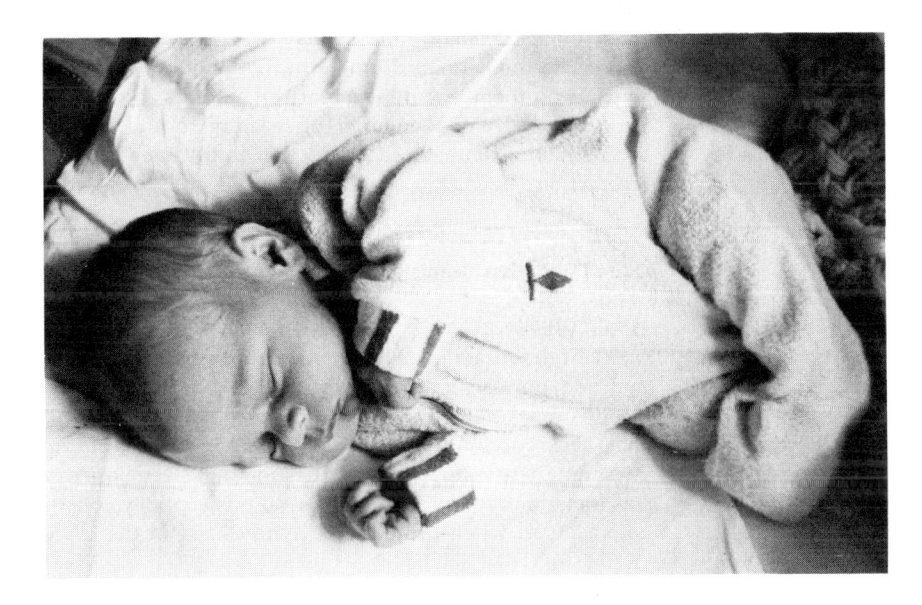

FIGURE 6-16. Quiet sleep.

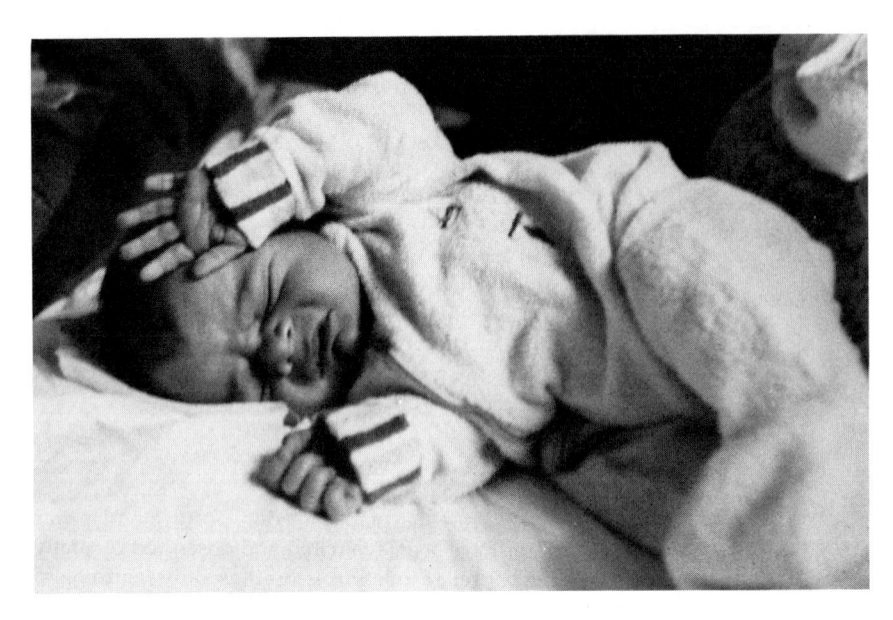

FIGURE 6-17. Active sleep.

cussed in "Gross Motor Development" and "Fine Motor Development."

HIGHER CORTICAL FUNCTIONING
The neonate is capable of more than reflex behavior; if evaluated in state 3, the neonate demonstrates orientation, attention, and habituation to visual, auditory, and tactile stimuli. These responses indicate beginning cognitive, language, and social development.

Neonatal assessment has also revealed purposeful motor behavior and affective behavior such as consolableness, ability to self-comfort, and degree of irritability. Evaluation of the neonate along these parameters has led to descriptions as variable, distinguishable, and individual.

INDIVIDUALITY
The individuality of the neonate in state profile and behavior is now appreciated. This individuality has implications for neonatal assessment. Assessment of state profile, reflex testing, and testing of higher-level, interactive behavior gives important data regarding neurological states as well as individual patterns of responding.

More importantly, the neonate's behavior will have an effect on his parents and thus the care giving he receives.

The neonate, by his individuality, shapes his environment. His manner of responding, level of nonresponse, ability to be consoled, and more will define one-half of the goodness of fit between himself and his parents.

Parents are reclaiming their neonates during and after birth, reestablishing their natural role as enablers of the child's development. As a result, parents are appreciating their impact on the infant's behavior; they may not fully appreciate the neonate's innate individuality or how this impacts on them as parents. Teaching parents about their neonate's individual manner of reacting to and coping with his environment may aid this understanding and interaction.

Sleep Clarissa Beardslee

OVERVIEW
Many of the functions of humans oscillate between maximal and minimal values once a day. It is thought that sleep is entrained to this so-called circadian rhythm and that sleep occurs during the depressed phase of the rhythm. There is no reason to question that sleep basically has a restorative function. One kind of sleep may constitute a phase when proteins are synthesized in the CNS.

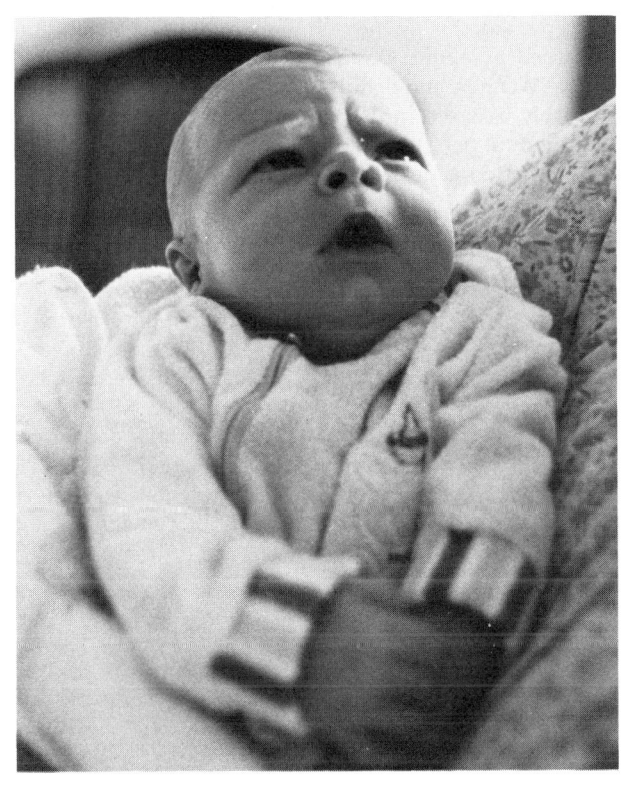

FIGURE 6-18. Quiet awake (alert).

Another kind of sleep may have a restorative function with respect to body systems involving processes of emotional adaptation to the environment and systems involved in consolidating learning.

Sleep might be defined as a period marked by closure of the eyelids, relaxed skeletal musculature, and an absence of goal-directed movements. Physiologically, sleep is marked by decreased metabolic activity, slowing of the heart rate, and decreased ventilation of the lungs. During sleep there is a shutdown of perception because the senses are not gathering information and communicating stimuli to the brain. This does *not* mean that the brain is resting.

From the time of Aristotle, sleep has been considered time taken from the important activities carried out during the waking state. Rather than a disturber of wakefulness, it is now considered to be a complement to the waking state. Wakefulness and sleep may be thought of as constituting alternate phases of a cycle, related one to the other as are the crest and trough of a wave. The absolute capacity for remaining awake gradually increases from a few minutes at birth to a continuous stretch of 15 to 17 h in the adult. A functioning cerebral cortex is essential for this evolution.

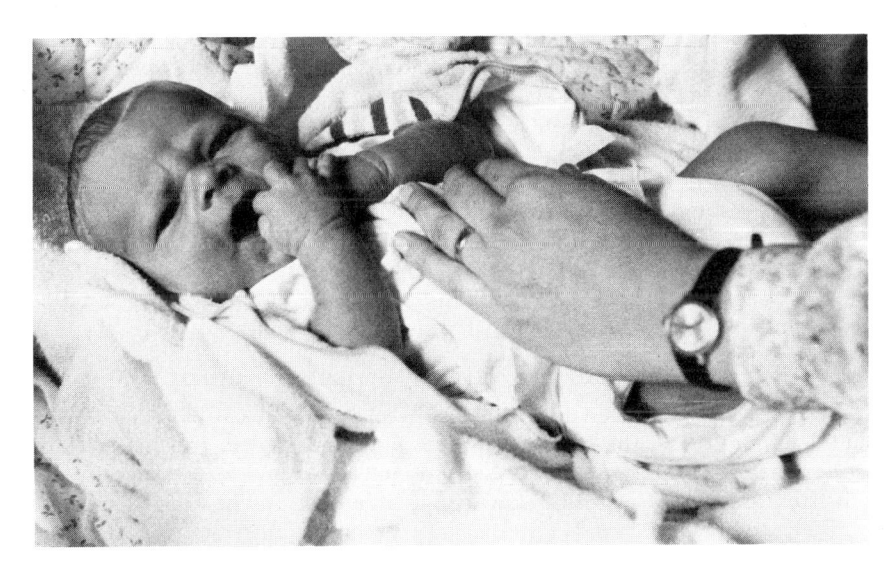

FIGURE 6-19. Active awake (alert).

WAKE AND SLEEP SYSTEMS

Knowledge concerning the mechanisms responsible for the sleep and wake systems is still incomplete. Currently, it is believed that the activity of the reticular formation is intimately involved in the induction and maintenance of wakefulness. Inactivity of this structure may induce sleep. What causes the inactivity of the reticular formation is not known. The cerebral cortex, as well as other structures of the brainstem, are thought to have some influence on the sleep-wakefulness system. An understanding of the way in which these or other brain structures exert their influence awaits further research.

FUNCTIONAL CHARACTERISTICS OF SLEEP

From birth on, every human being experiences two different kinds of sleep: non-rapid eye movement (NREM) and rapid eye movement (REM). These two kinds of sleep alternate rhythmically throughout the sleep period. The periods during which there are jerky, rapid eye movements beneath the closed lids are REM sleep. The movements occur in clusters several times during a night's sleep. During the periods of REM, small twitches of the facial muscles and fingertips can also be seen, but the muscles of the trunk and extremities cannot move. Dreaming is known to occur during REM sleep. A general absence of body movement and slow regular breathing characterize NREM sleep.

Sleep has been classified into several types of electroencephalograph (EEG) patterns called *stages* and numbered progressively from 1 through 4. Stages 2, 3, and 4 coincide with NREM sleep. In the course of a sleep period, stages 1, 2, 3, and 4 appear in succession. From stage 4 there is a reascent back to stage 1. This cyclic variation continues throughout the sleep period, with the sleeper passing through each stage several times each night. The amount of time spent in each stage is variable, depending on age among other things.

THE NEONATE

Neonates spend much of their time in sleep: probably an average of 17 h out of each 24. From the first through the fourth weeks of life the total amount of sleep decreases by less than 1 h. Information about the duration of sleep of prematurely born neonates is lacking, but the duration is undoubtedly longer for them than for full-term neonates.

During the first weeks of life both the distribution and duration of discrete sleep periods tend to be haphazard. For one group of neonates the average *longest* period of sleep per day during the first week of life was 4.08 h; this increased by about 30 min in the ensuing 3 weeks (Parmalee, Wenner, and Schulz, 1964). Sleep time varies considerably between individual neonates, both in terms of total amount per 24 h and length of discrete sleep periods. This variation is determined by the infant's own uniqueness as well as by his environment.

PHASIC CHARACTERISTICS

Even during the first month of life sleep does not have a unitary quality. Studies have revealed that the sleep cycle of neonates consists of two and possibly three different kinds of sleep. The first kind, *quiet sleep*, is defined as a neonatal sleep pattern which corresponds to NREM sleep in the adult. This is also state 1 in Prechtl's behavioral states. During quiet sleep the infant lies still except for irregularly occurring startles; the heart and respiratory rates are regular, and there are *no* movements of the eyeballs. Premature infants have very little quiet sleep; what they do have is ill-defined and of short duration.

The term *active sleep*, or state 2, has been given to the second kind of sleep manifested by neonates. This is defined as a sleep pattern equivalent to the REM sleep of adults. Active sleep has the following characteristics: Small movements of the face and limbs occur; breathing is both irregular and faster than that during quiet sleep; the pulse rate is increased; and there are movements of the eyeballs as well as of the lids and lashes. During the first week of life the neonate spends as much as 12 h/day in active sleep.

A third sleep phase, termed *intermediate*, has also been reported. This is a stage which occurs between the periods with and without eye movements. It may be a manifestation of the fact that cycling from quiet to active sleep and back again is still very irregular, rather than a discrete type of sleep.

Active sleep is thought to be a primitive sleep. For the full-term neonate, approximately 45 to 50 percent of total sleep is of this type; 35 to 45 percent of sleep is quiet, and the remainder is intermediate. This distribution changes with increasing age, with a gradual increase in the proportion of quiet sleep and a decrease in active sleep. The intermediate phase has usually disappeared by the time the full-term infant is 3 months old.

THE 24 h SLEEP-WAKEFULNESS RHYTHM

Even during the first weeks of life sleep time is not equally distributed between night and day. In the first week or two, infants sleep about two-thirds of the time from 8 P.M. to 8 A.M. and a little over one-half of the daytime hours. The disparity becomes greater during the latter half of the first month, with sleep accounting for nearly 70 to 80 percent of the nighttime and still just over one-half of the daytime.

ONSET OF SLEEP
Neonates frequently seem to be neither awake nor asleep but quasidormant. Direct, decisive transitions from waking to sleep are the exception rather than the rule. It is not unusual for the infant to fall asleep during a feeding as his hunger is appeased and comfort restored.

AWAKENING
Transition from sleep to wakefulness is still at a primitive level during the neonatal period. Premature infants are hard to rouse from sleep, and they return to sleep almost immediately when left alone. For the full-term neonate, shifting stages of wakefulness and drowsiness are apt to be interspersed with periods of sleep before a definitive waking period intervenes. During the course of awakening and neonate may exhibit brief spurts of writhing activity, and he may fret or cry from hunger or some other source of discomfort.

MODIFIABILITY OF SLEEP AND WAKEFULNESS
The neonate who is free of discomfort normally needs no help in falling asleep. Sucking, rocking, and softly sung lullabies are, however, effective promoters of sleep. Being rocked while held in a parent's arms may be more effective than rocking in a cradle because of the combined effect of tactile stimulation, body warmth, and motility.

Hunger, cold, or other forms of discomfort as well as sudden, loud noises may interfere with sleep. The less mature the infant, the less likely it is that he will be aroused by stimuli in the external environment. If the infant does rouse, the duration of wakefulness is likely to be brief unless he has some unsatisfied need.

The common beginnings of development, primitive reflex functioning, and higher-level responses of perception, all mediated by the neonate's state, will now be discussed in relation to specific areas of behavior.

Behavioral Development by Functional Area

Perceptual development Veronica A. Binzley

At one time the prevailing opinion held that the neonate had very little ability to make any sense out of the environment. However, research findings of the last 20 years have shown that this is not the case. On the contrary, infants, even neonates, have been found to be amazingly competent in making sense out of their environment. How does one determine what the neonate's capabilities are for organizing the information impinging on his senses? Investigators have devised some ingenious methods; however, these methods are not without problems, and this must be kept in mind when evaluating reports about the neonate's capabilities.

METHODS USED TO STUDY NEONATAL PERCEPTION
The experimental procedures most commonly used to study infant perceptual or sensory capacities are *reflex* and *habituation*. In the reflex procedure, one simply presents a stimulus of specified intensity or character and observes the neonate's response. Subsequent presentations of the stimulus might be given but only as a reliability check or procedural replication. Some behaviors frequently observed as response indicators in infant studies are listed in Table 6-6.

In the habituation procedure the effective stimulus is presented several times in sequence during which time the infant gradually decreases his response to the stimulus, which indicates that the infant has come to recognize the stimulus. The procedure is depicted in Fig. 6-20 in which heart rate is used as the observed response measure. In this figure the infant responds to both the onset and offset of the stimulus with a decrease in heart rate. However, when the stimulus is presented a second time, the infant responds with a smaller cardiac deceleration. If the stimulus is presented again, the response is even smaller yet. If one wishes to show that this behavior clearly indicates stimulus recognition and not just fatigue of the end organ, a new stimulus is usually presented. The infant responds to the new stimulus with a large cardiac deceleration, as he did to the first stimulus initially. This latter procedure is called *dishabituation*, and it frequently is used to study the neonate's discriminatory capabilities.

Each of the traditional sensory modalities have been studied using one or the other of these techniques, although vision and audition have been the most frequently studied senses. Figure 6-21 shows a neonate whose heart rate, respiration, nonnutritive sucking, and movement are being recorded in response to auditory stimulation.

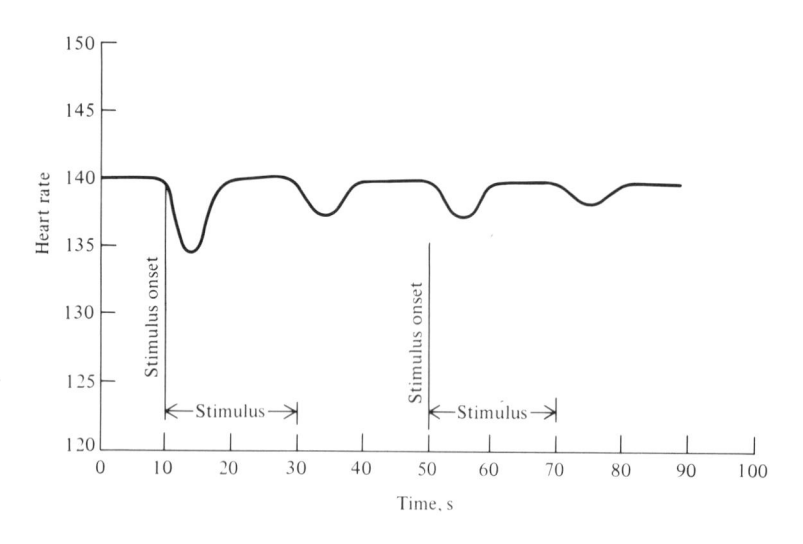

FIGURE 6-20. Habituation paradigm.

PROBLEMS ENCOUNTERED IN STUDYING PERCEPTION IN THE NEONATE

The major problem encountered in trying to study the neonate's perceptual capabilities is his changing state of alertness: his state. (The various states that have been identified are listed in Table 6-5.) The methods used to study perception require the neonate to be attentive, that is, in a state of quiet wakefulness. Unfortunately, the neonate spends little time in this state. According to Wolff, who studied a group of 10 neonates in their own homes, observing each for 30 h a week, the neonate spends only 11 percent of its time in quiet wakefulness during the first week. But this increases to 21 percent by the fourth week (MacFarlane, 1978).

If the investigator is fortunate enough to catch the neonate awake, the child may not stay in that state long enough to be studied because of the many factors other than internal biological rhythm that affect the state of alertness. Some of these factors are temperature of the surroundings, touch, amount of light, and presence of background noise. If the temperature of the surroundings is too hot, the neonate goes to sleep; if too cold, he starts to cry. Touch is important for, if tightly swaddled, he tends to go to sleep; but if he is totally naked, he may become distressed. Background noise frequently induces sleep in the neonate. Thus because of the problem with changing state, it is extremely difficult to accurately assess the neonate's perceptual capabilities. And much of what

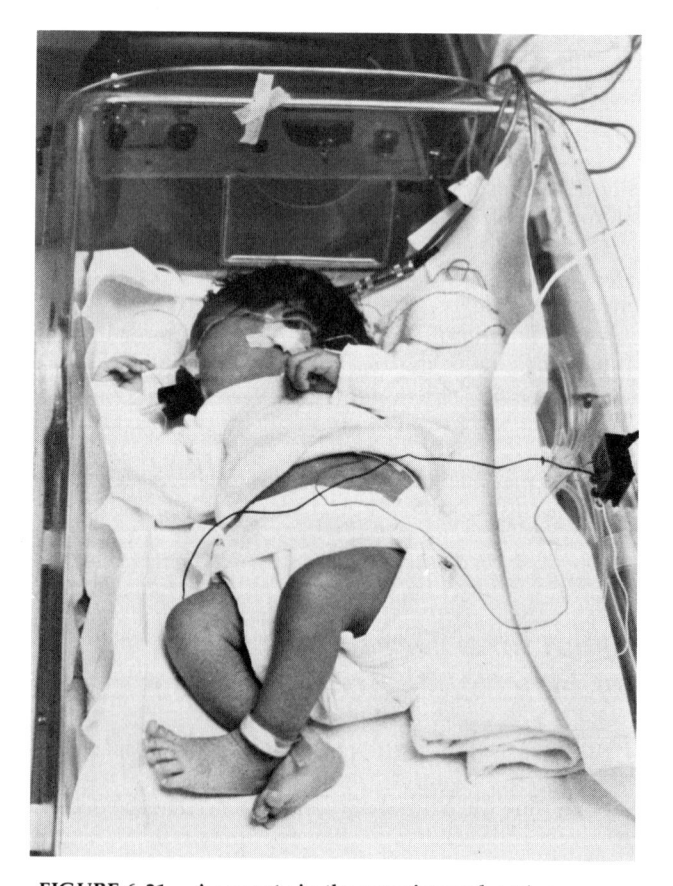

FIGURE 6-21. A neonate in the experimental setting.

TABLE 6-6 Infant behaviors frequently observed as response indicators

Behavior	Response
Sucking Nutritive or nonnutritive	Rate, duration
Eyes	Fixation direction, focal length of gaze, tracking arc
Eyelids	Opened, closed
Movement of extremities	Amount
Movement of trunk	Amount
Respiration	Rate, duration of cycle
Heart rate	Rate, duration of period
Pupillary	Dilation and constriction
Electroencephalogram	Pattern
Evoked responses	Amplitude, latency

is reported needs to be carefully scrutinized to be sure that state has been adequately controlled.

REPORTED PERCEPTUAL CAPABILITIES

Until recently it was commonly believed that the neonate's perceptual world was, in the words of William James, "a buzzing, blooming confusion." However, research findings of the last 10 years have shown that neonates do possess an ability to organize the information flooding in on their senses.

VISUAL PERCEPTION

Although some structures within the visual system are not completely formed, the general consensus is that at birth the eye is physiologically and anatomically prepared to respond differentially to most aspects of the visual environment. While this may be so, it should be pointed out that the processing going on must be subcortical because at birth the cortex is very little developed and its appearance suggests that little, if any, cortical functioning is possible (Tanner, 1970).

Nevertheless, it is well known that the neonate will fixate on a light, and several investigators (Kessen, Haith, and Salapatek, 1970) have reported differential fixation on targets varying in brightness. This would seem to indicate that brightness exists as a discriminable dimension of stimulation for the neonate. Visual acuity in the neonate has been reported to be approximately 20/150 Snellen, as determined by eliciting optokinetic nystagmus to moving stripes of different widths (Dayton, Jones, Aiu, Rawson, Steele, and Rose, 1964). However, values ranging up to 20/400 have also been reported using various testing procedures.

The question of whether the neonate can discriminate color has been studied since the late nineteenth century, and yet the evidence is still not clear because of the confounding of color and brightness. Evidence to date suggests, however, that color is not a discriminable dimension for the neonate.

MOVEMENT

Although it is well documented that movement, in the form of a moving edge or blinking lights, is a high attention getter for neonates, little research has been done to determine specifically the necessary conditions for eliciting pursuit of moving objects. A recent study reported finding stable individual differences in visual tracking ability at birth, some aspects of which correlate with tracking and attention at later ages (Haith and Campos, 1977).

SPACE: DISTANCE, DEPTH, AND DIRECTIONALITY

Several studies have reported eliciting partial, irregular eye blinks to a fast-approaching object at 3 weeks of age. This, however, is only evidence that on a reflex basis the neonate's system adjusts to variations in the distance of a stimulus. Obviously this is quite different from a true distance concept, for which at present there is no evidence in the neonate. Moreover, the fact that the neonate is not capable of sustained binocular convergence or variable accommodation of the lens, both of which could function as cues for distance, supports the conclusion that distance is not discriminated during this early period.

It was once thought that neonates had no sense of direction or location but that they presumably located the mother's breast or a light only through trial-and-error head-and-eye movements. Careful observation has found that this is not so. Neonates make directionally appropriate, if sluggish, eye movements to stimuli presented peripherally. By 1 month of age this directional response has become reasonably smooth and efficient.

PATTERN AND FORM PERCEPTION

Many investigators have commented that visual orienting in the neonate and very young infant is fixation rather than exploration. It has an obligatory quality to it, as though the infant were in some way captured by the stimulus or some aspect of it. Stechler, as reported by Gibson (1969), studied the development of visual orienting in infants from 6 days of age to 3 weeks. He presented black-and-white drawings of stylized faces, geometric forms, and living human faces for the infants to look at. He found attention to all objects was nearly 100 percent, and looking on occasion would continue for as much as 35 min at around the ninth or tenth day of life. At a later age, he found looking behavior took on a more "volitional" character. Others using measures of visual preference and detailed scanning have found that the neonate visually attends to high-contrast spots, edges, and corners within his view.

According to findings of scanning studies, the neonate scans primarily along the horizontal axis. Hence, the reported preference for some patterns over others may reflect differences in the location of critical elements with respect to a narrow vertical scanning window rather than differences in perceptual appeal. One should keep this in mind when evaluating reports of infant visual-preference studies. Notwithstanding this possibility, the evidence to date supports the general consensus that prior to $1\frac{1}{2}$ months infants process elements of form but are insensitive to visual organization or configuration (Haith and Campos, 1977).

Face perception Because it has long been recognized that the most complicated sight an infant sees after birth is his mother's face, considerable research has gone into trying to answer the questions of when and how the infant distinguishes his mother's face from all the others he sees. The number of studies done on this topic have been considerable and cannot be adequately reviewed here. The interested student is referred to Eleanor Gibson's thorough review in her book *Principles of Perceptual Learning and Development*. It is sufficient here to point out that the neonate finds the human face interesting, attends to high-contrast areas—eyes, external hair, skin, chin, and garment borders of the real face—but cannot yet distinguish his mother's face.

AUDITORY PERCEPTION

The neonate has been hearing sounds for at least 4 months prior to birth. The chief sensory stimuli during fetal life are, of course, the sounds of the functioning maternal viscera. However, for some time it was thought that

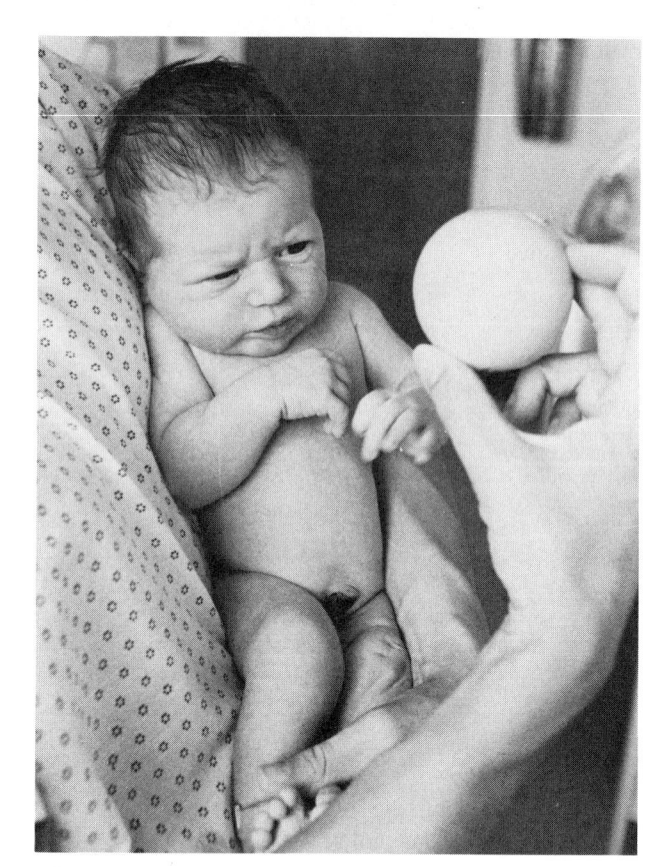

FIGURE 6-22. Visual orientation.

the neonate could not hear. The negative results apparently were due to the uninteresting stimuli that researchers were using and the neonate's high threshold for sound. Sounds reaching his ears are dampened by debris in the middle ear, which takes a day or so to be absorbed (see "Sensory System," in Sec. 1). Because of this, sounds must be presented at a high-intensity level in order to elicit a response.

Studies of auditory perception usually present the sound at intensity levels ranging from 60 to 90 dB, depending on the testing situation. This may seem unusually loud, but it is not when considered in relation to the noise level of the neonate's daily environment—sound levels of 70, 80, 90, and 100 dB have been recorded in the neonatal nursery (Northern and Downs, 1974). In utero, sounds of 72 dB have been recorded.

Auditory sensitivity Researchers have found that most neonates, even those with known central nervous system (CNS) abnormalities, can discriminate sound on the basis of frequency and intensity. And neonates a few hours old show a primitive auditory localization ability. Further, it has been reported that speechlike signals are remarkably effective in producing responses in neonates, and at 4 weeks of age beginning speech discrimination ability has been reported. Sensitivity to the consonant contrasts of ba/ga, pa/pi, and ta/ti as well as to the intonational contrast of ba+/ba− have been demonstrated. Reportedly the vowel sounds a/i and i/u are also discriminated (Haith and Campos, 1977).

Finding such ability in the very young infant has caused some theorists to speculate that the human organism has a biological predisposition for acquiring language, including a sort of built-in feature detector which is sensitive to the distinctive features of speech (Binzley, 1973).

OTHER SENSE PERCEPTIONS
Developmental studies of olfaction, taste, and temperature have been rather neglected despite the fact that the neonate has been found to be capable of perceptually discriminating among stimuli in each of these modalities. Hence, it is not known how a neonate's or young infant's response changes with variations in the dimension of stimuli employed.

Taste and smell The neonate probably is as sensitive to taste stimuli as he will ever be at any time in his life, although it is difficult to demonstrate this because of the practical difficulties encountered. The most important difficulty is that, in order to assess taste, the researcher must interfere with one of the vital activities of the neonate, his feeding routine.

One study using activity, breathing, and blood volume as dependent variables found quieting to sweet solutions (up to 5% sugar) and restlessness to sour (5% vinegar and 2% salt) solutions. Sucking rate was used to index a preference for sucrose over glucose (Haith and Campos, 1977).

Although taste and smell are usually considered together as the two chemoreceptors, smell might also be classed with vision and audition as it is a distance receptor. That is, the exciting stimulus, which is the volatile nature of some liquids and solids, is usually at a distance from the receptors. Because the neonate breathes through his nose from birth, the tiny filaments of his olfactory bulb are exposed to potential sources of stimulation. Infants only a few days old have been shown to respond differentially to asafetida, lavender, and valerian (Reese and Lipsitt, 1970). Also, some evidence was found that neonates can discriminate between aliphatic alcohols equated for subjective intensity and differing only in the length of the carbon chain.

Tactile and thermal sensitivity Although the skin is a growing organ and the specific receptors in the skin change their position as a result of growth, the neonate seems to know what part of his skin is being touched, and he will demonstrate this knowledge if the touch is irritating. For instance, the neonate can remove an irritant from his nose with his hand or get rid of an irritant on one leg with his other foot. Although these may seem minor accomplishments, as Bower (1977) points out, they actually imply an amazing amount of built-in organization.

The thermal regulator mechanism is not fully effective during the first day or so of life so that temperature changes in the environment do not elicit effective compensatory changes in the body. Therefore the neonate cannot maintain a constant internal temperature if the environmental temperature changes. This stability is reportedly reached by 1½ weeks of life (Reese and Lipsitt, 1970). Although it has been demonstrated that neonates respond both to warm and cold stimulation, they apparently have little ability to discriminate within the quality.

The neonate appears to have a number of built-in perceptual dispositions for responding to the significant aspects of its environment. However, the quality of these responses is for the most part reflexive and rather primitive. But rapid and rather dramatic changes occur in the infant's perceptual abilities as he develops motor control and starts actively exploring the environment.

Gross motor development Fay F. Russell and Beverly R. Richardson

On observation, the neonate evidently lacks gross motor skills. Essential to development and refinement of these skills is a maturing, intact neuromuscular system. The presence of such a system in the neonate is indicated by his muscle tone and motor behavior.

MUSCLE TONE
Muscle tone of a neonate is reflected by the firmness of his muscles and their resistance to pressure. Assessing range-of-joint movement is an easy, reliable means of assessing these factors. Two methods frequently utilized to assess range-of-joint movement and thus muscle tone are scarf sign and head rotation. For scarf sign, see Estimation of Gestational Age in "Maturation and Growth Deviation in the Neonate," in Sec. 1. In assessing degree of head rotation, the neonate's head is passively rotated. If he is 28 weeks' gestation conceptual age (ca) or less, his chin

will easily go well past the acromial tip. As his developmental age increases, the range-of-joint movement decreases until eventually his chin stops at the acromial tip as does a full-term neonate's.

While these indicators of range of joint movement are utilized most frequently, other tests, such as degree of head lag and the neonate's ability to touch his elbows behind his back, are also indicative of the firmness of his muscles and their resistance to pressure and thus his muscle tone overall.

GROSS MOTOR BEHAVIOR AT BIRTH

Gross motor activity of the neonate is essentially a continuation of his intrauterine activity and is controlled primarily by reflexes arising from the spine and midbrain. His movements are rapid, diffuse, nonproductive, and generalized, and most are either simple reflex actions or behavior prompted by reflex actions.

Several reflexes appear as early as the eighth to ninth week of gestation ca with several others appearing between that time and the date of birth. Major reflexes present at birth include the asymmetrical tonic-neck, Moro, neck-righting, traction, tonic labyrinthine, positive supporting, stepping, placing, trunk-incurvation (Galant's), plantar grasp, withdrawal, Babinski, crossed-extensor, and deep-tendon reflexes. Because these reflexes are responsible either directly or indirectly for the major portion of the neonate's motor activity and because their presence is indicative of the status of the neuromuscular complex, they are discussed in detail.

ASYMMETRICAL TONIC-NECK REFLEX

When placed in a supine position, the neonate may lie with his head turned to one side; the arm and leg on the side to which his face is turned are extended, and the arm and leg on the opposite side are flexed; both hands may be fisted (see Fig. 6-23). This asymmetrical tonic-neck reflex (ATNR) may be spontaneous or elicited by turning the neonate's head. The reflex is believed to appear between the twenty-fourth and twenty-eighth weeks of gestation ca and can be elicited for 12 to 18 weeks postnatally, although the infant may continue to assume this position while sleeping until he is 6 to 7 months old. The reflex is assumed to be abnormal if this posture is obligatory or asymmetrical (the neonate assumes this position when his head is turned to one side but not the other).

MORO REFLEX

The Moro reflex (which is often referred to as the *startle reflex*) is believed to be perhaps the most important neonatal reflex because of its correlation with gestational age and neurologic impairment. The reflex appears around the twenty-eighth week of gestation ca and can be elicited for 4 to 6 weeks postnatally.

Allowing the neonate's head to drop backward suddenly while his back is supported is the most reliable

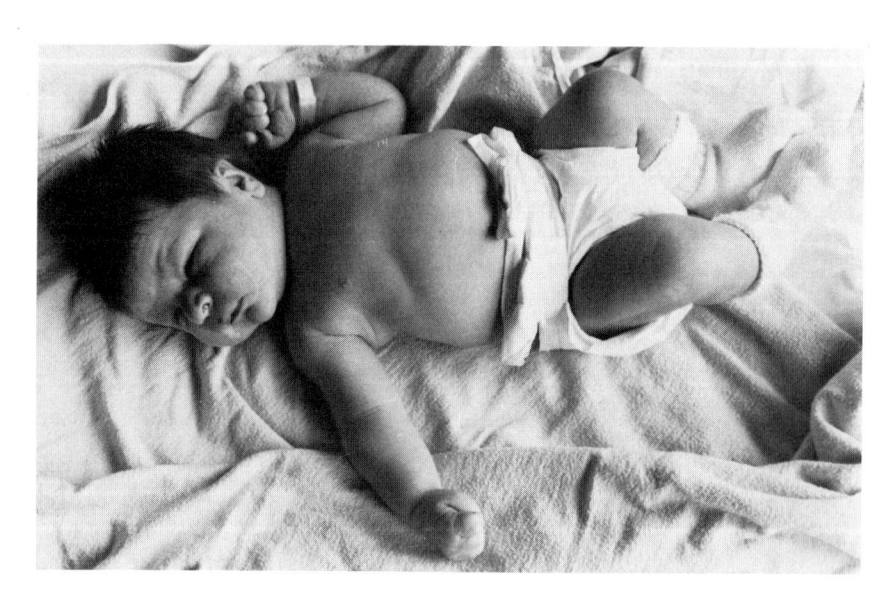

FIGURE 6-23. The asymmetrical tonic-neck reflex (ATNR) or "fencing position."

means of eliciting the Moro reflex. (The response is the result of the proprioceptive stimulus of stretching the neck muscles.) The neonate responds by abducting, extending, and supinating his arms and extending all digits except the thumb and forefinger, which remain in a C position; this is usually followed by a flexion and abduction of the arms, equal bilaterally, so that they appear to be in an embrace position and then a return to the resting position. There may be accompanying movements of the legs, but this response is less consistent than that of the arms and digits (see Fig. 6-24). Absence of this reflex has been associated with CNS depression, persistence associated with mental retardation and brain damage, and asymmetry with brachial palsy or fractured clavicle or humerus.

The true startle reflex may be elicited by a sudden noise or jarring of the surface on which the neonate is lying or by a sudden change in body posture such as in loss of support. The response of the neonate is predominately rapid flexion and does not have the initial extension pattern of the Moro. As the frequency of the Moro response decreases over time, the startle becomes increasingly predominant (Capute, Accardo, Vining, Rubenstein, and Harryman, 1978). However, it is often difficult to separate the two responses.

NECK-RIGHTING REFLEX

The primary neck-righting reflex usually appears between the thirty-fourth and thirty-sixth weeks of gestation ca and persists 9 to 10 months postnatally. It is a nonsegmental, hypertonic roll. As a measure of neurological maturation it is utilized in determining whether a low-birth-weight neonate is premature or SGA. The reflex is elicited by placing the neonate supine and flexing and turning his head to one side. The neonate responds by turning his shoulders, trunk, and pelvis in the same direction (see Fig. 6-25); this is commonly referred to as *logrolling* and will decrease as the neonate's capacity for trunk rotation increases. The neonate should respond approximately equally in either direction. The secondary or segmental (two-step) neck-righting reflex appears later in infancy.

TRACTION RESPONSE

The traction response, which appears between the thirty-second and thirty-sixth weeks of gestation ca, is elicited by placing the neonate supine and allowing him to reflexively grasp the examiner's fingers while the examiner lifts him. The response of the neonate, tonic in nature and believed to be evoked by the tonic labyrinthine righting reflex, consists of flexing his arms and pulling his trunk toward the erect position (see Fig. 6-26); his head lags depending on developmental age until 4 months of age, by which time he should be able to lift his head in line with his trunk. The grasp and arm flexion should be equal (with his head in midline).

Disappearance of the reflex can only be estimated as the response becomes voluntary when he is 4 to 6 months of

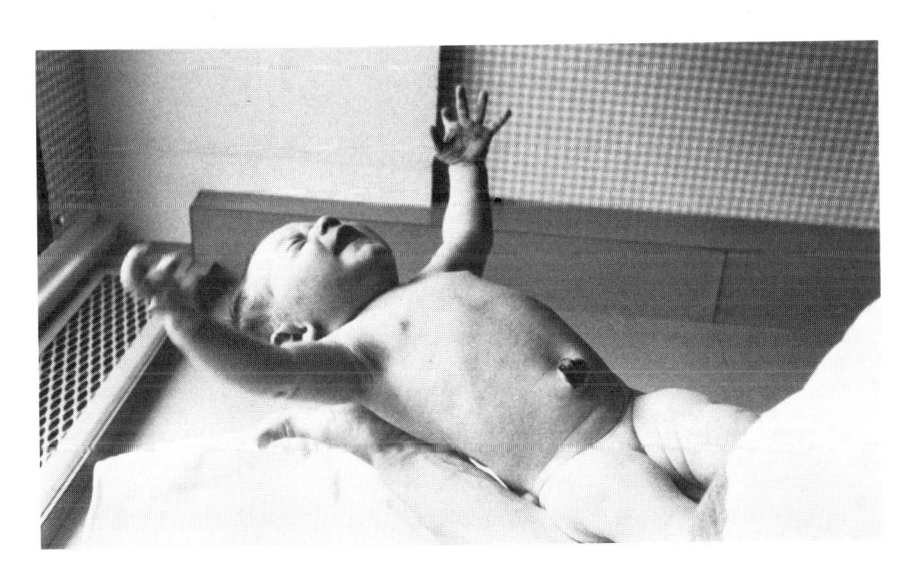

FIGURE 6-24. The Moro response.

340 THE NEONATE: BIRTH TO 1 MONTH

age. Absence of the response, marked head lag at 4 months of age, or increased tone resulting in extension of the legs are abnormal findings and may indicate CNS abnormality.

TONIC LABYRINTHINE REFLEX

When placed prone, the neonate assumes a flexion posture; when placed supine, however, the neonate assumes a posture in which the flexor tone decreases and extension increases (see Fig. 6-27). The tonic labyrinthine reflex is believed to be responsible for this behavior. While easily demonstrable in all neonates, it progressively becomes less pronounced until the infant is approximately 4 months of age, after which it is difficult to demonstrate. Persistence of this reflex and its effects on the infant's posture after he is 6 months old are associated with cerebral palsy.

POSITIVE SUPPORTING REACTION

Holding a neonate in an erect position and allowing the soles of his feet to touch a solid surface initiates the positive supporting reaction (see Fig. 6-28). The neonate's hips and legs extend and his ankles plantar flex or remain plantigrade so that he is able to support his weight with equal response bilaterally. There is a great deal of controversy over when the reflex emerges and when it disap-

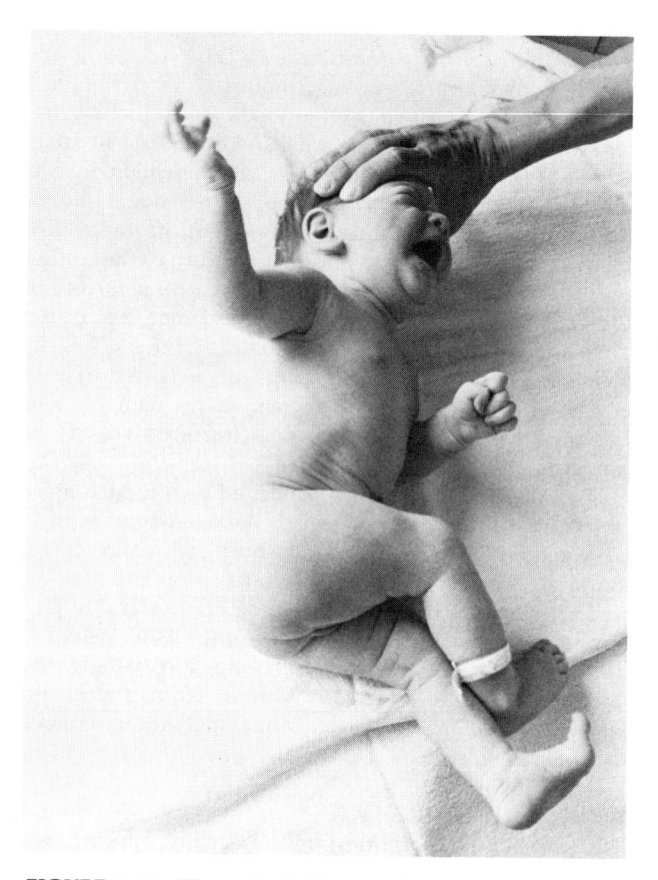

FIGURE 6-25. The neck-righting reaction.

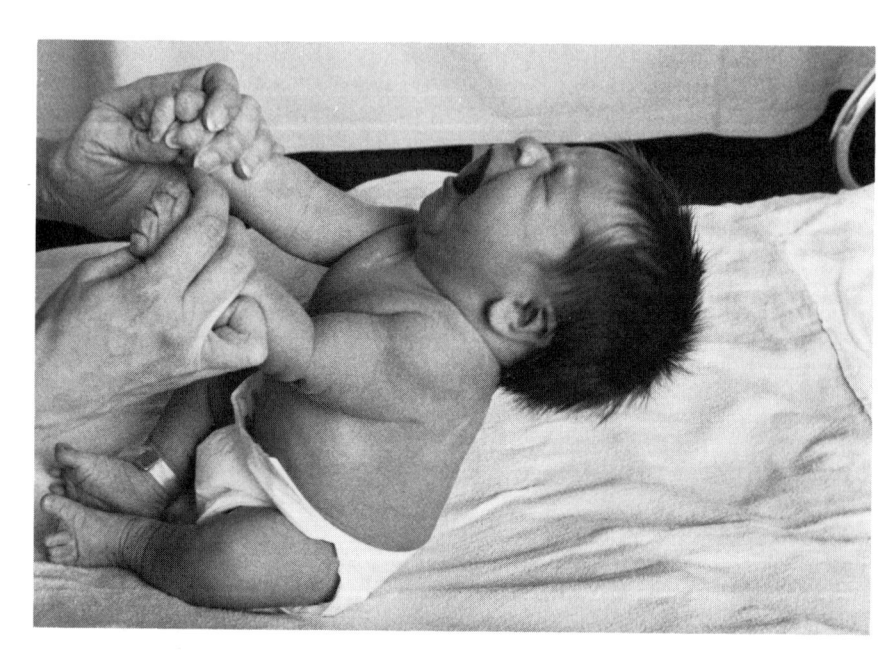

FIGURE 6-26. The traction response (pull to sit).

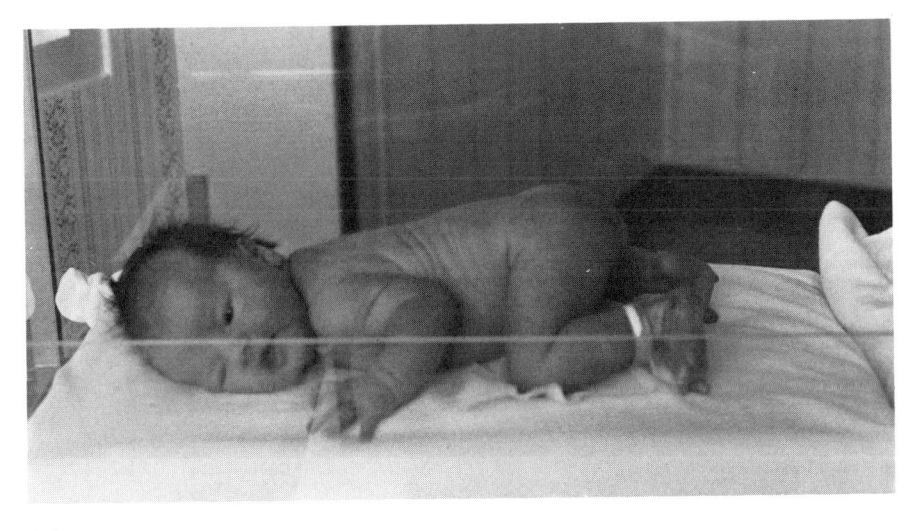

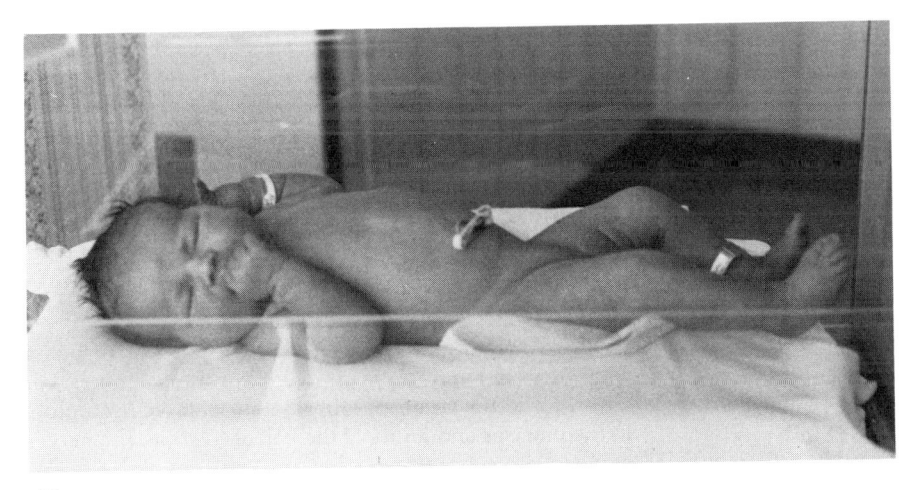

FIGURE 6-27. The tonic labyrinthine response: (a) prone; (b) supine. (Photos courtesy of Vincent Lanza.)

pears. It is generally believed that it emerges between the thirty-second and thirty-sixth weeks of gestation ca. Some authorities feel that it disappears 2 to 3 months postnatally, while others feel that it may last until voluntary standing occurs.

Because of conflicting opinion, more emphasis is placed on the quality of this reflex than on its presence or absence. For instance, the hips and knees of the neonate will often remain slightly flexed even under conditions described above because of increased flexor tone; consequently, complete extension of the hips and knees accompanied by marked plantar flexion suggests pyramidal or extrapyramidal motor dysfunction of the lower extremities, especially if it is present at 3 to 7 months of age. In addition, the legs of the neonate normally cross when he is suspended vertically because of increased adductor tone. However, persistence of this "scissoring" past 4 months of age is abnormal. It is believed that this reaction may be modified for use in standing by higher centers in the brain.

STEPPING REACTION

Holding the neonate in an erect position, moving him forward, and tilting him slightly to one side, so that one foot is pressed to the surface, causes him to make a stepping movement (leg flexion) on the other side; continuing the forward movement and alternating movement from side to side will prompt the neonate to exhibit a walking pattern (see Fig. 6-29). He "walks" rhythmically with a regular pace with his heel striking the surface on which he is walking first because of the increased dorsiflexion of his ankles. This reflex, the stepping reaction, begins to emerge at the thirty-fourth week of gestation ca and disappears by the third to fourth postnatal month. Although this reflex is often elicited, it appears to have limited value in assessing CNS maturity or abnormality at birth. However, abnormal findings, including early plantar flexion, persisting dorsiflexion, asymmetry, and persistence past 4 months of age indicate neuromotor dysfunction.

PLACING REACTION

Stimulating the dorsal side of a neonate's foot with light touch while holding him erect initiates the placing reaction (see Fig. 6-30). For example, positioning the neonate's foot against the edge of a table causes him to flex his leg at the knee and hip and appear to attempt to place his foot on top of the table. It is equal bilaterally. Motivation by a visual stimulus has been ruled out in this reaction. The reflex emerges around the thirty-sixth week of gestation ca and persists 10 to 12 months postnatally. Absence of the reflex is associated with spinal cord injury, and asymmetry is considered abnormal. Similar testing is conducted and similar response evoked with the hands.

TRUNK-INCURVATION (GALANT'S) REFLEX

The trunk-incurvation, or Galant's, reflex is elicited by holding the neonate prone, turning his head to one side, and stroking the skin in the lumboparavertebral area of the same side. The neonate responds by laterally flexing his trunk toward the side stimulated (see Fig. 6-31). When performed on the opposite side, the same response should be elicited. This reflex, which appears as early as the twenty-fourth week of gestation ca and persists 2 to 3 months postnatally, is often utilized to assess spinal integrity as its absence suggests a spinal cord lesion or general CNS depression.

PLANTAR GRASP REFLEX

When pressure is applied to the plantar surface of the sole of the neonate's foot with a finger, he plantar flexes all his toes: the plantar grasp reflex (see Fig. 6-32). This response continues as long as the pressure continues and is believed to be the result of stimulation of stretch receptors in the muscles and joints of the ball of the foot. It emerges between the sixteenth and twenty-fourth weeks of gestation ca and persists 8 to 12 months postnatally. The grasp should be equal bilaterally. Absence of this reflex may be indicative of spinal cord or nerve root damage or abnormality.

WITHDRAWAL REFLEX

The withdrawal reflex can be elicited by stimulating the sole of the neonate's foot as he lies in a supine position with his legs extended. He responds by flexing his hip, knee, and foot and by extending his toes. The response should be symmetrical bilaterally. The reflex may be weak or absent in a neonate whose presentation was breech with his legs extended. It is also absent when sciatic nerve damage exists.

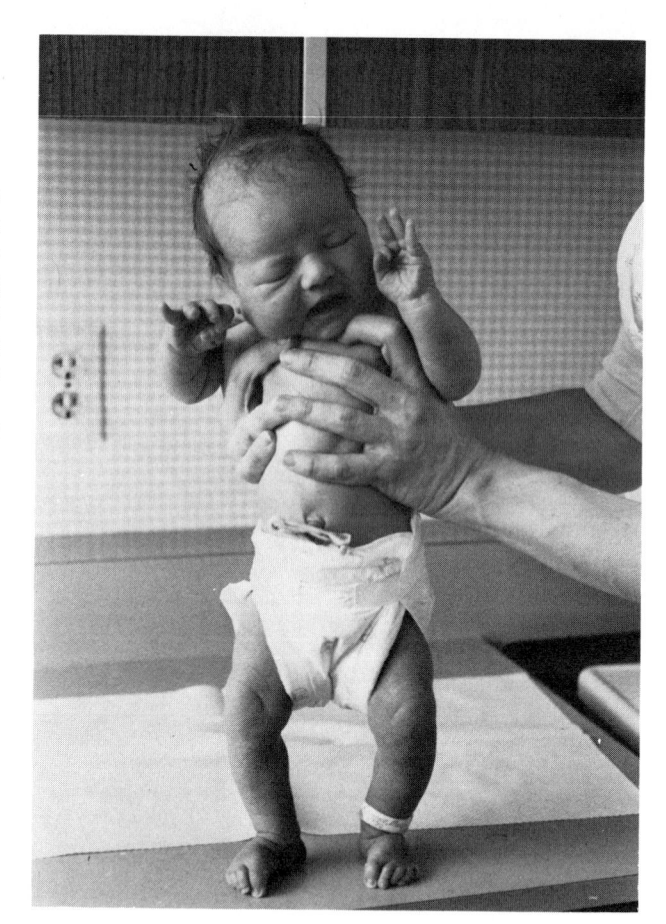

FIGURE 6-28. The positive-supporting reaction. (*Photo courtesy of Vincent Lanza.*)

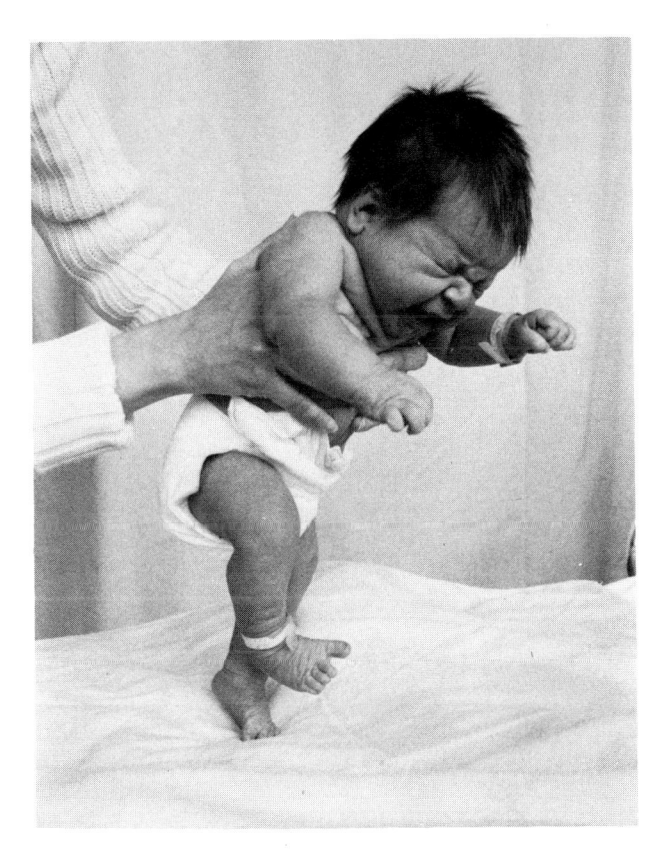

FIGURE 6-29. The stepping reflex.

FIGURE 6-30. The placing reflex. (*Photos courtesy of Vincent Lanza.*)

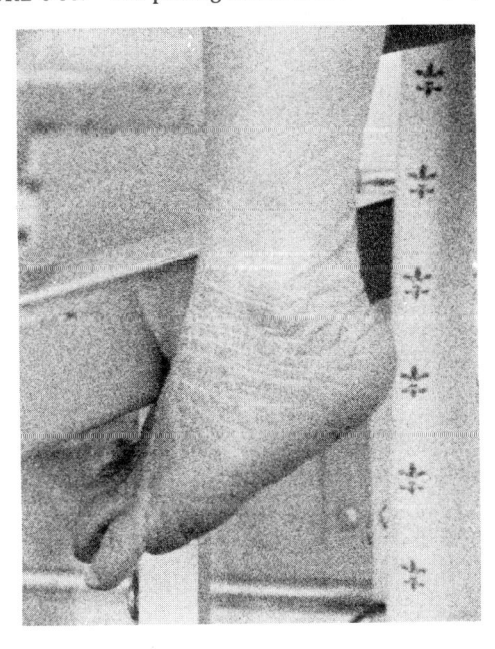

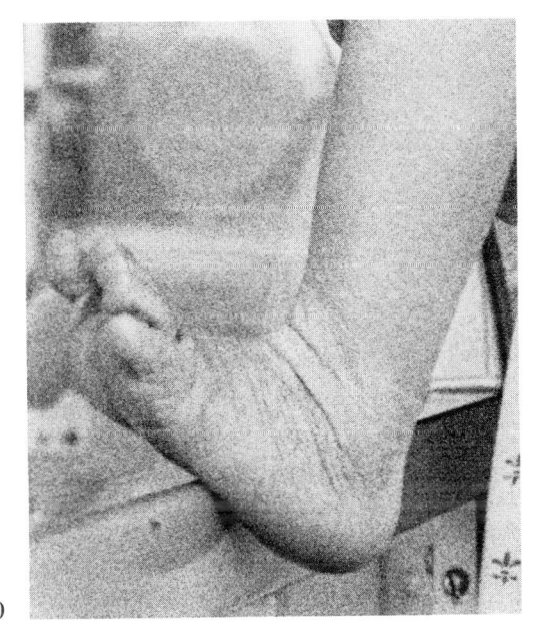

(a) (b)

BEHAVIORAL DEVELOPMENT 343

BABINSKI REFLEX

Stroking the lateral aspect of the sole of the neonate's foot in a heel-to-toes direction elicits the Babinski reflex (see Fig. 6-33). The response consists of dorsiflexing the great toe and fanning the other toes; he may also plantar flex one or more of the other toes, especially if too much pressure is applied. Again, the response should be equal bilaterally. This reflex emerges between the sixteenth and twenty-fourth weeks of gestation ca and persists in varying degrees for 12 to 18 months postnatally. This reflex has diagnostic value. Its presence or absence in the neonate reflects maturity or immaturity of the neuromuscular system; a strong positive response may indicate a pyramidal tract disorder; absence may suggest a lower spinal cord defect; persistence may be associated with spastic involvement of the lower extremities; and an asymmetrical response is often elicited with hemiplegia.

CROSSED-EXTENSOR REFLEX

The crossed-extensor reflex is elicited by placing the neonate supine, extending one leg, placing pressure on the knee of the extended leg, and stimulating the foot on that same side. The neonate will flex, extend, and abduct the contralateral leg and extend and fan his toes. The response should appear bilaterally equal. This reflex receives a great deal of attention because of the changes that occur with maturation.

Between the twenty-fourth and twenty-eighth weeks of gestation ca, a stimulus to the sole causes only a flexion withdrawal response, but by the thirty-second to thirty-sixth weeks of gestation ca, the flexion is followed by extension and often abduction. By term a stimulus evokes the mature response described above. The reflex disappears by the time the infant is 1 to 2 months of age. Absence of the reflex suggests a spinal cord defect at the level of the reflex arc or injury to peripheral nerves involved in the reflex; persistence may indicate a pyramidal tract lesion.

DEEP-TENDON REFLEXES

Finally, the group of reflexes known as the deep-tendon reflexes are present at birth. The biceps, triceps, brachioradialis, knee-jerk, and ankle-jerk reflexes are believed by many to be the most clinically significant reflexes of the group. Each of these reflexes is elicited by percussing a finger placed on an appropriate tendon or nearby structure, thereby resulting in stretching of muscle tissue. While degree of response (hyporeflexive or hyperreflexive) is significant, of particular importance is symmetry bilaterally. These reflexes are utilized to determine the nature of a motor disturbance—upper motor neuron or lower motor neuron—and to measure maturity of the nervous system. Significant findings include absence of the response, an exaggerated response, or an asymmetrical response. These reflexes persist throughout the life of the individual.

It should be remembered that the neuromuscular responses discussed above can most reliably be obtained after the second day of life and when the neonate is rested and comfortable. If hungry, tired, overstimulated, or otherwise uncomfortable, he also may respond differently; behavioral state influences response significantly.

SPONTANEOUS MOVEMENTS

The neonate does demonstrate gross motor behaviors which are not dominated by reflexes (see Figs. 6-34 and 6-35). For example, when placed prone, the neonate flexes his arms and legs as if attempting to creep, lifts his head slightly, and turns it from side to side. When crying, he slashes his arms and kicks his legs in addition to turning his head from side to side and arching his back. Recip-

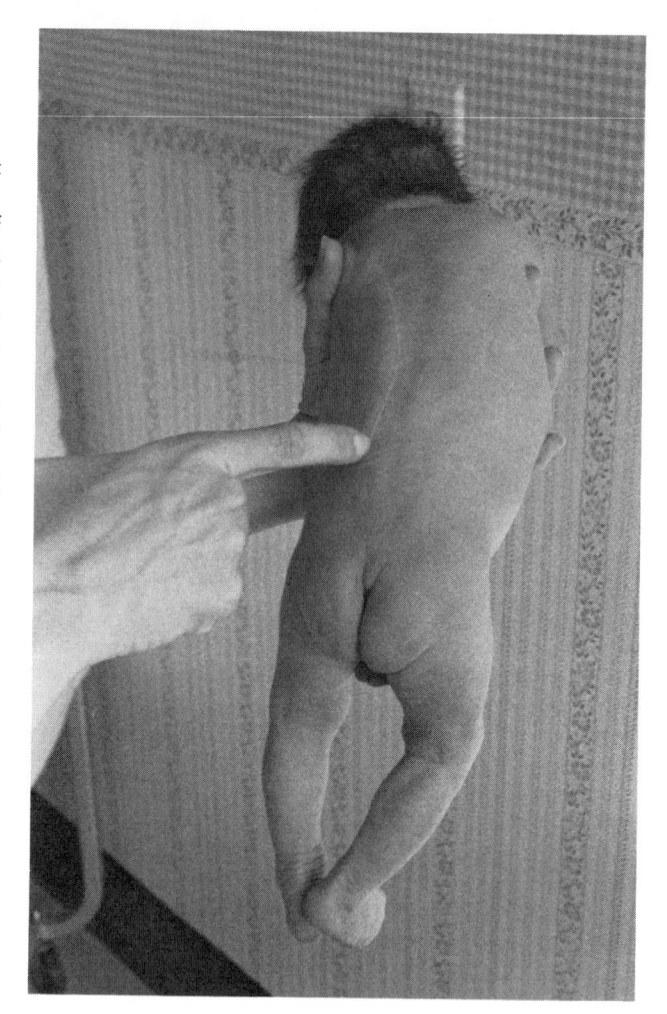

FIGURE 6-31. Galant's response (incurvation of the trunk).

rocal movement is detected at times, an obviously critical movement pattern.

When pulled to sit from supine, as noted in the discussion of the traction response, the neonate has little head control until he is more upright. As he is pulled to sitting, his head lags behind his trunk considerably. He is able to achieve some righting of his head as it comes to an upright position, and when it falls forward, he is able to lift it for a few seconds.

To comfort himself, he can turn his head and mouth his clenched fist. During the active-awake state, gross motor behavior generally interferes with full attentiveness. However, when arm and leg movements are at a minimum and the neonate is alert, he moves his head to track

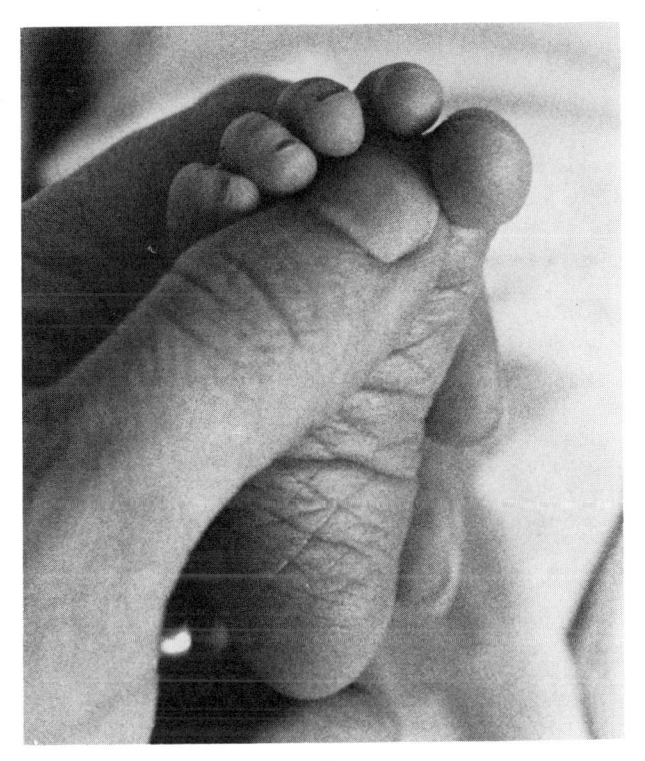

FIGURE 6-32. The plantar reflex.

an object. Thus, inhibiting gross motor movement is itself an important skill that the neonate must master.

GROSS MOTOR BEHAVIOR AT 4 WEEKS

At the end of the first month, the neonate continues to demonstrate all reflexes manifested at birth with the possible exception of the crossed-extensor reflex; no new reflexes have emerged by this time. He improves in his ability to lift his head while prone, the precursor and critical skill for further postural, gross motor skill development and beginning of the flexion-to-extension evolution.

By 1 month, further extension is seen as his knees are flexed under his abdomen only intermittently, and he is beginning to extend his hips. Although head lag is still considerable, it is not complete when he is pulled to a sitting position. When suspended in the prone position, his head is now raised slightly rather than hanging completely down, and his hips are partially extended.

Thus, though basic and limited, the neonate does demonstrate gross motor skill development as he begins to be less controlled by primitive reflexes and exhibits beginning extension. Acquisition of head control indicates cephalocaudal progression; utilization of abdominal muscles to pull to sitting position indicates ventrodorsal progression; and extension of arms and legs at the shoulders and hips, respectively, indicates proximodistal progression. While his motor behavior is still simple and random for the most part, he is showing early signs of acquiring purposeful behavior.

Fine motor development
Barbara Newcomer McLaughlin and Nancy L. Morgan

Fine motor development during the neonatal period involves a postural fixation and a coordination of eyes and hands. The asymmetrical tonic-neck reflex, discussed in "Gross Motor Development," allows for beginning prehensile ability. The neonate lies in this fencing position much of his waking hours, and this posture channels visual fixation on the extended hand. Gradually this leads to hand inspection, to active approach upon an object, and finally to manipulation of the object. The postural control of the head is an important feature of the asymmetrical tonic-neck reflex, and it is the basis for the development of prehension (White, 1975).

The primary fine motor characteristics of the neonatal period are a general flexion posture, generalized arm movements, hand-to-mouth movements, oral reflexes, the grasp reflex, and the predominantly closed position of the hands.

The neonate moves both arms equally, predominantly at the shoulder, resulting in gross whole-arm movements. Arm movement progresses from a more flexed posture with the hand close to the face to an extension position. The normal neonate has a grasp reflex that enables him to close his fist automatically around any object that touches his palm (see Fig. 6-36). This reflex is well developed and should be equal bilaterally. A neonate may be able to grasp an object strongly enough to be pulled to a standing position, as part of the traction response (also termed the *Darwinian reflex*). At this age, the hands clench on contact as the fisted hand fists more tightly when touched, though later it may open.

There is a great difference between the actual grasp reflex and prehensile ability, but the grasp reflex is very important to prehension as it involves use of the same musculature. The use of these muscles is preparatory to prehensile ability. The grasp may be elicited by placing

346 THE NEONATE: BIRTH TO 1 MONTH

an extended finger or rattle in the neonate's hand. The parent may interpret the neonate's grasp of an extended finger as a sign of affection, and the contact with the neonate is thus prolonged, a beneficial consequence.

Hand-to-mouth abilities are random and may elicit the oral reflexes. The rooting reflex occurs when the neonate is touched near his mouth—to either side, above, or below (see Fig. 6-37). The neonate will open his mouth and turn his head toward the stimulus; his movements are jerky initially, but in a few days he quickly orients. The asymmetrical tonic-neck reflex is not occurring with hand-to-mouth activity, thus making this behavior possible.

When the infant, by rooting, establishes oral contact with the object, breast or his own hand, he will reflexively suck. Sucking and swallowing, established prenatally, allow early hand-to-mouth behavior as well as initiate feeding and promote early fine motor development.

Cognitive development Virginia Pidgeon

The neonate, fixating on his parents with sober gaze from the depths of his bassinet, is an enigma. Is he the non-

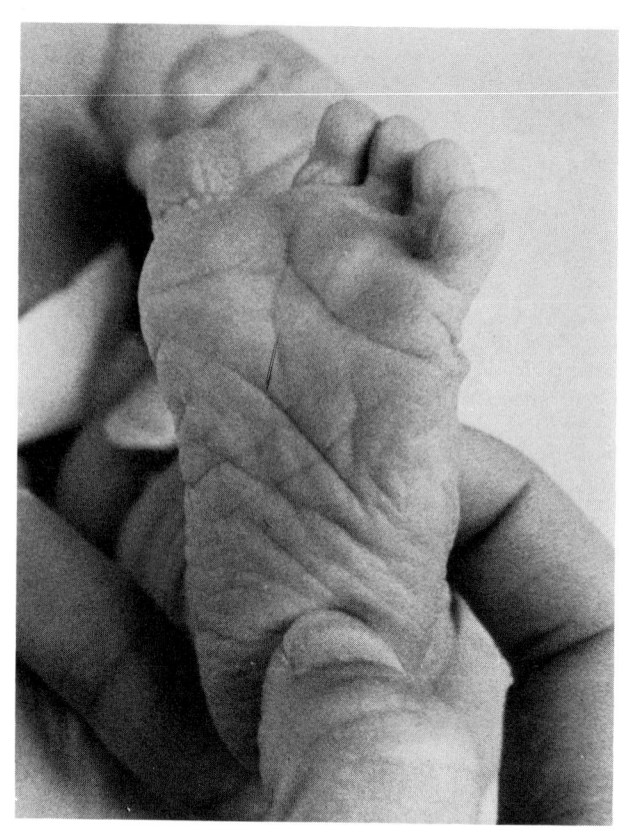

FIGURE 6-33. Babinski reflex.

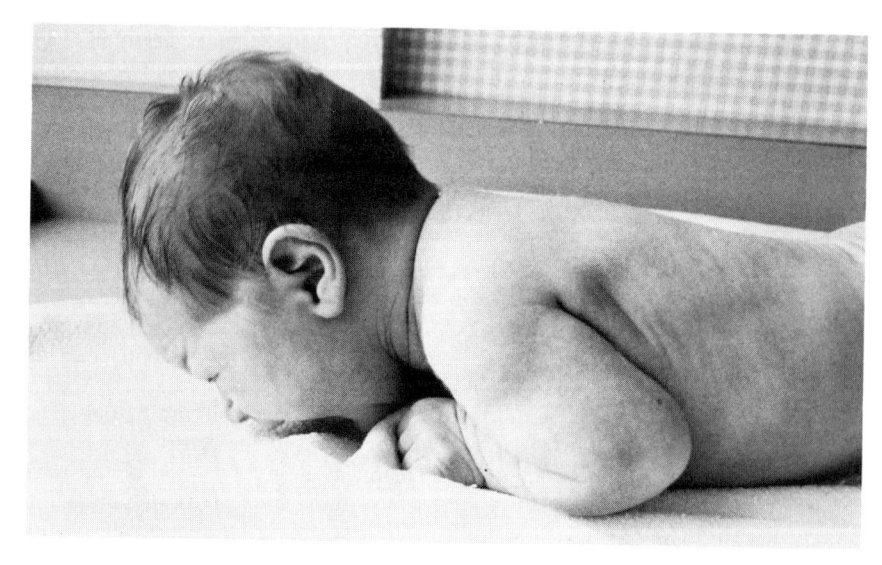

FIGURE 6-34. The neonate can raise his head slightly in the prone position.

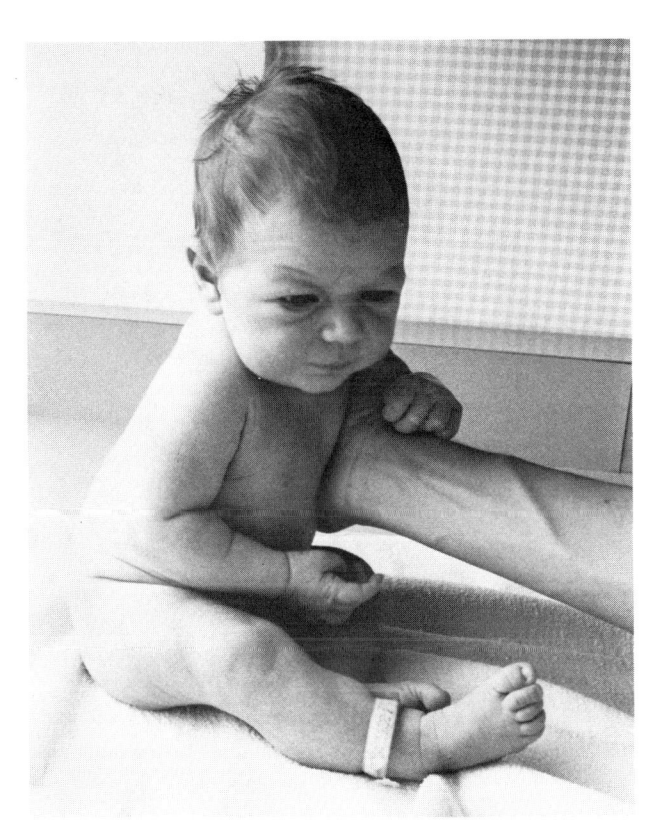

FIGURE 6-35. The neonate demonstrates some head control when held in the sitting position.

cerebrating creature of reflexes that has been described? Or does he ruminate philosophically over neonatal adjustments and life out of utero? Of the neonate Stone, Smith, and Murphy (1973) have this to say:

> Nowhere is the "new look" in infancy more evident than in our understanding of the human neonate, who until recently was considered to be a decerebrate creature, whose activities and experiences seemed both chaotic and unimportant, and whom so shrewd an observer as Piaget dismissed for a period of a month or more as involved merely in the exercise of reflexes. (p. 239)

To learn more of his cognitive status, we will review some of the research and Piaget's view of the neonate's cognitive development. Dimensions of neonatal cognitive development to be considered are attentiveness, responsiveness, learning, and schema development.

ATTENTIVENESS

The casual impression that the neonate slumbers his life away is misleading. Wolff (1965), in his 18-h vigils at the bedsides of neonates, identified seven different states of consciousness—regular, irregular, and periodic sleep; drowsiness; alert inactivity; waking activity; and crying. Among these states he singled out alert inactivity as that state in which the neonate is most accessible to external stimuli. In the state of alert inactivity he brightens in response to animate and inanimate stimuli, and his eyes take on a shiny appearance. His eyes fixate on a visual stimulus, and he follows it briefly with eye and head movements in the vertical and horizontal planes. Or he hears a sound and moves his eyes and head to discover its source. Alert inactivity is an attentive state in which the neonate can be intermittently interested in stimuli. It is almost the only state in which he responds to visual and auditory stimuli with tracking movements of the eyes. Wolff speculates that alert inactivity is a precursor of attention, or concentration. It is a state in which primitive cognitive activity seems to be taking place as the neonate, in brief respite from tension states, voluntarily takes in and responds to the world around him. As noted in "Perceptual Development," neonates are discriminating in their attentiveness to different kinds of visual stimuli.

Periods of alert inactivity regularly follow feeding and are longer than such periods at other times. Absence of hunger appears to be a precondition for alertness. Periods of alert inactivity and scanning behavior have been induced in crying neonates by picking them up and holding them over the shoulder (Korner and Grobstein, 1966).

Neonates differ in the frequency and length of periods of alert inactivity. The percentage of time spent in alert inactivity by neonates varied from 4 to 37 percent in a study by Brown (1964). The frequency and length of these periods is, according to Korner and Grobstein (1966), an index of the availability of the infant to external stimuli.

RESPONSIVENESS

Another dimension of early cognitive activity is the neonate's responsiveness to external stimuli. Neonates differ in the intensity of their response to external stimuli (Birns, 1965). Some neonates consistently respond vigorously to external stimuli, while others consistently display a moderate or mild response.

The responsiveness of the neonate is influenced by his internal state. Responsiveness varies in different states of consciousness and hunger, fatigue, and discomfort. In inactive states the neonate usually responds to a stimulus with an increase in activity, while in active states there is usually a decrease in activity (Wolff, 1965). Neonates differ in the degree to which they are subject to the influence of internal states, or are *state-bound*. Korner (1973) believes that state-boundedness is a constitutional variable arising from neurophysiologic, biochemical, and endocrine differences. Neonates who are very state-bound are less accessible to external stimuli.

LEARNING

It has been assumed that the neonate does not have the capacity to learn, but research today challenges that assumption. A simple form of learning is evident in the phenomena of habituation and recovery of response. As noted above, neonates have been observed to habituate to a repeated auditory stimulus by cessation of their initial startle reflex (Bridger, 1961) and to habituate also to repeated visual stimuli (Friedman, Carpenter, and Nagy, 1970). Neonates also differ in the extent to which they habituate.

Neonates who have habituated to a repeated stimulus will again recover responsiveness when exposed to a new stimulus. They also showed other qualitative changes in behavior on exposure to the new stimulus, such as active scanning, suppression of mouthing, and widening of their eyes.

The phenomena of habituation and recovery of response suggest a primitive form of learning in which the neonate learns not to respond to old and familiar stimuli and to respond when stimuli are novel. Many neonates, but not all, perceive and respond to novelty. Success in conditioning neonates is further evidence of rudimentary learning ability. Neonates learned to respond to an auditory stimulus with head turning or the rooting reflex when the auditory stimulus was presented in association with stimulation of the cheek (Papousek, 1967).

SCHEMA DEVELOPMENT

The neonate, according to Piaget, demonstrates little but reflex behavior in the first month of life. His behavior repertoire includes sucking, swallowing, crying, tongue movements, and mass body activity. The first 4 weeks of life are a cognitive hiatus in which there is no intelligent behavior. Essentially it is a practice period in which the neonate strengthens and consolidates his reflexes or schemata. He does so by assimilating an increasing number of objects to his schemata. He sucks on fingers as well as nipples and acquires a germinal sense of suckable nonnutritive and suckable nutritive objects. In addition, subtle and minor modifications of reflexes or accommodations to external reality occur. The neonate becomes more adept at localizing the nipple and distinguishing it from adjacent skin areas.

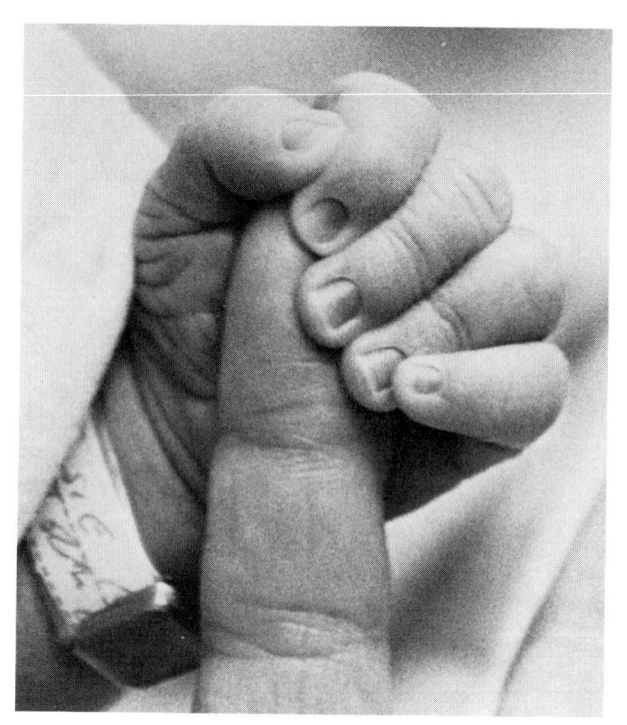

FIGURE 6-36. The grasp reflex results in the predominance of the fisted posture.

INFLUENCE OF THE CARE GIVER

The neonate is attentive at times to the human sounds and sights around him—the sound of the human voice and the sight of the human face hovering over him. In states of alert inactivity he is accessible and responsive to the rich variety of stimulation that can flow from a parent in interaction with the neonate. The variety inherent in human stimulation (changes in voice tone and in facial

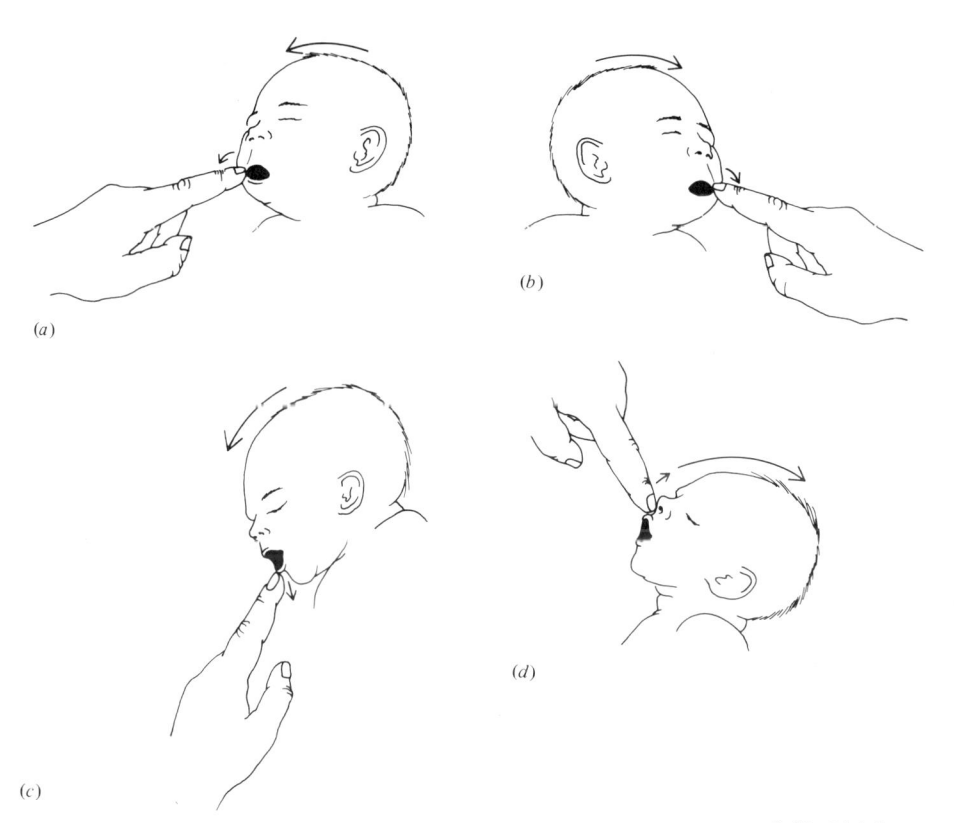

FIGURE 6-37. Rooting reflex of reaction of the four cardinal points. (a) and (b): Lightly stroking from the corner of the mouth toward the cheek results in the infant's head, mouth, and tongue turning toward the stimulus. (c) Stroking the lower lip toward the chin results in head flexion and downward movement of the tongue. (d) Stroking the upper lip toward the nose causes head extension and elevation of the tongue. These reactions are more easily elicited when the neonate is hungry. (Large arrows indicate movement of the neonate's head; small arrows indicate movement of the finger.) (*Adapted from Andre-Thomas, Y. Chesni, and S. Saint-Annne Dargassies, The neurological examination of the infant. London: Heinemann, 1960.*)

expression and simultaneous stimulation in several modalities) suggests that it is the method *par excellence* for capturing and prolonging the attention of the neonate. The efficacy of the shoulder position in inducing alert inactivity in crying infants suggests, along with other research, that stimulation by a parent can induce and prolong periods of attentiveness and influence early cognitive development.

The neonate, according to Piaget, is a creature of reflexes. The first 4 weeks of life are a practice period in which he strengthens and consolidates his reflexes. Recent research, in contrast, documents the attentiveness and responsiveness of the neonate and the presence of primitive forms of learning. It appears that parental stimulation can induce and prolong the attention of the neonate and enhance his responsiveness to stimuli.

Language development — Shirley Joan Lemmen

At birth, the neonate is a communicative being, and significant others begin to respond to him in a communicative way. Experts in infancy have alerted professionals to be aware of the neonate's own capacities to interact with the environment.

Even though the first month is predominantly governed by sleep and the repetitious activity of reflexive schemata of visual scanning, auditory scanning, sucking, and grasping, adaptations begin to be present because of the neonate's needs and environmental influences. The neonate is capable of responding to a modified stimulus. During the first month of life an observer can describe interpretable cues of the neonate in regard to orientation to auditory, visual, and tactile stimuli; as with cognitive development, development of language begins with perception.

Utilizing the neonatal assessment scale by Brazelton, one can observe the neonate's response to auditory stimuli. Brazelton uses two terms to describe a neonate's response to this sensory input: alerting and orientation. *Alerting* is defined as "brightening and widening of eyes" in contrast to *orientation*, which is defined as turning toward the direction of the stimulus (Brazelton, 1973). Each response is important in beginning communication.

Three other important aspects of behavior that facilitate interaction and reciprocity between neonate and parent are the neonate's consolableness, ability for self-quieting, and response to being held. The neonate's cries of discomfort are recognized as the earliest form of communication. Early sounds of comfort and vocalizations of pleasure are also communicative.

Three important aspects of such early signs of communication are discussed by Bloom (1978). The first is that early sounds and movements are the neonate's own; they are discovered by him as he moves, twists, and breathes. They are remarkably similar from one infant to another. Neonates do not learn these sounds and movements from the environment, they discover them on their own. The second aspect is that the sound and movements are part of the event being communicated. The third is that these behaviors in early infancy have their developmental counterpart later in more mature behaviors.

Neonatal communication behaviors are not forgotten or discarded; instead they gradually evolve into more complex forms of communication (Bloom, 1978). It is important for the parent to respond to these early vocalizations—to talk to the neonate, facilitating language acquisition and communication. As parents begin to attribute communicative function to differential cries or sounds that a neonate is emitting, they see the neonate beginning to communicate what he is experiencing.

Social development — Susan Blanch Meister

BASIS FOR SOCIALIZATION

Social development was discussed in Chap. 3 within the context of interaction. Applying the principles of interac-

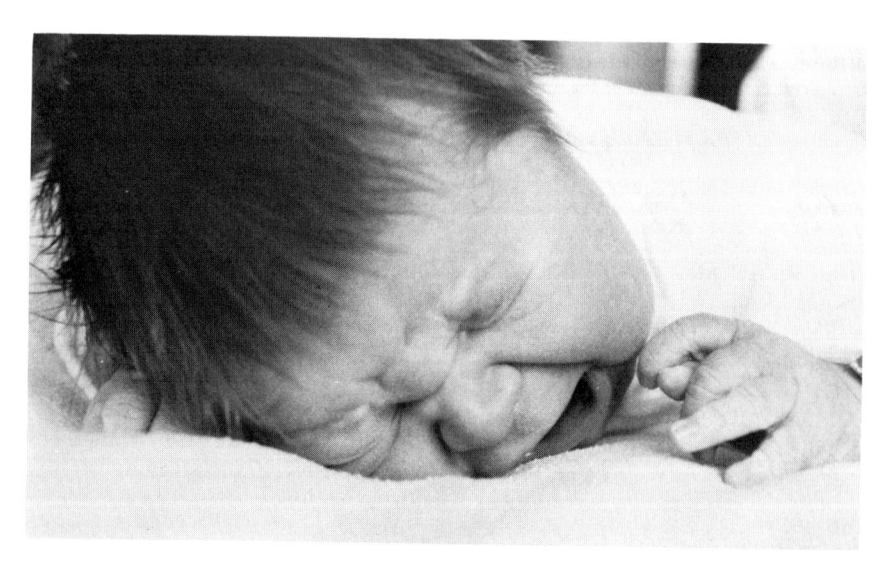

FIGURE 6-38.

tive experience to the neonate is difficult. The neonate requires an extended time period for cognitive processing, and yet his attention span is brief (Bayley, 1969). Neonates have, however, been observed in reciprocal behavioral interaction with their care givers (Brazelton, 1975). During face-to-face exchange, 3-week-olds demonstrated patterns of attention and response. It is known that neonates have social experiences and that they react to them. The actual impact of those experiences remains an uncertainty.

GOALS OF SOCIALIZATION

During this period of life, a great number of processes are initiated, and a great number are stabilized. Socialization processes fall into the category of initiation. The neonate's perception of social experiences is uncertain, but it is clear that those experiences occur and perhaps stand as a foundation for social development. The socializing agents provide a reliable, steady stream of social stimuli; the neonate's awareness of these stimuli and responses to them are areas for further study. It may well be that the neonate subordinates social learning in the service of survival and stabilization of physiology. However, the neonate may develop a sense of well-being within the context of ongoing, sensitive care giving.

PROCESSES INVOLVED IN SOCIALIZATION

ATTACHMENT

In Chap. 3, *attachment* was broadly defined as a process including an interactive relationship and powerful mechanisms of behavior. During the neonatal period, attachment is not achieved—rather, the foundation for that relationship is developed. One aspect of the foundation is care-giver sensitivity. Sensitive care-giver response will emerge as a crucial factor in attachment relationships (Ainsworth, 1972).

During this first month of life, the neonate is learning to use congenital signaling systems such as crying, sucking, and clinging. Each of these behaviors elicits adult protection and nurturance. Theorists propose that adults possess a bias to respond to infant cues, while infants possess a bias to respond to human stimuli. Neonate-parent contact results from this cue-giving and cue-responding exchange.

During the neonatal period, parents learn to recognize the infant's cues. The degree to which cues can be "read," the quality of the adult response, and the time frame are all factors related to parent sensitivity. They are also early factors in the development of attachment relationships (Ainsworth, 1972; Bowlby, 1969; Lamb, 1978).

GENDER IDENTITY

Although the neonate has not truly entered into the process of acquiring gender identity, the neonate's parents are certainly aware of the infant's gender. There are individual differences in responses to a boy or girl, but the impact of parental labeling of neonates has been emphasized (Mussen, 1969). *Parental labeling* is a term used for the parent's interpretation of the *meaning* of the infant's gender.

For example, in one study maternal care giving was much more likely to occur in response to an infant girl's cries than to a boy's (Moss and Robson, 1968). Considering the previous discussion of the importance of sensitive care giving, this gender-linked difference in response could be very significant. In this instance, the infant girls may have received more sensitive care.

Socialization processes during the neonatal period have been studied in a limited manner. It is likely that this period of social experience provides a foundation for future socialization. When theory and research are applied to individual neonates and parents, perspective must be employed. Future research may demonstrate particular variances in these processes or show how the processes are manifested. These variances may be bound to class, ethnic, or family-structure factors. Application of a normal standard must include provision for the broad range of normalcy.

Perception of behavioral competency and development of self-esteem
Judith Anne Ritchie

Awareness of the self as a separate entity is a necessary prerequisite to the child's developing a sense of a competent and worthy self. Important contributing factors to the delineation of the self and perception of self as competent and worthy are the child's motor, cognitive, and psychosocial development and the influence of others, particularly the parents, through the early years.

THE PARENT-CHILD BOND

There is general agreement that an effective parent-child relationship is of major importance in the development of a positive self-concept (Coppersmith, 1967; Erikson, 1963; Thomas, 1973). The foundation for the beginnings of self-awareness are laid during the prenatal and neonatal periods as the pregnant woman begins to "bind-in" to the child and to make significant others in the environment ready to accept the child (Thomas, 1973).

After the infant's birth, the process of binding-in continues and intensifies. According to Rubin (1977), the first aspect of the postpartal binding-in process is identification of the infant. Through the first weeks of life the mother comes to know her infant through every sensory modality—visual, tactile, olfactory, auditory, and even taste.

Rubin's theory of binding-in entails two further components of claiming and polarization. These activities establish the mother's perception of the neonate as an individual and competent being who exists as a separate person and who belongs to her and to her significant others. Such a process is essential if the mother is to be able to communicate to the child her own expectations that the infant is worthy and competent.

The reciprocal interactions of the neonate and parents during early hours and weeks of life extend the bond established through the maternal cognitive and tactile binding-in behaviors. Brazelton (1975) describes capacities of the neonate as contributing to the establishment of a cyclic reciprocity in parent-infant interactions within the first weeks of life. Brazelton suggests that it is this interaction which begins to structure the intrinsic motivation toward a "sense of competence" (White, 1959).

SYMBIOSIS

Except during the quiet-awake periods, when much of the behaviors described as facilitating the parent-infant bond occur, the neonate seems impervious to the external environment and is described as having an "autistic shell" (Mahler, 1975). Toward the end of the neonatal period, quiet-awake periods increase, and the autistic shell begins to "crack"—the period of symbiosis begins. Mahler describes this period as lasting through the first 6 months. The neonate is in a state of "undifferentiation, of fusion with the mother, in which the 'I' is not yet differentiated from the 'Not I' and in which inside and outside only gradually come to be sensed as in any way different" (1975, p. 44).

BEGINNING AWARENESS OF SELF

All the processes of binding-in and attachment provide the foundation for the neonate's expectations of parents and for the parents' expectations of the neonate. The child perceives touch, movement, position change, hunger, and pain and differentiates preferred visual patterns, smells, and direction of auditory stimuli. However, it is only gradually that the child learns which stimuli are internal or external in origin and that he exists as separate from the external sources of stimulation or satisfaction of needs. During the neonatal period, there is no perception of a separate self.

The neonatal period has been one of adjustment to extrauterine life and physiological stabilization. As he emerges from his sleep-eat cycles to increasing alert periods, the neonate begins to elaborate his role as change agent in the environment that surrounds him. The period of infancy, with major physical and behavioral progress, awaits.

Bibliography

PHYSICAL STATUS AND DEVELOPMENT
OF THE NEONATE

Avery, G. B.: *Neonatology: Pathophysiology and management of the newborn.* Philadelphia: Lippincott, 1975.

Fomon, S. J.: Body composition of the infant: The male "reference infant." In F. Falkner (Ed.), *Human development.* Philadelphia: Saunders, 1966.

Nellhaus, G.: Head circumference from birth to eighteen years. *Pediatrics,* 1968, *4,* 106.

Prechtl, H. F. R.: The behavioral states of a newborn (A review). *Brain Res.,* 1974, *76,* 185–212.

MATURATION AND GROWTH DEVIATION
IN THE NEONATE

Avery, G. B.: *Neonatology: Pathophysiology and management of the newborn.* Philadelphia: Lippincott, 1975.

Bard, H.: Intrauterine growth retardation. *Clin. Obstet. Gynec.,* 1970, *13,* 511–525.

Drillien, C. M.: The small-for-date infant: Etiology and prognosis. *Pediat. Clin. N. Amer.,* 1970, *17,* 9–24.

—— and M. B. Drummond: *Neurodevelopmental problems in early childhood.* Oxford: Blackwell Scientific, 1977.

Dubowitz, L. M., V. Dubowitz, and C. Goldberg: Clinical assessment of gestational age in the newborn infant. *J. Pediat.,* 1970, *77,* 1–10.

Fitzhardinge, P. M., and E. M. Stevens: The small-for-date infant: Part 2. *Pediatrics,* 1972, *50,* 50–57.

Klaus, M. H., and A. A. Fanaroff: *Care of the high risk infant.* Philadelphia: Saunders, 1973.

Korones, S. B.: *High risk infants; The basis for intensive nursing care.* St. Louis: Mosby, 1972.

Lubchenco, L. O.: Assessment of gestational age and development at birth. *Pediat. Clin. N. Amer.*, 1978, *17*, 125–145.

Miner, H.: Problems and prognosis for the small-for-gestational-age and the premature infant. *Amer. Maternal Child Nurs.*, 1978, *3*, 221–226.

Pape, K. E., R. J. Buncie, S. Ashby, and P. M. Fitzhardinge: The status at two years of low-birth weight infants born in 1974 with birth weights of less than 1,000 grams. *J. Pediatr.*, 1978, *82*(2), 253–260.

Toth, P.: Physical growth of children born small for gestational age. *Acta Paediat. Acad. Sci. Hung.*, 1978, *19*, 99–104.

SENSORY SYSTEM

Bordley, J. E., and W. G. Hardy: The special senses. In R. E. Cooke (Ed.), *The biologic basis of pediatric practice*. New York: McGraw-Hill, 1968.

Newell, F. W., and J. T. Ernest: *Ophthalmology, Principles and concepts* (3d ed.). St. Louis: Mosby, 1974.

Northern, J. L., and M. P. Down: *Hearing in children*. Baltimore: Williams & Wilkins, 1974.

Smith, J. L.: The eye in infancy and childhood. In R. E. Cooke (Ed.), *The biologic basis of pediatric practice*. New York: McGraw-Hill, 1968.

MUSCULOSKELETAL SYSTEM

Alexander, M. M., and M. S. Brown: *Pediatric physical diagnosis for nurses*. New York: McGraw-Hill, 1974.

Brown, M. S., and M. A. Murphy: *Ambulatory pediatrics for nurses*. New York: McGraw-Hill, 1975.

Malina, R. M.: Growth of muscle tissue and muscle mass. In F. Falkner and J. M. Tanner (Eds.), *Human growth 2, Postnatal growth*. New York: Plenum, 1978.

Popich, G., and D. W. Smith: Fontanels: Range of normal size. *J. Pediat.*, 1972, *80*(5), 749–752.

Rudolph, A. M. (Ed.): *Pediatrics* (16th ed.). New York: Appleton-Century-Crofts, 1977.

CARDIOVASCULAR SYSTEM

Nelson, N. M.: Respiration and circulation after birth. In C. A. Smith and N. M. Nelson (Eds.), *The physiology of the newborn infant* (4th ed.). Springfield, Illinois: Charles C Thomas, 1976.

RESPIRATORY SYSTEM

Auld, P. F.: Pulmonary physiology of the newborn infant. In E. M. Scarpelli (Ed.), *Pulmonary physiology of the fetus, newborn and child*. Philadelphia: Lea & Febiger, 1975.

Avery, G. B.: *Neonatology*. Philadelphia: Lippincott, 1975.

Avery, M. E., and B. D. Fletcher: *The lung and its disorders in the newborn infant*. Philadelphia: Saunders, 1974.

Brasel, J. A., and R. K. Gruen: Cellular growth: Brain, liver, muscle, and lung. In F. Falkner and J. M. Tanner (Eds.), *Human growth 2, Postnatal growth*. New York: Plenum, 1978.

Goss, R. L.: Adaptive mechanisms of growth control. In F. Falkner and J. M. Tanner (Eds.), *Human growth 1, Principles and prenatal growth*. New York: Plenum, 1978.

Guyton, A. C.: *Textbook of medical physiology* (5th ed.). Philadelphia: Saunders, 1976.

Kendig, E. L., and V. Chernick: *Disorders of the respiratory tract in children* (3d ed.). Philadelphia: Saunders, 1977.

Klaus, M. H., and A. Fanaroff: *Care of the high-risk neonate*. Philadelphia: Saunders, 1973.

Korones, S.: *High-risk newborn infant* (2d ed.). St. Louis: Mosby, 1976.

Marshall, W. A.: Puberty In F. Falkner and J. M. Tanner (Eds.), *Human growth 2, Postnatal growth*. New York: Plenum, 1978.

Murray, J. F.: *The normal lung*. Philadelphia: Saunders, 1976.

Nelson, N.: The onset of respiration. In G. B. Avery (Ed.), *Neonatalogy*. Philadelphia: Lippincott, 1975.

Pillitteri, A.: *Nursing care of the growing family*. Boston: Little, Brown, 1977.

Scarpelli, E. M. (Ed.): *Pulmonary physiology of the fetus, newborn and child*. Philadelphia: Lea & Febiger, 1975.

Strang, L. B.: *Neonatal respiration*. Oxford: Blackwell Scientific, 1977.

GASTROINTESTINAL SYSTEM

Agunod, M., N. Yamaguchi, R. Lopez, A. L. Luhby, and G. B. J. Glass: Correlative study of hydrochloric acid, pepsin, and intrinsic factor secretion in newborns and infants. *Amer. J. Dig. Dis.*, 1969, *14*, 400–414.

Ahn, C. I., and Y. J. Kim: Acidity and volume of gastric acid in the first week of life. *J. Korea Med. Ass.*, 1963, *6*, 948–950.

Ames, M. D.: Gastric acidity in the first ten days of life in the prematurely born baby. *Amer. J. Dis. Child.*, 1960, *100*, 252–256.

Crelin, E. S.: *Functional anatomy of the newborn*. New Haven, Connecticut: Yale, 1973.

Dancis, J., E. Grobow, and A. Boyer: The chloride concentration of saliva and sweat in infancy. *J. Pediat.*, 1957, *50*, 459–462.

Davidson, M.: Normal gastrointestinal function in children up to two years of age. In M. Sleisenger and J. Fortran (Eds.), *Gastrointestinal diseases*. Philadelphia: Saunders, 1973.

Ebers, D. W., D. I. Smith, and G. E. Gibbs: Gastric acidity on the first day of life. *Pediatrics*, 1956, *18*, 800–802.

Gothefors, L., B. Carlsson, J. Ahlstedt, L. A. Hanson, and J. Winberg: Influence of maternal gut flora and colostral and cord serum antibodies on presence of Escherichia coli in faeces of the newborn infant. *Acta Paediat. Scand.*, 1972, *65*, 225–232.

Gryboski, J. D.: Gastrointestinal function in the infant and young child. *Clin. Gastroenterol.*, 1977, *6*, 253–265.

——, W. R. Thayer, and H. M. Spiro: Esophageal motility in infants and children. *Pediatrics*, 1963, *31*, 382–395.

Lieberman, J.: Proteolytic activity in fetal pancreas and meconium. *Gastroenterology*, 1966, *50*, 183–190.

Polacek, M. A., and E. H. Ellison: Gastric acid secretion and parietal cell mass in the stomach of a newborn infant. *Amer. J. Surg.*, 1966, *3*, 777–781.

Rodbro, P., P. A. Krasilnikoff, and V. Bitsch: Gastric secretion of pepsin in early childhood. *Scand. J. Gastroenterol.*, 1967, *2*, 257–260.

Searcy, R. L., J. E. Berk, S. Hayashi, and B. D. Ackerman: Serum amylase activity in the newborn. *Pediatrics*, 1967, *39*, 294–296.

Timiras, P. S.: *Developmental physiology and aging*. New York: Macmillan, 1972.

Tyson, K. R. T.: Normal and abnormal physiology of the alimentary tract in infancy. *Amer. J. Surg.*, 1969, *117*, 876–880.

Walker, W. A.: Antigen absorption from the small intestine and gastrointestinal disease. *Pediat. Clin. N. Amer.*, 1975, *22*, 731–746.

——: Host defense mechanisms in the gastrointestinal tract. *Pediatrics*, 1976, *57*, 901–916.

ENDOCRINE SYSTEM

Korones, S. B.: *High-risk newborn infants, The basis for intensive nursing care*. St. Louis: Mosby, 1972.

Villee, D. B.: *Human endocrinology, A developmental approach*. Philadelphia: Saunders, 1975.

REPRODUCTIVE SYSTEM

Faiman, C., and J. S. D. Winter: Sex differences in gonadotropin concentrations in infancy. *Nature* (London), 1971, *232*, 130.

Kaplan, S. L., M. M. Grumbach, and T. H. Shepard: Gonadotropins in serum and pituitary of human fetuses and infants. *Pediat. Res.*, 1969, *3*, 512.

Root, A. W., G. P. Smith, A. P. S. Dhariwal, and S. M. McCann: Luteinizing hormone releasing activity of crude ovine hypothalamic extract in man. *Nature* (London), 1969, *221*, 570.

URINARY SYSTEM

Arturson, G. T., T. Groth, and G. Grottee: Human glomerular membrane porosity and filtration pressure: Pextan clearance data analyzed by theoretical models. *Clin. Sci.*, 1971, *40*, 137–158.

Edelmann, C. M., Jr., H. R. Barnett, and V. Troupkou: Renal concentrating mechanisms in newborn infants. Effects of dietary protein and water content, role of urea, and responsiveness to anti-diuretic hormone. *J. Clin. Invest.*, 1960, *39*, 1062–1079.

Guignard, J. P., A. Torrado, O. DaCunha, and E. Gautier: Glomerular filtration rate in the first three weeks of life. *J. Pediatr.*, 1975, *87*(2), 268–272.

Heller, H.: The renal function of newborn infants and animals. *Arch. Dis. Child.*, 1951, *26*, 195.

McCrory, W. W.: Renal excretion of inorganic phosphate in newborn infants. *J. Clin. Invest.*, 1952, *31*, 357.

Mott, J. C.: The place of the renin-angiotensin system before and after birth. *Brit. Med. Bull.*, 1975, *31*(1), 44.

Pitts, R. F., J. L. Ayer, and W. A. Schiess: The renal regulation of acid-base balance in man. III The reabsorption and excretion of bicarbonate. *J. Clin. Invest.*, 1949, *28*, 35–44.

Robillard, J. E.: Renal response of premature infants to administration of bicarbonate and potassium. *Pediatrics*, 1954, *13*, 4.

Tudvad, F. H., H. McNamara, and H. L. Barnett: Renal response of premature infants to administration of bicarbonate and potassium. *Pediatrics*, 1954, *13*, 4–16.

DEVELOPMENT OF BODY CONCEPT AND CONCEPTS OF ILLNESS AND WELLNESS

Benfeld, S.: *The psychology of infants* (R. Hurwitz, trans.). New York: Brentano's, 1929.

Bridger, W. H.: Sensory habituation and discrimination in the human neonate. In L. J. Stone, H. Smith, and L. B. Murphy (Eds.), *The competent infant*. New York: Basic Books, 1973.

Freytag, F.: *Hypnosis and the body image*. New York: Judian, 1961.

Greenacre, P.: Early determinants in the development of the sense of identity. *J. Amer. Psychoanal. Ass.*, 1958, *6*, 612–627.

Klaus, M. H., and Kennell, J. H.: *Maternal-infant bonding*. St. Louis: Mosby, 1976.

Kolb, L. C.: Disturbances of the body image. In S. Arienti (Ed.), *American handbook of psychiatry* (Vol. IV, 2d ed.). New York: Basic Books, 1975.

Langworthy, O. R.: Development of behavior patterns and myelinization of the nervous system in the human fetus and infant. Cited in L. C. Kolb, Disturbances of the body image. In S. Arieti (Ed.), *American handbook of psychiatry* (Vol. IV, 2d ed.). New York: Basic Books, 1975.

Oremland, E. K., and Oremland, J. D.: *The effects of hospitalization on children.* Springfield, Ill.: Charles C Thomas, 1973.

Poznanski, E. O.: Children's reactions to pain: A psychiatrist's perspective. *Clin. Pediatr.*, 1976, 15, 1114–1119.

Rich, E. O., R. E. Marshall, and J. J. Valpe: The normal neonatal response to pin-prick. *Develop. Med. Child Neurol.*, 1974, 16, 432–434.

Schilder, P.: *Contributions to developmental neuropsychiatry*, (L. Bender, Ed.). New York: International Universities Press, 1964.

Swafford, L. I., and D. Allan: Pain relief in the pediatric patient. *Med. Clin. N. Amer.*, 1968, 52, 131–136.

Wolff, P. H.: The Classification of States. In L. J. Stone, H. Smith, and L. B. Murphy (Eds.), *The competent infant.* New York: Basic Books, 1973a.

———: State and neonatal activity. In L. J. Stone, H. Smith, and L. B. Murphy (Eds.), *The competent infant.* New York: Basic Books, 1973b.

THE NEONATE: AWAKENING

Brazelton, T. B.: Neonatal behavioral assessment scale. *Clinics in Developmental Medicine* (No. 50). London: Heinemann, 1973.

Capute, A. J., et al.: *Primitive reflex profile.* Baltimore: University Park Press, 1978.

Lewis, M., and L. A. Rosenblum (Eds.): *The effect of the infant on its caregiver.* New York: Wiley, 1974.

Prechtl, H.: The behavioral states of the newborn infant (A review). *Brain Res.*, 1974, 76, 185–212.

———: The neurological exam of the full-term newborn infant (2d ed.). *Clinics in Developmental medicine* (No. 63). London: Heinemann, 1977.

Wolff, P. H.: State and neonatal activity. *Psychosom. Med.*, 1959, 21, 110–118.

———: The causes, controls, and organization of behavior in the neonate. *Psychological Issues*, 1966, 5(1), 7–11. (Monograph 17)

SLEEP

Dement, W.: *Some must watch while some must sleep.* San Francisco: San Francisco Book, 1976.

Dittrichova, J., K. Paul, and J. Vondracek: Individual differences in infants' sleep. *Develop. Med. Child Neurol.*, 1976, 18, 182–188.

Emde, R., and R. J. Harmon: Endogenous and exogenous smiling systems in early infancy. *J. Amer. Acad. Child Psychiat.*, 1972, 11, 177–200.

Hartmann, E. L.: *The functions of sleep.* New York: Yale University Press, 1973.

Jouvet, M.: Neurophysiology of the states of sleep. *Physiol. Rev.*, 1967, 47, 117–177.

Kleitman, N.: *Sleep and wakefulness* (rev. ed.). Chicago: University of Chicago Press, 1963.

Parmalee, A. H., H. R. Schulz, and M. A. Disbrow: Sleep patterns of the newborn. *J. Pediat.*, 1961, 58, 241–250.

——— and E. Stern: Development of states in infants. In C. Clemente, D. Purpura, and F. Mayer, (Eds.), *Sleep and the maturing nervous system.* New York: Academic, 1972.

———, W. Wenner, and H. Schulz: Infant sleep patterns: From birth to sixteen weeks. *J. Pediat.*, 1964, 54(4), 576–582.

Williams, R. L., I. Karacan, and C. Hursch: *Electroencephalography (EEG) of human sleep: Clinical applications.* New York: Wiley, 1974.

PERCEPTUAL DEVELOPMENT

Binzley, V.: An exploratory study of the orienting response of the newborn and the young infant to synthetic speech sounds. (Unpublished Ph.D. thesis, Case Western Reserve University, 1973.)

Bower, T. G. R.: *The perceptual world of the child.* Cambridge: Harvard University Press, 1977.

Dayton, G. O., Jr., M. H. Jones, P. Aiu, R. H. Rawson, B. Steele, and M. Rose: Developmental study of coordinated eye movements in the human infant I: Visual acuity in the new born human: A study based on induced optokinetic nystagmus recorded by electrooculography. *Arch. Ophthal.*, 1964, 71, 865–870.

Gibson, E. J.: *Principles of perceptual learning and development.* New York: Appleton-Century-Crofts, 1969.

Haith, M. M., and J. J. Campos: Human infancy. *Ann. Rev. Psychol.*, 1977, 28, 251–293.

Kessen, W., M. M. Haith, and P. H. Salapatek: Human infancy: A bibliography and guide. In P. H. Mussen (Ed.), *Carmichael's manual of child psychology* (Vol. I). New York: Wiley, 1970.

MacFarlane, A.: What a baby knows. *Hum. Nat.*, 1978, 1, 74–82.

Northern, J. L., and M. P. Downs: *Hearing in children.* Baltimore: Williams & Wilkins, 1974.

Reese, H. W., and L. P. Lipsitt: *Experimental child psychology.* New York: Academic, 1970.

Tanner, J. M.: Physical growth. In P. H. Mussen (Ed.), *Carmichael's manual of child psychology* (Vol. I). New York: Wiley, 1970.

Trehub, S. E., and M. Rabinovitch: Audio linguistic sensitivity in early infancy. *Develop. Psychol.,* 1972, *1,* 74–77.

GROSS MOTOR DEVELOPMENT

Capute, A. J., P. J. Accardo, E. Vining, J. E. Rubenstein, and S. Harryman: *Primitive reflex profile.* Baltimore: University Park Press, 1978.

Egan, D. F., R. S. Illingsworth, and R. C. MacKeith: *Developmental screening 0–5 Years.* London: Spastics International, 1969.

Fiorentino, M. R.: *Normal and abnormal development.* Springfield, Ill.: Charles C Thomas, 1972.

———: *Reflex testing methods for evaluating C.N.S. development.* Springfield, Ill.: Charles C Thomas, 1973.

Gordon, N.: *Paediatric neurology for the clinician.* London: Spastics International, 1976.

Hellmuth, J. (ed.): *Exceptional infant* (Vol. 1). New York: Brunner/Mazel, 1967.

Illingworth, R. S.: *The development of the infant and young child.* New York: Churchill Livingstone, 1975.

Prechtl, H.: *The neurological examination of the full-term newborn infant.* London: Spastics International, 1977.

Sheridan, M. D.: *Children's developmental progress.* London: NFER, 1973.

Touwen, B.: *Neurological development in infancy.* London: Spastics International, 1976.

FINE MOTOR DEVELOPMENT

Gesell, A., H. M. Halverson, H. Thompson, F. L. Ilg, B. Castner, L. B. Ames, and C. S. Amatruda: *The first five years of life.* New York: Harper & Brothers, 1940.

Knobloch, H., and B. Pasamanick: *Gesell and Amatruda's developmental diagnosis.* New York: Harper & Row, 1974.

White, B. L.: *The first three years of life.* Englewood Cliffs, N.J.: Prentice-Hall, 1975.

COGNITIVE DEVELOPMENT

Birns, B.: Individual differences in human neonates. *Child Develop.* 1965, *36,* 249–256.

Bridger, W.: Sensory habituation and discrimination in the human neonate. *Amer. J. Psychiat.,* 1961, *117,* 991–996.

Brown, J.: States in newborn infants. *Merrill-Palmer Quart.,* 1964, *10,* 313–327.

Fantz, R.: Pattern vision in newborn infants. *Science,* 1963, *140,* 296–297.

Flavell, J.: *The developmental psychology of Jean Piaget.* New York: Van Nostrand, 1963.

Friedman, S., G. Carpenter, and A. Nagy: Decrement and recovery of response to visual stimuli in the newborn human. *Proceedings, 78th Annual Convention, American Psychological Association,* 1970, *5,* 273–274.

Hershenson, M., H. Musinger, and W. Kessen: Preference for shapes of intermediate variability in the newborn infant. *Science,* 1965, *147,* 630–631.

Korner, A.: Some hypotheses regarding the significance of individual differences at birth for later development. In L. J. Stone, H. Smith, and L. Murphy (Eds.), *The competent infant.* New York: Basic Books, 1973.

——— and R. Grobstein: Visual alertness as related to soothing in neonates: Implications for maternal stimulation and early deprivation. *Child Develop.,* 1966, *37,* 867–876.

Papousek, H.: Conditioning during early postnatal development. In Y. Brackbill and G. G. Thompson (Eds.), *Behavior in infancy and childhood.* New York: Free Press, 1967.

Stone, L. J., H. T. Smith, and L. B. Murphy (Eds.): *The competent infant.* New York: Basic Books, 1973.

Wolff, P.: The development of attention in young infants. *Ann. New York Acad. Sci.,* 1965, *118,* 815–830.

LANGUAGE DEVELOPMENT

Bloom, L., and M. Lahey: *Language development and language disorders.* New York: Wiley, 1978.

Brazelton, T.: *The neonatal behavioral assessment scale.* Philadelphia: Lippincott, 1973.

Erickson, M. L.: *Assessment and management of developmental changes in children.* St. Louis: Mosby, 1976.

Louis, M., and L. A. Rosenblom: *The effect of the infant on its caregiver.* New York: Wiley, 1974.

SOCIAL DEVELOPMENT

Ainsworth, M. D.: Individual differences in the development of some attachment behaviors. *Merrill-Palmar Quart.,* 1972, *18,* 123–143.

Bayley, N.: *Bayley scales of infant development.* New York: Psychological Corporation, 1969.

Bowlby, J.: *Attachment and loss.* New York: Basic Books, 1969.

Brazelton, T. B.: Early mother-infant reciprocity. *Parent-*

Infant Interaction, Ciba Foundation Symposium 33. New York: Associate Scientific Publishers, 1975.

Lamb, M. (Ed.): *Social and personality development.* New York: Holt, 1978.

Moss, H. A., and K. S. Robson: Maternal influence on early social visual behavior. *Child Develop.,* 1968, *39,* 401–408.

Mussen, P. H.: Sex-typing and acquisition of sex-role identity. In D. A. Goslin (Ed.), *Handbook of socialization theory and research.* Chicago: Rand McNally, 1969.

PERCEPTION OF BEHAVIORAL COMPETENCY AND DEVELOPMENT OF SELF-ESTEEM

Brazelton, T. B.: Early parent-infant reciprocity. In V. C. Vaughn and T. B. Brazelton (Eds.), *The family—Can it be saved?* Chicago: Year Book, 1975.

Coppersmith, S.: *The antecedents of self-esteem.* San Francisco: Freeman, 1967.

Erikson, E. H.: *Childhood and society* (2d ed.). New York: Norton, 1963.

Klaus, M. H., and J. H. Kennell: Parent-to-infant attachment. In V. C. Vaughn and T. B. Brazelton (Eds.), *The family—Can it be saved?* Chicago: Year Book, 1975.

———, and ———: *Maternal-infant bonding.* St. Louis: Mosby, 1976.

Mahler, M. S., F. Pine, and A. Bergman: *The psychological birth of the human infant.* New York: Basic Books, 1975.

Rubin, R.: Maternal tasks in pregnancy. *Maternal-Child Nurs. J.,* 1975, *4,* 143–153.

———: Binding-in in the postpartum period. *Maternal-Child Nurs. J.,* 1977, *6,* 67–75.

Thomas, J. B.: *Self-concept in psychology and education.* Great Britain: NFER, 1973.

White, R. W.: Motivation reconsidered: The concept of competence. *Psychol. Rev.,* 1959, *66,* 297–333.

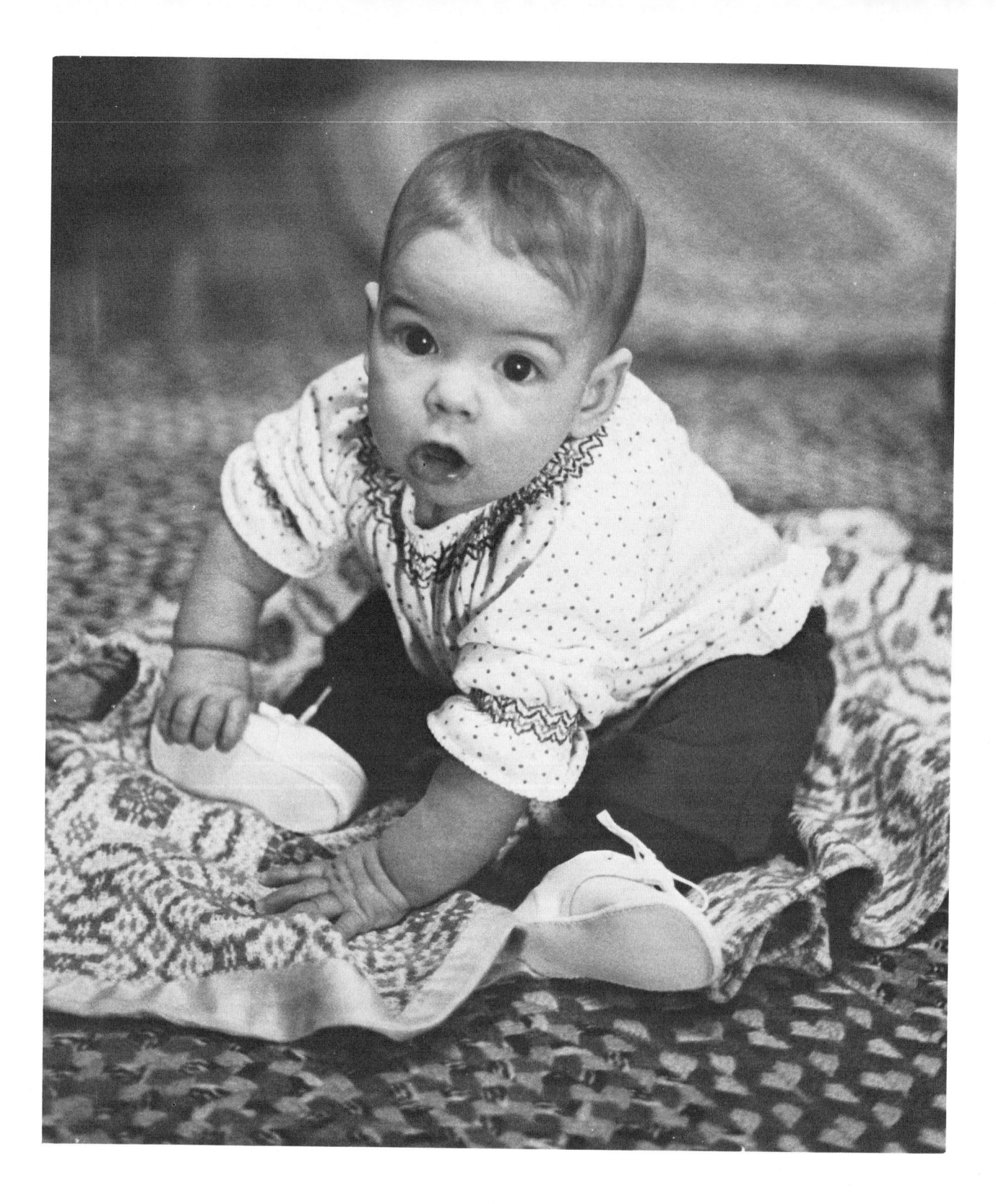

CHAPTER 7
The Infant: 1 Month to 12 Months

Introduction

The infant is the changeling of the years of childhood; the 1-year-old barely resembles the tiny infant of 1 month. The developmental strides made between 1 and 12 months will never be equaled in later life.

Growth during infancy, although slower than prenatally, is tremendous, and by 1 year the infant has doubled in length and tripled in weight. The infant will begin to find his genetically determined growth channel before the first year is over. Physiological stability is no problem for the infant; all body systems are functional and appropriate for age and size.

Despite the neonate's large head relative to body size, he soon lifts it to look about, thus initiating the progression to upright stature. The infant discovers objects in his world, both animate and inanimate, and his knowledge about them increases daily through exploration.

No one is more important to the infant in daily interaction than his parents. He comes to know them, demand them, and communicate with them.

The period of infancy inspires awe and respect for the measure of development achieved.

FIGURE 7-1. *(Photo courtesy of Cynthia St. Clair Taylor.)*

SECTION 1
Physical Development

Physical development of the infant
Marilyn A. Chard and Martha Underwood Barnard

DEVELOPMENTAL APPROACH TO PHYSICAL ASSESSMENT

Approaches to physical assessment of the infant must be based on the developmental changes which the infant is experiencing. There are as many different approaches for the first year of life as there are for 1- to 16-year-olds. The important thing to remember is that because there is such a wide variety of developmental tasks accomplished during infancy, the systematic approach is not governed by the specific age in months but, rather, by the stage of development and present behavior. For example, evaluation of the heart, of respirations, of the abdomen, and of the anterior fontanel should take place while the infant is quiet. Thus, the most propitious time for examination may be while the infant is sleeping in his parent's arms or nursing. The remainder of the examination can take place during times when the infant might be crying.

Another example concerns the infant who is between 6 and 10 months of age. During these months, the infant may exhibit fear of strangers. He may even resist direct eye contact. In order to accustom the infant to the nurse's presence, several techniques can be utilized. Giving him instruments or toys to play with before the actual examination takes place is important. The nurse can sit on the floor or away from the infant while eliciting the history so that the infant can become accustomed to this person as part of his environment. This "submissive" position is maintained until the infant makes eye contact as his first step in initiating closer contact with the nurse.

It is important that, during the first 6 months of the infant's life, as much of the examination as possible be done with the infant in his parent's lap. This technique enhances the infant's feelings of security and provides for less jostling. During the latter 6 months, after the infant is sitting up and crawling, he is allowed to explore the environment actively while his behavior is observed and historical data are obtained from the parent. Toys, a stethoscope, or any other tool which cannot harm the infant or be damaged by him can be offered to him for exploratory purposes. Many attempts should be made to develop rapport with the infant during the latter 6 months so that he does not become increasingly fearful of the examiner.

Parents are invited to participate in the physical examination. For example, the parent may be asked to pat the infant's abdomen (light palpation) to determine the presence of tenderness. Should the infant cry, deep palpation can be accomplished each time the infant inspires deeply during the crying process. Certain procedures have to be done with the infant's safety kept in mind. Those procedures should be carried out last, and appropriate restraints should be applied.

PHYSICAL STATUS

NORMAL GROWTH PARAMETERS

Height, weight, and head circumference The first year of life is a rapid-growth period. The infant's growing body mass is particularly evidenced in changes in his length and weight, which exhibit a simple curvilinear pattern (see Figs. 7-2 and 7-3). Weight reflects growth of body tissues (muscle, bone, fat, and organs). Average weight gain in early infancy is 19 g ($\frac{2}{3}$ oz) per day and in mid- and late infancy is 14 g ($\frac{1}{2}$ oz) per day. The infant's weight is doubled by 4 to 5 months and tripled by 10 to 12 months. Length represents bony growth (spine and long bones). Length is increased approximately 25 percent at 4 months and 50 to 56 percent in 1 year.

Head circumference reflects brain growth. The infant's head circumference increases about 2 cm (0.8 in) per month the first 2 months of life, then approximately 1.5 cm (0.6 in) per month for the next 2 months, and 1 cm (0.4 in) per month for the following 2 months. During the last 6 months of the first year of life, it grows by approximately 0.5 cm per month (see Fig. 7-4).

The National Center for Health Statistics (NCHS) charts provide up-to-date, reliable data by which to assess the infant's physical growth serially if measurement techniques are correct (see Chap. 2). Health care providers are becoming increasingly aware of the importance of triceps-skinfold measurements in indirectly estimating the amount of body fat as an indication of growth. Measurements which fall between the 15th and 85th percentiles are thought to be normal for age and sex (Frisancho, 1974). Although there are stated means, body length,

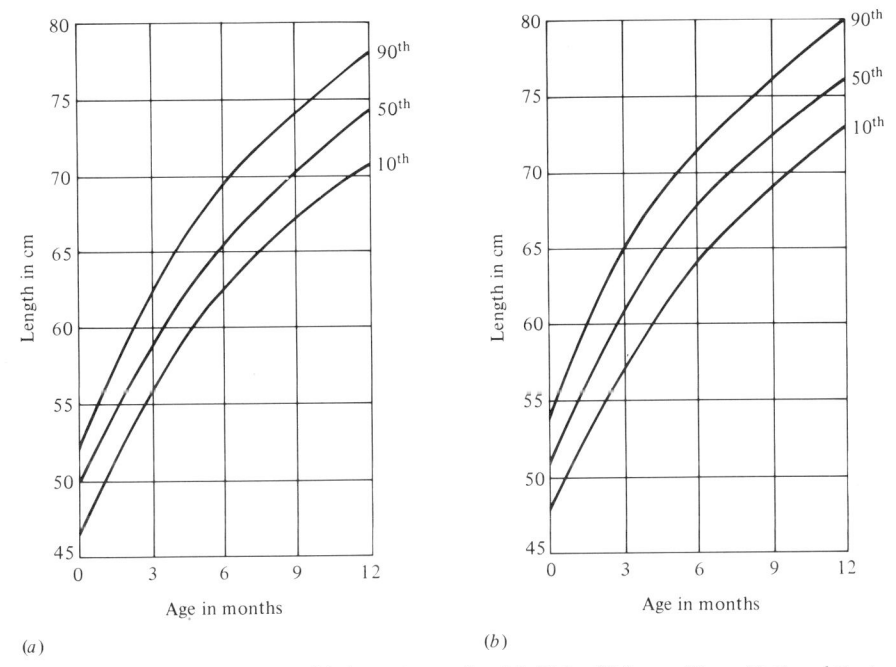

FIGURE 7-2. Length by age, birth to 12 months. (a) Girls; (b) boys. [From National Center for Health Statistics, NCHS growth charts, 1976. Monthly Vital Statistics Report (HRA) 76–1120 (Vol. 25, No. 3). Rockville, Maryland: U.S. Health Resources Administration, 1977 (supplement).]

weight, and head circumference are polygenic and thus vary between infants. The characteristics of a racial group reflect the gene pool.

Body proportion Throughout infancy, the child's head is large in relation to the rest of the body (see Fig. 7-5). The shape of the head is usually symmetrical. Sutures, which remain as slight ridges throughout the first 6 months of life, are considered normal. Complete closure does not occur until early in adulthood. Closure of the fontanels begins during infancy (see "Calvarium and Face").

The vault of the skull is large to accommodate rapid brain growth. At birth, the brain accounts for 12 percent of total body weight, and it doubles its weight by 1 year of age. The infant's neck is short, and his chest rounded. The xiphisterum may protrude due to the loose attachment between the xiphoid and the body of the sternum. The attachment strengthens with growth. His barrel-shaped chest explains why the infant is an abdominal breather. The purpose of thoracic respiration is to raise the ribs to a more horizontal position. Yet the ribs are already in a horizontal position because of the shape of the chest. In order to increase the anteroposterior and lateral diameters of the chest wall, the infant must be a diaphragmatic (abdominal) breather. Respirations gradually become a mixture of abdominal-thoracic movements until 7 years of age, when they are mostly thoracic. The infant's chest and head have approximately the same circumference. His abdominal circumference is larger than that of his chest and head until 2 years of age because his liver is large in relation to the abdominal cavity and the pelvis.

During infancy, the bladder is an abdominal organ. It is little wonder, then, that the infant's neck is short, since the thorax and shoulder girdle are pushed up by his overcrowded abdomen (Sinclair, 1978). The infant's upper limbs are further developed than his lower limbs, but the peripheral parts of his extremities are more advanced than the central parts. Thus, his hands seem large in proportion to his arms, and his feet seem large in proportion to his legs.

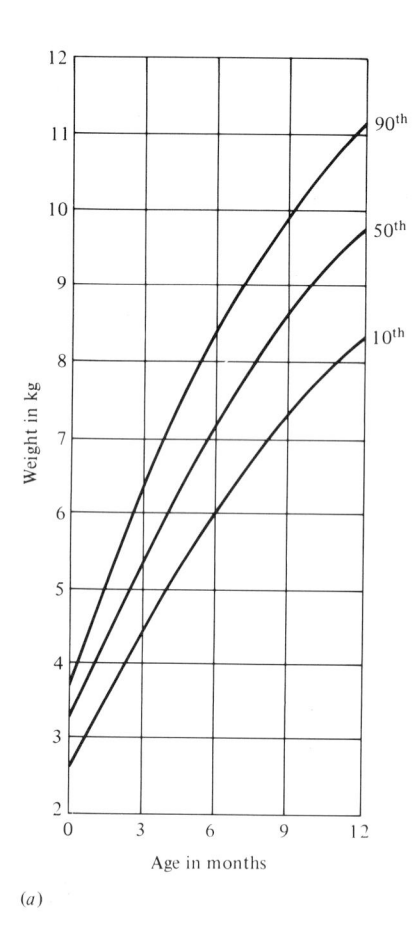

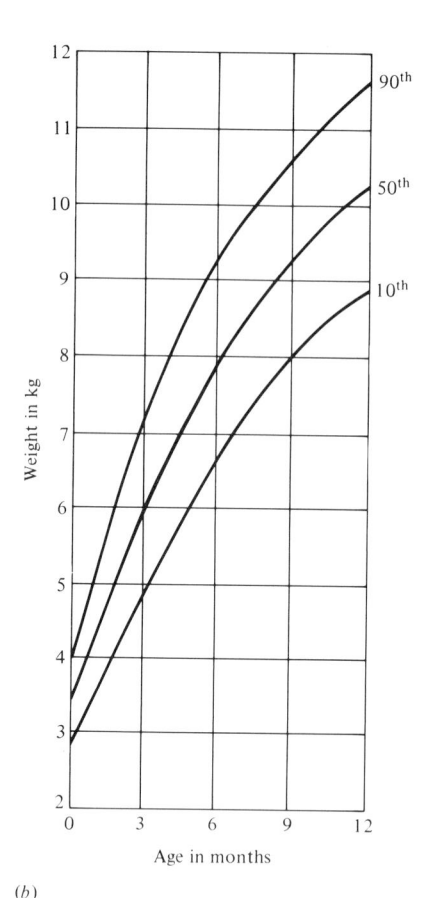

FIGURE 7-3. Weight by age, birth to 12 months. (*a*) Girls; (*b*) boys. (*From NCHS, 1977.*)

Body posture At birth, the neonate has two primary curvatures of the vertebral column: thoracic and sacral. During the first 6 or 7 months of life, two secondary curvatures appear. The first to be noted, at approximately 3 months of age, is the cervical, and the second is the lumbar. With the advent of the cervical curvature, the infant advances from flexion to extension of the neck. He can now hold up his head. Following the appearance of the lumbar curvature, the infant progresses from flexion to extension of the back.

When prone, the 1-month-old infant holds his pelvis high and his knees drawn up toward his abdomen. Intermittently, he will partially extend his hip and knee. By 6 weeks, the infant's knees are no longer under his abdomen when he is prone, and he increasingly extends his hip. Between 3 and 4 months of age he lifts his head and chest off a flat surface and holds his limbs in extension.

By 6 months of age, the infant is capable of maintaining a sitting position without benefit of environmental support. He now takes the first symbolic step toward becoming an independent being. The progress of his anterior-to-posterior development is indicated as his back becomes straighter. The center of gravity is found at the twelfth thoracic vertebra. Thus, he has a broad-based stance when he assumes an upright posture. His large liver is responsible for an exaggerated lumbar lordosis as he strives to bring his thorax into a vertical position.

General posture evolution, as all of development, proceeds from flexion to extension in cephalocaudal, anterior-to-posterior, and proximal-to-distal directions.

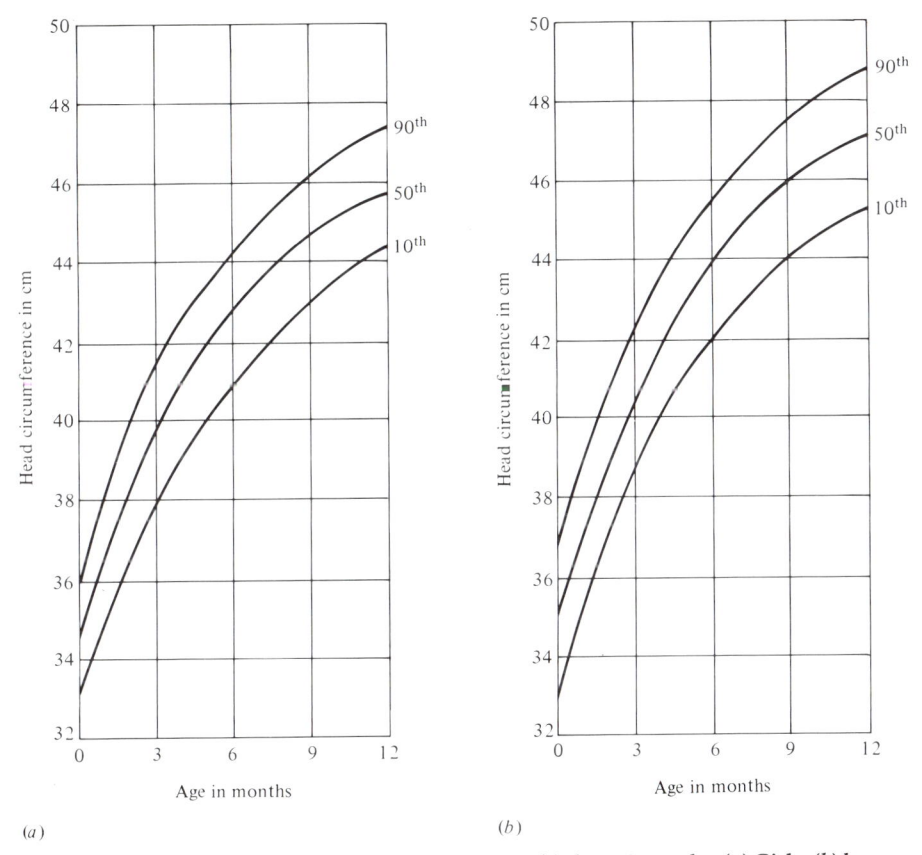

FIGURE 7-4. Occipital-frontal circumference by age, birth to 12 months. (*a*) Girls; (*b*) boys. (*From NCHS, 1977.*)

Postural orientation progresses from lateralization to midline orientation. Position evolves from horizontal to vertical posture.

Plantar fat pads, which gradually disappear during the first and second years of life, account for the infant's seemingly flat feet. During this same time period the lower extremities are in the genu varum (bowlegged) position with the feet externally rotated. Some infants begin walking as early as 7 months, while others do not start until 14 to 15 months of age. The gait is broad-based and somewhat unstable. Lumbar lordosis is prominent.

Negro infants are advanced in skeletal growth. In the United States their general postural evolution is ahead of Caucasian infants.

Body composition The body composition is divided into fat and lean body mass. Lean body mass is equivalent to fat-free body weight. According to Holliday (1978), the major organs (brain, liver, heart, and kidneys) constitute 15 percent of body weight at 3 months of age and 14 percent at 18 months of age. Muscle mass reflects 22 percent at 3 months and 23 percent at 18 months. Extracellular fluid (ECF) accounts for 32 percent at 3 months and 23 percent at 18 months. Connective tissue and bone are generally stable at about 15 percent. In 3-month-old infants, body fat constitutes 11 percent of body weight, and in 18-month-olds, 20 percent (Holliday, 1978, pp. 123–125).

Organs and muscle mass grow proportionately with

body weight. After 18 months, muscle mass increases at a more rapid rate than organs or body weight. In relation to body weight, ECF decreases, particularly in the first year of life. Fat is a major growth variable during this period and thus deserves further discussion.

Two types of adipose tissue are present: brown and white. Brown fat is important for thermogenetic function in the neonate and is active early in this growth period. Its function is thought to cease early in infancy. White fat provides a major store of energy, insulates and protects the body, is important in thermogenesis, and provides energy.

The most rapid growth period of fat cells in size and number is postulated to be between the seventh month of gestation and the end of the first year of infancy. It may begin slightly earlier and may be slightly greater in male infants. Measurement of skinfold thickness provides an estimate of fat-cell growth (Brook, 1975, p. 23).

Although genetic factors are thought to have a strong influence on this growth, little is known of their role. Environment is important in that fat cells may become hypertrophic and hyperplastic with overnutrition and decrease in size with undernutrition. Hormonal influences also are thought to be present; that is, insulin can cause an increase in size and growth hormone an increase in number of fat cells (Brook, 1975, pp. 26–31).

COMMON VARIATIONS IN NORMAL GROWTH PARAMETERS

Serial measurements, using growth charts such as those developed by the NCHS, are important in assessing the infant's growth parameters. Short stature is the most common growth variation. Macrocephaly may be familial and thus a normal variant. In preterm infants whose development is appropriate for gestational age (AGA), a more rapid head growth seemingly is present. When correction for age is included, the preterm infant's head grows at the same rate as a full-term infant's once the AGA infant has reached 40 postmenstrual weeks. The same is true for length and weight. Most small-for-gestational-age (SGA) infants can experience catch-up growth in head circumference during the first 6 to 8 months of life if they are given early and high caloric feeding. Catch-up length and weight growth may occur at later ages but not in infancy (Brandt, 1978). The NCHS growth charts do not correct for age.

Flattening of the head can occur on one side as a result of the infant's lying in one position for prolonged pe-

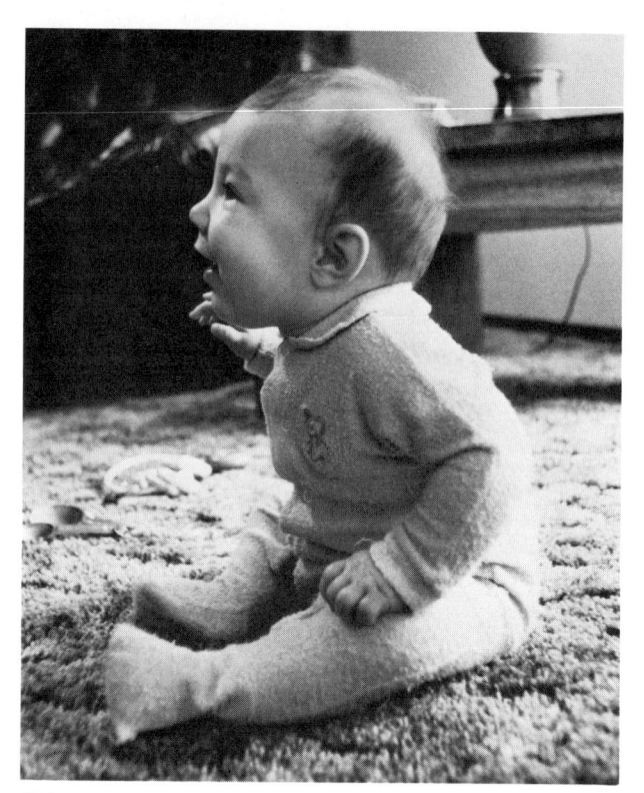

FIGURE 7-5. The infant's head is still large relative to the rest of the body.

riods. Flattening of the occiput may be found in the young infant who spends a major portion of each day in his crib, lying on his back. Such findings may be clues that the infant is stimulated infrequently. In some infants, anterior fontanels up to 4 or 5 cm in length and width, in the absence of other signs and symptoms, can be considered normal; however, they should decrease in size by 6 months of age. Early closure of the anterior fontanel between 4 and 9 months of age is considered normal if head-circumference growth proceeds along the same percentile. A full anterior fontanel which increases when the infant cries is a common variant. A third fontanel along the sagittal suture between the anterior and posterior fontanels may be a normal variant but is also frequently found in infants who have Down syndrome. Fibrous closure of the anterior fontanel may occur early in an infant's life and is considered equivalent to an open fontanel. It usually precedes bony closure by 1 to 2 months. Intracranial bruits, representing normal vascular turbulence, can occasionally be auscultated in the infant and child up to 5 years of age.

Length and weight, as plotted on the NCHS growth charts, are considered normal if they fall within the 25th to 75th percentiles. The 10th to 25th or 75th to 90th percentiles may be normal or may be a deviation. Family stature, dietary intake, development, pattern of growth, and general health must be considered in conjunction with these measurements. For occipital-frontal circumference (OFC), any measurement above the 75th or below the 25th percentiles, changes in percentiles between visits, and a head circumference which is markedly disproportionate to length and weight are suspicious.

VITAL SIGNS

The vital signs most commonly monitored in infancy are body temperature, pulse rate, and respiratory rate. Blood pressure determinations are not recommended unless the infant has a specific disorder, such as a heart abnormality. Usually blood pressure readings become a part of the routine physical assessment at 3 years of age.

Body temperature normally is 37.6°C (99.6°F) rectally, but it may be higher in hot, humid weather or following vigorous activity or crying. Pulse and respiratory rates will decrease from the beginning of the first year to the latter part of the first year. Generally, the average pulse rate in the first 6 months is 130 bpm with a range of 85 to 175 bpm, while in the second 6 months it is 115 bpm with a range of 75 to 175 bpm. The respiratory rate varies from 30 to 50 breaths per minute. Since the infant's chest wall is thin, his breath sounds on auscultation seem loud in comparison with those of older children and adults.

Fifty percent of children from infancy to early school age may have innocent heart murmurs which are not associated with actual defects. They are generally soft (grade I or II), short in duration, occur early in systole, do not radiate, and may be transient in nature. These murmurs do not affect physical development. Transiency may be associated with a change in position or activity, e.g., crying or, in the older infant, crawling. Some common causes of innocent murmurs in infancy are the physiologic anemia which occurs between 3 and 4 months of age, fever, or a change in hemodynamics due to rapid growth of the infant in his first year of postnatal life.

Tachycardia, or rapid heart beat, in infants can be related to change in activity and to fever. A rate of 160 to 170 bpm in a young infant or 120 to 140 bpm in an older infant who is crying, fretful, or hungry or who has been busily moving about can be considered normal. Changes in rate also occur with respirations; that is, an increase on inspiration and a decrease on expiration. A third heart sound is a normal variant which can occur, but a distinction between this variant and a gallop rhythm must be made (Pasternak and Lybarger, 1979).

DEVIATIONS IN PHYSICAL DEVELOPMENT

If the infant's measurements have been following a pattern and then fall either progressively or suddenly, the infant needs to be evaluated nutritionally, socially, and emotionally, as well as for a congenital disorder or disease state. Length, weight, and OFC percentiles between the 5th and 10th or the 90th and 95th are suspicious, and those below the 5th and over the 95th are cause for concern. Changes from one visit to another which reveal crossing of two channels or more on growth grids are deviant. A length/weight ratio below the 10th percentile may indicate failure to thrive, and one over the 95th percentile may indicate obesity. Generally, if length for age and sex is above the 10th percentile while weight for length is below the 5th, further investigation is warranted (National Center for Health Statistics, 1977).

Triceps-skinfold measurements greater than the 95th percentile in conjunction with weight for length beyond the 95th percentile are thought to be indicative of overnutrition, and those less than the 5th percentile in conjunction with weight for length below the 5th percentile are considered to represent undernutrition (Frisancho, 1974).

Nutritional status interacts with physical activity and health. Studies regarding overnutrition are not as clear as those for undernutrition, in which a direct relation has been established between nutrition and growth. The relation of illness to growth is unclear since other factors also interact, e.g., nutrition and available oxygen supplied to cells. Environmental factors, such as socioeconomics, culture, and parenting, are important considerations regarding growth (Johnston, 1978, pp. 107–112).

States of undernutrition and overnutrition are reflected in changes in body composition. In undernutrition, both muscle mass and adipose tissue decrease because the body's energy is derived from muscle protein (glucose for the brain) and fat. Extracellular fluid may be unchanged, or in the instance of chronic caloric undernutrition, it will increase. The resultant edematous state is reflected in weight gain. In overnutrition, a gain in body fat content occurs. Muscle mass usually remains the same, as does ECF (Holliday, 1978, pp. 119–122).

Cultural food patterns can affect body composition. In the United States, undernutrition, overnutrition, and iron deficiency are common. Undernutrition is more prevalent in the low-income population, but the other two know no socioeconomic barriers.

Parenting is an important variable related to body

composition. Infants who suffer deprivation of sensory and emotional needs fail to thrive.

As total body growth continues at a rapid rate, significant growth and maturational changes also occur in body systems during infancy. Through this physical development, further stabilization and adaptation to extrauterine life are accomplished.

Calvarium and face Mary Tudor

CALVARIUM

At the time of birth, the neonate's calvarium allows for overriding of the flat bones for passage through the birth canal. During the first year, five of the six fontanels of the calvarium will close, including the posterior at 2 to 4 months.

During the first few months of postnatal life, the anterior fontanel actually enlarges with cranial growth (Nelson, Vaughn, and McKay, 1975; Popich and Smith, 1972). By the sixth month, however, it has begun to diminish in size and will close by 18 months of age. Mean fontanel size, which is determined by taking one-half the sum of the anteroposterior length and the transverse width, has been determined for Caucasian infants birth to 11 months of age (Popich and Smith, 1972) (see Fig. 7-6). Comparing changes in head size and anterior fontanel size can give clues regarding normal growth versus increasing head size due to increasing intracranial pressure.

There is tremendous growth of the calvarium during the first 12 months, 40 to 50 percent of total growth, reflecting rapid brain growth. The mastoid processes are small at birth and develop during infancy and later childhood. The temporal bone is also incomplete. The cranial base is flat, giving a short-head appearance. The frontal and parietal bones are prominent relative to other structures. The sinus cavities are not present at birth.

FACE

Facial growth is slower than growth of the calvarium during the first year. However, it results in a decreasing of the calvarium/face ratio from 6:1 at 1 month to 4.5:1 by 12 months (Israel, 1978). The relatively large eyes and orbits, nearly adult-sized, give the large-eyed look that more than any other feature connotes childhood. The eyes appear hyperteloric compared with those of the older child and adult.

Growth of the jaws, alveolar processes, and teeth cause a significant change in facial contour during the last half of the first year. This process will continue into adulthood. The two halves of the mandible fuse during infancy as it grows down and forward.

TOOTH FORMATION

Tooth emergence into the oral cavity usually begins between 5 and 8 months, at 6 months as an average. However, variations, from birth to 12 months, are seen in normal children. The mandibular central incisors are usually first to emerge. Continuing calcification of the root causes the eruption and emergence of the deciduous tooth. Root formation is complete when the tooth reaches the occlusal level.

By the end of the first year, typically, the four lower and four upper incisors will have emerged as well as the mandibular primary molars (see Fig. 7-7).

Central nervous system Mary D. Guthrie

As the maturing central nervous system continues to add myelin to the neurons, sensory and motor skills become more mature and integrated. It is now that the infant be-

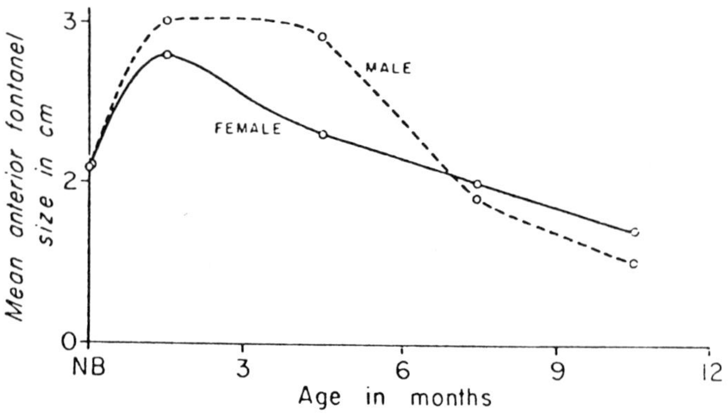

FIGURE 7-6. Mean anterior fontanel size by sex plotted against age. [From G. A. Popich and D. W. Smith, Fontonels: Range of normal size. *J. Pediat.*, 1972, 80(5), p. 751. Reprinted by permission of C. V. Mosby Company.]

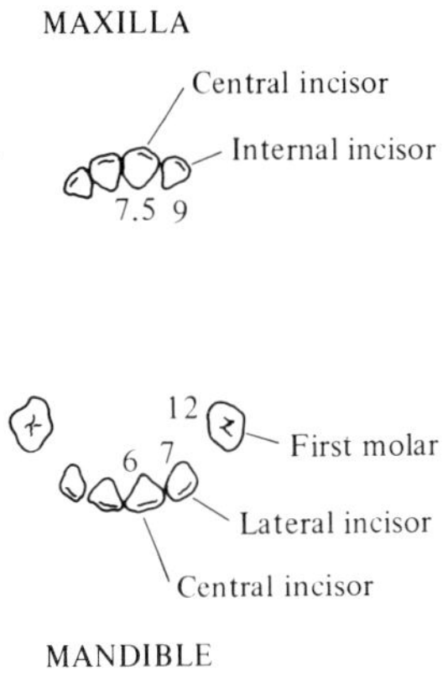

FIGURE 7-7. Deciduous dentition at 12 months of age with mean age of emergence in months.

gins to integrate functionally his two brains, two eyes, two ears, two arms, and two legs.

All head and hand activities are more nearly midline after 4 months. At this time the infant is able to see small objects, but for lack of dexterity he is not able to pick them up until he is about 10 months old. Between 7 and 9 months he uses his hands in a pawlike fashion for transfer of objects. At 10 months he can handle smaller objects, but it is not until he is 1 year old that he has good forefinger-thumb movements and grasp. It is only after 1 year that he displays spatial concepts. Just as the upper-extremity muscles were innervated before those of the lower extremity, coordinated movement and dexterity appear in the hands before the feet.

Sensory system Anna M. Tichy

VISUAL SYSTEM

Evidence of sophisticated eye-brain function becomes apparent in infancy. The time lag for this development is not caused by physiological immaturity of the eye but is the result of the evolvement of the requisite cortical connections for appropriate interpretation and response to visual input.

The eye, still hyperopic, continues to grow in size. Pupillary diameter also increases, and the lens continues to grow. The macula is mature by the end of the first year, and the transverse diameter of the cornea reaches adult size. Eye muscles are mature in their movement by 12 months of age as well. Tear glands begin to secrete, and by 3 months the child will tear with crying. The blue iris of the neonate becomes gradually pigmented during the first 6 months of life. True blinking is also established at 6 months of age.

During the first year of life there is a gradual increase in visual acuity, so that by 12 months of age it is approximately 20/100. The neural elements necessary for dichromatic color vision and for brightness discrimination are present in the 2-month-old infant.

During the first 3 months, esotropia is frequently seen. However, conjugate gaze with binocular vision is fairly well established by 4 months of age, and after 6 months there is normally no deviation. Strabismus may be assessed by noting a deviation in the position of a light reflection in the pupils; the reflection should be seen at the same point on each pupil. Monocular esotropia, or disconjugate fixation, results in two images being received by the optic cortex. The double images will cause diplopia, or more commonly, one of the images will be suppressed. The latter condition may lead to strabismic amblyopia in which one eye stops functioning to full capacity. Visual acuity in that eye is markedly reduced because of suppression of central vision. Alternating esotropia is less significant and has a good prognosis before 2 years of age.

AUDITORY SYSTEM

The external, middle, and inner ears continue to grow during infancy. The external ear maintains the same relative position on the head. The position of the external ear to the internal ear changes, however, as the child grows. Examination of the ear in the infant reveals a diffuse light reflex on the tympanic membrane. The bright cone-shaped light reflection from the umbo becomes apparent at several months of age. The tympanic membrane is adult-sized at birth, but it is set obliquely. As the external auditory canal lengthens, the tympanic membrane assumes an erect position by 2 years of age.

Knowledge of the direction of the external auditory canal is necessary for proper placement of the otoscope. In the infant, the canal is directed upward; therefore, it is necessary to pull the auricle downward to visualize the tympanic membrane. In the older child, the canal is directed downward, reflecting the change in relative position.

Otitis media is particularly prevalent in the infant and toddler. In infancy, the eustachian tube is wider, shorter, and straighter than in the older child. This anatomical factor predisposes the young child to the spread of infectious materials from the respiratory tract.

TACTILE SYSTEM

By 1 month of age, most of the lanugo which was prevalent on the shoulders and back has disappeared. Simultaneously, some of the tactile receptors continue differentiation, a process which may not be completed for several months. Continued development of tactile receptors may partially account for increased responsiveness to cutaneous tactile and pain stimuli in the first year of postnatal life. Myelination of spinal cord fibers, which began in midfetal life, continues during the first postnatal year, and myelin formation in the brain continues until adolescence.

The first year of postnatal life is characterized by increasing ability to respond more appropriately and specifically to stimuli. This behavioral change is the result of further maturation of the sensory receptors, increased myelination of corticospinal pathways and the cortex, and the beginning ability to coordinate and integrate stimuli. These structural and functional developments are preparatory for the infant's future participation in the complex environment of the toddler.

Musculoskeletal system Sherrilyn Passo

During the first 12 months of life, rapid growth of the infant reflects development of the skeletal system, as length increases 50 percent. The major portions of the ends of the long bones are still cartilage in the infant. Several epiphyseal centers do appear, particularly in the tibia, fibula, femur, and humerus. All bones of the skeleton are rapidly growing. As the infant begins to stand, this weight bearing, as other physical activity, stimulates bone growth, notably density and diameter (Roche, 1978).

The face and skull grow and change relative proportion (see "Calvarium and Face"). The lower limbs and pelvic girdle remain shorter and less advanced than the upper limbs and shoulder girdle, although the former are growing more rapidly and catching up. By 1 year of age the ilia has become thicker and stronger, and the acetabulums are deeper.

A secondary curve appears in the cervical area of the spine around 3 to 4 months when the infant begins to lift his head in prone. As the infant learns to sit well, his back continues its evolution from this C curve. By 10 months, the infant sits with straight lower spine, and by 12 months upright posture results in the mature S curve.

Muscular activity not only stimulates bone growth but also causes limb muscle hypertrophy, increasing the size and length of fibers. Muscle strength increases as well, although there is no significant difference between girls and boys of the same size. As the infant gains control over smaller muscles, more refined, finite movements replace the gross, large-muscle movements of infancy.

Gastrointestinal system
Anna M. Tichy and Dianne Chong

FUNCTIONAL MATURATION

The characteristic breathing-feeding pattern of the neonate, with periodic glottic opening and closure for the purpose of breathing during sucking, continues for 6 to 8 months. After that time the infant must interrupt sucking to breathe. The rooting and sucking reflexes, which are important for feeding in the early months of life, persist for approximately 6 months, when sucking becomes voluntary.

The infant can swallow semiliquid foods, such as strained fruits and vegetables, early in life. However, any semisolid food introduced into the infant's mouth before 4 to 5 months of age is treated in the same manner as the nipple. The food, as it is pressed against the hard palate, is partially passed to the pharynx and partially pushed anteriorly through the lips and out the mouth. This extrusion reflex is not an indication of dislike for the new diet but a normal developmental phase of swallowing. At 4 to 5 months, the infant treats materials placed in the mouth selectively, sucking a nipple but transferring solid foods to the pharynx for swallowing.

GROWTH AND MATURATION

Drooling becomes apparent at 3 months of age. The salivary glands steadily increase in size, tripling in weight in the first 6 months of life. The structural change is accompanied by an increased production of saliva, which is difficult for the infant to handle. Until swallowing of this secretion becomes automatic, the infant drools considerably.

In the first 6 months a considerable amount of air is swallowed during sucking. Swallowing of air, the poor tone of the lower esophageal sphincter, and the pressure gradient between the stomach and esophagus explain the need for "bubbling" the infant and the postfeeding regurgitation characteristic of this age group. As sphincter tone improves during the first year, the incidence of esophageal reflux and regurgitation after feedings diminishes. In addition to peristaltic propulsive waves, small, nonpropagative peristaltic waves are present during infancy. These nonpropagative waves are nonexistent in the adult (Gryboski, Thayer, and Spiro, 1963).

STOMACH

Stomach capacity of the infant increases progressively, and gastric emptying time varies from 1 to 4 h following a feeding. Milk is evacuated at a uniform rate for the first two-thirds to nine-tenths of the feeding, after which the rate diminishes. The infant's peristaltic waves, induced by stretching stomach musculature, are shallow and identifiable only in the distal portion of the stomach. The same factors which affect gastric emptying in the neonate are operative in the infant. The 4-h average length of time for gastric emptying is the basis for the customary 4-h feeding schedule in young infants.

Secretory activity of the fundic glands in infants has been studied, and though findings are not uniform, the developmental pattern of secretion suggests that the output of hydrochloric acid, pepsin, and intrinsic factor continue to rise in the second and third months (Agunod, Yamaguchi, Lopez, Luhby, and Glass, 1969). This steady rise follows the transient drop at the end of the neonatal period. Despite this pattern of early increase in gastric secretion, the infant, by adult standards, remains markedly hypochlorhydric for the first 6 to 9 months of postnatal life (Tyson, 1969).

A study of gastric pH and microflora of bottle-fed, breast-fed, and diarrheic infants has shown that bottle-fed infants have low gastric-pH values and bacterial concentrations. In contrast both breast-fed and diarrheic infants have higher gastric-pH values; however, the former group did not develop the bacterial overgrowth of the infants with diarrhea. This finding suggests that some factor other than gastric acidity regulates bacterial growth in the gastric contents of breast-fed infants (Maffel and Nobrega, 1975). By the third month, intrinsic factor output, when calculated on the basis of body weight, approximates adult levels.

SMALL INTESTINE

Anatomically, the arrangement of the intestinal tract in the abdominal cavity of the infant differs significantly from the older child or adult. Whereas the greatest diameter of the intestinal mass is vertical in the adult, it is transverse in the infant due to the infant's relatively large liver mass and abdominal width. During infancy the intestinal tract increases about one-third in length.

Transit time through the small intestine continues to be extremely variable; the normal range is 1 to 6 h, although exceptions are common. As in the neonate, transit time is affected by a number of factors including size of the meal and amount of feces in the colon. Motor activity in the region of the duodenum in infancy continues to be less than that of the adult.

DIGESTION AND ABSORPTION

As in the neonate, the low amylase activity within the duodenal fluid of the young infant may be primarily of salivary origin. With increasing age, duodenal aspirates show gradually increasing activity, but by 1 year of age amylase activity has not attained adult levels (Andersen, 1942). The ability to hydrolyze starch in infancy may be deficient; an alternate pathway of starch digestion may be operative. It is postulated that glucamylase activity of the intestinal mucosa has a role in starch hydrolysis during infancy (Alpers and Solin, 1970). Disaccharidase activity of maltase and sucrase are at or slightly in excess of adult values during infancy. Lactase activity of the small intestine, which is high at birth, may decline somewhat during infancy, though the activity level still exceeds adult values.

Lipase activity increases throughout the first 2 to 3 years of life (Zoppi, Andreotti, and Pajino-Ferrara, 1972). Age related changes have been shown in bile acids in the small intestine of normal infants: with increasing age, the concentration of bile acids increases correspondingly (Challacombe, Edkins, and Brown, 1975). Short- and medium-length-chain triglycerides may be absorbed without micelle formation, so that their absorption is unimpaired in early infancy. However, the absorption of long-chain, unsaturated fatty acids and cholesterol is impaired in early infancy, when bile acids are not present in adequate amounts; adult levels of lipid absorption are achieved by 4 to 6 months of age. Studies of the absorptive process of lipids have not been conducted in the infant; however, it is believed the transport process for fat is functional in this age group.

Activity of the proteolytic enzyme trypsin is lower in early infancy than it is in older children. This activity gradually increases, and by 9 months of age the volume responses to stimulation increase tenfold. Data involving peptidase activities in the intestinal mucosa of the infant are not available. Protein digestion and absorption are fairly well developed in the infant. Protein breakdown to amino acids and absorption occurs primarily in the upper areas of the small intestine. The absorption of intact proteins, which occurs in many infant mammals, has not been identified in the healthy human infant.

LARGE INTESTINE

The colon during infancy is characterized by a high position, a cone-shaped cecum with the appendix arising from the apex of the cone, and a sigmoid colon that extends into the right abdomen. The infantile appendix is less likely to obstruct than the appendix of the older child. Motility of the large intestine of the infant is similar to the adult with both propulsive and resting motor-activity patterns and contraction of the external sphincter and relaxation of the internal sphincter in response to distension of the rectum.

The intrinsic nerve plexus of the colon continues to develop during infancy. Defecation in the infant occurs reflexively; the number of stools passed per day is dependent upon the nature of the feeding (see Chap. 6, "Development of the Gastrointestinal System"). The nature of the diet also affects pigmentation and composition of the stool. The stool weight varies between 75 and 100 g/day in late infancy. The coloration of the infant's stool is subject to much greater variation than in later childhood. The intestinal flora that results from a milk diet affects the reducing power of the intestinal contents. Thus, bile bilirubin may be incompletely reduced, and the excreted bilirubin may be oxidized causing the yellow stool to become green on standing.

Endocrine system Norma J. Briggs

Although the endocrine system is functional early in postnatal life, dysfunction of some part of the endocrine system may occur theoretically at any point in time affecting growth. Trauma, tumors, autoimmune responses, and viral infections are only a few of the etiological factors which may disrupt normal functioning of endocrine tissues. A subsequent failure of control mechanisms or of endocrine tissue to respond appropriately to control mechanisms results in excesses or deficits of the hormones produced by these tissues. Excesses or deficits of hormones produce symptoms in the child related to the original functions of each specific hormone. An understanding of the functions of each hormone will readily facilitate recognition of health deviations in the child.

THYROID

During the first 6 months after birth, normal brain development is dependent upon thyroxine. If the infant is hypothyroid during this time, permanent defects in brain structure and function may occur. Diagnosis of hypothyroidism during this critical time is not always easy; however, the sooner the diagnosis is established and therapy started, the better the prognosis regarding brain development.

The most common cause of hypothyroidism is autoimmune destruction of the thyroid. Failure of the thyroid to migrate from the area at the base of the tongue during fetal development of the gland results in a lingual thyroid. Such a gland is small and unable to sustain adequate function for the growing child and leads to a gradual onset of hypothyroidism. Delayed growth and development with retarded bone age are significant symptoms.

PANCREAS

The infant is born nondiabetic, but there is a slow-rising curve in the incidence of diabetes mellitus with peaks at 3, 6, and 12 years of age. Juvenile, or insulin-dependent, diabetes usually occurs before the age of 15 and has a more rapid onset than the maturity-onset diabetes which occurs in adults. The symptoms of diabetes are essentially the same regardless of when it develops, as the underlying defect in carbohydrate metabolism is the same. However, diabetic children who have not achieved their growth potential fail to grow and thrive and are thin due to the unavailability of glucose for cellular metabolism.

IMMUNE SYSTEM

An infant is more susceptible to infection than a toddler. While both the humoral, or immunoglobulin (IgG), and the cellular immunity systems are continuing to mature, at birth the infant immunoglobulin is primarily IgG which has been acquired from the mother. At about 3 months of age, the maternal IgG disappears, and the infant begins to manufacture his own. Not until adolescence are adult levels of immunoglobulins achieved. There is little known about cellular immunity in infancy. Deficiencies of either system produce an increased number of infections which are unusually severe.

Development of body concept and concepts of illness and wellness
Judith Anne Ritchie

BODY CONCEPT, CONTENT, AND FUNCTION

Early in the first year the hand emerges as the tool for building the body image (Freud, 1952). Following the twelfth week, the hand-to-mouth relationship is well established. The infant now begins to use his hands to discover and organize information about his own body and other persons' bodies as well as other objects.

Increasing visual acuity permits further discovery of information concerning body parts. Usually the mouth becomes involved in expanding the infant's knowledge base about texture, resistance, and boundaries of new objects such as hands and feet. The infant is described as behaving "toward its own body exactly as it does to foreign objects" (Bernfeld, 1929). However, the unique position of the body as both the perceived and the perceiver eventually permits the infant's discovery that this "foreign object" is a part of "me."

During the infant's second 6 months, movement in space and contact with other objects provide information about size, shape, texture, boundaries, and function of his body parts and his own separateness of himself from the outer world. The mobile infant is deluged with tactile, kinesthetic, and proprioceptive impressions about his body parts and his position in space.

The infant expands his awareness of body parts through intense visual examination of those around him. This visual examination is supplemented by careful, often vigorous manual examination through touching, prodding, pinching, and pulling.

Body games, such as this little piggy or knock on the door, increase the infant's awareness of body parts and provide interesting tactile and kinesthetic sensations that seem to delight the infant. The attitudes of parents during hygienic care and body games teach the infant to perceive various body parts as "good or bad, pleasing or repulsive, clean or dirty, loved or disliked" (Kolb, 1975).

By the end of the first year the infant has constructed a "provisionally organized" (Freud, 1942) concept of the discrete parts of the body and their functions. The child must now establish those parts as "interrelated and joined in a definite structure" (Witken, 1965, pp. 27–28).

WELLNESS, ILLNESS, AND HOSPITALIZATION

Infants' responses to feeling unwell are as variable as their responses to any event or change in their environments. An infant may become extremely restless and irritable or may seem to withdraw, become affectless, and be much less active than usual.

The young, hospitalized infant is described as exhibiting a "global reaction" (Prugh, 1965). Parents and care givers report alterations in the infant's behavior patterns in eating, sleeping, elimination, and activity patterns.

PERCEPTION OF PAIN

During the first year of life the infant's response to painful stimuli gradually becomes more specific. He seems more able to localize the source of perceived pain and rub or "pull at" the painful area. Extreme pain from an unidentifiable source, such as incisional pain, may produce global but unmistakable pain behavior of screaming and holding the body in a rigid posture.

Pain, even for the infant, is accompanied by a high degree of anxiety and is said to be remembered for a long time after its occurrence (Freud, 1952). It is theorized that recurrent painful sensation in any body part may result in distortions of body image in which that part occupies a disproportionate degree of the body concept (Schilder, 1964).

REACTIONS TO RESTRAINT AND PROCEDURES

Unless very ill, most infants react to any infringement on their mobility with protest and attempted escape (Mittleman, 1960). Heavy casts produce facial expressions of confusion and puzzlement, and the infant may make attempts to remove the cast.

However, even after brief restraints the infant no longer protests and becomes passive. For example, an infant 9 months of age had been restrained for intravenous therapy for 3 days. When restraints were reapplied after periods of play, his response was to cry briefly and then lie passively quiet with a sad facial expression.

The infant under 6 months whose arms are restrained for long periods appears to "forget" his usual motor responses. He often leaves his arms at his sides and needs stimulation to bring his hands to midline.

Infants' responses to hurtful procedures are typically a surprised expression followed by loud protest. If the procedure recurs, the infant learns to recognize the preceding events and to respond with fear as soon as the sequence is recognized. The very ill infant needs to conserve energy and may passively submit to procedures. However, as he recovers, he begins to resist procedures, especially if they place him in the vulnerable back-lying position or are intrusive.

REACTIONS TO HEALTH CARE WORKERS AND SEPARATION

As infants receive health care, they are exposed to numerous health care workers. The infant's age, sex, state of health, cognitive developmental level, and motor abilities all affect his responses. Even very young infants apparently recognize unfamiliar handlers. However, it is not until the sixth to eighth month that the infant consistently reacts to strangers and health workers with careful, sober searching of the stranger's face. Later the infant's responses tend to become more fearful with active return to the familiar person and crying if the stranger approaches too closely (Spicher, 1976).

While the classical behaviors of *separation anxiety* may not be fully demonstrated until the end of the first year, it is apparent that even much younger infants watch for the parent, are disturbed by the separation, and undergo a period of adjustment. On his third hospital day, a 9-month-old infant lay in bed passively and watched other infants or nurses in the room or rolled his head from side to side whimpering with a blank facial expression. When given the opportunity, he could play quite happily, but when returned to bed he cried and quickly reverted to his previous behavior. On the fourth day he appeared sad, depressed, and rejecting. Only after an hour of play did he begin to react with more enjoyment.

By the fifth day the infant appeared settled in, with considerable interest in activity, food intake, and the environment. He did laugh and smile at times; however, when his mother visited late in the afternoon, he could be described as truly happy, with very lively play, sparkling eyes, and frequent laughing.

The major effect of hospitalization as perceived by the infant is separation. His behavior at the time of hospitalization demonstrates the degree to which he finds separation distressing. Douglas' research (1975) suggests that separation through hospitalization between ages 6 and 12 months has long-term behavioral effects.

DEATH

The infant does not have a cognitive understanding of death. However, it has been suggested that some behaviors and experiences of even young infants lay the foundations for the development of a concept of death. Peekaboo and other games of disappearance and return are described as beginning experiences of nonbeing, separation, or death (Maurer, 1966). It is difficult to assess the ill infant's awareness of his own death. However, it has been suggested that the dying infant's affective responses are significantly affected by those about him (Schowalter, 1970).

SECTION 2

Behavioral Development

The major percentage of growth and morphological development has been achieved during the prenatal, neonatal, and infancy periods. Physical changes of the same magnitude will not be seen again until puberty.

Evidence of physical development in behavioral skills exists prenatally but is most vigorous in infancy. As the structures have evolved and the environment surrounds the infant with stimuli and opportunity, functional growth and adaptation flourish.

The infant: Outward and upward
Mary Tudor

Just as the embryological period is the time of morphogenesis, the infancy period represents the same stage in behavioral development: establishment of the *form* of adaptive functioning. During the first to twelfth months, major accomplishments are observed in all areas. More than these separate milestones, there is an overall quality change in behavior, and it establishes a mature form.

The child, in behavioral development, is transformed in an outward and upward progression from an inward-directed, flexed, and horizontal infant to an outward-directed, extended, and upright toddler.

Major outward evolution results as primitive reflexes are integrated to the purpose of functional motor behavior and the infant moves from nonfunctional flexion to extension posture. He begins with head lifting in prone in response to environmental stimuli. This can occur as a result of the infant advancing from being reflex-bound to exhibiting volitional behavior secondary to higher central nervous system maturation.

Another outward movement is seen in the infant's longer wakeful periods which allow the infant to utilize well-developed sensory capabilities. He is no longer "state-bound." The sensory system, precocious in maturation, seems to lead the way, and sensory perception initiates the unfolding process. The infant "latches on" to the world through tactile, visual, and auditory modes and begins to covet the stimuli available in his environment.

Thus, sensory stimuli not only prompt the outward orientation of flexion to extension but also the evolution of being focused inward to orientation to the environment outside himself. With intact and improving visual perception, the infant catches hold of novel stimuli. Initially, he responds with general excitement evidenced by total body wriggling and kicking. He smiles at the surprise of discovery outside himself. He is capable of and primarily interested in recapturing motor experiences.

Soon, with more outward (extended) body posture and movement and outward direction of attention, the infant works to integrate these sensory and motor experiences. He acts on objects and then acts again to recapture novel effects. The infant has now begun a lifelong interaction with the world. Before long, the infant is not content to discover this world in a static position but becomes mobile in exploration, rolling, crawling, creeping, and cruising. From his motor actions on the world, the infant learns.

The infant directs most of his attention to his parents and responds to the visual, tactile, and auditory experiences they provide. A social being from the start, the infant's cognitive development allows progression from indiscriminate attachment to attachment with specific, recognized persons. The infant rewards these trusted and important others with smiles and squeals. Soon the infant is vocally communicating pleasure and displeasure and in the latter half of the first year is making needs known through gestures.

Because the infant can stay awake longer and adopts the diurnal pattern of the family, he progresses from being unscheduled or "out of sync" with the rest of the world to adopting an acceptable daily pattern. He also takes on more responsibility for himself during this first year; he can feed himself and comfort himself to a limited extent. He is capable of playing to entertain himself. By his preferential social responses, increased independence, and civilized daily routine, he becomes more of an integral part of the family unit, socially directed outward.

Assumption of an upright posture often marks for parents the end to the period of infancy. The infant has worked for this status since he first raised his head and looked about. From that point on he is directed upward. By the end of the first year he is extended and upright and able to continue to move outward in the world.

Behavioral Development by Functional Area

Perceptual development Veronica A. Binzley

**METHODS USED
TO STUDY INFANT PERCEPTION**

The methods used to study the perceptual abilities of the infant are more sophisticated than those used during the neonatal period. This is necessary in order to adjust methods to the infant's rapidly increasing abilities. Instead of a reflex model, the habituation paradigm is used more often.

For example, in a *visual-discrimination study*, time spent looking is usually used as the response measure. But the paradigm remains the same. That is, as the infant becomes familiar with the stimulus, there is a decrease in looking time. But if the infant is then shown a new stimulus and as a consequence looking time increases, the assumption is that the infant has discriminated the stimuli. He recognizes that in some way they are different. However, if the two targets differ in a number of ways, the basis for the infant's discrimination is not clear. This can only be stipulated when two targets differ in only one dimension.

Two other procedures used in studying infant perception are the *stimulus-preference method* and *conditioning*. In the preference method, if an infant looks at one stimulus significantly longer than another or responds with more sucking or more of a cardiac response, the assumption is that the infant can discriminate the two stimuli. On the other hand, failure to demonstrate a preference for one stimulus over another cannot automatically be interpreted as evidence that the infant cannot discriminate them. The infant may simply not find either stimulus attractive or may find them equally so.

In the conditioning paradigm, a response, such as sucking or reaching in the presence of a stimulus, is rewarded a sufficient number of times so that just the presentation of the stimulus will elicit the conditioned response. Then one presents another stimulus similar to the first but presumably discriminable to the older child. If the infant responds with the conditioned response to the second stimulus, then it is assumed that he cannot discriminate them.

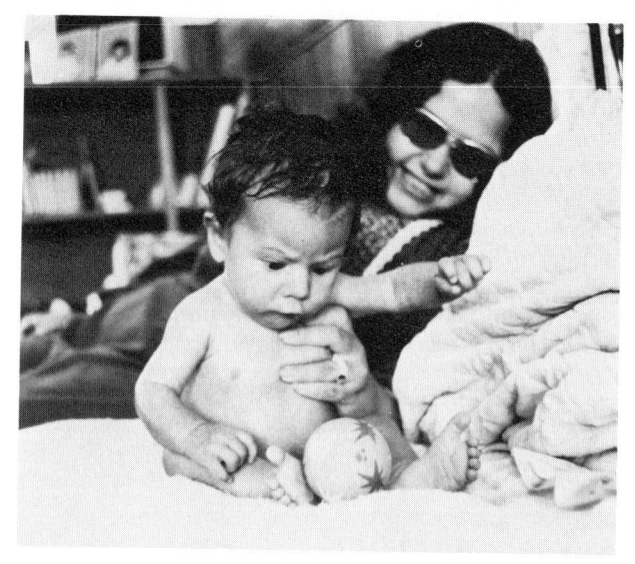

FIGURE 7-8.

CHANGES IN RESPONSE MEASURES

The response measures one uses also must change to accommodate the infant's growing capabilities. For instance, even at 3 months of age, many infants begin to prefer their own thumbs to a pacifier. Later when they begin to teethe, they will chew and/or mouth the nipple; so the response measure is no longer usable as it is not the same reflex response elicited in early infancy. Moreover, there is even some question as to whether nonnutritive sucking indexes the same behavior at 3 months as it did during the first month (Binzley, 1974). During the neonatal period, sucking is associated with cardiac acceleration and seems to reflect excitement, but in the older infant this is not so. There is not significant cardiac acceleration, and sucking appears to index interest and/or pacification rather than excitement.

Smiling, which usually begins to be elicited at about 6 weeks, is added to the list of response measures along with vocalization and reaching. State becomes less and less of a problem during the first year as states become more stable and individual states longer in duration. Hence, there are longer periods of quiet wakefulness.

REPORTED PERCEPTUAL ABILITIES

VISUAL PERCEPTION
The young infant's visual acuity improves significantly during the first year and continues to do so through childhood. Recent data place visual acuity of the 12-month-old child at 20/100 (Ellis, 1978). Binocular vision

begins at 6 weeks and is fairly well established by 4 months. At about the same time, the infant begins to show evidence of accommodation (change of lens focus) to the changing distance of targets.

Color vision and movement Whether the neonate can see color is not known even though there has recently been a number of studies of color vision in the young infant. According to those who labor in this area, testing color vision in any organism is difficult because of the confounding of intensity and wavelength. These recent studies indicate that color vision is functional at least by 2 to 4 months of age. And at 4 months the infant's color vision is similar to that of the adult (Haith and Campos, 1977).

In the young infant little is known about movement other than the fact that it continues to be an attractive stimulus and reportedly enhances the attractiveness of real faces for older infants.

Space: Distance, depth, and directionality As the infant begins to crawl, he is exposed to a more varied environment, and as a result of this practice, space becomes better differentiated for him. However, even before then, there is evidence for visual sensitivity to depth cues.

Infants after 2 months of age show fixation preferences for a sphere over a circle, which is evidence that they can discriminate some of the cues which specify depth (Gibson, 1969). In this case the cues appeared to be texture and shading. Depth perception has also been studied using the visual cliff technique developed by Walk and Gibson (Pick and Pick, 1970). This technique consists of placing an infant on a centerboard between two glass surfaces onto which he can crawl. The typical depth test consists of placing a surface directly under the glass on one side and a surface at some distance below the glass on the other side. Of course this technique is applicable only to infants who can locomote, which usually means infants 6 months and over. In a careful study using this technique, it was found that 90 percent of the infants at all ages (6½ to 15 months) who responded in the situation avoided the deep side of the cliff. However, a number of infants who initially chose the shallow side were able to be coaxed across the deep side. Again the cue for depth appeared to be *visible* texture as many infants were reluctant to crawl on a perfectly safe, heavy glass surface that could be touched and tested unless the surface looked safe. That is, texture must be apparent (Gibson, 1969).

In regard to directionality, it has been reported that 2-month-old infants learn a vertical-horizontal discrimination, and by 6 months infants respond to or ignore a new orientation of an object depending on whether they had seen it in varying orientations or not (Haith and Campos, 1977).

Pattern and form perception By 3 or 4 weeks of age the young infant watches his mother's face intently as she speaks to him; by 4 to 6 weeks he begins to smile at her as she speaks to him. However, he will also smile at a face-sized card with two eye dots—and still more at one with six dots. A finding such as this demonstrates the difficulty in trying to identify what it is the infant is responding to when he shows a preference for one target over another. This is precisely the problem with many of the studies in pattern and form perception.

Prior to 8 weeks of age, infants reportedly prefer a red, horizontal, striped pattern over a bull's-eye. But after 8 weeks of age and until 6 months, the red bull's eye is preferred over the horizontal, striped pattern. So presumably the infant can discriminate the pattern characteristics of linearity and curvilinearity. Other form differentiations that have been reported in the young infant include regularity and irregularity, concentricity, number of line directions, and orientation of elements. Yet a 2- or 3-month-old infant does not discriminate an odd element in a matrix, something which immediately attracts the adult's attention as well as that of the 2½- and 3½-year-old child (Haith and Campos, 1977).

Face perception There have been many studies on the development of face perception, and some of the findings are contradictory; so it is difficult to specify unquestionably what features of the face the infant discriminates at which time. However, Gibson (1969) has thoroughly reviewed these studies, and in her opinion the data support the following conclusions: At 2 months the real face features begin to be differentiated, beginning with the eyes. At 3 months the eyes remain dominant, but a mutilated face (cut off below the eyes) is noticed. By 5 months the differentiation includes the mouth as a feature and an oval head shape. However, individual faces are not yet differentiated; nor are expressions. After 5 months, living and animate faces are clearly differentiated from solid dummies, even when the latter are moving. The uniqueness of individual faces is appreciated sometime around 6 to 7 months. And after 8 months, the infant's ability to differentiate faces is quite refined and specific.

AUDITORY PERCEPTION

The young infant's sensitivity to sound increases as a function of age. If one presents a sound to the 3-

month-old at the same loudness necessary to evoke a response from the neonate, he would be distressed. Also with increasing motor control, the infant is able to move his head around, scanning the environment for information about sound localization. Normal values for auditory threshold as well as sound-localization ability during the first year are given in Table 7-1.

SPEECH PERCEPTION

Until very recently little attention was paid to the fairly sophisticated perception which must precede the production of language in the young child. However, the flurry of studies that have been stimulated by the recent focus on perception have not been systematic; nor have they been guided by any specific theory of speech perception. Aside from these shortcomings, the studies have demonstrated two important things: first, that the growing infant is very sensitive to the phonemic contrasts of speech and, second, that infants have listening preferences which change with age as the infant's abilities increase.

In addition to listening to the speech sounds of others, the infant soon begins to monitor his own vocalizations which, in some form or another, he has been making since birth. In the neonatal period, these vocalizations are described as chirps, but by 1 month they begin to sound like cooing and later like babbling. These early sounds are apparently not tied into the auditory feedback system yet as the same kind of vocalizations are found in otherwise-normal deaf infants until 5 or 6 months of age, at which time the deaf infant stops babbling. The normal-hearing infant on the other hand begins to show at this time elementary control of rhythm, intonation, and duration, as well as control of the frequency range of sounds.

Although all the data are not yet complete, it seems fairly clear that by the end of the first year the infant can discriminate all the significant phonemic features of his language. For it is at this time that his first meaningful word is uttered, and that achievement takes much careful listening.

OTHER SENSES

There have been few studies of the changes, if any, in the other senses of the infant during the first year of life. However, it can be observed that the first year of life is increasingly characterized by oral and manual exploration of the environment. Objects are placed in the mouth for exploration by the richly innervated lips and tongue. Tactile feedback, along with vision, directs and refines pre-

TABLE 7-1 Normal values for auditory threshold and sound localization

Age, months	Threshold, dB	Localization ability
3–4	50–60	Begins to turn head to the side at which the sound is heard
4–7	40–50	Turns head directly toward the side of a signal but cannot locate a sound above or below
7–9	30–40	Directly locates a sound source to the side and indirectly below
9–13	25–35	Directly locates a sound source to the side and below

hension skills. Tactile stimulation, proprioception, and kinesthesia are gained from the infant's gross motor activity. Through this feedback, movements are adjusted and repeated. These sensations, along with vestibular input, direct gross and fine motor development.

A Russian investigator reported that both cold and warm stimuli showed broad generalization gradients, and infants even up to 6 months of age had difficulty differentiating among thermal stimuli (Kessen, Haith, and Salapatek, 1970). A rare study on the vestibular system examined the effective parameters of vestibular stimulation on the activity of the 2-month-old infant (Peterson and TerVrugt, 1973). They found infants were quieted most by maximum acceleration. That is, high-frequency and high-amplitude rocking had the most effect on decreasing activity.

EFFECTS OF EXPERIENCE ON PERCEPTION

What information we have on the importance of experience in perceptual development comes from two kinds of studies: enrichment and deprivation. In most instances, data come from animal studies, particularly in the case of deprivation studies. In such studies, one hopes to determine (1) if altering the environment will have a specific effect on perceptual development, (2) if there are critical periods for the effect, and (3) what, if any, are the long-term consequences.

ENRICHMENT

Many of the enrichment studies, particularly those with animals, have failed to specify the nature of the enhanced sensory information to which the subjects have been exposed. And indeed, there is some question as to whether the environment from the animal's point of view is even enriched. Thus, one must be cautious generalizing from the results of these animal studies to the human situation.

A series of studies done by White (1971) in which he provided massive stimulation to infants born and reared in an institution found some evidence that exploratory behavior and visual attention were facilitated. One group of infants who were only given 20 min a day of extra handling later were found to be more visually attentive than a control group. Another group at 37 days had pacifiers surrounded by a red and white pattern mounted on their cribs, and at 68 days a multicolored stabile was suspended above the cribs. This group developed sustained hand regard at the same age as the control group. However, the enriched group achieved skilled reaching earlier than the controls and also showed more consistent visual attention. Gibson (1969), in reviewing White's studies, concluded that there was little evidence to support the idea that perceptual development could be speeded up by sensory enrichment.

DEPRIVATION STUDIES

According to the results of a number of animal studies, rearing in a barren, unchanging environment does appear to affect perceptual development. The effect, however, is not a specific deficit but rather a maladaption of attention and of perceptual motivation. However, in several studies in which self-produced movement was restricted in the presence of pattern stimuli, depth and movement perception were found to be impaired (Pick and Pick, 1970). If the visual system is deprived of light for a sufficient length of time, neural degeneration occurs.

Additional insights regarding the effects of sensory deprivation on perceptual development have been gained from careful observation of those with congenital deficits. Fraiberg (1977), in a longitudinal study of 10 blind but neurologically intact infants, made some interesting observations about the importance of vision for gross motor development. Her blind infants did not smile as much as their sighted counterparts. All of them were delayed in crawling because in the absence of a visual stimulus there is not a strong incentive for the infant to creep. Ironically, the blind child who needs the augmented sound and tactile experiences which mobility would bring to construct his world is motorically delayed. Fraiberg concluded that it was not blindness alone that imperiled the infant but the effect of the visual deficit upon other modalities that must serve adaptation. Fraiberg's blind infants were also delayed in sound localization ability and in the development of language.

Congenital deafness can have an equally devastating effect on the child's development. If a child is to acquire language, he must be able to hear in order to monitor his attempts at vocalization. Therefore it is imperative that children with a hearing loss be detected early so that remediation with amplification, if practical, can be instituted. For in audition there is some evidence for critical, or sensitive, periods, that is, a limited period of time in which stimulation is necessary if a skill is to develop normally. For language, the period appears to be the first 2 years of life.

Gross motor development Fay F. Russell and Beverly R. Richardson

At no other time in his life does a human being experience a faster rate of progression in gross motor development than in the period of infancy. During this period, the infant attains those skills basic to all future gross motor functioning.

NEUROLOGICAL MATURATION AND CHANGES IN REFLEX PATTERNS

Fundamental to this skill development is neurological maturation. Specific changes in this area which influence acquisition of these skills include changes in the reflexive patterns demonstrated by the infant and the continuation of the process of myelinization.

INTEGRATION OF PRIMITIVE REFLEXES

By the end of the first year most primitive reflexes demonstrated by the neonate have been integrated and, consequently, can no longer be elicited. For example, the crossed-extensor reflex may disappear as early as the end of the first month of life; if not, however, it should not persist beyond the end of the second month, which also marks the end of the normal duration of the withdrawal reflex. The positive supporting reaction and trunk-incurvation (Galant's) reflex disappear around the second or third postnatal month.

The asymmetrical tonic neck reflex and stepping reaction do not normally persist beyond the third or fourth month, and the tonic labyrinthine reflex is also normally integrated by the end of the fourth month. During the fourth to sixth months, the Moro reflex should disappear, and the traction response becomes voluntary.

The plantar grasp reflex should be integrated between the eighth and twelfth months; the neck-righting reflex

378 THE INFANT: 1 MONTH TO 12 MONTHS

disappears by the ninth or tenth month and the placing reactions by the tenth to twelfth month. The only neonatal reflex which may persist beyond 12 months without being considered abnormal is the Babinski reflex, which may be elicited until the child is 12 to 18 months of age. The effects of these and other reflexive changes are discussed below.

As the above reflexes are integrated, several new ones emerge. The *Landau reflex* emerges between the third and sixth months and may persist until the infant is 12 to 24 months of age. This reflex is responsible for the infant's extending his legs and spine when he is suspended horizontally in a prone position with his head raised either actively or passively; conversely, he flexes his legs and spine when held in the same position with his head flexed against his chest (see Fig. 7-9). The symmetrical extension of his trunk and hips is believed by some to prepare the child for standing. Absence of this reflex may be associated with spinal cord abnormalities and labyrinthine defects, as in cerebral palsy.

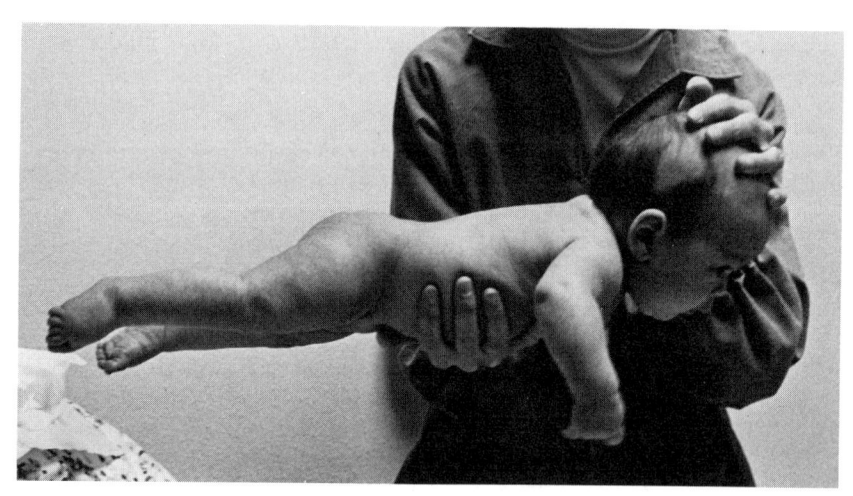

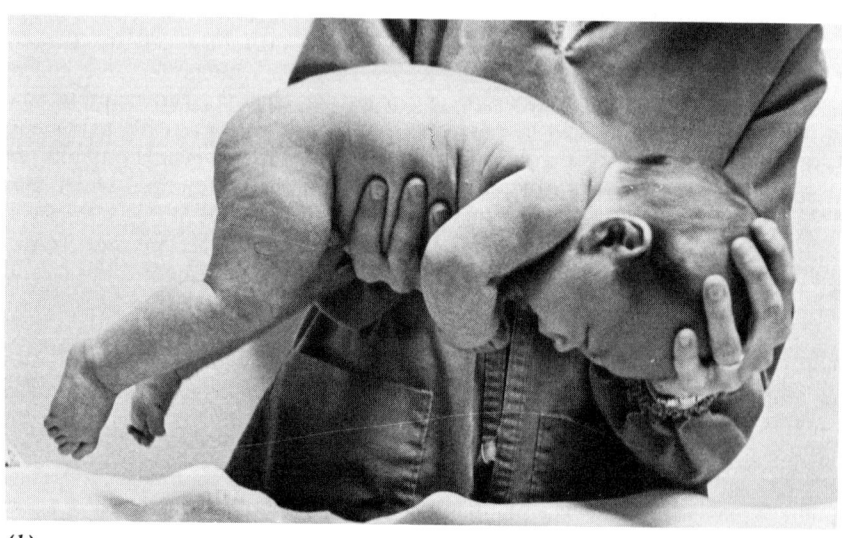

FIGURE 7-9. The Landau reflex showing (*a*) leg and spine extension with extension of the neck and (*b*) leg and spine flexion with neck flexion.

EMERGENCE OF POSTURAL REFLEXES

During infancy, several automatic, or postural, reflexes emerge at the same time that the primitive reflexes disappear (see Fig. 7-10). These reflexes are involved with righting, protective, and equilibrium reactions of the infant. The righting reactions enable the infant to roll from prone to supine and supine to prone, get on his hands and knees, sit, restore the normal position of his head in space, and maintain the proper postural relation between his head, trunk, and extremities during motor activities. Included among these righting reflexes are the labyrinthine righting reaction on the head, the optical righting reaction, and the body-righting reactions.

The labyrinthine righting reaction on the head emerges around the second month when the infant, suspended horizontally in prone and blindfolded, is able to raise his head so that his face is in a vertical position. When the infant is approximately 6 months of age, he is able to lift his head in the same manner when blindfolded and suspended horizontally in a supine position. Finally, between 6 and 8 months of age, the infant is able to right his head so that again his face is in a vertical position when he is blindfolded, held upright, and tilted to one side. This reaction persists throughout life with the response gradually becoming voluntary.

The optical righting reaction appears soon after the labyrinthine righting reaction on the head and enables the infant to lift his head in the same manner when placed in the same position *without* being blindfolded. He can lift his head so that his face is in a vertical position when suspended in a prone position when he is approximately 2 months old, when suspended in a supine position when he is approximately 6 months old, and when held vertically and tilted to one side when he is 6 to 8 months old. This reaction persists throughout life and increases in importance as the role of vision increases in maintaining the normal position of the head and body (see Fig. 7-11).

Body-righting reaction on the head usually appears about the sixth month and results in righting of the head when some part of the infant's body touches a firm surface. This reflex interacts with the labyrinthine righting reaction on the head to ensure maintenance of normal position of the head in space. The reflex persists with the response gradually becoming voluntary.

Body-righting reaction on the body modifies the neck-righting reflex and allows rotation of the trunk between the shoulders and pelvis to occur. Whereas previously the infant's body turned as a whole in response to an active or passive turning of his head, log rolling, the body-righting reaction, enables him to turn segmentally with one portion of his body initiating the movement and the others following. This reflex also appears about the sixth month and persists with the response gradually becoming voluntary. Trunk rotation is essential for normal movement patterns such as getting to sitting and walking.

Protective reflexes are reflexive attempts by the infant to

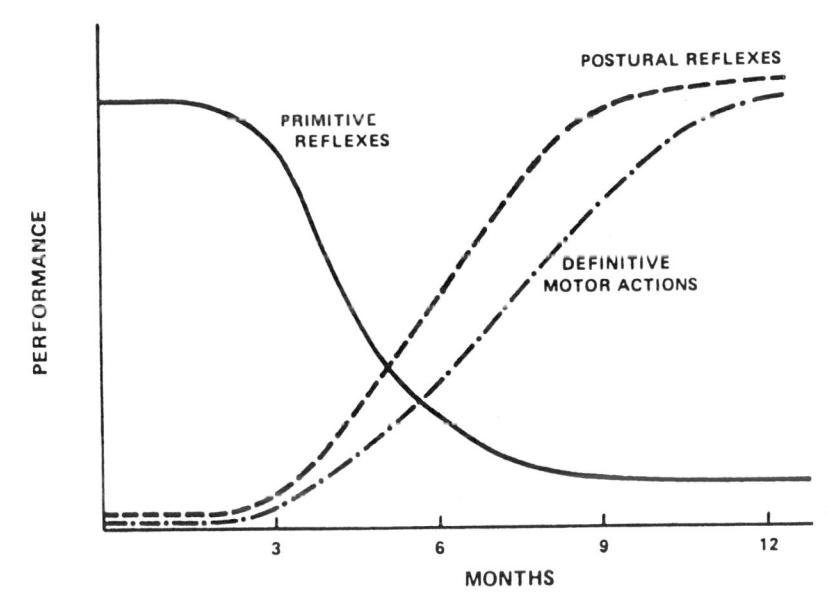

FIGURE 7-10. Reflex curves showing the declining intensity of primitive reflexes and increasing strength of postural reflexes and definitive motor actions (skills). [From A. J. Caputo, P. J. Accardo, E. P. G. Vining, J. E. Rubenstein, and S. Harryman, *Primitive reflex profile. Monographs in Developmental Pediatrics* (Vol. 1). Baltimore: University Park Press, 1978, p. 10. Reprinted by permission of University Park Press.]

break a fall. The parachute reaction and the protective extension (propping) reactions are important protective reflexes.

The *parachute reaction* appears at about 7 to 9 months and is elicited by suspending the infant horizontally in the prone position and suddenly thrusting him downward. The infant responds by extending his hands and arms as if to protect himself. This response normally persists throughout life. An asymmetrical response may suggest an orthopedic or neuromuscular disorder.

Protective extension, or *propping, reactions* enable the child to sit supporting his weight on his arms in order to prevent falling. The infant is able to support himself in this position with his arms extended forward at 6 months of age, sideways at 8 months of age, and backward at 10 months of age (see Fig. 7-12). These reactions also normally persist throughout life.

Equilibrium reactions enable the infant to maintain a given posture independent of mild changes in his position. These reactions begin appearing about the fourth to sixth month and are gradually perfected over the next few years. Equilibrium reactions appear for prone, supine, sitting, kneeling, standing, and walking in this order with the reaction for each position appearing around the time the infant attains the next skill. For example, equilibrium reactions appear in sitting around the time the infant begins to kneel. These reactions, too, persist throughout life.

In summary, the automatic responses of righting, protective, and equilibrium reactions are a group of reflexes which emerge primarily during the first postnatal year and which are vital to development of gross motor skills because of their influence on balance, coordination, and movement. The effects of these and other reflexive changes are discussed below.

GROSS MOTOR SKILL DEVELOPMENT

As stated above, skill development during infancy is dependent on maturation of the nervous and musculoskeletal systems. The maturational changes of reflex behavior have been investigated; now, the effects of these changes in terms of gross motor skill development will be considered.

HEAD CONTROL

In the prone position, the neonate can lift his head only slightly and intermittently and turn it to one side. The infant, however, demonstrates great strides in achieving and maintaining control of his head. At about 8 weeks of age the infant lifts his head so that the plane of his face is at a 45° angle to the surface on which he is lying. Rewarded by visual experiences and with strength resulting from practice, the infant lifts his head so that his chin and shoulders do not touch the surface; by 12 weeks he can maintain this position for several seconds.

Prone position soon becomes a favorite, and the 16-week-old infant lifts his head and chest so that the plane of his face is at a 90° angle to the surface. By 20 weeks he lifts his head and chest and supports his weight on his

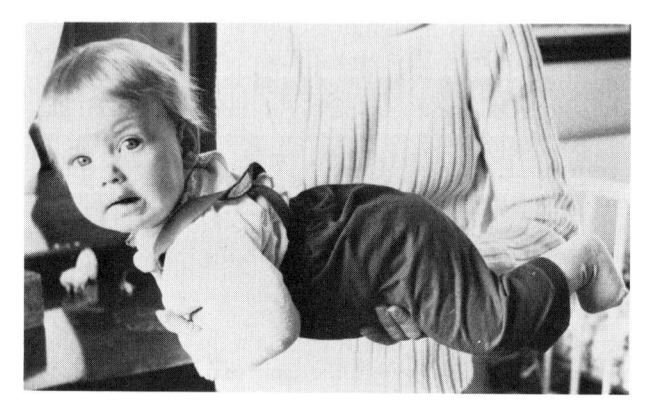

(a)

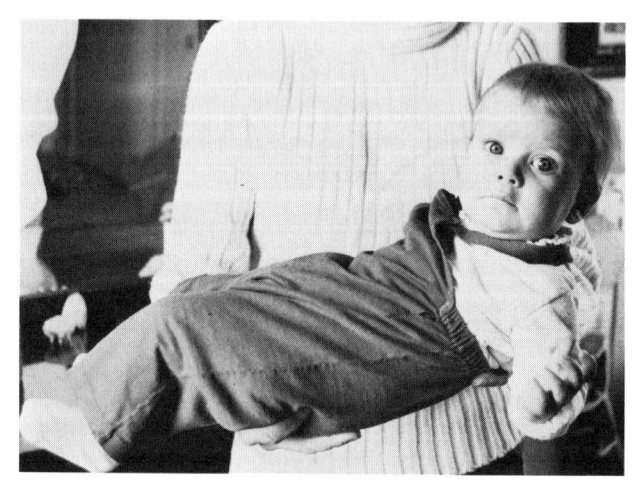

(b)

FIGURE 7-11. The optical righting reflex. (*a*) Prone; (*b*) supine; (*c*) tilted in vertical suspension.

(c)

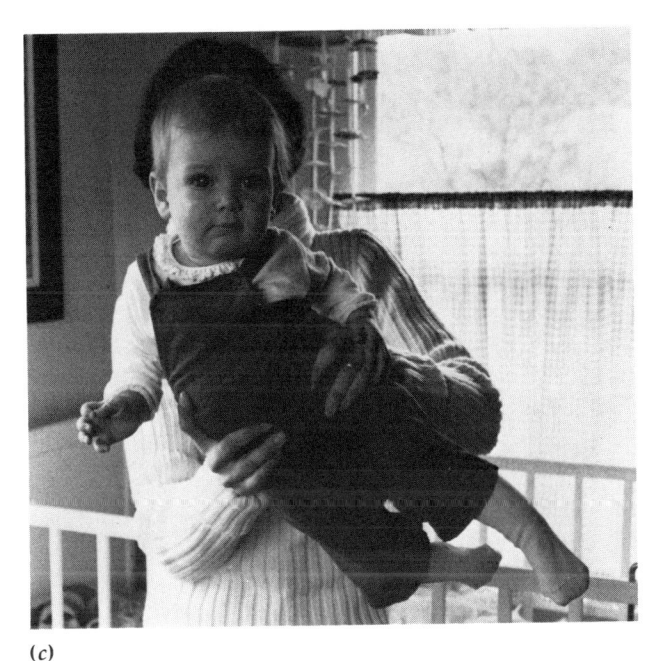

FIGURE 7-11. (*Continued*)

forearms, requiring extension of the trunk and upper extremities. Finally, at about 24 weeks, full head control in prone is exhibited as the infant lifts his head, chest, and upper abdomen and supports his weight on his palms with his arms fully extended (see Fig. 7-13).

This progression is assisted by the emergence of the labyrinthine righting reaction on the head and the disappearance of the tonic labyrinthine and asymmetrical tonic neck reflexes. The emergence of the Landau reflex assists the infant in developing the ability to extend his trunk and extremities.

In addition to developing the ability to lift his head in prone, the infant also develops the ability to lift his head in supine. As discussed above, the neonate's head still lags at 4 weeks of age. However, the infant demonstrates great strides in achieving and maintaining control of his head in supine (see Fig. 7-14). At 12 weeks of age, the infant lifts his head with only slight head lag when pulled to a sitting position. By 16 weeks of age, he lifts his head with only a slight head lag upon initiation of movement. The infant lifts his head with no head lag when pulled to sitting at 20 weeks of age. Finally, full head control in supine is evidenced as the infant lifts his head spontaneously when he is about to be pulled to sitting at 24 weeks of age. The infant can be observed to lift his head in supine spontaneously at 28 weeks.

This progress, as with head control in prone, is contributed to by emergence of the labyrinthine righting reaction on the head and disappearance of the tonic labyrinthine and asymmetrical tonic neck reflexes. The ability to lift his head in prone and supine is the first critical step in development of the ability to sit and stand.

Disappearance of the tonic labyrinthine and asymmetrical tonic neck reflexes and emergence of the Landau reflex also assist the infant in the attainment of reaching. Reaching is initially a whole-arm movement originating from the shoulder. Later reaching is refined to elbow, wrist, and finger movement. These skills are discussed in detail in "Fine Motor Development."

TRUNK CONTROL

Rolling Using the head control recently attained, the infant develops the ability to roll from a prone to a supine position and vice versa (see Fig. 7-15). At 4 weeks the infant turns from supine to side lying by turning his head with the neck-righting reflex causing his trunk to follow. Later, the entire sequence is voluntary. At 8 weeks of age the infant turns from a prone position to a side-lying position. Finally, at 5 to 7 months, the infant, by first raising his head, rolls from prone to supine and then from supine to prone. Good head control is essential to the normal sequence of rolling.

Development of this skill is also assisted by emergence of the labyrinthine righting reaction on the head and the body-righting reaction and disappearance of the tonic labyrinthine and asymmetrical tonic neck reflexes. As the infant's skill in rolling improves, he uses more and more trunk rotation and can stop his rolling progress at any point, demonstrating equilibrium in prone and supine.

Sitting When held in a sitting position at 4 weeks of age, the neonate sits with his entire back rounded and his head erect only momentarily. The infant, however, progressing from a flexed to an extended posture in a cephalocaudal direction, gains head and trunk control in the upright position. He sits supported with his head erect but bobbing at about 8 weeks of age. At 16 weeks, the infant sits supported with his head steady but slightly forward and his upper back erect.

By 24 weeks he sits supported with his head steady and all but his lower back erect. By 6 months he can usually be

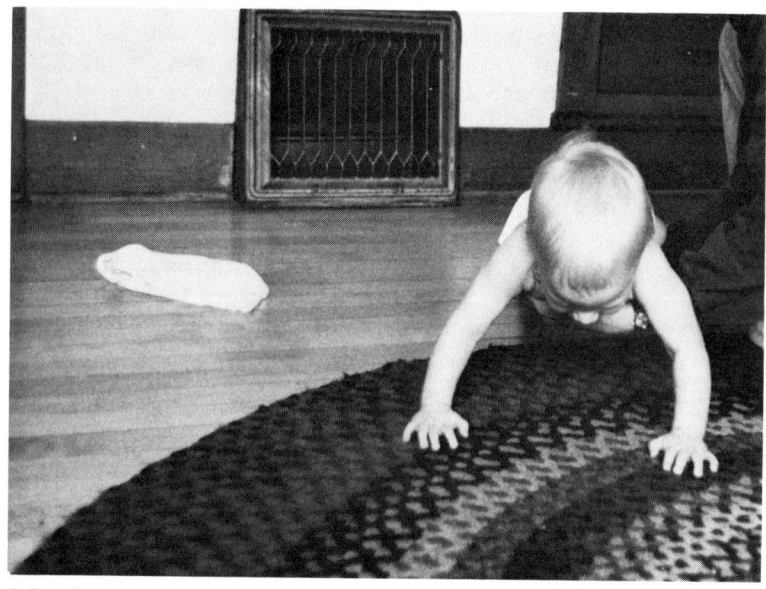

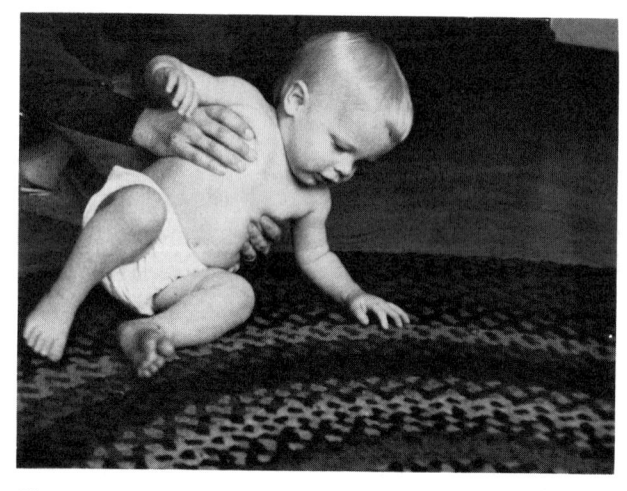

FIGURE 7-12. Protective extension. (a) Forward; (b) to the side.

safely propped in the corner of a chair, and he sits in a high chair. Soon afterward, at 6 to 7 months, the infant will sit unsupported with his arms propped forward and even sits erect momentarily. By 8 to 9 months of age he will sit erect without support and lean forward without losing his balance for several minutes. With a fully extended back and good equilibrium in sitting, the infant of 10 to 12 months can sit, rotate, and pivot without losing his balance (see Fig. 7-16). The infant delights in his newly acquired skill of sitting independently and strongly resists being laid down, even for quick diaper changes. In sitting his arms are free for play and his eyes

BEHAVIORAL DEVELOPMENT **383**

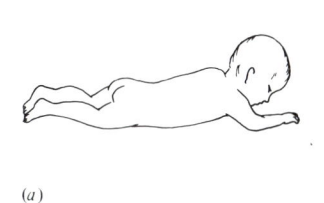

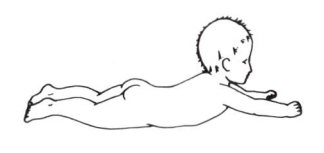

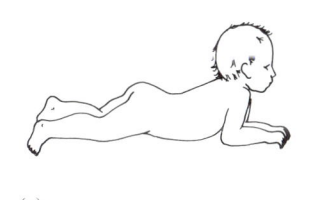

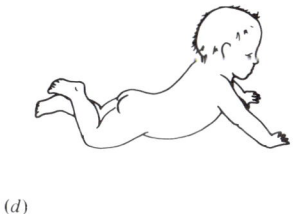

FIGURE 7-13. Progressive head control. (*a*) 8 weeks, 45°; (*b*) 16 weeks, 90°; (*c*) 20 weeks, propped on forearms; (*d*) 24 weeks, arms extended, weight on palms.

can quickly scan his surroundings.

Presence of the labyrinthine righting reaction on the head and the body-righting reaction enables the infant to maintain an upright posture while protective extension reactions counteract any abrupt changes in position and the equilibrium reactions counteract any subtle changes in position. Development of this skill is also assisted by disappearance of the tonic labyrinthine and asymmetrical tonic neck reflexes and emergence of the Landau reflex.

CRAWLING AND CREEPING

Crawling is generally accepted to mean reciprocal arm and leg mobility with the child's abdomen on the floor. Creeping is true four-point mobility with only hands and knees (or feet) on the floor (see Fig. 7-17). For either skill,

FIGURE 7-14. Progressive attainment of head and trunk control when pulled to sitting. (*a*) The neonate is unable to maintain his head in alignment with his trunk. (*b*) The infant of 16 to 20 weeks is able to maintain his head in alignment with his trunk when pulled to sitting. He cannot maintain an upright position, however. (*c*) By 28 weeks the infant anticipates coming to sitting by lifting his head in supine and using his trunk and legs to assist in coming to a sitting position. (*From M. B. McGraw, The neuromuscular maturation of the human infant. New York. Columbia, 1945. Reprinted by permission of Columbia University Press.*)

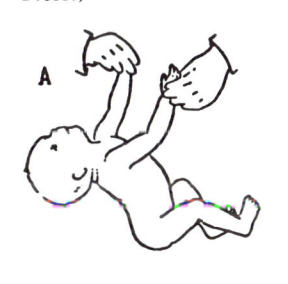

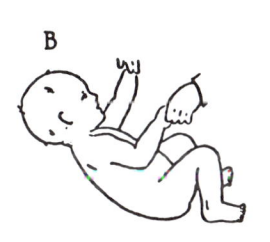

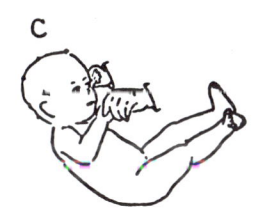

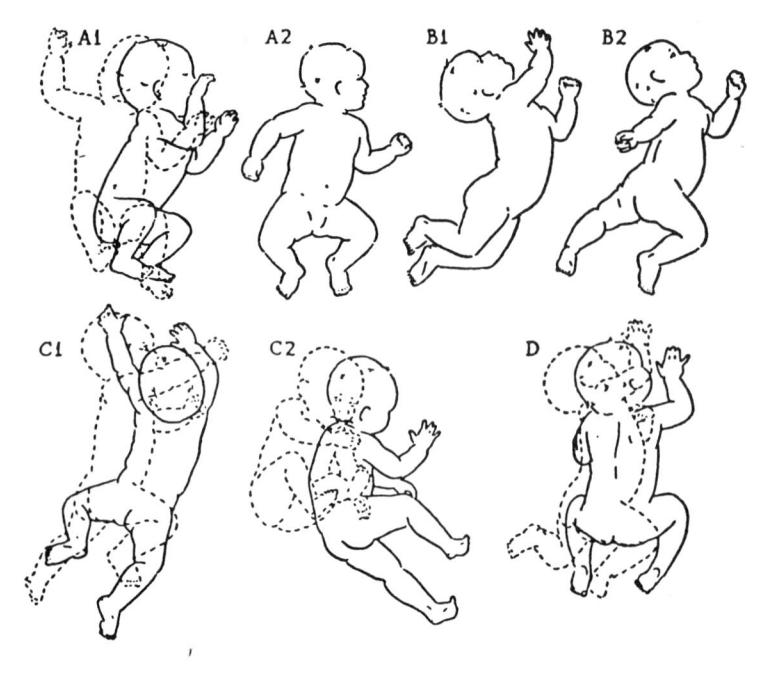

FIGURE 7-15. Four positions involved in rolling from supine to prone: (*a*) The neonate appears to roll from back to side with random movements. (*a2*) The neonate will turn his head to one side as an isolated movement not involving the rest of his body. (*b*) The 1-month-old extends his neck after turning his head to the side. The extremities on the top are then brought over. (*b1*) Initially the shoulder girdle leads. (*b2*) Later the initial movement may be in the pelvic region, throwing the leg over. (*c*) Automatic rolling: 28 to 34 weeks, with (*c1*) spinal extension or (*c2*) spinal and leg flexion. The infant uses no caution in executing the automatic roll. (*d*) Deliberate rolling: 42 to 52 weeks. The child rolls over as part of a deliberate performance. As soon as he turns he goes into creeping or sitting. (*From M. B. McGraw, 1945, p. 45. By permission of Columbia University Press.*)

reciprocal movement of arms and legs is important, although variations of movement are seen.

There is some disagreement as to when the infant achieves these skills. Crawling begins with reciprocal kicking movements at about 12 weeks of age. Later, at about 7 to 8 months of age, the infant crawls backward on his abdomen accidently; soon afterward he crawls forward on his abdomen. Often the child uses one arm to pull himself along. The infant will get up on his hands and knees and rock, experimenting with posture change and equilibrium on all fours. But he often plops down to his abdomen to make actual progress forward and then gets up on all fours again once he has stopped. Finally, feeling more secure, he creeps on his hands and knees with his abdomen up at 10 to 11 months of age with movement of his arms and legs gradually becoming smoothly and consistently reciprocal.

Reciprocal limb movements in crawling and resulting trunk flexibility and rotation are important for the pattern of walking. Emergence of the equilibrium reactions and disappearance of the asymmetrical tonic neck and tonic labyrinthine reflexes as well as positive supporting reflexes assist the infant in development of crawling and creeping. The infant becomes quicker and more flexible in his creeping and soon creeps as fast as others walk. He can look over his shoulder as he creeps, creep with one or both legs extended in a hands-feet fashion, and creep backward or forward with his head down. There is no end to his experimentation and versatility. Knees of coveralls and tops of shoes are quickly worn through.

TRANSITION SKILLS
Gross motor skills that enable a child to get from one major position to another are often overlooked. However, without these transition skills, the infant is less than fully functional. Equilibrium and trunk flexibility or rotation are essential for these skills. At about 8 to 10 months, the infant goes from sitting to prone. He first props forward on his extended arms (as he often did in early sitting), and then with one leg flexed he shifts his weight forward and lands prone. Later, at about 10 to 12 months of age, he reverses the process. He moves from prone to all fours by backing up with his arms over a flexed leg and then can drop into sitting (see Fig. 7-18).

By 12 months the infant is expertly moving from sitting to a creeping or prone position and back. Often he will stop somewhere in between and, like the amateur acrobat he is, experiment with his balance reactions. The ability

BEHAVIORAL DEVELOPMENT **385**

(a)

(b)

(c)

(d)

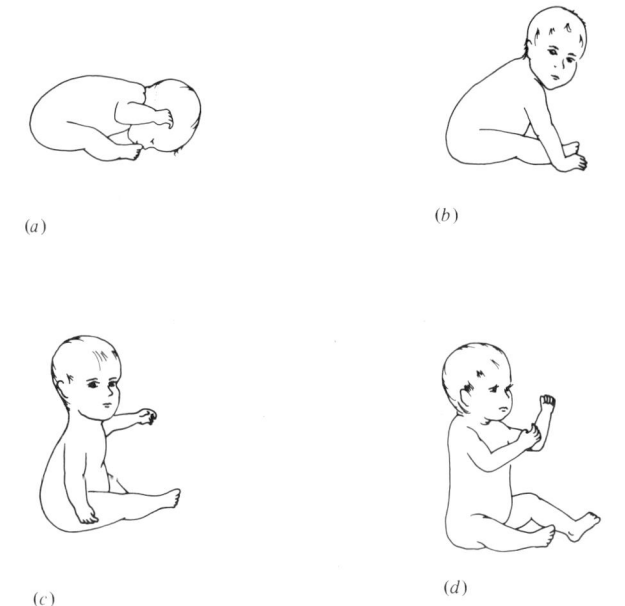

FIGURE 7-16. Progressive head and trunk control in sitting posture in a cephalocaudal direction. (*a*) The neonate has a fully rounded back in sitting. By 8 weeks the infant can lift his head erect in sitting but it will bob up and down. At 4 months the upper back is erect and at 6 months all but the lower back is erect. (*b*) By 6 to 7 months the infant can sit unsupported propped forward on his arms. (*c*) By 8 to 9 months sitting balance, protective extension, and equilibrium improve allowing the child to sit erect with only the lower back rounded. (*d*) Fully erect sitting is achieved by 10 to 12 months. (*Adapted from M. B. McGraw, 1945, p. 64. Used by permission of Columbia University Press.*)

to move into and out of these positions makes them truly functional for the infant. Later, the infant moves upward as he reaches and pulls himself to half-kneeling and kneeling and then to standing. Again, with practice, he soon becomes expert in moving from an upright to a sitting position and back.

STANDING
In developing the ability to stand, the infant of 6 months bears a large fraction of his weight on his extended legs. At about 10 months he can achieve and maintain a kneeling position largely by pulling with his arms and to a lesser extent by reciprocally "walking" forward on his knees. He can also move sideways on his knees along a piece of furniture. Much of the infant's interest is now focused upward, reinforcing his drive to stand and walk. His parents are learning to place untouchables higher than was previously necessary.

By 9 to 10 months the infant pulls to stand and stands holding on. His toes are clenched in the standing position as if to grip the surface. Thus, bare feet or thin slippers are least inhibiting to him. This correlates with disappearance of the Babinski reflex. By 12 months he stands for a few minutes without holding on with his hands. Unsure of himself, he will often lean his trunk against the object he used to pull to stand. As he perfects this skill, he uses his arms less and his legs more.

Protective and equilibrium reactions assist the infant in developing this skill while persistence of the asymmetrical tonic neck and tonic labyrinthine reflexes along with a strong positive supporting reaction would interfere.

WALKING
While the infant does not typically develop the ability to walk well independently by 12 months, he does attain skills basic to independent walking. For example, at 10 months he will walk with two hands held. He also will independently cruise (sidestep) the length of a piece of furniture. These two ways of walking are different in form. The first is a high-stepping, forward movement of his feet. The second is a slide-stepping to the side. Neither allows full use of the arms for balance and protective extension.

By about 12 months, the infant has sufficient upright balance to walk with one hand held. As in development of the ability to stand, the ability to walk is assisted by the emergence of the protective and equilibrium reactions and the disappearance of the asymmetrical tonic neck and tonic labyrinthine reflexes and the positive supporting reflexes.

Once the infant begins to move from creeping to learning to walk, the sequence of skills usually evolves quickly. Some children, however, are happy moving from standing holding on and cruising back to creeping. Others give up creeping almost immediately after discovering upright mobility, and they walk soon after learning to pull to stand. No doubt coaxing from parents has an effect on the infant's desire and opportunities to practice walking.

The infant demonstrates remarkable progress in gross motor development, not only in terms of the multiplicity of skills he acquires, but also in the nature of these skills. Whereas much of the gross motor behavior of the neonate is simple, generalized, and random, gross motor behavior of the infant is progressively more complex, specific, and purposeful. The infant demonstrates the extension pattern and cephalocaudal development as he progresses from

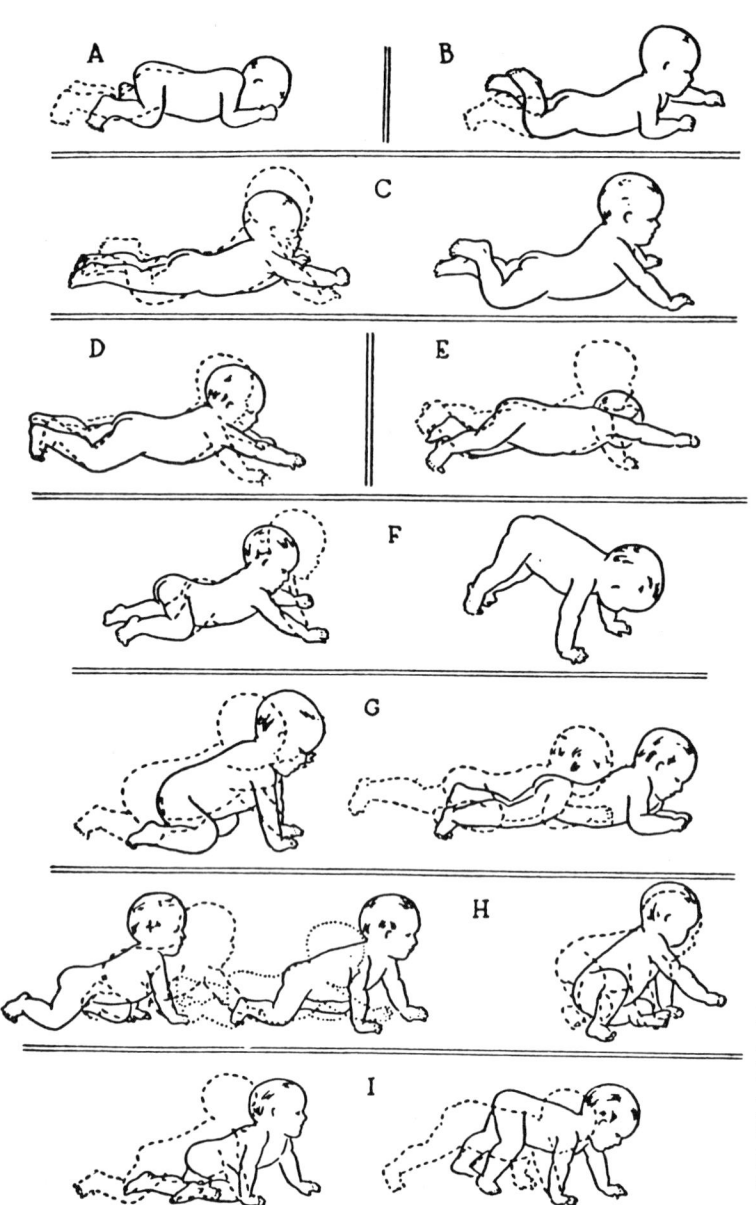

FIGURE 7-17. Nine phases in development of prone progression. (a) The neonate assumes a flexed posture. Rapid bilateral or alternating flexor-extensor leg movements are present, probably due to lack of inhibition from cortical centers. (b) Beginning spinal extension (10 to 14 weeks). (c) Advanced spinal extension (18 to 22 weeks); the infant can easily raise and lower his upper body. (d) Attempt at propulsion using the upper body (22 to 28 weeks). (e) The lower body begins more active involvement in the attempt to move forward (22 to 28 weeks). (f) The infant practices attaining the creeping posture (28 to 34 weeks). (g) Deliberate but unorganized forward progression using all of body (32 to 36 weeks). (h) Organized creeping progression in a contralateral pattern of hands and knees (8 to 10 months). Some infants creep on their bottom. (i) Integrated creeping progression, smoothly coordinated (10 to 14 months). (*From M. B. McGraw, 1945, p. 51. Reprinted by permission of Columbia University Press.*)

lifting his head to sitting, reaching, and creeping and then to pulling to a standing position and cruising. He demonstrates ventrodorsal progression as he pulls himself to sitting before he can sit well unsupported and proximodistal progression as he reaches and misses before he reaches and makes contact. The conclusion of the period of infancy marks the end of the most dramatic progress the child will experience in gross motor development.

Fine motor development
Barbara Newcomer McLaughlin and Nancy L. Morgan

Fine motor ability during the first year proceeds at an accelerated rate as maturation and exploration give rise to highly individual, coordinated, functional patterns. One of the special developmental tasks of infancy is the ability to reach with the hand, grasp, and manipulate objects in the environment. Eye-hand coordination is essential as prehensile ability develops. Reaching must be visually guided, and the visual portion of the pattern, possible through maturation and exercise of the visual mechanism for space perception, is preliminary to the actual grasp of an object (Stott, 1974).

Fine motor development is based upon the grasp reflex, but voluntary movements begin to replace this reflexive behavior. The young infant's fine motor ability soon develops to the point that he can purposefully get his hand to his mouth, and he engages in clutching and scratching movements. Also, the infant begins to reach to the sides of his body, a preliminary step to being able to reach forward. The infant progresses to reaching and grasping as the uncoordinated movements of the hand and arm begin to diminish.

The age of exploration with eyes, fingers, hands, and mouth begins; the infant can hold and manipulate objects, and his hands appear coordinated in this process. The ability to use both hands equally well, to examine toys, and to learn about objects with the mouth is characteristic, as coordination and curiosity have increased. Soon the infant is able to pick up small objects with finger motions as opposed to using his entire hand. Thus, by 12 months of age, the infant is skillfully manipulating his environment.

1 TO 6 MONTHS

Fine motor development in the neonatal period is characterized by the grasp reflex and the predominantly closed position of the hands. At 8 weeks the hands are often open or loosely closed (see Fig. 7-19). By 12 weeks, the infant looks as if he would like to grasp an object held out to him. He will grasp the object placed in his hand; however, he soon drops it. Grasp should be equal bilaterally.

The asymmetrical tonic neck reflex is diminishing by 16 weeks, though it has served the important function of channeling the visual pathways from fleeting periods on the extended arm to more prolonged inspections of the

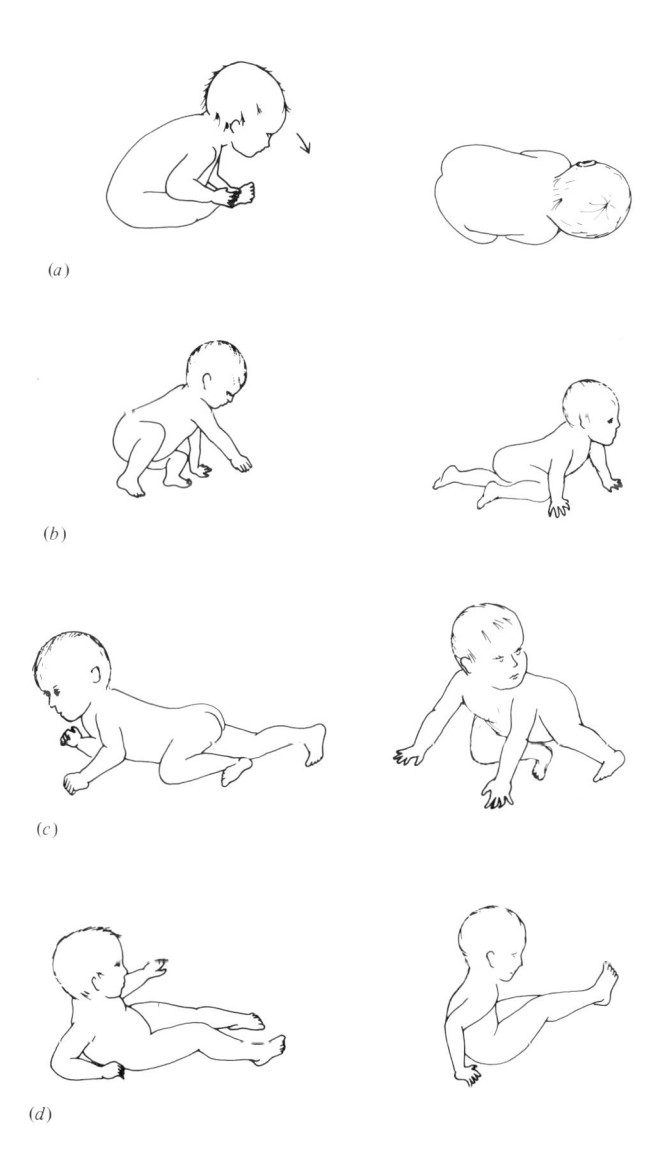

FIGURE 7-18. Transition movements. (*a*) Initially the infant moves from sitting to prone by falling forward and to the side. (*b*) Later, increased trunk control and integration of protective extension of the arms results in the infant moving smoothly from sitting to prone or all fours. (*c*) The infant moves to sitting by pushing up from the prone position over his legs (ventral push). (*d*) The child will get to sitting from supine pushing off with one arm (dorsal push). (*Adapted from M. B. McGraw, pp. 64 and 51. Used by permission of Columbia University Press.*)

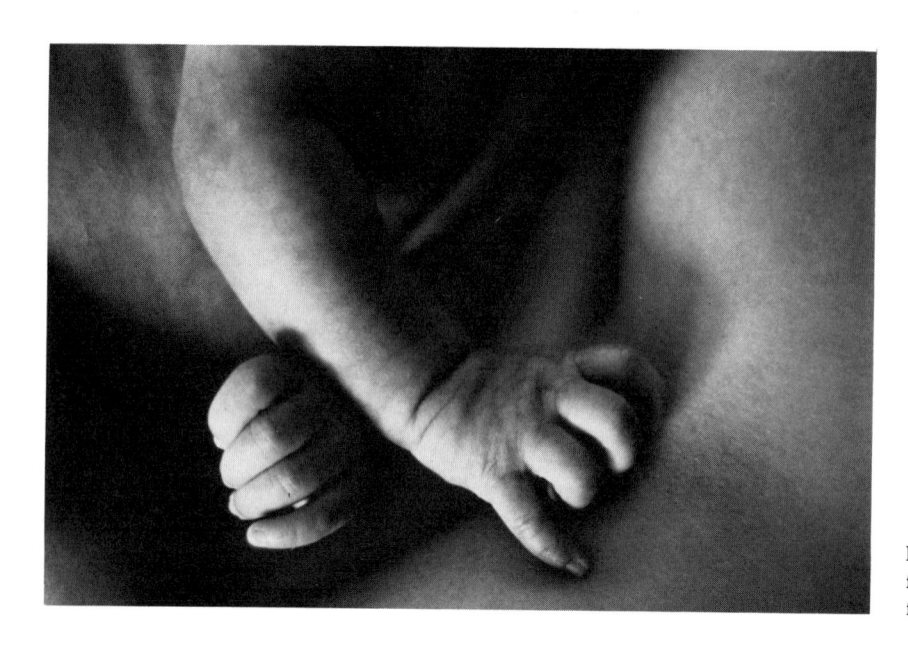

FIGURE 7-19. The 1-month-old infant's hands are more open, not tightly fisted like the neonate's.

FIGURE 7-20. (a) The 3-month-old visually "grasps" the mobile and then (b) observes her hands, which are together at midline. Soon swiping and grasping skills emerge. (*Photos courtesy of Betsy Smith.*)

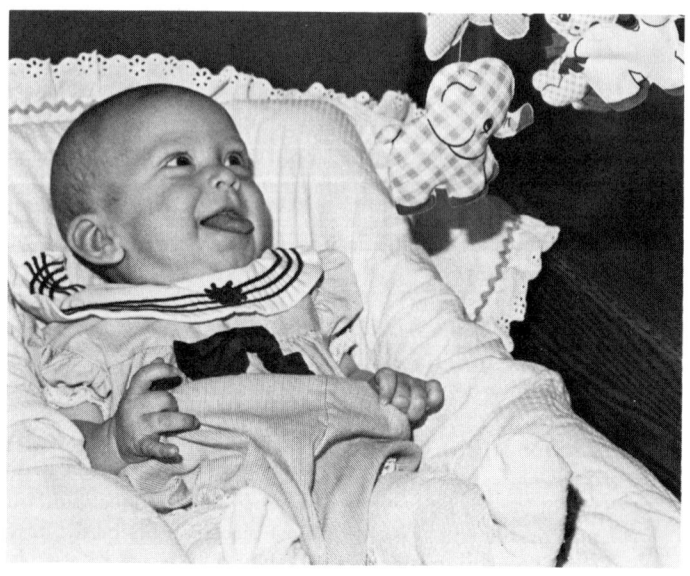

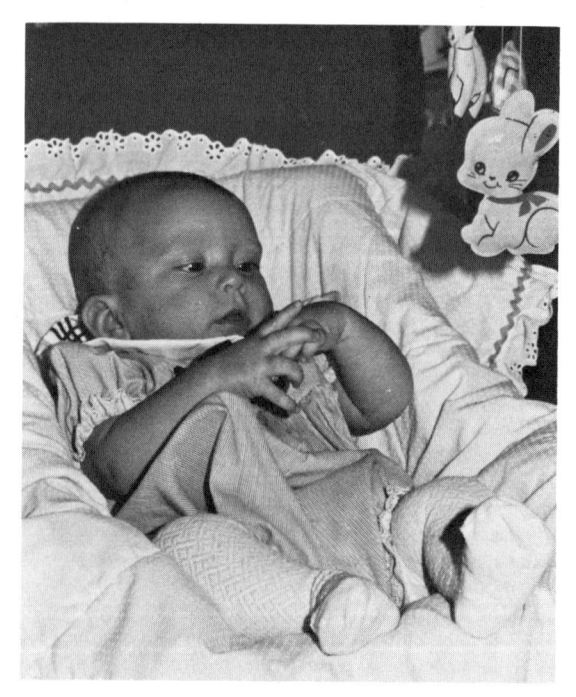

(a)

(b)

hand. The hands come together, and the infant tries to reach for objects but usually overshoots the target.

The infant is soon ready to grasp an object on visual cue, as now his free hand will come toward the rattle in an attempt to grasp and manipulate it. Selectively the infant will regard, not only his own hands, but also those of an adult caring for him (see Fig. 7-20).

About 20 weeks of age, the ability to grasp becomes voluntary, and the infant exhibits a bidextrous approach to objects. He will begin by reaching out to objects in his view and batting them with circular movements. This action quickly progresses to taking objects that are touching or held near his hands. The infant explores objects held in his hands with his mouth and eagerly explores his toes with his fingers at every given opportunity. Activities to aid in natural exploration include selecting several objects that share the same general characteristics, such as being hard or soft, presenting them to him, and talking about the toys as he plays. The safety of objects is always important as the infant will inevitably put them in his mouth (Gesell et al., 1940; Gordon, 1970).

FIGURE 7-21. **The 8-month-old easily transfers, using a radial-digital grasp.**

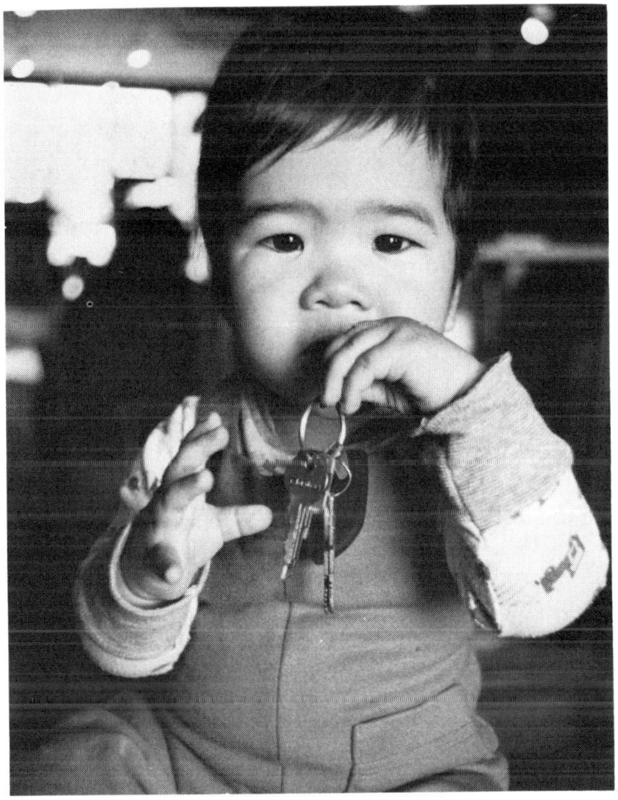

6 TO 12 MONTHS

By the time the infant has reached 6 months of age, he is able to hold his bottle independently, though it is still important for his social development to be held for feedings. He will repetitively shake and pound objects in the air and on a surface. The infant first develops a palmar grasp of smaller objects. At this point, the infant will drop one cube when offered another one due to the mirror function of the hands; one hand reaches, and the other opens, too, thus dropping the object. Opportunity to feel objects of varying textures is important as the infant continues to manipulate objects with his fingers and with his mouth.

At 6 to 7 months the infant is readily able to transfer objects from hand to hand as he reaches with one hand, obtains an object with a palmar grasp, and then transfers to the other hand (see Fig. 7-21). At first, the infant "pushes" the object into the other hand, which grasps the object. This is an early transfer versus a free transfer, which is a simultaneous release and grasp at a later stage. The infant is initially able to release onto a surface and later develops the ability to release in the air. He utilizes a unidextrous approach and is able to feed himself a cracker.

The infant is now able to retain one object when offered a second one. He sees a toy, grasps and clenches it, bangs it repetitively, brings it to his mouth, feels its characteristics, withdraws it and looks at it, rotates it as he continues to look, places it back in his mouth, and repeats the sequence (or variations thereof) numerous times. His fine motor behavior is full of versatility as objects in his reach are soon in his busy, busy hands. Practice in reaching and transferring a variety of objects is predominant at this stage as the infant picks up objects quickly and precisely (Gesell et al., 1940) (see Fig. 7-22).

The beginning of thumb finger apposition is the major characteristic of fine motor development around 9 to 10 months. The early thumb finger grasp, also termed the *lateral pinch*, marks the start of the ability to pick up objects with the fingers as opposed to the entire hand. At this point, the infant has a great deal of interest in tiny objects, and he is able to pick up a very small object between his thumb and finger.

The infant will go after and is able to retrieve a dropped toy and also delights in dropping toys for others to retrieve. Prehension skills at 9 months also include the ability to take one object in each hand and to bang them together at the midline, an important cognitive as well as fine motor milestone.

390 THE INFANT: 1 MONTH TO 12 MONTHS

(a)   *(b)*

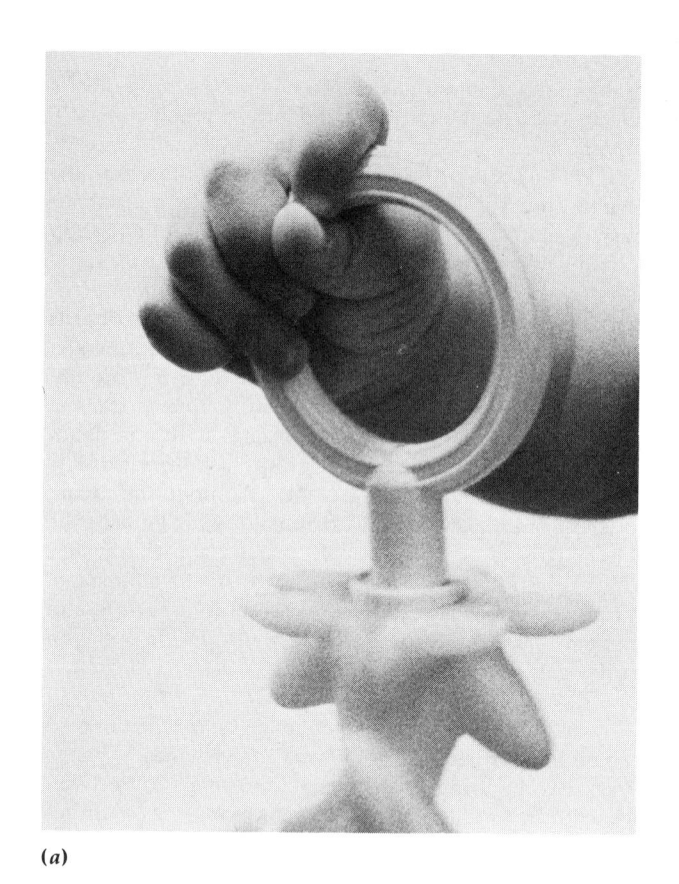

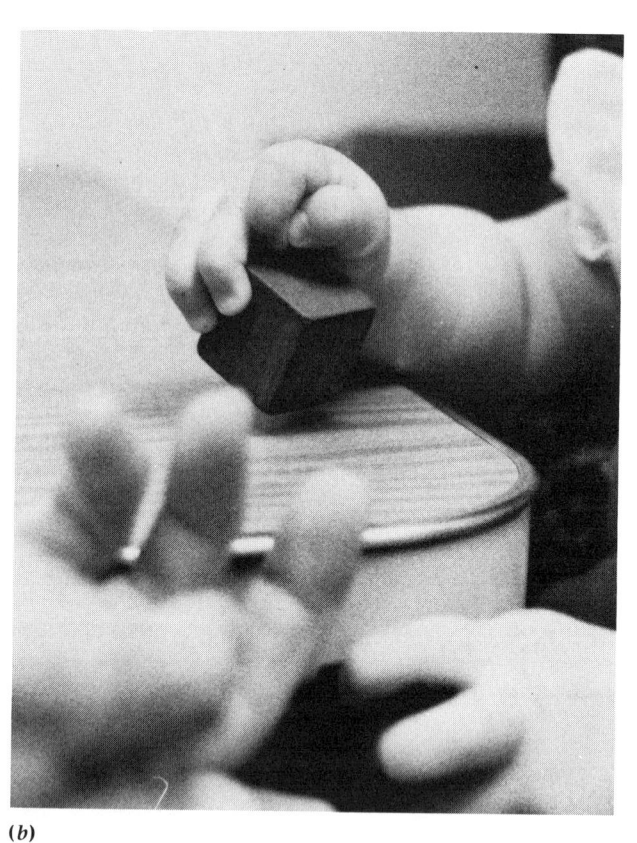

FIGURE 7-22. The sequence of prehension skills is demonstrated. *(a)* Whole-hand, active grasp, 3 to 4 months; *(b)* ulnar-palmar grasp, 4 to 6 months; *(c)* midpalmar grasp, 6 to 7 months; *(d)* radial-digital grasp, 7 to 8 months; *(e)* index finger approach and inferior pincer grasp, 9 to 10 months; *(f)* neat pincer grasp, 11 to 12 months.

At about 10 months of age, the infant engages in a probing behavior with his index finger. He displays a strong interest in detail and is able to isolate a single detail for his attention or to react successively to two details or objects. The continual palpation and prying with the index finger opens the world of dimension.

The infant has the ability to release objects, though he will usually offer an object to another person and not release it. It is important for the infant to have a variety of objects with detail to explore; however, it is essential that small pieces or parts be nonremovable by the infant. Having perfected equilibrium reactions in the sitting position allows the older infant to freely use his hands for manipulation while sitting. He is also now able to reach and secure objects in a sitting position without tumbling over.

A neat pincer grasp develops by 11 to 12 months of age. The infant is able to engage in interactive fine motor games such as pat-a-cake and peekaboo. Stacking large blocks and boxes of various sizes is an enjoyable activity. The infant is also able to put one object after another into a basket or container; he particularly enjoys filling a container, dumping out the contents, and refilling over and over again (Gesell et al., 1940). This activity is especially important to cognitive development.

By 1 year of age, voluntary release (and cognition) develops to the extent that the infant will release an object to

(c)

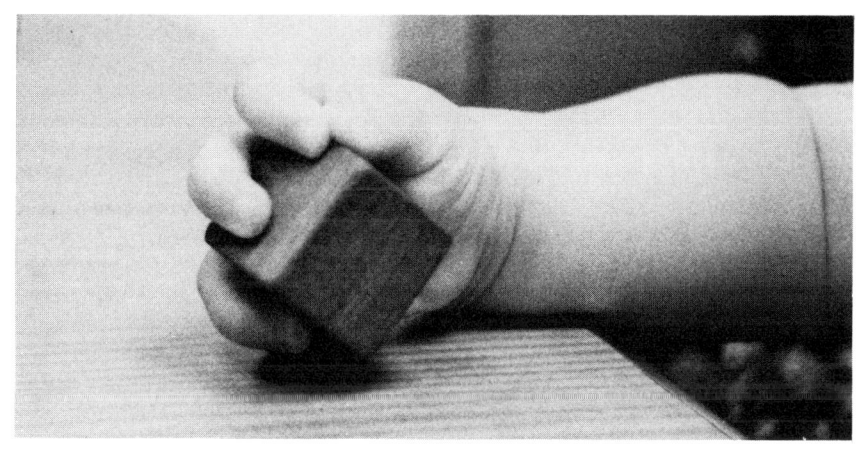

(d)

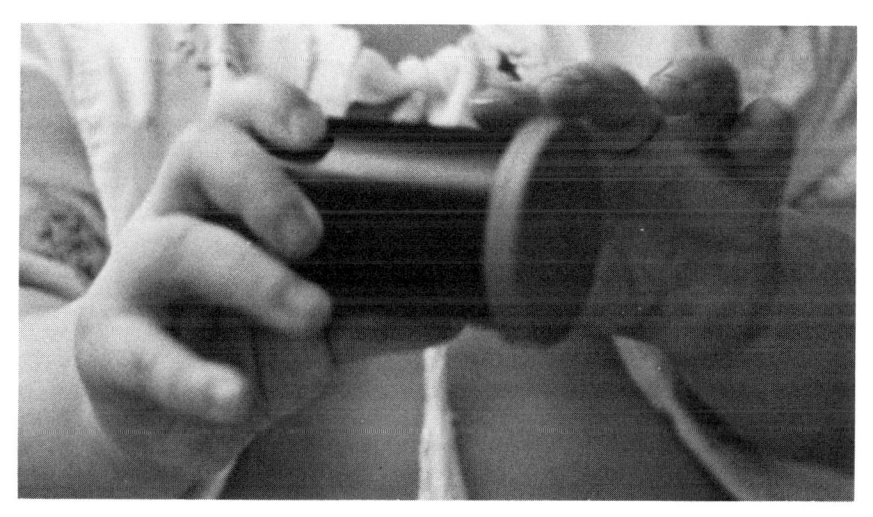

FIGURE 7-22. (*Continued*)

another person when requested. Also, the infant will release an object and then go after the object himself. The infant can easily manipulate small objects into a container with a slot or hole in the lid; this is an activity that he is likely to practice and repeat, usually trying both hands until he can go faster and faster (Gordon, 1970).

By the end of the infant's first year, hand dominance is evident. He uses the dominant hand primarily for exploration and the nondominant hand to carry objects. The infant is able to thrust a finger in a hole and, utilizing his increasingly skilled power of release, place articles in a container.

He has the beginnings of the ability to geometrize space, and he is able to momentarily bring one object above another. The infant has a manual orientation to spatial relationships (he experiences relative distances in space and sees the space within a container in relation to object size) since he is able to manipulate a bottle, to expel a pellet, and to place one cube after another on a flat surface. His fine motor behavior reaches a sensitiveness to

(e)

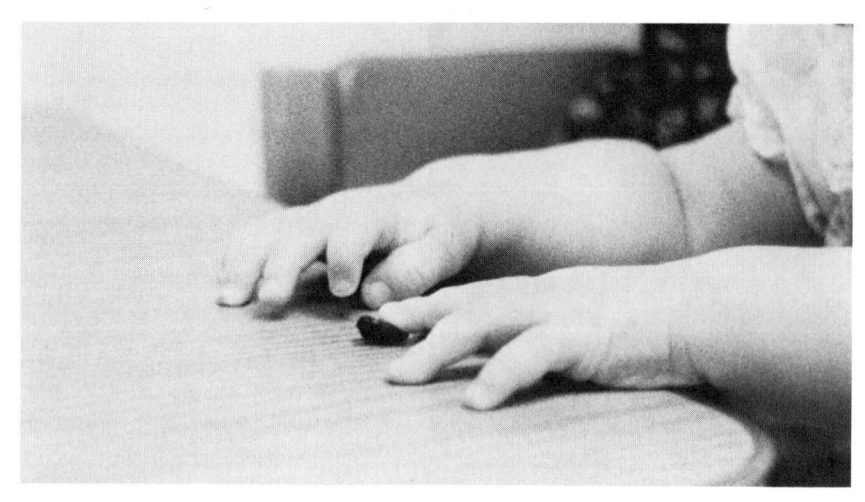

(f)

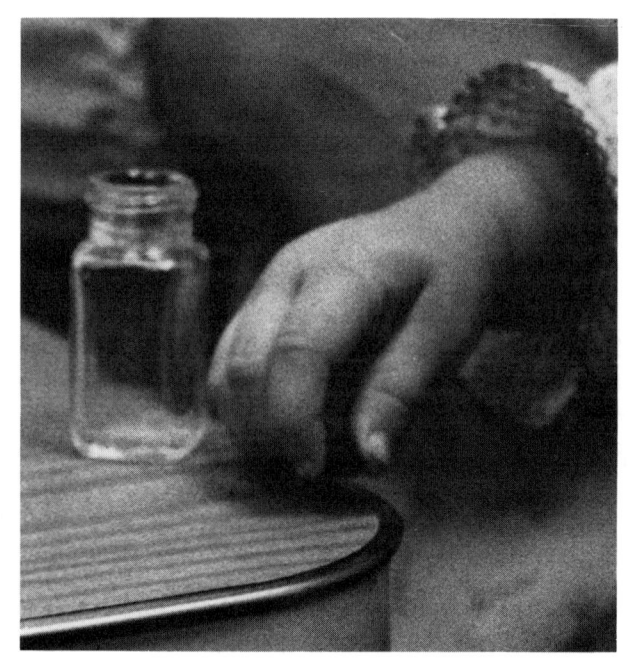

FIGURE 7-22. (*Concluded*)

imitation since he will bring a crayon to a piece of paper, though his behavioral response increases when a scribble is demonstrated (Gesell et al., 1940).

The basis for the fine motor development of a 1-year-old infant has been rapidly developed over the first year. The level of fine motor skill, from the clenched fist of the neonate to the hand dominance of the 1-year-old infant, continually increases through sequential development and refinement. Each change serves as the precursor for the next developmental step in the sequence, and all the changes in the first year of life form the foundation for further refinement during childhood.

Cognitive development Virginia Pidgeon

What are the characteristics of cognitive development in infancy? What would the infant tell, if he could, of his world and himself? The infant remains inarticulate and inaccessible to the probing of his mind. The best way to learn more about infant cognition is to seat the child in his parent's lap and administer a developmental examination. But this attempt is confounded by the impossibility of separating cognitive and motor development. Piaget reminds child-development students that this is the age of sensorimotor intelligence, or intelligence in action. Keep the impediments to understanding infant cognitive development in mind while the current research and Piaget's theory is reviewed. Aspects of infant cognitive development to be considered include attentiveness, learning, schema development, and object concept.

ATTENTIVENESS
Infants are attracted and pay more attention to stimuli that are novel and unfamiliar (Fantz, 1965; Saayman, Ames, and Moffett, 1964). Older infants appear to lose visual interest in the familiar aspects of their environment and direct their visual attention to the unfamiliar. They express surprise when they encounter the unexpected. Their preference for novel stimuli suggests that infants have memory traces of old stimuli.

The presence of a memory trace (or mental schema) enables the infant to recognize a familiar stimulus or event, recall information about it, and distinguish between familiar and unfamiliar stimuli. Kagan (1973) found that infants pay more attention to stimuli that are moderately different from their schema than to stimuli that are either familiar or extremely different. Infants ignore or are fearful of stimuli that are too unfamiliar or different.

LEARNING
Infant learning may take several forms: learning by imitation, learning through reinforcement, and learning through problem solving in interaction with the environment. Imitative learning has been reported as early as 20 days of life in the form of tongue protrusion in imitation of an adult. These stages in the development of imitative learning are described by Užgiris (1973). In the first stage (up to 3 to 4 months) when an adult performs a familiar act, it elicits the same act in the infant. When the adult coos, the infant coos. Infants continue to coo without regard for whether or not the adult is cooing and do not seem to distinguish between their own acts and those of the adult. In the second stage (5 to 7 months) the infant watches the vocal or gestural act of the adult as a spectacle but does not imitate it. In the pauses between the adult's acts the infant vocalizes or gestures as if seeking to elicit a repetition of the act. The infant seems to have learned to take turns.

In the third stage (toward the end of the first year) the infant imitates unfamiliar acts and deliberately tries to approximate his performance to that of the adult. An infant, watching an adult spin a top, at first pushes, shoves, and wiggles it and then finally turns it. He seems to recognize his failure to accurately imitate the act and actively tries to approximate his performance to that of the adult. Basic to the development of imitative learning is the infant's increasing differentiation to himself from others.

Infant learning is also seen in problem-solving behavior. Problem-solving behavior implies the ability of the infant to anticipate a goal. It also implies the ability to select a means, to sustain means activity toward the goal, and to modify means activity so that it will lead more directly to the goal.

Problem-solving behavior in infants is described in several studies of infant conditioning. Infants in the process of being conditioned displayed facial expressions of pleasure, displeasure, tension, concentration, disappointment, and surprise, which were interpreted as evidence of their involvement in the problem-solving process (Papousek and Berstein, 1969). Infants were being trained to turn their heads to the left at the sound of a bell and to the right at the sound of a buzzer. Correct behavior was rewarded with milk. Infants developed common strategies to solve the problem. These strategies included turning the head to the side on which the milk had come on the last trial and turning the head to the side from which milk had most frequently been given. Infants who experienced incongruence when the actual outcome was not what they expected displayed an increase in searching eye movements and motor activity. Infants who experienced congruence when the actual outcome was what they expected often displayed signs of pleasure and relief.

Young infants (5 to 12 weeks old) were shown a blurred motion picture in another experiment (Kalnins and Bruner, 1973). Under one condition the picture could be made clear by sucking on a nipple. Infants learned to suck and look at the picture at the same time and to avert their gaze when they were not sucking and the picture became blurry. Under a second condition sucking produced blurring, and the picture could be made clear by not sucking. Infants learned to look when not sucking and to avert their gaze due to the blurriness of the picture when sucking. Babies learned these strategies and increased the amount of time they spent in viewing clear pictures.

From early problem-solving experiences infants derive a sense of mastery. The infant experiences himself as an agent of change—a shaker of rattles, a creator of sounds, a pursuer and capturer of desired objects. These conquests enhance his awareness of his own separateness as an actor from that which is acted on or the environment. Mastery activity marks a turning point in which the infant shifts from a passive mode of using cognitive abilities (responsiveness to stimulation) to an active mode of using them in manipulation and mastery of his environment.

SCHEMA DEVELOPMENT

The infant in the first 12 months of life, according to Piaget, alters or adapts his reflex schemata and acquires a secondary class of schemata that produce interesting effects in his environment. Lastly, toward the end of the first year he coordinates schemata in instrumental or problem-solving behavior. The stages of cognitive development through which he passes are: stage 2, the first acquired adaptations and the primary circular reaction; stage 3, the secondary circular reaction and procedures for making interesting sights last; and stage 4, the coordination of secondary schemata and their application to new situations (see Fig. 7-23).

The stage 2 infant (1 to 4 months) alters or modifies his reflex schemata as a result of experience. These altered reflex schemata (*acquired adaptations*) are evidence of the infant's beginning ability to accommodate his schemata to the requirements of external reality. The infant's behavior in this stage is not intentional but is characterized by groping that accidentally leads to new results. A chance hand-to-mouth contact leads to the discovery and establishment of finger- and thumb-sucking.

In addition, in stage 2 the *primary circular reaction* emerges. The infant accidentally stumbles upon an act or behavior that produces new and unexpected effects. He repeats the act again and again to recapture the experience. These repetitions constitute the primary circular reaction and consolidate the new act. The infant, moving his arms randomly, accidentally encounters his mouth and sucks his fingers. A circular reaction of finger-sucking ensues in which he learns to direct his fingers to his mouth and shape his mouth to fit his fingers and his

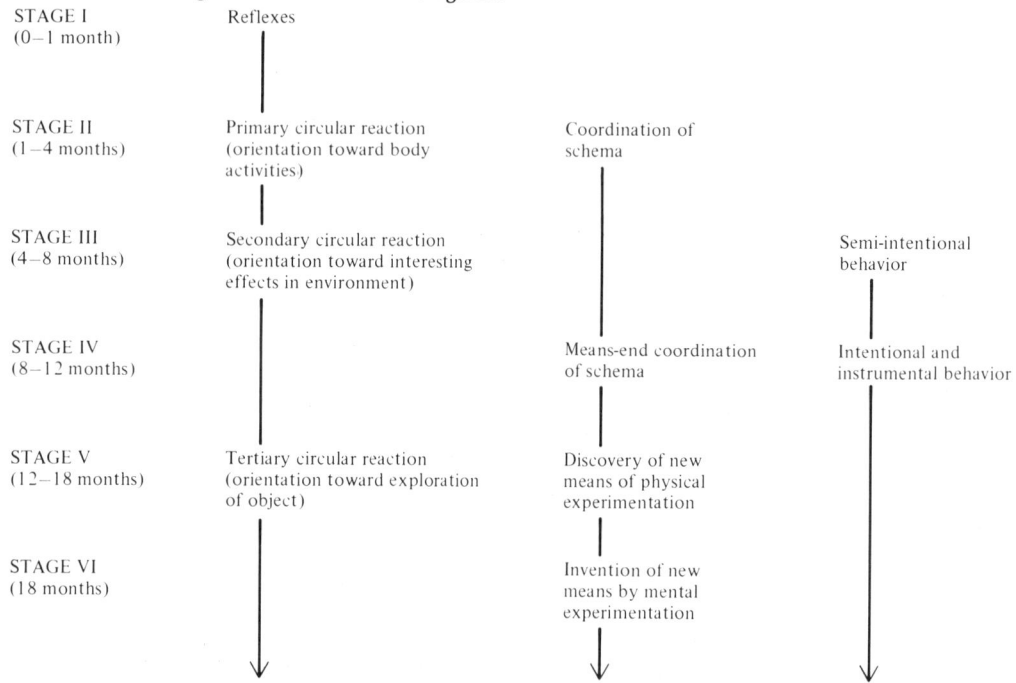

FIGURE 7-23. Stages in sensorimotor intelligence.

STAGE I (0–1 month)	Reflexes		
STAGE II (1–4 months)	Primary circular reaction (orientation toward body activities)	Coordination of schema	
STAGE III (4–8 months)	Secondary circular reaction (orientation toward interesting effects in environment)		Semi-intentional behavior
STAGE IV (8–12 months)		Means-end coordination of schema	Intentional and instrumental behavior
STAGE V (12–18 months)	Tertiary circular reaction (orientation toward exploration of object)	Discovery of new means of physical experimentation	
STAGE VI (18 months)		Invention of new means by mental experimentation	

fingers to fit his mouth. Primary circular reactions are oriented toward bodily activities of the infant rather than toward the environment.

The stage 3 infant (4 to 8 months) moves beyond alterations of reflex behaviors to discover motor acts that produce interesting effects on his immediate environment. He discovers that shaking a rattle produces a sound and that hitting a suspended ring makes it swing. He repeats the act (shaking or hitting) again and again to recapture the interesting effect he has produced. His repetitions constitute the *secondary circular reaction* and consolidate this new behavior. From the secondary circular reactions there emerges a new class of behaviors to make interesting sights last that includes banging, shaking, swinging, and rubbing. When the infant encounters a new object, he rapidly runs through this repertoire of new behaviors.

In contrast to primary circular reactions, secondary circular reactions are centered on the changes or effects produced by one's actions on the environment. The infant is intensely interested in the sights and sounds that he produces. His interest is, however, primarily in the application of his schemata rather than the discovery of the novel features of an object. Assimilation of objects to his schemata still predominates. Behavior in stage 3 is semi-intentional, or transitional between unintentional and intentional behavior. The infant initially has no goal. By accident he discovers an act that produces an interesting effect and then sets as his goal the replication of that act.

In stage 4 (8 to 12 months) we see the emergence of truly intentional behavior. The older infant coordinates two schemata in instrumental, or problem-solving, behavior. He uses one schema as a means to achieve another schema, or goal. He perceives an obstacle in the form of a pillow between him and a ball. He pushes and shoves the pillow out of the way and retrieves the ball. More precisely, the infant tries to achieve an immediate goal (grasping the ball) and discovers obstacles. He then looks for an intermediate act that will help him achieve the goal. Implicit in this behavior is the ability of the infant to keep the goal in mind while turning his attention to the intermediate act and adapting it to achieve the goal. The secondary schemata of grasping, shaking, pushing, and pulling are now used flexibly in different combinations to solve a variety of problems.

The interest of the stage 4 infant centers on the discovery of the novel features of a new object rather than on application of his schemata. Encountering a new object, he spends more time looking at it and commences a series of exploratory actions: touching, poking, mouthing, and turning it to survey its different facets. In contrast to the stage 3 infant he subordinates his schemata to the exploration of external reality.

OBJECT CONCEPT

The infant is developing embryonic concepts of objects in his environment. At first he does not distinguish between his action, or schema, and the object to which he applies it. Objects exist only in terms of his actions on them and are things of action. The young infant may conceive of bottles and fingers simply as suckables and blankets and rattles as graspables. The older infant conceives of objects in terms of his actions on them and the effects they produce. A rattle may be a "shake and make noise"; a suspended ring, a "push and make swing." The older infant, as he coordinates schemata, comes to perceive the visual and tactile as well as the action properties of objects. He discovers that a block, as well as being graspable and suckable, is also hard, angular, and shiny.

INFLUENCE OF PARENTS

What is the influence of the parent or care giver on the cognitive development of the infant? The several parental roles in furthering the cognitive development of the infant include stimulator, catalyst, and promoter of a sense of mastery.

As a stimulator, the parent has a duel function. She or he serves as a buffer or shield by modulating strong and aversive stimuli and reducing stimulation when the infant becomes overexcited or fatigued. The parent also serves as a provider and enhancer of stimuli as she or he repeats and intensifies playful actions that elicit pleasure in the infant and introduces variations in the actions to sustain his attention. The care giver's function as a stimulator becomes increasingly important in the critical period beginning at 8 weeks, when the infant is increasingly vulnerable to overstimulation and stimulus deprivation (Murphy, 1973). Infants in playful interactions with their mothers have shown more complex and sustained behavior than when they were playing alone with a variety of objects (Escalona, 1968). Minimal research has focused on fathers.

The parent has been described as a catalyst whose presence and interactions are essential to the emergence of cognitive abilities in the infant. This catalytic role appears to consist of the components of reassurance and reinforcement. According to Escalona (1968) the infant interacting with his mother is immersed in a tide of social responsiveness that embraces reassurance in the face of difficulty and affection and recognition in response to accomplishments.

The parent is also a promoter of a sense of mastery on

the part of the infant. Parental responsiveness to infant wants fosters in the infant a sense of mastery or agency, of being able to affect the environment by one's actions (Lewis and Goldberg, 1969). The unresponsiveness of institutional environments to infant wants may dilute or negate the sense of agency.

The individuality of the infant is a factor influencing the amount of attention and stimulation he receives. Infants who loudly and clearly pronounce their needs are more likely to receive attention from parents and nurses than those who express their needs more subtly. Infants who soothe themselves by sucking their fingers or rocking are less likely to attract attention, as adults often assume they will quiet down if left alone.

There has been much speculation about social-class differences in mothering. In a study of mother-infant interaction in middle- and working-class mothers, there was no difference in time spent in proximity to infants (Tulkin and Kagan, 1972). There were also no differences in the frequency of holding, physical contact, kissing, prohibitions, or maternal responsiveness to contacts initiated by the infants. Middle-class mothers did more often talk to and entertain their infants and also more often held them in the *en face* position. They also responded more often and more quickly to infant fretfulness. There appeared to be little difference between the classes in the affective component of maternal care, but differences did exist in the components of verbal interaction and cognitive stimulation.

Cause for concern is the cognitive deficit reported in infants placed either briefly or at length in hospitals and institutions. Concern has been expressed about the stimulus deprivation and social isolation of prematures and other infants in isolettes. In an experiment premature infants in isolettes, handled for 5 min every hour both day and night, were more active than those who received routine care (Solkoff, 1969). Young infants (3 or 4 months of age) in home and institutional settings were found to spend similar amounts of time in play (Rheingold, 1961). Home infants played more often with toys, and institution infants played with their hands, bed clothes, crib bars, and bottle holders. Older institutionalized infants lacked interest in toys and other objects and seldom approached or manipulated them. In addition vocalization was meager and language development severely retarded.

Recent enrichment programs designed for hospitalized and institutionalized infants are intriguing. An enrichment program for hospitalized premature infants included 10 min of mothering daily, holding and handling during two feedings, and brief periods of stimulation whenever they opened their eyes (Sinqueland, 1973). Enriched prematures were more successful at a cognitive task than those who received routine care.

Another enrichment program was inaugurated in an institution where neonates were kept in cribs with covered sides and received only essential physical care. Measures included 20 min of handling daily, lying prone for 15 min after three feedings with crib sides uncovered, suspension of a mobile in the crib, and the use of colored and patterned crib sheets and bumpers. At first the visual interest of enriched infants in the environment declined and then rapidly increased as they began to reach for and grasp mobile objects and bed bumpers (White, 1971).

In summary, infancy is the period of sensorimotor intelligence. In this period the infant alters or adapts his reflex schemata, acquires a secondary class of schemata that produce interesting effects in his immediate environment, and lastly coordinates schemata in instrumental, or problem-solving, behavior. Both imitative learning and problem solving are seen in infancy. The parent influences the cognitive development of the infant as stimulator, catalyst, and promoter of mastery.

Language development Shirley Joan Lemmen

During the first year, the infant's prelinguistic behaviors depend upon maturation in motor and cognitive development with special regard for emerging concepts of object permanence, imitation of motor acts and vocalization, and means-to-end activity (see "Cognitive Development"). The impact of the environment includes sensory input and social interaction, very important processes during the first year.

BEHAVIORAL COMMUNICATION

Very early in the first year the infant demonstrates skills at communicating or signaling to others. He communicates effectively through a variety of behaviors: head and body movements, tone, gaze, facial expressions, and vocalizations. These early vocalizations and motor behaviors (before 10 months) are not intentionally communicative. In other words, the infant is not apparently aware of the communicative value of his signals to others.

It is important that parents are aware of and respond to this gestural language. By the age of 3 or 4 months, all these behaviors can be integrated to form recognizable, complex, expressive acts. The distinction between vocalization and motor acts is less compelling at this point and, in fact, if designated too sharply, obscures a view of early vocalization (Stern, Jaffe, Beebe, and Bennett, 1978). According to Halliday (1975), there is no form or structure in such vocalization, but there is expression and meaning in the function that such vocalizations serve.

In regard to vocalization of infants with their mothers, Stern et al. (1978) noted some interesting phenomena: Mothers not only vocalize with their infants in alternation, they also vocalize simultaneously. Their study suggests that vocalizing together, especially in conjunction with mutual gaze, is a form of establishing group membership, or bonding, particularly under conditions of heightened arousal. This coaxial vocalization between parent and infant may be considered early attachment behavior. Vocalizing in unison as a mutual expression of joy or excited delight in being with someone may be central to the creation of a positive experience or relatedness and should in this regard be added to a growing list of human behaviors that bond a parent and infant together. It is also suggested that alternating modes transform into the conversational dialectic pattern to function later in the exchange of symbolic information. The coaction mode transmits emotional communication expressive of the nature of the ongoing interpersonal relationship as well as contributing to the formation of the relationship.

By 4 months of age, the infant has volitional movement which results in novel experiences that happen quite by chance and are very interesting to the infant and worthy of recapturing. The infant will repeat the movement to repeat the novel experience, the secondary circular reaction discussed earlier in this section. Likewise, the infant makes a sound and then attempts to recreate it.

EARLY VOCALIZATIONS

Vocalizing is not forgotten but becomes more extensive. Playing by vocalizing vowel sounds and some consonants occurs. The infant enjoys vocal play and attempts to repeat his own sounds by 5 or 6 months. The syllables that can be recognized by the listener as units of sounds, morphemes, or words are interspersed with gurgling, guttural sounds, clicks of the tongue, and rashing (motor sound with lips together). What is most intriguing for parents is the infant's interest in vocalizing and his ability to listen and reciprocate the communicative interchange.

Before the onset of single words, vocalization and motor behavior are described as predominantly prelocutionary acts, unintentional communicative acts. The child also begins to use pitch and stress in vocalizations to gain attention. Behaviors that the infant imitates facilitate communication and interaction from the listener. It is generally thought that the infant's communication becomes intentional at about 10 months; however, rudiments of intentional behavior can be observed much earlier. Some examples of intentional acts are smiling to initiate social contact, reaching for an object or person, and maintaining close physical contact. The infant may also look directly at the person while vocalizing.

When the infant's interaction with objects becomes intentional, the rudiments of play begin. Mobility, comprehensive exploration of objects, and awareness that objects have permanence introduce a whole new world to explore and are important for language development. The child's intentional behavior from 8 to 12 months includes intentional vocalization. With the advent of intentionality, subtle but important differences arise in the mental processes that the infant uses to cope with reality. The capacity to form mental representations prepares the way for symbolic function.

Parents usually report that the child's first two words are heard when he is 1 year of age; however, there is wide variation within the normal population. One child may have one word at 10 months and 10 to 15 words at 1 year, and another child may not have a true word until 14 months of age. First words are related to concrete experience and are always expressed in the context of the reference (object or person). These words are often close approximations of the adult model. However, the utterances may have substitutions in the initial position or an omission of consonants in the final position. They also are simple monosyllables, such as "ba" for bottle, "da" for dog, "uh" for up, or simple polysyllables, such as "dada" for daddy.

ENVIRONMENTAL FACTORS INFLUENCING LANGUAGE

Language development during the first year of life is critical. An infant's readiness to handle a symbolic system can best be observed in a naturalistic setting; language development is a dynamic process that occurs throughout the infant's entire waking hours but more readily in his own environment.

The following are environmental factors critical to determining the infant's prelinguistic behaviors and influencing his opportunity for communication:

- Home environment
- Variation of experiences for the infant in daily living
- Parents' teaching styles
- Parents' education levels

- Parents' perceptions of the infant
- Parents' understanding of development, particularly language acquisition
- Expectations of the parents regarding communication of the infant
- Parents' understanding of how the infant influences their communicative style

Direct observation and description of the child's communication skills are useful methods of obtaining objective data, especially over time. The change in receptive and expressive language skills in the first year is very important. Some questions to direct the observation of expressive language are listed below:

- What are the sounds that the infant is making?
- How does the infant initiate social interaction or express needs?
- As the infant gets older, can a variety of sounds be heard? Are strings of syllables apparent?
- Does the infant smack his lips together or make clicking sounds?
- Does the infant repeat his own sounds?
- Does the infant use inflection and stress in vocalization?
- Does the infant imitate pat-a-cake?
- Does the infant hold out his arms to be lifted up?

In observation of receptive language skills one can ask these questions:

- How does the infant attend to sounds that are familiar to him?
- What does the infant do in response to sound?
- What does the infant recognize in the environment when named?
- What words does the infant understand with appropriate or without appropriate gestures?
- How does the infant respond to single commands like "Look at the ball," or "Give me the spoon."

The first year is extremely important for the readiness to understand and to use language for communication and learning about the environment. Infants must learn about relations between objects, begin to learn the rules of the native language, and learn what the communicative environment is like. The three components of language acquisition—cognitive, social, and motor—are important during the first year; the most obvious are cognitive and social. The infant engages in activity that has communicative value to the parent. The infant is also exploring his environment and bringing attention to himself from his environment.

Self-help skill development   Doris Julian

FACTORS INFLUENCING SKILL DEVELOPMENT

During the first year of life, the infant typically achieves a level of neuromotor maturation which sets the stage for beginning self-care skills. The ability to coordinate head and eye movements with purposeful use of the hands for reaching and grasping is a significant achievement. This ability, accompanied by trunk and arm control, makes it possible for the infant to assume beginning autonomy in self-feeding and to assist with the dressing process. Postural control, including independent sitting and achieving an upright position, is established in the first year. These skills are prerequisites for bladder and bowel control.

Self-help skills in infancy are built on progressive steps following typical developmental patterns. Although the pattern is predictable for all infants, individual variations in achievement of a particular ability can be expected. Schedules correlating ages with specific accomplishments need to be viewed as rough estimates only. Infants will tend to follow the progression identified in such a schedule but at a rate unique to the child.

Family and cultural expectations for skill development influence timing and the method of providing opportunities for the infant to learn self-care skills. Size of the family and birth order may also contribute to specific expectations. In some Euro-American families emphasis may be placed on early skill achievement by firstborn children (McDonald, 1967). In subsequent children, less emphasis may be placed on early accomplishment with the relaxed expectation that the infant learns by observing siblings.

FEEDING SKILL DEVELOPMENT

SENSORIMOTOR CONSIDERATIONS

The first major self-help skill achieved in infancy is that of feeding. Beginning with the reflex activities of rooting, sucking, and swallowing, the infant gradually develops a repertoire of abilities leading to independence in feeding. The significance of these early reflex behaviors has been explored by a number of researchers. Wolff (1967; 1968) describes patterns of sucking behavior in both nutritive (food present) and nonnutritive situations. He observed that sucking occurred in bursts ranging from 4 to 12 sucks in nonnutritive situations with the infant resting from 2 to 10 s between bursts. When fluid was provided by breast or bottle, the duration of sucking bursts increased, and pauses decreased. This pattern of behavior reflects the infant's competency in food seeking (Dubignon and Campbell, 1969; Wolff, 1968) (see "Gastrointestinal System").

As the infant progresses in oral pharyngeal musculature control, sucking increases in vigor, and swallowing patterns become refined. The rooting and bite reflexes have disappeared by 6 months, and sucking, using negative pressure, is volitional. By $6\frac{1}{2}$ months of age ability to coordinate the tongue and pharynx has progressed so that pureed foods can be handled with ease. At approximately $7\frac{1}{2}$ months, chewing has begun, and the infant can be observed to have substituted biting for mouthing in feeding and play situations.

The infant of $8\frac{1}{2}$ months has the ability to bite off a piece of cracker, chew, and swallow. At $9\frac{1}{2}$ months, increased tone and control of lips, tongue, and jaws reduce drooling. This, in turn, permits increased efficiency in swallowing fluids, and the infant of 10 months can be expected to handle liquids from a cup without difficulty. Development of specific oral skills is outlined in Table 7-2.

The preceding maturational skills are major accomplishments in the infant's first year of life. Accompanied by head, eye, hand, and trunk control, a foundation for self-sufficiency in feeding is well established. During the first 16 weeks of postnatal life, the infant has developed increasing ability to focus on an image or object and can enjoy observing and playing with hands. Approach of the bottle (if familiar to the infant) can result in generalized arm movements but not grasping.

Between the fifth and sixth months, the infant will reach for an object and can hold a bottle if assistance is provided. During the eighth and ninth months these abilities are further refined. A bottle and finger foods can be handled without help. A spoon, cup, or glass may require some assistance. With increasing trunk, head, eye, arm, and hand control, the infant of 10 to 12 months exhibits the precise skill of pursuing a small piece of food, securing it in a neat pincer grasp, and bringing it to his mouth.

SOCIALIZATION AND BEHAVIOR FACTORS

The feeding situation in infancy is recognized as a very significant opportunity for development of a reciprocal relationship between parent and child. Smart and Smart (1967) note that this first cooperative venture promotes a feeling of trust and confidence in the infant and enhances the parent's sense of nurturing and generativity. If the feeding activity is perceived as satisfactory, parent and child can expand the cooperative approach to other activities as well.

The issue of bottle versus breast-feeding is frequently raised as a consideration in infant feeding. Although arguments supporting both sides are available, the relationship established between parent and child during the process is of primary concern. Close contact, involving holding and cuddling, and awareness of the child's cues of comfort and satiety are significant in either breast- or bottle-feeding. Certainly individual differences in parent and infant and contemporary and societal values will influence choice of method (Brazelton, 1969). The logistic problem of choosing breast-feeding and yet providing opportunities for father-infant closeness can be solved in various ways.

Weaning from the breast is influenced by a variety of factors with child and mother readiness a major consideration. In some families, the advent of the infant's first teeth and/or ability to chew solids are used as criteria for weaning. These events typically occur between 6 and 12 months; however, many mothers choose to breast-feed longer. Weaning from the breast or bottle also represents a significant psychological event by identifying the infant as an individual capable of assuming some self-care responsibility.

Recognition of this critical period in an infant's life requires attention to emerging self-feeding abilities and provision of environmental adaptations to support them. Infant seating arrangements which provide good trunk and head control and free mobility of arms and hands are essential. A solid surface (tray) provides the infant with a working surface on which to practice skills. The most useful utensils for the young infant attempting early hand-to-mouth skills are his own fingers.

For the infant 10 to 12 months and older, utensils which can be easily grasped and are resistant to biting and breaking, such as a Teflon-coated, short-handled spoon and a small plastic or metal cup, are appropriate. A bowl which adheres to the tray with a suction device or a bowl set on a moistened towel will provide the infant with some measure of success in scooping. For the infant, however, plates are often an impediment or an object to throw on the floor. Finger foods can simply be placed directly on the tray.

It is relatively easy to smile and verbally reward the infant who demonstrates skill in self-feeding. Ignoring the spills and messes which inevitably accompany early attempts may be more difficult but is an equally desirable strategy. Parents often unintentionally discourage experimentation, and thus self-feeding, because of a strong aversion to sticky hands, hair, and surrounding environment! The infant's pleasure in accomplishment can serve as a reward to both parent and child and as an inducement to proceed to the next level of skill in self-feeding.

TOILETING SKILLS

SENSORIMOTOR CONSIDERATIONS

Achievement of bladder and bowel control requires significant maturation of the central and peripheral nervous systems. During the first year of life the infant accomplishes a major part of this necessary maturation. Typically, however, this process is not complete until well into the second year. Further refinement, permitting complete voluntary control—diurnal and nocturnal—may extend into the early school years.

During the first year, the infant achieves postural control, permitting independent sitting and pulling to stand. Some infants will have started walking by the end of the first year. Bladder capacity, maturation of the renal system, and sphincter control will have progressed so that the infant of 8 or 9 months may wake up dry from a nap and occasionally have intervals of dryness extending up to 2 h. Maturation of the gastrointestinal system, dietary changes, and anal sphincter control have progressed so that the child of 10 to 12 months may have regular elimination patterns and occasionally be able to hold the stool until placed on the toilet. These abilities are prerequisites for achievement of voluntary control by the infant.

SOCIALIZATION OR BEHAVIORAL FACTORS

Of all the self-help skills, that of independent toileting has acquired the most emphasis and concern. Control of elimination has had significance above and beyond a developmental task. Issues of cleanliness, status, and meeting criteria for nursery school enrollment have created additional conflicts.

Contemporary views have reduced some of the pressure on parents to institute toilet training in the first year of life. Some families may still, however, attempt to introduce this task as soon as there is evidence of any regularity in bowel habits or the infant is perceived as

TABLE 7-2 Progression of oral skill development

Age, months	Oral skills, reflex activity
1–3	Root, suck, bite, and gag reflexes are present Initial sucking in short bursts; by 48 h bursts of 10 to 30 sucks are present Simultaneous sucking-breathing pattern
4–6	Rooting reflex disappears at about 4 months; bite reflex disappears by 6 months; gag reflex is less pronounced True negative-pressure sucking pattern is present with a tight, lateral seal; suck is volitional Infant sucks food from spoon with same sucking pattern; pureed food is pushed out of mouth because of sucking motion of tongue Initial volitional biting seen at 6 months
7–10	Simultaneous sucking and breathing disappears Lateral tongue movements; volitional tongue protrusion and retraction Vertical chewing begins Bites off food Early cup drinking; losing some liquid at corners of mouth at 10 months
11–12	Beginning rotary chewing Drinks well from cup with consecutive swallowing

having some volitional control. A classic study by Sears, Maccoby, and Levine (1957) described a group of mothers, 50 percent of whom began bowel training before the child was 9 months old. The study demonstrated that total time for completion of bowel training was less for the older infant.

Sears and associates also evaluated the training methods of these mothers in terms of severity, ranging from mild disapproval to severe punishment. They reported that warm, permissive mothers were more successful in achieving bladder control and night dryness. This was without relevance to the age of beginning bladder training.

From this discussion it is seen that a number of variables are significant in laying the foundation for bladder and bowel control. The first year of life is a fruitful period for establishing communication and trust between parent and infant. Parents who respond with sensitivity to cues presented by the infant, both physiological and temperamental, can build on this understanding and reduce much of the conflict underlying toilet-training stress. Par-

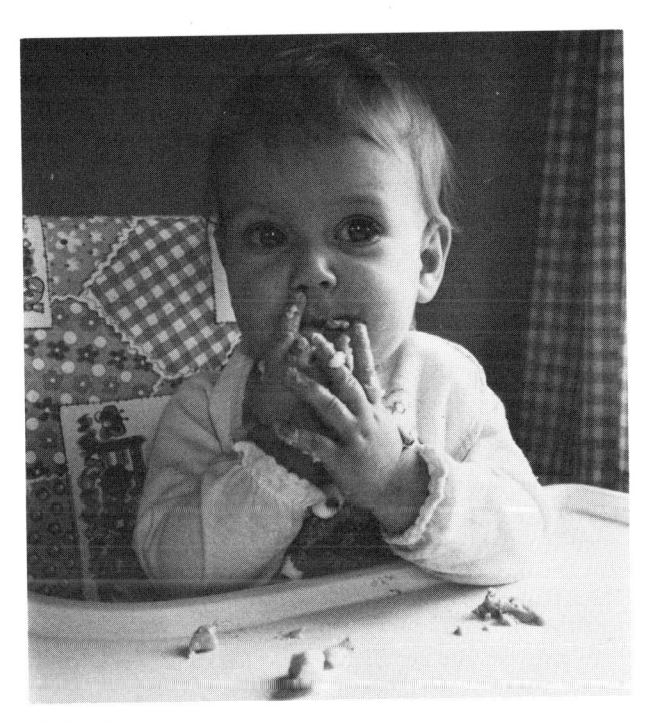

FIGURE 7-24.

ents, in identifying individual characteristics in their infants, will also be aware of their own unique needs (for cleanliness, order, freedom from laundry chores) and may wish to effect compromises to meet these needs (such as disposable diapers or laundry service).

An occasional infant may achieve bowel and bladder control by the end of the first year. Night dryness has also been reported in some 1-year-olds (MacKeith, Meadow, and Turner, 1973). These instances are rare, however, and the parent will do well to recognize that the infant's readiness is a key factor in instituting plans for bowel and bladder control. Further discussion of preparation for autonomy in elimination is presented in relation to the toddler age group.

DRESSING SKILLS

MOTOR OR MATURATIONAL FACTORS
Dressing and undressing skills require a combination of gross motor and fine motor abilities. Acquisition of these abilities during the first year of life provides the infant with a foundation for assisting with undressing. Further fine motor maturation is required before dressing is feasible. In addition, equilibrium must be such that sitting, stooping, reaching, and grasping can be accomplished without loss of balance.

Gesell, Ilg, Ames, and Rodell's (1974) behavior profile of the 1-year-old describes the infant's pleasure in practicing taking off garments. Items of clothing may also become favorite play objects, which can lead to a continuing process of taking off. Motor skills involved in this activity are also useful for cooperating in dressing. The infant of 1 year is able to extend arms and legs while the parent puts on the garment. It is interesting to note that maturation and cognitive growth frequently allow the infant to make a correct association of body part with the appropriate item of clothing.

SOCIALIZATION AND BEHAVIOR FACTORS
In most cultures the nonambulatory infant is not expected to initiate dressing. Sitting still and cooperative behavior may be expected, however, as soon as independent sitting occurs. This behavior, if rewarded with smiles or praise from the parent, will facilitate continued compliance. As previously noted, however, the infant's exploratory needs will lead to repeated removal of garments. Although the two behaviors seem incompatible with compliance on the one hand and garment removal on the other, both are useful in increasing the diversity of the infant's skills.

In 1 year's time the infant has come a long way in moving toward independent functioning. The neonate, as a dependent recipient of complete care, has been replaced by an alert, upright individual with needs, wants, and abilities that are distinctive and separate from the parent.

Social development Susan Blanch Meister

BASIS FOR SOCIALIZATION
The interactive context of socialization changes during the period of infancy. An important change is the steady decrease of nonspecific social input (parent) and social output (infant). The interactive context of infancy is one which becomes increasingly specific (Escalona, 1973).

GOALS OF SOCIALIZATION
The goal of socialization was defined in Chap. 3 as promotion of the natural tendency to become social. During infancy, the child experiences development of cognitive,

affective, and physiological parameters as well as socialization: the infant's capacities and capabilities expand. Simultaneously, the parent is motivated to achieve the goal of socialization. The result of these factors is an increase in specific social input and an increase in the child's understanding of that input. The infant learns more about the consistency and reliability of the parent. As the parent proves trustworthy, the infant gains a generalized sense of trust and well-being (Erikson, 1963).

PROCESSES INVOLVED IN SOCIALIZATION

ATTACHMENT

Early in infancy, the child acquires a differential social response. Specific adults receive specific crying, vocalizations, clinging, and smiling. During early infancy, multiple care givers are still of survival value, and infants remain accepting of substitute care givers.

In the middle of infancy, attachment becomes less flexible. The infant is learning to discriminate the attachment figure and becomes less accepting of substitutes. The attachment system is increasingly sophisticated, and maintaining optimal proximity to care givers is an ever-expanding infant capability.

The attachment is now solidified. The infant has formed an affective, interactive relationship with a specific care giver, usually a parent. Individual differences in the quality of this relationship are readily found. Indeed it is the *quality* of the relationship that is of importance. A securely attached infant acquires essential foundations for further development. That infant has a secure base from which to explore the world as well as a reliable and sensitive relationship with the person who is that secure base. Once again, the importance of sensitivity in care giving emerges. The parent who is adept at reading infant cues responds to those cues appropriately and permits safe exploration, is "sensitive," and plays an essential role in fostering social development (Ainsworth and Bell, 1974; Lamb, 1978).

Strangers are now discriminated by the infant. Wariness and gaze aversion are typical infant responses. Some infants respond to a stranger with wariness and increased heart rate followed by gaze aversion and decreased heart rate. This stranger reaction has been interpreted as a stress response (increased heart rate) followed by a period of cognitive processing (gaze aversion) (Waters, Matas, and Sroufe, 1975). Actual displays of wariness vary widely among normal, attached infants.

EMPATHY

Components of empathy have been identified as social cognition, learning affective cues, and developing altruistic motivation. Social cognition and affective cues are of importance during the period of infancy.

Essential elements in social cognition are the realization that others are separate from self and that others exist even when they are absent. These cognitive developments are called *person permanence:* learning that others are separate from self. This learning occurs during infancy.

Learning affective cues implies that someone provides those cues. During infancy, adults give cues to the infant. Siblings may also provide cues, but an infant experiences differences in social contact with mother, father, and siblings. The three relationships are far from redundant: each offers a unique set of experiences to the infant. When an infant has the opportunity to interact with more than one of the three possible people, the intensity of the interactions will decrease, but their differences remain salient (Lamb, 1977; 1978). During infancy, the child has three different sources of affective cues, and social learning occurs at these different levels.

GENDER IDENTITY AND SEX ROLE

During the infancy period, parental treatment of infants is likely to be gender-linked. Individual interpretations of the meaning of being male or female exist; parents foster the acquisition of sex roles in many ways. Whether parents foster feminine, masculine, or androgynous sex roles is irrelevant to the fact that parents play an active role in gender-identity socialization.

What is the role of the infant? The infant is not yet aware of gender in the context of its social meaning. The categories of male and female and their associated stereotypes are not salient to the infant. In sum, the child works within an undifferentiated gender framework (Parsons and Bryan, 1978).

On the other hand, each parent engages in some degree of gender-role "training," and certainly the infant is responsive to this parental tuition. Currently, rigid and restrictive sex-role expectations are beginning to fade, which will affect gender-role training. As parents become differentiated in the child's eyes (Lamb, 1978), the strength of their tuition changes. The infant begins to demonstrate parental preferences, and it follows that the impact of each parent's gender-linked training may be affected by the infants' preferences.

Gender-role development during infancy is a process of social development which occurs on two levels: parent and child. The child is attached to each parent and engages in social interaction with them. The parents are each attached to the infant and take part in social interaction. Parental labeling and gender-linked tuition occur (Mussen, 1969), and the infant learns from each parent in a nonredundant manner (Lamb, 1978).

Socialization during infancy is a period of increasing specifics; concurrent development of the child contributes to his ability to absorb those specific inputs.

Perception of behavioral competency and development of self-esteem
Judith Anne Ritchie

THE PARENT-INFANT BOND
As the infant's quiet-alert periods increase in length and frequency and his behavioral capacities increase, the parent-infant bond is strengthened. The infant's increasing behavior repertoire elicits favorable response from parents, and he begins to learn which behaviors are most likely to evoke positive reactions.

The degree to which a strong and positive bond is established has major impact on the development of an environment which is conducive to the infant's development of behavioral competence. The parent who is strongly attached to the infant is said to be more likely to be interested in, sensitive to, and respectful of the child's needs (Appleton, Clifton, and Goldberg, 1975).

PHASES OF SEPARATION-INDIVIDUATION
Mahler, Pine, and Bergman (1975) have described in great detail the process by which the child establishes the self as a separate and autonomous functioning individual. They refer to these developmental phenomena as the phases of separation-individuation and note three interrelated developments which contribute to the process. "These are the rapid body differentiation from the mother; the establishment of a specific bond with her; and the growth and functioning of the autonomous ego apparatuses in close proximity to the mother" (p. 65).

At about 4 to 5 months of age the symbiotic infant begins to indicate awareness of an "out there" separate from self. As the infant "hatches" from the symbiotic phase into the phase of differentiation, he becomes aware that his need satisfaction is dependent on someone other than himself, and he appears more alert and outer directed during his longer wakeful periods.

Playful exploration of his own body and his parent's body and clothing permits gradual differentiation of his own body boundaries and provides the basis for perception of self as a separate individual. Peekaboo games provide experimentation with separateness.

Motor development permits the 7- to 8-month-old infant to move away from the parent, to view her or him from a distance, and to become aware of the capacity to function alone. The onset of creeping or crawling marks movement into the *practicing period*, the second subphase of separation-individuation. During this phase, the infant explores and manipulates his environment and is content as long as he can easily "refuel" by reestablishing physical contact with the parent.

The infant's developing view of self as separate is also observed in the development of the phenomena of transitional objects and stranger anxiety. As the infant hatches from the symbiotic phase, he begins to internalize some of the parent's satisfying activities. Tolpin (1967) suggests that as an aid to the process of internalization, the infant "transfers" the maternal satisfying actions to a blanket or some other significant object, which then is a vehicle for the child to soothe himself. "The treasured 'not-me' possession . . . preserves the soothing effects of the last symbiotic merger" (p. 347).

The advent of some degree of stranger anxiety marks awareness of a separate, vulnerable self. When the infant has become sufficiently individuated to recognize parents' faces, he begins to explore the faces of others with varying degrees of interest and apprehension. There appears to be an "inverse relationship between basic confidence and stranger anxiety" (Mahler et al., 1975, p. 58).

The study of the infant's capacity to recognize his own mirror image is complex. Recent research indicates that recognition of the self-mirror-image emerges in a predictable developmental sequence of stages. This developmental sequence begins at approximately age 6 months and is completed by age 24 months (Bertenthal and Fischer, 1978).

AWARENESS OF MOTOR FUNCTION AND ABILITY
As the infant learns about his body parts and how to coordinate their movement, there emerges a wide range of activities in interaction with the environment. White (1959) theorizes that, from infancy onward, there is an "effectance motivation" toward a sense of competence. This sense of competence provides the "inner root" of self-esteem and must be coordinated with the component of self-esteem derived from the perceptions of others' opinions about the self.

The older infant clearly finds pleasure in experimentation with what his body can do and in persistence at attempts for motor control and achievement. It appears that there is an intrinsic motivation to mastery of motor control and that such learning is self-rewarding (White, 1959). Even the high rate of failure and painful falls does not result in cessation of attempts to master new skills. However, it is also essential that the environment provide positive response for motivation to be "maintained as the infant learns new and better ways to affect the objects and surrounding events" (Appleton et al., 1975, p. 158).

The infant has progressed from a helpless, horizontal being to a multiskilled, upright toddler. The infant is capable in all areas: motor, cognitive, language, and social. The infant knows his family and is a person in his own right to them.

The infant, however, is more on a brink than on a pinnacle. As the infancy period ends, adaptive abilities which were covertly being assembled and implemented on himself are about to burst forth onto the world outside himself.

Bibliography

PHYSICAL DEVELOPMENT OF THE INFANT

Brandt, I.: Growth dynamics in low-birth-weight infants with emphasis on the perinatal period. In F. Falkner and J. M. Tanner (Eds.), *Human growth 2, Postnatal growth*. New York: Plenum, 1978.

Brook, C. G. D.: Cellular growth: Adipose tissue. In F. Falkner and J. M. Tanner (Eds.), *Human growth 2, Postnatal growth*. New York: Plenum, 1978.

Frisancho, A. R.: Triceps skinfold and upper arm muscle size norms for assessment of nutritional status. *Amer. J. Clin. Nutr.*, 1974, 27, 1052–1058.

Holliday, M. H.: Body composition and energy needs during growth. In F. Falkner and J. M. Tanner (Eds.), *Human growth 2, Postnatal growth*. New York: Plenum, 1978.

Johnston, F. E.: Somatic growth of the infant and preschool child. In F. Falkner and J. M. Tanner (Eds.), *Human growth 2, Postnatal growth*. New York: Plenum, 1978.

National Center for Health Statistics: NCHS growth charts, 1976. *Monthly Vital Statistics Report*, (HRA) 76-1120 (Vol. 25, No. 3). Rockhill, Maryland: Health Resources Administration, 1977. (Supplement)

Pasternak, S. B., and P. M. Lybarger: The cardiovascular system. In G. M. Scipien, M. U. Barnard, M. A. Chard, J. Howe, and P. J. Phillips (Eds.), *Comprehensive pediatric nursing*. New York: McGraw-Hill, 1979.

Sinclair, D.: *Human growth after birth* (3d ed.). New York: Oxford University Press, 1978.

CALVARIUM AND FACE

Demirjian, A.: Dentition. In F. Falkner and J. M. Tanner (Eds.), *Human growth 2, Postnatal growth*. New York: Plenum, 1978.

Enlow, D. H.: *Handbook of facial growth*. Philadelphia: Saunders, 1975.

Israel, J.: The fundamentals of cranial and facial growth. In F. Falkner and J. M. Tanner (Eds.), *Human growth 2, Postnatal growth*. New York: Plenum, 1978.

Nelson, W., V. Vaughn, and J. R. McKay: *Textbook of pediatrics* (10th ed.). Philadelphia: Saunders, 1975.

Popich, G. A., and D. W. Smith: Fontanels: Range of normal size. *J. Pediat.*, 1972, 80(5), 749–752.

Sullivan, P. G.: Skull, jaw, and teeth growth patterns. In F. Falkner and J. M. Tanner (Eds.), *Human growth 2, Postnatal growth*. New York: Plenum, 1978.

SENSORY SYSTEM

Avery, G. B.: *Pathophysiology and management of neonatology*. Philadelphia: Lippincott, 1975.

Bordley, J. E., and W. G. Hardy: The special senses. In R. E. Cooke (Ed.), *The biologic basis of pediatric practice*. New York: McGraw-Hill, 1968.

Conway, B. L.: *Pediatric neurologic nursing*. St. Louis: Mosby, 1977.

Murray, R., and J. Zenter: *Nursing assessment and health promotion through the life span*. Englewood Cliffs, N.J.: Prentice-Hall, 1975.

Newell, F. W., and J. T. Ernest: *Ophthalmology: Principles and concepts* (3d ed.). St. Louis: Mosby, 1974.

Northern, J. L., and M. P. Down: *Hearing in children*. Baltimore: Williams & Wilkins, 1974.

Smith, J. L.: The eye in infancy and childhood. In R. E. Cooke (Ed.), *The biologic basis of pediatric practice*. New York: McGraw-Hill, 1968.

MUSCULOSKELETAL SYSTEM

Alexander, M. M., and M. S. Brown: *Pediatric physical diagnosis for nurses*. New York: McGraw-Hill, 1974.

Malina, R. M.: Growth of muscle tissue and muscle mass. In F. Falkner and J. M. Tanner (Eds.), *Human growth 2, Postnatal growth*. New York: Plenum, 1978.

Nelson, W., V. Vaughn, and J. R. McKay: *Textbook of pediatrics* (10th ed.). Philadelphia: Saunders, 1975.

Roche, A. F.: Bone growth and maturation. In F. Falkner

and J. M. Tanner (Eds.), *Human growth 2, Postnatal growth*. New York: Plenum, 1978.

Rudolph, A. M. (Ed.): *Pediatrics* (16th ed.). New York: Appleton-Century-Crofts, 1977.

Sinclair, D.: *Human growth after birth* (3d ed.). London: Oxford University Press, 1978.

GASTROINTESTINAL SYSTEM

Agunod, M., N. Yamaguchi, R. Lopez, A. Luhby, and G. B. J. Glass: Correlative study of hydrochloric acid, pepsin, and intrinsic factor secretion in newborns and infants. *Amer. J. Dig. Dis.*, 1969, 14, 400–414.

Alpers, D. H., and M. Solin: The characterization of rat intestinal amylase. *Gastroenterology*, 1970, 58, 833–842.

Andersen, D. H.: Pancreatic enzymes in the duodenal juice in the celiac syndrome. *Amer. J. Dis. Child.*, 1942, 63, 643–658.

Challacombe, D. N., S. Edkins, and G. A. Brown: Duodenal bile acids in infancy. *Arch. Dis. Child.*, 1975, 50, 837–843.

Crelin, E. S.: *Functional anatomy of the newborn*. New Haven, Conn.: Yale University Press, 1973.

Grybooki, J. D., W. R. Thayor, Jr., and H. M. Spiro: Esophageal motility in infants and children. *Pediatrics*, 1963, 31, 382–395.

Maffel, H. V. L., and F. J. Nobrega: Gastric pH and microflora of normal and diarrhoeic infants. *Gut*, 1975, 16, 719–726.

Timiras, P. S.: *Developmental physiology and aging*. New York: Macmillan, 1972.

Tyson, K. R. T.: Normal and abnormal physiology of the alimentary tract in infancy. *Amer. J. Surg.*, 1969, 117, 876–880.

Zoppi, G., G. Andreotti, and F. Pajino-Ferrara: Exocrine pancreas function in prematures and full-term infants. *Pediat. Res.*, 1972, 6, 880–885.

ENDOCRINE SYSTEM

Krueger, J. A., and J. C. Ray: *Endocrine problems in nursing, A physiologic approach*. St. Louis: Mosby, 1976.

Spencer, R. T.: *Patient care in endocrine problems*. Philadelphia: Saunders, 1973.

Villee, D. B.: *Human endocrinology, A developmental approach*. Philadelphia: Saunders, 1975.

DEVELOPMENT OF BODY CONCEPT AND CONCEPTS OF ILLNESS AND WELLNESS

Bernfeld, S.: *The psychology of infants* (R. Hurwitz, trans.). New York: Brentano's, 1929.

Douglas, J. W. B.: Early hospital admission and later disturbances of behavior and learning. *Develop. Med. Child Neurol.*, 1975, 17, 456–483.

Freud, A.: The role of bodily illness in the mental life of children. *Psychoanal. Stud. Child*, 1952, 7, 69–80.

Freud, S.: *The ego and the id* (3d ed., J. Riviere, trans.). London: Hogarth Press and Institute of Psychoanalysis, 1942.

Hoffer, W.: Mouth, hand and ego-integration. *Psychoanal. Stud. Child*, 1949, 3–4, 612–627.

Kolb, L. C.: Disturbances of the body image. In S. Arient, (Ed.), *American handbook of psychiatry* (Vol. IV, 2d ed.). New York: Basic Books, 1975.

Maurer, A.: Maturation of concepts of death. *Brit. J. Med. Psychol.*, 1966, 39, 35–41.

Mittleman, B.: Intrauterine and early infantile motility. *Psychoanal. Stud. Child*, 1960, 15, 104–127.

Prugh, D. G.: Emotional aspects of the hospitalization of children. In M. F. Shore (Ed.), *Red is the color of hurting*. Washington, D.C.: Government Printing Office, 1965.

Schilder, P.: *The image and appearance of the human body*. New York: Wiley, 1964.

Schowalter, J. E.: The child's reaction to his own terminal illness. In B. Schoenberg et al. (Eds.), *Loss and grief*. New York: Columbia University Press, 1970.

Spicher, C.: Infant affective responses during interactions with health worker strangers in a child health conference. *Matern. Child Nurs. J.*, 1976, 5, 131–150.

Witken, H. A.: Development of the body concept and psychological differentiation. In S. Wapner and H. Werner (Eds.), *The body percept*. New York: Random House, 1965.

PERCEPTUAL DEVELOPMENT

Binzley, V.: Relationship between infant cardiac rate and nonnutritive sucking as a function of sex, stimulus and state factors. (Unpublished paper, 1974.)

Ellis, P. P.: Eye. In C. H. Kempe, H. K. Silver, and D. O'Brien (Eds.), *Current pediatric diagnosis and treatment* (5th ed.). Los Altos, Calif.: Lange, 1978.

Fraiberg, S.: *Insights from the blind: Comparative studies of blind and sighted infants*. New York: Basic Books, 1977.

Friedlander, B. Z.: Receptive language development in infancy: Issues and problems. *Merrill-Palmer Quart.*, 1970, 16, 7–51.

Gibson, E. J.: *Principles of perceptual learning and development*. New York: Appleton-Century-Crofts, 1969.

Haith, M. M., and J. J. Campos: Human infancy. *Ann. Rev. Psychol.*, 1977, 28, 251–293.

Illingworth, R. S.: *The development of the infant and young child*. Baltimore: Williams & Wilkins, 1962.

Kessen, W. H., M. M. Haith, and P. H. Salapatek: Human infancy: A bibliography and guide. In P. H. Mussen (Ed.), *Carmichael's manual of child psychology* (Vol. I). New York: Wiley, 1970.

Northern, J. L., and M. P. Downs: *Hearing in children.* Baltimore: Williams & Wilkins, 1974.

Pederson, D. R., and D. Ter Vrugt: The influence of amplitude and frequency of vestibular stimulation on the activity of 2 months-old infants. *Child Develop.*, 1973, 44, 122–28.

Pick, H. L., and A. D. Pick: Sensory and perceptual development. In P. H. Mussen (Ed.), *Carmichael's manual of child psychology* (Vol. I). New York: Wiley, 1970.

White, B. L.: *Human infants: Experience and psychological development.* Englewood Cliffs, N.J.: Prentice-Hall, 1971.

GROSS MOTOR DEVELOPMENT

Capute, A. J.: *Primitive reflex profile.* Baltimore: University Park Press, 1978.

Egan, D. R., R. S. Illingworth, and R. C. MacKeith: *Developmental screening 0–5 years.* London: Spastics International, 1969.

Fiorantino, M. R.: *Normal and abnormal development.* Springfield, Ill.: Charles C Thomas, 1972.

——: *Reflex testing methods for evaluating C.N.S. development.* Springfield, Ill.: Charles C Thomas, 1973.

Gordon, N.: *Paediatric neurology for the clinician.* London: Spastics International, 1976.

Hellmuth, J. (Ed.): *Exceptional infant* (Vol. I). New York: Brunner/Mazel, 1967.

Illingworth, R. S.: *The development of the infant and young child.* London: Churchill Livingstone, 1975.

Paine, R. S., and T. E. Oppe: *Neurological examination of children.* London: Spastics International, 1966.

Sheridan, M. D.: *Children's developmental progress.* London: NFER, 1973.

Touwen, B.: *Neurological development in infancy.* London: Spastics International, 1976.

FINE MOTOR DEVELOPMENT

Gesell, A., H. M. Halverson, H. Thompson, F. L. Ilg, B. Castner, L. B. Ames, and C. S. Amatruda: *The first five years of life.* New York: Harper & Brothers, 1940.

Gordon, I. J.: *Baby learning through baby play.* New York: St. Martin's, 1970.

Illingworth, R. S.: *The development of the infant and young child—Normal and abnormal.* London: Churchill Livingstone, 1975.

Knobloch, H., and B. Pasamanick: *Gesell and Amatruda's developmental diagnosis.* New York: Harper & Row, 1974.

Kopp, C. B.: Fine motor abilities of infants. *Develop. Med. Child Neurol.*, 1974, 16, 629–636.

Stott, L. H.: *The psychology of human development.* New York: Holt, 1974.

COGNITIVE DEVELOPMENT

Church, L. J., H. T. Smith, and L. B. Murphy (Eds.): *The competent infant.* New York: Basic Books, 1973.

Escalona, S.: *The roots of individuality: Normal patterns of development in infancy.* Chicago: Aldine, 1968.

Fantz, R.: Visual perception from birth as shown by pattern selectivity. *Ann. N.Y. Acad. Sci.* 1965, 118, 793–814.

Flavell, J.: *The developmental psychology of Jean Piaget.* Princeton: Van Nostrand, 1963.

Kagan, J.: The determinants of attention in the infant. In L. J. Church, H. T. Smith, and L. B. Murphy (Eds.), *The competent infant.* New York: Basic Books, 1973.

Kalnins, I., and J. Bruner: Infant sucking uses to change the clarity of a visual display. In L. J. Church, H. T. Smith, and L. B. Murphy (Eds.), *The competent infant.* New York: Basic Books, 1973.

Lewis, M., and S. Goldberg: Perceptual cognitive development in infancy: A generalized expectancy model as a function of the mother-infant interaction. *Merrill-Palmer Quart.*, 1969, 15, 81–100.

Murphy, L. B.: Development in the first year of life: Ego and drive development in relation to the mother: infant tie. In L. J. Church, H. T. Smith, and L. B. Murphy (Eds.), *The competent infant.* New York: Basic Books, 1973.

Papousek, H., and P. Berstein: The functions of conditioning stimulation in human neonates and infants. In A. Ambrose (Ed.), *Stimulation in early infancy.* New York: Academic, 1969.

Rheingold, H.: The effect of environmental stimulation upon social and exploratory behavior in the human infant. In B. M. Foss (Ed.), *Determinants of infant behavior.* New York: Wiley, 1961.

Saayman, G., E. Ames, and A. Moffett: Response to novelty as an indicator of visual discrimination in the human infant. *J. Exp. Child Psychol.*, 1964, 1, 189–198.

Siqueland, W.: Biological and experiential determinants of exploration in infancy. In L. J. Church, H. T. Smith, and L. B. Murphy (Eds.), *The competent infant.* New York: Basic Books, 1973.

Solkoff, N.: Effects of handling on the subsequent development of premature infants. *Develop. Psychol.*, 1969, 1, 765–768.

Tulkin, S. R., and J. Kagan: Mother-child interaction in the first year of life. *Child Develop.*, 1972, 43, 31–41.

Užgiris, I.: Patterns of vocal and gestural imitation in infants. In L. J. Church, H. T. Smith, and L. B. Murphy (Eds.), *The competent infant.* New York: Basic Books, 1973.

White, B.: An analysis of excellent early educational practices: Preliminary report. *Interchange*, 1971, 2(2), 86–87.

LANGUAGE DEVELOPMENT

Halliday, M. A. K.: Learning how to mean. In E. Lenneberg and E. Lenneberg (Eds.), *Foundations of language development.* New York: Academic Press, 1975, pp. 239–264.

Kriegsman, E.: *Providing an optimal language environment for the young child.* (Unpublished paper, Seattle, Wash., 1978.)

Stern, D. V., J. Jaffe, B. Beebe, and S. L. Bennett: Vocalizing in unison and in alteration: Two models of communication within the mother and infant dyad. In *Readings in language development.* New York: Wiley, 1978.

SELF-HELP SKILL DEVELOPMENT

Brazelton, T. B.: *Infants and mothers: Differences in development.* New York: Dell, 1969.

Dubignon, J., and D. Campbell: Sucking in the newborn during a feed. *J. Exp. Child Psychol.*, 1969, 7, 282–298.

Gesell, A., F. Ilg, F. Ames, and J. Rodell: *Infant and child in the culture of today* (rev. ed.). New York: Harper & Row, 1974.

Knobloch, H., and B. Pasamanick (Eds.): *Gesell and Amatruda's developmental diagnosis.* Hagerstown, Md.: Harper & Row, 1974.

MacDonald, A. P. Jr.: Birth-order effects in marriage and parenthood: Affiliation and socialization. *J. Marriage Family*, 1967, 29, 656–661.

MacKeith, R., R. Meadow, R. K. Turner: How children become dry. In I. Kolvin, R. C. MacKeith, and R. Meadow (Eds.), *Bladder control and enuresis.* Philadelphia: Lippincott, 1973.

Sears, R. E. Maccaby, and H. Levine: *Patterns of child rearing.* New York: Row, Peterson, 1957.

Smart, M., and R. Smart: *Children—Development and relationships.* New York: Macmillan, 1967.

Wolff, P. H.: The role of biological rhythms in early psychological development. *Bull. Menninger Clin.*, 1967, 31, 197–218.

———: The serial organization of sucking in the young infant. *Pediatrics*, 1968, 42, 943–956.

SOCIAL DEVELOPMENT

Ainsworth, M. D., and S. Bell: Mother-infant interaction and the development of competence. In K. J. Connolly and J. S. Bruner (Eds.), *The growth of competence,* New York: Academic, 1974.

Erikson, E.: *Childhood and society.* New York: Norton, 1963.

Escalona, S.: Basic modes of social interaction: Their emergence and patterning during the first two years of life. *Merrill-Palmer Quart.*, 1973, 19, 205–232.

Lamb, M.: The development of parental preferences in the first two years of life. *Sex Roles*, 1977, 13, 495–497.

———: The father's role in the infant's social world. In J. H. Stevens and M. Mathews (Eds.), *Mother/child, father/child relationships.* New York: National Association for the Education of Young Children, 1978.

Mussen, P. H.: Sex-typing and acquisition of sex-role identity. In D. A. Goslin (Ed.), *Handbook of socialization theory and research.* Chicago: Rand McNally, 1969.

Parsons, J., and J. Bryan: Adolescence: Gateway to androgyny. *Occasional Papers Series.* Ann Arbor: University of Michigan Women's Study Program, 1978.

Stayton, D. J., R. Hogan, and M. D. Ainsworth: Infant obedience and maternal behavior: The origins of socialization reconsidered. *Child Develop.*, 1971, 42, 1057–1069.

Waters, E., L. Matas, and L. A. Sroufe: Infant's reactions to an approaching stranger: Description, validation and functional significance of wariness. *Child Develop.*, 1975, 46, 348–356.

PERCEPTIONS OF BEHAVIORAL COMPETENCY AND DEVELOPMENT OF SELF-ESTEEM

Appleton, T., R. Clifton, and S. Goldberg: The development of behavioral competence in infancy. In F. D. Horowitz (Ed.), *Review of child development research* (Vol. IV). Chicago: University of Chicago Press, 1975.

Bertenthal, B. I., and K. W. Fischer: Development of self-recognition in the infant. *Develop. Psychol.*, 1978, 14, 44–50.

Klaus, M. H., and J. H. Kennell: *Maternal-infant bonding.* St. Louis: Mosby, 1976.

Mahler, M. S., F. Pine, and A. Bergman: *The psychological birth of the human infant.* New York: Basic Books, 1975.

Robson, K. S.: The role of eye-to-eye contact in maternal infant attachment. *Child Psychol. Psychiat.*, 1967, 8, 13–25.

Tolpin, M.: On the beginnings of a cohesive self: An application of the concept of transmuting internalization to the study of the transitional object and signal anxiety. *Psychoanal. Stud. Child*, 1967, 26, 316–352.

White, B.: An analysis of excellent early educational practice. In L. J. Stone, H. Smith, and L. B. Murphy (Eds.), *The competent infant.* New York: Basic Books, 1973.

White, R.: Motivation reconsidered: The concept of competence. *Psychol. Rev.* 1959, 66, 297–333.

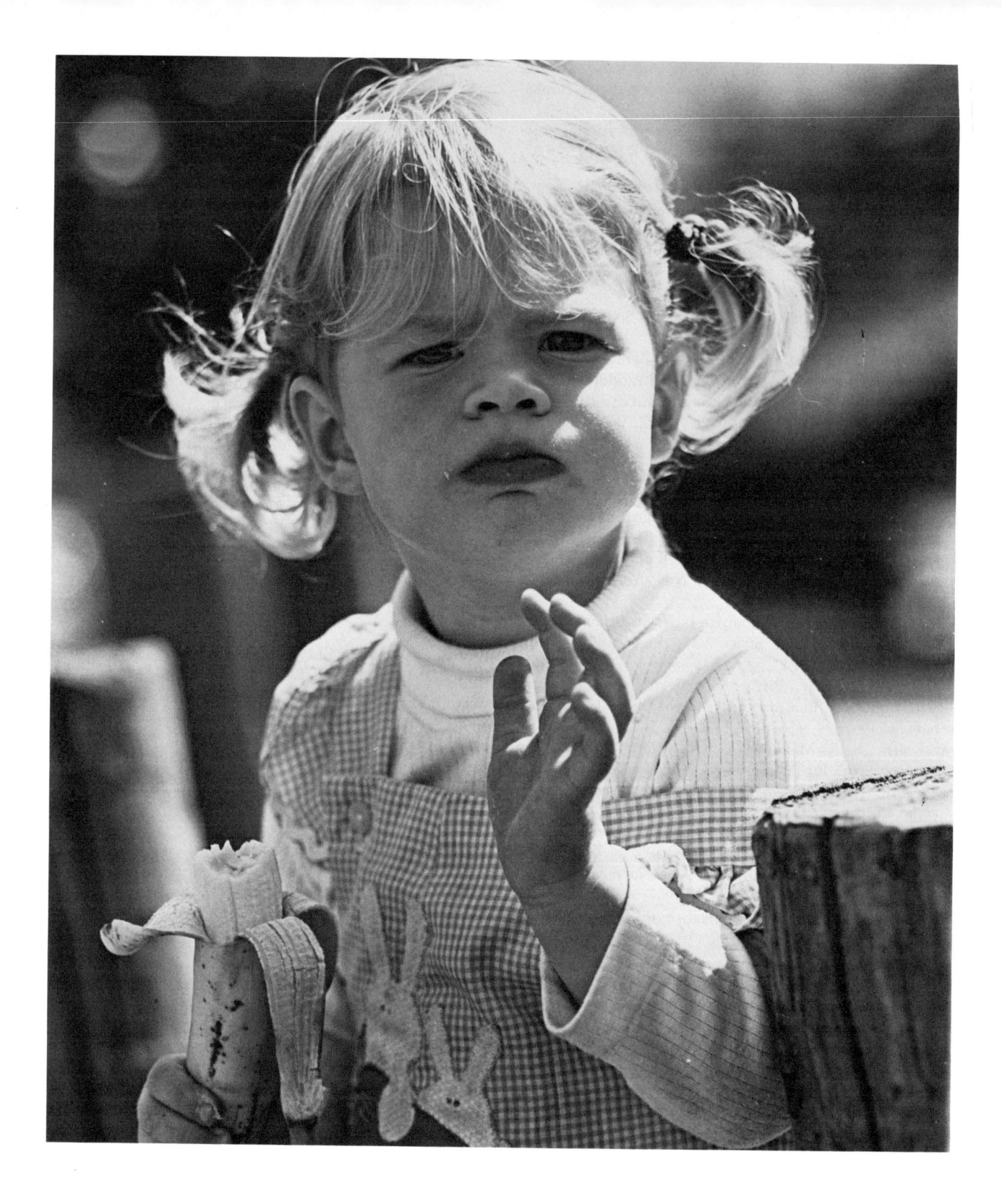

CHAPTER 8

The Toddler: 1 Year to 3 Years

Introduction

The toddler is an upright wonder, and his parents are left wondering what he will do next. Although energy level seems to escalate, growth rate continues to gradually slow from 1 to 3 years of age. There are no major physiological transformations, but steady maturational change in body proportion and neuromuscular maturation is evident. The child looks less like a rotund, short-legged infant and hints of a lanky build to come.

The toddler has earned the right to have his autonomy respected; during these years, the child becomes capable of self-care, self-expression, and self-entertainment. Self-regulation, however, is lacking, and the drive behind relentless practicing of skills seems boundless. Accomplishments are barely acknowledged by the toddler in the rush to do more.

"Me do it!" says the toddler to his arch adversaries—those within his own home. And do it he will, developing into a capable and autonomous individual.

FIGURE 8-1. *(Photo courtesy of Betsy Smith.)*

SECTION 1
Physical Development

Physical development of the toddler
M. Colleen Caulfield

DEVELOPMENTAL APPROACH TO PHYSICAL ASSESSMENT

Assessment of the toddler brings to mind memories of instant delight—and instant dismay! One minute this child is playful and cooperative; the next minute, the lexicon of the "terrible twos" is joined. Every attempt at interaction is met with an assertive "No." How is this child, who refuses to be touched, to be approached? The traditional format of history first, followed by head-to-foot examination, simply will not work. Instead, a developmental approach that is unstructured and opportunistic is used.

UNSTRUCTURED AND OPPORTUNISTIC

History, physical, and developmental assessment are blurred together and integrated into a series of games that are used to gain cooperation and elicit data. Opportunities are both presented and taken advantage of. Presenting the toddler with colorful cubes will provide tools for play and an opportunity to examine him. Observation while playing provides information about gross and fine motor skills, problem-solving abilities, attention span, and more. Placing physical-assessment equipment within his sight will elicit curiosity; giving him the stethoscope to play with will diffuse its unfamiliarity and decrease fear when used. The same equipment can be transformed into magical toys that delight. The otoscope can become a light that goes on and off as the toddler blows or follows its beam. The stethoscope can become a telephone that calls the child's name.

The nurse learns to move rapidly; cues are responded to as presented by the toddler. While sitting quietly in the parent's lap is an excellent time for heart and lung auscultation; gait, coordination, and range of motion are observed while he explores the examining room. If asked, the toddler may proudly display his "belly button," and the abdomen is palpated. An unhappy moment provides an excellent opportunity to observe the parent's ability to console.

Beginning with least threatening or intrusive aspects will gain trust and decrease fear. The toddler's attention span and ability to tolerate frustration are very limited; those aspects of the examination which require cooperation are best done early, before trust is lost. Intrusive procedures and examinations of any part of the head are usually met with resistance and should be done last.

DEVELOPMENTALLY BASED

All the tricks and games in the world will not gain cooperation if the toddler is not approached from a framework that has behavioral development as the cornerstone. In addition to gaining cooperation, such an approach will foster development of a healthy self-concept and attitude toward health care providers.

According to Erikson, the toddler's developmental task is autonomy versus shame and doubt. Inherent in this stage is the child's need to feel in charge of himself for most activities. Take away this control, and the toddler will resist with his whole being. Instead, let the child set the pace, all the while giving opportunities for exhibiting graduated amounts of self-control and assertion.

Immobility, or restraining motor activity, is viewed as a significant threat. Allowing the toddler to choose his position during the examination will not take away his needed mobility. This position will usually change frequently. The 18-month-old who violently reacts to being placed on the examination table may be responding to the imposed immobility rather than to the table itself.

Another issue central to the development of autonomy is the distinction between self and nonself. Initially egocentric, the toddler refers every event to himself. The origins of separation anxiety are founded as he becomes aware of self and nonself. The social, outgoing infant of a few months earlier may now eye the nurse with suspicion. Trust must be regained, and the toddler's need to keep the nurse at a safe distance must be respected. The distance should be slowly and imperceptibly closed; offering toys will often entice the toddler to move closer.

The toddler's newly acquired autonomy is very fragile, and security is still determined by the presence of the parent. Ability to explore the world and tolerate anxiety is impaired when the parent is not present; thus the parent should be present during an examination. Most toddlers can be completely examined while sitting in the parent's lap, a position of security.

PHYSICAL STATUS

The pudgy, top-heavy infant begins to take on a more adultlike appearance after the first year. With locomotion and with a tremendous activity level, the toddler begins to lose "baby fat," resulting in a general slendering. He stands upright and becomes more proportionate. His abdomen is protuberant, and his posture lordotic (see Fig. 8-2).

NORMAL GROWTH PARAMETERS

Height, weight, and head circumference As if consolidating energy to maintain a high activity level, the growth rate of the toddler is much less dramatic than that of the infant. In fact, there is an abrupt shift downward in velocity (see Fig. 8-3).

Weight, which roughly tripled from an average of 3.4 kg to 10 kg (7½ lb to 22 lb) in the first year, will only quadruple to 12.6 kg (28 lb) by age 2. By age 3, another 1.8 kg (4 lb) will be added (see Fig. 8-4).

FIGURE 8-2. *(Photo courtesy of Andrea Netten Sechrist.)*

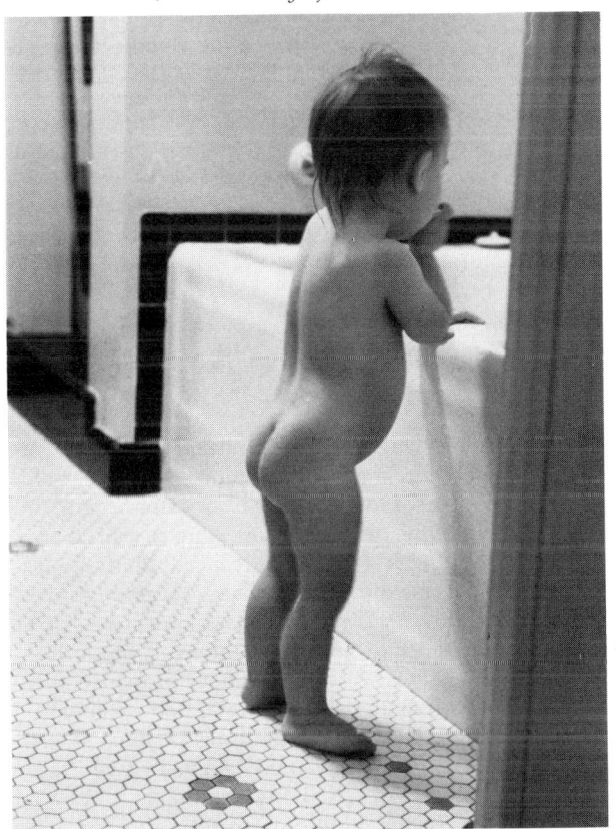

Growth in length shows a similar trend. For the average neonate an increase of about 26.5 cm (10½ in) can be expected by age 1. This is a 50 percent increase. In contrast, the whole of the second year shows an increase of only 11.5 cm (4½ in). This is less than one-half the first year's increase. From age 2 to 3 another 10 cm (4 in) is added (see Fig. 8-5).

Stature is one of the most heritable of morphological characteristics. After the first year, growth has changed from a pattern that is determined mainly by maternal size to a pattern that is genetically controlled.

A diminution of growth rate is also observed in head circumference. During the first year, the brain grows at a very rapid rate, increasing about threefold in weight; most of myelinization is completed by the beginning of the toddler period. During the second year, myelinization is completed, and the brain reaches 80 percent of adult size. (Peripheral myelinization, however, continues until about age 8 years.) This is accompanied by about a 1-in increase in circumference. Very little growth, about 1.25 cm, occurs from age 2 to 3 (see Fig. 8-6).

Channelization of growth With advancing age, linear growth becomes increasingly related to the child's genetic background. This genetic influence tends to be self-stabilizing, target seeking, and channelized (Smith et al., 1976). A shifting of linear growth may occur as the child seeks his genetically determined growth channel. In order to determine the timing and nature of these shifts, Smith et al. conducted a study of 90 otherwise-normal full-term infants who were either at or below the 10th percentile or at or above the 90th percentile for length and who had moved up or down to the 50th percentile.

A shifting of linear growth rate in the first 2 years of life was demonstrated for the majority of the studied children. For the neonates at or below the 10th percentile, acceleration of growth occurred early, and a new growth channel was achieved by a mean age of 11½ months (see Fig. 8-7a). Neonates who were large (90th percentile or greater) but with a genotype for smaller size tended to maintain fetal growth rate for the first 3 to 6 months and then decelerate. A new channel of growth was obtained by the mean age of 13 months (see Fig. 8-7b).

By 2 years of age, the average toddler has joined the genetic curve which will basically determine his eventual adult height. For this reason, perusal of parental height will provide the best correlation of the appropriateness of the height of the child with respect to his genetic back-

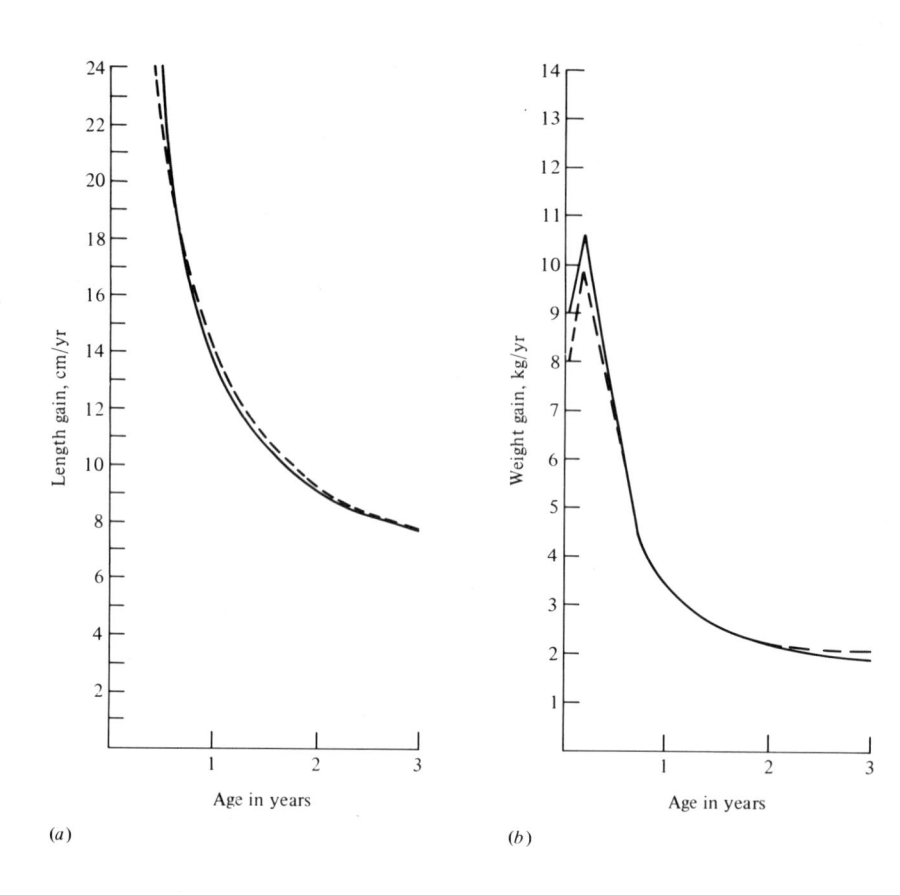

FIGURE 8-3. Length (*a*) and weight (*b*) velocity curves for girls and boys birth to 3 years showing the abrupt downward shift during this period. (*Modified from J. M. Tanner, R. H. Whitehouse, and M. Takaishi, Standards from birth to maturity for height, weight, height velocity, and weight velocity: British children, 1965, Part I. Arch. Dis. Child., 1966, 41, 454, p. 466.*)

ground. Tanner, Goldstein, and Whitehouse (1970) have utilized mean parental height in the development of charts which determine this relation for children between the ages of 2 and 9.

These charts can provide valuable information in the growth assessment of any child. The significance is best illustrated by an example of a hypothetical boy who measures 87 cm at 30 months of age. This places the child at the 25th percentile for height on the Tanner height charts. [National Center for Health Statistics (NCHS) growth grids are used in this textbook. However, comparison of standard deviations is more meaningful if the same measurement standards are used. For this reason, Tanner's growth grids were used. It is recognized that there are differences between the NCHS grids of U.S. children and Tanner's grids of British children, with U.S. children being slightly larger.] This would not in itself arouse suspicion. But if the child has tall parents, with a mean height of 175 cm, his true percentile drops below the 3d percentile. The child is now considered small, perhaps pathologically so.

Body proportions Figure 8-8 illustrates the body proportions of the toddler relative to the neonate and 6-year-old. The cephalocaudal and proximodistal patterns are followed. Growth of the head is always more advanced than the trunk; the trunk is more advanced than the extremities. Transverse dimensions change; the midpoint of the body descends. By 2 years of age, the relative size of the trunk and upper extremities is of adult proportion. The head and neck are still large but have proportionately decreased from 30 to 20 percent of total body volume.

Development of the lower extremities is much slower. After the first year they develop rapidly; by age 2 they constitute 20 percent of total body volume, as compared with 30 percent in the adult. An exception to the prox-

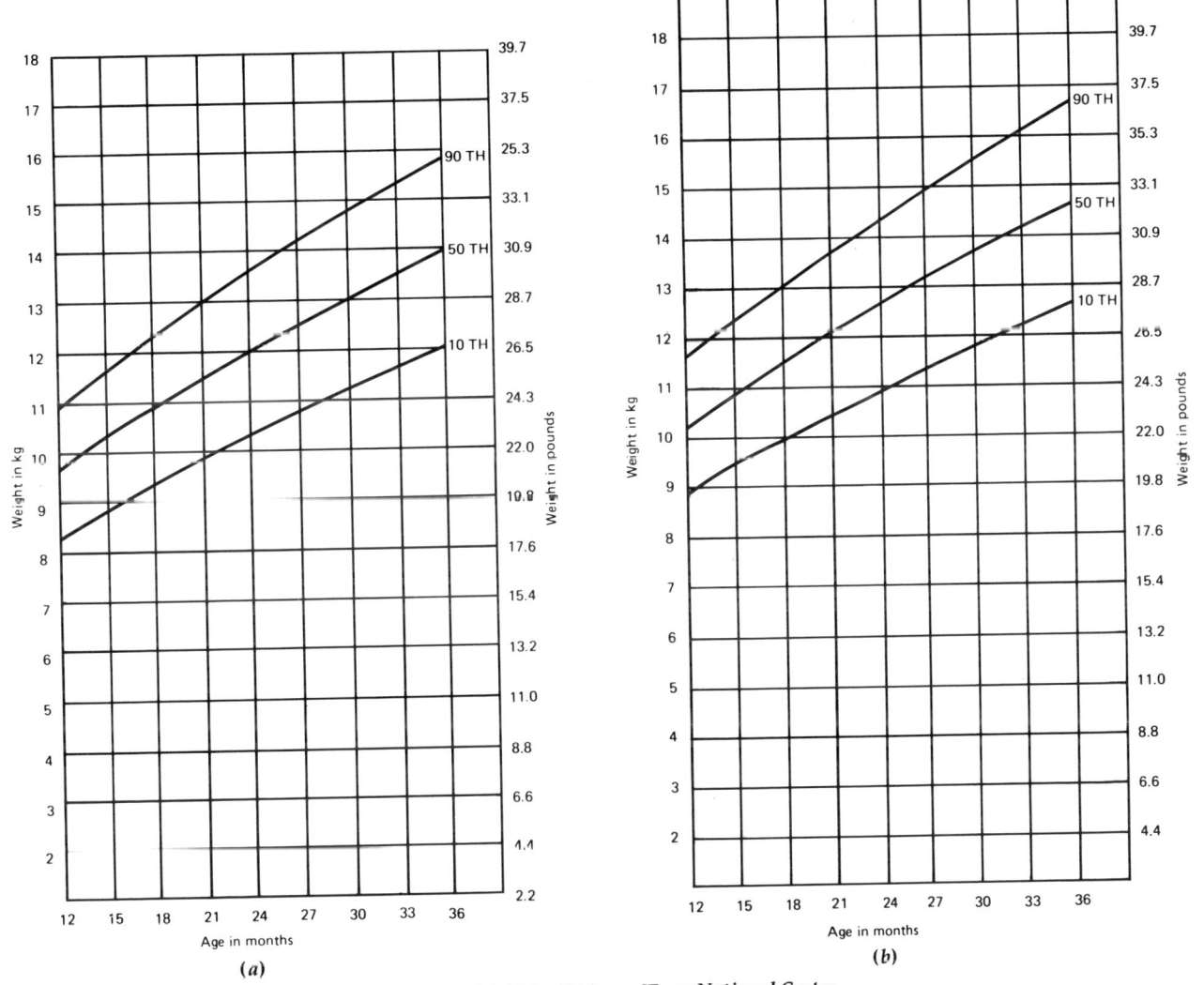

FIGURE 8-4. Weight by age, 12 months to 3 years. (*a*) Girls; (*b*) boys. [*From National Center for Health Statistics, NCHS growth charts, 1976. Monthly Vital Statistics Report HRA 76-1120 Vol. 25, No. 3, Rockville, Maryland: U.S. Health Resources Administration, 1977* (supplement).]

imodistal principle of growth is seen in this part of the body. By 18 months, the foot is one-half adult size, whereas the femur will not attain the same proportion until 4 years of age. Thus, the distal portion of the legs matures more rapidly than the proximal segment.

The protuberant abdomen of the toddler is a reflection of changing body proportions. Abdominal circumference continues to be greater than either head or chest circumference until about 2 years of age. This is due, in part, to a large liver and, in part, to a relatively small pelvis, which cannot completely contain the abdominal contents. With growth of the pelvis, the abdominal contents shift down

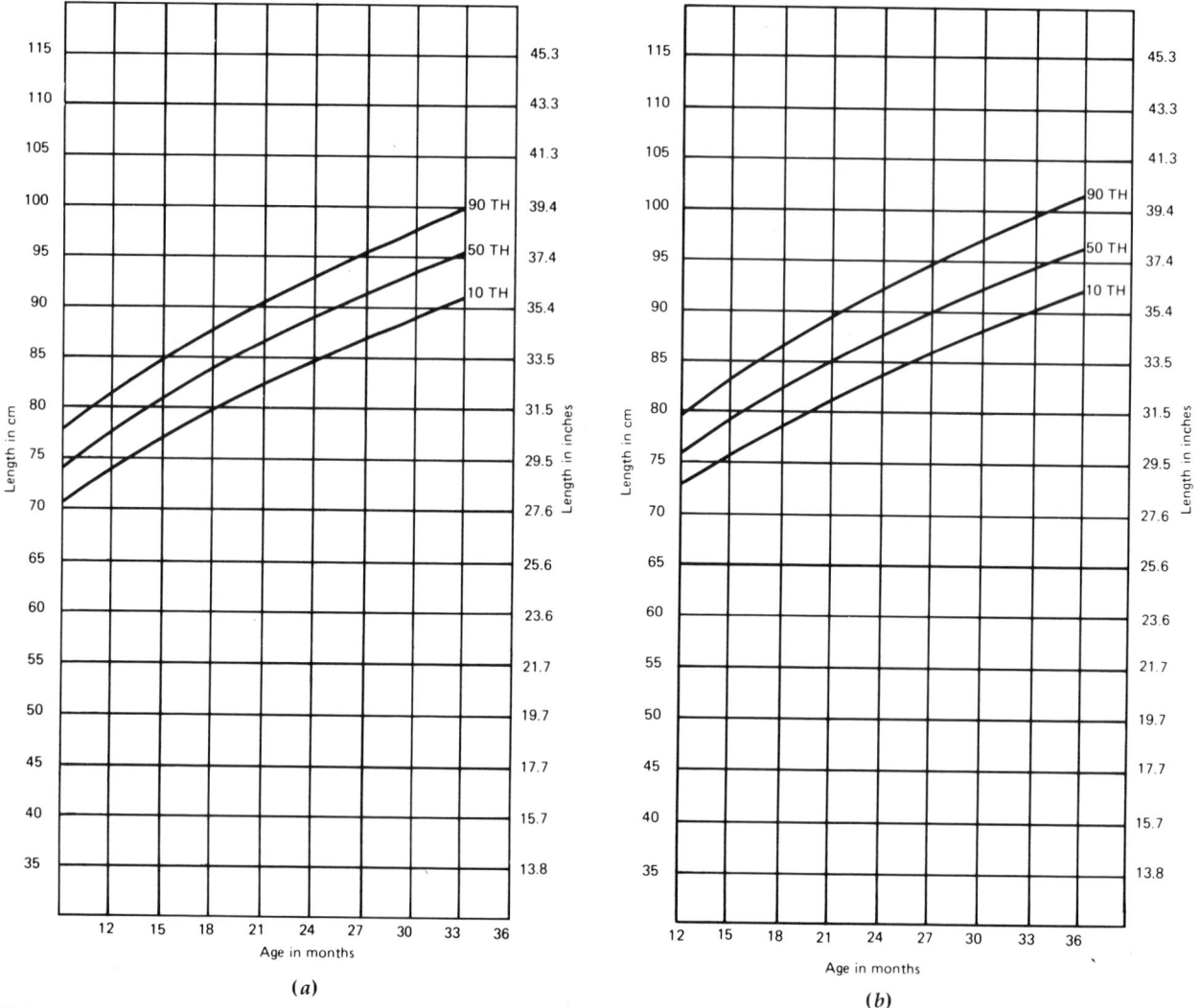

FIGURE 8-5. Length by age, 12 months to 3 years. (a) Girls; (b) boys. (*From NCHS, 1977.*)

into the pelvis, and a flattening of the abdominal wall occurs.

Body posture The toddler's changing body proportions have an impact on development of stance and posture (see Fig. 8-9). The center of gravity of the top-heavy older infant and gaining toddler is quite high; in order to balance securely, the legs are rotated outward, and the feet point out. With inward rotation of the hips, the feet come closer together. A temporary stage of pigeon-toes and bowlegs may occur, followed by a period of knock-knees.

In addition to being high, the toddler's center of gravity is forward because of his larger abdomen and forward pelvis. The lumbar spine compensates for this with exaggeration of curvature, and the upper part of the body is brought into vertical position. Thus, the posture of the toddler is lordotic. As the pelvis rotates backward and the abdomen slims, this compensatory lordosis is no longer

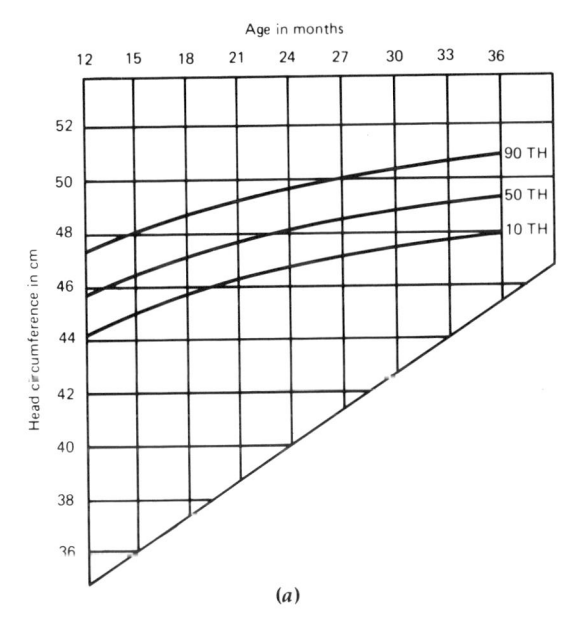

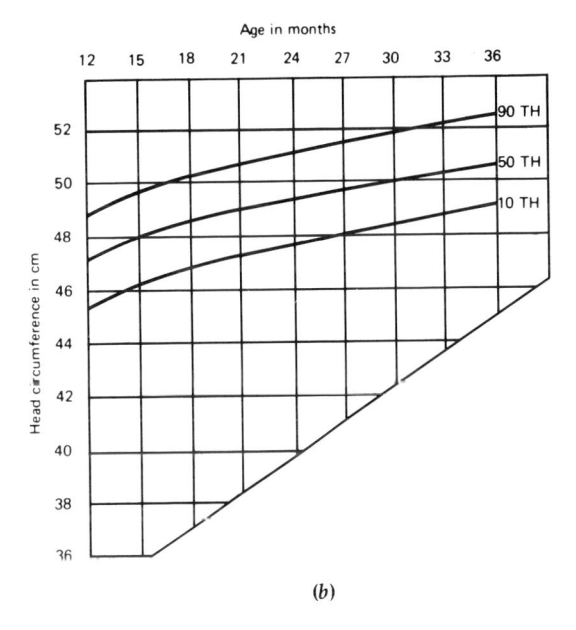

FIGURE 8-6. Occipital-frontal circumference by age, 12 months to 3 years. (a) Girls; (b) boys. (*From NCHS, 1977.*)

needed; thus, the preschooler stands straight and tall. However, adultlike posture is not achieved until adolescence.

VITAL SIGNS

Vital signs steadily decrease throughout childhood. Between the ages of 1 and 2, pulse rates average 80 to 140 bpm. They average 80 to 130 bpm at age 2 and 80 to 120 bpm at age 3. Respiratory rate at rest is approximately 25 breaths per minute between 1 and 3 years. Blood pressure is 96/65 (±27/27) at age 1 to 2 and 96/61 (±24/24) age 2 to 3.

The toddler period marks the end of the early, most rapid, and most significant era of growth. The late fetal period and infancy demonstrate marked growth. However, velocity drops dramatically during the second and third years. The toddler's size reflects that of his parents, and thus his genetic background in stature is notable. His growth, of course, will continue at a slowed rate through childhood, and he will continue to apply his increasing size and upright posture to tasks in his broadening world.

Calvarium and face Mary Tudor

Growth of the calvarium is significant but less rapid than during infancy. The anterior fontanel closes by 18 months, and the skull becomes thicker. The parietal eminence becomes less prominent, and the skull becomes taller due to growth of the base as well as to maxillary and mandibular growth.

More facial contour change is notable with remodeling accompanying growth. The child begins to "grow into" his eyes; the sucking fat pads of infancy are lost during the toddler period also adding to the loss of the round infant face.

TOOTH FORMATION

During the second year of life, the child's deciduous teeth complete eruption and emerge into the oral cavity. The maxillary primary molars, mandibular and maxillary cuspids, and mandibular and maxillary second molars appear, usually in that order (see Fig. 8-10). Calcification of the roots of the deciduous teeth is not complete until about 3 years of age.

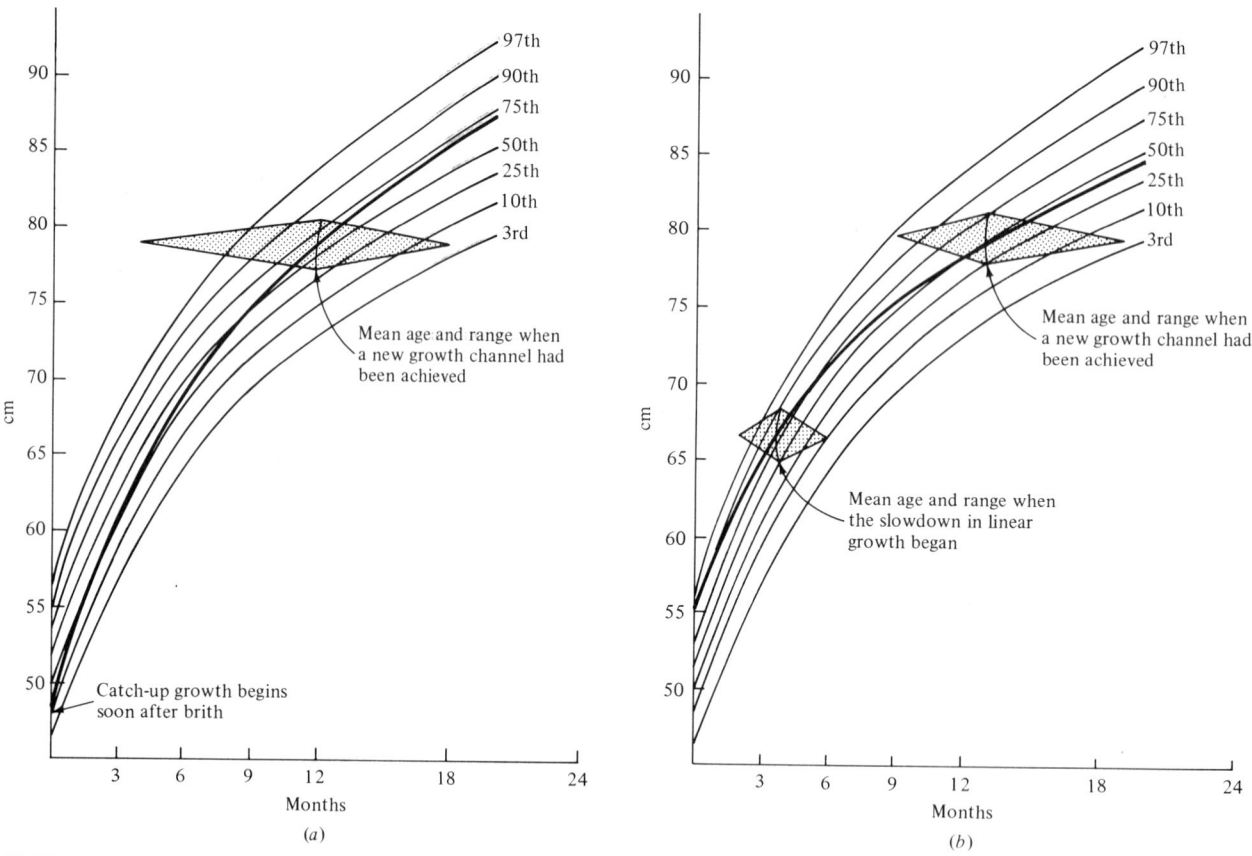

FIGURE 8-7. (a) Mean growth curve for 16 infants who were close to the 10th percentile in linear size at birth and who had shifted growth to near the 70th percentile by age 2 years. (b) Mean growth curve for infants who were close to the 90th percentile in linear size at birth and who had shifted growth down to near the 40th percentile by age 2 years. (From D. W. Smith, W. Truog, J. E. Rogers, L. J. Greitzer, A. L. Skinner, J. J. McCann, and M. A. Harvey, Shifting linear growth during infancy: Illustration of genetic factors in growth from fetal life through infancy. J. Pediat., 1976, 89, 225.)

Thus, the child will have 20 deciduous teeth from approximately 2 years until approximately 6 years, when shedding of the deciduous teeth begins. During this time, the permanent teeth continue to calcify under the gum line, and as the root of the permanent tooth grows, it will gradually erupt.

Sensory system Anna M. Tichy

Visual acuity improves steadily in the toddler years so that by 2 years of age it is approximately 20/60 and at the end of the third year visual acuity is 20/40 to 20/30.

The sensitive period of the development of human binocular vision is between 1 and 3 years of age. This period is defined as the critical time during which a child is not only more affected by sensory deprivation but can make new connections more readily, adapting to variations in sensory stimulation. The structure and function of the visual system are greatly affected by abnormal visual experiences during the sensitive period.

Experimental animal research has evaluated effects of visual experiences on subsequent development of visual corticoneural processes. Gross impairment of vision in kittens results if both eyes are sutured or covered during

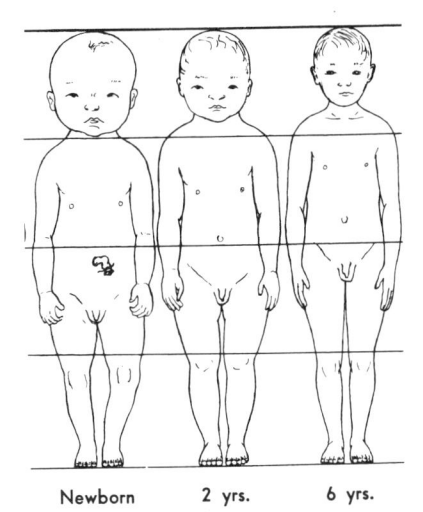

FIGURE 8-8. Body proportion of the toddler (2 years of age) compared with the neonate and the 6-year-old.

the first 3 months of life, the critical period for the cat. Abnormal neurophysiological and histological findings in visually deprived cats have been confirmed with behavioral studies. Findings indicate that the change in cortical visual neurons following absence of stimulation is due to some type of a degenerative process rather than to a developmental failure.

An analogous critical period for binocular vision, which is necessary for fusion and depth perception, exists in the child. The major clinical implication of this finding is that early identification and surgical correction of strabismus are indicated for the development of cortical binocularity.

With increased mobility leading to an expanded environment for the toddler, the sensory system assumes a major role in the child's ability to understand the external world and to maintain some degree of constancy of the internal environment.

Musculoskeletal system Sherrilyn Passo

Although overall growth of the toddler is not as rapid as that of the infant, important changes occur in the musculoskeletal system. Ossification of bone continues during the second and third years, although at a slower rate and in fewer ossification centers. In the second year, the bones in the lower limbs finally become longer than those in the upper limbs, corresponding to their greater functional significance in ambulation. Weight-bearing and gross motor activities requiring increased muscle movement stimulate long-bone growth in the legs.

Muscular development is also rapid in the lower limbs. The child's ability to walk produces changes in his lower spine, causing the appearance of the lower S curve, the lumbar curve, around 12 to 18 months.

FIGURE 8-9. Development of stance: (a) 18 months old, bowlegs; (b) 3 years old, knock-knees; (c) 6 years old, legs straight. [From D. Sinclair, Human growth after birth (3d ed.). London: Oxford University Press, 1978, p. 49. Reprinted by permission of the publisher.]

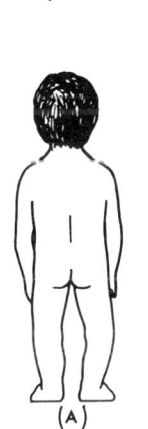

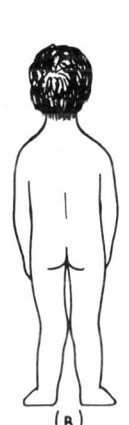

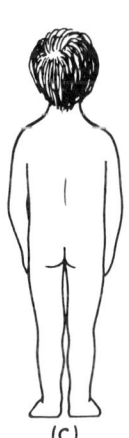

Gastrointestinal system Anna M. Tichy and Dianne Chong

Though the first year after birth is associated with maximal growth of the digestive system, further growth and development of the system continues at a gradual rate throughout childhood. At 1 year of age the length of the intestinal tract has increased by one-third of the birth length. The secretory and absorptive surfaces were for the most part functioning adequately during the neonatal period; data regarding physiological developmental changes in these areas during childhood are minimal.

A number of significant developmental changes occur in the mouth during the toddler period. The salivary glands acquire adult histological characteristics and undergo a fivefold increase in weight since the age of 6 months. Functional changes accompany the anatomical ones. The aqueous parotid gland secretion of the 3- and 4-year-old is much greater than that in older children.

The anatomical capacity of the stomach is approximately 500 mL by the end of the second year. With increasing maturation, peristalsis and contractions assume adultlike characteristics. The number of gastric glands progressively increases, and the musculature continues to develop. In infancy the stomach lies in the transverse plane of the body, but by the second to third year it assumes the common "cow's horn" configuration. Hydrochloric acid and pepsin secretions, when corrected for body weight, are within the normal adult range by 2 years of age.

Motility in the small intestine is not of the quality or variety of wave forms characteristic of the adult. However, the colon has an adult-type motor function in the toddler. Digestion of fats, carbohydrates, and proteins proceeds efficiently in the child, though there are some age-related changes in pancreatic enzyme activity. Recent work has shown that lipase activity in the young child is independent of age (Hadorn, Zoppi, Schmerling, Prader, McIntyre, and Anderson, 1968). Adult levels of small intestine fat absorption are attained in the beginning of the toddler period. Amylase activity steadily increases, whereas sucrase, maltase, and lactase activity levels remain constant at the adult value throughout the remainder of childhood. Trypsin activity, which is adequate from birth, is positively correlated with age and body weight. By school age, gastric transit time, emptying, and secretion are as in the adult.

Though functionally mature in its digestive functions at an early age, the liver continues to grow throughout childhood. The weight of the liver increases 10 times its birth weight by puberty. The left lobe of the liver decreases in relative size, composing one-third to one-fourth of the liver mass in childhood as compared with one-half to one-third of the liver mass in the neonate.

The small and large intestinal tracts are functionally mature in this age period. The digestive system, as a whole, descends with growth and continues to increase in length, musculature, and amount of total absorptive surface area. A fourfold increase in the surface area of the intestinal tract occurs between birth and adulthood.

DEFECATION

By 1 to 2 years neurological pathways necessary for voluntary sphincter control are developed. With attainment of physiological maturity, defecation becomes voluntary. In the continent child the act of defecation is initiated when (1) some feces enter the rectum increasing intraluminal rectal pressure, (2) rectal sensory nerve fibers transmit signals to the spinal cord, (3) descending parasympathetic fibers transmit signals that initiate strong peristaltic contractions that may effectively empty the colon, (4) the higher central nervous system accepts the information provided by the reflex responses of the rectum, and (5) the environment is deemed socially acceptable for this function.

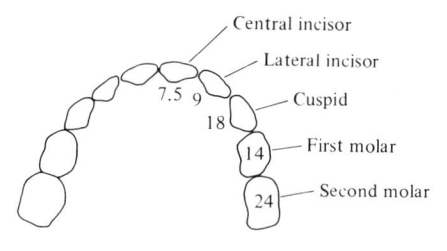

During the toddler period, the gastrointestinal tract reaches functional maturity; growth continues to adulthood.

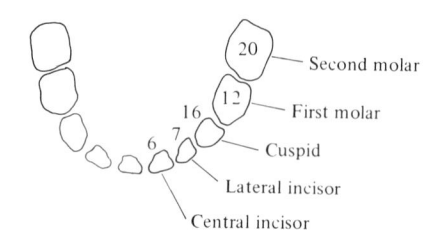

FIGURE 8-10. Deciduous dentition at 24 months of age with mean age of emergence (in months) illustrated.

Development of body concept and concepts of illness and wellness
Judith Anne Ritchie

BODY CONCEPT, CONTENT, AND FUNCTION

The toddler's upright posture and increased visual acuity permit the child to perceive his body structure more accurately. Body play with his own and others' bodies helps to locate and organize names of body parts. Mirror play makes unseen parts, such as the face, more familiar. The toddler recognizes the mirror image as his own although he may at times look behind the mirror for the other child.

EXPLORATION OF BODY ORIFICES

During the second year the body orifice of dominance becomes the anus (Fisher and Cleveland, 1958). In the later toddler period the oral area and head regain important positions in the body concept, but they are in competition with increased genital feeling (Cohn, 1960; Greenacre, 1958; Linn, 1955). The toddler seeks information about his own and others' genitalia through observing naked siblings and parents and handling his own genitals (Gesell, Ilg, and Ames, 1974). Any orifice is explored manually and, if possible, visually.

CONCEPT OF CONTENT AND FUNCTION
Advance in motor abilities during the toddler years provides considerable information about the body, its boundaries, and its functions. The acts of standing and walking alone help the toddler to learn the separateness of the body from external objects. Experiments with motor activities clarify perceptions of body mass and center of gravity. Sometimes painful collisions with door frames, tables, chairs, and other objects define body boundaries, size, density, and constancy.

The beginning concept of the content of the body relates to feces. The toddler who becomes upset or waves bye-bye while watching his feces being flushed away demonstrates the perception that whatever "emanates out of our body will still remain a part of the body-image" (Schilder, 1964, p. 213).

WELLNESS, ILLNESS, AND HOSPITALIZATION
From infancy onward the child learns about health and health practices primarily from the parents or major care giver. Their constant input increases the toddler's awareness of the value of the body, the need to maintain its intactness, and the means of doing so. The toddler often appears confused and alarmed when anything interrupts the body's intactness; the older toddler quickly learns to avoid such situations.

The toddler's developmental task of achieving autonomy greatly influences his perception of illness. Respiratory distress or diarrhea and vomiting represent frightening loss of control of the body and loss of body contents. The recently toilet-trained toddler is upset by the loss of ability to control elimination and by the soiling of clothing and linens (Freud, 1952). The ill toddler often is quieter and more easily irritated than usual. He exerts his need for closer contact with the parent in clinging and demanding behavior. However, unless the illness is severe, he usually refuses to remain resting in bed.

PERCEPTION OF PAIN
The child over 2 years begins to locate painful sensations more accurately. The toddler frequently points to a painful body part or holds up a cut finger and repeats "boo boo" or some other word to signify hurt. More intense pain or visceral pain seems to confuse the toddler and to be difficult to locate.

The toddler's inability to understand and his lack of vocabulary seriously limit the capacity to communicate presence or location of pain. Many toddlers seem to cope with pain in a manner similar to one child, aged 14 months, who had surgery for a pilonidal sinus. For several postoperative days he had little appetite and was content to lie or play very quietly in bed or a carriage. Once a pressure dressing was removed, he resumed more autonomous behavior in eating, was much more active in play, and had considerable interest in walking.

The amount and context of prior painful experiences and the reactions of parents will also influence the toddler's perception of a painful event and reactions to it. Under 2 years of age, the child's ability to understand pain seems limited to the sensation itself (McCaffery, 1969).

PERCEPTION OF RESTRAINT AND PROCEDURES
Mobility is the toddler's major means of discovery of the body and the environment and of coping with stress. Any attempt to restrain movement is met with fear, resistance, and protest. Children over 18 months fight restraints less, possibly because of learning that such struggle is not successful or understanding that struggle causes increased pain (Dowd, Novak, and Roy, 1977). The back-lying position seems to be experienced as highly vulnerable, and children restrained in this position for painful or nonpainful procedures struggle immediately to regain the upright position.

Toddlers who are restrained for long periods often seem to withdraw and to become depressed, perhaps because they experience distortion or monotony (O'Grady, 1969). Because the toddler uses mobility as an active coping device, any restriction in mobility often results in lowering ability to tolerate stress.

Their inability to verbally express concerns and feelings renders toddlers particularly vulnerable to being overwhelmed by the sights, sounds, and sensations of procedures. Reactions are highly individual and depend on previous experiences and whether the procedure involves separation from a familiar person. Toddlers respond tearfully to loud noises, such as that made by cast cutters, and to unfamiliar sensations, such as application of pressure or cold solutions. Some toddlers become frantic in such situations and can be soothed only with considerable effort—usually after completion of the procedure. Others may use wary vigilance or withdrawal as a coping mechanism.

HOSPITALIZATION

For the hospitalized toddler, separation from parents becomes the major focus of behavior. There are three phases in the typical response of the toddler subjected to separation without a consistent care giver and/or frequent visits from parents (Bowlby, 1960; Robertson, 1970). The initial reaction is protest with loud crying and struggle to regain the lost parent. Attempts to comfort are often rejected. In the second phase of despair, the toddler becomes quiet, anorexic, and appears depressed. In the third phase of detachment or denial, the toddler appears to have settled in and to be adjusted to the separation. However, careful observation reveals little engagement in play and social responses that are indiscriminate and shallow. When parents visit for a considerable time daily or adequate substitute parenting is provided, the toddler is not so overwhelmed, and while showing some stress, he is able to manage his anxiety and cope with the separation (Robertson and Robertson, 1971).

While coping with unfamiliar sensations of illness, the strange environment, and separation, it is not uncommon for the toddler to display feelings of anger, rage, and frustration. Temper tantrums may increase in frequency, and there may be sudden outbursts of aggression. For example, being examined by his familiar physician while sitting on his mother's lap, one toddler, aged 28 months, suddenly vigorously lashed out, hitting the doctor and pulling the stethoscope down and out of his ears.

The absence of familiar rituals of meals, baths, and bedtime contributes to the toddler's degree of upset. The toddler frequently reacts with marked behavioral changes such as regression to bottle feeding or loss of bladder and bowel control. He may also evidence poor appetite and inability to cooperate with baths or bedtime.

If the toddler is securely accustomed and adapted to brief separations from parents, he may adjust to hospitalization with less difficulty. Decreased short- and long-term behavioral disturbances have been demonstrated in children whose mothers had started working more than 6 months prior to the child's hospital admission (Douglas, 1975).

When a previous hospitalization has been a growth experience through successful coping and mastery, the toddler may have less difficulty coping with a second hospitalization. However, hospitalizations are noted to have

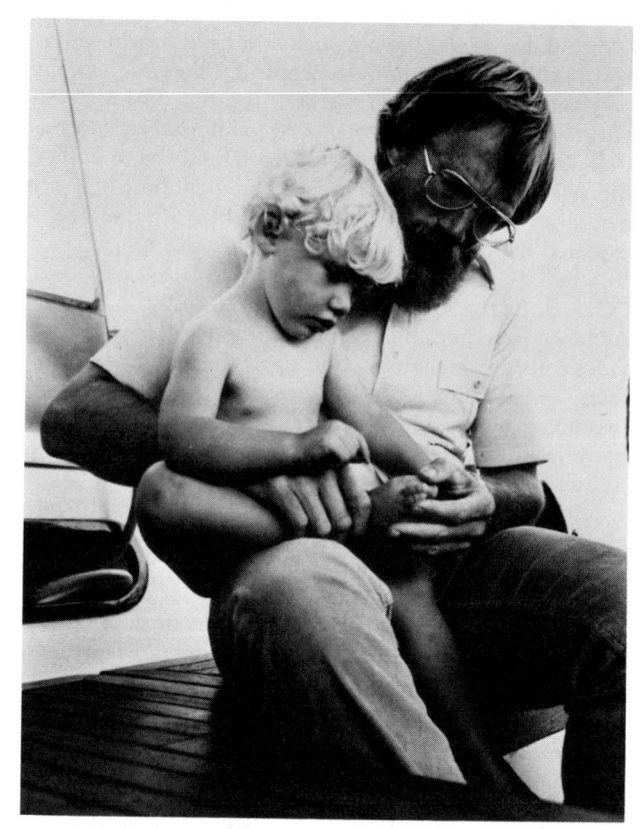

FIGURE 8-11.

the most effect on the toddler under 3, and it has been noted that multiple hospitalizations in the early years are associated with adverse behavioral ratings in the adolescent years (Douglas, 1975).

DEATH

The toddler between 2 and 3 years does not have a realistic concept of death but does continue to experiment with separation and with being and nonbeing (Grollman, 1967). The very ill toddler perceives the difference in his parents' interaction and the growing separation from them. The dying toddler, or one who is critically ill, often becomes withdrawn and apathetic unless a parent or parent substitute is emotionally available on a consistent basis (Schowalter, 1970).

According to Furman (1964), the 2- to 3-year-old can master death in the course of day-to-day experiences. However, the child is said to interpret death as a separation and to have no clear understanding of the inevitability or irrevocability of death (Nagy, 1948; Natterson and Knudson, 1960).

Physical development is relatively less significant in the toddler period than infancy. Slowed growth rate is notable on measurement as well as in food consumed. The cephalocaudal pattern will be less apparent in physical development after the toddler period as bladder and bowel control is gained.

The toddler is determined to experience his body and physical prowess primarily through mobility. Through mobility comes physical separation from parents. The toddler appears determined to establish himself as being as emotionally and behaviorally independent as he perceives himself to be physically. Behavioral development is discussed in the following section.

SECTION 2

Behavioral Development

Rapid development of behavioral skills during the toddler period cannot be denied. In all areas of functioning the ages from 1 to 3 years mark the transition from infancy to childhood.

The toddler moves from relative dependency to relative independence. He no longer has the primary drive of action for action's sake but can pause to redirect his energy to the outside world. He is transformed from being primarily a mover into a sayer and doer. The degree to which the toddler has practiced and accomplished the behavioral tasks of this period will be evident as the child moves to apply them in the broader world as a preschool-age child.

The toddler: Demanding recognition
Mary Tudor

Who has not seen the young toddler, arms in high, wing-flapping posture, short legs taking quick, short strides, squealing and running away from a pursuing parent? The toddler is consumed by his demand for recognition. This recognition will come from establishment of autonomy and individuality.

The toddler wants autonomy in the world that he just learned as an infant is "out there." Thus he has a drive to be in control, leading to the toddler's infamous negative behavior. In order to earn this autonomy, the toddler must first gain control of his body, mastering those skills so rapidly accumulated in infancy. This mastery is achieved from repetition and experimentation.

Through repetition of behaviors, such as climbing into the box, out of the box, into the box, and so on, the toddler develops proficiency and integrates skills. The child experiences success in self-initiated tasks, and when he does, he can be delightful to behold; not all toddlerhood is negative! Yet the toddler is unable to set limits on his repetition and may drive himself to a point of emotional disintegration. The toddler also demands repetition from his environment asking for the same book, same song, same food, same blanket, and so on. In this way, ritualistic patterns emerge.

The toddler is an explorer. In his explorations he experiments with the world, applying his trial-and-error approach within ever-widening boundaries. His joy is evident as he discovers the world. But again, he can carry exploration too far, lose control through exhaustion, and experience frustration from this loss.

The toddler seeks autonomy in every area of behavioral development. Motorically, he is walking and running, and this affords a tremendous sense of power. The toddler demonstrates autonomy from parents as he motorically moves away from them. This is easier in the early stages, perhaps because the "out there" is an exciting unknown; he merely wants to escape.

The toddler soon discovers that the out there can mean falls and bumps, inability to find parents, strangers, and failures. An element of ambivalence colors his motoric conquest for autonomy from parents. He wants their protection while he seeks freedom from their influence. As if to remedy this conflict through language, self-help endeavors, and in play, the toddler finds ways to be in control of, but not physically removed from, parents.

The young toddler's all-encompassing one-word phrases are demands and refusals as well as labels. Later, two- and three-word phrases are substituted, but many needs are still made known nonverbally. As the toddler masters the art of self-feeding, he uses food throwing and refusal as a potent statement of autonomy. Sleep patterns, a success of infancy, become disrupted, and staying in bed and *whose* bed become bargaining grounds for the issue of control. Perhaps the most memorable struggle is over toilet training. Although praise for success in bowel and bladder control is important for self-esteem, the toddler learns that it can be another area for exerting autonomy.

The toddler gains strength for this scrimmage and copes with the results through play. The toddler motorically and later mentally acts through the important autonomy issues at hand. He also imitates those he perceives to be in control. When failures confront him and his quest for autonomy is thwarted, he can retreat to "play it out." With sensitive parental guidance and appropriate boundaries, in the end the toddler will experience more success than failure and can gain control of the environment without losing control of himself in the effort.

In his autonomy, the toddler displays his individuality: those characteristics that determine *how* each particular toddler carries out those generally observed behavioral skills. Terms such as *personality* or *temperament* are used to describe these differences in children. Nine characteristics have been described by Thomas and Chess (1977): activ-

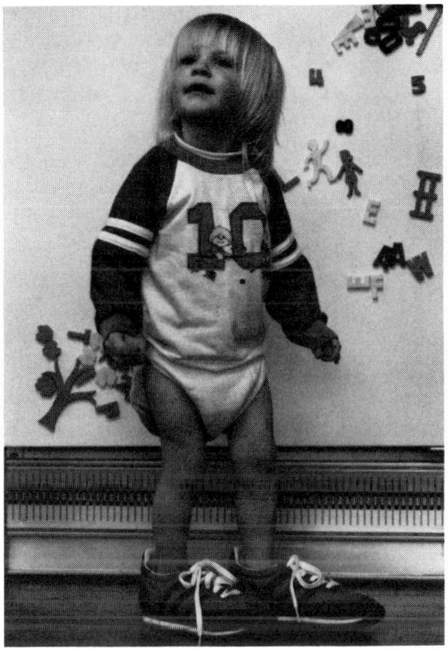

FIGURE 8-12. *(Photo courtesy of Grant Allen.)*

ity level, rhythmicity, degree of approach or withdrawal to new situations, adaptability to change, threshold of responsiveness, intensity of reaction, quality of mood, distractibility, and persistence and attention span. These individual characteristics can be noted beginning early in infancy but often come into sharper focus due to parent-child interaction during the stormy toddler period.

The particular constellation of characteristics determines a child's temperament. Three temperamental constellations have been identified by Thomas and Chess (p. 23): the easy child, the difficult child, and the slow-to-warm-up child (see Chap. 4).

A child's temperament characteristics determine half the quality of the parent-child interaction. Parents expectations of and attitudes toward the child and themselves as well as their behavior toward the child are affected.

In the preschool years the temperamental constellation of the Easy or Difficult child can continue to affect the parents' responses as new demands for adaptation and self-mastery arise. In addition, these new demands and expectations, combined with the child's ever expanding range of activities and capabilities, enhance the significance of other temperamental attributes in the developmental process. Here, too, as in the earlier period, temperament can affect the parents' attitudes and behavior toward the child. (Thomas and Chess, p. 73)

The high-energy tasks of mastery of skills and quest for control meet with parental frustration but also with success as they are reinforced in the broader environment. Finally, with consolidated skills and with a sense of autonomy and self-competency, the toddler is able to move on and to delight in his world and himself.

Behavioral Development by Functional Area

Perceptual development

With the beginning of independent walking, sometime between 12 to 18 months of age, the toddler's environment is greatly enlarged through exploration. As the toddler moves about actively seeking out and investigating things in his environment, he develops certain expectations about his world. And as Bower has noted (1977), after 1 year of age the toddler is less dominated by his direct perceptual experiences and more by his developing knowledge of how things are ordered. In addition, the toddler is more actively exploratory in his movements and search for information than the infant. However, he is less systematic in this than the older child.

CONTINUING PROBLEMS IN STUDYING PERCEPTION

The toddler's increased mobility and sense of self-direction cause problems for the would-be investigator of perceptual development. Now the investigator must capture the toddler's interest in order to get him to cooperate. Because of this difficulty, many areas of perceptual development have not been explored during this age period. For example, it is probable that *object constancy* is well developed by 3 years of age; that is, the toddler recognizes that an object remains the same object even though it is viewed from different angles, which produces a different image on the retina. However, the data to substantiate this are lacking because of the inappropriateness of methods for testing for this age group.

Most information about perception at this age comes from careful observation of the toddler in various situations. The toddler is a great imitator of visual and auditory happenings in his surroundings, and it is assumed that anything he can imitate must first be perceived. Hence, this is one way of studying how the toddler perceives events. One must be cautious using this method because in the normal toddler productive or motor abilities usually lag behind perceptual abilities. Therefore the extent of a child's perceptual ability is not always reflected in his performance.

Another way to study the toddler's perceptual expectations is to set up perceptually discrepant situations and observe the toddler's response. For example, the toddler is shown a motion picture of his mother with someone else's voice dubbed in. Or, as Bower (1977) has done, the toddler is presented with a situation which seems to violate perceptual laws: A solid object appears to disappear into thin air. The toddler is usually filmed, and then behaviors, such as eye opening, facial expressions, and looking persistence, are scored.

REPORTED FINDINGS

VISUAL PERCEPTION

Most of the basic visual abilities are fairly well established by this time: brightness discrimination, color vision, binocular vision with the resultant stereopsis, pattern differentiation, and movement recognition. What happens of most note during this time, other than the further improvements in some basic abilities, is the differentiation of space. As a result of this the child develops object constancy and an appreciation of distance.

Prior to walking, most of the infant's experience with space differentiation involved reaching for things within view. But now with increased mobility, the toddler is able to explore in order to detect the invariant (sameness despite change) properties of objects as they undergo perspective transformations in space. And it is this experience, according to E. Gibson (1969), that is necessary for the development of object constancy. Also as a result of increased mobility, there is the integration of proprioceptive and vestibular stimulation with visual input which guides reaching or movement toward a target in the spatial layout.

Symbolic thought begins at around 18 to 24 months, and at approximately the same time the toddler develops the ability to identify representations of things, such as pictures. This ability, according to a study done by Hochberg and Brooks (1962), is an unlearned ability. They tested a 19-month-old child who learned his vocabulary by reference to solid objects alone and had absolutely no instruction or training as to pictorial meaning. Yet when tested with pictures, both outline drawings and photographs of a number of the objects known to him, he was able to recognize them. Thus, it would seem that the ability to pick two-dimensional pictures as representations of three-dimensional objects is not the abstract task it was once thought to be.

AUDITORY PERCEPTION

Basic auditory abilities are well established by the end of the first year. What is seen during this period is a seeking of repetitive stimulation. Every parent who has ever read to a toddler is familiar with this behavior: the child's request that the same nursery rhyme be read over and over, much to the dismay of the adult. Some studies on listening preferences also provide evidence of this kind of behavior (Friedlander, 1970). Friedlander devised an automated "toy" which he attached to the toddler's crib or playpen for the purpose of recording the child's listening preferences.

The toy, called a Playtest, consisted of a pair of large response switches that the toddler could operate at will, a loudspeaker, an electrical control-and-response recording unit, and a stereo tape player with a preprogrammed selection of two-channel audio tapes. When the toddlers were offered a choice between tape recordings of ebullient family conversations that differed only in the amount of redundancy, they initially chose the high-redundancy selection. But after several days of this, followed by a period of lower overall listening, the toddlers switched to the low-redundancy message.

In addition to demonstrating listening preferences that require close attention and good discrimination ability, Friedlander's studies provide additional evidence for the potency of even abstract voices coming out of a loudspeaker for the young child. This was clearly evident by the amount of listening time some of the children produced.

Additional evidence for the toddler's tendency to seek repetitive auditory stimulation comes from the vocal self-stimulating behavior observed at this time. Weir (1966) studied this behavior in her own children when they were between the ages of 2 and 5 years. She found that this self-stimulating behavior that frequently occurred in the evening was not mere aimless play. On the contrary, the child endlessly repeated sounds and grammatical structures that he had previously heard as if trying to perfect them. J. J. Gibson (1966) views the self-stimulating aspects of speech as an important form of proprioception which provides guidance information to the speaker about the quality of the unfolding performance. Other people have also commented on the apparent usefulness of self-stimulating behavior for organizing the speech input to which the child is continually exposed.

And judging by his speech, the average 3-year-old has done an amazing job of making sense out of the language he hears. He combines two words to form grammatical utterances, follows simple directions, and uses the plural form correctly. How this is achieved remains a mystery. None of the theories so far suggested, mimicry, social modeling, or creative synthesis, begins to account for this amazing accomplishment.

OTHER SENSES

Tactile input, proprioception, and kinesthesia play a role in development of gross motor and fine motor skills. Whether these sensations are determinative or facilitative is still debated. Independent walking, a major milestone as well as ongoing amusement for the toddler, is directed by tactile input. Proprioceptive sensations monitor body positions, and kinesthesia monitors movement. All work in an intricate feedback system.

Tactile input also continues to help the toddler define and redefine the limits of his growing body. Development of body concept is primarily a function of tactile and motor experience.

Gross motor development Fay F. Russell and Beverly R. Richardson

Although the rate of developmental progression is not as rapid during the toddler period as during the period of infancy, the child continues his acquisition and refinement of gross motor skills. This developmental progression also remains contingent upon neuromuscular maturation. Truly a "toddler," walking and later running dominate the child's gross motor activity. During the second year, much of the time is spent trying to satisfy this drive.

NEUROMUSCULAR MATURATION

Specific changes involved in neuromuscular maturation are primarily a continuation of events which began during infancy. As described earlier, the primitive Babinski reflex is gradually integrated during the early toddler period, while the Landau reflex continues to persist until the child is 12 to 24 months of age. It is thought that the Landau reflex assists the toddler in developing the ability to stand with stability through the promotion of the symmetrical extension of his trunk and hips.

The automatic reflexes—righting, protective, and equilibrium—are refined during the toddler period and continue their vital role in gross motor skill development. Specifically, the labyrinthine righting reaction on the head allows the toddler to assume and maintain an erect posture, while the other righting reflexes act to maintain proper alignment of the head and body. Protective reactions allow the toddler to break a fall by rapid arm extension, and the equilibrium reactions permit him to automatically respond to shifts in posture.

In addition to the important reflexive maturation occurring during this period, the process of myelinization continues. As this process unfolds, more peripheral nerve pathways become functional resulting in progressive gross motor development and refinement.

Muscular maturation continues as the fibers increase in size and muscles increase in strength. While the toddler may lack a great deal of strength, coordination, and control early in this period, he demonstrates considerable progress in these areas during the second and third years.

GROSS MOTOR SKILL DEVELOPMENT

WALKING

When considering the toddler's development of locomotion skills, progression in walking is a major component which is based on skills acquired during infancy. The age these skills are acquired is variable. As an average, the toddler of 12 to 13 months stands with stability without support and takes one or two steps independently. Soon he will walk short distances and fall by collapsing. By 13 to 15 months the toddler walks independently with a wide-based gait, unequal steps, and high guard (hands at shoulder height, ready to break a fall). At 15 months he walks with stability with a narrow base and full-sole step, and he can start and stop suddenly. Gradually the toddler uses medium and then low guard as balance improves allowing more subtle equilibrium responses (see Fig. 8-13).

The toddler of 13 to 15 months is able to stoop to pick up an object and rise again to standing without holding on (see Fig. 8-14). The 18-month-old is often seen maintaining a squatting position to play. Later, when the toddler develops an adult-type heel-toe gait and his arms are no longer necessary for protective extension, he can carry, pull, or push objects while walking. At about the same time, the toddler can run stiffly with a flat-footed gait. By 24 months, practice allows a smoother, looser run with heel-toe gait. The toddler delights in trying to outrun his parents and can soon look over his shoulder and make wide turns while running: good avoidance tactics.

Protective and equilibrium reflexes are prerequisite to walking. An intense positive supporting reaction or persistence of the asymmetrical tonic neck or tonic labyrinthine reflexes may interfere. Another important factor in

426 THE TODDLER: 1 YEAR TO 3 YEARS

FIGURE 8-13. Seven phases of erect locomotion. (*a*) The neonate exhibits the stepping reflex, birth to 3 or 4 months. (*b*) Inhibition or static phase: the stepping reflex is inhibited, the extremities are less flexed, and the head is in line with the body plane, 5 months. (*c*) Transition phase: the infant is more active with the balance response beginning, 6 months. (*d*) Deliberate stepping: stepping movement and equilibrium responses improve. The shoulder girdle is more in line with the pelvic girdle. The infant may observe his feet, 8 to 10 months. (*e*) Independent stepping: the child holds his arms in extension and abduction (high guard). A wide-based gait with marked hip and knee flexion and high steps is seen. The leg movements are isolated and staccato but not separate from whole-body movements. The extension and abduction in arms decreases, and so they are held more at the side with forearms at right angle to the body (medium guard). The base becomes more narrow, and less hip and knee flexion is seen, 10 to 13 months. (*f*) Heel-toe progression: the toddler walks in a heel-toe pattern, arms at sides, 11 to 15 months. (*g*) Integration or maturity of erect locomotion: the toddler walks with synchronous arm swings with contralateral, well-coordinated leg movement. (From M. B. McGraw, *The neuromuscular maturation of the human infant.* New York: Columbia University Press, 1945, p. 77. Reprinted by permission of the publisher.)

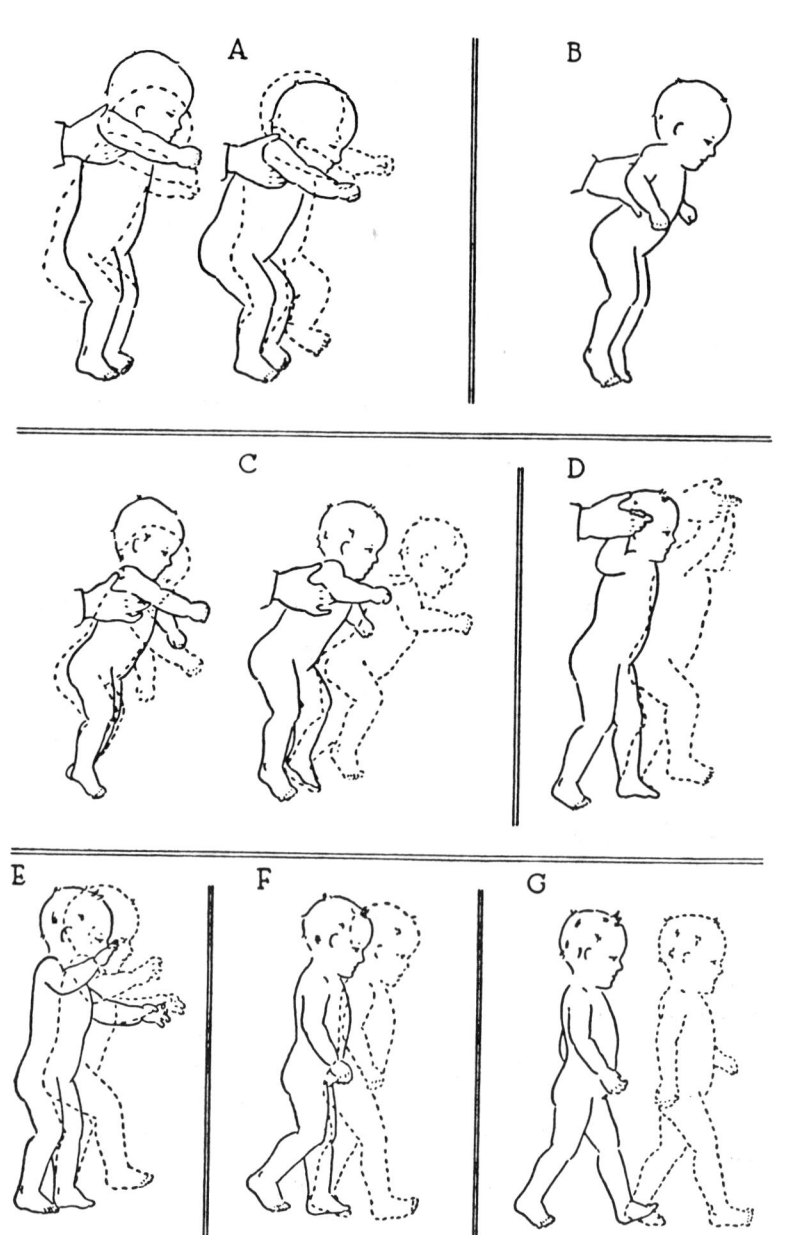

development of this skill is the toddler's ability to visually scan his environment while mobile. Initially, he must visually monitor his leg movements. As visual-motor and visual-spatial skills evolve, he becomes able to walk without this visual monitoring.

CLIMBING

The toddler is an avid climber. Initially he is content to climb into adult chairs or onto parents' laps. Later, he attempts to scale greater heights. Acquiring the ability to ascend and descend stairs is also a climbing skill that is

BEHAVIORAL DEVELOPMENT **427**

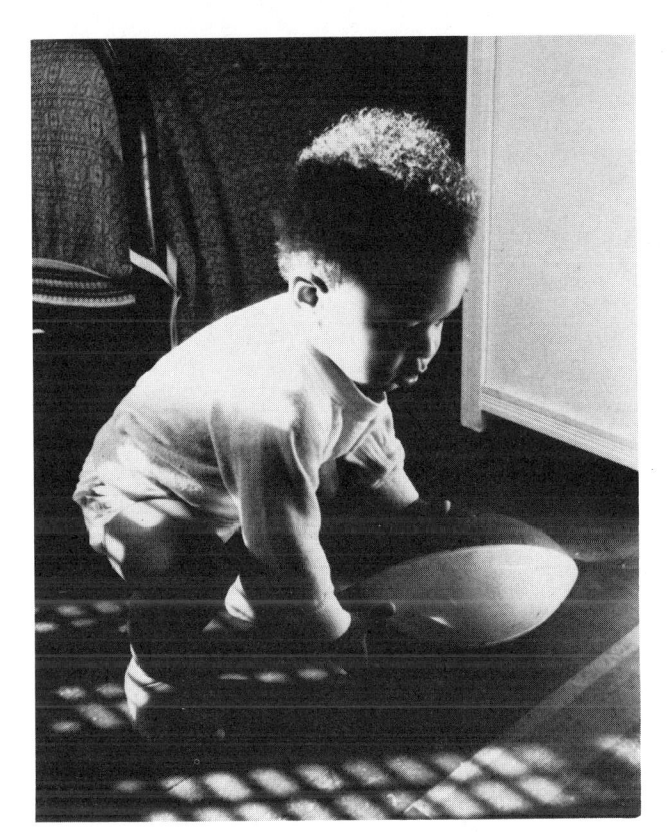

FIGURE 8-14.

acquired during the toddler and preschool years. The child builds on the locomotion skills he acquired earlier and utilizes his improving strength, control, balance, coordination, and visual-spatial perception as well as his drive for independence to learn these skills.

The toddler will (if stairs are available) creep upstairs by about 15 months and turn around to creep down by 18 months. At about the same time he learns to walk upstairs with one hand held, two feet on each step. By about 21 months, he can walk downstairs with one hand held, again two feet on each step. Finally, at 3 years of age the toddler can walk upstairs independently, alternating feet.

OTHER GROSS MOTOR SKILLS
Important in gross motor development of the toddler is refinement of skills he began acquiring prior to this period. Variations of previous skills and experimentation with movement are the toddler's theme. For example, he develops the ability to jump, kick, walk backwards, seat himself in a small chair, throw objects, and ride a tricycle. The basic motor skills developed in the first 3 years as well as perfected equilibrium reactions form the basis of the more complex gross motor skills of older children. The toddler will often attempt to imitate older siblings in play; acrobatics, such as headstands, somersaults, whirling around, and other gross motor movements he sees older children perform are crudely imitated. Laughter generally reinforces his attempts.

Like the infant, the toddler needs an environment which is safe and secure both physically and emotionally and parents who are aware of means to promote developmental advance in order to maximize his potential for gross motor development. Providing the toddler with the opportunity to practice these skills is one way of promoting such advance.

The basic principles of gross motor development discussed in Chap. 7 remain operant during the toddler period. For example, the principle of cephalocaudal development is demonstrated in increased control of the lower extremities achieved during this period following the previously developed head and trunk control. The principle of proximodistal development is demonstrated as the ability to reach precedes the ability to throw and the ability to stand precedes the ability to kick. By the end of the toddler period, the child is in a fully upright (extended) posture and has acquired a multiplicity of purposeful, specific, complex skills which prepare him for future elaboration of gross motor development.

Fine motor development
Barbara Newcomer McLaughlin and Nancy L. Morgan

Fine motor development during the toddler years consists primarily of progressive refinement of hand and finger movements. The child's coordination becomes smoother, and he develops a high degree of thumb, finger, and hand precision as he manipulates small objects with dexterity. Fine motor movement by the end of the toddler period represents a significant integration of cognitive and motor abilities.

The 1-year-old child begins to discriminate perceptions of form and space, probing the third dimension with his index finger. He also has a rudimentary concept of above and vertical as well as of a container and the contained. The toddler begins to feed himself with gross hand-to-mouth movements, frequently turning over the spoon before he gets the food to his mouth. As his coordination becomes smoother, he is able to insert the spoon into his

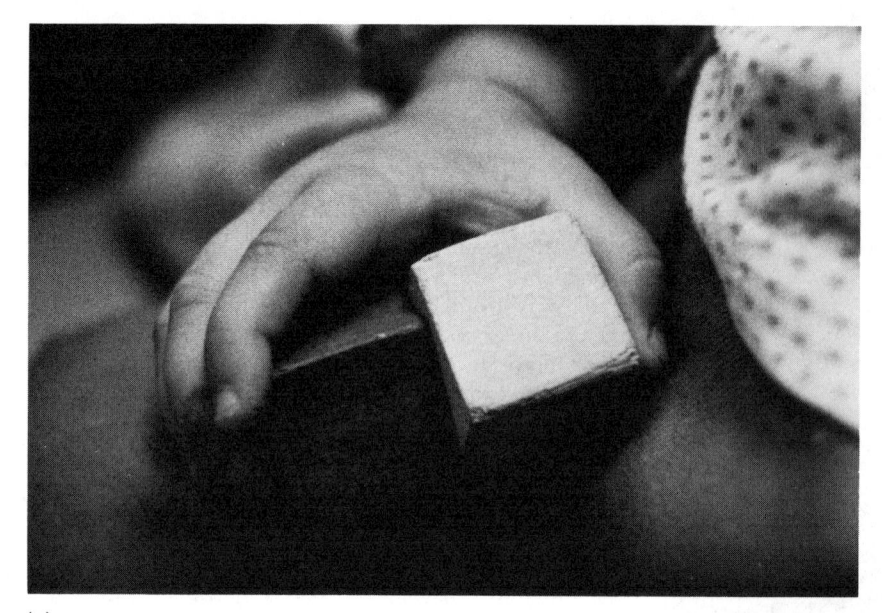

FIGURE 8-15. Development of prehension skills in the toddler. (*a*) The toddler holds two objects in one hand, 13 to 15 months. (*b*) The toddler dumps raisins from bottle demonstrating unilateral movement and hand supination, 16 to 18 months. (*c*) Scribbling with palmar grasp of a pencil, 13 to 15 months. (*d*) More complex skills are now possible, such as fitting related objects together, by using all previously developed skills.

mouth without spilling. The 12- to 15-month-old child reaches for objects by coordinated, continuous movement and demonstrates refined spatial awareness. He enjoys casting objects to the floor and frequently makes a social game of this activity.

The 15-month-old is able to hold two objects in one hand (see Fig. 8-15*a*). He can coordinate his hands and begins to use them together in complementary functions. He is able to hold a container with one hand while probing for or releasing objects into the container with the other hand. He can also turn and empty a container (see Fig. 8-15*b*). He can fit related objects together, a type of grasp-release combination demonstrating cognitive development.

By this age the child attempts to scribble with a whole-hand grasp of the writing implement (see Fig. 8-15*c*). He is able to build a tower of two or three blocks (see Fig. 8-15*d*). The child finds picture books particularly intriguing as he constantly pats or manipulates the book though he is usually unable to point to specific pictures when asked. Parents can plan activities so that the 12- to 15-month-old child has the opportunity to build with blocks, scribble, play with fit-together toys, release objects into containers, and manipulate books with easily recognizable pictures (Gesell, Halverson, Thompson, Ilg, Castner, Ames, and Amatruda, 1940).

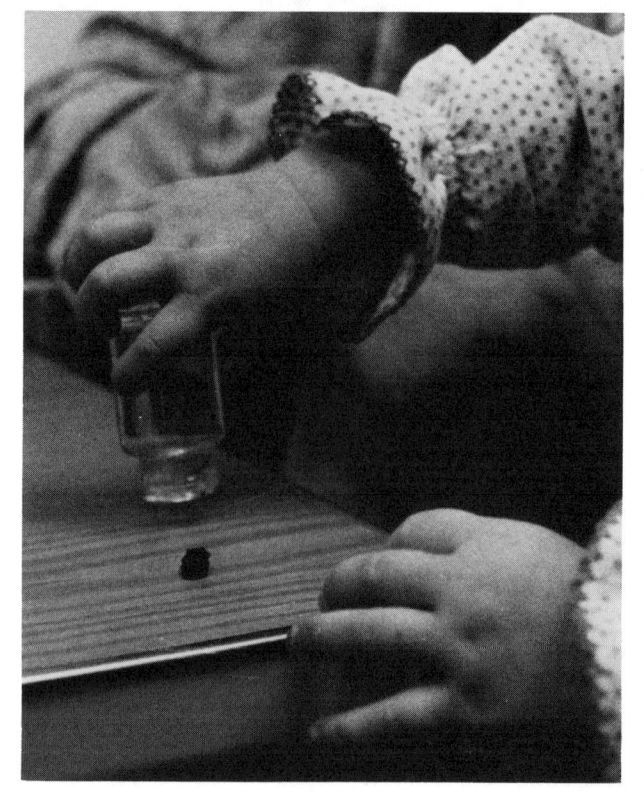

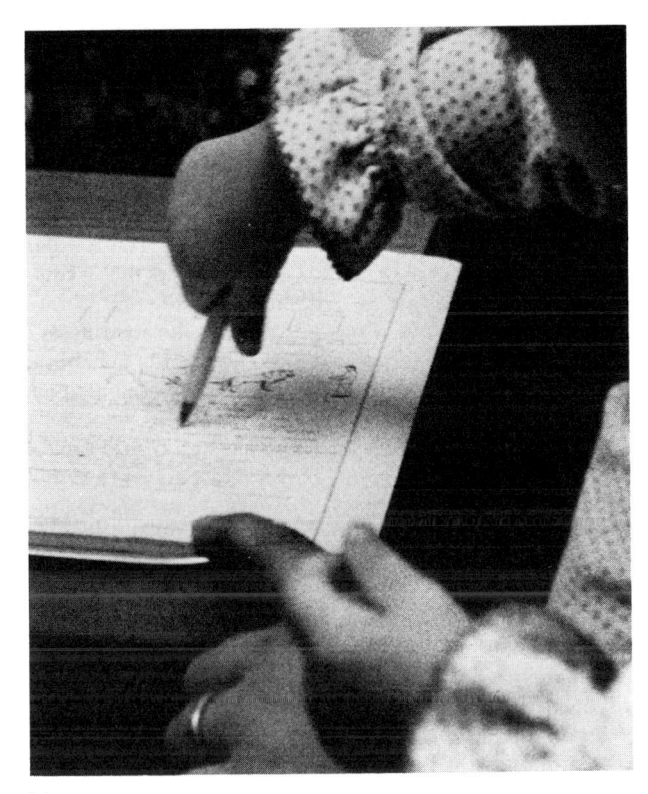

BEHAVIORAL DEVELOPMENT **429**

a vertical line holding the pencil between finger and thumb.

The 18-month-old has an increased scope of attention as he displays an interest in "many" and "more." Whereas the 1-year-old child takes and then discards one block after another, the 18-month-old child likes to hold and keep several blocks in his possession. He is able to stack three to four blocks in a tower at this time. Practice with the above skills in play will increase the child's dexterity in his fine motor development (Gesell et al., 1940).

The period from 18 months to 2 years of age represents less change in fine motor development than from 1 year to 18 months, though the changes that occur are significant because of the interdependence of motor and mental development in the 2-year-old. The 2-year-old is able to build a tower of 8 to 10 blocks, which represents a real gain in attention span. The child will stay with confining tasks for longer periods of time and adapts well to fine motor activities at a table.

There is now a finer discrimination in his perceptual and imitative behavior; he has progressed from matching a round block and round hole at 18 months to inserting a square block edgewise through a rectangular hole. The formativeness of his manipulatory geometry is inept because he is not able to free his hands to move with versatility in different directions. The 18-month-old shows facility with vertical control, but the 2-year-old has progressed to imitation of a horizontal stroke and has already mastered a horizontal row of blocks. Horizontal and vertical are equal in precision of coordination; however, in configuration, horizontal is more difficult.

The 2-year-old uses basic grasping skills to perform more and more complex activities. He is able to assemble separated puzzles of one to three pieces and is usually able to work most latches, doorknobs, hooks, slide bolts, and screw lids. He is also able to put on his shoes, socks, and pants (Gesell et al., 1940).

The time between 2 and 2½ years of age primarily represents a continuous refinement of the skills that the child began to develop at 2 years. The 2½-year-old displays an overgrasp and an overrelease of objects. He develops the ability to hold a pencil in his hand as opposed to his fist, and he is content for an extended period of time utilizing this newly learned skill of beginning to draw. The toddler also masters the task of pouring liquids from one container into another (Gesell et al., 1940).

The toddler years bring much in the way of refinement to the child's hand and finger movements. Coordination improves, and there is a high degree of thumb, finger,

(c)

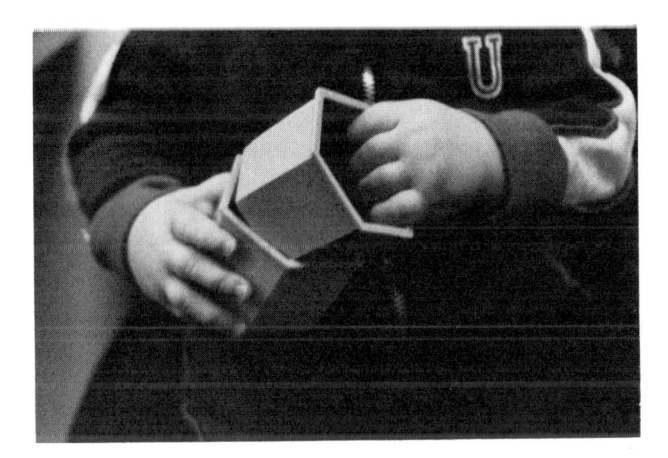

(d)

FIGURE 8-15. (*Continued*)

The 18-month-old child readily makes geometric discriminations as he learns where things are and where they belong. The child turns pages of a book in a precise manner and points to pictures of common items—car, dog, eyes, ears—on verbal command. His sense of vertical has progressed so that he can align two to three objects vertically with little effort. Likewise the child is able to imitate and hand precision even when the toddler manipulates very small objects. Skills have progressed from an imitative scribble to a deliberate copy of a line in a purposeful, directed manner. Fine motor movements are smooth and continuous and are enacted with a high degree of dexterity.

Cognitive development Virginia Pidgeon

What of cognition in the toddler years? The thinking of the toddler remains remote and inaccessible in the transition period from sensorimotor intelligence to representational thought and symbolic thinking. The toddler is a relentless explorer off on countless expeditions to discover the intracacies and novelties of objects in his world. He gazes with intense interest and awe at the underpinnings of a chair as he sits on the floor and completes his scientific exploration by poking, prodding, and sampling flavor and texture. Returning to his mother, he excitedly reports his findings. The miracle of embryonic language is witnessed in his loud and imperious utterances—"mook," "bell buoy"—yet an interpreter is needed to communicate with this little person.

Intelligence in this transition period is increasingly liberated from actions. With development of the ability to represent objects, actions, and events in his mind, the toddler is now able to contemplate his actions and the mysteries of the world of objects and persons. Schema development, the development of symbolic thinking, and object concept during the toddler period are considered.

SCHEMA DEVELOPMENT

Changes in cognitive structure occur in the second year of life that mark the completion of the period of sensorimotor intelligence. The toddler in this period becomes more proficient as a problem solver. He discovers new means to solve problems by physical experimentation and then by mental experimentation. The stages of cognitive development through which he passes include stage 5, the *tertiary circular reaction* and the discovery of new means by active *experimentation,* and stage 6, invention of new means through *mental combinations.*

Like the stage 3 infant, the stage 5 toddler (12 to 18 months) stumbles across an unexpected and intriguing effect produced by a familiar action on an unfamiliar object. As before, he enters into a series of repetitions or repeated encounters with the phenomenon. The stage 3 infant, however, seeks simply to recapture the initial effect by stereotyped repetition of his actions. In contrast the stage 5 toddler introduces variations into the action with repetition and studies the effect of the variations on the object. He subordinates his actions to exploration of the object as a thing apart from himself and to experimentation to discover the novelty of the object. The toddler presses his finger on a matchbox and discovers that it tilts. He then exerts pressure with his finger at different points on the matchbox and discovers that it tilts in different ways. He presses his finger on the center of the matchbox and discovers that it does not tilt but is displaced. This is a tertiary circular reaction.

The young child in this stage is interested in and preoccupied with the object itself. This interest stems from his developing concept of *object permanence* and his awareness of objects apart from himself (Flavell, 1963). Encountering novelty in objects, the toddler now explores their properties instead of repeating his actions on them. Assimilation and accommodation are now differentiated and used in a complementary manner. The toddler initially assimilates the object to his schema or action. When he discovers an unexpected effect, he then performs a series of accommodations of his schema designed to discover the uniqueness of the object.

In addition, the stage 5 toddler is able, through a process of trial-and-error experimentation, to discover new means to solve problems. The stage 4 infant in contrast used only familiar schemata as means to solve problems. The stage 5 toddler discovers that by tilting an object he can pass it through the bars of his crib. He learns that he can obtain an out-of-reach ring by pulling the attached string.

The stage 6 toddler (18 to 24 months) is able to discover and invent new means to solve problems by mental rather than physical experimentation. He invents new solutions through covert, inner mental experimentation rather than overt physical experimentation. A toddler inadvertently pushes a doll carriage against the wall. He walks backward pulling the carriage but finds this difficult. He pauses and then goes to the wall and pushes the carriage backward. Implicit in mental experimentation are the two processes of *representation* and *invention.* The child is now able to represent mental images of schemata in his mind. In addition, he can mentally combine different schemata in means-end sequences and discover a solution.

SYMBOLIC THINKING

The toddler years mark the inception of *symbolic thinking.* The young child can now represent in his mind objects, actions, and events. As a result he is able to perform mental manipulations of reality in his mind rather than physically through trial-and-error motoric actions. In addition he can recall the past, anticipate the future, and represent the present. He is also able to contemplate his actions and their consequences rather than simply to act on them. Also symbolic thinking with the advent of language makes possible the socialization of thought through an exchange of thoughts and sharing.

The toddler represents objects and events in his mind first in terms of actions, then images, and finally symbols or words (Bruner, 1968). These three modes of mental representation are the *enactive mode* (by actions), the *iconic mode* (by images), and the *symbolic mode* (by words). The toddler first acquires a mental schema of throwing in terms of the actions involved (grasping, lifting arm, and letting go). He then acquires a mental image of throwing (a child throwing a ball). Finally he acquires the word *throw*, which he learns to associate with the mental schema of throwing and with the mental image. An adult's mental representation of a car includes his experience in driving it and the effect of habitual actions (braking or shifting) upon it. It also includes visual images of different kinds of cars and words descriptive of different categories or classes.

The hallmark of symbolic thinking to Piaget (1962) is the ability to distinguish between a *signifier* (an image, gesture, or word) and the *significate* (that which it represents). The toddler learns the symbolic function, or that signs represent, or stand for, objects and events. He learns to recognize hand waving as a sign signifying that the departure of someone is imminent. He learns to recognize the word *kitty* as a sign signifying a soft, furry creature.

According to Piaget, there are two kinds of signifiers—signs and symbols. *Signs* (words and scientific symbols) have socially accepted and consensual meanings. In addition they do not resemble their significates. The word *boat* bears no resemblance to an actual boat. In contrast symbols are uncodified and private in meaning and often bear a resemblance to their significates. They include dream symbols, play props (the piece of wood that the child represents as a gun), and the first concepts and first words of the toddler. The first concepts and first words of the toddler carry highly personal and idiosyncratic meanings that have little correspondence with social and conventional meanings.

The first signifiers acquired by the toddler are symbols that are nonverbal and private in meaning. He learns to use objects and gestures symbolically before the advent of language. A cloth may be used in play to represent a pillow. The first words uttered by the toddler are technically signs but have more of the flavor of symbols. They are invested with private and unconventional meanings and often refer to action schemata rather than to objects or persons. The word *mommy* may carry implicit meanings like mommy play with me or mommy feed me.

The functions of language parallel the different modes of representation (enactive, iconic, and symbolic). Words can be used enactively as a guide for action (a recipe or instructions). Young children often use words enactively to guide or influence the actions of others and obtain their own wants. According to Luria (1968), young children also use words to guide and regulate their own actions. ("Now I will draw a line down here and color this yellow.") Words are also used iconically to describe images or states. Young children often use words iconically to describe objects and events. ("There was this black cat. And he was big. And he scratched me.") Lastly words are used symbolically by adolescents and adults to express abstract concepts (e.g., detente or fission), variables, and their relations.

OBJECT CONCEPT

The toddler's concepts of objects evolve from concepts that are action-ridden (rattle = shake and make noise) to concepts that are imagistic and relatively free of his actions on them (rattle = an object with a handle that makes a noise). These early object concepts are global and diffuse. Bruner believes that the toddler is engaged in a matching process by which he detects congruence or incongruence between an object or event and his concept of it. Seeing a fur coat, a small child pronounced "kitty," as he detects congruence with his concept of cat. A hospitalized child detects incongruence when he notes, "This bed is high."

The toddler also develops a concept of object permanence. The concept of object permanence implies an awareness that objects are separate entities and that they continue to exist when not seen by the viewer. It also includes awareness that objects exist apart from one's actions on them. Clues to the development of object permanence can be derived from infant and toddler behavior in response to vanishing objects. A young infant appears not to miss or search for a vanished object. At the most he may stare briefly at the point where it disappeared. Objects out of sight cease to exist.

Between 5 to 8 months the infant leans over his high chair to look for an object he has dropped. The older infant now actively searches for a vanished object. Hide an object in sight of a toddler, and then out of his sight switch it to a different hiding place. The young toddler, failing to find the object at the original site, abandons his search. In the latter part of the second year the toddler, not finding the object at the original site, now searches actively in several possible hiding places. Piaget infers at this point the presence of a concept of object permanence. Objects now are seen as separate entities and continue to exist when out of sight. In a similar manner the parent is now seen as a separate person with an independent existence who is missed in his or her absence.

The toddler in the second year becomes proficient as a problem solver and uses both physical and mental experimentation to find solutions. He also acquires symbolic thinking and represents objects in his mind in terms of actions, images, and finally words. Symbolic thinking enables the toddler to manipulate reality in his mind, to recall the past and anticipate the future, and to contemplate his actions and their consequences.

Language development Shirley Joan Lemmen

In a discussion of the language of the toddler, it is important to note the development of symbolic behavior that has occurred during the first year; language is one aspect of symbolic behavior. In order for toddlers to use language as a symbolic system, they must learn the rules of language. Rules are learned in the following areas:

- Sound production: phonological development
- Acquisition of words: lexicon
- Using word order: syntax
- Using words in a meaningful way to express feelings and experiences and to gain new information: semantics

SINGLE-WORD UTTERANCES

Toddlers usually use one-word utterances from about 12 months until 24 to 30 months of age. They begin to combine words as early as 18 months of age. One cannot talk about the form of language until the child begins to use two- or three-word sentences.

What is apparent in one-word utterances, however, is content and function. The toddler is able to produce words that are intelligible to the listener. The words contain *phonemes* (sounds) that are familiar and closely approximate the phonemic structure of adult speech. In other words, the groups of sounds making up one-word utterances are perceived by the adult as closely approximating standard words in the native tongue. However, in order to determine what the toddler is saying, the listener must have additional cues from the context (situation) in which the utterance occurs. In relation to the toddler's first words, what will be discussed in this article are phonological development, vocabulary growth, and how

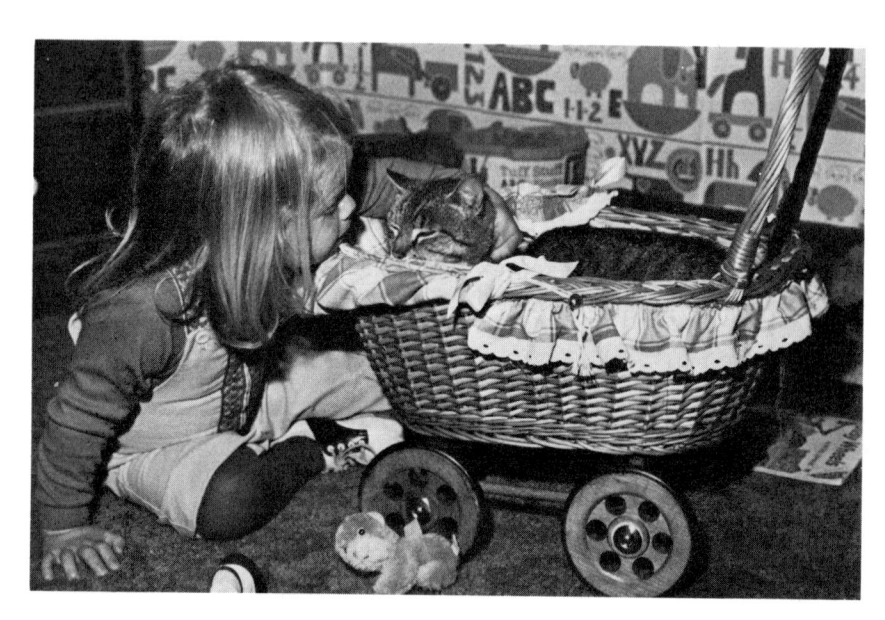

FIGURE 8-16. (*Photo courtesy of Betsy Smith.*)

he comprehends relations between words that relate to experience.

PHONEMIC DEVELOPMENT

Until the 1970s, studies focused on isolated phonemes or separate speech sounds. This was most often done with tests of articulation. Also, auditory discrimination studies were done in order to determine whether the child could discriminate between sounds in words such as *cat* and *bat*. More recent studies have suggested that toddlers do not learn individual sounds but learn words and sounds according to the strategies or rules for their language.

For analysis, the units to attend to have become syllables and words; toddlers learn phonology according to the features they perceive and discriminate in the words they hear and first attempt to say (Bloom and Lahey, 1978). Production of sounds in words, then, is dependent on what the toddler hears in the environment: the adult model. However, learning words is not a passive process, and words are not learned only to acquire a vocabulary. Toddlers first learn words that are useful to them and relate to their concrete experiences.

Sound production also has physiological (neuromotor) constraints. Toddlers must learn to combine the features of friction, nasality, and voicing with particular placement of the tongue and lips and with jaw movement. How he is able to produce a word depends on auditory perception and the ability to manipulate these articulators in an integrative and smooth fashion.

VOCABULARY GROWTH

Most toddlers initially develop a vocabulary (lexicon) containing nouns, adjectives, and self-invented words. These are words which refer to a large number of objects and, to a lesser extent, action words, modifiers, and grammatical function words. Words which refer to objects, classes of objects, and events based on perceptual features of the objects are *substantive* words. *Functional* words are modifiers or action words, noting particular relationships or behaviors of objects (Bloom and Lehay, 1978).

Some toddlers have initial vocabularies which contain significantly fewer action words but more words expressing feelings, needs, and social relationships. Prior conceptual development, experiences, and parent-child interactions may influence the makeup of initial vocabulary (Coggins and Carpenter, 1978). Nelson (1973) reports that toddlers do not use their initial vocabularies in the same way, reflecting these differences.

At 13 to 15 months of age a toddler should have about 10 words (Coggins and Carpenter, 1978). This seems to be a more important indicator of beginning word acquisition, as the onset of the first word is difficult to pinpoint.

First words may be close approximations to the adult model and predominately two or three syllables.

Examples of first words which relate to a specific object are *mommy* and *doggy;* words which relate to a class of objects are *juice* and *ball;* action words are *up* and *bye-bye;* modifier words are *pretty* and *hot;* and function words are *more, what,* and *that.* Also, a toddler may have nonsense words like *feda fodder* for a specific object in his environment. The word has symbolic meaning for the child; however, it does not have meaning to the listener until the child uses his word consistently in relation to the object or experience and the listener understands the word in this familiar context.

Words that appear early in a vocabulary may be used by a child and then disappear (Bloom, 1973; Nelson, 1973). This instability may reflect the toddler's shifting attention to various aspects of his daily experiences. It is substantive words that change and have an attrition. Once the toddler has functional words, they remain in the lexicon.

By adult standards, a toddler's early vocabulary may be an *overexpansion* of objects or activities under one word. For example, he might have the word *moon* in his early vocabulary and use this word in relation to any object that is the same shape, such as using *moon* for *ball* or *circle*. Thus, the toddler begins to perceive similarities and regularities in objects.

Another phenomenon observed in the toddler is the beginning of *change association* of words (Bloom and Lahey, 1978). He may first say *wa* for *water* from a faucet and later, seeing water in the bathtub, in a puddle, or in rain on the window, use the word *wa* for each.

During the time that single words are used, toddlers begin to reflect *semantical meaning.* The meaning of a toddler's earliest communication indicates that he has some understanding of behaviors of objects, that objects do disappear and reappear and exist even when not seen (see "Cognitive Development"). In other words, the actions that toddlers name most often are concepts of existence, nonexistence, disappearance, and reappearance. Words like *all gone, high, go, come,* and *bye-bye* are heard. For example, a toddler putting blocks into a container might say, "Boc all gone."

The first single-word utterances are the most difficult to study in regard to comprehension (Dale, 1976). They seem to be attempts to express complex ideas and are called *holophrastic speech.* For instance, when a toddler says, "Milk," he may not simply be indicating the white liquid. He may mean that he wants milk or that he spilled his milk. Holophrastic utterances are strongly linked to action, particularly the toddler's own action.

During the single-word stage it is also important to note that the toddler still uses jargon. *Jargon* is a series of sounds or strings of words, such as sentences in conversation, with intonation and inflection.

COMPREHENSION

Shortly after his first birthday, a toddler begins to respond to commands and conversation when accompanied by gesture. It has been well documented that parents tend to adapt their vocalizations to the toddler's level of competence, such as making shorter phrases, using gestures, and using situational cues to facilitate appropriate response by the toddler to the communicative interaction. As he approaches his second birthday, the toddler should be able to follow a simple command without gestures.

TWO- AND THREE-WORD UTTERANCES

From 18 months to 2 years, the transition from single words to two- and three-word phrases begins. Two-year-old children talk about their experiences in the here and now. If one were observing a 2-year-old child for his communicative behavior, it would be more successful to observe him in a naturalistic setting than to place him in a test environment and attempt to elicit communicative behavior. However, a testing situation is necessary when there are serious questions about a child's communication and a cross-sectional sample of his communicative skills is needed to determine whether there is a lag.

At about 2 years of age, there is a tremendous growth in vocabulary; the child has about 270 words in his lexicon. This does not imply that he verbalizes all 270 words; some words are understood, or *receptive* language, and some are both understood and verbalized, or *expressive* language. It is well documented that children's understanding of communication, or receptive language, is slightly higher than or at the same level as their verbal communication, or expressive language. As stated above, some words are dropped from the lexicon when they are no longer useful to the toddler; other words will stay in his vocabulary.

Again, the content of these two- and three-word phrases is primarily present events that the toddler is experiencing. When looking at the context from which the toddler is speaking, a rich variety of relationships or structural meanings are being expressed. Some examples are listed below:

- Nomination: That book. That car.
- Notice: Hi, Mommy. Hi, Baby.
- Recurrence: More.
- Object: More milk. More cookie.
- Nonexistence: Milk all gone.

Some combinations that include attributive adjectives are the following:

- Noun: Big ball.
- Possessive: Mommy's sock.
- Locative: Sweater, chair.
- Agent and action: Boy walk. Frog jump.
- Noun plus verb: Mommy read. Baby cry.

It is important to remember that the 2-year-old child's language, as with the younger child, is dependent on many variables: his conceptual development, his motor development, his environment, and his motivation to use language.

SYNTAX DEVELOPMENT

The emergence of *syntax* (word order) in a toddler's communication begins to be apparent to the listener when he uses two- and three-word phrases. It has not been documented clearly how a child learns the syntax of language. Brown (1973) describes the simple index of mean length of utterance as a guideline for linguistic maturity. The sampling of a child's spontaneous speech is laborious and usually done on a few children over a longitudinal study. In contrast, the mean length of utterance is an excellent simple index of grammatical development because almost every kind of linguistic knowledge increases the length of utterances.

FORM

What grammatical forms do children between 2 and 3 years of age use? Some of the most important changes in a toddler's communication are length of utterance, word order, and the inclusion of pronouns, prepositions, articles, conjunctions, and auxiliary verbs. These words include *my, has, and, I have, to, me, at, in, the,* and *on.* The words in a toddler's sentences may not be grammatically or phonetically perfect; however, he soon learns correct word order. A toddler may say, "Baby no sit," between $2\frac{1}{2}$ and 3 years of age, but at about $3\frac{1}{2}$ years he uses *can't.* Between 2 and 3 years of age, toddlers also add articles such as *a, the, this,* and *that* to their sentences.

SENTENCE ELABORATION

The two linguistic structures that subsume under the heading of sentence elaboration are the noun phrase and the verb phrase. Both noun and verb phrases may be elaborated on and are governed by linguistic rules of the language being spoken. Words are combined with definite form, and the form allows for more explicit information to the listener. For example, "I am going to the store" implies very explicit information and is understood because of word order. "Store going I am to" confuses the listener; it does not follow the rules of English grammar.

The reason that toddlers' earliest sentences are difficult to interpret is that obligatory cues present in adult speech are absent in the child's utterances. The 2-year-old child may say, "Daddy car." He may be making a comment in relation to possession, "That is Daddy's car," or location, "Daddy is in the car." Until the toddler begins to inflect the nouns and verbs used to encode such relational meanings, the intent often has to be inferred from the immediate nonlinguistic (situational) context.

INFLECTIONAL DEVELOPMENT

Development of *inflection* may span from 2½ to 6 years or older. Inflections are used to modify the meaning of major content words in the sentence, nouns and verbs, or to indicate the relation between content words more accurately. Inflections that emerge between 2½ and 3½ years of age include the present progressive *-ing* (the boy is running), the plural *-s*, (blocks, cookies); and the possessive *-'s* (Daddy's) at 3 to 3½ years.

The development of grammatical inflections used to specify the relations between content words is also a long process which begins with the use of the preposition *in* at 2½ years and *on* at 3 to 3½ years. The comprehension of these linguistic forms precedes consistent use of the form (Coggins and Carpenter, 1978).

INTERROGATIVE SENTENCES

In a toddler's first utterances at 12 to 14 months, *interrogative* structures (questions) differ only from declarative sentences by the intonation. The question is expressed by the rise of inflection at the end of the utterance. Children at this age may also add *no* to the structure, which makes a negative question. By simply adding *no* and intonation at the end of the sentence, as in "no milk," he is able to ask a question (Dale, 1976).

At 24 to 30 months, articles (a, the) and modifiers (big, little, three) are used, inflections appear, and occasionally a prepositional phrase may be heard: Mommy fix it? Daddy in house? Toddlers also begin to answer questions at 24 to 30 months of age. The parent may notice responses to questions much earlier; however, these responses are most likely turning toward the speaker, making an attempt to respond by either yes or no gestures, or motorically demonstrating what he is doing. Questions from the child facilitate the gaining of new information, alert the parents to focusing their attention on the interest of the child, and are powerful initiators of social exchange.

PARENT-CHILD INTERACTION

Parents are the most significant persons in the toddler's environment and provide experiences to enrich his use of verbal communication. Probably more important than the absolute quality of parents' speech is the nature of the linguistic interchange between parent and toddler (Dale, 1976). Before their child is 2 years of age, parents often use longer phrases than they do later when the toddler actively participates with words, phrases, and gestures that more closely approximate the adult model. It is thought that the parents initially talk for themselves and will talk at their child.

Between 2 and 3 years, the toddler is able to become a more active participant in verbal interchange, and so a parent's speech becomes more a function of the child's specific demands; the parent begins to talk with and in response to the toddler. This has only been demonstrated with middle-class mothers (Ramey, Farren, Campbell, and Finkelskin, 1976).

Frequency of mother's questions has been positively related to receptive language scores at 20 months and vocabulary scores at 30 months. In verbal interaction, middle- and lower-class mothers appear to use different sentence types. Lower-class mothers use more imperative statements, and middle-class mothers use more questions. Questions are important in language development as they provide a means to elicit a child's speech and encourage him to focus on aspects of the environment. It has also been documented that, in addition to questions, maternal vocalizations which expand or elaborate on the child's vocalizations appear to be facilitative of language development and communication.

Although some research has been done in relation to styles of language teaching, such as asking questions, expanding the toddler's vocalizations, and exact repetitions, more research is needed on parent-child dyads (especially with fathers) where the parents are of varying linguistic styles and abilities. It appears that the most facilitative verbal interaction for future linguistic ability in the child is one in which the child's developing capabilities are matched by the parent's changing vocal input.

The parameters that Dale (1976) discusses with respect to linguistic interchange between mother and toddler predominately describe mothers' behaviors in relation to a child's vocalizations. These are prompting, echoing, and expansion.

The parent asks a question, such as, "What do you want?" If the child does not respond, the parent tries again, "You want what?" In other words, the parent tries another sentence that might be easier for the child to understand. This is *prompting*.

Echoing occurs when the toddler utters a sentence that is in part unintelligible. For example, a 2-year-old might say, "I going owa noa." The parent imitates the child as best as possible and replaces the unintelligible part with *what, where,* or *who:* "You are going where?" The parent is asking the question pertinent to what the toddler has said, which helps him respond more clearly.

By *expansion* the parent imitates the toddler but does not reproduce the utterance exactly. Instead, he adds something to it. For example, the toddler might say, "kitty box." The parent may reply, "The kitty is in the box." There are many possible expansions on a toddler's vocalizations, but the parents' expansion should be appropriate to what the toddler is attempting to communicate. Usually parents' approval of toddlers' vocalizations is not contingent on the fact that the utterances are grammatically correct, but most often the toddler is reinforced for truthfulness in the statement: how it relates to the reality of the experience that is being communicated.

One does not decide to teach a child language specifically; rather the richness of the environment gives the child multiple opportunities every day to learn language. By 2½ years of age a child can increase language skills through planned activities of listening, verbal exchange with another person, watching children's television programs, and hearing stories.

Kriegsmann (1978) has provided ideas for clinicians and parents that would facilitate a child's communication. The parents can extend their toddler's vocalizations and play by allowing him to make decisions about play, initiate verbal interactions, and control his activities whenever possible. Young children talk about what they are doing or what interests them; the parent can follow and attend to this verbalization. As a general guideline, parents should respond to what the child says with additional information and praise the toddler for communicative attempts.

Children develop communication skills in early infancy and by age 3 have the basic skills of language in terms of function, form, and content. Language does not proceed at an even rate; there are many hesitations, plateaus, and spurts in the toddler's mastery of language. However, the overall growth in language is tremendous during these 2 years and will continue to expand with the expanding world of the child.

Self-help skill development Doris Julian

At the end of the first year the infant has acquired many of the prerequisite skills, especially fine motor ones, essential for autonomy in self-care. Ability to use the hands as tools is an essential component of self-care. Further maturation of the nervous system has inhibited reflexive responses, permitting postural and sphincter control. The 1-year-old now has beginning skills in self-feeding and control over elimination.

These skills, accompanied by a strong drive to exercise motor abilities, explore the environment, and interact with parents, set the stage for the toddler period. The toddler has become an upright, freely mobile individual. In both a motoric and psychologic sense, he is motivated to explore his relation to both the animate and inanimate environment and does so in an assertive manner (Caplan and Caplan, 1977; Gessel, Ilg, Ames, and Rodell, 1974; White, 1975).

The toddler's need for increasing self-direction can facilitate building self-care skills. The attentive parent can arrange the environment in a manner permitting the safe practice of emerging motor abilities. The toddler's exploratory activities will include observation and imitation of the people in his world. Adults and children, particularly preschoolers, can provide useful models for desirable behavior in a variety of skills: eating, toileting, dressing, and household chores. The delightfully assertive toddler has many of the skills but little of the judgment of the older preschooler, so that expectations must be carefully geared to the individual child's actual abilities.

EATING SKILLS

MOTOR OR MATURATIONAL FACTORS
The child entering the toddler period has achieved considerable control over both gross and fine motor abilities. It is now possible for the child to take all meals in a sitting position and to handle finger foods with ease. Beginning

skills with cup, glass, and spoon are present. Assistance is often needed and may be tolerated for a part of the meal.

Skills are progressively refined during the succeeding months so that by 18 months the toddler can manage feeding with a minimum of spilling. The intricacies of handling a spoon require a longer interval of time, but usually by the end of the second year food can be scooped and carried successfully to the mouth.

SOCIALIZATION OR BEHAVIORAL FACTORS

For the busy toddler intent on exercising strong motoric drives, constraints and contingencies imposed by parents may be both a challenge and a frustration. In the feeding situation there will be as much variation in parent's behavior as in child's. Many a busy parent will prefer to feed the child in order to speed the process and eliminate the messes of the novice self-feeder. Others will heed the toddler's demands to practice newly developing skills recognizing the significance of the activity to feelings of competence. Toddlers with older siblings may be particularly insistent on imitating the behavior of brothers and sisters. Patience and tactfully offered assistance can alleviate some of the mutual frustration experienced in the early toddler period.

Typically, by 18 to 21 months, the essential feeding skills are handled with acceptable finesse. Since mealtimes are a major socializing activity and an excellent opportunity for practicing communication skills, inclusion of the toddler for at least part of the meal is helpful in facilitating socially appropriate behavior. Parental expectation of appropriate eating behavior will be influenced by prior experience in child rearing, family and societal pressures, and contemporary views obtained from reading, television, radio, and adult peer groups. The child-rearing practices of the parents' own family are frequently used as models in the feeding situation.

One of the feeding practices most subject to the influences described previously is that of weaning the child from the breast or bottle to the cup. Parents, in their desire to do the right thing for the child, may be torn between encouraging early independence and supporting the child's need for oral gratification through sucking. Studies of Chess, Thomas, and Birch (1965) note that there is no one best age for a child to be weaned. The infant may spontaneously initiate the process before the end of the first year in imitation of older siblings or wait for cues from care givers at a much later time. In these studies, most middle-class families delayed the process until well after the second birthday. Studies from other cultures identify specific times and practices (Munroe and Munroe, 1977).

TOILETING SKILLS

MATURATIONAL FACTORS

During the second year, nervous system maturation will have progressed so that control of the anal and urethral sphincters is under beginning voluntary control. This ability, accompanied by increased bladder capacity, permits the toddler to experience occasional freedom from wetting and soiling (MacKeith, Meadow, and Turner, 1973). At a cognitive level, this association is essential for the toddler to have awareness that control over this body function is indeed his responsibility.

Other related physiologic changes are maturation of locomotive and postural skills. The toddler of 15 months is typically able to stand independently and to walk without assistance. Dynamic postural changes, such as stooping, squatting, and going from a sitting to a standing position and back again, are also possible (Espenschade and Eckert, 1967; Knoblock and Pasamanick, 1974). These are requisite abilities for independent toileting. Fine motor dexterity is also improving during the second year and has a role in the clothing manipulation needed in toileting. To be independent, the toddler needs the skill to grasp pants around the waist, pull them down to the knees, and pull them up again.

SOCIALIZATION OR BEHAVIORAL FACTORS

In addition to motor and physiologic maturation, independent toileting requires corresponding cognitive and language development. The toddler, within this second postnatal year, has developed a useful communication system. Communication of the need to use the toilet may be present early in the second year with single words, gestures, and sounds. For the most part, however, this ability is a later-developing skill. Typically, by the age of 20 to 22 months, the toddler understands a consistent word or sound for urination and defecation and can also remember and respond to a two-part direction. These clues to level of understanding are a major asset in identifying the child's readiness for self-care in toileting (Murphy, 1975).

Because elimination is under the toddler's voluntary control, a willingness, or motivation, for socially desirable behavior must be present. Parents who can respect and enjoy the busy "me do" toddler will create an atmosphere of trust and affection. The toddler's desire for approval will encourage him to imitate behavior of significant people and to repeat activities that result in praise and affection. Brazelton (1974) describes the mixed dependency-independency feelings and drives that accompany the toddler period. Awareness of the normalcy of the toddler's alternately clinging and pushing-away behavior may reduce parental frustration in responding to conflicts around toilet training.

Although it is not a consistent finding, girls are frequently reported to be easier to toilet-train, and many do achieve control of elimination before boys. This is attributed to more rapid nervous system maturation as well as to parental expectations (Stehbens and Silber, 1971). Sex role is well established by the toddler period (Fein Johnson, Kosson, Stork, and Wasserman, 1974). Cultural values of compliance and modesty may be stressed for girls and play a subtle but significant part in toileting expectations.

For both girls and boys the toileting process may present the parent with an opportunity or a perceived obligation to introduce the sexual values and taboos of society. Infants and toddlers in exploratory play with their own bodies may wish to repeat pleasurable sensations by masturbation, a behavior which some parents may tolerate in infants but not in toddlers. This overt behavior may trigger adult responses in the form of attempting to control masturbation, reducing the possibility of sex play with other children, and keeping genitalia covered with diapers or pants. The older toddler may be expected to understand or at least to heed the concept of privacy during elimination for himself and others.

Training about appropriate sexual and elimination behavior is closely linked in many cultures. The method and timing of this information will vary, however, from culture to culture. A contemporary trend of relaxation of rigid views about early toilet training places emphasis on individual readiness. This change in attitude has had carry-over to perceptions of the needs of the toddler for sex training.

DRESSING SKILLS

MATURATIONAL FACTORS
The infant has enjoyed patting, pulling, and tugging at clothing as an exploratory play activity. For the toddler, these activities become tasks in their own right. As a skill, removal of clothing articles is an easier task and precedes dressing by a few months. Both dressing and undressing require sufficient postural balance so that hands can be used as tools rather than for support.

With increased refinement of pincer grasp ability, the toddler of 18 to 21 months is able to handle large zippers and large buttons. By the end of the second year many have mastered the abilities needed for removing and putting on simple garments. Discrimination of the front and back and the inside and outside of a garment requires further cognitive development.

SOCIALIZATION OR BEHAVIORAL FACTORS
Independent dressing is a particular challenge to the busy toddler and the adult interested in introducing the task. For the toddler, the entire body is involved in the dressing activity. In addition, an association of article of clothing with the correct body part is required.

A useful approach involves determining both the toddler's level of readiness and the parent's level of patience. If the toddler has the motoric abilities necessary, can imitate motion directions, and can attend to a simple task for a few minutes, undressing can be practiced. In the beginning phases, toddler and parent may find it useful to have all the process completed except for the final step. As the toddler's skills increase, preceding steps can be added.

Successful undressing establishes a feeling of competence so important to the toddler as a motivating factor. Dressing, using simple garments, can then be introduced in progressively difficult steps. Emphasis is placed on the parent's readiness, too. Patience and ample time are required to match the toddler's abilities with his motor distractibility and desire to assert his individuality.

GROOMING

MATURATIONAL FACTORS
Beginning early in the second year the toddler makes a marked transition from passive recipient of care to active participant. The specific age will vary with the child. During this second year, abilities and motivation allow beginning steps in self-grooming, which can be fun for the child. The delight comes primarily from imitation of a significant other rather than from the task itself. The toddler can enjoy bathing and participate by taking swipes at his mouth with the washcloth. The same approximation of a skill is evident in attempts to comb hair and brush teeth.

By the end of the second year, abilities will have been refined so that washing and drying hands can be a routine expectation, along with wet floors and clothing! Often, however, the novelty of imitation of self-care ac-

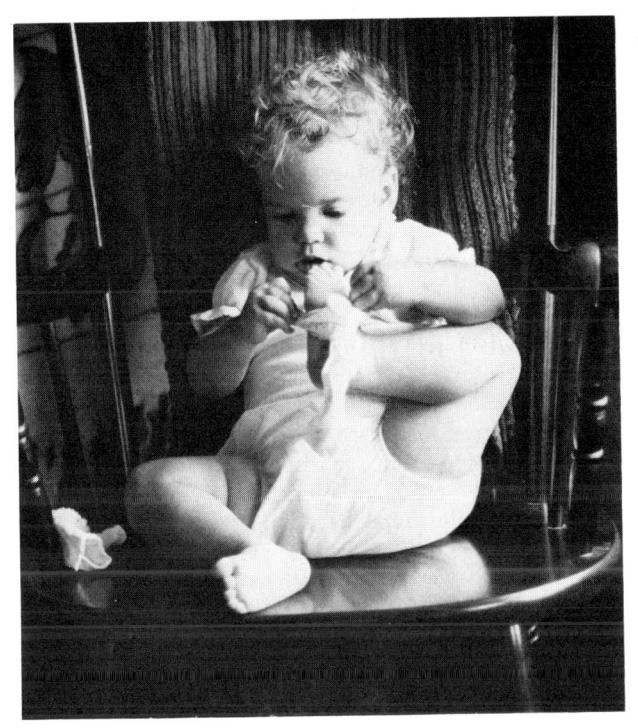

FIGURE 8-17. *(Photo courtesy of Cynthia St. Clair Taylor.)*

tivities disappears, and the independent, often negative attitude prevails. Parents can be advised to delay further independence training until the preschool years, when the child takes pride in such skills.

SOCIALIZATION FACTORS

Parents need to recognize the ambivalence of the toddler in both wanting help with frustrating tasks and demanding the right to test his own abilities. Careful staging of a task so that the skill level is appropriate for the toddler and will result in success is a useful strategy. Children who could not be expected to complete a head-to-toe bath can be handed a washcloth and told: "Now, you wash your face."

The toddler's increasing awareness and responsiveness to the environment makes all his observations a learning experience. He may follow and observe family members as they perform routine activities, such as brushing hair or shaving, and repeat the activity to the best of his ability. Dolls and stuffed animals are appropriate recipients for the toddler's emerging skills in grooming.

Self-care skills in grooming can be further facilitated by clear identification of tasks in which the toddler has a choice about performing and those for which the parent assumes responsibility. The parent's sensitivity to the toddler's emerging abilities can make this a dynamic process reducing frustration of both toddler and adult. The toddler's development of rituals, as in bathing and getting ready for bed, enhances a matter-of-fact, orderly approach to routine expectation. The adult maintains responsibility for the task, and the toddler has the prerogative of insisting on the ritual.

ENVIRONMENTAL CARE

Parents observing their busy toddler emptying wastebaskets and removing items from one shelf and putting them on another may express dismay at pending household disorder. These activities, however, indicate that the toddler has combined perceptual observations with motor skills and is ready to take on a sharing role in the care of the household environment.

Activities at age level for the toddler include dusting or mopping of safe surfaces, sweeping with a small broom, and fetching and putting away frequently used household items. By approximately 20 months, the toddler has a fairly good idea of where things belong and delights in maintaining order by seeing that they are properly stored. With encouragement, the interest and ability carry over to toys. Parents can be prepared to assist, model, and praise the toddler's beginning efforts at helping with household chores.

During this second year the child has progressed from dependent infant to independent toddler. The foundation for skills essential to this independence has been established.

The most significant accomplishment of this period, however, is recognition by the toddler of his potential for control of his own needs. The feeling of self-worth generated by this recognition will provide motivation for continued striving toward independence.

Social development *Susan Blanch Meister*

BASIS FOR SOCIALIZATION

The interactive context of socialization takes on a new nature during the second and third years. During the second year, social input becomes predominantly initiatory rather than reactive. Parents are initiating behaviors that are directed toward decreasing the spontaneous, self-directed behaviors of the toddler. Recognizing the new motor skills and exploration capabilities of toddlers, this initiatory social input (parent) is adaptive. The initiatory input of parents is accompanied by a reactive output by the child. In other words, as the child becomes increasingly subject to intrusion upon self-initiated behaviors, the child's self-directed behaviors give way to reactive behaviors (Escalona, 1973).

This behavioral change does not imply that the toddler is no longer interested in self-initiated behavior. Quite the opposite. And the conflict between the toddler's interest and the parents' initiatory social input is a hallmark of this period in social development.

GOALS OF SOCIALIZATION

The nature of parental social input is clearly concordant with promoting the tendency to become social. The nature of the toddler's response is related to a struggle to be autonomous in the face of social input which prevents such self-direction. Unfortunately, it is possible for this struggle to instill self-doubt in the toddler. Erikson (1963) has aptly labeled the struggle of this period "autonomy versus shame and doubt."

PROCESSES INVOLVED IN SOCIALIZATION

ATTACHMENT

The attachment relationship was solidified during infancy, but some of its major effects emerge during the toddler period. It is during this period of increased motor abilities and cognitive function that the effects of the quality of the attachment relationship can be seen.

Quality of attachment is global in the sense of its impact upon the child. A secure attachment will foster development of clear and varied communication, an expectation of appropriate responses, and the desire as well as the ability to explore the world. Avoidance or an ambivalent attachment relationship fosters development of a set of very different characteristics.

In some sense, the attachment relationship shapes the nature of the child. It also affects the openness of the child to new experiences and the child's responses to those experiences (Ainsworth, 1974; Bowlby, 1969; Lamb, 1978C; Matas, Arend, and Sroufe, in press).

MORAL INTERNALIZATION

During the toddler period, the context of socialization acquires a greater proportion of disciplinary encounters.

Parent socialization behaviors are somewhat subject to child effect. The energy, inquisitiveness, and impulsiveness of the toddler affect the activation, intensity, and reinforcement of parent behaviors.

A greater issue, in terms of moral internalization, is the effect of parental discipline techniques. Discipline techniques that are primarily inductive are most highly associated with development of optimal moral internalization. In other words, discipline which points out the consequences of the child's behavior (especially the consequences for others) is more likely to promote moral standards which will become an integral part of the child. Many disciplinary encounters involve both parental power assertion and induction. Power assertion is best utilized as an arousal technique—to engage the child's attention prior to inductive discipline (Hoffman, 1975).

Parental patterns of discipline are an important contribution to early moral development and therefore an important component of developmental assessment of a toddler and his context of socialization.

EMPATHY

A major component of empathy is social cognition. During the toddler period, several aspects of development contribute to growth in precursors of social cognition. One such aspect is attention. Over the 2 years of toddlerhood, the child's attention span and awareness of surroundings rapidly increase (Bayley, 1969). The child is now in a position to absorb more of the content of social interaction. As described in Chap. 7, the child experiences different aspects of social contact in interaction with the mother, father, and siblings.

The toddler is also likely to experience social contact with peers. In many instances, peers are a source of distal social contact: The interaction occurs over space rather than during physical contact. In this regard, the toddler encounters a very new context of social stimulation.

Toddlers also evidence growth in another component of empathy: learning affective cues. The toddler acquires new abilities to recognize the emotional quality of situations. He is often adept at identifying happy situations, and although this is not equivalent to identifying that another person is in a happy situation, it is an advance toward that ability (Shantz, 1975).

GENDER IDENTITY AND SEX ROLE

Near the end of the toddler period, children often progress from the undifferentiated gender role of infancy and acquire differentiation of sex role. This second stage has been called *hypergender role* and involves the child in rigid stereotyping of social gender categories. A set of studies (Hetherington, 1965) suggests that the father may play a crucial role in this process. The central hypothesis is that a child identifies with a role *relation* with the father. In this instance, the father's gender-linked tuition will shape the child's role relation and affect gender-role development.

This differentiation may operate to varying degrees in individuals. Parental values, parental training, and the context of socialization are factors in individual differences. The quality of attachment to each parent will also affect the saliency of that parent's input (Lamb, 1978b).

Perception of behavioral competency and development of self-esteem
Judith Anne Ritchie

COMPLETION OF THE SEPARATION-INDIVIDUATION PROCESS

The process of separation-individuation parallels the child's motor, language, and cognitive development. By the end of the third year the child has an awareness of the self as an individual who functions independently of the parents and whose parents continue to exist when they disappear from the area in which the child is (Mahler, Pine, and Bergman, 1975). However, the toddler is not able to function at the level of abstract thinking necessary to formulate a full self-concept (Coopersmith, 1967).

During the *practicing phase proper,* from the onset of upright locomotion until about the age of 18 months, the toddler enthusiastically explores, expands, and tests his environment. Independent walking is highly significant for the child as it permits a considerably increased sense of autonomy (Erikson, 1972) and is a major step toward identity formation (Mahler et al., 1975). The toddler's delight and concentration in discovery of his own abilities and objects in the environment have led Greenacre to describe the toddler as having a "love affair with the world" (1957). During this period, the toddler tolerates frustrations and falls, accepts substitute adults well, and while still needing to "refuel," is able to do so by visual or auditory contact with the parent (Mahler et al., 1975).

During the *rappochement phase,* from approximately 18 to 24 months, the toddler becomes more aware of his own separateness, is more concerned about the whereabouts of the parent, and more actively seeks physical contact with her or him. The toddler, who has so recently been delightfully independent, now is more easily frustrated and much more demanding of a parent's involvement with him. At the same time battles with parents begin as the toddler struggles with ambivalence about his relationship with them. The process of individuation is facilitated when parents are able to encourage their toddler toward independence while remaining emotionally available as the child needs them (Mahler et al., 1975).

As the toddler moves into the third year and the phase of *consolidation of individuation,* he has achieved the first level of identity—being a separate, individual entity. Through the third year the toddler's rapidly differentiating cognitive functions of verbal communication, fantasy, and reality testing permit tremendous development of individuation. During this period the toddler achieves a measure of self-consistency, including self-boundaries and gender identity, and a "relatively stable internal image of mother" (Mahler et al., 1975, p. 112).

CONCEPTION OF AUTONOMOUS POWER AND MASTERY

While the toddler's motor development is highly significant in helping to differentiate self as a separate being, feelings of skillfulness and power derived from independent exploration and manipulation of the environment provide a sense of competence. The toddler seems to exercise abilities in walking, partially for the delight of functioning, but also from a need to master the skill (Erikson, 1963). This inner drive toward a sense of competence is satisfied through "activities which though playful and exploratory in character, at the same time show direction, selectivity, and persistence in interacting with the environment" (White, 1959, p. 329). The sense of self as competent derives from intrinsic rewards of having an effect on the environment through ability to create and master novel situations and from external rewards of positive parental response to the toddler's accomplishments (Harter, 1978).

During the toddler years, it appears that sense of mastery and competence is approached through play. Play permits continual restructuring and repeated mastery of the environment. The beginnings of symbolic play in the older toddler permit identifications with "omnipotent" or "all-competent" adults. Play serves the purpose of helping the toddler to learn, not only what is possible and imaginable, but also what is effective and permissible (Erikson, 1972). In addition, fantasy play permits the toddler to become more comfortable with reality and promotes a sense of being able to master difficult situations (Murphy, 1972).

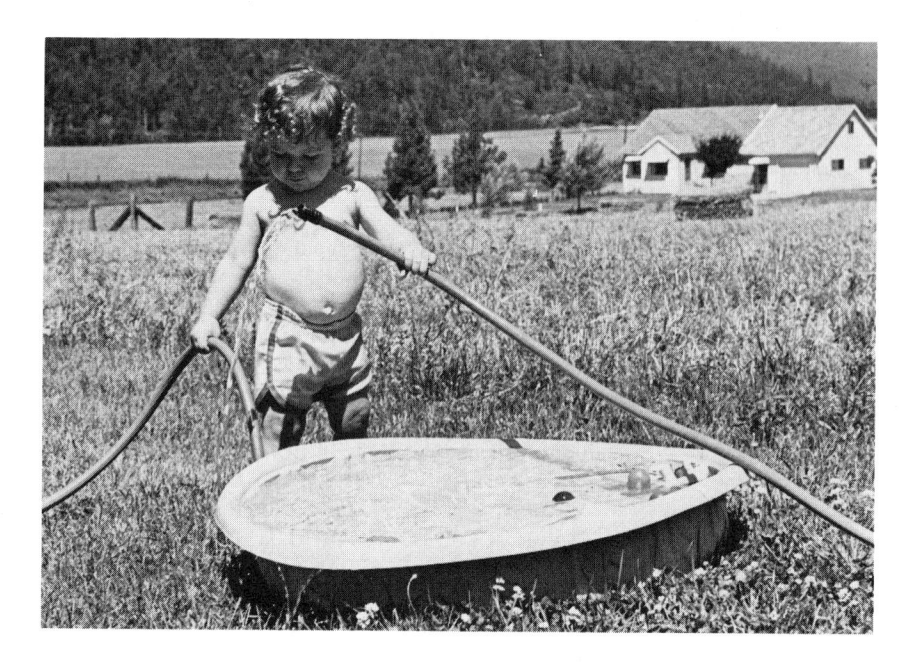

FIGURE 8-18. (*Photo courtesy of Betsy Smith.*)

ROLE OF OTHERS IN DEVELOPMENT OF FEELINGS OF COMPETENCE AND SELF-ESTEEM

The toddler's ability to exert his autonomous power to make decisions about his own actions is an essential component of developing a concept of self as competent and worthy (Brandon, 1969). However, while there is no definition of the specific parental behaviors correlating with positive self-esteem, there is agreement that the toddler is dependent on positive responses of other individuals, particularly parents, toward him and his actions (Coopersmith, 1967; Yamamoto, 1972). Competency motivation was initially described as intrinsic, but it is clear that the sense of competence can be destroyed by the external environment. The development of a sense of competence is said to be "the result of a transaction with the social environment" (Franks, 1974, p. 80).

In the early years it is predominantly parents who supply the external portion of such transactions. The child learns from their responses which behaviors and competencies are expected, appropriate, and valued.

The toddler who successfully achieves the developmental tasks of the second and third years has a sense of a separate self and a sense of autonomy. The ability to exercise self-control contributes, Erikson says, to a "lasting sense of good will and pride" (1963, p. 254). Erikson goes on to say that loss of self-control, usually resulting from overcontrol by parents, results in a lack of self-esteem and a "lasting propensity for doubt and shame."

Bibliography

PHYSICAL DEVELOPMENT OF THE TODDLER

Bayer, L. M., and N. Bayler: *Growth diagnosis* (2d ed.). Chicago: University of Chicago Press, 1976.

Rudolph, A.: *Pediatrics* (16th ed.). New York: Appleton-Century-Crofts, 1977.

Sinclair, D.: *Human growth after birth* (3d ed.). London: Oxford University Press, 1978.

Smith, D. W.: *Growth and its disorders*. Philadelphia: Saunders, 1977.

——— and E. L. Bierman: *The biological ages of man*. Philadelphia: Saunders, 1973.

———, W. Truog, J. E. Rogers, L. J. Greitzer, A. L. Skinner, J. J. McCann, and M. A. Harvey: Shifting linear growth during infancy: Illustration of genetic factors in growth from fetal life through infancy. *J. Pediat.*, 1976, 89, 225–230.

Tanner, J. M., H. Goldstein, and R. H. Whitehouse: Standards for children's height at age 2–9 years allowing for height of parents. *Arch. Dis. Child.*, 1970, *45*, 755–762.

———, R. H. Whitehouse, and M. Takaishi: Standards from birth to maturity for height, weight, height velocity, and weight velocity: British children, 1965, Part I. *Arch. Dis. Child.*, 1966a, *41*, 454–471.

———, ———, and ———: Standards from birth to maturity for height, weight, height velocity, and weight velocity: British children, 1965, Part II. *Arch. Dis. Child.*, 1966b, *41*, 613–635.

CALVARIUM AND FACE

Israel, H.: The fundamentals of cranial and facial growth. In F. Falkner and J. M. Tanner (Eds.), *Human growth 2, Postnatal growth*. New York: Plenum, 1978.

Sullivan, P. G.: Skull, jaw and teeth growth patterns. In F. Falkner and J. M. Tanner (Eds.), *Human growth 2, Postnatal growth*. New York: Plenum, 1978.

SENSORY SYSTEM

Banks, M. S., R. N. Aslin, and R. D. Leston: Sensitive period for the development of human binocular vision. *Science*, 1975, *190*, 675–677.

Bordley, J. E., and W. G. Hardy: The special senses. In R. E. Cooke (Ed.), *The biologic basis of pediatric practice*. New York: McGraw-Hill, 1968.

Gesell, A., R. L. Ilg, and G. E. Bullis: *Vision, Its development in infant and child*. New York: Hoeber-Harper, 1949.

Smith, J. L.: The eye in infancy and childhood. In R. E. Cooke (Ed.), *The biologic basis of pediatric practice*. New York: McGraw-Hill, 1968.

Wiesel, T. N., and D. H. Hubel: Single-cell responses in striate cortex of kittens deprived of vision in one eye. *J. Neurophysiol.*, 1963, *26*, 1003–1017.

——— and ———: Comparison of the effects of unilateral eye closure on cortical unit responses in kittens. *J. Neurophysiol.*, 1965, *28*, 1029–1040.

MUSCULOSKELETAL SYSTEM

Alexander, M. M., and M. S. Brown: *Pediatric physical diagnosis for nurses*. New York: McGraw-Hill, 1974.

Brown, M. S., and M. A. Murphy: *Ambulatory pediatrics for nurses*. New York: McGraw-Hill, 1975.

Rudolph, A. M. (Ed.): *Pediatrics* (16th ed.). New York: Appleton-Century-Crofts, 1977.

GASTROINTESTINAL SYSTEM

Hadorn, B., G. Zoppi, D. H. Shmerling, A. Prader, I. McIntyre, and C. M. Anderson: Quantitative assessment of exocrine pancreatic function in infants and children. *J. Pediat.*, 1968, *73*, 39–50.

Rodbro, P., P. A. Krasilnikoff, and V. Bitsch: Gastric secretion of pepsin in early childhood. *Scand. J. Gastroenterol.*, 1967, *2*, 257–260.

———, ———, P. M. Christiansen, and V. Bitsch: Gastric secretion in early childhood. *Lancet*, 1966, *11*, 730–731.

DEVELOPMENT OF BODY CONCEPT
AND CONCEPTS OF ILLNESS AND WELLNESS

Bowlby, J.: Grief and mourning in infancy and early childhood. *Psychoanal. Stud. Child*, 1960, *15*, 9–54.

Cohn, R.: *The person symbol in clinical medicine*. Springfield, Ill.: Charles C Thomas, 1960.

Douglas, J. W. B.: Early hospital admission and later disturbances of behavior and learning. *Develop. Med. Child Neurol.*, 1975, *17*, 456–483.

Dowd, E. L., J. C. Novak, and E. J. Roy: Releasing the hospitalized child from restraints. *Amer. J. Matern. Child Nurs.*, 1977, *2*, 370–373.

Fisher, S., and S. Cleveland: *Body image and personality*. Princeton, N.J.: Van Nostrand, 1958.

Freud, A.: The role of bodily illness in the mental life of children. *Psychoanal. Stud. Child*, 1952, *7*, 69–80.

Furman, R.: Death and the young child: Some preliminary considerations. *Psychoanal. Stud. Child*, 1964, *19*, 321–328.

Gesell, A., F. L. Ilg, and L. B. Ames: *Infant and child in the culture of today*. New York: Harper & Row, 1974.

Greenacre, P.: Early determinants in the development of the sense of identity. *J. Amer. Psychoanal. Ass.*, 1958, *6*, 612–627.

Grollman, E. A.: *Explaining death to children*. Boston: Beacon, 1967.

Linn, L.: Some developmental aspects of the body image. *Int. J. Psychoanal.*, 1955, *36*, 36–42.

McCaffery, M.: Brief episodes of pain in children. In B. Bergerson et al. (Eds.), *Current concepts in clinical nursing* (Vol. II). St. Louis: Mosby, 1969.

Nagy, M.: The child's theories concerning death. *J. Genet. Psychol.*, 1948, *73*, 3–27.

Natterson, J. M., and A. G. Knudson: Observations concerning fear of death in fatally ill children and their mothers. *Psychosom. Med.*, 1960, *22*, 456–465.

O'Grady, R. S.: Restraint and the hospitalized child. In B. Bergerson et al. (Eds.), *Current concepts in clinical nursing* (Vol. II). St. Louis: Mosby 1969.

Robertson, J.: *Young children in hospital* (2d ed.). London: Tavistock, 1970.

———, and J. Robertson: Young children in brief separa-

tions: A fresh look. *Psychoanal. Stud. Child*, 1971, 26, 264–315.
Schilder, P.: *The image and appearance of the human body.* New York: Wiley, 1964.
Schowalter, J. E.: The child's reaction to his own terminal illness. In B. Schoenberg et al. (Eds.), *Loss and grief.* New York: Columbia University Press, 1970.

THE TODDLER: DEMANDING RECOGNITION
Thomas, A., and S. Chess: *Temperament and development.* New York: Brunner/Mazel, 1977.

PERCEPTUAL DEVELOPMENT
Bower, T. G. R.: *The perceptual world of the child.* Cambridge: Harvard University Press, 1977.
Friedlander, B. Z.: Receptive language development in infancy: Issues and problems. *Merrill-Palmer Quart.*, 1970, 16, 7–53.
Gibson, E. J.: *Principles of perceptual learning and development.* New York: Appleton-Century-Crofts, 1969.
Gibson, J. J.: *The senses considered as perceptual systems.* Boston: Houghton Mifflin, 1966.
Hochberg, J. E., and V. Brooks: Pictorial recognition as an unlearned ability: A study of one child's performance. *Amer. J. Psychol.*, 1962, 75, 624–628.
Pick, H. L., and A. D. Pick: Sensory and perceptual development. In P. H. Mussen (Ed.), *Carmichael's manual of child psychology* (Vol. I). New York: Wiley, 1970.
Weir, R.: Some questions on the child's learning of phonology. In F. Smith and G. A. Miller (Eds.), *The genesis of language.* Cambridge, Mass.: MIT, 1966.

GROSS MOTOR DEVELOPMENT
Banus, B. S.: *The developmental therapist.* Thorofare, N.J.: Charles B. Slack, 1971.
Corbin, C. B.: *A textbook of motor development.* Dubuque, Iowa: Wm. G. Brown, 1973.
Egan, D. R., R. S. Illingworth, and R. C. MacKeith: *Developmental screening 0–5 years.* London: Spastics International, 1969.
Gesell, A., H. M. Halverson, H. Thompson, F. L. Ilg, B. M. Castner, L. B. Ames, and C. S. Amatruda: *The first five years of life.* New York: Harper & Brothers, 1940.
Illingworth, R. S.: *The development of the infant and young child.* London: Churchill Livingstone, 1975.
Knobloch, H., and B. Pasamanick: *Gesell and Amatruda's developmental diagnosis.* New York: Harper & Row, 1974.

FINE MOTOR DEVELOPMENT
Gesell, A., H. M. Halverson, H. Thompson, F. L. Ilg, B. Castner, L. B. Ames, and C. S. Amatruda: *The first five years of life.* New York: Harper & Brothers, 1940.
Gordon, I. J.: *Baby learning through baby play.* New York: St. Martin's, 1970.
——, B. Guinagh, and R. E. Jester: *Child learning through child play.* New York: St. Martin's, 1972.
Illingworth, R. S.: *The development of the infant and young child—Normal and abnormal.* London: Churchill Livingstone, 1975.
Knobloch, H., and B. Pasamanick: *Gesell and Amatruda's developmental diagnosis.* New York: Harper & Row, 1974.

COGNITIVE DEVELOPMENT
Bruner, J.: *Studies in cognitive development.* New York: Wiley, 1968.
Flavell, J.: *The developmental psychology of Jean Piaget.* New York: Van Nostrand, 1963.
Fraiberg, S.: *The magic years.* New York: Scribner, 1959.
Luria, A.: The directive function of speech in development and dissolution. In R. C. Oldfield and J. C. Marshall (Eds.), *Language.* Baltimore: Penguin, 1968.
——: *The role of speech in the regulation of normal and abnormal behavior.* Bethesda, Md.: U.S. Department of Health, Education, and Welfare, 1960.
Piaget, J.: *The language and thought of the child.* New York: Harcourt, Brace, 1962.
Wenar, C.: *Personality development from infancy to adulthood.* Boston: Houghton Mifflin, 1971.

LANGUAGE DEVELOPMENT
Bloom, L.: *One word at a time: The use of single word utterance before syntax.* The Hague: Mouton, 1973.
—— and M. Lahey: *Language development and language disorders.* New York: Wiley, 1978.
Brown, R.: *A first language,* Cambridge, Mass.: Harvard University Press, 1973.
Coggins, T. E., and R. L. Carpenter: Developmental changes in language and communication: What children acquire from eight months to eight years. In M. Cohen and P. Gross (Eds.), *Developmental pin points.* New York: Grune & Stratton, 1978.
Dale, P.: *Language development: Structure and function.* New York: Holt, 1976.

Kriegsmann, E.: *Providing an optimal language environment for the young child.* (Unpublished paper, Seattle, 1978.)

Nelson, K.: Structure and strategy in learning to talk. *Monographs of the Society for Research in Child Development,* 1973, *38* (Serial no. 149).

Ramey, C. T., D. C. Farran, F. A. Campbell, and N. W. Finkelskin: *Observation of mother-infant interactions; Implications for development.* Chapel Hill, N.C.: Frank Porter Graham Child Development Center, University of North Carolina, 1976.

SELF-HELP SKILL DEVELOPMENT

Brazelton, T. B.: *Toddlers and parents: A declaration of independence.* New York: Dell, 1974.

Caplan, F., and T. Caplan: *The second twelve months of life.* New York: Grosset & Dunlap, 1977.

Chess, S., A. Thomas, and H. Birch: *Your child is a person.* New York: Viking, 1965.

Espenschade, A., and H. Eckert: *Motor development,* Columbus, Ohio: Merrill, 1967.

Fein, G., D. Johnson, N. Kosson, L. Stork, and L. Wasserman: Sex stereotypes and preferences in the toy choices of 20-month old boys and girls. *Develop. Psychol.,* 1974, *10*(4), 554–558.

Gesell, A., F. Ilg, L. Ames, and J. Rodell: *Infant and child in the culture of today* (rev. ed.). New York: Harper & Row, 1974.

Knobloch, H., and B. Pasamanick (Eds.): *Gesell and Amatruda's developmental diagnosis* (3d ed.). Hagerstown, Md.: Harper & Row, 1974.

MacKeith, R., R. Meadow, and R. K. Turner: How children become dry. In I Kolvin, R. C. MacKeith, and R. Meadow (Eds.), *Bladder control and enuresis.* Philadelphia: Lippincott, 1973.

Munroe, R., and R. Munroe: *Cross-cultural human development.* New York: Jason Aronson, 1977.

Murphy, M: Toilet training—When and how. *Pediat. Nurs.,* November/December 1975, 22–27.

Stehbens, J. A., and D. L. Silber: Parental expectations in toilet training. *Pediatrics,* 1971, *48*(3), 451–454.

White, B. L.: *The first three years of life.* New York: Avon, 1975.

SOCIAL DEVELOPMENT

Ainsworth, M. D.: Infant-mother attachment and social development: "Socialization" as a product of reciprocal responsiveness to signals. In M. P. Richards (Ed.), *The integration of the child into a social world.* London: Cambridge University Press, 1974.

———, and S. Bell: Mother-infant interaction and the development of competence. In K. J. Connolly and J. S. Bruner (Eds.), *The growth of competence.* New York: Academic, 1974.

Bayley, N.: *Bayley scales of infant development.* New York: Psychological Corporation, 1969.

Bowlby, J.: *Attachment and loss.* New York: Basic Books, 1969.

Erikson, E.: *Childhood and society.* New York: Norton, 1963.

Escalona, S.: Basic modes of social interaction: Their emergence and patterning during the first two years of life. *Merrill-Palmer Quart.,* 1973, *19*, 205–232.

Hetherington, E. M.: A developmental study of the effects of sex of the dominant parent on sex-role preference, identification and imitation in children. *J. Personality Soc. Psychol.,* 1965, *2*, 188–194.

Hoffman, M.: Moral internalization, parental power and the nature of parent-child interaction. *Develop. Psychol.,* 1975, *11*, 288–239.

Jacobs, B. S., and H. Moss: Birth order and sex of sibling as determinants of maternal-infant interaction. *Child Develop.,* 1976, *47*, 315–322.

Lamb, M.: The father's role in the infant's social world. In J. H. Stevens and M. Mathews (Eds.), *Mother/child, father/child relationships.* New York: National Association for the Education of Young Children, 1978a.

———: Interactions between 18 month olds and their preschool aged siblings. *Child Develop.,* 1978b, *49*, 51–59.

———: *Social and personality development.* New York: Holt, 1978c.

Matas, L., R. Arend, and L. Sroufe: Continuity of adaptation in the second year: The relationship between quality of attachment and later competence. *Child Develop.* (in press).

Parsons, J., and J. Bryan: Adolescence: Gateway to androgyny. *Occasional Papers Series.* Ann Arbor: University of Michigan Women's Study Program, 1978.

Shantz, C.: The development of social cognition. In E. M. Hetherington (Ed.), *Review of child development research* (Vol. 5). Chicago: University of Chicago Press, 1975.

PERCEPTION OF BEHAVIORAL COMPETENCY AND DEVELOPMENT OF SELF-ESTEEM

Brandon, N.: *The psychology of self-esteem.* Los Angeles: Nash, 1969.

Coopersmith, S.: *The antecedents of self-esteem.* San Francisco: Freeman, 1967.

Erikson, E. H.: *Childhood and society* (2d ed.). New York: Norton, 1963.

———: Play and actuality. In M. W. Piers (Ed.), *Play and development.* New York: Norton, 1972.

Franks, D. D.: Current conception of competency motivation and self-validation. In D. Field and D. Mills (Eds.), *Social psychology for sociologists.* Ontario: Nelson, 1974.

Greenacre, P.: The childhood of the artist: Libidinal phase development and giftedness. *Psychoanal. Stud. Child,* 1957, *12,* 27–72.

Harter, S.: Effectance motivation reconsidered: Toward a developmental model. *Hum. Develop.,* 1978. *21,* 34–64.

Kuhn, D., S. C. Nash, and L. Brucken: Sex-role concepts of two- and three-year-olds. *Child Develop.,* 1978, *49,* 445–451.

Mahler, M. S., F. Pine, and A. Bergman: *The psychological birth of the human infant.* New York: Basic Books, 1975.

Murphy, L. B.: Infants' play and cognitive development. In M. W. Piers (Ed.), *Play and development.* New York: Norton, 1972.

White, R. W.: Motivation reconsidered: The concept of competence. *Psychol. Rev.,* 1959, *66,* 297–333.

Yamamoto, K.: *The child and his image.* Boston: Houghton Mifflin, 1972.

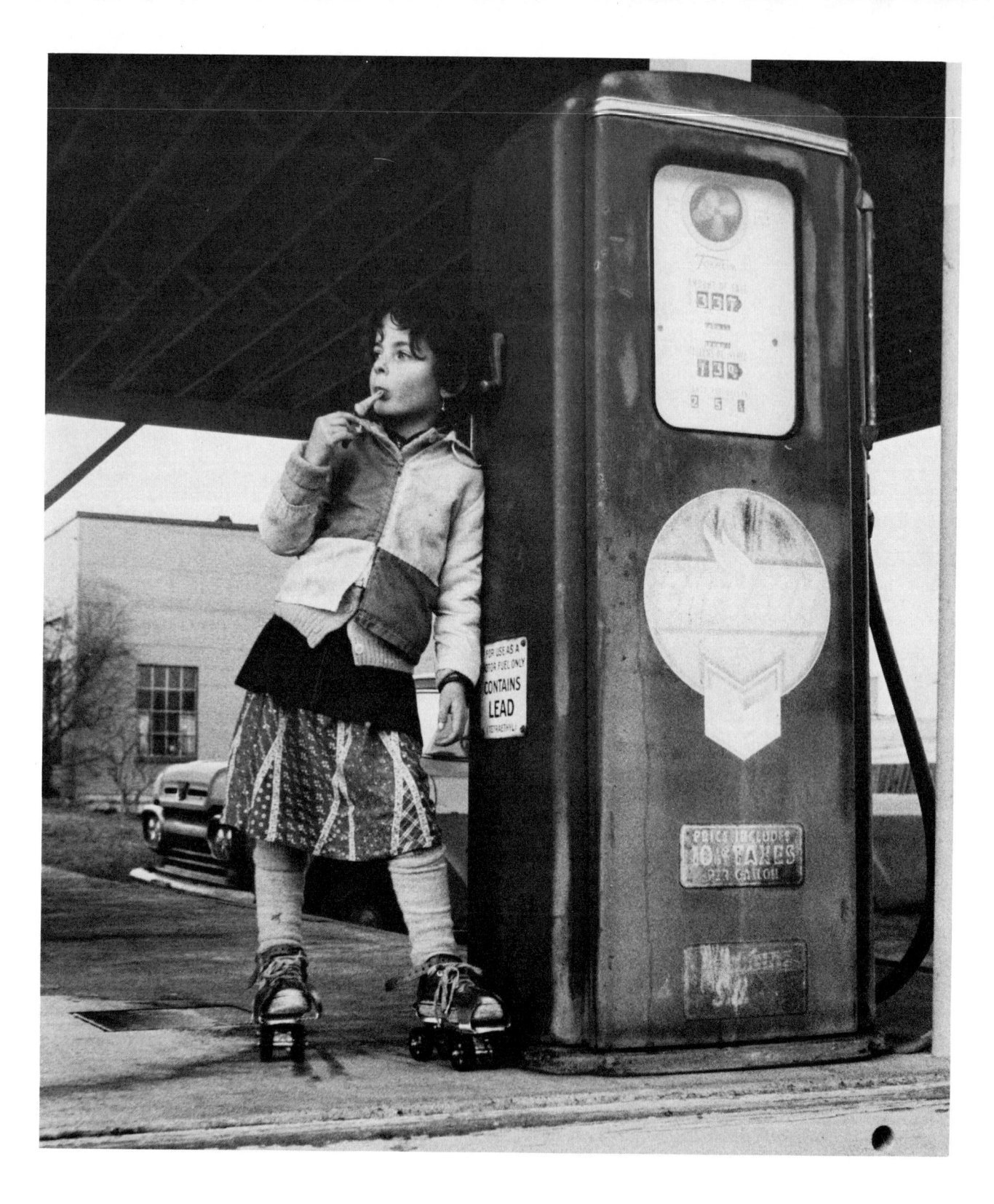

CHAPTER 9
The Preschool Child: 3 Years to 5 Years

Introduction

The preschool child, from 3 to 5 years of age, is competent, skilled, quite verbal, and very egocentric! Physically he is well in control of himself, and growth is steady; nothing disrupts his physiological equilibrium. His own body as well as others', however, has the preschooler's attention and is the subject of his unending curiosity.

The preschool child is anxious as well as prepared to apply his many skills in worldly exploration. Spinner of a thousand questions and magical theories, he knows himself to be all-powerful and all-important. The child is not, however, immune to fears and doubts, but his openness, curiosity, eagerness, and helpfulness make the preschool-age child's love affair with life contagious.

FIGURE 9-1.

SECTION 1
Physical Development

Physical development of the preschool child M. Colleen Caulfield

DEVELOPMENTAL APPROACH TO PHYSICAL ASSESSMENT

The preschooler's response to health appraisal is more predictable and less variable than that of the toddler. Having successfully completed the tasks of autonomy, the child enters the stage of initiative versus guilt. This stage builds upon autonomy and adds the ability to plan, undertake, and complete a task. Eager to work cooperatively and share obligations, the child is very ready to learn. The preschooler is proud of accomplishments. Thus, the unstructured, opportunistic approach that was needed with the toddler is no longer totally appropriate. The preschooler can be an active participant in the examination; structure is added by making clear what is expected of the child.

Walking, running, and climbing are now effortless activities. Immobility or the restraint of physical activity is no longer viewed as a significant threat in itself. If given clear expectations and asked for help, the preschooler will demonstrate pride in sitting still while the ears are examined.

The toddler fought hard to gain control of the body and its functions; the preschooler will fight equally hard to maintain *body integrity*. Mutilation fears are at a peak during this stage, and any intrusive procedure is viewed as a hostile invasion. All aspects of the assessment must be explained and assurance given that the body will remain intact following any procedure. The preschooler who violently reacts to heart auscultation may be doing so because of a fear that the stethoscope tube is siphoning from the body.

At times, the preschooler can become overwhelmed by a frightening sense of power. Security must be provided and limits clearly defined. Prolonged bargaining is to be avoided—this is both frustrating and frightening to the child because no one is in control.

Play is the preschooler's occupation; through play, unfamiliar objects and situations are explored, dealt with, and placed in proper perspective. An accurate perception of the meaning of the assessment tools is enhanced if the preschooler is given the opportunity to play with them before they are used. The stethoscope may be a marvelous toy for listening to everything—parent, self, a toy, or the abdomen. The otoscope can be an especially fearful item because of its intrusive quality. If played with prior to use, an immeasurable amount of relief is given to the child. An excellent way to decrease fear is to demonstrate first on the parent or a doll. The child can then imitate the procedure in play.

PHYSICAL STATUS

The trend of decreasing adiposity and increasing muscularity that began in the toddler continues in the preschool years. The general appearance becomes increasingly adultlike; the head is no longer so large in relation to the rest of the body (see Fig. 9-2). The abdomen flattens, and the postural lordosis of the toddler disappears. The 3-year-old may be slightly knock-kneed. (Refer to Chap. 8 for a discussion of posture and stance.)

NORMAL GROWTH PARAMETERS

Height, weight, and head circumference By age 2, the major shifts in growth rate are completed, and the preschool child grows at a genetically (as well as environmentally) determined, fairly constant rate. The abrupt downward shifts in height and weight velocity that began early in life have stabilized (see Fig. 8-3).

Head circumference increased very rapidly during the early years; 80 percent of the growth of the brain was completed by age 2 years. By age 5 years, adult size is nearly reached. Head circumference is not routinely measured after 3 years of age; the National Center for Health Statistics (NCHS) growth charts give values only up to age 3 years.

Height increases by 7.6 cm (3 in) per year during the preschool years (see Fig. 9-3). Mid-parental height charts development by Tanner (see "Physical Development of the Toddler," Chap. 8) can be used to assess the appropriateness of the child's height with respect to genetic background. Prediction of adult height is possible by age 3 years; boys will have attained 53 percent of eventual adult height, and girls will have attained 57 percent (Bayer and Bayley, 1976). Starting at age 3, standing height (stature) rather than length is obtained, and the 3- to 18-years height curves are used.

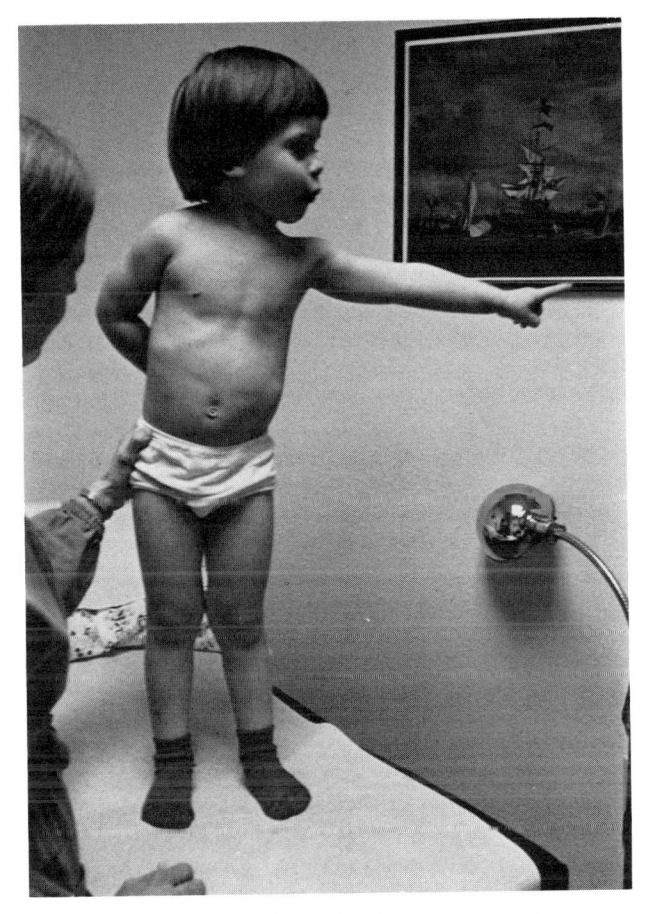

FIGURE 9-2. The preschool child's growth in stature is reflected in changing body proportions. The head does not make up as great a percentage of height, and the legs are longer.

Weight gain is also slow and steady (see Fig. 9-4). At age 3, weight is about five times birth weight. The preschooler will gain approximately 1.8 kg (4 lb) per year, a trend which began at age 2. Weight is also plotted on the 3- to 18-year curves.

Body proportions The preschooler continues with the changes in body proportions that began in the toddler. The head and neck continue to decrease in proportion to the rest of the body. The lower extremities increase their relative proportion as they continue to grow faster than the head, trunk, and arms. Ossification centers appear in the epiphyses of the wrist, elbow, ankle, and knee during the preschool years. Overall, the typical preschooler looks even more adultlike than the toddler due to skeletal maturation.

Vital signs The trend of gradually diminishing heart and respiratory rates and blood pressure continues. Pulse rate is approximately 95 bpm in the 3-year-old, 92 bpm in the 4-year-old, and 90 bpm in the 5-year-old. Average respiratory rate from 3 to 5 years is 25 to 24 breaths per minute, respectively. Blood pressure is 85 to 90/60. It is recommended that blood pressure be routinely taken starting at age 3 years (Recommendations of the Task Force, 1977).

Sensory system   Anna M. Tichy

During the first 3 years of postnatal life, a number of anatomical changes have occurred which are associated with functional development of vision. The cornea and the relatively small pupils of birth have assumed a greater diameter. The sclera now thickens, becoming characteristically white and less cellular, and the ciliary processes assume a more posterior position as the eye grows.

Visual acuity in the preschool-age child improves from 20/40 at age 3 years to near the adult level, approximately 20/30, at 4 years. Adult visual acuity level of 20/20 is attained at 5 to 7 years of age (Ellis, 1978). Assessment of visual acuity in the preschooler is reliable with the Snellen E chart. A child of this age, of normal intelligence, will quickly respond to this test if it is presented in the form of a game. A nine-letter Stycar can also be used and may detect astigmatism.

Assessment of visual acuity in this age group is important for the early identification of refractive errors. Hyperopia (farsightedness), which is common in infancy and in most preschoolers, is characterized by a short eyeball with a decreased distance from the lens to the retina (see Fig. 9-5). This causes the image of a distant object to be formed behind the retina in a resting eye. A deficiency of the refractive power of the optical system in which the lens system is too weak when the ciliary muscle is completely relaxed may also cause hyperopia. The latter refractive problem will persist into adulthood; however, the hyperopia associated with growth of the eyeball diminishes as the child matures.

Myopia (nearsightedness) is caused by an abnormality of the curvature of the optical elements or elongation of the eyeball, increasing the lens-to-retina distance. Physiological myopia is relatively common with a familial tendency.

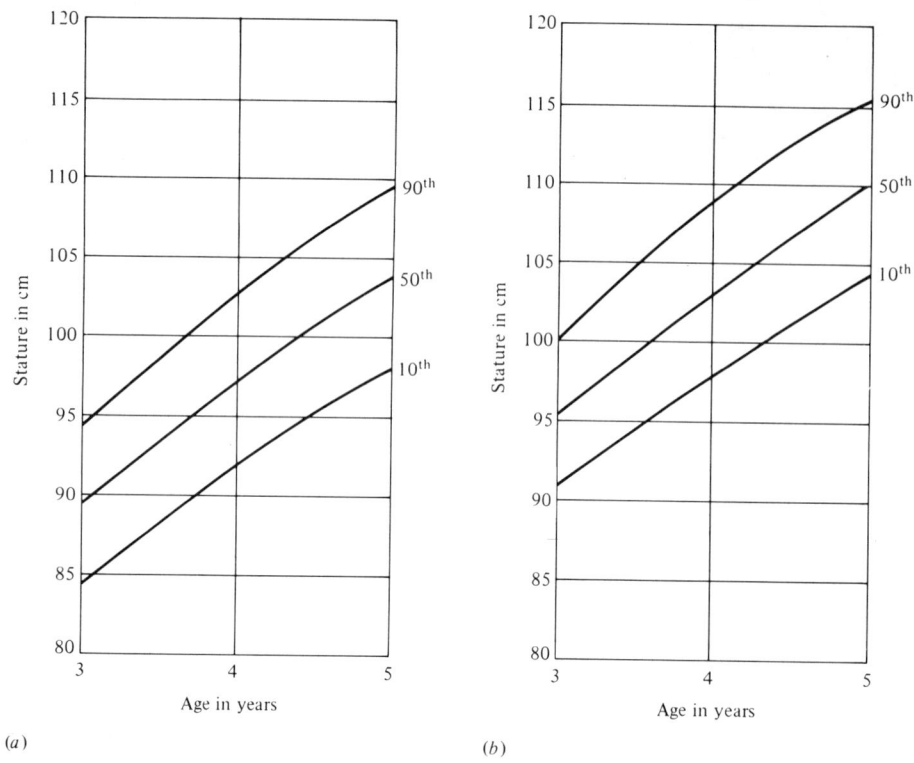

FIGURE 9-3. Height by age, 3 to 5 years. (*a*) Girls; (*b*) boys. [*From National Center for Health Statistics, NCHS growth charts, 1976. Monthly Vital Statistics Report (HRA) 76–1120 (Vol. 25, No. 3). Rockland, Maryland: U.S. Health Resources Administration, 1977. (Supplement.)*]

Development of the visual system is essentially complete by age 7 years. It does not undergo significant structural or functional changes following the early school-age period.

Development of body concept and concepts of illness and wellness
Judith Anne Ritchie

BODY CONCEPT, CONTENT, AND FUNCTION

BEGINNING STABILITY OF THE BODY CONCEPT

The child at age 4 years has a relatively stable percept of the relations between his body and its parts and between the body and the outer world. However, there remain remarkable inconstancies in the body concept and a great tendency to transformation (Ausubel, 1958; Simmel, 1966). This is apparent in the preschool child's play activities involving mirrors, body movement, and clothing.

The preschool child displays considerable interest in the differentiation between the sexes and clarifies his perception of his own naked body and its function through comparisons with others (Dillon, 1934). A girl, age 4 years, visited two boys, 4 and 3 years of age, while they were having their bath. She chatted very briefly and then came quickly downstairs announcing in amazement, "Mummy, Mummy, guess what? David and Andrew have tails!" The boys soon afterward managed a similar excursion and expressed equal surprise at the girl's lack of a penis. Another preschool girl, aged 3 years, asked about an infant boy, "How come he has what they call a peanut [penis]?" Girls this age who have seen boys voiding are

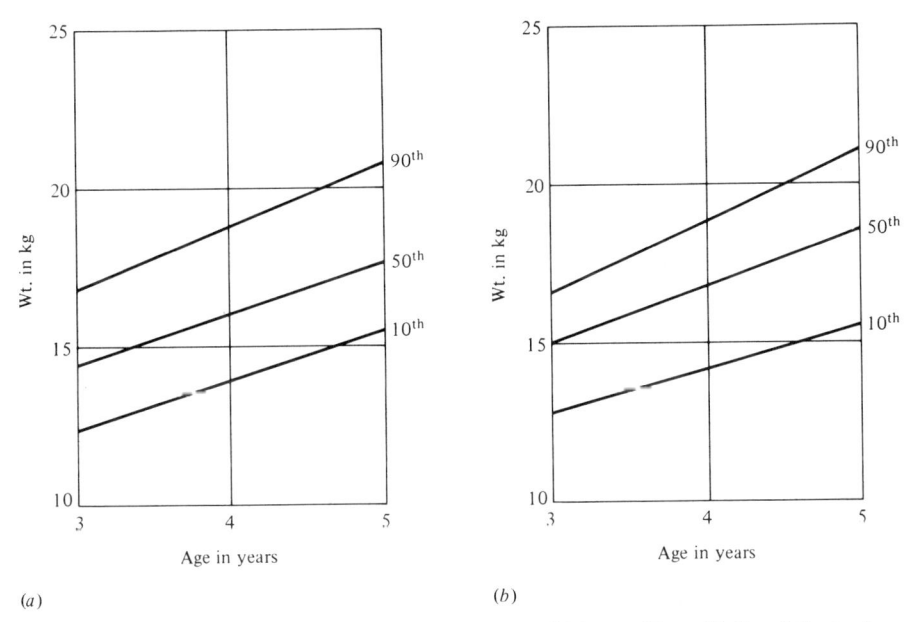

FIGURE 9-4. Weight by age, 3 to 5 years. (*a*) Girls; (*b*) boys. (*From National Center for Health Statistics, NCHS Growth Charts, 1976.*)

frequently observed trying to void while standing up in front of the toilet.

The preschool child's body concept is strongly influenced and reinforced by parental ideals and teaching, interaction with peers, and the culture in which he develops (Kolb, 1975; Schilder, 1964). Differences in values and attitudes toward the body in boys and girls are apparent even in the preschool years. Boys are expected to be strong and athletic, and girls, as early as 3 years, associate smallness with femininity (Levy, 1932). More girls than boys at age 4 to 5 years place emphasis on comparative body size (Katcher and Levin, 1955).

CONCEPT OF THE INSIDE OF THE BODY

The concept of the contents of one's body is developed much more slowly than the concept of the body's outer appearance. The young child is aware of the inside of the body as a heavy mass (Schilder and Wechler, 1935). Most preschool children are able to list one or two internal parts—most frequently bones, food and/or drink just consumed, and blood (Gellert, 1962). The internal body is seen as a hollow organ encased in skin (Fraiberg, 1959).

Conceptions of internal functions of the body are as vague and inaccurate as the conceptions of the body content. Most verbalized comments, questions, and fantasies about internal function relate to where babies come from and how babies get in and out of mother's "stomach" (Fraiberg, 1959; Gesell, Ilg, and Ames, 1974).

WELLNESS, ILLNESS, AND HOSPITALIZATION

Four- and five-year-old children have assimilated many beliefs about health and how to remain healthy. They need supervision and reminders as their drive for exploration overrules their knowledge of "health rules" (Freud, 1965). Children at this age have begun to learn that they are at least partially responsible for their own health.

MAJOR CONCERNS AND REACTIONS TO ILLNESS AND HOSPITALIZATION

Body integrity The preschool child's perception of body concept, knowledge of self as an individual, and egocentric thought processes contribute to his awareness of the vulnerability of the self with predominance of fears about body integrity. Minor injuries are often reacted to as if

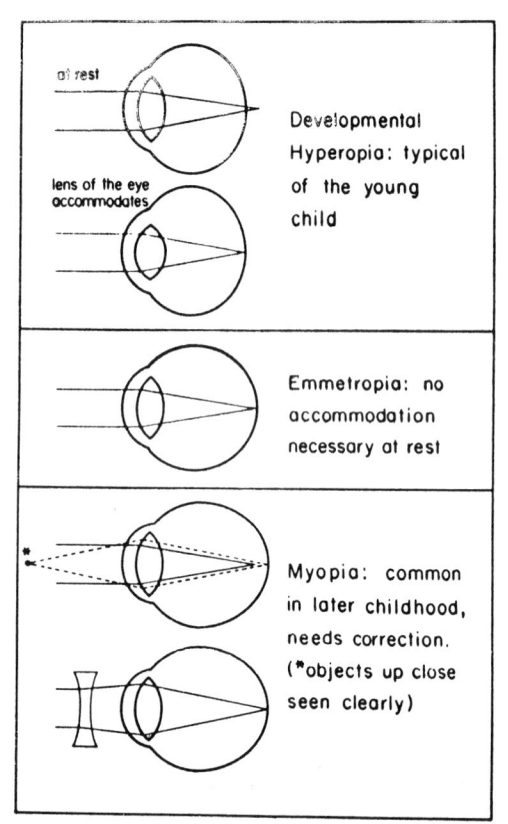

FIGURE 9-5. Changes in the eye showing developmental hyperopia, emmetropia, and myopia. (*From D. W. Smith and E. L. Bierman, The biological ages of man, from conception through old age. Philadelphia: Saunders, 1963, p. 117. Reprinted by permission of the publisher.*)

catastrophic. Small scratches require some form of bandage so that "all my blood won't fall out."

Changes in sensation, function, or appearance of the body may result in reactions which adults feel are out of proportion to the threat posed. During venipunctures for blood samples, children often react with terror and panic, expressing fear that all their blood will be taken. Incisions, drain sites, and burn wounds that ooze body fluids or leave body surface "uncovered" are threatening for similar reasons. Casts precipitate a variety of concerns. For example, a 3-year-old child, crying and frightened because of x-rays and cast application to a fractured arm, expressed his concerns very clearly:

I was scared the doctor would put a cast on my mouth. I want this cast off. Take this cast off now. It makes me all wet. It's too hot. My bed will get wet. I can't take a bath. I have to clean my body. I can't feed myself. I can't go to potty—I can't take my pants down with one hand.

Pain is interpreted as a punishment and a threat to body integrity (Freud, 1952). It has been stated that children tolerate discomfort well and do not relate discomfort to pain (Swafford and Allan, 1968). However, Eland and Anderson found that young children can, by placing an X on a body outline, "localize the source of their discomfort even though they may be unable to verbalize how bad they feel" (1977, p. 453). If previous pain experience has been limited to bumps and bruises, preschool children may be confused by more intense pain (McCaffery, 1969).

Some preschool children may have insufficient language or may confuse terminology and therefore be unable to communicate verbally. For example, a 4-year-old had a shoulder disarticulation and complained afterward of her knee hurting. When asked which knee, she pointed to the area where her elbow would have been. She agreed she had the words elbow and knee mixed up.

Intrusive procedures The study of hospitalized preschoolers' play reveals that areas of greatest concern are intrusive events such as injections, procedures, and tests (Erikson, 1958). Events which intrude on the body's interior or boundary and on the child's autonomy are repeated frequently during play. For some preschool children, play materials that closely represent the reality of hospital equipment may evoke such strong feelings of anxiety as to cause play disruption.

Preschool children intensely dislike rectal thermometers or examination of the ears and react by vigorous protest or by rigid, tight control of the entire body. They react with fear to even the presence of a person regarded as likely to carry out an intrusive procedure.

Separation Separation anxiety decreases in intensity for the preschool child as concerns with integrity and intrusion predominate (Prugh, 1965). The preschool child's awareness of the continued existence of the absent parent permits some hope of reunion, and therefore the degree of distress is not usually as great as in the younger child. However, because of feelings of acute loneliness, loss of protection, and abandonment, the preschool child continues to find separation a major concern.

Verbal and cognitive skills permit the preschool child to ask about and discuss parental whereabouts. Skills in

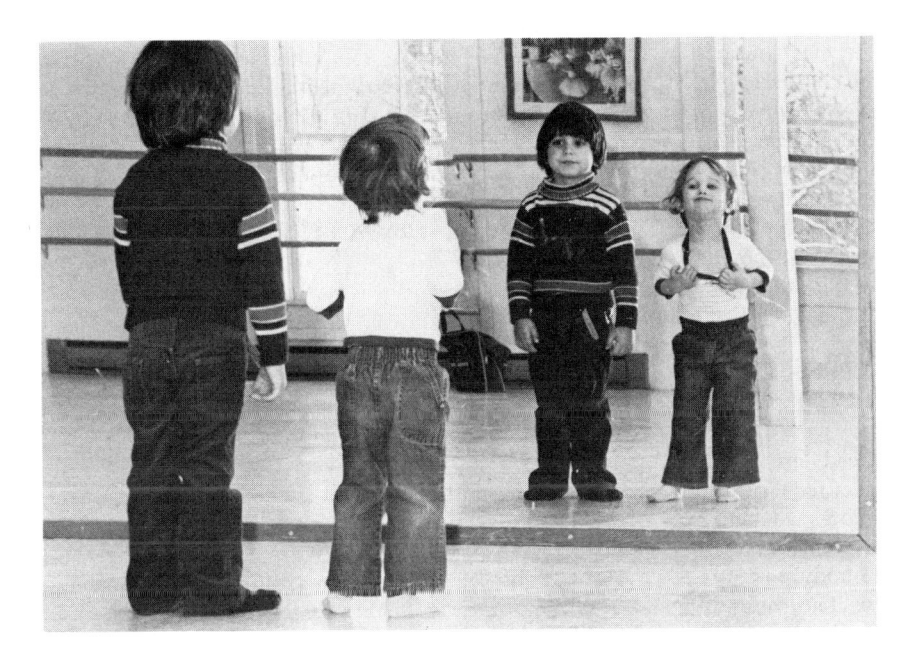

FIGURE 9-6. (Photo courtesy of Betsy Smith.)

play and fantasy make it possible to use these activities as defenses against overwhelming feelings of aloneness.

Lack of prior experiences with separation from parents and the presence of multiple concurrent stressors may alter the preschool child's expected ability to cope with separation. One child, aged 5, had several previous illnesses and hospitalizations. Separation constituted 52 percent of her communicated concerns—a proportion much higher than that expected of a 5-year-old. Another preschool child, aged 4 years, had never previously been separated from family members. By her third hospital day, her ability to play virtually ceased, and she constantly cried for her mother, "I want my mom. I *need* my mom."

Punishment The preschool child's egocentric thinking, awareness of partial responsibility for health, and fantasies of omnipotence and retaliation contribute to the child's feelings of guilt when ill or injured and his interpretation of illness as punishment (Fraiberg, 1959; Prugh, 1965). At times this interpretation may have been stimulated or reinforced by adults through such threats as, "If you cry, I'll tell the nurse to give you a needle."

A boy, aged 4 years, was immobilized in traction and plaster cast for a fractured elbow sustained in a fall from a snowmobile. His feelings of treatments and hospitalization as punishment were clear in his statements about the hospital: " 'This is a bad place for boys and girls to be.' He paused, and continued, 'I don't like it here.' He wrinkled his face and shifted his body nervously. 'Ohhh, oh. My fingers will never wiggle again. I'll never go on a 'mobile again. I promise.' He then started to sob."

Unfamiliar environment A further source of concern for the hospitalized preschool child is the strangeness of the environment with presence of unfamiliar furniture and equipment and very large rooms and absence of familiar household furnishings. The practice of placing the preschool child in a crib alarms and confuses the child who has long since given up the shameful "baby" bed and moved into a "big" bed.

Much hospital equipment has unusual functions and sounds and may contribute to alarming fantasies. For example, most children are unfamiliar with intercom systems. When his name was called over the intercom, a 4-year-old boy remained silent but wide-eyed. When his name was called again, he replied shakily, "What do you want, wall?"

The preschooler's literal interpretation of explanations and his egocentrism contribute to many fearful fantasies about the threats in the environment. He may interpret phrases such as *ICU* to mean *I can see you,* or *special picture of the inside of you* as including pictures of what he is thinking. When procedures are carried out on other children, the preschool child appears to wonder if he is to be the next victim. Most children can manage their anxiety and become comfortable if given truthful and age-appropriate explanations of the purpose of equipment, the meaning of strange words, and why the other child requires events or equipment that they do not require.

MEANS OF COMMUNICATING CONCERN

In contrast to the younger child, the preschool child has more extensive coping skills and can give very specific verbal and nonverbal cues to what his needs are and to what he finds upsetting. When the reality of the illness or hospital experience is overwhelming, the preschool child may be verbally unable to express concerns and resort to nonverbal cues of facial expressions and body postures. The child of this age effectively eliminates disturbing experiences or conversations by changing the subject or turning away to other activities.

The preschool child who finds it impossible to listen or talk about the reality of his own illness and therapy may use fantasy to deal with such disturbing material. The use of fantasy is a mechanism the child uses to adjust to, adapt to, and learn about himself and reality (Pitcher and Prelinger, 1963). A 5-year-old child used fantasy to communicate her concerns and feelings about separation and illness. Her familiar stuffed toys could "state" precisely how they felt about being hospitalized. When discussion of her illness was broached through puppets and a favorite stuffed toy, she tolerated a detailed explanation and discussion for almost 25 min and was intently interested and involved (Ritchie, 1972).

The preschool child's means of coping with the stresses of illness and hospitalization are varied, individual, and dependent on a number of factors. Regression to earlier behavioral patterns may occur as a positive and beneficial coping resource (Freud, 1952). Other coping mechanisms used by preschool children include identification with or ability to relate to health care personnel, development of cognitive understanding of illness or hospitalization, unsublimated expression of emotions, and mastery of anxiety through verbalizations or acting out in play (Blom, 1958; Erickson and Holt, 1964; Langford, 1961; Prugh, 1965).

DEATH

Preschool children begin to be much more aware of death. Death play is prevalent through crashes of airplanes and motor vehicles and in fantasies of being shot. Death is perceived as separation or departure (Nagy, 1948) and, as other trips, voluntary. A 4-year-old child spoke angrily about her grandfather who had died 6 months previously: "He's dead. He went away—and he never said goodbye."

The preschooler sees death as a different form of living and as temporary or reversible (Nagy, 1948). The child may be capable of mourning (Furman, 1970) but seems to be mourning the separation and to believe the person is still capable of eating and breathing and returning. Another preschool child, aged 4, cried when told her mother had died in the same accident in which she had been injured. However, she later said, "I know she's dead, but when I get home, then she'll come back." It is not until ages 5 and 6 years that the denial of death disappears. Even at that stage, degrees of death are perceived, and death is still not recognized as a definite and inevitable fact (Kastenbaum, 1967; Nagy, 1948).

Preschool children with fatal illnesses rarely ask if they are dying. Their behavior tends to focus on fears of mutilation and separation and the perception of illness as punishment.

SECTION 2
Behavioral Development

Physical development in the preschool period marks the end of most rapid growth which began during fetal development. This period of physiological stabilization allows a basis and time for continued rapid behavioral adaptation. As the preschool child applies his body in learning encounters with the larger world, he seems to learn its importance to him. Knowing, too, his vulnerability, he zealously protects himself from possible bodily harm.

The successes and satisfactions of preschool behavioral development are discussed in this section.

The preschool child: "Here I am!"
Mary Tudor

The preschool child has established himself as an intact, complete, and competent person. Having gained control over his body function and mastery over himself, he now consolidates and elaborates on his behavioral skills during the preschool period.

The preschool child is notoriously egocentric. This is understandable when one recognizes cognitive limitations as well as the fact that his developmental tasks so far have of necessity been learning about and teaching himself. And although he has had a great deal of exposure to self, the world outside is just now opening to include him, cognitively and geographically. The toddler's need was to say, "I am!" The preschooler delightedly and egocentrically pronounces, "Here I am!"

Motor control has progressed in a cephalocaudal, proximodistal pattern to the outer boundaries by the preschool years. Elaboration of these abilities for the purpose of new experiences occurs. The preschool child easily runs; now he will master simple motor games, riding toys, and backyard gym sets. His skills of prehension are artistically applied, and he begins to express his cognitive maturation with materials at hand. He enters a symbolic world of art, play, and thinking.

Cognitive development of the preschool child is limited by egocentric thinking. He can reason but with limitations. He sees cause-and-effect relationships where none exist and explains happenings in the world by human actions or psychological influences, particularly his own.

The preschool child is extremely verbal, and he enjoys this verbal fluency. The communication skills learned and practiced during infancy and toddler years are now a tool to express thoughts and feelings and to gather information and cooperation. The preschooler is quite self-sufficient in all aspects of care—feeding, bathing, and dressing—and even extends these tasks with pride to family chores.

Because of his many abilities and limited frustrations, the preschool child is truly in love with the world. And why not? From his egocentric point of view, the world exists for and centers around him. He is eager to apply his abilities and is an avid explorer both motorically and mentally. Unlike the toddler, the preschool child can freely explore, feeling secure in not losing sight of himself.

As the preschool child announces "Here I am," he says it to a new audience: his peers. The preschool period is a time of moving beyond family boundaries for short intervals. This experience is preparatory for school years and later dependence. The 3- to 5-year-old is quite curious about other children and adults: what they look like; what they do. He peeks, asks about, and role-plays these differences. Having been exposed to many variations on himself, he tries them on to see how they fit.

No longer are motor, language, and other skills practiced only in solo but more often in unison (harmonious or discordant) with another child. Behavioral skills are used in social play, and the preschooler begins to learn the rules and boundaries the "hard way" in interacting with others. Yet again, egocentrism will limit the give and take of the interchange.

The preschool child sees parents more as allies than as those who thwart him, as the toddler perceived them to be. The child may call his parents by their first names, reflecting this feeling of equality and role playing as the parent's "best friend." The preschooler can move away from his parents for short periods of time and know that they will not desert him.

The preschooler, in his outward excursion, can cognitively appreciate the power of others, especially adults, and thus learns of his own vulnerability and limits.

Through these experiences and this recognition come fears of bodily harm. He perceives himself as capable of large horizons but is knowledgeable of powers greater than himself.

These limitations, however, do not discourage the preschool child's cooperative, eager, and hopeful spirit. As he knows himself to be competent and complete, he is proud to demonstrate this strength and delights those around him.

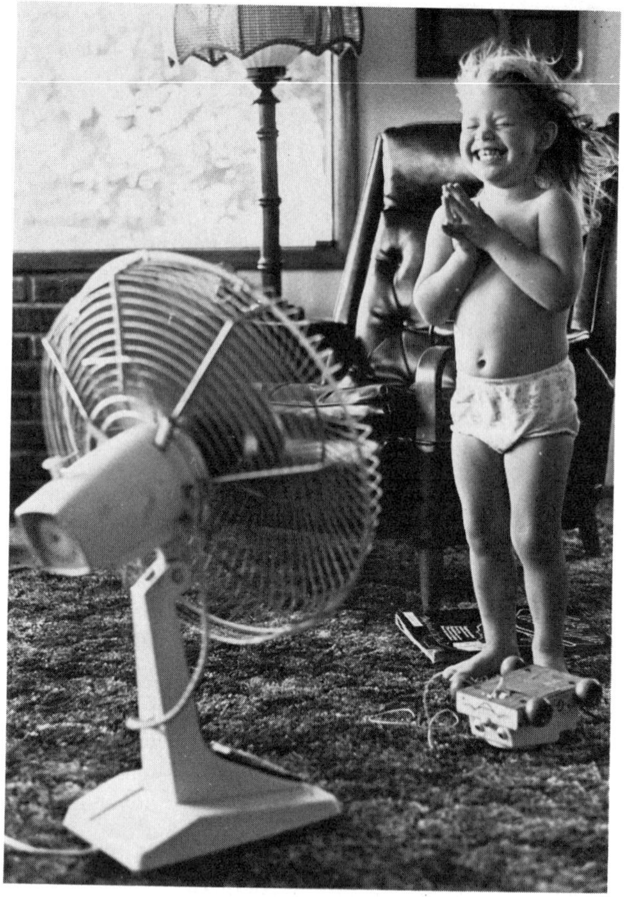

Behavioral Development by Functional Area

Perceptual development Veronica A. Binzley

The primary perceptual task of the preschool child in Western civilization is the perception of symbols, such as speech sounds and letters. This differs from the kind of perceptual processing the child has primarily been doing in two ways. First, after the symbols themselves have been perceptually discriminated, then mapping from the symbol set to the set symbolized must be learned. For example, after the child has discriminated the word *ma ma*, he has to learn that the word refers to his mother. Secondly, the child must learn the rules for how symbols may be put together in a sequence to convey information and, similarly, be able to perceive these same structural constraints in a sequence. That the preschool child does this can be shown by his language. Even though emerging language consists of only two- to three-word utterances, these utterances are grammatical and semantically meaningful. The child may say "big ma ma" and "bad ma ma" but never "green ma ma." The last statement would be nonsensical. The perceptual abilities the child brings to this task are presented below.

VISUAL PERCEPTION
A number of studies have examined the child's perceptual strategy by observing eye movements while looking at a stimulus. This is done by using a technique which superimposes on a picture being looked at a photographic record of eye movements made while looking at the picture (Gibson, 1969). These studies found that children as young as 5 years are still relatively unskilled in visual

FIGURE 9-7. (*Photo courtesy of Betsy Smith.*)

exploration; they do not scan systematically, nor do they sample as widely as the task requires.

WHOLE VERSUS PART PERCEPTION
Older research on this question indicates that children perceive in a diffuse or global manner without much attention to detail. This view originated in the notion of primacy of the whole over the part, which represents a central tenet of the Gestalt theory of perception that was highly influential in earlier work on perceptual development.

Recent research has resulted in contradictory results indicating that the question is unanswerable in an absolute sense. That is, the child's response depends on the nature of the stimulus. The young child will respond to detail in a stimulus configuration if the whole is complex or weakly structured, but he will respond to the whole if it is simple or strongly structured (Reese and Lipsitt, 1970).

DIRECTIONALITY

Contrary to popular opinion, children, even those as young as 3½ years, do discriminate among objects on the basis of directionality. They can distinguish vertical and horizontal lines but have difficulty discriminating two diagonal lines. Preschool children tend to have difficulty discriminating right-left mirror images such as one encounters in certain letters of the alphabet: *b, d, p, q*. In one such study, 4-year-olds reportedly made such confusions in approximately 45 percent of the relevant cases. Up-down mirror images also cause discrimination problems but not as much as right-left mirror images. Most children no longer have problems with letter reversals by age 7 or 8.

SUSCEPTIBILITY TO ILLUSION

Among those who study illusions developmentally, it is generally agreed that there are two types of illusions. The first type decreases in magnitude with increasing age, while the second type increases. According to Piaget, the child's scanning technique is the basis for change in both. The first type depends on field effects occurring in a single glance before the perceptual activity of exploration and results from over- and underestimation of elements of the display. However, there are some investigators who do not agree with Piaget's classification, although they agree that there are two types of illusions. The 5-year old, regardless of whose classification system is employed, is generally found to be quite susceptible to visual illusions.

AUDITORY PERCEPTION

SPEECH PERCEPTION

In addition to discrimination tasks, one can also obtain information about units of auditory perception of speech by requiring subjects to attempt some type of analysis of words or groups of words. One such study required children to isolate and pronounce only the first or last sound of individual words. Findings indicate that children in general had more difficulty isolating the final sound than the first. The 3- to 5-year-olds first had to pronounce the whole word before giving only the requested sound. The 6- and 7-year-olds did the task as outlined (Pick and Pick, 1970).

Another study using 5- and 9-year-olds asked the child to respond with the word remaining after a particular sound had been deleted. The 5-year-olds could not do the task at all, but the 9-year-olds could. On yet another task involving reversal of two-word utterances of various types, it was found that 4- and 5-year-olds had difficulty if the utterance was a grammatical sequence. But they were able to do the task when the utterances were pairs of letters or numbers and words of the same part of speech.

These findings indicate that young children, whose mastery of language is not yet complete, have difficulty moving from one level of analysis to another. And as expected, the 4- and 5-year-olds do not yet analyze common grammatical sequences; but this is a high level of structure for a preschool child to detect and process (Pick and Pick, 1970).

OTHER SENSES

It is an ancient and unfortunately seldom-scrutinized notion that vision gains its meaning from touch; that is, that the hand teaches the eye. Recent studies have found that *haptic perception* is much later in maturing than comparable visual ability. However, the developmental trend in haptic perception is much the same as that encountered in vision. The child progresses from a fixed grasp with passive, global exploration to active, orderly search. The specific stages that have been suggested are shown in Table 9-1 (Gibson, 1969).

Thus, it would seem that evidence does not support the idea that touching is necessary for form perception. On the contrary, even in older children vision is found to be far superior in form-learning studies. Many educators, particularly those concerned with remedial reading, claim that tactile exploration is necessary in order for the child to recognize letters. This is not the case. But that is not to say that once the preschool child's hands are under control so that he is utilizing them to gather information about objects and things tactile information cannot be

TABLE 9-1 Haptic perception

Age	Hand movement and haptic ability
3½ to 4 years	Tactile exploration which is global and relatively passive
4 to 5 years	Crude differentiation of linear from curvilinear shapes but no differentiation within these classes; later progressive differentiation of shapes according to angles and dimensions with some searching for clues
6 years and older	Methodical exploration and search for distinctive features with the ability to distinguish between complex forms

used to supplement visual input. Indeed it can and probably does naturally.

Gross motor development
Fay F. Russell and Beverly R. Richardson

During the preschool years, gross motor development consists primarily of refinement and elaboration of previously acquired skills. There is little basic change in neuromuscular development; reflexive patterns remain essentially the same, myelinization continues, and muscle fibers increase in size and strength with use. The child, however, is much more directed in his activity than he was in the past. He enjoys gross motor games rather than moving only for the sake of movement, as the toddler. His coordination and ability to voluntarily control his movements increase significantly, thereby increasing his capacity for refinement of gross motor skills.

GROSS MOTOR SKILL DEVELOPMENT
As indicated above, the developmental progression of the 3-year-old is primarily reflected in the refinement of skills he acquired during the toddler period. His major accomplishments include the ability to walk a straight line; walk backward; walk on tiptoes; run paying little attention to his feet (but lacking full control in starting, stopping, and turning); throw a ball while standing without losing his balance; catch a ball on or between extended arms; kick a ball; jump from a height of several inches; and ride a tricycle using the pedals and turning wide corners.

The 4-year-old builds further on these skills as reflected in his ability to run on tiptoes and with more control in starting, stopping, and turning; to bounce a ball and catch a ball with his arms flexed; to balance on one foot for 3 to 5 s; to kick a ball with more accuracy; to jump from greater heights with more skill; to ride a tricycle pedaling quickly and turning sharp corners; to hop on his preferred foot; and to climb such things as ladders, trees, and playground equipment.

Play is the chief facilitator of gross motor skill development as well as the major social experience during the preschool years. The preschool child uses his gross motor skills for more complex, interactive play rather than for solitary mastery of skill.

By providing the child with a stimulating environment and proper equipment, the parent can enhance the preschool child's play, thereby increasing his opportunity to refine gross motor skills through repetition and interactive play. Praise and attention may be used to reinforce the child's efforts as he takes pride in his accomplishments.

By the time he reaches the preschool years, the child has acquired his basic gross motor skills according to the

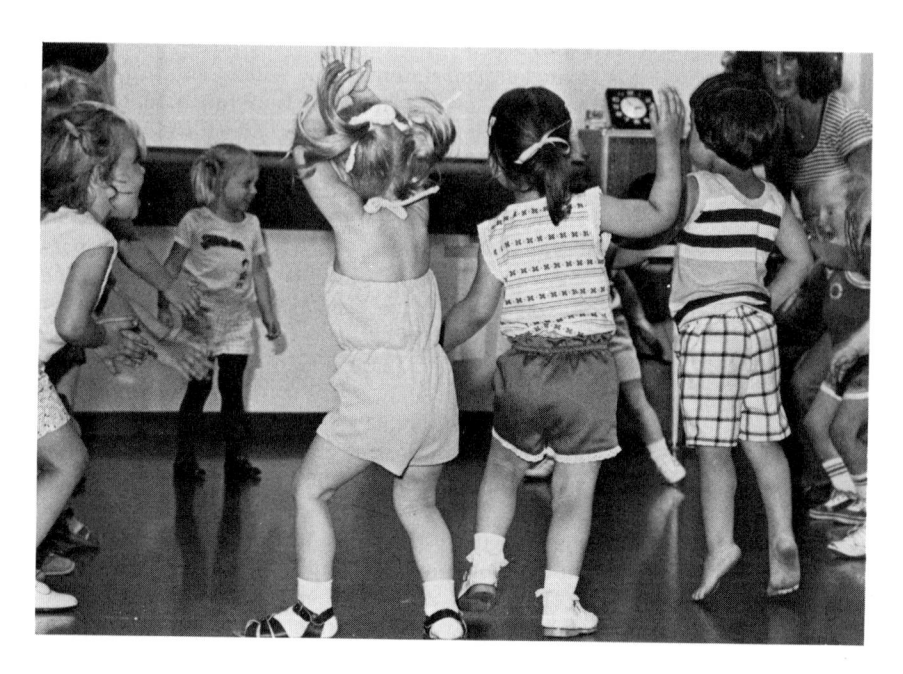

FIGURE 9-8. (*Photo courtesy of Betsy Smith.*)

principles of gross motor development. This does not, however, signify the end of developmental progression in this area as the child now turns his attention to the refinement and specialization of previously acquired skills.

Fine motor development
Barbara Newcomer McLaughlin and Nancy L. Morgan

The toddler years brought much in the way of refinement in coordination and precision of the child's thumb, finger, and hand movements. During the preschool period the child continues to complete basic skills and refine them as he replaces the previous clumsy behavior with ease and economy of effort. Fine motor-adaptive behavior is dependent at this age on the child's previous establishment of basic relationships and his perceptual abilities of dimension, shape, depth, and memory of sequencing. Fine motor play takes on new social significance as the child draws, glues, and constructs with peers. Imitation of others occurs, improving prehension skills.

Pencil and paper take on new meaning to the child as his meaningless scribbles give way to purposeful attempts to copy and repeat specific forms. Drawings are characteristically subjective, assuming meanings to each particular child. The child needs freedom to draw unguided so that he may draw things that are significant to his conceptualization of them. Providing the child with proper materials will prompt him to express his feelings and conceptions in a way not yet permitted by verbal language (Gesell, Halverson, Thompson, Ilg, Castner, Ames, and Amatruda, 1940).

The 3-year-old is content for extended periods in more sedentary activities. He uses crayons appropriately and is more interested in the finer manipulation of play materials. His fine motor behavior indicates more discriminative ability as he makes more controlled marks which are better defined, less diffuse, and less repetitive. The 3-year-old can build a tower of 9 to 10 blocks, which is an improvement over the 6 to 7 block tower of the 2-year-old. This increased ability in the vertical plane is more directly due to neuromotor maturation than to increased attention span.

The 3-year-old can fold a piece of paper lengthwise and crosswise but is unable to fold diagonally. When asked, a preschooler at 3 years can copy a circle but still requires a demonstration to draw a cross. The child can readily insert a circle, square, and triangle into a three-hole form board; he is also able to put together separated halves of a picture even when one piece has been rotated 180°.

Dressing and undressing fully reflects the fine motor skills of the 3-year-old. By 3½ years the child may exhibit a mild tremor in his fine motor coordination; he may also begin to use his nondominant hand or even shift handedness. The parent should allow the child to use whichever hand he prefers and not require him to use a particular hand (Gesell, et al., 1940).

The 4-year-old finds pleasure in fine motor coordination. He begins to button his clothes and lace his shoes. In drawing, he depicts objects with few details, though he may give concentrated effort to the representation of one specific detail. He characteristically draws a circle in a clockwise direction, and his circle is more circumscribed than at 3 years. He is able to copy a cross but unable to copy a diamond from a model. A typical drawing of a person consists of a head, two appendages, and maybe two eyes. Frequently the child will draw a circle around the parts to achieve a unity.

Imitating a demonstration, the 4-year-old can fold a piece of paper three times, making the last crease a diagonal one—a definite advance from 3 years. The preschooler begins to make crude designs and letters. He enjoys having his name printed on his drawings, and he begins to copy the letters. The 4-year-old can also use scissors with a degree of success (Gesell et al., 1940).

Basic skills are refined as the child continues to make use of his previous knowledge of basic relationships and of his perceptual abilities of dimension, shape, depth, and memory of sequencing. He expresses his feelings and conceptions through fine motor abilities and behaviors in a way which is not yet possible through his verbal ability.

Cognitive development Virginia Pidgeon

The preschool child is a fluent conversationalist and readily recounts a blow-by-blow description of an experience. His feet appear firmly planted in the world of reality, and he overflows with information. Ten minutes later he is a miniature fireman holding a hose and climbing a ladder. Ten minutes later he jumps off a stool into an imaginary lake that, according to him, is infested with crocodiles that are going to eat him. Is he a faithful student and chronicler of reality? Or is he a spinner of prolific fantasies? What are the cognitive abilities of the preschool child? How can the poles of fantasy and reality coexist within him?

The preschool years are the preoperational period in cognitive development (see Fig. 9-9). The young child's conceptualization of reality in these years is subjective and colored by his egocentric thinking. He tends to assimilate objects and events to his own personal and private mental schemata. Toward the end of the preschool years he displays an intuitive intelligence that leads him to question and correct some false assumptions. Egocentrism, object concepts, precausal thinking, and mental operations in the preschool period are considered.

EGOCENTRISM

The preschool child is egocentric in the sense that he is only aware of his own point of view. He is not yet aware that others have points of view or that points of view may differ. Consequently he is unconcerned with proof or logical justification of his point of view and does not seek validation of his point of view by others. Egocentric thinking presents a barrier to the intrusion of other opinions.

The young child's egocentrism permeates his thinking. Using himself as a model, he does not distinguish between animate and inanimate objects and attributes to the latter some of his own human qualities of consciousness and intentions. It leads him also into precausal thinking in the conviction that all causality is psychological, or willed and intentional. It is also evident in egocentric speech in which the young child talks aloud as if to himself and does not adapt his speech to his listener. Basic to the young child's egocentrism is lack of differentiation between himself and the world.

OBJECT CONCEPTS

The preschool child's concepts of objects are *preconcepts* (Piaget, 1965; 1947) and are vague and global. They incorporate one or two striking features of an object rather than its multiple characteristics and do not distinguish between characteristics that are essential and nonessential. Contributing to the diffuseness or fuzziness of the young child's object concepts is centration, or the tendency to focus on a single striking feature of an object rather than its multiple characteristics. A young child seeing a dog for the first time notes the tail and a black spot over the eye and forms a concept of a dog based on these characteristics. He does not recognize the black spot as a nonessential characteristic. Consequently he experiences difficulty in recognizing objects in the presence of perceptual changes or variations in their appearance. This lends an instability to the identity of objects in the world around him.

The vagueness of the preschool child's preconcepts leads him to recognize and label objects correctly and incorrectly. Given the concept that a car is any wheeled vehicle, he labels cars accurately but also subsumes to this category bicycles, trains, and planes. He may categorize as sick all persons with fever and stomachache and exclude those with bleeding or broken bones. In time he will be able to define "carness" and order the characteristics of cars in a hierarchy of essential and nonessential characteristics.

Sensory impressions of objects, rather than reason or logic, dominate his object concepts and lead him to believe that objects are as they appear to him in his perceptions. The absence of a concept of conservation, or the knowledge that the mass, weight, and volume of objects remain constant despite perceptual variations in their appearance, is an example. Shown two identical tall flasks containing equal amounts of fluid, the preschool child agrees that the amounts of fluid are equal. Before his eyes, fluid is poured from the tall flask into a short, broad flask. Asked if the amount of fluid in the flasks is now equal, he replies either that there is more or less fluid in the short container. Centering on the greater width of the short flask, he may conclude that there is more fluid. Or centering on the lesser height of the short flask, he may conclude that there is less fluid. Centration introduces distortions

FIGURE 9-9. Schematic representation of preoperational thought and the various components making up this cognitive process.

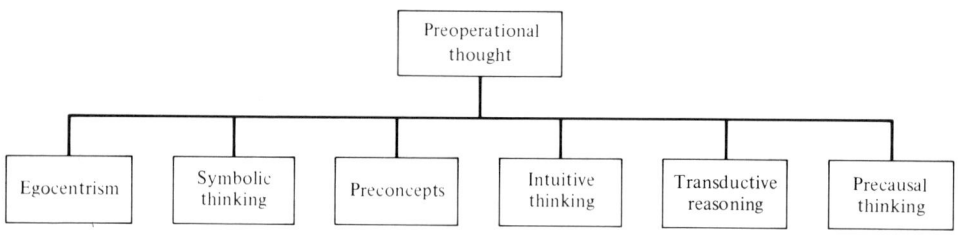

into his reasoning and thinking. Also compounding his error is his tendency to focus on successive states of an event rather than on transformations.

PRECAUSAL THINKING

The preschooler's reasoning is transductive and precausal. It is *transductive* in that he does not reason from the particular to the general nor from the general to the particular but simply links one particular event with another and assumes a cause-and-effect relation. Events that are contiguous in time or space are often linked by him in a cause-and-effect relation. He appears to assume an association between the linked events rather than a true causal relation.

The young child's thinking is precausal in that he is unaware of physical or mechanical causes of natural phenomena and events and assumes that all causes are psychological, or motivational. On the basis of his own experience that people make things happen, he adopts a human-action, or psychological, model of causation. He assumes that all natural phenomena and events are caused either by persons (self or others) or by a supernatural being (a god or a master planner). Seeing fallen leaves on the ground, a young child asks "Who put them there?" and upon encountering a grape seed wonders "Why do they put seeds in grapes?" Generalizing the human-action model, the young child sees intention and purpose in everything and cannot conceive of accidents, coincidences, and impersonal physical and mechanical forces.

Among the different types of *precausal* thinking described by Piaget are participation, phenomenism, and finalism. In *participation* the young child believes that there is a mutual influence or interaction between himself and an object in the environment. He may believe that the moon follows him or that his motion makes the moon move. In *phenomenism* he perceives two objects or events that are contiguous in time or space and assumes that they are connected in a cause-and-effect relation. Seeing a train engine and a fire in proximity, a young child explains that the fire made the engine go. The young child in the hospital who was naughty harbors the belief that hospitalization is a punishment.

In *finalism* the young child believes that each object has a function and that the existence or properties of the object are explainable in terms of that function. Asked why there are lakes, he answers lakes are to swim in. Asked why boats float, he replies boats float to carry people. Finalism reflects a concept of an ordered world arranged by someone for the convenience of human beings. When young children in isolation were asked why they were in a room alone, they often answered " 'Cause I'm supposed to be" or " 'Cause I have to be." These answers have a finalistic ring that suggests an unquestioning acceptance of the ordering of the hospital world. The young believer in finalism seeks no further explanation.

The child's egocentrism and his precausal thinking lead him to misinterpret and personalize the causation of events in his life—separation from one parent through divorce or separation from parents in the hospital. The young child readily implicates himself and his wrongdoing as the causal factor.

MENTAL OPERATIONS

The preschool child does not yet carry out systematic mental operations (subtraction, seriation, and composition and decomposition of classes) like the school-age child. He may perform an isolated operation, like counting pennies, but does not yet perceive the reversibility of this operation that pennies can be added and taken away, or subtracted. He acknowledges that he has a brother but denies that his brother has a brother. In the years from 4 to 7 he begins to acquire three basic mental operations—to think in terms of classes, to deal with numbers, and to perceive relations. He can now sort or classify objects according to a single criterion like angularity or color.

The evolution of sorting or classification of objects can be glimpsed in the young child's changing behaviors. Asked to sort a set of blocks that vary in shape, size, and color, the very young child forms heaps or unorganized groupings that somehow coalesce in his mind. He may also sort blocks into clusters in which one block is a nucleus around which others are grouped because of a resemblance regardless of whether or not they resemble each other. If the nucleus block A is a large blue triangle, he adds B due to triangularity, C due to blueness, and D due to largeness. Later the young child learns to sort blocks into complexes according to a single criterion or attribute (red blocks, tall blocks) or a theme (mommy block, daddy block, and baby block). The young child remains unable in the preschool years to sort objects simultaneously by two criteria (red triangles, blue triangles, red squares, and blue squares).

Intuitive intelligence emerges in the later preschool years and supplements mental experimentation, or problem solving. The young child now has sudden flashes of insight in which he takes a second look at and questions his conclusions. As a result he makes regulations or corrections in the errors in his thinking. In the experiment with the flasks he centers on one characteristic of the flask (its width) and then pauses to take in other characteristics (its height and fluid level) and may or may not arrive at the correct answer.

INFLUENCE OF THE PARENT

There has been much controversy over differences in parent-child (especially mother-child) interaction and their impact on the young child's cognitive development, often in terms of social-class differences. The language and the teaching strategies used by mothers or other care givers have been cited as important factors. It appears that the use of the restricted language code, or language that is terse, nonspecific, and condensed in meaning, and the control of children through appeals to power ("shut up"; "stop it") hinder cognitive development. Conversely, cognitive development is favored when the elaborated language code, or language that is specific, explicit, and individualized to the child and the situation, is used and when control of children is mediated through appeals to rationality. ("You can't go outside because it is raining, and you don't have your rubbers.")

Differences in teaching strategies used by parents with small children also influence cognitive development. Teaching strategies that inform the child in advance about what the task is and how to go about it and provide freedom for trial-and-error experimentation favor cognitive development. Teaching strategies that do not provide advance instruction but instead provide specific step-by-step instruction or instruction that is reactive to the child's right or wrong actions hinder cognitive development (Bernstein, 1962; Hess, 1964). Adults' unwillingness to allow children to make errors, overspecific help, and lack of encouragement all adversely influence cognitive development.

In summary, the preschool child is egocentric in the sense that he is only aware of his own point of view for which he seeks no logical justification. His concepts of objects are preconcepts, and perceptions or sensory impressions rather than reason or logic dominate these concepts.

The reasoning of the young child is transductive and precausal. Although the preschool child does not carry out systematic mental operations, he develops an intuitive intelligence that leads him to correct errors in his thinking.

Language development Shirley Joan Lemmen

The dramatic development of language implies that a child not only learns rules of pronunciation and grammar as well as meanings and relations of words, but he also learns the rules of usage. The most important communication task for the preschooler is how to use the language that has been acquired to best interact with the environment. Language can now be used to communicate with others in a much more explicit manner than the child was able to do before 3 years of age.

The rules for using language vary from culture to culture, and the child learns to communicate differently in different settings. The broader environment shapes learning about communication in the preschool child; however, the family is still an important influence on developing communication skills.

By the time a child is 5 years old and ready for school, he is expected to be able to ask questions, carry on a conversation with adults and peers, follow complex directions, and speak alone in the presence of a group. How does the preschool child develop these communication skills that help to integrate the experiences necessary for all aspects of development, especially socialization, self-esteem, and cognition? Children learn language in their natural setting, even though neither the child nor the parent is seen to focus attention on the language-learning process.

Allen (1976) and Brown (1973) state that both children and adults think about meanings and motives and only subsidiarily about syntax (word order), rules of grammar, or phonology as they speak. It would seem that children learn rules about communication and how to employ the language code to meet the demands of communication situations.

There seem to be two dynamic processes being developed in the child: one of language acquisition and development, the other of communication patterns. The most significant, immediate communicative environment for the child is the family. "If family communication patterns coincide with the larger units of society, the child's communication is reinforced by contacts outside the home. If communication roles and language patterns learned at home vary markedly from settings in the larger culture, these children are likely to encounter communication difficulties in the school" (Allen, 1976, p. 155).

In the early years of a child's development, language acquisition is very much dependent on cognition, motor development, and motivation. During the preschool years, as the child develops an awareness about himself, the relationships he has with others will influence how the child uses language. The responsiveness of significant others to the communicative interaction will provide the child with opportunities for learning. Nonverbal as well as verbal behavior of others will affect the child's attempts for communication, his feelings of self-worth, and his attempts for social interaction.

How language develops, how a child develops communication, is still largely unknown. What have been considered to be important factors in language and communication have undergone drastic changes in the last 20 years. In the 1970s, many studies focused on the development of interaction strategies. In interviewing mothers about child strategies in eating, sleeping, and playing, it is found that 3- to 4-year-olds integrate verbal with nonverbal strategies and employ psychological tactics such as withdrawing affection, expressing loneliness, appealing to fear, expressing desires to be held, and using the father to get around the mother (Allen, 1976; Brown, 1973).

The following is found when preschool children are observed in unstructured play settings:

- Child dyads contain abundant verbal behaviors with clear, grammatically well-formed language and adaptation to the listener's perspective.
- Talk was related to the activity of the potential listener. Speakers revealed an interest in the listener's reaction to what was said.
- Younger children (3½ years) performed as well as older children; therefore, processes in maintenance of verbal exchanges emerges at younger ages. These processes include producing technically good utterances (grammar and syntax), displaying social intent when speaking, and maintaining mutual engagement between children.

It has been noted in recent studies that significant persons, especially mothers, modify their speech when they are talking to their young child to aid the child in learning language. Snow (1972) reported in her study of mothers' speech that the modification mothers produce for young children may be valuable in at least two ways. The first way is to keep the speech simple, interesting, and comprehensible to the young child and, secondly, that simplified speech is designed to aid children in learning language. The willingness of the child's parents to produce simplified and redundant speech combined with the child's own ability to attend selectively to simple, meaningful, and comprehensible utterances provides the child with tractable, relatively consistent, and relevant linguistic information from which to formulate the rules of grammar.

The child's mastery of a sufficient amount of skill in form, content, and use of language involves the following developmental functions:

- Phonetic development: sound production
- Lexicon: acquisition of words
- Semantics: use of words and their relations to each other
- Ability to understand language (verbal) and express language (verbal communication)
- Mean length of utterance
- Syntax: rules of grammar
- Intention of the communication: social interaction, to gain information, to give information, to express needs and feelings
- Parent-child interaction
- Communication of norms and rules of a culture
- Communication of rules of a situation
- Intonation and stress patterns of speech

These functions are specifically related to the child's ability to communicate in an explicit manner to the listener as well as to understand language.

FORM OF LANGUAGE: 3 TO 4 YEARS OF AGE

PHONOLOGICAL DEVELOPMENT

All vowel sounds are correctly articulated by this age. Consonants of *m, n, ng, f, p, l, w, b, t,* and *h* can be articulated in the beginning, middle, and end of words that the child consistently uses. There is always a wide variability in the intelligibility of speech of 3-year-old children; generally, however, research indicates that children of 3 years should have mastered most vowels and the above-stated consonants. Over 90 percent of the 3-year-old's speech should be readily understood (Von Riper, 1978).

LEXICON

By 3 years, the child has an expressive vocabulary of about 900 words and may have a receptive vocabulary of approximately 1500 words.

MEAN LENGTH OF UTTERANCE

Mean length of utterance for the 3- to 4-year-old child is 2.7 to 4 words (Brown, 1973).

SYNTAX

Sentence structure is well established. The complex noun phrase + verb phrase + verb phrase is seen: "I want more cookie and then I'm gonna drink milk." The child begins to use pronouns: *them, you, your, she.* Use of the prepositions *in* and *on* is seen. The child has consistent use of *-s* to express plurality: book*s*, toy*s*, block*s*. At this age the child begins to coordinate phrases with conjunctions: *and* and *then.* The child begins to ask questions with *what* at the beginning of sentences. This language development gives more explicit information to the listener decreasing the need to rely so heavily on situational cues.

CONTENT OF LANGUAGE: 3 TO 4 YEARS OF AGE

The child begins to seriate events in time: temporal relations and sequences of ideas or events. He can return to previously discussed topics. The child responds to explanations with additional questions. The child is also able to establish relations and classify information: "I want a Band-Aid 'cause I hurt my finger." "I want a cracker 'cause I like it." He begins to increase descriptive terms regarding size, shape, and color: "I want to play with the little doggie." "The giraffe has a big, tall neck."

By his fourth birthday, the child can discuss a wide number of topics. The child can verbalize what he is doing or past experiences with specific descriptions that are understandable to the listener: "I saw a big white bear at the zoo yesterday." "Daddy works on big airplanes that fly in the sky."

Perhaps the most significant change during the third to fourth year is that the child can use language to ask about events and to give information; he begins to maintain a dialogue with adults and children and can express mode or feelings with words.

FORM OF LANGUAGE: 4 TO 5 YEARS OF AGE

PHONOLOGICAL DEVELOPMENT

Most consonant sounds are articulated correctly with the most common exceptions being *r, s,* and *l.* In certain contexts of sentence structures, the sound will be distorted or substituted, and many times speech may be nonfluent and halted. However, the child at this age is usually fluent and speech is intelligible (Lillywhite, 1958).

LEXICON

The child at 4 to 5 years of age has approximately 1500 words in his expressive vocabulary. He comprehends about 1500 to 2500 words (Lillywhite, 1958).

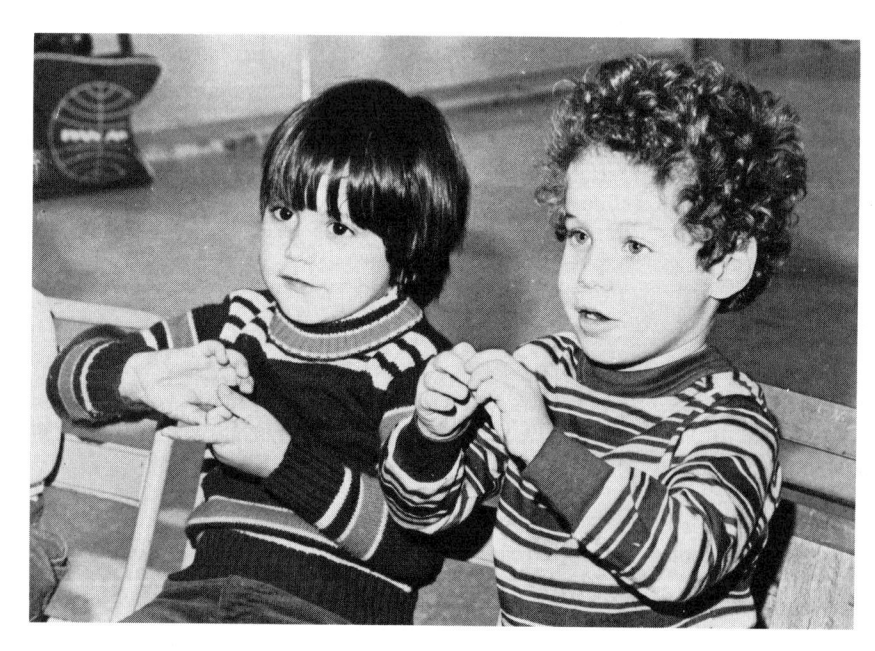

FIGURE 9-10. (*Photo courtesy of Betsy Smith.*)

SYNTAX

The 4- to 5-year-old child uses complex sentence structures. Pronouns, prepositions, auxiliaries, and conjunctions are well established. Articles *a* and *the* are also well established.

Children of 4 to 5 years of age have a variety of ways to express questions: "Am I going to have a birthday party?" "When is my birthday?" "Will you come to my birthday?" "Can I have a birthday cake?" "Can't I go to the birthday party?" "Where will I have my birthday party?"

USE

The child of this age can begin to narrate a story or series of events. He pairs imaginative play with dialogue. He can also maintain a dialogue around a topic. Preschool children often pair motor gestures and responses to define words and describe activities. The child can tell the listener about an event, for example, how he created a picture or made an object, using speech and complex gestures. The child can describe differences and similarities in objects.

During the first 5 years, a tremendous accomplishment in establishment of communication has occurred. Over the remainder of the child's lifetime, new words and complex language skills as well as refinement of basic skills occur. One may learn a foreign language or a specialized technical language or writing ability. However, the foundation for all communication has been firmly established by age 5 years. Language is now a tool for social and work experiences, education, and, of course, daily living.

Self help skill development   Doris Julian

The toddler period is characterized by a number of significant achievements. Motor skills have developed and matured so that basic self-care needs in feeding and elimination can be managed by the child. Skills in communicating thoughts, needs, and feelings are present. The toddler's increasing social awareness encourages responsiveness to cues provided by the environment.

The preschool period builds upon accomplishments of the preceding months. In the United States, the preschool child is typically expected to care for his own basic needs. Tasks requiring both discrete motor skills and discrimination will be possible by the end of the preschool period. Increased cognitive and language ability also facilitate skill building.

The preschool child's desire to please significant people, as well as his delight in successful achievement, will continue to be a motivating factor. Erikson's (1950) concept of a "sense of initiative" as a dominant feature of the preschool period is particularly appropriate.

EATING SKILLS

MOTOR OR MATURATIONAL FACTORS

Improvement in coordination of hand and eye is a major gain in the preschool period. By the age of $2\frac{1}{2}$, self-feeding with a spoon is well established. If the opportunity is provided, use of a fork for spearing is also within the preschool child's capabilities. At 3 years, the fork can also be used for cutting. Increasing motor control is also evident in ability to pour fluids without spilling and to serve individual portions from a serving dish.

SOCIALIZATION OR BEHAVIORAL FACTORS

The preschool child is particularly responsive to the positive attention of parents and other adults. Parental approval of behavior is very helpful in reinforcing socially desirable eating skills or table manners (Prugh, 1964). A child of this age is also increasingly aware of siblings and peers and their reaction to his abilities. The desire to emulate "big girl" or "big boy" behavior and thus gain peer approval is a significant motivating factor for skill improvement.

Since meals and eating are typically tied into family and cultural practices, the preschool child's degree of independence depends on the family. In many U.S. families, as noted by Brazelton (1974), early independence is greatly valued. Measures to support this independence could include modeling, contingency approval, skill expectations appropriate for the child, and learning opportunities. For the older child, nursery school or kindergarten provide further exposure to peer modeling and social expectations.

TOILETING SKILLS

MATURATIONAL FACTORS

The young child begins the preschool period with all the prerequisite skills for elimination control. These are further consolidated and refined during this period. Typically, the 3-year-old has sufficient sphincter control to remain dry during the day and will have both the skills and the awareness of internal cues so that he can take care of daytime toileting. Girls may achieve this ability earlier than boys, as a general rule. Brazelton (1962) reported a series of observations of preschoolers and noted that 98.5 percent of his study group were dry by the age of 5 years. Bowel control frequently precedes bladder control.

Although the ability to communicate toileting needs is present, adults may have to assume responsibility for reminding and being prepared to offer assistance. Complete independence in toileting requires neurological maturation, cognitive awareness, and specific motor skills. This can be expected of most 4-year-olds. Parents must recognize that occasional accidents may occur if the child is under stress, is ill, or "forgets."

SOCIALIZATION OR BEHAVIORAL FACTORS
Additional significant factors relate to the preschool child's increased awareness of societal expectations in terms of privacy, sex segregation in use of bathrooms when not at home, and increased curiosity about elimination. Parents need to respond to the child's search for information and to demonstrate socially appropriate behavior in the use of the bathroom. Independence in all aspects of toileting is an expectation for the child entering school. Encouragement of the child's emerging abilities in self-care will greatly facilitate the socialization required in school and other group settings.

The preschooler's curiosity about his body and its functioning typically extends to a similar interest in the bodily functions of other children or family members. Some parents may make use of this opportunity to provide information about sexuality issues as well as bodily function. Cues provided by the child will be helpful in identifying the timing and the information desired.

DRESSING SKILLS

MATURATIONAL FACTORS
At the beginning of the preschool period, the child can remove and put on simple garments. Tasks such as buttoning and use of zippers and snaps are often feasible by the third year. Postural control must be well established so that balance can be maintained for a period of intensive concentration. At a perceptual and cognitive level the child needs to be able to plan and carry out a motor scheme for identifying the appropriate sequence of tasks in dressing. This ability also requires discrimination of front and back, inside and outside, and left and right.

Because of the complexity of dressing, parents may find it useful to introduce it in carefully graduated phases. Presentation of simple garments in the proper order for dressing is helpful to the young child. Some children achieve independent dressing by age $3\frac{1}{2}$. For many preschoolers, however, some assistance will be required until age $4\frac{1}{2}$ to 5 years. Tying shoes is a more difficult task and typically will not be possible until the child is 6 or 7 years of age.

SOCIALIZATION OR BEHAVIORAL FACTORS
The preschooler typically has accepted the family's approach to clothing and works diligently at mastering skills needed for dressing. Dressing and undressing dolls, family pets, and younger siblings provide opportunities for practice. Neatness and orderliness are influenced by family modeling and cultural sex-role expectation. Researchers have observed that children as young as 2 years of age may be aware of the sex typing of some clothing articles. This awareness increases with age (Thompson, 1975).

The child of 4 or 5 years will typically have a clear idea of appropriate clothing and family expectations on degree of orderliness. An expectation that girls are consistently clean and tidy and boys are not may be part of the acculturation of the preschool years. Most families will find, however, that the preschooler, girl or boy, is responsive to approval and will modify or learn behavior to receive that approval.

Beginning skills in clothing care are possible at this age, and the preschooler can be quite helpful in picking up clothing, sorting for laundry, and folding simple items. Although identifying clothing appropriate for climate and weather is culturally assigned to mothers ("Don't forget your hat!"), most preschoolers can begin to discriminate and make choices as a further progression toward independent self-care.

GROOMING

MATURATIONAL FACTORS
Fine motor coordination is essential for the more precise skill of brushing teeth. The preschool child may not have the hand control needed to perform this task adequately. Thus, it is appropriate for the parent to brush the child's teeth after the child's attempts. The preschooler of 4 years will be able to wash and dry his face and hands without supervision. Independent bathing involves several steps, including discrimination of water temperature and level as well as concept of total body cleanliness, and may not be possible until the youngster is 5 or 6 years. Hair brushing and combing, although perfunctory, can be expected of the older preschooler. Again, individual variation should be noted.

SOCIALIZATION OR BEHAVIORAL FACTORS

A major contributor to achievement in the area of grooming is the preschool child's pleasure in imitating older children, family members, and friends. The provision of personal items of grooming and adapting equipment encourages the child's cooperative participation in grooming. The parents' positive response to the preschooler's attempts at grooming will increase the likelihood of continued efforts. Play equipment, such as miniature grooming aids, and facilities that encourage practice of grooming skills, such as step stools and low mirrors, are useful in assisting the preschooler with mastery of abilities.

The parent also needs to be aware that large-muscle activity and environmental exploration are important to the developing preschooler. Such activities may be incompatible with fastidious grooming. The adult can assist the child in discriminating times when a casual appearance is appropriate and other times when cleanliness and order are required. In all self-help skills, social awareness is as significant an accomplishment as mastery of motor skills.

ENVIRONMENTAL MAINTENANCE

Simple housework chores are within the capability of the preschooler. Beginning with activities such as picking up and putting away toys, the young child can become increasingly responsible for belongings and personal space. Sweeping, dusting, setting the table, and drying and putting away silverware are examples of contributions the older preschool child can make to care of the general household. Some chores can be routine expectations, while others would require assistance and supervision.

The foundation for competence in self-care skills has been laid down in the preschool years. The child is now able to care for all his basic physical needs. Increased social awareness has stimulated the preschool child's interest in the environment of home and immediate neighborhood. Although continued guidance and supervision are essential, the preschool child is now prepared to enter the next developmental phase with many of the prerequisite skills needed for survival in the broader environment.

Social development Susan Blanch Meister

BASIS FOR SOCIALIZATION

The interactive context of socialization continues to change during the preschool years. Peers become an increasingly greater source of social contact. The frequency of discipline encounters also increases (Escalona, 1973). The child is now able to utilize newfound motor, language, and cognitive abilities. In sum, the preschooler is an enthusiastic initiator and recipient of rich social stimuli. *Initiative* is Erikson's (1963) key word for this age group. The preschooler is often the intruder, the beguiler, and the interrupter.

GOALS OF SOCIALIZATION

The primary goal of this period in our society is attainment of school-readiness. Socialization and other facets of development are directed toward channeling the preschooler's increasing capacities and initiative so that he will be approaching school readiness at the end of this age period. Socialization is directed toward ensuring that the preschool child's abilities, motivation, and knowledge reach an optimal level for school entry.

PROCESSES INVOLVED IN SOCIALIZATION

ATTACHMENT

Attachment relationships may well become an ongoing, internalized source of security for preschoolers. The quality of the attachment relationship has affected the nature of the child in terms of developing a social style: a manner of approaching and reacting to social experience (Lieberman, 1977). The preschooler's social style affects approaches to social contact with peers, siblings, and adults. The potential experiences and their effect upon the child are influenced by the individual nature of the child.

MORAL INTERNALIZATION

Moral internalization continues to develop in relation to parental discipline techniques. When preschool development of moral internalization is measured, the child often demonstrates uneven behavior. It is essential to remember that although the preschool child may have absorbed the content of inductive discipline, application of the content involves another process. Application may require cognitive processes which are beyond the preschooler's abilities. In other words, actual development of moral internalization may be masked by a current cognitive limitation of behavior (Hoffman, 1970). Fluctuation in the child's behavior, in regard to learned standards, is related to the ability to understand situations.

EMPATHY

Preschool children acquire a particular form of social cognition. When the situation of the other person involves

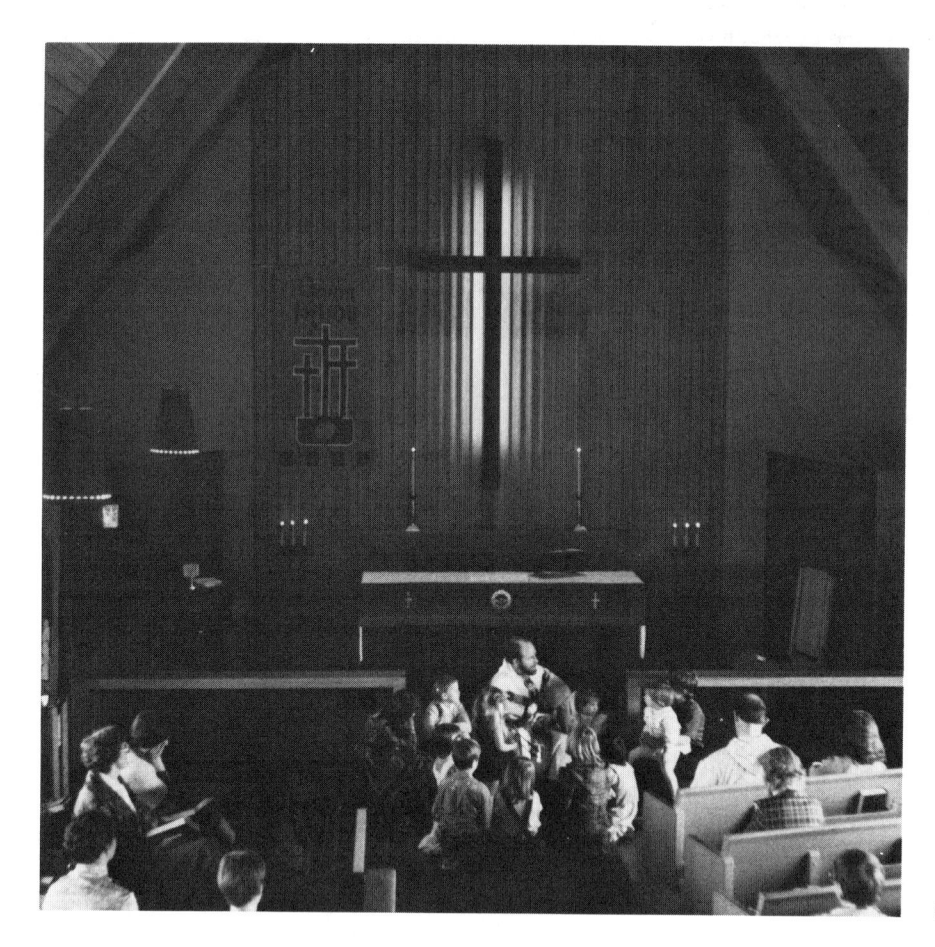

FIGURE 9-11.

fairly simple emotions, when the situation is familiar to the child, and/or when the other person is similar to the child, *then* the preschooler can make a fairly accurate appraisal of the other's perspective (Shantz, 1975).

The preschooler is beginning to understand that others' perspectives differ from his own, but he is often uncertain of what those perspectives are. In other words, preschoolers experience empathic distress but often offer inappropriate assistance (Hoffman, 1975).

It is likely that the egocentrism and limited cognitive judgment of this age group contribute to this level of empathic development. Social cognition is bound to simple and familiar contexts, and this characteristic affects the scope of affective cues which are salient to the child (Bryan, 1975).

GENDER IDENTITY AND SEX ROLE

The preschooler is a clear example of the difference between gender identity and sex role. The rigid gender stereotyping (which began at the end of the toddler period) continues to develop. It is important to note that this development is basically in the cognitive realm. Sex-role behavior may not be as sharply differentiated as is the conceptualization of gender identity. The preschooler has not yet attained the necessary degree of developmental integration between cognitive abilities and social behavior (Parsons and Bryan, 1978).

It might be expected that preschool children would demonstrate similarity to their same-sex parent. Often this similarity will not emerge until early school age. During the preschool period, a child is more likely to display similarity to whichever parent assumes a more dominant role.

Comparing both parents in this light, the father may play an especially crucial role. Fathers of preschoolers have been found to be more aware of gender identity development and more active in their promotion of that development. They also demonstrate greater discrimination between sons and daughters (Johnson, 1971). These factors suggest that the father may often assume a dominant role, or particular salience, in the area of gender-identity development during this stage of development.

Perception of behavioral competency and development of self-esteem
Judith Anne Ritchie

DEVELOPMENT OF A SENSE OF COMPETENCE

The preschool child has developed verbal, cognitive, and motoric capacities that permit imagination and vigorous direct exploration and testing of objects, situations, and people in his environment. This tremendous curiosity about the environment, the need to explore and manipulate, and the need to create novel situations are components of a theorized drive toward a sense of competence (White, 1959).

PHYSICAL ABILITIES

The preschool child, well aware of body parts and himself as a separate individual, now seems intent on establishing a sense of self as physically competent. There is tremendous activity aimed at developing and experimenting with physical abilities. A major feature of the preschool child's self-concept is perception of action competencies (Keller, Ford, and Meacham, 1978).

Perceptions of the self as intact, complete, and competent are developed through manipulation of the body in dance, gymnastics, climbing, jumping, and dramatic play. Clothing such as "grown-up clothes," "Indian suits," and construction or fireman helmets seem to transform the child's perception of the self from small, insecure, and vulnerable to the idealized "big" person—strong, all powerful, and impenetrable.

Most 4-year-old children observed in dance sessions enjoyed experimenting with rhythm and bodily expressions of the leader's expression. Other children seem unable to relax their armor enough to participate in such expressions of self. Hartley, Frank, and Goldenson (1952), writing about dance, movement, and music, say this:

The effect of releasing emotion and achieving order and self control through rhythm is to give the child "harmonious contact with himself", and through this, increasing integration of body and mind and enhanced self-acceptance. (p. 299)

Attempts at mastery of climbing, building, pushing, and pulling seem to be undertaken to prove, to others and the self, the completeness and competence of the body. The fact that much of this activity is displayed by boys is said to be a symbolic expression of masculinity (Freud, 1963). One 4-year-old boy, whose parents placed emphasis on athletic qualities, constantly drew attention to his skill and seemed almost desperate to prove these abilities. Two other 4-year-old boys repeatedly, but reluctantly, attempted to climb a Junglegym as if they had an inner drive to master these activities.

ACHIEVEMENT MOTIVATION

The preschool child's level of preconceptual thought permits beginning awareness of competence in cognitive skill areas of symbolic speech and play, imitation, and fantasy (Harter, 1978; Piaget, 1952). Development of a sense of cognitive competence is dependent on some degree of success (Brandon, 1969; White, 1959). However, the preschool child is said to have considerable energy to explore new, desirable areas with a sense of direction even in the face of failure (Erikson, 1968). Harter (1978) suggests that the development of a sense of competence is dependent on interaction of success and failure. While failure provides negative feedback, it gives the child information about the boundaries of his competence.

EXPECTATION OF PARENTS

External sources of approval are necessary for the young child to develop a sense of competence (Franks, 1974; Gale, 1969; White, 1959; Yamamoto, 1972). The expectations and particular areas of emphasis of parents and teachers strongly influence which aspects of competence or effectance motivation will be developed in the individual child (Harter, 1978; Schilder, 1964a, 1964b; Yamamoto, 1972).

SOURCES OF SELF-ESTEEM

While the preschool child continues to have a rather haphazard abstraction of self, increasing behavioral capacities permit him to begin to develop three of the four sources of self-esteem—competence, power, and signifi-

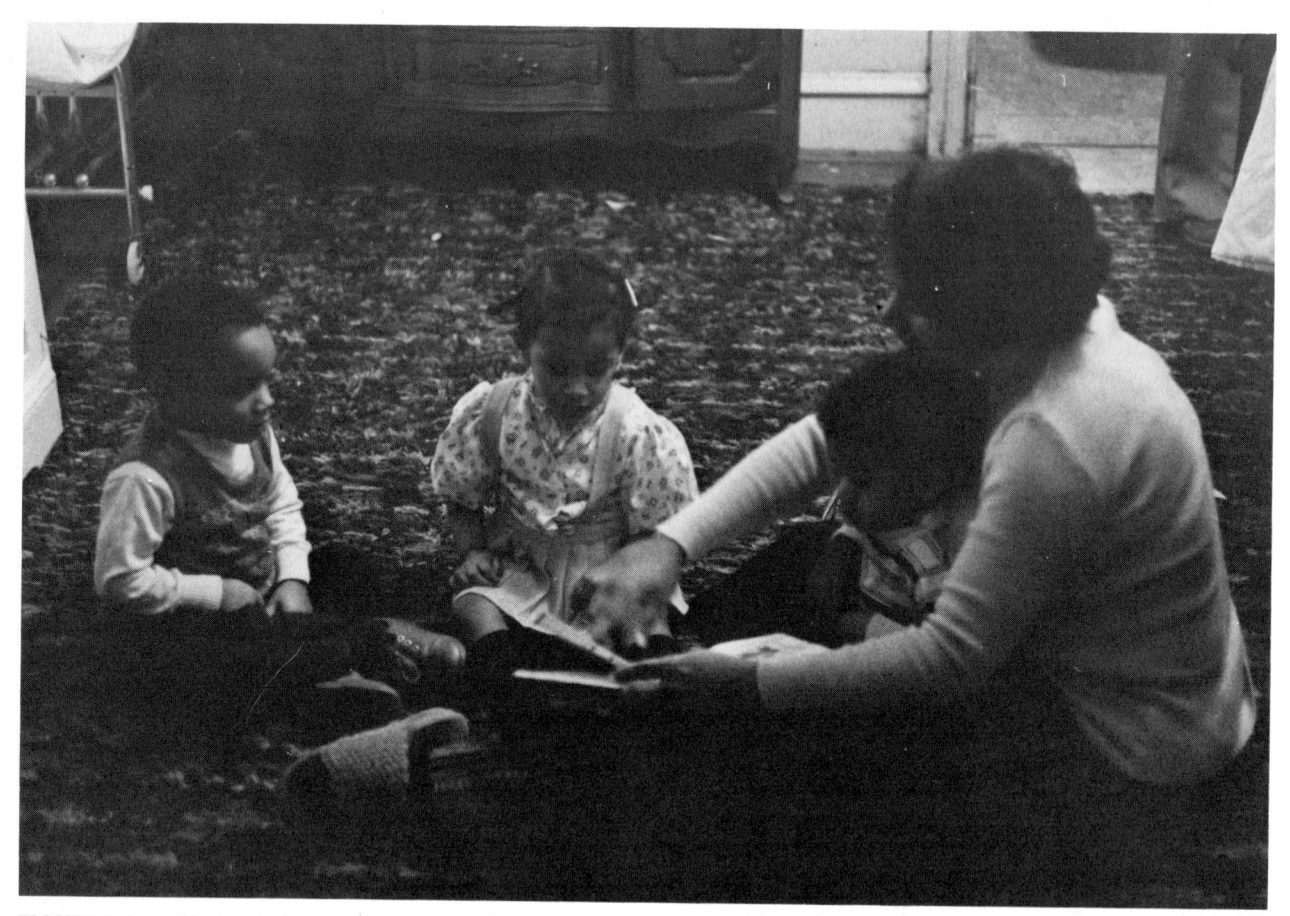

FIGURE 9-12. *(Photo courtesy of Armand Seavo.)*

cance (Coopersmith, 1967). The cognitive ability to use imagination and to begin to classify enable the preschool child to experiment with the kind of person he could be (Erikson, 1968).

LEARNING OF POTENTIAL ROLES
In role-play enactment of roles, such as parent, "airplane driver," or disciplining adult, the preschool child experiments with his conceptualization of roles and role expectations (Sarbin, 1954). Within the child's skillful role play he often assigns qualities to the self (Sarbin, 1968). Beginning attempts at self-evaluation follow the preschool child's identification with and introjection of the capacities and authority of these adult, often parental, roles.

Such self-evaluation may lead either to feelings of well-being and self-esteem or feelings of guilt (Freud, 1965). Role playing serves the child in many ways but, overall, contributes to a more realistic self-esteem (Erikson, 1963).

FAMILIAL EXPERIENCES AND LIMIT SETTING
The family's consistent and sincere encouragement and positive reinforcement of the preschool child are important elements in developing a sense of self-esteem (Coopersmith, 1967; Erikson, 1963; Thomas, 1973; Yamamoto, 1972). Equally important aspects are the family's interest and concern and the parents' ability to provide an environment that encourages exploration and

mastery of motor and cognitive skills. The nature of the child's self-concept and the degree to which self-esteem is developed are also affected by the parents' provision of information and limit setting in relation to expectations and appropriateness of various behaviors (Coopersmith, 1967; Harter, 1978).

SOCIAL EXPERIENCES
As the preschool child's world expands to include peers and teachers, he receives further information regarding others' opinions about his own adequacy. The child's ability to master social situations contributes to his sense of esteem or worthiness. The social situations themselves provide further opportunities for experimentation with the self-concept. The adequacy of the self-concept will be significantly influenced by such experiences (Thomas, 1973).

The preschool years result in a broadening and higher-level integration of behavioral skills and the consolidation of these skills in the extended social environment. The preschool child begins to recognize the value of his competency through the eyes of others, especially those outside his family. The 3- and 4-year-olds are in love with life and with their ability to impact daily events as well as important others around them.

Bibliography

PHYSICAL DEVELOPMENT
OF THE PRESCHOOL CHILD
Bayer, L. M., and N. Bayley: *Growth diagnosis* (2d ed.). Chicago: University of Chicago Press, 1976.
Erikson, E.: *Childhood and society* (2d ed.). New York: Norton, 1963.
Recommendations of the task force on blood pressure control in children. *Pediatrics,* 1977, *59*(5), 797–820. (Supplement)
Rudolph, A.: *Pediatrics* (16th ed). New York: Appleton-Century-Crofts, 1977.
Sinclair, D.: *Human growth after birth.* New York: Oxford University Press, 1969.
Smith, D. W.: *Growth and its disorders.* Philadelphia: Saunders, 1977.
———, and E. L. Bierman: *The biological ages of man.* Philadelphia: Saunders, 1973.

SENSORY SYSTEM
Bordley, J. E., and W. G. Hardy: The special senses. In R. E. Cooke (Ed.), *The biologic basis of pediatric practice.* New York: McGraw-Hill, 1968.
Ellis, P. P.: Eye. In C. H. Kempe, H. K. Silver, and D. O'Brien (Eds.), *Current pediatric diagnosis and treatment* (5th ed.). Los Altos, Calif.: Lange, 1978.
Gesell, A., R. L. Ilg, and G. E. Bulis: *Vision, its development in infant and child.* New York: Hoeber-Harper, 1949.
Newell, F. W., and J. T. Ernest: *Ophthalmology: Principles and concepts* (3d ed.). St. Louis: Mosby, 1974.
Smith, J. L.: The eye in infancy and childhood. In R. E. Cooke (Ed.), *The biologic basis of pediatric practice.* New York: McGraw-Hill, 1968.

DEVELOPMENT OF BODY CONCEPT
AND CONCEPTS OF ILLNESS AND WELLNESS
Ausubel, D.: *Theory and problems of child development.* New York: Grune & Stratton, 1958.
Blom, G. E.: The reactions of hospitalized children to illness. *Pediatrics,* 1958, *22,* 590–600.
Dillon, M. S.: Attitudes of children toward their own bodies and those of other children. *Child Develop.,* 1934, *5,* 165–176.
Eland, J. M., and J. E. Anderson: The experience of pain in children. In A. K. Jacox (Ed.), *Pain: A sourcebook for nurses.* Boston: Little, Brown, 1977.
Erickson, F.: *Play interviews for four-year-old hospitalized children.* Lafayette, Ind.: Child Development, 1958.
———, and J. Holt: *Play interviews for preschool children.* (Unpublished research report, University of Pittsburgh, 1964.)
Fraiberg, S.: *The magic years.* New York: Scribner, 1959.
Freud, A.: *Normality and pathology in childhood.* New York: International Universities, 1965.
———: The role of bodily illness in the mental life of children. *Psychoanal. Stud. Child,* 1952, *7,* 69–80.
Furman, R. A.: The child's reaction to death in the family. In B. Schoenberg et al. (Eds.), *Loss and grief.* New York: Columbia, 1970.
Gellert, E.: Children's conception of the content and function of the human body. *Genetic Psychology Monographs,* May 1962.
Gesell, A., F. L. Ilg, and L. B. Ames: *Infant and child in the culture of today.* New York: Harper & Row, 1974.
Kastenbaum, R.: The child's understanding of death: How does it develop? In E. A. Grollman (Ed.), *Explaining death to children.* Boston: Beacon Press, 1967.
Katcher, A., and M. Levin: Children's conception of body size. *Child Develop.,* 1955, *26,* 103–110.
Kolb, L. C.: Disturbances of the body image. In S. Arienti

(Ed.), *American handbook of psychiatry* (Vol. IV, 2d ed.). New York: Basic Books, 1975.

Langford, W.: The child in the pediatric hospital: Adaptation to illness and hospitalization. *Amer. J. Orthopsychiat.*, 1961, *31*, 667–682.

Levy, D. M.: Body interest in children and hypochondriasis. *Amer. J. Psychiat.*, 1932, *89*, 295–315.

McCaffery, M.: Brief episodes of pain in children. In B. Bergerson et al. (Eds.), *Current concepts in clinical nursing* (Vol. II). St. Louis: Mosby, 1969.

Nagy, M.: The child's theories concerning death. *J. Genet. Psychol.* 1948, *73*, 3–27.

Pitcher, E. G., and E. Prelinger: *Children tell stories: An analysis of fantasy.* New York: International Universities, 1963.

Prugh, D. G.: Emotional aspects of the hospitalization of children. In M. F. Shore (Ed.), *Red is the color of hurting.* Washington, D. C.: Government Printing Office, 1965.

Ritchie, J. A.: Fantasy in communicating concerns about body integrity. *Matern. Child Nurs. J.* 1972, *1*, 117–126.

Schilder, P.: *The image and appearance of the human body.* New York: Wiley, 1964.

——, and P. Wechler: What children know of the interior of the body. *Int. J. Psychoanal.*, 1935, *16*, 355–360.

Simmel, M. L.: Developmental aspects of the body scheme. *Child Develop.*, 1966, *37*, 83–95.

Swafford, L. I., and D. Allan: Pain relief in the pediatric patient. *Med. Clin. N. Amer.*, 1968, *52*, 131–136.

PERCEPTUAL DEVELOPMENT

Ellis, P. P.: Eye. In C. H. Kempe, H. K. Silver, and D. O'Brien (Eds.), *Current pediatric diagnosis and treatment* (5th ed.). Los Altos, Calif.: Lange, 1978.

Gibson, E. J.: *Principles of perceptual learning and development.* New York: Appleton-Century-Crofts, 1969.

Pick, H. L., and A. D. Pick: Sensory and perceptual development. In P. H. Mussen (Ed.), *Carmichael's manual of child psychology* (Vol. I). New York: Wiley, 1970.

Reese H. W., and L. P. Lipsitt: *Experimental child psychology.* New York: Academic, 1970.

GROSS MOTOR DEVELOPMENT

Corbin, C. B.: *A textbook of motor development.* Dubuque, Iowa: Wm. C. Brown, 1973.

Cratty, B. J.: *Perceptual and motor development in infants and children.* New York: Macmillan, 1970.

Illingworth, R. S.: *The development of the infant and the young child.* London: Churchill Livingstone, 1975.

Knobloch, H., and B. Pasamanick: *Gesell and Amatruda's developmental diagnosis.* New York: Harper & Row, 1974.

FINE MOTOR DEVELOPMENT

Gesell, A., H. M. Halverson, H. Thompson, F. L. Ilg, B. M. Castner, L. B. Ames, and C. S. Amatruda: *The first five years of life.* New York: Harper & Brothers, 1940.

Gordon, I. J., B. Guinagh, and R. E. Jester: *Child learning through child play.* New York: St. Martin's, 1972.

COGNITIVE DEVELOPMENT

Bernstein, B.: Linguistic codes, hesitation phenomena and intelligence. *Lang. Speech*, 1962, *5*, 33–36.

Bruner, J., R. Olver, and P. Greenfield: *Studies in cognitive growth.* New York: Wiley, 1966.

Flavell, J.: *The developmental psychology of Jean Piaget.* New York: Van Nostrand, 1963.

Hess, R.: Educability and rehabilitation: The future of the welfare class. *J. Marriage Family*, 1964, *25*, 424.

Phillips, J. L.: *The origins of intellect: Piaget's theory.* San Francisco: Freeman, 1969.

Piaget, J.: *The child's concept of physical causality.* Totowa, N.J.: Littlefield, Adams, 1965.

——: *The psychology of intelligence.* London: Routledge, 1947.

Pidgeon, V.: Child thought and counseling implications in the hospital. *Patient Counseling and Health Education.* Princeton, N.J.: Excerpta Medica, 1978. (To be published.)

——: Characteristics of children's thinking and implications for health teaching. *Matern. Child Nurs. J.*, 1977, *6*, 1–8.

——: Children's concepts of the rationale of isolation technics. *A.N.A. Clinical Sessions,* 1966. New York: Appleton-Century-Crofts, 1967.

Sigel, I.: The attainment of concepts. In M. Hoffman and L. Hoffman (Eds.), *Review of child development research* (Vol. 1). New York: Russell Sage, 1964.

LANGUAGE DEVELOPMENT

Allen, R. R.: *Developing communication competence in children.* Skokie, Ill.: National Textbook, 1976.

Brown, R.: *A first language.* Cambridge: Harvard, 1973.

Lillywhite, H.: Doctors' manual of speech disorders. *J. A. M. A.*, 1958, *67*(7), 850–58.

Snow, C. E.: Mothers' speech to children learning language. *Child Develop.*, 1972, 549–565.

Van Riper, C.: *Speech correction.* Englewood Cliffs, N.J.: Prentice-Hall, 1978.

SELF-HELP SKILL DEVELOPMENT

Brazelton, T. B.: *Toddlers and parents: A declaration of independence.* New York: Dell, 1974.

———: A child oriented approach to toilet-training. *Pediatrics*, 1962, *29*, 121.

Erikson, E. H.: Growth and crises of the healthy personality. In *Problems of infancy and early childhood*. New York: Josiah Macy, Jr. Foundation, 1950. (Supplement II)

Gesell, A., F. Ilg, L. B. Ames, and J. Rodell: *Infant and child in the culture of today* (Rev. ed). New York: Harper & Row, 1974.

Largo, R. H., and W. Stutzle: Longitudinal study of bowel and bladder control by day and at night in the first six years of life. In epidemiology and interrelations between bowel and bladder control. *Develop. Med. Child Neurol.*, 1977, *19*(5), 598–613.

MacKeith, R., R. Meadow, and R. K. Turner: How children become dry. In I. Kolvin, R. C. MacKeith, and R. Meadow (Eds.), *Bladder control and enuresis*. Philadelphia: Lippincott, 1973.

Prugh, D. G.: The preschool child. In H. Stuart and D. Prugh (Eds.), *The healthy child*. Cambridge: Harvard, 1964.

Thompson, S. K.: Gender labels and early sex role development. *Child Develop.* 1975, *46*, 339–347.

SOCIAL DEVELOPMENT

Bryan, J. H.: Children's cooperative and helping behaviors. In E. M. Hetherington (Ed.), *Review of child development research* (Vol. 5). Chicago: University of Chicago Press, 1975.

Erikson, E.: *Childhood and society*. New York: Norton, 1963.

Escalona, S.: Basic modes of social interaction: Their emergence and patterning during the first two years of life. *Merrill-Palmer Quart.* 1973, *19*, 205–232.

Hoffman, M.: Developmental synthesis of affect and cognition and its implication for altruistic motivation. *Develop. Psychol.*, 1975, *11*, 607–622.

———: Moral development. In P. H. Mussen (Ed.), *Carmichael's manual of child psychology*. New York: Wiley, 1970.

Johnson, M.: Sex-role learning in the nuclear family. In G. C. Thompson (Ed.), *Social development and personality*. New York: Wiley, 1971.

Lieberman, A.: Preschooler's competence: Relations with attachment and peer experience. *Child Develop.* 1977, *48*, 1277–1287.

Parsons, J., and J. Bryan: Adolescence: Gateway to androgyny. *Occasional Papers Series*. Ann Arbor: University of Michigan Women's Study Program, 1978.

Shantz, C.: The development of social cognition. In E. M. Hetherington (Ed.), *Review of child development research* (Vol. 5). Chicago: University of Chicago Press, 1975.

PERCEPTION OF BEHAVIORAL COMPETENCY AND DEVELOPMENT OF SELF-ESTEEM

Brandon, N.: *The psychology of self-esteem*. Los Angeles: Nash, 1969.

Coopersmith, S.: *The antecedents of self-esteem*. San Francisco: Freeman, 1967.

Erikson, E. H.: *Identity: Youth and crisis*. New York: Norton, 1968.

———: *Childhood and society* (2d ed.). New York: Norton, 1963.

Franks, D. D.: Current conception of competency of motivation and self-validation. In D. Fields and D. Mills (Eds.), *Social psychology for sociologists*. Ontario: Nelson, 1974.

Freud, A.: *Normality and pathology in childhood*. New York: International Universities, 1965.

———: The concept of the developmental lines. *Psychoanal. Stud. Child*, 1963, *18*, 245–265.

Gale, R. F.: *Developmental behavior*. London: Collier-Macmillan, 1969.

Harter, S.: Effectance motivation reconsidered: Toward a developmental model. *Hum. Develop.*, 1978, *21*, 34–64.

Hartley, R. E., L. K. Frank, and R. M. Goldenson: *Understanding children's play*. New York: Columbia, 1952.

Keller, A., L. H. Ford, and J. A. Meacham: Dimensions of self-concept in preschool children. *Develop. Psychol.*, 1978, *14*, 483–489.

Piaget, J.: *The origins of intelligence in children*. New York: International Universities, 1952.

Sarbin, T. R.: Role theory. In G. Lindsay (Ed.), *Handbook of social psychology* (Vol. I). Cambridge: Addison-Wesley, 1954.

———, and V. L. Allen: Role theory. In G. Lindsay and E. Arensen (Eds.), *The handbook of social psychology* (Vol. I, 2d ed.). Reading: Addison-Wesley, 1968.

Schilder, P.: *Contributions to developmental neuropsychiatry* (L. Bender, Ed.). New York: International Universities, 1964a.

———: *The image and appearance of the human body*. New York: Wiley, 1964b.

Thomas, J. B.: *Self-concept in psychology and education*. Great Britain: NFER, 1973.

White, R. W.: Motivation reconsidered: The concept of competence. *Psychol. Rev.* 1959, *66*, 297–333.

Yamamoto, K.: *The child and his image*. Boston: Houghton Mifflin, 1972.

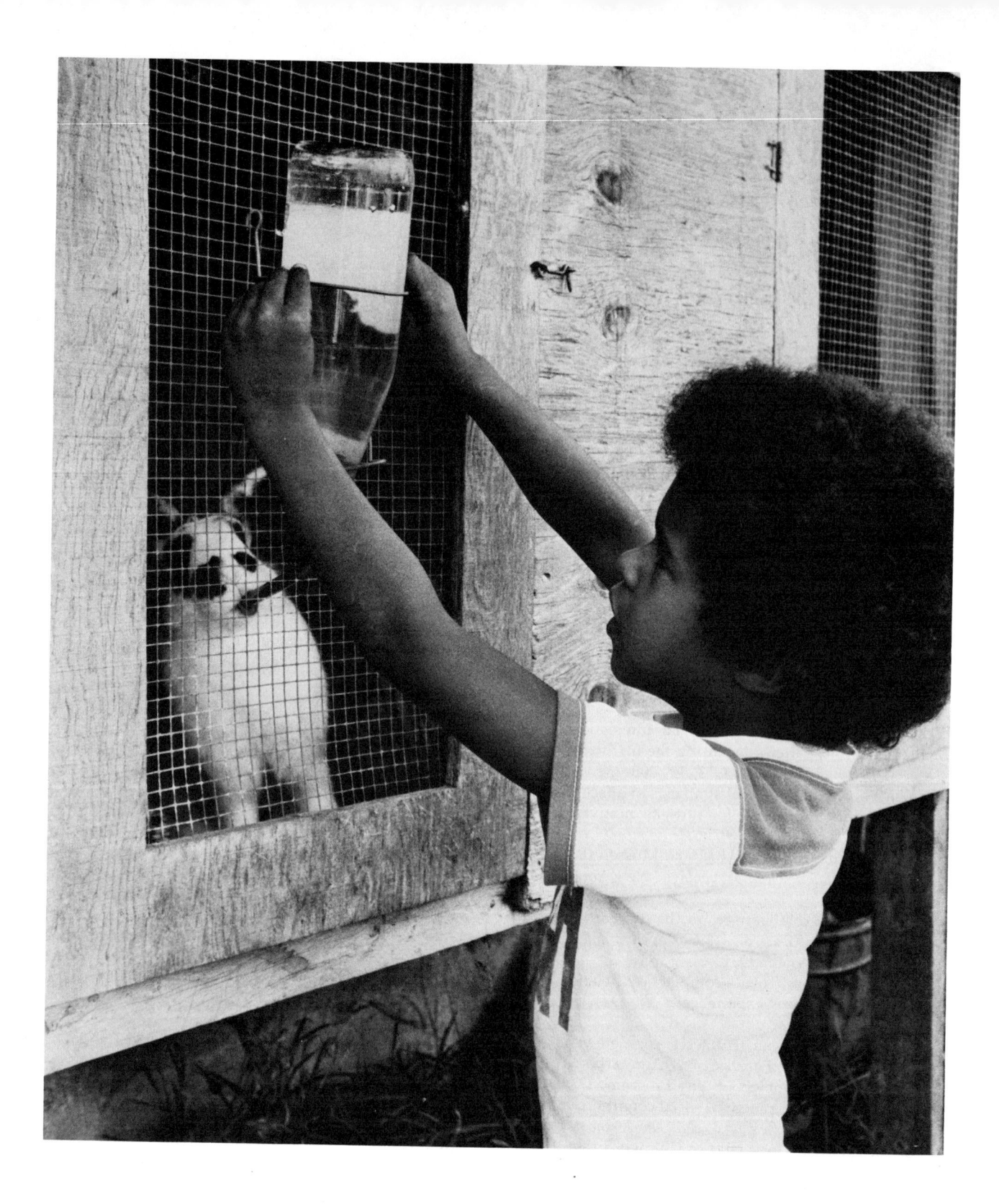

CHAPTER 10

The School-Age Child: 5 Years to Puberty

Introduction

The school-age period, age 5 years to the onset of puberty (at 10 to 12 years), is an important time of stability prior to the era of adolescence. This time of childhood is not physically remarkable (with the exception of losing and gaining teeth). Soon, however, prepubertal changes begin; by the end of childhood, the growth spurt is seen and sexual maturation has started.

The young school-age child is unconcerned about this impending physical transformation; with the onset of school, a new, exciting period has begun in social and academic realms. Carefree days of play and creation and collection are at hand.

The school-age child, recently exploring the backyard on hands and knees, now disappears down the street on his bicycle. The child is outward-bound, and childhood is drawing to a close.

FIGURE 10-1.

SECTION 1
Physical Development

Physical development of the school-age child Maija S. Ljunghag

DEVELOPMENTAL APPROACH TO PHYSICAL ASSESSMENT

The school-age child is a curious human being who is interested in learning and is in the process of developing independence from home and parents. The 5-year-old who has just started kindergarten can still be shy, afraid of strangers and unfamiliar procedures, even when explanations are offered. By the time the child starts first grade, he has gained enough confidence and independence to meet unknown adults with equanimity and a willingness to become acquainted easily. When approaching a school-age child, the nurse or other health care professional should take time to get to know the child, making observations in play or other spontaneous-activity situations.

Any child should be treated as an individual human being. Not only should he be called by his name, but he should also know the adult's name and the role that the adult will play in his care. The conduct of the nurse and the level of conversation must be appropriate for the age of the child. Yet, the adult must also remain natural because children sense very quickly any hypocritical attitudes adults might assume in their presence.

The conversation with a school-age child is directed toward discovering the child's feelings, fears, and needs. Allowing him to ask questions and then redirecting these questions to the child enables him to tell the nurse his own ideas and feelings regarding these questions. Using the third-person technique, such as, "You know, lots of times kids with your problems think (whatever you believe he is feeling). Does that make sense?" gives the child an opportunity to explore his feelings and ideas and an opening to express them. It is very important for the school-age child to know that the nurse is willing to listen and talk to him and that what the nurse says to him is truthful.

The school-age child has a need for privacy, whether he is getting a physical examination or wants to communicate his feelings. Girls seem to have an innate sense of modesty at a much earlier age than boys, and baring their chests even before breast development has started is very embarrassing to some. A school-age child should never be asked to undress in front of peers or a group of adults.

PHYSICAL STATUS OF THE PREPUBERTAL CHILD

GENERAL APPEARANCE

The expression, "well developed, well nourished," when describing a child's appearance, is nonspecific and ambiguous. Only after much experience can a health professional state, based on knowledge of physical growth and development and comparisons with mental images of children of the same age and sex, that a particular child is well developed. The state of nutrition cannot be stated unless a nutrition history is completed. When defining general appearance, direct observations and descriptions of behavior, whether verbal or nonverbal, are recorded. Some of the following can be included:

Age Age should be stated to the month, for instance, 7,9 would describe a child who is 7 years and 9 months old. This gives a more accurate description, especially during school age, when children change so rapidly. Sex and race of the child are also noted.

Body build Body build, or physique, should be described as short, medium, tall, slender, obese, stocky, or other terms. Trying to classify the somatotype of the typical school-age child is difficult because variations of the body build become infinite during these years and are on a continuum rather than being clear-cut and distinct.

After this introductory statement it should be noted whether the child looks well or ill. A physically well school-age child has good skin color, is alert to the surroundings instead of lethargic, is physically active and maintains good posture when sitting or standing instead of slouching or supporting his head in his arms on the table, is curious and asks questions after overcoming initial shyness instead of accepting any and all procedures without reactions, and is free of any overt signs of illness. It is important to note the child's reaction to the nurse. A child who feels at ease maintains eye contact or returns to

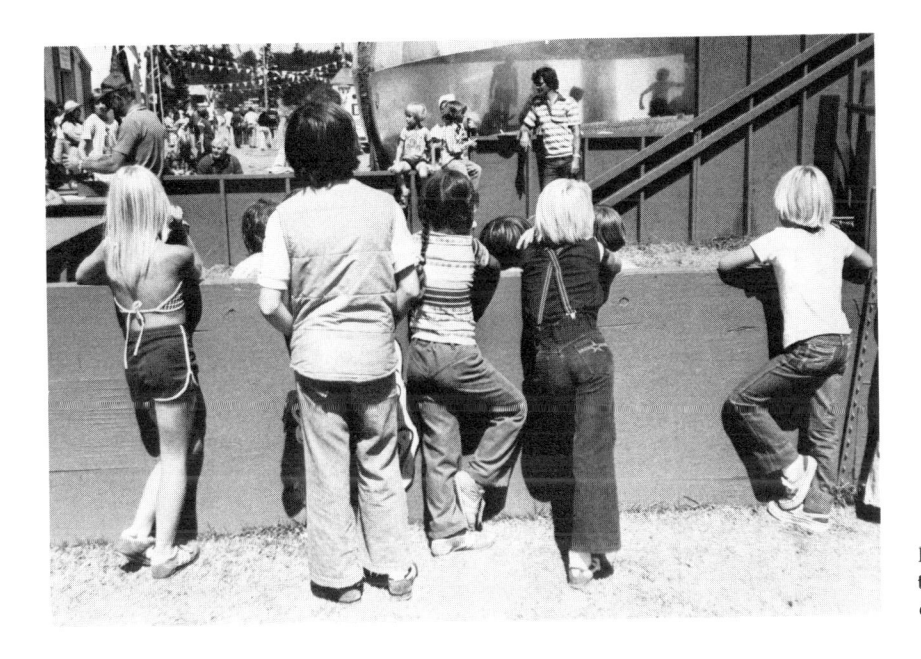

FIGURE 10-2. The physique (body type) as well as size of the school-age child is quite variable.

it after exploring the environment. A description of facial expressions or facies is helpful. The school-age child expresses his emotions endlessly, openly, and very clearly by smiling, frowning, and crying and by showing fear, anger, resentment, and hurt as well as pleasure, joy, and pride in achievement.

NORMAL GROWTH PARAMETERS

Height and weight The body as a whole and the various tissues and organs have characteristic growth patterns that are the same in all children. Yet the variability among normal school-age children, within this growth pattern, is significant in size as well as in the length of time that growth is completed. Factors influencing growth, both hereditary and environmental, have been discussed in previous chapters.

Rate of growth is more important in the school-age population than actual size. A series of measurements of height and weight, recorded as absolute figures and percentiles, is the best indicator of the rate of growth and the status of health in the school-age child. Height increases at a slowly declining rate until the pubertal spurt, and the birth length is usually tripled by the age of 13 years (see Fig. 10-3). The average rate of growth for the school-age child is about 5.1 to 7.6 cm per year. The male and female mean rates of growth are equal until the child enters puberty. (The measurement of height in a school-age child is usually done in inches when done in the school since most school scales are not yet metric.)

The weight of a 5-year-old child should be double his 1-year-old weight, and at 10 years it should have increased to 10 times the birth weight (see Fig. 10-4). According to Weeche's formula, the school-age child should add 6 lb to his weight yearly from 6 to 9 years and 9 lb during his tenth year. Another way to evaluate weight gain would be the addition of the birth weight yearly from the age of 5 to 10. (The measurement of weight in a school-age child is often done in pounds and fractions of them since school scales do not have metric measurements.) The measurements of height and weight are compared with one another, using the height-for-weight–ratio curve, and should be within normal limits (see Figs. 2-18 and 2-19).

Head circumference The rate of growth of the head after the age of 5 years is very slow, only 1.27 cm ($\frac{1}{2}$ in) per 5 years, until full maturity at puberty, and thus is not a valuable indicator of growth in the school-age child. If

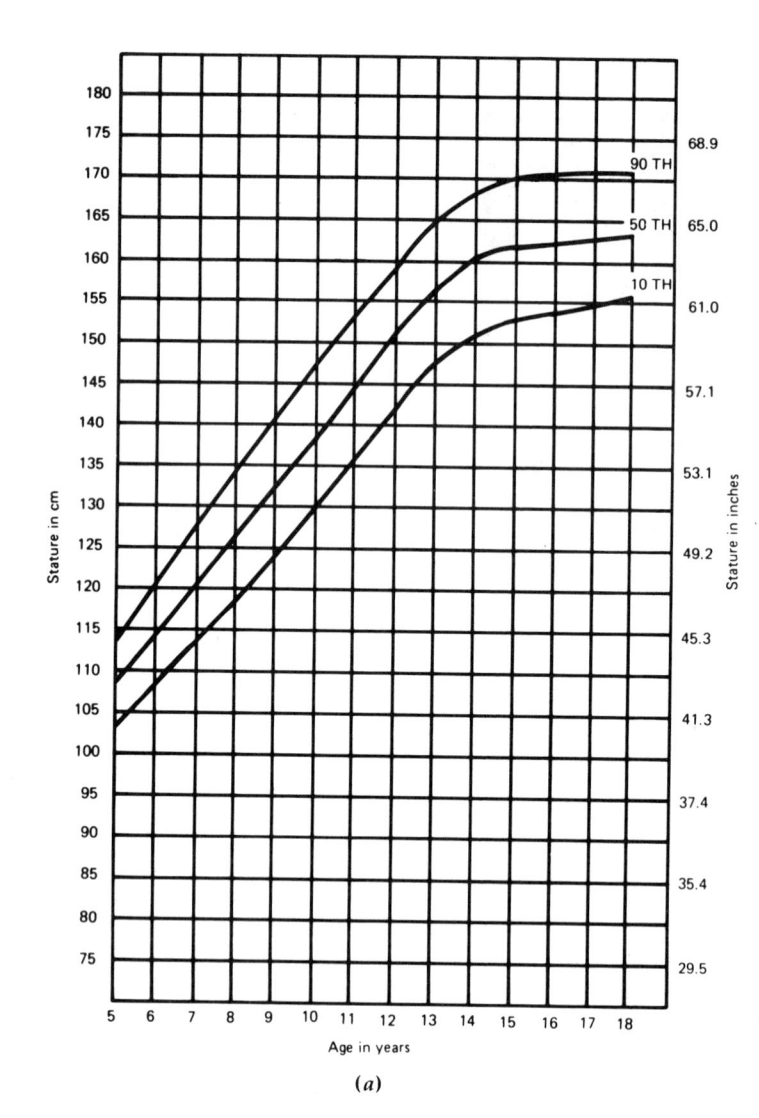

FIGURE 10-3. Height by age, 5 to 18 years. (*a*) Girls; (*b*) boys. [*From National Center for Health Statistics, NCHS growth charts, 1976. Monthly Vital Statistics Report (HRA) 76-1120 (Vol. 25, No. 3). Rockland, Maryland: U.S. Health Resources Administration, 1977. (Supplement.)*]

there are no head-circumference measurements on record from birth to 5 years of age, then measurement should be done. The head circumference could vary from 49.2 to 52.1 cm (19½ to 20¾ in) at the age of 5 years and from 52.1 to 55.1 cm (20¾ to 22 in) at puberty when the head is adult-sized.

BODY PROPORTIONS
The school-age child continues an uneven growth of body parts, differential growth, with the legs growing the most rapidly. The leg growth accounts for 66 percent of the height increase from the age of 1 year to the onset of puberty (see Fig. 10-5). Both boys and girls of school age are long-legged, with the relation of the shoulder width to the pelvic breadth remaining the same in both sexes. The midpoint of the height lowers steadily from the umbilicus to halfway between it and the symphysis pubis. The proximodistal pattern of growth is broken by growth of the feet. A sudden increase in foot length is the initial indication of the pubertal growth spurt.

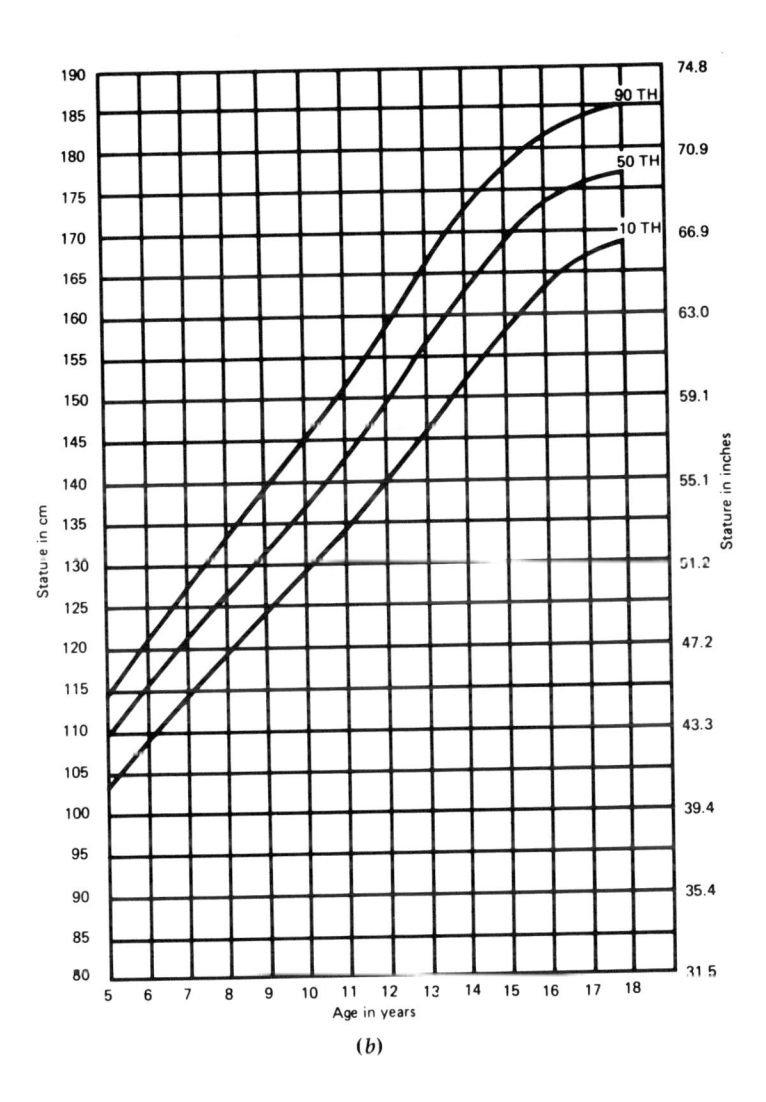

FIGURE 10-3. (Continued)

BODY COMPOSITION

The gain in musculature during childhood equals the growth of all other organs, systems, and tissues combined. Muscle mass actually constitutes the largest percentage of the body. Although the number of striated muscle fibers remains about the same in all humans, the difference in size and the changes in muscle size and mass occur because of an increase in the size of the individual muscle fibers. During school age there are no noticeable differences in muscle mass in boys and girls; increased size in muscle fibers creates increased strength in all school-age children. The increase in strength becomes greater in boys than in girls, especially when they approach puberty.

There is a gradual decrease of fat stored in the body from 1 to 6 years of age. Girls tend to retain more fat even at this age, but both sexes reaccumulate it at an even rate from the age of 7 until puberty. Thereafter girls continue to accumulate adipose tissue while the boys stop at puberty.

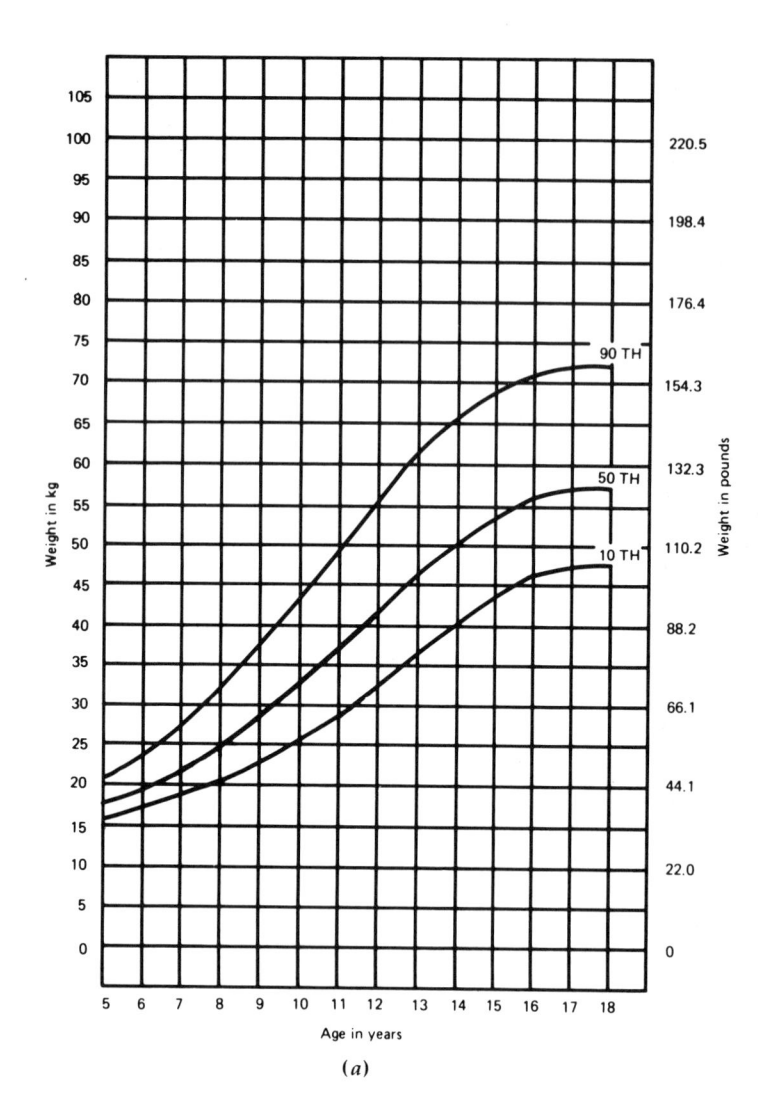

FIGURE 10-4. Weight by age, 5 to 18 years. (a) Girls; (b) boys. (*From National Center for Health Statistics, NCHS growth charts, 1976.*)

VITAL SIGNS

The mean temperature for school-age boys and girls is about the same, and no differentiation occurs until puberty. There is a slow lowering of the body temperature all through the school years at the rate of about 0.2°C (0.4°F) per year. The temperature in children is affected by environmental temperature, physical exertion, emotional excitement, eating, and time of day. The normal oral temperature varies from 35 to 37°C (95 to 99°F).

Heart rate falls steadily throughout childhood. The lower limits of pulse rates at rest are about 75 for the 6-year-old and 70 for 8- to 10-year-olds. The upper limits of normal are 115 and 110 for the corresponding ages. Heart rate varies greatly with respirations, accelerating with inspiration and lowering with expiration.

Blood pressure becomes a more significant measurement during the school-age years. At least three of the Korotkov sounds should be recorded; the point at which the sounds are first heard (phase I), which is the systolic pressure; the point at which the sounds become muffled

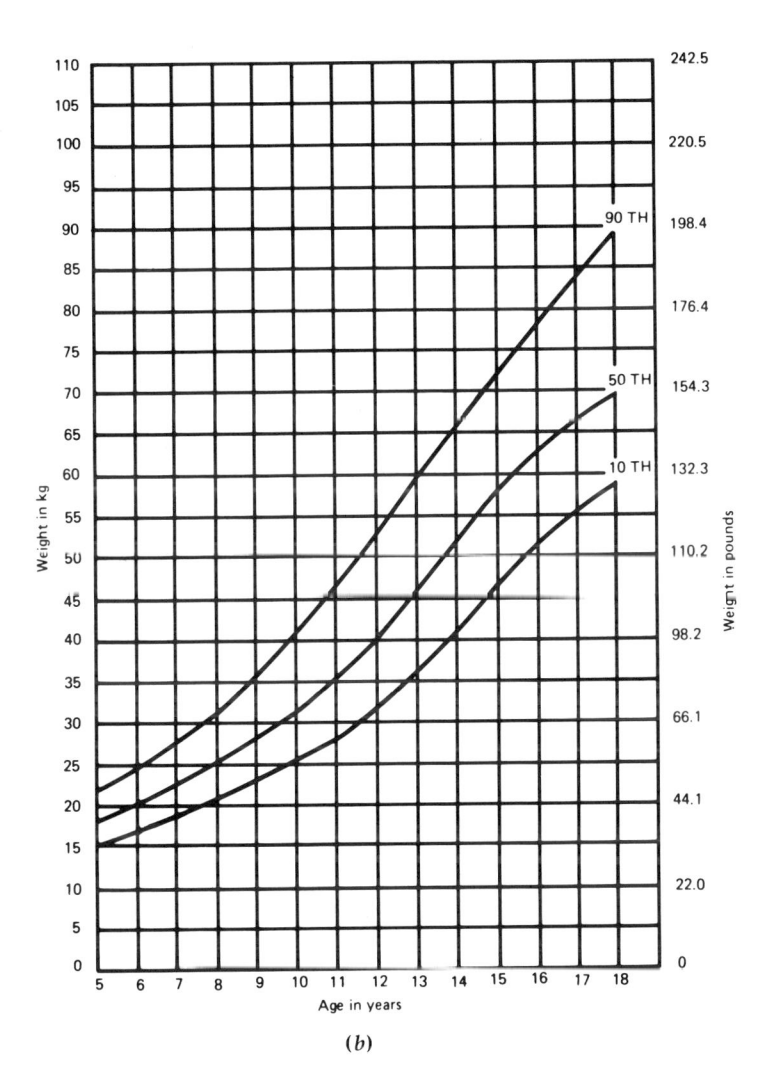

FIGURE 10-4. (Continued)

(b)

(phase IV); and the point at which the sounds disappear (phase V). The muffling sound is the diastolic pressure in the school-age child. The nurse should also compare the systolic and diastolic readings. Normally the difference between these two readings is from 20 to 50 mmHg in the school-age child. A wider or narrower difference warrants repeated measurements on subsequent visits to ensure accurate readings.

The blood pressure shows a slow increase during the school years and beyond, from 98/62 at 6 years to 115/75 at 12 years (mean). *The Report of the Task Force on Blood Pressure Control in Children* (1977) recommends comparing blood pressure readings to percentile charts (see Fig. 2-49). This allows the nurse to follow a pattern over a period of time. Blood pressure values do not follow the percentile channels exactly as weight and height values do in the school-age children.

Boys and girls in the same age group have essentially the same blood pressure readings until the onset of puberty. Also, there is no significant difference in black children when compared to children of other races even though black adults have a higher rate of hypertension than the rest of the population. The nurse is encouraged to measure blood pressure during physical examination of children above the age of 3 years.

Lung growth continues until the age of about 8 years, and this occurs because of the increased alveolar size and the branching of the terminal bronchioles and respiratory units. The diameter of the airway also continues to expand until puberty. Respirations of a young school-age child are mixed abdominal and costal, becoming predominantly costal by the age of 7 years. With this increased efficiency of muscle use the respiratory exchange becomes gradually more efficient, being about the same in boys and girls until puberty. This efficiency shows in decreased amounts of oxygen and increased amounts of carbon dioxide in the expired air.

As the size of the lungs increases with physical growth, inspiratory volume increases also, the increase being about the cube of the increase in height. Thus, if a child grows 2 in in height per year, his volume of air inhaled increases $(2 \text{ in})^3$ or 8 in^3. The respiratory rate continues to decrease very slowly in the school-age child, the averages for boys and girls being the same and decreasing from about 22 to 19 breaths per minute from 5 years to age 10.

PHYSICAL SCREENING

VISION

Vision impairment is the fourth most common disability in the United States and the leading cause of handicapping conditions in childhood. Approximately 20 to 30 percent of school-age children have visual problems, but only about 25 percent of these will manifest enough symptoms to elicit an eye examination without prior screening. The rest, or 75 percent, will go undetected for long periods of time unless screened in the school setting.

Most school-age children undergo a superficial screening for far-vision acuity, near-vision acuity, and color vision. Few parents are asked to give visual history, especially as it relates to behaviors indicating visual difficulties. Such behaviors may include inattentiveness, facial contortions, squinting of the eyes, closing of one eye, and cocking of the head. The child may also rub his eyes often, blink, or complain of blurring. He might have a tendency to sit close to the television.

A 20/30 vision acuity bilaterally is adequate for a school-age child until the age of 7 to 8; thereafter the acuity should be on the adult 20/20 level. Any child who fails to see the required-sized letters but sees equally well

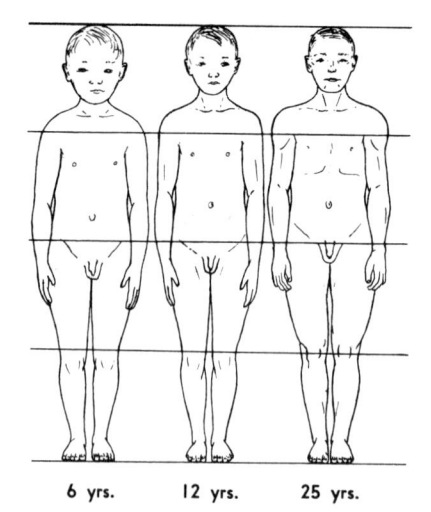

FIGURE 10-5. Body proportion during the school years and in comparison with the adult.

with each eye should be rescreened carefully, have visual history taken, and be observed in the classroom. A child who has a two-line difference between eyes, regardless at what level he sees, and any child who fails rescreening should be referred for an eye examination. A difference in visual acuity between the eyes can cause the child to suppress the vision in the poorer eye.

Problems in visual perception can cause a young school-age child to respond incorrectly to the Snellen E chart. He may reverse the right and left and/or the up and down E's very easily when he is not sure of the directionality of his hand and what he visually perceives. The Snellen test discovers faults in far-vision acuity, such as myopia, somewhat severe astigmatism, and also amblyopia.

A school-age child not only must have good visual acuity but must also have coordinated binocular vision. *Heterotropia* is an obvious defect in focusing the eyes together; *heterophoria* is a tendency toward the same problem. Obvious nonbinocularity causes double vision, suppression of vision in one eye, and eventual loss of vision in the suppressed eye. There is normally no awareness of this problem on the child's or the parents' part. For perfect binocular vision this problem should be discovered before the child reaches school age. Yet, many kindergarten and first-grade children never have a vision screening until they enter school.

Normally, all young children are farsighted, or hyperopic, but in a lessening degree when advancing through the early grades. An abnormal degree of farsightedness should also be detected as soon as possible.

Awareness of color-vision deficiencies in a school-age

child is also important to protect him from failures in color-coded tests, which are increasingly popular in reading. The nurse should screen all kindergarten children, first graders, and new students for color deficiencies and also educate teachers as to the presence of this defect.

HEARING

As the child grows, the lower part of the face grows proportionately more than the upper, causing the eustachian tube to become longer, narrower, and more slanted. This makes it harder for any disease organism to invade the middle ear. Yet it is estimated that about 3 to 5 percent of all school-age children have serious hearing defects that interfere with schoolwork. This figure is higher, about 19.8 percent, in children who live in poor socioeconomic conditions.

Hearing and language development are very closely associated, and a positive history of frequent otitis media is associated with both expressive and receptive language delays. The hearing screenings done in this age group by the nurse can become a highly effective tool in making the school-age child and his parents aware of any intermittent or permanent hearing loss, resulting in better control and prevention of further loss.

The most common hearing loss in children in kindergarten and first grade is conductive peripheral loss due to respiratory airway congestion blocking the eustachian tubes and causing the collection of fluid in the middle ear, serous otitis media. This fluid can also become viscous causing a "glue ear," which prevents the movement of the otic bones. Poor or no management will result in permanent hearing loss due to ruptured or scarred, stiff tympanic membranes.

Some school-age children have minor hearing loss which is genetic and progressive. This usually starts in the high frequencies. There is no treatment or prevention program for this type of hearing loss.

PUBERTY

Puberty is defined as all "morphological and physiological changes which occur in the growing boy or girl as the gonads change from their infantile to their adult state" (Marshall, 1978, p. 141). It is a significant period of transitional development, marking the beginning of the end of childhood and the start of adolescence, another maturational period of several years duration. Marshall (1978) lists the following principal manifestations of puberty:

- Growth spurt: acceleration followed by deceleration of musculoskeletal growth as well as some body systems, especially the cardiovascular and respiratory
- Development of the gonads
- Development of secondary sex characteristics and secondary accessory reproductive organs
- Changes in body composition, specifically lean/fat body-mass ratio.

Thus, there are broad functional as well as structural changes.

Although these changes are generally age-related, as with other areas of development, variability between children is normal. Age of pubertal onset, length of time to complete the process, and sequence of maturation of body structures vary. For each child, these are genetically determined and highly environmentally modified. Girls are approximately 2 years ahead of boys of the same chronological age. Racial differences are not clear as they are compounded by environmental factors. Health status, nutrition, and geography—particularly altitude—do affect puberty.

As puberty is principally represented by activity of the reproductive system, specific manifestations of puberty are discussed in "Reproductive System and Pubertal Changes." It is full maturation of this system, resulting in the ability to reproduce another life, that determines the completion of puberty—and the end of childhood. Maturational changes in the craniofacial and musculoskeletal systems are also presented.

Calvarium and face Mary Tudor

By age 7 years, 90 percent of brain growth is achieved, and it is essentially completed by 10 to 12 years of age; thus, the same is true of the calvarium. However, minimal growth, 1 percent per year, will continue for life. The cranial base continues to grow until 17 to 20 years (Sullivan, 1978).

The calvarium/face ratio is 3.5:1 by 6 years, 3:1 by adolescence, and finally 2.5:1 in maturity. Thus it is obvious that the face continues to grow after calvarium growth is essentially completed.

Significant facial changes accompany puberty. There is slight growth in head length and breadth which occurs during the pubertal growth spurt. Whether this represents soft-tissue, bone, or cranial-vault growth is unclear (Marshall, 1978).

Facial growth peaks a few months after peak stature velocity of puberty. The frontal sinus and brow ridges develop, and the nasal bridge becomes more prominent. Nasomaxillary and mandibular growth continue, accommodating the permanent teeth and giving the child a longer, more adultlike face. A significant portion, 25 percent, of mandibular growth occurs between 12 and 20 years (Marshall, 1978). Increase in thickness as well as length of the mandible is achieved by about 23 years of age, completing facial development.

TOOTH FORMATION
The school-age child has had all deciduous teeth since he was 2 to 2½ years old. During the following 4 years, the underlying permanent teeth continued to calcify. As the root of each permanent tooth develops and it emerges toward the gum surface, reabsorption of the root of the corresponding deciduous tooth occurs. Thus, when the deciduous tooth is shed, it consists only of the crown and a small portion of the root.

Emergence of the permanent tooth usually closely follows loss of the deciduous tooth. Emergence of the third molar is later, highly variable, and may never occur in some individuals. Girls are 1 to 6 months ahead of boys of the same chronological age in permanent-tooth eruption. Calcification of the permanent teeth is completed (except for the third molar) by 14 to 15 years of age.

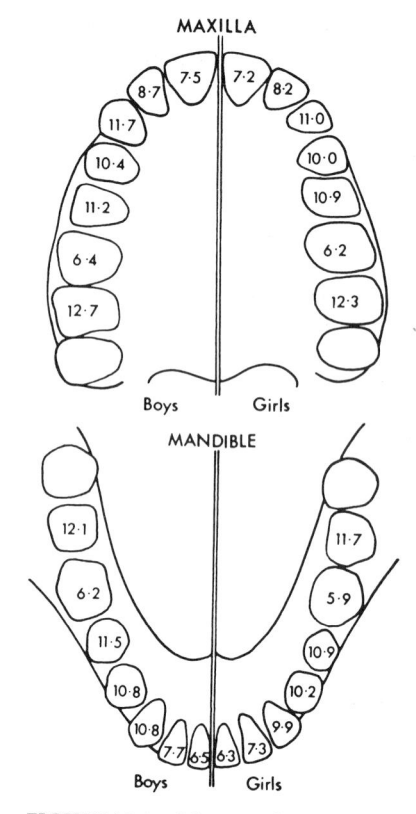

FIGURE 10-6. Mean age in year and month of emergence of the permanent teeth for boys and girls. (From D. Sinclair, *Human growth after birth*. London: Oxford University Press, 1978, p. 103. Reprinted by permission of the publisher.)

Musculoskeletal system Sherrilyn Passo

SKELETAL GROWTH
The school-age child continues to grow in height secondary to regular increases in long-bone growth. Most of the bones of the skeleton are complete, although some epiphyseal centers are still being formed. Ossification of the ends of small and long bones continues throughout the school-age period. Much growth in height remains, as illustrated in Fig. 10-7, and most of this growth will take place during adolescence (see "Reproductive System and Pubertal Changes"). At that time, the boy will double his skeletal mass, with maximal growth between 12 and 14 years. Girls begin this skeletal growth earlier, with maximal growth usually taking place between the ages of 10 and 14 years.

The pubertal growth spurt results in significant increase in shoulder and hip breadth and increase in trunk length. Leg, foot, and hand lengths gain final relative size sooner than the trunk as the pubertal growth spurt is first evident in the distal portion of the limbs.

There is "no clear relationship between skeletal maturation, represented as bone age, and the development of secondary sex characteristics in normal children" (Marshall, 1978, p. 169). Skeletal age appears to be as variable as chronological age at the onset of puberty. In other words, puberty does not commence at a particular bone age.

MUSCULAR GROWTH
Muscular growth continues in a linear relation to body weight and parallels the increase in skeletal growth. There is a significant increase, over average, of muscle mass in taller persons; however, this increase is much less marked in females. Between 5 years and the end of adolescence, muscle mass accounts for an increased percentage of total body weight.

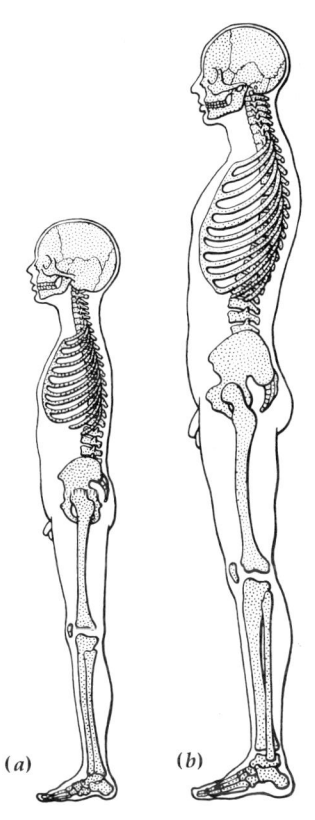

FIGURE 10-7. Difference in skeletal development between (*a*) 8 years and (*b*) adult. [*From J. P. Schaeffer, Morris' human anatomy (11th ed.). New York: McGraw-Hill, 1953, p. 50. Reprinted by permission of the publisher.*]

As children of both sexes mature, the increase in muscle strength in various portions of the body proceeds at uneven rates. For example, shoulder-flexion strength has been found to accelerate to the age of 8 years; back-lift strength improves throughout the school-age period and then becomes less pronounced at 12 years of age; and ankle-flexion strength improves regularly at all ages in childhood (Cratty, 1970). During school-age years, boys are somewhat stronger than girls; however, this difference is not significant until adolescence. Increased muscle density and power are evidenced in both sexes.

As increase in muscle mass parallels the increase in skeletal growth, there is a spurt of growth in muscle tissue during the pubertal growth spurt which is more pronounced for males than females (see "Reproductive System and Pubertal Changes"). The girl reaches her maximal muscle growth in the twelfth year, after which this growth slows. In the thirteenth year the rate of growth of muscle in boys will triple the rate of growth in girls. Muscle growth will reach a maximum for boys in the fourteenth year, followed by less remarkable slowing growth (Grumbach, Grave, and Mayer, 1974). Thus, after puberty, males have significantly more muscle mass than females due to the greater relative proportion of muscle to body size.

The school-age child also develops increasing control and strength of the muscles. As myelination is completed about the eighth year, control of increasingly complex tasks becomes possible. The child's capabilities increase as he practices motor activities. Increased strength results from increased muscle density and is evidenced in both boys and girls. During the early part of the school-age period, boys begin to move ahead in most tasks involving simple applications of force and power. Girls often catch up or surpass the boys in late childhood, reflecting the hormonal changes which occur earlier in girls than in boys. Maximum strength occurs just after peak growth in height and just before peak growth in weight. At puberty, male strength increases; however, female strength levels.

Reproductive system and pubertal changes Nancy Reame

PREPUBERTAL CHANGES IN REPRODUCTIVE HORMONES

The younger school-age child is similar to the infant in terms of reproductive development. Both internal and external reproductive organs are comparable in size and function. Gonadotropin levels in the blood are low in both sexes, but girls have higher plasma concentrations of FSH than boys (Lee, Midgley, and Jaffe, 1970).

After age 8, however, subtle changes begin to occur that will lay the foundation for the onset of sexual maturation. Long before any visible signs of maturation occur in the reproductive organs, hormonal activity begins to change. In both boys and girls, concentrations of adrenal androgens rise progressively from age 8 to about age 15 (Ducharme et al., 1976).

These androgens are steroid hormones that exert testosterone-like effects and are believed responsible for the deepening of the voice and production of acne in girls. The growth of pubic and axillary hair may be related to this increased adrenal activity, since removal of the ovaries in prepubescent girls can inhibit breast development but does not interfere with axillary or pubic hair growth. The early increase in adrenal androgens may also play a role in the maturation of the hypothalamic-pituitary-ovarian axis (see Chap. 2), since children with adrenal tumors exhibit precocious luteinizing hormone (LH) activity (Boyar, Jordan, David, Roffward, Kapen, Weitzman, and Hellman, 1973).

Shortly after the prepubertal increase in adrenal activity occurs, gonadal and gonadotropic hormone concentrations in the blood also begin to rise. There is a progressive increase in levels of follicle-stimulating hormone (FSH) at age 9 in both boys and girls; LH levels in the blood also rise after age 9 in girls but not until age 11 or 12 in boys (Lee et al., 1970; Lee, Jaffe, and Midgley, 1974). Interestingly, changes in secretory activity for LH are first seen only during sleep as pulsatile surges in both boys and girls who are in the early stages of puberty (Boyar, Finkelstein, Roffwarg, Kupen, Weitzman, and Hellman, 1972). Once puberty is well established, the sleep-related surges disappear in girls but not in boys and continue during adult male life.

What causes these changes in secretory activity is presently unknown, but it is believed that the onset of puberty is associated with an increase in the set point of hypothalamic "gonadostat" resulting in higher and higher levels of both pituitary and gonadal hormones which finally trigger reproduction-related growth and function (Grumbach, 1975). Puberty, then, encompasses those biologic events which transform a reproductively immature individual into a mature one. All the manifestations of puberty discussed above involve quantitative changes such as the skeleton, muscles, and lungs growing larger. Even some sexual functions, such as the ability to have an erection, may precede puberty. But the capacity to reproduce is a qualitative change that has no prepubescent counterpart.

THE PUBERTAL GROWTH SPURT AND THE REPRODUCTIVE SYSTEM

After age 5 and until age 10 years, girls and boys are very similar in height, weight, strength, and body composition. Then girls take a temporary lead over boys, as they enter puberty earlier, so that girls in the sixth and seventh grades tend to be taller and heavier than their male schoolmates (see Fig. 10-8).

This period of rapid general growth, the pubertal growth spurt, starts in girls about $10\frac{1}{2}$ years, peaks at age 12 years, and ends by age 14 (Marshall and Tanner, 1969). Total gain in height during the year of peak velocity is 6 to 11 cm (Marshall, 1978). In boys, this growth spurt does not usually begin until age 12 or 13 years, peaks at age 14, and ends at about age 16, resulting in a 1- to 2-year lag behind girls (Marshall and Tanner, 1970) (see Fig. 10-9). Total gain during the peak velocity year is 7 to 12 cm (Marshall, 1978). Sex differences in somatic growth at puberty are summarized in Table 10-1.

Skeletal growth is influenced by the main type of sex steroid produced by the gonad. Although both estrogens and androgens have anabolic effects on bone, males have a larger bone mass due to a thicker cortical layer when compared with females (Gryfe, Exton-Smith, Payne, and Wheeler, 1971). Estrogen has a special effect on the pelvis, changing the pelvic outlet from the narrow, funnellike outlet of the male into a broad, oval outlet which favors spontaneous birth. Estrogen is believed to exert its effect by decreasing the responsiveness of bone to parathyroid hormone, thus favoring osteoblast function.

Since sex steroids also stimulate the cessation of growth by stimulating epiphyseal closure, the earlier sexual maturation of females is one reason why males are about 10 percent taller as adults. Because they mature later, boys have time to continue growing. The cause of this difference in onset of sexual maturation is not known. Sex differences in body size are much larger after puberty than before since the boys' adolescent spurt is greater than the girls' (Tanner, Whitehouse, and Takaishi, 1966). Sex dimorphism differs from one population to another, both before and after puberty. The age of girls taller than boys is much less variable in European countries compared with African and Asiatic nations (Tanner and Eveleth, 1975).

The pubertal growth spurt starts with feet and hands, followed by hips, chest, shoulders, and trunk. Most of the increase in the height occurs in the trunk rather than the lower limbs due to growth of the vertebral column. In the earliest stage of puberty there is increase in body fat in girls and boys. With the growth spurt there is a loss of fat, especially from the limbs. The loss of fat is not nearly as dramatic in girls as in boys, especially in the region of the pelvis, breasts, upper back, and backs of the arms. As adolescence proceeds, girls gain more fat. Increase in lean body mass (LBM), which also is a function of stature, is much greater in boys. Final percentage of LBM is therefore greater in boys; in fact, the sex difference in LBM is even more pronounced than that for either height or weight (Forbes, 1975) (see Fig. 10-10). Because of this genetically and hormonally determined fat distribution, female bodies are more rounded and their skeletal muscles and surface blood vessels appear less prominent.

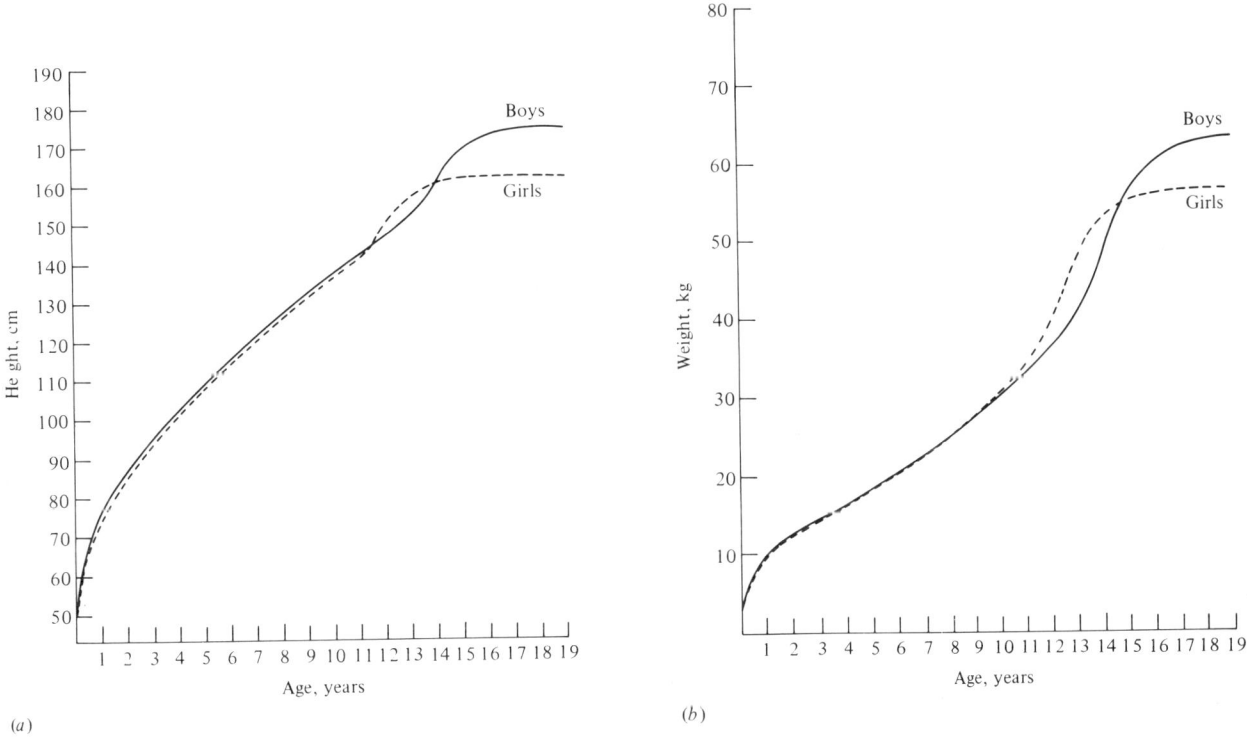

FIGURE 10-8. Sex differences in height and weight during childhood and adolescence. Girls are heavier and taller at age 13. (*From J. M. Tanner, R. H. Whitehouse, and M. Takaishi, Standards from birth to maturity for height, weight, height velocity and weight velocity. Arch. Dis. Child., 1966, 41, 467. Reprinted by permission of the British Medical Association.*)

With puberty, sex differences appear for muscle mass and strength, which may be attributable in part to cultural influences as well as hormonal factors (Katchadourian, 1977). Because testosterone has significant effects on the production of muscle protein, postpubertal boys have about 56 percent more muscle tissue than girls (Falkner, 1975). This effect on protein anabolism is also believed responsible for a higher basal metabolic rate (BMR) in boys than girls after puberty (Guyton, 1976).

The heart, also a muscle, reflects sex difference in terms of size, pulse pressure, systolic blood pressure, and blood volume, all being greater in males (Beach, 1974; Maresh, 1948). Pulse rate, however, is higher in females (Tanner et al., 1966) (see Figs. 10-11 and 10-12). Males have an average of 500,000 to 1 million more red blood cells per cubic millimeter than females. This difference may be due in part to the increased metabolic rate rather than to a direct effect on red blood cell production. The respiratory system is also influenced to a greater extent by testosterone than estrogen resulting in enhanced respiratory function in males (see Fig. 10-13). Respiratory rate, however, does not appear to be significantly different between sexes.

CLINICAL INDICATORS OF THE ONSET OF PUBERTY

Because the internal reproductive organs cannot be readily evaluated in terms of growth and development, changes in the outward appearance of the genitals, body hair, and breasts have been used as clinical indexes of normal reproductive maturation. Tanner is credited with providing a description of the progressive pubertal stages in both boys and girls and identifying the normal age

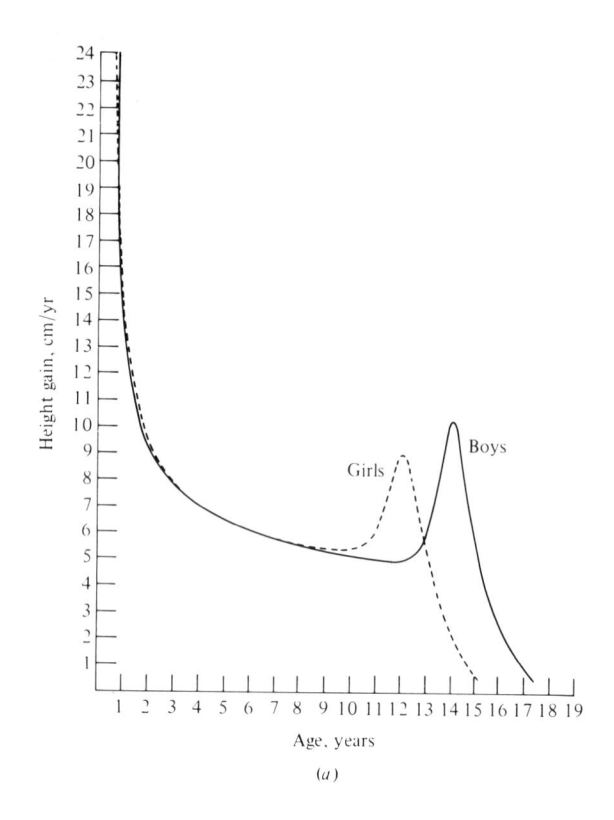

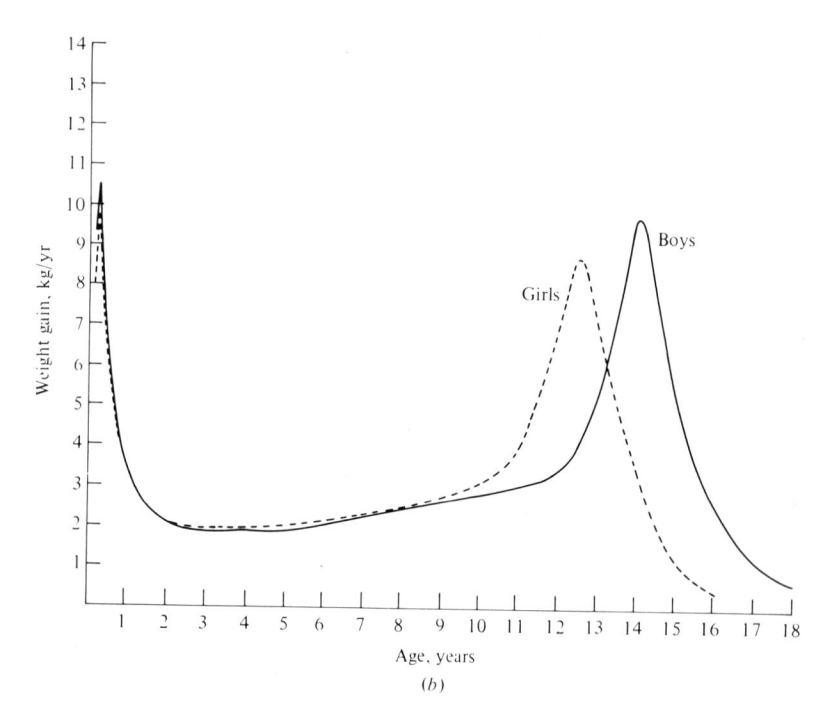

FIGURE 10-9. Sex differences in the onset of the adolescent growth spurt for height and weight. Girls reach their peak rate of growth about 2 years sooner than boys. (*From J. M. Tanner et al., 1966. Reprinted by permission of the British Medical Association.*)

PHYSICAL DEVELOPMENT **491**

range within which these stages occur (Marshall and Tanner, 1969, 1970; Tanner, 1962).

FEMALE
Female reproductive maturation is usually described in terms of three sets of events which follow a predictable sequence: (1) *thelarche*, or breast development, (2) *adrenarche*, or growth of body hair, and (3) *menarche*, or the onset of menstruation.

Thelarche Usually breast development is the first visible sign of puberty and starts between the ages of 8 and 13 years (on the average at about 11). Five maturational stages have been described which are generally completed between the ages of 13 and 18, with age 15 being the average age of attainment of stage 5, the adult breast (see Fig. 10-14). It is not unusual for one breast to develop faster than the other resulting in asymmetry and causing anxiety on the part of the young adolescent who is very much aware of her changing body and its social signifi-

TABLE 10-1 Pubertal changes in somatic organ systems

Organ system	Change at puberty	Sex difference
Central nervous system		
Cell number, cell size	No puberty-specific changes known	Biphasic in girls, monophasic in boys
Basal body temperature	Decline to adult levels is reached by age 12 in girls but later in boys	
Musculoskeletal		
Stature	Adolescent growth spurt	Earlier in girls, greater in boys
		Boys are 10% taller
Dry skeletal weight	Increases	Greater in boys
Thickness of bone cortex	Increases	Greater in boys
Muscle-cell number	Increases	Fourteenfold increase in boys; tenfold in girls
Muscle-cell size	Increases	Increases until age 40 in males, age 10½ in females
Cardiovascular		
Heart size	Doubles in weight	Larger in males
Systolic blood pressure	Progressive rise	Higher in males
Resting heart rate	Slowing down of the gradual decline with age and may even increase	Faster in males
Red blood cells, hemoglobin, blood volume	Dramatic increase in males but no puberty-specific changes in females	
Respiratory		
Lung mass	Increases	Larger in males
Vital capacity	Increases	Greater in males
Respiratory rate	No puberty-specific changes in gradual decline	None
Efficiency of O$_2$ exchange	Increases	Greater in males
Inspiratory volume	Dramatic increase in males but no puberty-specific changes in females	
Basal metabolic rate	Temporary slowing of the gradual decline with age	Higher in males
Lymph system	Regression of the thymus after age 12	None
	Decreased susceptibility to infection	

Source: Summarized from H. Katchadourian, *Biology of adolescence*. San Francisco: Freeman, 1977, and A. C. Guyton, *Textbook of medical physiology* (5th ed.). Philadelphia: Saunders, 1976.

cance. Any difference in size is usually corrected by the time development is completed.

Andrenarche In girls, the appearance of pubic hair (between the ages of 11 and 12) generally occurs after the onset of breast budding, but it can appear before. Pubic hair growth and distribution have also been classified into five developmental stages (see Fig. 10-15). The adult pattern is established by about the age of 14. Axillary hair growth begins about 1 year later than pubic hair growth.

Menarche The first menstrual period occurs from 2 to 5 years after the onset of breast development. In contemporary society, the average age at which menarche occurs is 12⅔ years but ranges from 9 to 18 years (Zacharias, Rand, and Wurtman, 1976). In relation to other events of puberty, menarche fits into the picture toward the end of the process, which points out the common misconception that menarche marks the onset of puberty. In reality, a 10- or 11-year-old who begins menstruating has already undergone some significant somatic and hormonal changes, perhaps beginning as early as age 7 or 8 years.

After about age 10, the uterus will double in length and increases tenfold in weight. This growth is due to an increase in the size of the muscle layers as well as of the endometrium. With the pubertal growth spurt, the shape of the uterus as well as the cervix/corpus ratio changes so that the corpus (body) grows much more in proportion to the cervix, becomes more flexed, and lies more at an angle instead of being upright in the pelvis, as it is in the young child.

The first menstrual period may be prolonged if the endometrium has been building up for a long period of time, or it may be only a day or 2 of spotting if estrogen levels are still fairly low. The first cycle is usually anovulatory so that only 20 to 30 percent of cycles at age 12 are ovulatory, but 50 percent of cycles in a 16-year-old are ovulatory. It takes an average of 15 months to complete the first 10 menstrual cycles.

In the first year after menarche, which is considered the first gynecologic year, cycles may vary in length by as much as 58 days. Even when ovulatory cycles occur, progesterone production by the resulting corpus luteum may be abnormally low and endometrial development insufficient to maintain a pregnancy. Full fertility is therefore usually not achieved until 1 to 2 years following menarche. This period of frequent anovulation or incomplete uterine maturity is known as the period of *adolescent*

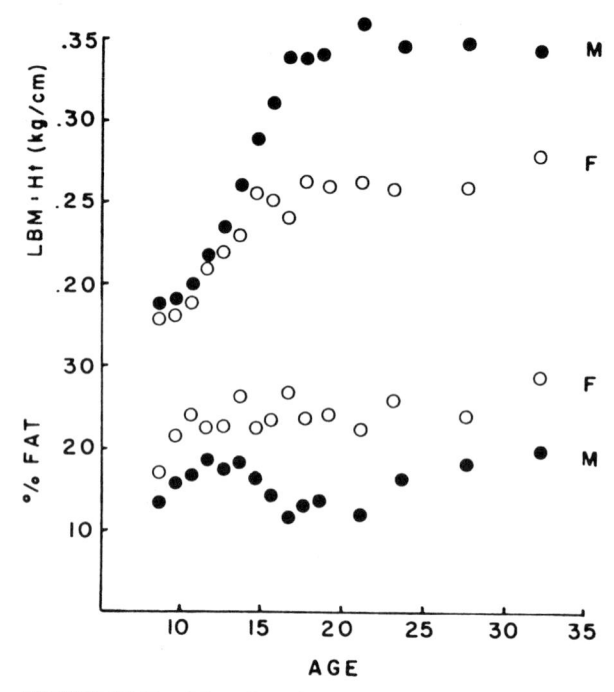

FIGURE 10-10. Mean lean-body-mass–to–height ratio of the upper portion in kg/cm and percentage of body fat of the lower portion. [From G. B. Forbes, Body composition in adolescence. In F. Falkner and J. M. Tanner (Eds.), *Human growth 2, Postnatal growth*. New York: Plenum, 1978, p. 257. Reprinted by permission of the publisher.]

infertility. Since dysmenorrhea is believed to be more commonly associated with ovulatory menstrual cycles, menstrual cramps should not be a significant complaint during this period of infertility. However, cultural influences may again color biologic events, especially if cramps are looked upon as a sign of "growing up."

Other changes Under the influence of rising levels of estrogens, the external genitalia increase in size and sensitivity to stimulation. The vagina becomes larger, longer, and thicker. The cells of the vaginal epithelium have been shown to be the first cells to respond to estrogen as a target organ even before the initial signs of puberty are observed in the breast. Vaginal cells are stimulated by estrogen to undergo typical maturational changes, characterized by an enlargement and flattening of the cytoplasm and progressive degeneration of the nucleus (cornification).

Impending puberty may also be indicated by the production of profuse, acidic vaginal secretions due to increased glycogen synthesis, which in the younger child

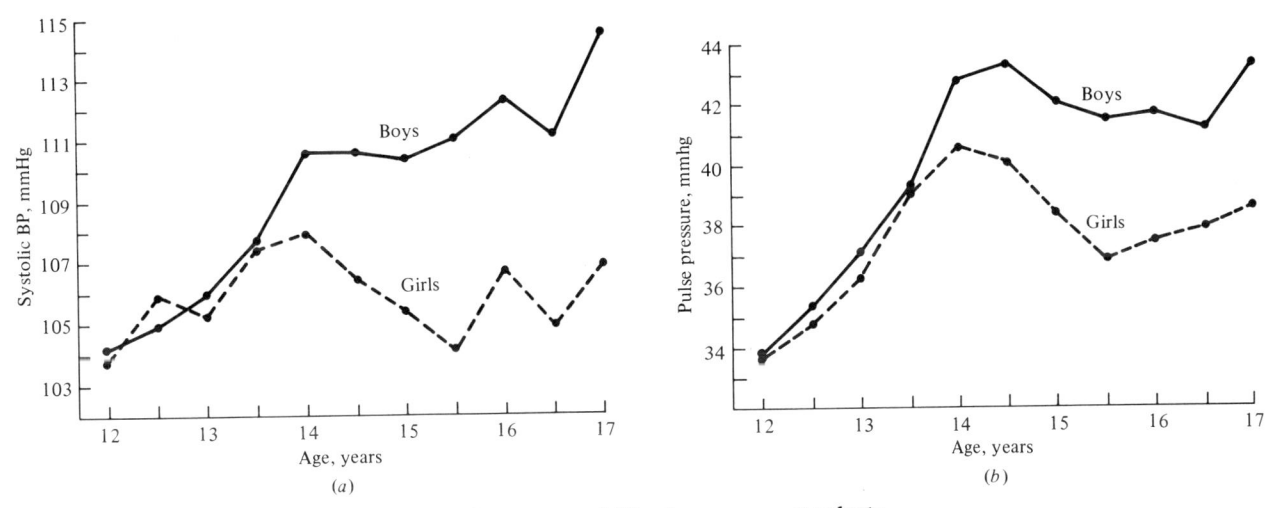

FIGURE 10-11. Rise of (a) basal systolic blood pressure and (b) pulse pressure at puberty, showing development of sex differences. [From J. M. Tanner, *Growth at adolescence* (2d ed.). London: Blackwell Scientific, 1962, p. 159. Reprinted by permission of the publisher.]

FIGURE 10-12. Change in basal heart rate (bpm) showing development of sex differences at adolescence. (From J. M. Tanner, 1962, p. 161. Reprinted by permission of Blackwell Scientific Publications.)

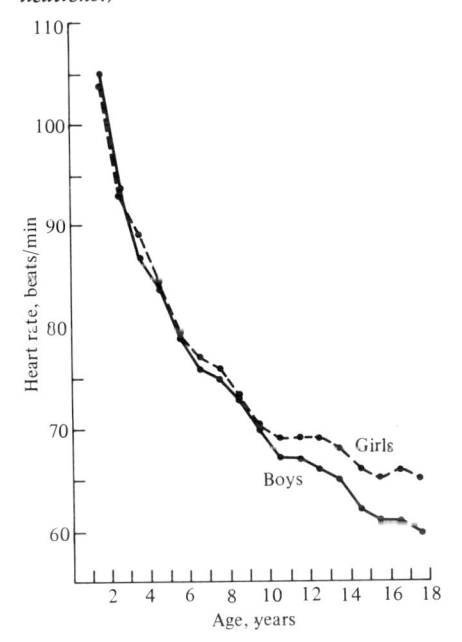

FIGURE 10-13. Change in vital capacity from ages 5 to 17 in boys and girls in relation to age. (From J. M. Tanner, 1962, p. 166. Reprinted by permission of Blackwell Scientific Publications.)

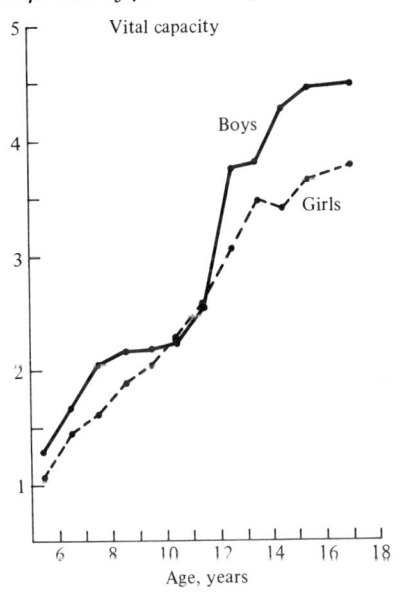

were scanty and alkaline. Tight-fitting nylon underwear may contribute to an increased incidence of nonspecific vaginitis.

The hymenal membrane, thin and delicate in early childhood, doubles in diameter and thickness under the influence of increasing estrogens. The base as well as the leaves of the membranous cuff vary in thickness and distensibility. It is very vascular and bleeds easily if traumatized. By the onset of menarche the hymenal opening is approximately 1 cm in diameter.

The ovary, which contains oocytes arrested in the diplotene stage of meiosis since birth, increases in size and weight. Variations in the appearance of the ovary between infancy and maturity are largely due to the growth, maturation, and senescence of follicles. The ovary in childhood is sensitive to pituitary hormones, and considerable numbers of oocytes in growing follicles attempt to mature precociously under the influence of FSH. Developing follicles are present at all ages before puberty. In the absence of a mature hypothalamus, this development is often abnormal, rarely culminating in ovulation, and resulting in degeneration. Thus, about 300,000 oocytes are present at age 7, of which an estimated 40 percent show signs of degeneration (Baker, 1963). The atretic process further reduces the number of oocytes to approximately 21,000 at the time of menarche (Morrow and Hart, 1975). The final stages of maturation are controlled by a critical concentration of gonadotropins, especially LH, and the resumption of meiosis, which occurs 36 to 48 h prior to ovulation. Once initiated, this process of maturation may require several cycles to result in consistent ovulations.

MALE

As noted above, boys tend to begin their sexual maturation from ½ to 2 years later than girls, even though prepubertal rises in some reproductive hormones occur at about the same age for both sexes. The primary clinical indicators of puberty in males include growth of the genitals, ability to ejaculate, and appearance of pubic hair.

Genitals In the child, the testes are nonfunctional. The seminiferous tubules contain no lumen and are lined by immature Sertoli cells and primitive germ cells which are not capable of differentiating into sperm. After about age 6 years, the tubules show the first signs of developing a lumen.

Testicular-volume increase is the first clinical sign of

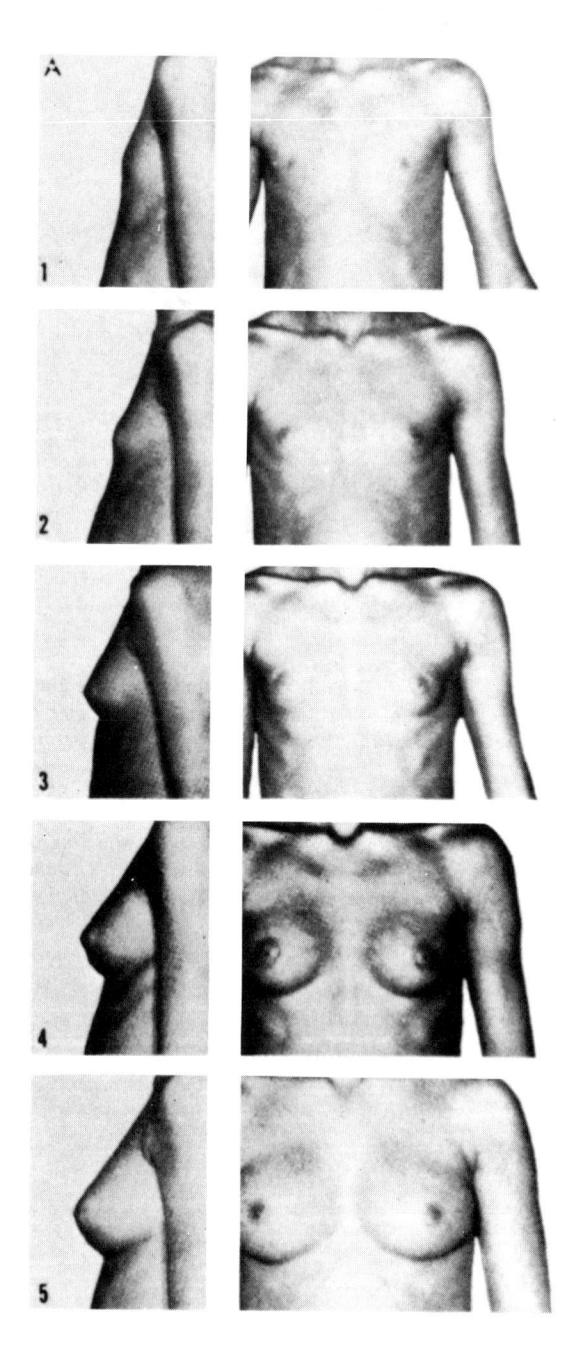

FIGURE 10-14. Tanner's five stages of breast development: (1) The infantile stage from immediate postnatal to onset of puberty. (2) The bud stage: the breast and papilla are slightly elevated, and areola diameter is increased. (3) The breast and areola are further enlarged. (4) The breast is further enlarged, and the areola forms a secondary mound above the breast. (5) Adult stage is reached in size and contour. (From J. M. Tanner, 1962, p. 37. Adapted by permission of Blackwell Scientific Publications.)

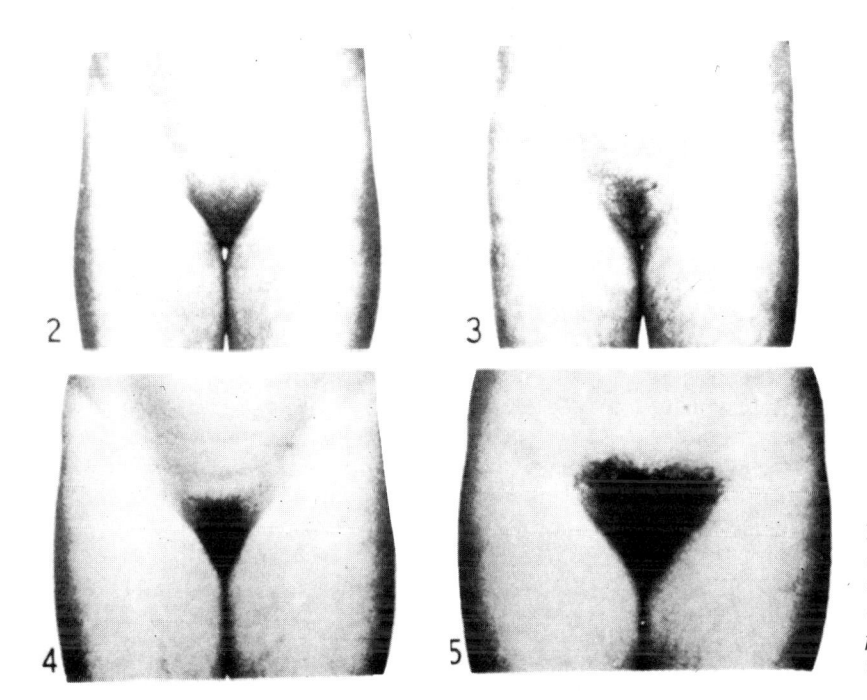

FIGURE 10-15. Pattern of growth and distribution of pubic hair in girls from the first appearance (stage 2) to the adult type (stage 5). (*From J. M. Tanner, 1962. Used by permission of Blackwell Scientific Publications.*)

puberty and occurs at about age 10 years, approximately 1 year before the appearance of pubic hair or any other secondary sex characteristic (Prader, 1975). This occurs under the influence of rising levels of FSH. In addition, the seminiferous tubules enlarge and the gonocytes undergo a series of divisions to form mature forms of spermatogonia. Testicular volume can be estimated clinically by means of an orchidometer, a measuring instrument consisting of 12 ellipsoids with volumes ranging from 1 to 25 ml. Testicular volume of less than 10 mL is abnormal in adolescent boys who already show some evidence of secondary sex characteristics.

The pubertal development of the testis is a rather long process lasting for 5 or 6 years, with the fastest growth occurring between 13 and 14 years of age. During this time, it is normal for one side of the scrotum to be larger than the other. This is at a time when LH plasma levels have begun to rise rapidly and are stimulating testosterone production by the Leydig cells, which in turn function to initiate meiotic division and the final stages of spermatogenesis. All adult types of spermatogonia appear at this time, followed by primary and secondary spermatocytes at the successive stages of meiosis and eventually by spermatids, which complete their development into spermatozoa at the end of puberty. Full spermatogenic activity in terms of morphology and quantity is usually not attained until about 15 years of age.

Because growth of the penis depends on testosterone production, its size increases slowly during infancy and childhood. In the child, the stretched penis ranges from 5 to 11 cm. Pubertal enlargement and lengthening of the penis occurs about a year after the onset of testicular growth and requires a much shorter time to reach adult proportions. Five stages are described by Tanner (see Fig. 10-16).

Pubic hair Pubic hair growth is usually an early event of puberty in boys but may normally begin anytime between the ages of 10 and 15 years. Its pattern of distribution is characteristic of the male genotype. It generally appears after testicular growth has begun and in association with penile enlargement, at approximately age 13 (see Fig. 10-17). The pigmentation and wrinkling of the scrotal skin also becomes more extensive with the onset of pubic hair growth. Axillary and facial hair usually appear 2 years after the first growth of pubic hair.

Ejaculation Although the ability to have an erection may be present at birth, the capacity to discharge semen during orgasm is a pubertal event. Most boys will have this experience for the first time between the ages of 11 and 15 (Kinsey, Pomeroy, and Martin, 1953). In a study by Kinsey, spontaneous nocturnal emissions occurred almost 1 year after ejaculatory ability had been achieved through masturbation, contradicting the belief that nocturnal emission is early evidence of pubertal onset.

Other secondary sex characteristics A transient breast enlargement may occur in boys aged 10 through 16 which may be restricted to the nipple area or extend to the subcutaneous fat deposits but generally dissipates within a year or 2 (Nydick, Bustos, Dale, and Rawson, 1961). During puberty, the areola darkens in both sexes but to a greater extent in adolescent males than in females prior to pregnancy. The diameter of the areola, which is equal in both sexes before puberty, increases considerably, though less in boys than in girls. The acceleration of the growth of the larynx does not occur until near the termination of the penile growth spurt and is presumably due to a direct stimulation by testosterone of the cells of the laryngeal cartilages.

Only when physical signs of puberty have not appeared by age 16 is puberty considered delayed. Factors which have been shown to affect age of onset of puberty include sex, heredity, climate, altitude, season, light, illness, and socioeconomic level; nutritional status appears to be the most influential factor determining growth and development (Katchadourian, 1977). Figure 10-18 illustrates variations in reaching pubertal stages.

Development of body concept and concepts of illness and wellness
Judith Anne Ritchie

BODY CONCEPT, CONTENT, AND FUNCTION

STABILITY OF THE BODY CONCEPT
The perception of body parts as a constantly interrelated unit is achieved between 8 and 11 years, coinciding with such cognitive concepts as left-right connotation and perceptual constancy (Schilder, 1964; Simmel, 1966). Body-

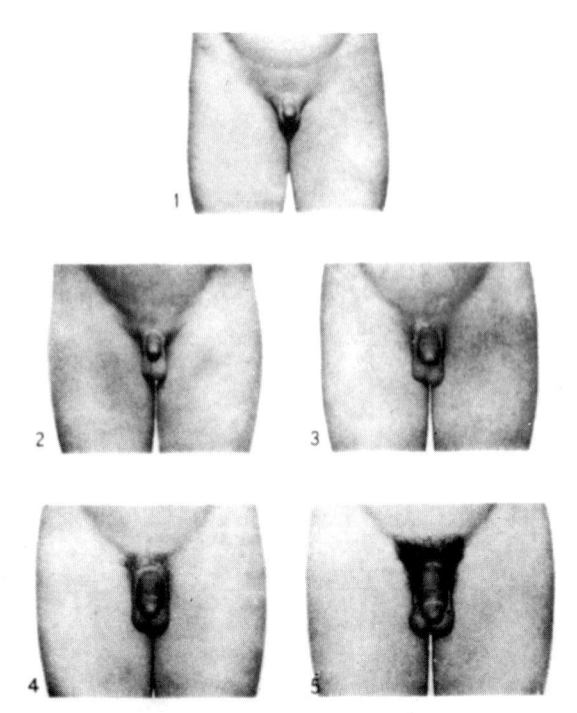

FIGURE 10-16. Stages of male genital growth. (1) The infantile stage which persists until puberty begins. (2) The scrotum has begun to enlarge and become reddened and textured. (3) The penis has increased in length and, to a lesser extent, in breadth. The scrotum has enlarged further. (4) Penile length and breadth have increased further, and the glans has developed. The scrotum has enlarged further and darkened. (5) The genitalia reach adult size and shape. (*From J. M. Tanner, 1962. Used by permission of Blackwell Scientific Publications.*)

boundary awareness increases between ages 5 and 10 years (Fisher and Cleveland, 1958). However, variation in the definiteness of the perceived boundary remains (Fisher, 1973).

Throughout the school years certain body features or changes in the body may provoke concern or be valued. For example, the shedding of deciduous teeth may evoke short-lived fears of loss of integrity. Family attitudes may precipitate overevaluation or derogation of particular body features such as beauty, freckles, or athletic ability (Kolb, 1975). Children from 5 to 12 years reject a child whose body differs from their own and are threatened by confrontation with obvious body deformity (Centers and Centers, 1963; Richardson, 1971).

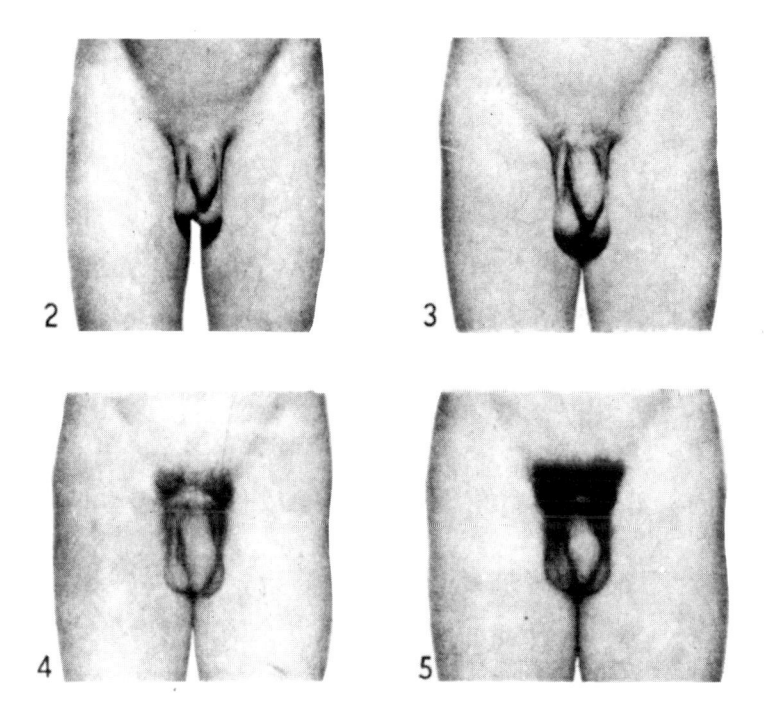

FIGURE 10-17. Stages of pubic hair growth and distribution in boys during puberty from first appearance (stage 2) to adult type (stage 5). (From J. M. Tanner, 1962. Used by permission of Blackwell Scientific Publications.)

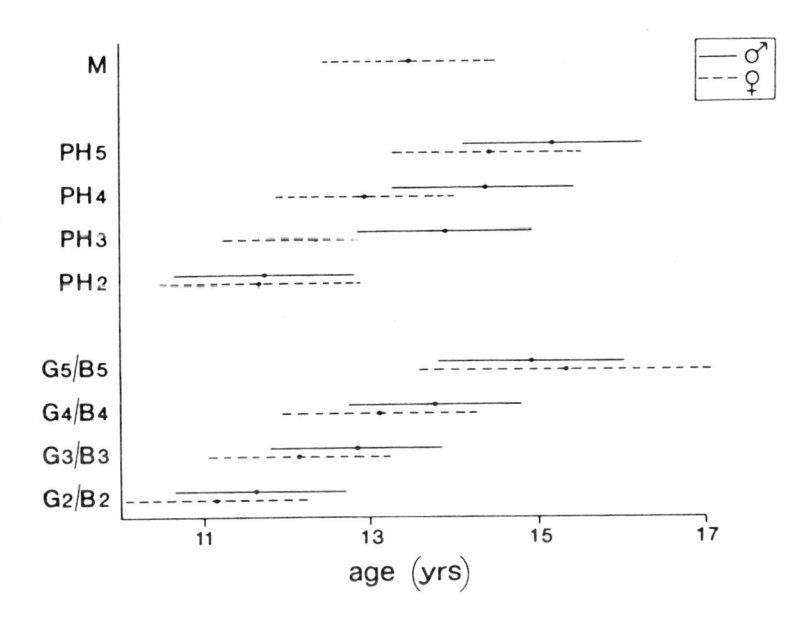

FIGURE 10-18. Variation in age on reaching stages of puberty in boys and girls. PH-2, PH-3, etc., stand for the pubic hair stages; B-2, B-3, etc., stand for the stages of the penis and scrotum; G-2, G-3, etc., stand for the female breast stages; M is menarche. Each horizontal line extends for one standard deviation on either side of the mean. [From W. A. Marshall, Puberty In F. Falkner and J. M. Tanner (Eds.), Human growth 2, Postnatal growth. New York: Plenum, 1978, p. 154. Reprinted by permission of the publisher.]

AWARENESS OF THE CONTENT AND FUNCTION OF THE BODY

By age 10 to 11 years, the child is able to name or draw more than twice as many internal body parts as the 6-year-old. Most frequently named internal body parts are portions of the musculoskeletal, cardiovascular, and central nervous systems (Gellert, 1962; Porter, 1974; Smith, 1977). It is not unusual for a child to give unexpected answers to the question, "What is under your skin?" One 9-year-old boy replied, very seriously, "Rocks. Daddy told me I have rocks in my head!"

Defining the location and structure of internal body parts is more difficult than naming them (see Figs. 10-19 and 10-20). Bones may be drawn by younger children as horizontal lines, circular structures, or long lines with no joints. The heart is usually depicted as a valentine-shaped structure somewhere in the chest. Blood is usually not perceived as contained in blood vessels until the tenth or eleventh year (Porter, 1974).

Children tend to see each part as having an independent and singular function. The purpose of the brain is frequently said "to help you think" (Smith, 1977); the heart, typically believed the most important body part, is "to keep you alive" or "to pump blood"; and the digestive system is a receptacle for food and drink (Gellert, 1962).

Illness experiences may affect the parts of the body named. A 10-year-old boy with chronic renal disease and renal transplantation could name only "blood, urine, and kidneys." Sinuses were included by another 10-year-old who had just had sinus x-rays.

WELLNESS, ILLNESS, AND HOSPITALIZATION

CONCEPT OF HEALTH AND HEALTH BEHAVIOR

The child between 7 and 10 years perceives health differently from the older child. It is suggested that "the general concept of health may be too abstract for the younger child" (Gochman, 1970). The average school-age child continues to need adult supervision in health-maintenance practices regardless of the amount of effort parents have devoted to teaching about such matters. However, when children are separated from their parents, they often proceed to carry out such preventive health behaviors (Freud, 1952).

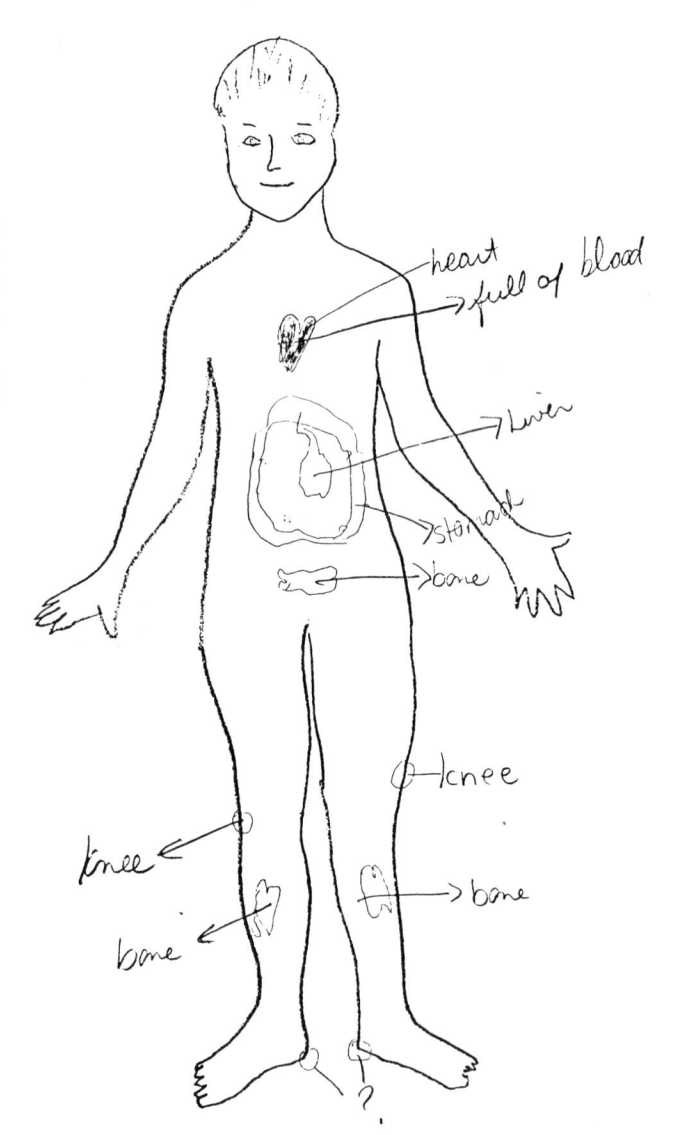

FIGURE 10-19. A 7-year-old boy's drawing in response to, "Draw a picture of what is under your skin."

CONCERNS AND REACTIONS TO ILLNESS AND HOSPITALIZATION

The line between illness and health is poorly defined. Campbell (1975) has demonstrated that children aged 6 to 12 years and their mothers view the same symptoms as indicators of illness, while perception of self as well or ill is a function of increasing maturity. Even the hospitalized child may deny being a sick person while indicating that a particular body part is ill (Shontz, 1975).

The young school-age child's precausal cognition con-

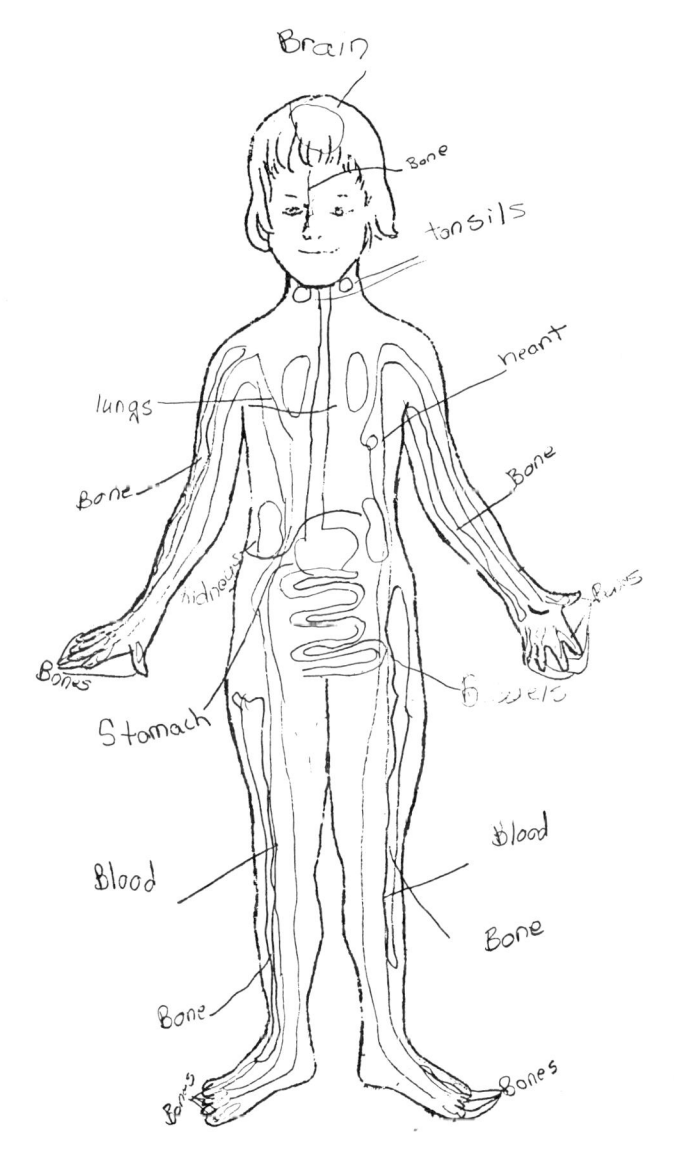

FIGURE 10-20. A 10-year-old girl's drawing in response to, "Draw a picture of what is under your skin."

tributes to his misconceptions that the cause of illness is human misbehavior and illness and treatment are punishments (Nagy, 1951). With increasing age, the child becomes more objective and begins to recognize that there are multiple causations of illness (Nagy, 1951; Peters, 1978).

Mutilation Fears of loss of body integrity and fantasies of mutilation and annihilation are prominent in the hospitalized school-age child (Prugh, 1965). The child can clearly express his expectations, whether or not they are realistic. A 7-year-old's screaming behavior ceased when the nurse corrected the child's misconception that broken legs were treated by "cutting them off." Similarly, children being prepared for surgery frequently verbalize the expectation that the type of knife used is a "butcher knife," that they will waken during surgery, and that too much anesthesia will result in death. Drawings of hospitals often depict expectations of pain, disagreeable procedures, mutilation, and even hostility of health professionals (see Fig. 10-21).

Research indicates that white males are more disturbed by threats to integrity than are females (Fisher, 1973). Boys tend to act out their anxieties in very active and aggressive play, whereas girls may verbalize questions and fears or become very quiet and withdrawn. Both boys and girls sometimes assume the role of "joker" as a means of disguising and managing their anxiety.

School-age children seek opportunities to assure themselves that their bodies are intact. Careful inspection of the part follows any procedure. Often progress toward recovery is measured by the intactness and appearance of the body. For example, a chronically ill 10-year-old demanded a mirror, scrutinized himself for several minutes, and announced he was "gettin' better. My face is gettin' fat and my arms ain't thin like a baby's anymore."

Control of body by self and others Illness, hospital rules, or treatments such as casts or traction may interfere with or prohibit independent functions in areas such as toileting, dressing, and feeding. Loss of such abilities represents an earlier level of function and may be passively accepted or vigorously resisted (Freud, 1952). For example, following his hip disarticulation, a child aged 9 years became extremely passive. For more than a week he insisted that his mother feed him. When he wanted a drink, he folded his arms across his chest and ordered his mother to lift his head and hold the cup for him to drink.

Multiple examinations, treatments, and strange hospital clothing clash with the school-age child's strong sense of modesty. Children whose bodies are frequently exposed for examination or therapy or who have some type of body-altering procedure are often described as having lost their modesty or being exhibitionistic. Actually, their

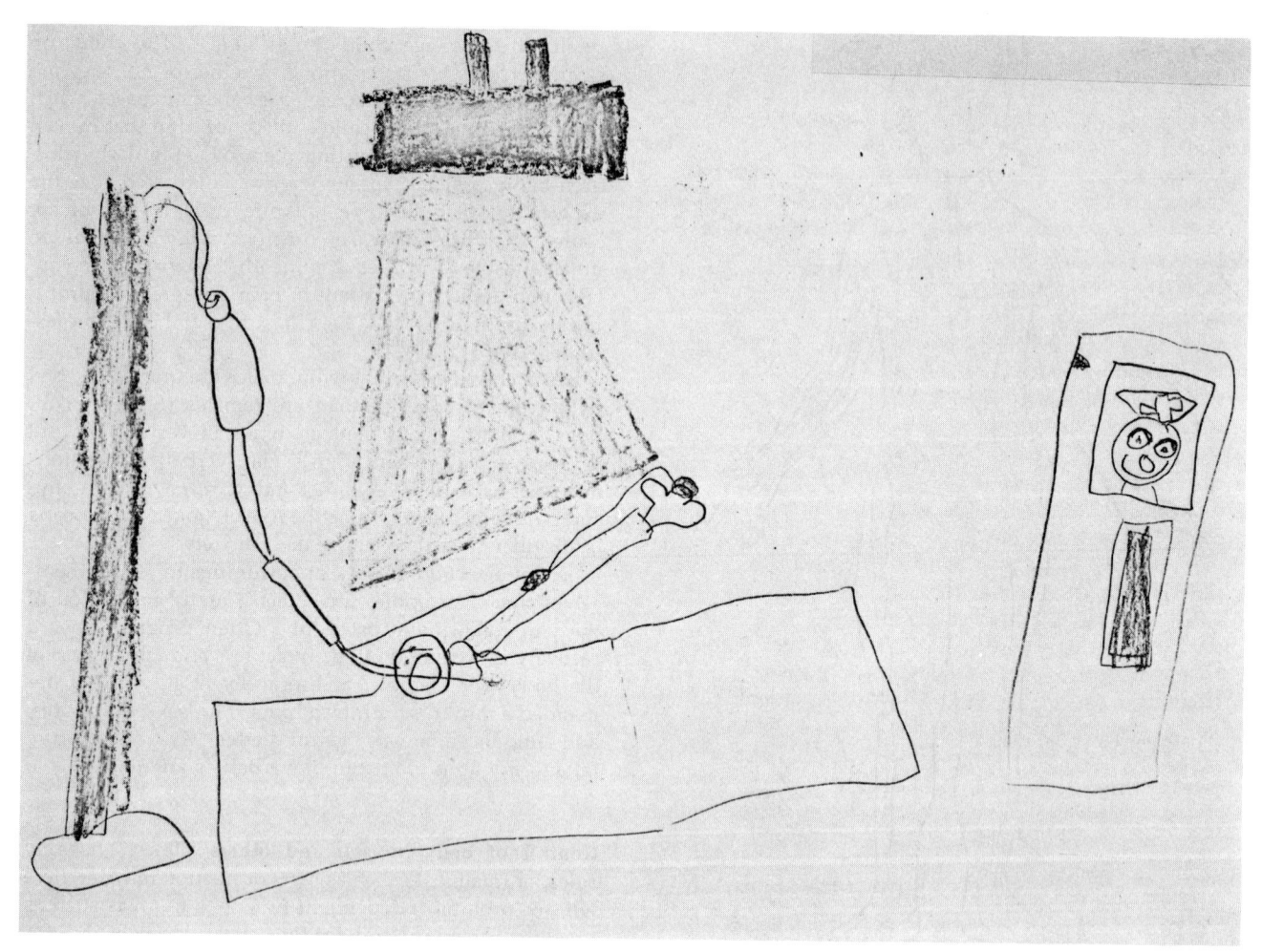

FIGURE 10-21. A 6-year-old boy's school drawing in response to, "Draw a picture about what you think a hospital is like."

behaviors seem to be directed at "testing" the reactions of society in an effort to reestablish a body image.

Mobility Through the school years the child uses vigorous motor activities as outlets for feelings of joy, anger, and fear. Situations which prevent mobility and which threaten future mobility arouse tremendous anxiety.

Core reactions of children who suffered paralytic poliomyelitis have been described as frustration, anxiety, and rage (Bernabeu, 1958). Children subjected to long-term or permanent loss of, or altered, mobility may display similar responses. A 9-year-old boy faced permanent alteration in motor ability through leg amputation. When he was told about the surgery, he screamed "No, no, no, no!" wailed, and quite vigorously protested. Thereafter, he found it almost impossible to tolerate any discussion of the impending surgery. His play was most often with toy soldiers or a plastic knight in armor and involved extremely aggressive fighting and killing.

Predominance of the child's need for mobility is frequently depicted in drawings with many portrayals of motion and wheeled vehicles. The immobilized child's behavior may reflect his feelings of hostility and revenge against adults who are mobile as he begins to use the adults in the environment to render services—"to fetch and carry" (Bernabeu, 1958).

Defense mechanisms seem particularly prevalent in situations which threaten body image and mobility. Denial is most frequently used by younger children who deny negative feelings such as anger or sadness. A 9-year-old boy and a 10-year-old girl responded to leg amputation with these comments: "The leg was no good anyway—all brown and icky" (referring to radiation burns); and "It was God's will."

Withdrawal and suppression are often particularly apparent when mobility is compromised. Television watching becomes a means of withdrawing from situations which stimulate thoughts of loss of mobility. Extensive use of defense mechanisms typically results in the child's affect becoming pleasant but shallow. The distress he feels may break through these defenses in other behaviors. For example, a 10-year-old child, in traction as treatment for a fractured femur, was "pleasant and cooperative." However, his distress seemed to be portrayed in his persistent sitting up and doing exercises, scratching until his leg bandages disintegrated, and being unable to independently play or study at age level.

Disruption of normal activities Illness or hospitalization results in disruption of the child's usual daily patterns and separates him from the increasingly important peer group. In contrast with hospitalized children, healthy children seem not to perceive an illness as a disruptive event which would interfere with social relationships or learning (Brodie, 1974).

Efforts to restore some of the usual activities to the child's daily schedule often result in marked behavioral change. Children seem to interpret routine scheduling of schoolwork or efforts to ensure age-appropriate activity as signals of recovery or at least of staff's expectations that recovery is possible. Following amputation of her leg, a school-age girl was very dependent and fearful, cried or whined frequently, and preferred to remain in bed. Following her involuntary attendance at the hospital school, she showed much less regressive behavior, was more independent, and began "mothering" another very frightened school-age child in the room—telling her what things were or were not reasonable to fear!

Strange environment That the hospital is a strange and frightening place is clear in children's drawings and written material. Frequently the hospital is depicted as a huge building with many windows and occasionally with sad-faced people looking out. A child age 8 years, in a detailed diary of her trip to an outpatient clinic appointment, scrawled: "I HATE to go to Children's Hospital," and "I like Children's Hospital (sometimes)." Children strive to make hospitals more familiar through exploration and observation. Even when recovering from major surgery, they "take in" and remember minute details about such unfamiliar places as intensive care units (Barnes, 1975).

DEATH

The concept of death as permanent and universal develops gradually through the sixth to tenth years. The child tends to personify death and conceives of some external source as causing death (Nagy, 1948). Some seriously or fatally ill children behave as though they fear "someone coming to get them" if they are left alone. An 8-year-old girl with terminal leukemia repeatedly pleaded, "Please don't leave—there's someone out in the hall." On the day of his death, a 10-year-old boy repeatedly referred to an "old man" being on the windowsill or under his bed.

While school-age children can define death as "not alive," they have notions of the dead person living on in some manner underground (Nagy, 1948). Only after age 8 or 9 does the child conceive of death as an inevitable process with complete cessation of body functions (Nagy, 1948; Kastenbaum, 1967). In a discussion about her brother's recent death, a 7-year-old girl and her 8-year-old classmate speculated about what it might be like to be dead. Both expressed opinions that the earth would be cold and itchy and asked, "How can you breathe underground?"

It is during the school years that children with serious illness begin to ask if they are dying. Recent studies have demonstrated that fatally ill children have significantly higher levels of anxiety than other ill children and include more themes of loneliness, separation, and death in their stories. They even attribute their supposedly unknown diagnoses to characters in their stories (Waechter, 1971; Spinetta, Rigler, and Kavon, 1973).

SECTION 2
Behavioral Development

As in the embryologic period and early childhood, physical development of the school-age child is advanced over behavioral development. While final processes of growth, sexual development, and other processes of physical maturation are major physiological occurrences, even more significant behavioral changes must occur from ages 5 to puberty to attain adolescent status of adaptive functioning.

This tremendous development in behavioral competency is discussed in this section.

The school-age child: Age of achievement Mary Tudor

The middle school years, from age 5 to puberty, is an era of achievement. Relatively free from the developmental stress and struggles for autonomy of younger ages, the school-age child has solidified abilities and now applies these to more complex but enjoyable activities at school and play. The major challenge is adaptation to the broader social realm of the school where the child learns about himself through comparison with others and where he is judged by them.

Peer interaction as well as cognitive maturation dispel the egocentric view of the young child, and the school-age child is able to be more objective, to see others' points of view. The school-age child must learn cooperation in peer interaction; at the same time he learns competition in educational, sports, and social areas. And through daily frustrations he must learn to cope, without parental intervention.

Gender identity is more sharply defined and more important. School-age children play in same-sex groups and determine many of their interests along sex-stereotyped dimensions. The child also matures in the greater realm of social interaction as he internalizes society's moral codes.

The school-age child's quest for achievement dominates these years. The child at this age is a doer. He is engaged in multiple activities alone, with one or two friends, or in a club, formal or "secret." His refined motor skills allow endless elaboration and experimentation. Skateboarding, top-speed bicycling, swimming, and playing baseball are abilities that will be developed during these years. Cooperative games, such as tag, hide-and-seek, and kick the can, are also favorites of younger children. Soon, formal sports with agreed-upon rules and logic will have more interest.

The school-age child is a maker and a collector. Constructing models, cutting out snowflakes, and making a pencil holder for mom or a birdhouse for dad consume much time. How well his projects are received by others is important to the child's self-esteem. Collections are also a source of great pride and energy; baseball cards, comic books, beer cans, and stamps are treasures to the school-age child. Prehension skills are smoothed during the school years, allowing more rapid and precise movements.

The school-age child meets intense demands in formal education; the academic process is a new challenge. The child is capable of logical thinking but remains reality based. His mental processing is concrete and systematic. The verbal language skills, so easy as a preschooler, take on new meaning and form as they are read and written.

Immersed in activities in peer company, the school-age child uses relative successes and failures to judge his competency. He compares himself with others in terms of his motor and educational achievements. Can he run as fast, draw as well, or read aloud as rapidly? He also validates himself through the reactions of other children. How well is he liked? How many other children consider him their friend? Who wants to sit with him at lunchtime? School years are a time for these discoveries.

More and more, the school-age child seeks time away from parents: time with peers. The child no sooner arrives home from school than he is off to play with neighborhood children. Later, he may leave just to "mess around." Alone time is also sought as the school-age child pursues a hobby or escapes in reading or television. The doors to separate places are often closed behind him.

Soon, the school-age child will be catapulted by bodily changes into a new era with emotional and social stresses not experienced since the toddler ages. In comparison with adolescence, the middle school years may be seen as the calm before the tempest.

In the meantime, the child is an endless achiever, and in the successes he experiences, he begins to discover who he is.

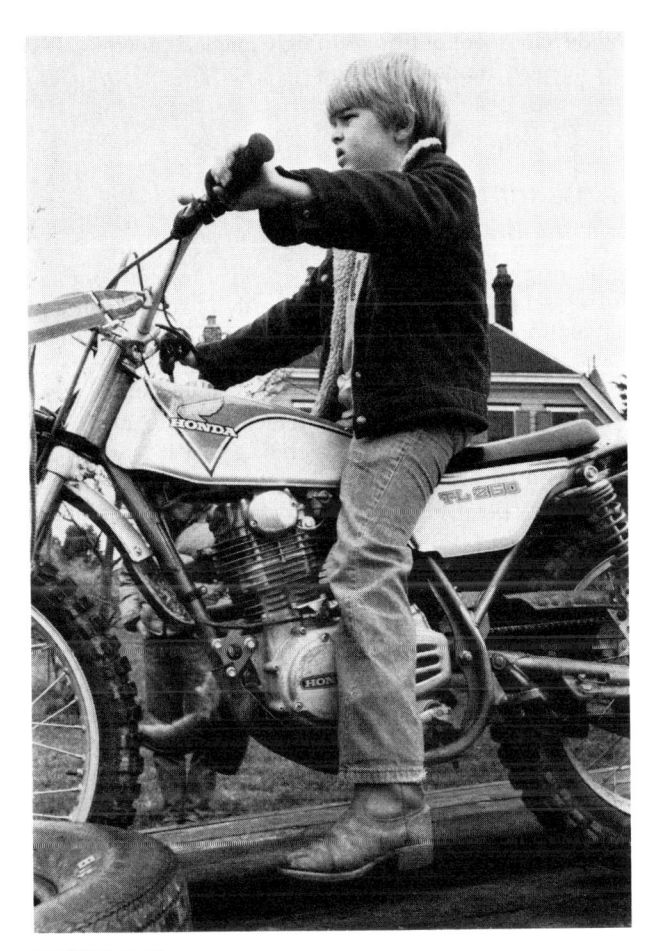

FIGURE 10-22.

Behavioral Development by Functional Area

Perceptual development   Veronica A. Binzley

Success in school requires a good deal of perceptual control and sophistication from the child. First and most important, the child must be able to focus his attention for sustained periods of time, and often this must be done in the face of attractive and distracting stimuli. Second, if the child is ever to experience any kind of academic success, he must learn to read. To do so requires a good deal of complex perceptual processing which the adult reader often fails to appreciate.

The complexity of this task has only recently come to the attention again of experimental psychologists who have begun to study the many subtasks involved in successfully learning to read (Gibson and Levin, 1975). At the very least, the child must learn to identify the letters of the alphabet, learn the rules for how letters are put together to make words, and then learn how words are sequentially ordered into sentences and paragraphs. In addition there are symbols which are specific to the written code, such as periods, commas, and exclamation points, that the child must learn to recognize and must respond to appropriately. The following discussion on perceptual processing in reading draws heavily on the findings of Gibson and Levin.

PERCEPTUAL PROCESSING IN READING

EYE MOVEMENT

Studies of eye movements in reading have found these movements to be specific to reading and not predictive of strategies used in other visual tasks. In reading the eyes move across the page in a "hopping" fashion, temporarily fixating on various words as the text is read. These eye movements are called *saccadic* and are usually analyzed into two components: the movement itself and the pause or fixation. Another ocular variable in reading is the regression movement, which is a saccade to a previously read part of the text. Hence, readers can vary in terms of number of pauses, length of pauses, length of movements between pauses, and number of regression movements they make while reading.

It has been reported that an average reader spends 6 percent of his time in eye movements and 94 percent in fixation pauses. Of course, these values differ depending on the nature of the reading material as pauses in reading are reflective of the difficulty of the text. Notwithstanding these differences, eye-movement behaviors do show a developmental trend. Fixation frequency, duration of pauses, and number of regressions decrease markedly from the first to the fourth grades, but thereafter few changes are noted. Good readers differ in almost all measures of eye movements from their less skilled peers.

DETECTION OF GRAMMATICAL STRUCTURE

Until fairly recently, most teachers and even the few interested researchers have viewed a beginning-reader's errors as perceptual inaccuracies or lack of knowledge rather than an indication of the reader's expectations based on his knowledge of grammatical constraints. When the reading errors of two classes of first-grade children were examined for their grammatical structure and preservation of meaning up to the point of error, the sentences with errors were found to be grammatical 90 percent of the time. The few ungrammatical errors were found to be graphically more similar to the printed text than errors that maintained the meaning to the point of error. Thus, it seems that the beginning reader is sensitive to both the grammatical and graphic constraints of a text but, at the beginning stages of reading, is unable to integrate the two sources of information. Presumably, with experience the child is able to integrate the two strategies: graphic and grammatical constraints.

Studies using the eye-voice span (EVS) method have also provided evidence about perceptual processing of written texts. The EVS is the distance, usually measured in words, that the eyes are ahead of the voice. The EVS is determined by covering the text at some predetermined point and asking the child to report as much of the text in advance of his voice as he can. Consistently these studies have reported that the EVS increases with age and is readily affected by the difficulty of the material. When unstructured word lists are used, the EVS is fairly small and remains constant across all ages. wbut when structured grammatical material is used, it is significantly larger.

A study (Levin and Turner, 1968) using this technique examined responses to determine the unit of decoding in reading. It was found that all ages except second graders end their EVSs at phrase boundaries well beyond the chance level. In addition the tendency to chunk oral reading in phrase units did not significantly increase between the fourth grade and adulthood.

To summarize, the data from the EVS studies indicate that the detection of grammatical and syntactical structure is an important perceptual task in learning to read, and this perceptual task appears to be fairly well mastered by fourth grade (9 years of age). However, exactly how a reader progresses toward processing higher-order and more complex material is not clear.

By 10 years of age the average child has become very adept and efficient at extracting information from his surroundings. He can focus his attention, filtering out irrelevant information in order to rapidly detect the meaningful, sometimes complex patterns of stimulation, and he has essentially mastered the written and spoken communication systems of his culture. However, much about the development of this seemingly magical process called *perception* remains unknown.

Gross motor development
Fay F. Russell and Beverly R. Richardson

As during the preschool years, gross motor development during school years consists primarily of refinement and elaboration of previously acquired skills. Neuromuscular maturation continues but to a much less dramatic degree with changes being few and subtle. Reflexive patterns remain essentially the same, and the process of myelinization continues with many theorizing that it is generally completed by about 8 years.

The nervous system does demonstrate maturation as nerve impulses resulting in unwanted movements can be inhibited, thereby increasing the child's ability to control his movements. This improvement in control along with the increase in muscle size and strength enables the child to further refine his gross motor skills.

How he performs in organized sports as well as unstructured play with peers is critical to the school-age child. Because of the tremendous variety of rate of maturation, body build, and basic ability in the school-age population, children are slower or faster, more clumsy or more agile, and weaker or stronger. Bicycle races, climbing or running, competitive sports such as softball or football, or other tests of others' and one's own abilities are often seen in these years. Those who are good in gross motor skills are picked first when choosing teams. Being poor in these skills and being chosen last is a difficult social experience for the school-age child.

GROSS MOTOR SKILL DEVELOPMENT
The school-age child builds further on those skills he acquired during the preschool years and earlier periods. As skill acquisition is based on past skill development and provides the foundation for future skill development, gross motor development of the child is considered during each year through the school-age period.

The 5-year-old possesses greater strength, coordination, and balance than the 4-year-old. This, in combination with his improved ability to reason, enables him to perform gross motor tasks with greater skill and precision. He uses many of his skills in organized sports or informal play. Major accomplishments include the ability to run up and down stairs, run skillfully, throw a ball well assuming an adult stance, balance on one foot for 8 to 10 s, jump from greater heights with more skill, hop well on one

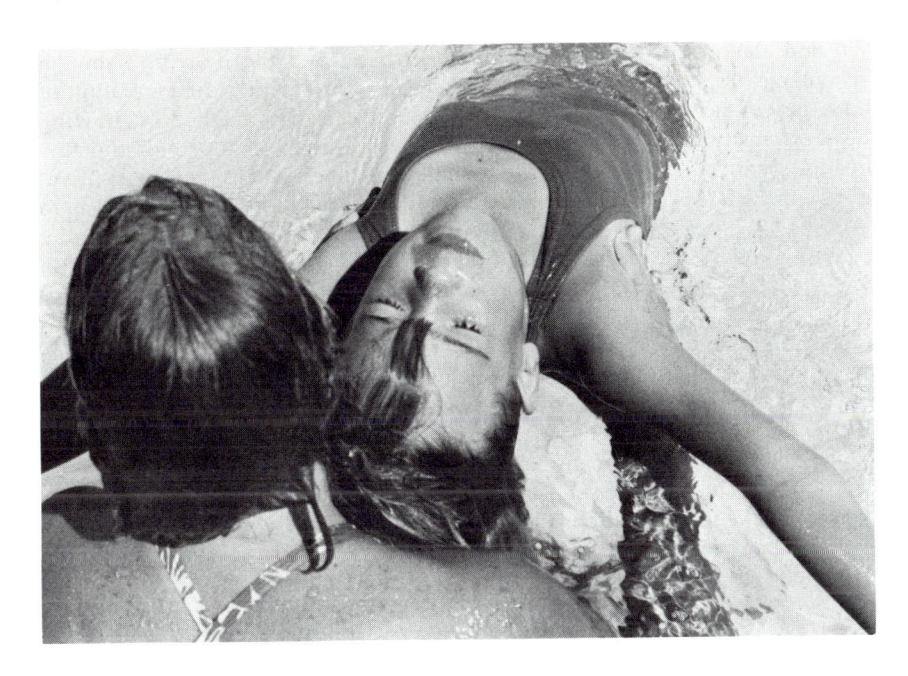

FIGURE 10-23.

foot, climb skillfully, skip alternating feet, jump rope, and roller-skate.

Constant motion is characteristic of the 6-year-old; he enjoys physical activity immensely but may demonstrate some clumsiness due to fatigue. There is noticeable improvement in his balance, and his arm and leg movements are well coordinated. The 6-year-old continues to demonstrate increased skill in climbing, hopping, jumping, skipping, and throwing and catching a ball. Increased opportunity to practice such skills in structured recreation as part of his education facilitates this development. He may begin performing more complex stunts such as high jumping and broad jumping; he may learn to ride a bicycle and a skateboard.

The 7-year-old is graceful, speedy, and agile. He enjoys games which allow him to sit and rest, but he also experiences sudden spurts of active behavior. Sex differentiation, primarily in muscle size and strength, will not occur until puberty; thus, differentiation in activities is social, both peer- and parentally influenced.

The 8-year-old enjoys playing ball, jumping rope, hiking, swimming, dancing, climbing trees, riding bicycles, and organized games and sports. The 9- and 10-year-olds demonstrate great skill in their performance of gross motor activities and enjoy displaying this skill. They are very competitive and demonstrate improved timing and well-developed hand-eye coordination.

By his twelfth birthday, the child has perfected all basic gross motor skills. The pubertal growth spurt may result in temporary loss of some agility. Hands and feet enter the growth spurt first, possibly resulting in some clumsiness. Increased body size must be rapidly adapted to as must the self-consciousness which usually accompanies such changes.

The school-age child needs regular exercise; participation in gross motor activities, such as those mentioned above, promotes development of strength, balance, and coordination resulting in perfection of basic gross motor movements by the end of the school-age period. Supervised games with his peer group are of prime value in terms of gross motor skills as well as being socially important to the school-age child. Now, many avenues of gross motor refinement are open: gymnastics, ballet, and organized sports, as well as vocational skills to name only a few. Thus, some adolescents will continue gross motor "development"; others will not.

During the first 3 years of life, the child acquires most of the basic gross motor skills according to the principles of gross motor development with refinement and elaboration occurring during the preschool and school-age years. By the time he reaches his twelfth birthday he has perfected most gross motor skills and made the transition from helpless neonate to independent preadolescent.

Fine motor development
Barbara Newcomer McLaughlin and Nancy L. Morgan

The preschool period brought ease and economy of effort in fine motor skill development. Previous knowledge of basic relationships and perceptual ability became more meaningful as the child expressed feelings and conceptions through fine motor activity in ways which were not yet possible through the child's verbal abilities. Fine motor development that occurs during the school years reflects changes indicative of what previously has occurred and what will occur in adolescence (Gesell and Ilg, 1946).

The 5-year-old's coordination has reached a new maturity as he approaches an object directly, prehends it precisely, and releases it with dispatch. The child shows good precision with tools and is readily able to brush his teeth, comb his hair, and wash his face. By this time the child can manipulate those buttons on clothes which he can see, and can lace his shoes.

Likewise, he is able to utilize a crayon with greater assurance and definite movement. He begins to draw a recognizable human figure, and the drawing shows a completeness from head to feet with a differentiation of parts including eyes and ears. His method of drawing aims at realism and something definite with the first stroke of the pencil. The 5-year-old is more executive, more sensible, more accurate, more relevant, and more practical than the younger child. He has the least difficulty with vertical strokes and the most with oblique. He still has difficulty copying a diamond, but a square and triangle are done easily. The child at this age enjoys manipulating sand and molding objects with clay. He likes to color within lines and to cut and paste simple things, but he is not yet adept with these skills. As the 5-year-old progresses to $5\frac{1}{2}$, he may still appear awkward in many of his manipulations. He usually shows an interest in learning to print his own first name and in underlining capitals and words in a familiar book (Gesell and Ilg, 1946).

The 6-year-old child makes a good start in many performances, but he needs some assistance and direction to complete the activity. The child performs eye-hand functions with less speed at 6 than at 5. Though the 6-year-old usually makes a more deliberate approach and tries to work more accurately, at times he will work with a careless approach. He often asks, "What do you do with

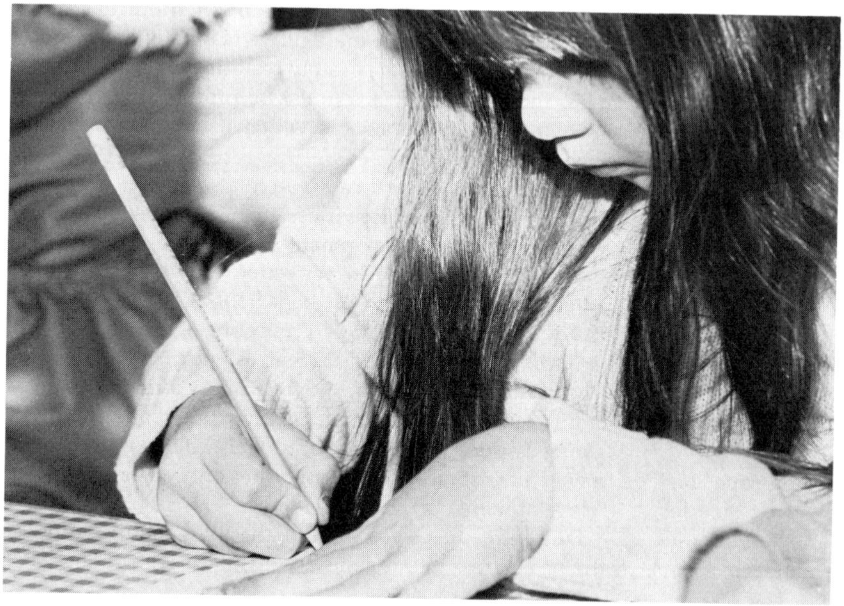

FIGURE 10-24. (*Photo courtesy of Betsy Smith.*)

this?" as he handles and explores materials and wants to do everything.

The 6-year-old is easily distracted by the environment in the process of utilizing tools and materials. He enjoys cutting and pasting as he makes books and boxes. At this age he can learn to print capital letters, though he commonly reverses them. He has the ability to attempt sewing with a large needle, making large stitches. In carpentry the child can make crude structures, though he needs plenty of assistance because saws will jam and bend and the hammer will often miss the head of the nail (Gesell and Ilg, 1946).

By 7 years, the child's manipulation of tools is somewhat more tense than at 6, but there is also more persistence evident. He grips the pencil tightly and often close to the point; the pressure is variable but apt to be heavy. The 7-year-old develops interest in comparative sizes; the height of capital and small letters is becoming more uniform though they may taper uniformly as he proceeds across a page. The child can print several sentences with the letters getting smaller toward the end of each line. There are individual differences in the size of printing—some children print very small, while others continue to make very large letters. The 7-year-old has much less problem staying with his task in spite of the environment than does the 6-year-old as he becomes more absorbed in what he is doing. However, the 7-year-old is still likely to touch and manipulate everything he sees (Gesell and Ilg, 1946).

By 8 years of age there is an increase in speed and smoothness of eye-hand performance. The approach and grasp are rapid, smooth, and sometimes even graceful, and the release is sure and easy. The child now holds pencils, brushes, and tools less tensely than at 7 years. By 8 years the child writes or prints all letters and numbers accurately, maintaining fairly uniform alignment, slant, and spacing. He is also beginning to develop perspective in drawing; he is able to draw action figures in good proportion (Gesell and Ilg, 1946).

The eyes and hands are well differentiated in 9- to 12-year-olds, and they can generally use their two hands quite independently. There is, by this time, a wide individual variation in skills, and the child is usually definitely either skillful or awkward with his hands. The child knows how to use garden tools and is able to handle them appropriately. Handwriting has now become a tool for expression, and the child will write for long periods, particularly enjoying making extended lists and categorizing his collections.

The 9-year-old begins to sketch in his drawings, which are often quite detailed. Movements tend to be more restrictive than at 8 years of age, and the 9-year-old enjoys still life, portrait, or poster painting. Maps and designs also hold particular intrigue at this age. He sketches lines with short strokes and much detail, and there is an atmosphere of concentration about his work (Gesell and Ilg, 1946).

During the school years, the child's fine motor development reflects the ability to use "tools" in a manner of meaningful personal expression and also reflects changes indicative of what previously has occurred and what will occur in adolescence.

Cognitive development Virginia Pidgeon

The school-age child at his desk pouring over his homework with pursed lips seems immersed in cognitive activity. He appears to be a scientific and orderly young thinker whose mind yields surprising and illuminating items of information. The horizons of his world are large, and he ponders outer space and the colonization of his country.

What changes in cognitive development occur in the school-age years? What explains the metamorphosis into ordered, objective thinking from the egocentric, fantasy-ridden thought of the preschool child? The school-age child is remarkable for his systematic concrete thinking. Reason and logic now dominate his perceptions, and he no longer believes whatever he sees.

The school-age child is immersed in actual, concrete reality and is not yet able to deal with the hypothetical, or theoretical. The metaphorical meanings of proverbs escape him. Asked to interpret the proverb "A stitch in time saves nine," a 9-year-old responded: "Like if you had a broken hand, you stitch it, like if someone got hurt, say, like a 9-year-old he needed stitches" (Church and Stone, 1973, p. 392).

Various facets of the cognitive development of the school-age child—the development of objectivity, logical operations, object concepts, and causal thinking—will be considered below.

OBJECTIVITY
The school-age child moves from egocentric to objective thinking. He becomes aware of his own thought processes and his subjectivity. He also becomes aware of and values the points of view of others and realizes that they may differ from or coincide with his own. Repeated social interactions and arguments with other children force him

into awareness of his own and others' points of view. Now taking into account his own subjectivity, he questions and seeks to validate and clarify his beliefs. Reality is now conceived as that which is consensual or common to all points of view. As he takes in the points of view of other children, he becomes capable of social cooperation and teamwork.

LOGICAL OPERATIONS

The school-age child acquires a set, or system, of concrete, logical mental operations which he applies to the process of understanding and organizing reality. These mental operations are concrete in the sense that they are directed toward the organization of actual reality rather than hypothetical or theoretical reality. They are organized in a system of mental operations that are integrated and related. Among other mental operations they include addition, subtraction, multiplication, division, ranking or seriation, setting two series of objects into a one-to-one correspondence, and operations on classes of objects.

By contrast the mental operations of the preschool child are isolated, intuitive, and unsystematic. Counting his pennies, he performs an isolated mental operation. The school-age child intending to buy a comic book counts his capital and the cost, subtracts the cost, and calculates the remainder. He perceives addition and subtraction as related and reciprocal mental operations within a system that includes other mental operations.

The school-age child performs a set of logical mental operations on the elements of a group in the knowledge that a group possesses the properties of *associativity, composition, reversibility,* and *identity*. These group properties are essentially algebraic concepts. According to Piaget (1965), the school-age child understands these concepts and is able to apply them. He understands that associativity means that the elements of a group can be combined in any order and the final result is the same.

$$a \times (b \times c) = (a \times b) \times c$$

He understands that identity means that within a set of elements there is only one element, the identity element, that when combined with any other element of the group, does not change that element.

$$a \times 1 = a \quad \text{and} \quad a + 0 = a$$

The school-age child can also perform another set of logical mental operations on groups which he knows have a *lattice structure* and lattice properties (a logic concept). A group has a lattice structure when a particular relation exists between two or more of its elements. That relation is that there is a smallest element that includes both elements and a largest element that is included in both. Consider this hierarchy:

Trees = deciduous + others

Trees is the smallest element that includes both, and *deciduous* is the largest element that is included in both.

Given an understanding of lattice properties, the school-age child can combine classes to form a supraordinate class and break down a supraordinate class into its

FIGURE 10-25.

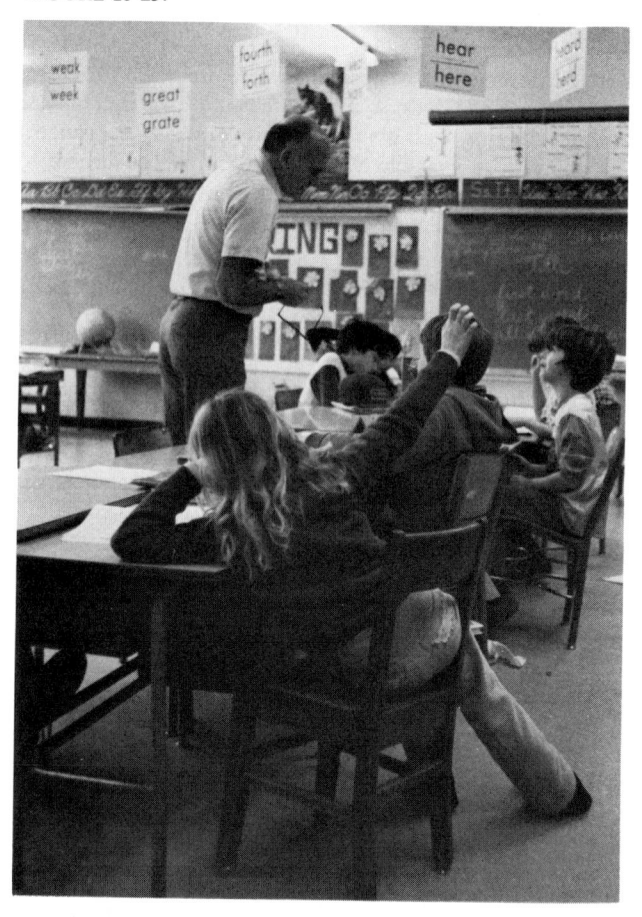

subclasses. He understands a hierarchy like

> Humans + anthropoid apes = anthropoids

and

> Anthropoids + others = primates

Given the problem

> Primates − others = ?

he can figure out the answer: anthropoids or humans and anthropoid apes. The school-age child also understands the equivalence of different subgroupings of elements within a group. He realizes that

> Spaniels + nonspaniels = terriers + nonterriers
> = beagles + nonbeagles
> = domestic dogs

Basic to these operations is the ability of the older child to grasp a classificatory structure. Notable also is the ease with which he composes and decomposes classes.

The older child's ability to compose and decompose classes is reflected in the strategy he uses in playing the game of twenty questions. Six-year-olds playing the game of twenty questions in an experimental situation used the strategy of hypothesis scanning almost exclusively. They simply asked a series of unrelated questions each of which tested hypothesis, or guess, about what the object was ("Is it a hammer?"). Eight-year-olds first asked constraint-seeking questions and then quickly switched to questions testing hypotheses. A constraint-seeking question is a general question that groups a large number of possibilities into two classes in one of which lies the correct answer ("Is it a tool?"). Eleven-year-olds used many constraint-seeking questions before venturing final hypothesis guesses. The use of constraint-seeking questions by older children reflects their ability to organize objects into a hierarchy and to narrow down the possibilities by ruling out whole classes of objects.

OBJECT CONCEPTS

The school-age child develops object concepts that embrace the multiple characteristics of objects and distinguish between their essential and nonessential characteristics. His object concepts reflect his increasing ability to decenter, or perceive the multiple characteristics of objects rather than one or two striking features. He may define a germ as something small, like a dot, that is everywhere, that may or may not make you sick, and against which your tonsils protect you. Consequently he recognizes objects despite perceptual changes or variations in their appearance, and the object world is to him more stable than to the preschool child.

Reason and logic rather than perception now dominate his conceptualization of objects in the physical world. His acquisition of the concept of conservation—that the mass, weight, and volume of objects remain constant despite perceptual variations in their appearance—is an example. Roll one of two identical Plasticine balls into a sausage shape, and ask the child if the balls are the same or if one is larger. The 6- to 8-year-old replies either that it is larger or smaller. The older child answers that they are the same. Contributing to his understanding of conservation is decentration and the ability to focus on transformations rather than on successive states of a phenomenon.

CAUSAL THINKING

School-age children slowly shift from precausal to causal thinking and now differentiate between physical, or mechanical, and psychological, or motivational, causes of natural phenomena and events. Though their theories about the causation of natural phenomena and events increasingly involve physical, or mechanical, causes, overtones of psychological causation linger on. Asked why the clouds move, some children said that the clouds set themselves in motion and then were driven by air produced by their movement. Other children replied that the wind pushed the clouds. The following explanation by a 10-year-old boy of the causation of diabetes is tinged with remnants of precausal thinking:

> When I was about 4, I went to visit my grandfather. He usually gave me candy. The shock of his dying and my grandmother dying is partly the cause, I think. Sometimes my dad would have candy on the table. Sometimes I'd take a piece.

School-age children also form and describe chains of intermediary events between cause and effect in which there is implicit the recognition that each event is the result of the preceding and the cause of the following event. Creeping into the older child's causal thinking is the realization that cause-and-effect sequences are reversible, for example, that a stone is made of particles of dirt and can be decomposed again into earth.

In summary, the thinking of the school-age child is systematic, concrete, and logical. He has developed objectivity and is aware of his own and others' points of view. He has acquired an integrated system of logical and reciprocal mental operations which he applies to elements in a group and to class hierarchies. These mental operations are concrete and focus on actual reality rather than the domain of the hypothetical, or theoretical. He can perform mental operations on the elements of a group using algebraic theorems and can also combine classes to form a supraordinate class and break down a supraordinate class into its subclasses.

The object concepts of the school-age child incorporate the multiple characteristics of objects and their essential and nonessential features. Reason and logic rather than perception now dominate his concepts of objects, and he perceives their constancy despite perceptual variations. The school-age child shifts from precausal to causal thinking and distinguishes between physical, or mechanical, and psychological causation, though remnants of precausal thinking remain.

Self-help skill development Doris Julian

The school-age period marks the transition from home to a broader environment with school becoming the significant influence on the child. This period will provide the child with an opportunity and expectation of practicing and adapting self-care skills to a situation outside the home.

The 5-year-old child has some proficiency in basic self-help skills of eating, eliminating, dressing, and grooming; self-direction will be beginning, but not complete, in terms of initiating these skills. The ability to contribute to maintenance of individual possessions and to help with household chores is present. Of significance, also, is the child's acquisition of essential survival skills. The 6- to 7-year-old has within his repertoire of behavior strategies skills for assisting himself or manipulating the environment to meet primary needs of food, clothing, and shelter. Further refinement of these skills and of the ability to discriminate dangers or threats will continue during the school-age period.

Discussion of the self-help skills of this age group focuses on progress in basic skills of eating, toileting, dressing, and grooming. Preparation for puberty, specifically menstrual hygiene for girls, is also a grooming task. In addition, the contribution of chores in the home, school, and community as preparation for independent functioning is presented.

MOTOR OR MATURATIONAL FACTORS

Middle-childhood years are characterized by slow, steady growth ending in a pubertal growth spurt. This relatively stable period permits consolidation of maturational gains of earlier years and qualitative refinement of earlier skills. Gains in stature, strength, and motor performance are significant during childhood years. The school-age period is especially characterized by development in language and cognition.

Children of this age are also able to withhold or delay immediate responses to situations. This permits weighing alternatives and making discriminations. This ability provides a strong basis for acquisition of self-help skills in later school years.

SOCIALIZATION OR BEHAVIORAL FACTORS

As noted by Strommen, McKinney, and Fitzgerald (1977), neurophysiological maturation is a prerequisite for the development of certain behaviors but does not guarantee their appearance. The importance of such factors as experience, motivation, and practice is stressed. The significance of these factors is borne out in the school years.

Entry into a setting outside the home provides both opportunity and motivation to practice self-care skills that require independent initiation and implementation. Peers and teachers expect and reinforce the school-age child's self-direction in caring for himself. Peers as reinforcing agents have been the subject of numerous studies. Hetherington and Parke (1975) noted home and background factors contributing to reinforcement patterns of children. In the United States, parental reinforcement patterns were carried over in their children's behavior. Fishbach (1973) compared social-class differences noting that middle-class Caucasian children used a greater amount of positive reinforcement than children from lower-economic-status families.

Modeling social behaviors and skills is another valuable contribution of a peer group. As Piaget (1951) has inferred, capacity for imitation of others is related to age and will show an increase over time. The child encountering difficulties with complex tasks, such as tying shoes, may find great value in a skill demonstration by a peer.

Teachers are significant adults, and their guidance and approval encourage the child's continuing development in self-care. It has been recognized, however, that girls may fare better than boys in securing this approval in the school setting, possibly because the teacher is more likely to be female. If the teacher is male, encouragement provided boys may be improved, according to a study by Lee and Wolinsky (1973).

The sex of adults in the child's environment has relevance to the home and wider community as well as to the school. During the school years, the child is frequently involved in youth organizations such as the YMCA, the YWCA, the Scouts, and church groups. Although studies of parent-child relationships cannot be specifically applied to group situations outside and home, the mode of interaction which has been established contributes to an understanding of children's task learning.

Some studies identify differential behavior between child-to-father and child-to-mother interaction (Osofsky and O'Connell, 1972). In one study, girls of 4 to 6 years spent more time working on an activity with their fathers and with their mothers spent more time talking and requesting help. Elementary school children of both sexes described their father as teacher, disciplinarian, and protector in a study by Thomas (1968).

PROGRESS IN SELF-CARE SKILLS

FEEDING
By the age of 7 or 8 years, the child has the ability to use a knife for cutting meat. All tools for eating can be used efficiently and neatly. Simple meals, such as sandwiches, soup, or cereal, can be prepared for self and others. The child by age 9 or 10 can follow recipes for baking and cooking.

TOILETING
For most children, probably 90 percent, bowel and bladder control for both day and night have been achieved by the age of 6. Toileting includes other skills such as manipulating clothing, wiping, flushing, and hand cleansing. These are within the 6-year-old's capabilities. Continued awareness of male-female differences are present in these years; parents need to provide simple and accurate information.

DRESSING
Children entering school typically have mastered the skills required in dressing and undressing if simple garments are provided. Motor planning and coordination for fine movements continue to improve throughout the school years. The complex skill of tying shoes requires further maturation and may not be accomplished until the child is 6½ years or older.

Later-developing skills include ability to select clothing appropriate for activities and weather conditions. This discrimination and judgment appear late in the middle school years. Caring for clothing can range from helping with laundry to mending and can be introduced to a child in graduated steps. Assisting a parent in making clothing purchases is a useful activity for school-age children.

GROOMING
Although attention and motivation for careful grooming will vary considerably in the period between 6 and 12 years of age, hand skill and discrimination abilities are present. The 6- to 7-year-old might be expected to give himself a complete bath. The 7- to 8-year-old can use brush, comb, and toothbrush with competence. Because of the importance of permanent teeth, parents may wish to offer occasional toothbrushing assistance or provide "disclosure tablets" to ensure thoroughness.

ENVIRONMENTAL MAINTENANCE
The school-age child has abilities and knowledge which can make him a helpful assistant to the parent. Gesell, Ilg, Ames, and Rodell (1974) note that the 8-year-old may do tasks if rewarded but not for the sake of helping or home upkeep. Thus, an allowance or special privileges may increase interest in tasks. Children of this age may also seek jobs in the neighborhood with the intent of earning money. As he receives money, the child also learns to spend it. This is an important self-help skill for the school-age child, and the opportunity should be given. Purchases cannot always be judged by adult standards, and choices should not be ridiculed.

The 9- or 10-year-old child may be helpful with younger siblings and occasionally assume brief responsibility for them. The ability to plan and carry through a task with minimal guidance is an expectation of middle childhood. The attitudes and skills established during this period are prerequisites for future vocational success.

The preceding summary of self-care skills presents some of the highlights of accomplishments of this developmental period. It is by no means inclusive, and wide variation can be expected in all children. Individual abilities, opportunities, and family and societal expectations are variables affecting skill acquisition.

PREPARATION FOR NEXT LEVEL OF SKILL
As each level of skill in self-care is achieved, it serves as a foundation for the next. Adults working with the school-age child have the dual responsibility of assisting in age-level task accomplishments and preparing for the needs of

the next developmental period. For the school-age child such preparation will include anticipation of puberty for both girls and boys. Typically, girls and boys of 9 and 10 have displayed interest in physiological and anatomic changes in themselves and other youngsters. This can serve as a cue for the provision of appropriate information about sexual development. Changing needs in the area of grooming can be introduced at this time.

The school-age years can provide excellent preparation for skills needed for survival in society. Survival requires knowledge and ability in meeting basic physical needs, avoiding dangers, and finding a means for self-maintenance. A child who can care for himself completely, communicate intelligibly, and demonstrate knowledge of the purchasing or bartering system of society has acquired basic survival skills.

The years between 5 and 12 provide time and opportunity for refinement of skills essential for self-care. Knowledge and understanding of application of skills to environments outside the home are acquired during this period. Further development of skills receives significant support and encouragement by peers, teachers, and youth leaders. During the middle school years, the child is able to demonstrate competence in tasks of home and school. These abilities provide the foundation for independent functioning within society.

Social development Susan Blanch Meister

BASIS FOR SOCIALIZATION
During these years, the context of socialization acquires an entirely new component: school. The child has a new source of approval and direction: the teacher. Peer relations now involve longer periods of time as well as an element of social comparison. Relations with parents continue, but the nature of those relations changes.

Parents of school-age children experience a shift of position. Prior to school entry, they were the central source of approval, direction, and social comparison. When the child enters school, the parents are no longer in a position to control and validate a large proportion of social experience. They assume a role of coaching; the child must now stand as an individual and independently participate in many social processes while the parents become advisers and directors.

GOALS OF SOCIALIZATION
The social context of school places a premium upon achievement and mastery, or what Erikson (1963) calls industry. The continuing social context of the family places a premium upon types of ethnic and cultural characteristics. The school attends primarily to the goals of the larger society, and the family attends primarily to those of the smaller society. The goals of socialization of school-age children are to mediate the two realms in a manner which will promote attainment of abilities, motivation, and capabilities useful to life cycle development.

PROCESSES INVOLVED IN SOCIALIZATION

MORAL INTERNALIZATION
Several principles of moral internalization are relevant to this age group. Disciplinary encounters communicate

FIGURE 10-26.

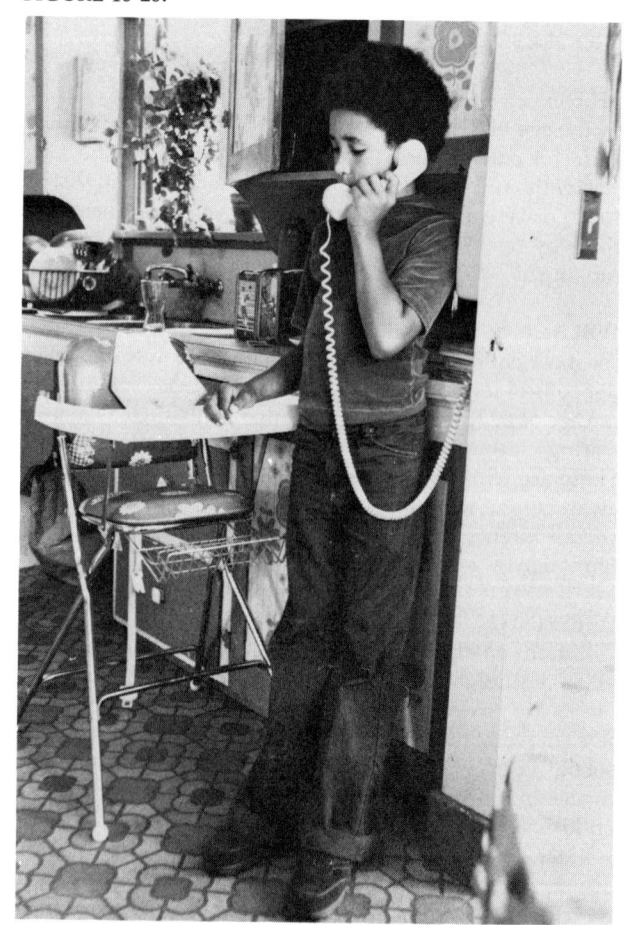

disapproval and arouse anger in the child. Discipline techniques provide the learning focus, and learning is affected by the child's emotional and motivational states.

The school-age child achieves the cognitive ability to recognize self as a causal agent. Concurrent development of social cognition also occurs. In short, the school-age child is highly responsive to inductive discipline techniques and therefore to moral internalization development.

During this period, children can demonstrate two major perspectives of moral internalization. They may have internalized institutional norms, which are the norms of social agencies such as school or family. They may have internalized humanistic norms which are the norms of interpersonal relations and human concerns (Hoffman, 1970). These two perspectives are an interesting focus in developmental assessment of school-age children.

EMPATHY

School-age children surpass the simple and familiar social cognition of preschoolers. These older children are capable of fairly accurate appraisal of the situations of others in unfamiliar situations and when the other is dissimilar to self. They also begin to attempt an explanation of the other's perspectives. The school-age child makes significant progress in the development of social cognition (Shantz, 1975).

FIGURE 10-27. (*Photo courtesy of Betsy Smith.*)

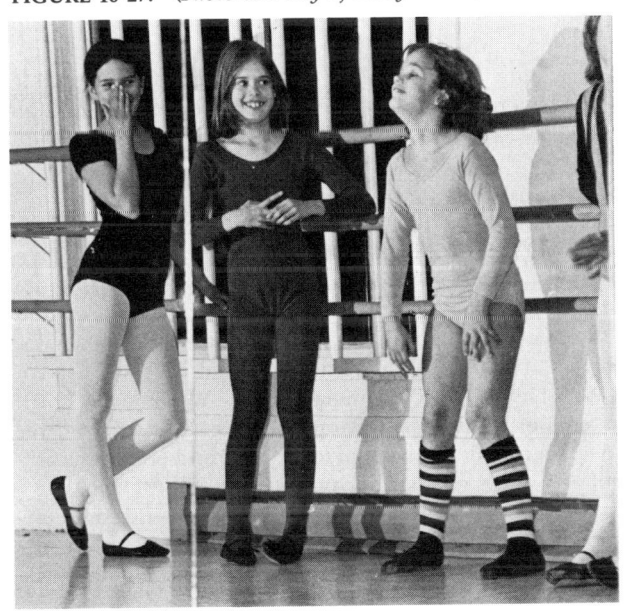

Advances in learning affective cues occur during this period. The school-age child is less egocentric and has cognitive capacities which promote an increased awareness and understanding of the affective cues of others (Bryan, 1975).

Altruistic motivation is the desire to help even when no recognition or reward is likely. School-age children have been found to demonstrate increasing altruistic helping and rescuing behaviors. These children have developed a sense of their own continuing identity: that their existence continues over time. They learn to recognize the continuing identity of others. As they learn that others exist continuously and therefore have unique experiences, role taking becomes possible. Role taking of others promotes awareness of the situation of others. Unpleasant or unhappy states of others are recognized, altruistic motivation and empathic distress are aroused, and school-age children begin to act effectively to help or rescue others (Hoffman, 1975).

GENDER IDENTITY AND SEX ROLE

Learning gender identity during this period becomes intertwined with peer groups. School-age children are in extended contact with other children in the school setting. The combination of messages from the setting and from peers becomes a strong factor in development of gender identity and sex role. These messages may or may not match the messages from parents. The school-age child may well experience conflicts between what was learned at home and what is enforced at school; thus, the learned concept of "appropriate" gender roles may be tested during the school years.

A term has emerged in theories and research pertaining to gender identity: *androgynous,* referring to a gender identity which is not totally bound to established male or female gender roles. A child who has been taught an androgynous gender identity is a child who has acquired some degree of both stereotypical masculine and feminine characteristics. There are many variables in androgynous gender identity. For example, the amount of masculine characteristics learned by a girl may vary. The particular characteristics which are learned may also vary.

The effect of androgynous socialization is still uncertain. Some theorists predict that it will eventually cause major confusion within the self-concept. Other theorists predict that it will afford the child a valuable degree of flexibility. One can expect a life-style effect of androgynous socialization. The nature of that effect remains to be determined. Androgynous socialization represents an essential concept in socialization of children. It is clearly related to the social values of today and brings the discussion back to the introductory concept of the context of social development (see Chap. 3).

This context with its dynamic nature is perhaps the core principle of social development. Social development must be relevant to the child and the adult that child will become. The nature of socialization must be flexible and responsive to social changes. When used in assessment of the social development of children, one must always consider the relevance of normal parameters to the current and future social world of the child. It may be more useful to focus on the adaptive potential of a child's social development than to focus on normal parameters of that development.

Perception of competency and development of self-esteem
Judith Anne Ritchie

PERCEPTION OF BEHAVIORAL COMPETENCE

With movement into formalized learning experiences demanded of the school-age child, there is sudden and drastic change in society's expectations of the child's behavior. In most instances, the child is expected to meet much higher demands in cognitive and social or interpersonal competencies than in physical competence. The school-age child's ability to function within the demands is dependent on self-concept which has been obtained largely through reacting to and internalizing values of family members (Lidz, 1968).

For most school-age children, there is considerable pressure to achieve successfully in the cognitive domain. However, individual peer groups, families, and schools may place increased emphasis on other areas such as physical appearance, musical ability, or athletic prowess. The child's perception of behavioral competence in any area may be influenced by social expectations, developmental level, actual competence, perception of control, and the specific situation (Harter, 1978).

During the school years, the child develops a sense of industry—the need to produce things successfully (Lidz, 1968). It is from positive achievement and recognition in this area that the child formulates the basis for a lasting feeling of competence. Failure to produce successfully results in a sense of inferiority—the feeling that he will never be capable (Erikson, 1968).

DEVELOPMENT OF SELF-ESTEEM

Self-esteem consists of two interrelated aspects: a sense of personal competence and a sense of personal worth (Brandon, 1969). Coopersmith defines self-esteem as "the extent to which the individual believes himself to be capable, significant, successful, and worthy" (1967, p. 3).

Because of the young child's limited experience and lack of cognitive ability for abstract conceptualization, there is a very limited self-concept. It is in later childhood that there is cognitive capacity for reflective appraisal and building of self-esteem (Arieti, 1967). The school-age child now can begin to develop some strong foundations in all areas defined as sources of self-esteem:

- Adherence to moral and ethical standards—virtue
- Successful performance in meeting demands for achievement—competence
- Ability to influence and control others—power
- Acceptance, attention, and affection of others—significance (Arieti, 1967, p. 38)

ABILITY TO SUCCEED IN SCHOLASTIC AND OTHER ENDEAVORS

The child's perception of behavioral competence is a major factor in his development of self-esteem. Successful school experiences are likely to result in the child's positive self-concept (Yamamoto, 1972). One dimension of personality is said to be a *scholastic self-concept,* which consists of three factors: certainty, attitude, and accuracy. The young child's positive self-image and academic achievement are closely related to the child's perception of the teacher's positive feelings toward him (Yamamoto, 1972).

PARENTAL, FAMILIAL, AND SOCIAL INFLUENCES

Feelings of power and significance are derived mainly from interaction with the social environment. Parental influence is generally acknowledged to have the major impact on the child's development of self-esteem (Coopersmith, 1967; Thomas, 1973; Yamamoto, 1972). Parents of children with high self-esteem accept and respect their children's behavior and set and enforce clearly defined limits on that behavior (Coopersmith, 1967).

The effect of sibling relationships on self-esteem is unknown. It is felt that if there is competition between siblings or if parents engage in comparative evaluation, the effect on self-esteem is negative (Yamamoto, 1972).

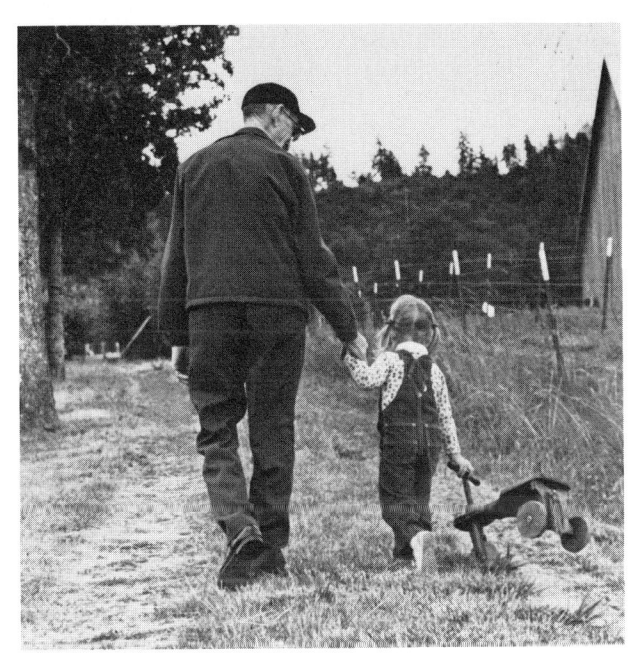

FIGURE 10-28. (*Photo courtesy of Betsy Smith.*)

Evaluations of parents, peers, and teachers provide the child with external criteria of what is correct, worthy, and appropriate. Positive evaluations eventually lead to feelings of high self-esteem, while negative evaluations result in lack of perceived competence and low self-esteem. One study indicates that the 6-year-old child almost entirely bases self-judgment on social feedback. By the age of 10 years, self-judgment is based both on dimensions of social feedback and the objective evidence of the child's success or failure (Harter, 1978).

Effects of race and social class on development are not well defined. It appears that prestige of social group is not a major influence on self-esteem (Rosenberg, 1965). Self-esteem is more dependent on experiences within the family and social groups.

As the school-age child passes through the physiological processes of sexual maturation, lasting several years, childhood gradually ebbs into adolescence. Puberty is considered the final stage of childhood and the embryological stage of adulthood as reproductive structures rapidly grow, mature, and become functional.

Achievement of full behavioral or adaptive maturation is a lifelong process. However, the child has, in the first 12 years of life, achieved all major milestones which serve as tools to be used throughout life. Soon after puberty, a significant scattering occurs due to differing interests, abilities, and ambitions as well as environmental reinforcement and constraints. Yet the same fundamentals of cognitive, social, and motor function serve as underpinnings for all adult endeavors.

Adolescence, then, is the infancy stage of adulthood during which early adult behaviors gradually mature to accompany the already mature physique, and development continues. Thus, growth and maturation and functional adaptation continue throughout life. The foundation prepared in childhood, prenatally and postnatally, will determine the quality of this continuing human development.

Bibliography

PHYSICAL DEVELOPMENT
OF THE SCHOOL-AGE CHILD

Alexander, M. M., and M. S. Brown: *Pediatric physical diagnosis for nurses.* New York: McGraw-Hill, 1974.

Barness, L. A.: *Manual of pediatric physical diagnosis* (4th ed.). Chicago: Year Book, 1972.

Brown, M. S., and M. A. Murphy: *Ambulatory pediatrics for nurses.* New York: McGraw-Hill, 1975.

Marshall, W. A.: Puberty. In F. Falkner and J. M. Tanner (Eds.), *Human growth 2, Postnatal growth.* New York: Plenum, 1978.

Report of the task force on blood pressure control in children. *Pediatrics,* 1977, *59*(5). (Supplement.)

Smith, D. W. (Ed.): *Introduction to clinical pediatrics.* Philadelphia: Saunders, 1977.

Tanner, J. M.: *Growth at Adolescence* (2d ed.). Oxford: Blackwell Scientific, 1962.

Vander-Bogert, F., and C. L. Moravec: Body temperature variation in apparently healthy children. *J. Pediat.* 1937, *10*(4), 466–467.

CALVARIUM AND FACE

Demirjian, A.: Dentition. In F. Falkner and J. M. Tanner (Eds.), *Human growth 2, Postnatal growth.* New York: Plenum, 1978.

Israel, J.: The fundamentals of cranial and facial growth. In F. Falkner and J. M. Tanner (Eds.), *Human growth 2, Postnatal growth.* New York: Plenum, 1978.

Marshall, W. A.: Puberty. In F. Falkner and J. M. Tanner (Eds.), *Human growth 2, Postnatal growth.* New York: Plenum, 1978.

Sullivan, P. G.: Skull, jaw, and teeth growth patterns. In F. Falkner and J. M. Tanner (Eds.), *Human growth 2, Postnatal growth.* New York: Plenum, 1978.

MUSCULOSKELETAL SYSTEM

Cheek, D. B.: Body composition, hormones, nutrition, and adolescent growth. In M. Grumbach, G. Grave, and F. Mayer (Eds.), *Control of onset of puberty.* New York: Wiley, 1974.

Cratty, B.: *Perceptual and motor development in infants and children.* London: Macmillan, 1970.

Grumbach, M., G. Grave, and F. Mayer (Eds.): *Control of onset of puberty.* New York: Wiley, 1974.

Malina, R. M.: Growth of muscle tissue and muscle mass. In F. Falkner and J. M. Tanner (Eds.), *Human growth 2, Postnatal growth.* New York: Plenum, 1978.

Marshall, W. A.: Puberty. In F. Falkner and J. M. Tanner (Eds.), *Human growth 2, Postnatal growth.* New York: Plenum, 1978.

REPRODUCTIVE SYSTEM AND PUBERTAL CHANGES

Baker, T. G.: A quantitative and cytological study of germ cells in human ovaries. *Proc. Roy. Soc. [Biol.],* 1963, *158,* 417.

Beach, F. A.: Human sexuality and evolution. In W. Montagna and W. A. Sadler (Eds.), *Reproductive behavior.* New York: Plenum, 1974.

Boyar, R., J. Finkelstein, H. Roffward, S. Kupen, E. Weitzman, and L. Hellman: Synchronization of augmented luteinizing hormone secretion with sleep during puberty. *New Eng. J. Med.,* 1972, *287,* 582.

———, W. F. Jordan, R. David, H. Roffward, S. Kupen, E. D. Weitzman, and L. Hellman: Twenty-four hour patterns of plasma luteinizing hormone and follicle stimulating hormone in sexual precocity. *New Eng. J. Med.,* 1973, *289,* 282.

Ducharme, J. R., M. G. Forest, E. De Peretti, M. Sempe, R. Collu, and J. Bertrand: Plasma adrenal and gonadal sex steroids in human pubertal development, *J. Clin. Endocrinol. Metab.,* 1976, *42,* 468.

Falkner, F.: Body composition. In S. R. Berenburg (Ed.), *Puberty. Biologic and psychosocial components.* Netherlands: Stenfert Kroese, 1975.

Forbes, G. B.: Puberty: Body composition. In S. R. Berenburg (Ed.), *Puberty. Biologic and psychosocial components.* Netherlands: Stenfert Kroese, 1975.

Grumbach, M. M.: Onset of puberty. In S. R. Berenburg (Ed.), *Puberty. Biologic and psychosocial components.* Netherlands: Stenfert Kroese, 1975.

Gryfe, C. I., A. N. Exton-Smith, P. R. Payne, and E. F. Wheeler: Pattern of development of bone in childhood and adolescence. *Lancet,* 1971, *1,* 523–526.

Guyton, A. C.: *Textbook of medical physiology* (5th ed.). Philadelphia: Saunders, 1976.

Katchadourian H.: *The biology of adolescence.* San Francisco: Freeman, 1977.

Kinsey, A. C., W. B. Pomeroy, C. E. Martin, and P. H. Gebhard: *Sexual behavior in the human female.* Philadelphia: Saunders, 1953.

Lee, P. A., A. R. Midgley, and R. B. Jaffe: Regulation of human gonadotropins. *J. Clin. Endocr.,* 1970, *31,* 248.

———, R. B. Jaffe, and A. B. Midgley: Serum gonadotropin, testosterone and prolactin concentrations throughout puberty in boys. *J. Clin. Endocr.* 1974, *39,* 664.

Maresh, M. M.: Growth of the heart related to bodily growth during childhood and adolescence. *Pediatrics,* 1948, *2,* 382–404.

Marshall, W. A.: Puberty. In F. Falkner and J. M. Tanner (Eds.), *Human growth 2, Postnatal growth.* New York: Plenum, 1978.

———, and J. M. Tanner: Variations in the pattern of pubertal changes in girls. *Arch. Dis. Child.,* 1969, *44,* 291–303.

———, and ———: Variations in the pattern of pubertal changes in boys. *Arch. Dis. Child.,* 1970, *45,* 13–23.

Morrow, C. P., and W. R. Hart: The ovaries. In S. L. Romney et al. (Eds.), *Gynecology and obstetrics, The health care of women.* New York: McGraw-Hill, 1975.

Nydick, M., J. Bustos, J. H. Dale, and R. W. Rawson: Gynecomastia in adolescent boys. *J. A. M. A.,* 1961, *178,* 449.

Prader, A.: Testicular growth in puberty. In S. R. Berenburg (Ed.), *Puberty. Biologic and psychosocial components.* Netherlands: Stenfert Kroese, 1975.

Tanner, J. M.: *Growth at adolescence* (2d ed.). Oxford: Blackwell Scientific, 1962.

———, and P. B. Eveleth: Variability between populations in growth and development at puberty. In S. R. Berenburg (Ed.), *Puberty. Biological and psychosocial components.* Netherlands: Stenfert Kroese, 1975.

———, R. H. Whitehouse, and M. Takaishi: Standards from birth to maturity for height, weight, height velocity and weight velocity. *Arch. Dis. Child.,* 1966, *41,* 454–471.

Zacharias, L., W. M. Rand, and R. J. Wurtman: A prospective study of sexual development and growth in American girls: The statistics of menarche. *Obstet. Gynec. Survey,* 1976, *31,* 325.

DEVELOPMENT OF BODY CONCEPT AND CONCEPTS OF ILLNESS AND WELLNESS

Barnes, C.: Levels of consciousness indicated by responses of children to phenomena in the intensive care unit. *Matern. Child Nurs. J.*, 1975. (Monograph 4.)

Bernabeu, E.: Effects of severe crippling on the development of a group of children. *Psychiatry*, 1958, *21*, 169–194.

Brodie, B.: Views of healthy children toward illness. *Amer. J. Public Health*, 1974, *64*, 1156–1159.

Campbell, J.: Attribution of illness: Another double standard. *Health Soc. Behav.*, 1975, *16*, 114–126.

Centers, L., and R. Centers: Peer group attitude toward the amputee child. *J. Soc. Psychol.*, 1963, *61*, 127–132.

Fisher, S.: *Body consciousness*. Englewood Cliffs, N.J.: Prentice-Hall, 1973.

———, and S. Cleveland: *Body image and personality*. Princeton, N.J.: Van Nostrand, 1958.

Freud, A.: The role of bodily illness in the mental life of children. *Psychoanal. Stud. Child*, 1952, *7*, 69–80.

Gellert, E.: Children's conceptions of the control and function of the human body. *Genetic Psychology Monographs*, May 1962.

Gochman, D.: Children's perceptions of vulnerability to illness and accidents. *Public Health Rep.*, 1970, *85*, 69–73.

Kastenbaum, R.: The child's understanding of death: How does it develop? In E. A. Grollman (Ed.), *Explaining death to children*. Boston: Beacon Press, 1967.

Kolb, L. C.: Disturbances of the body image. In S. Arienti (Ed.), *American handbook of psychiatry* (Vol. IV, 2d ed.). New York: Basic Books, 1975.

Nagy, M.: The child's theories concerning death. *J. Genet. Psychol.*, 1948, *73*, 3–27.

———: Children's ideas of the origin of illness. *Health Ed. J.*, 1951, *9*, 6–12.

Peters, B.: School-aged children's beliefs about the causality of illness: A review of the literature. *Matern. Child Nurs. J.*, 1978, *7*, 143–154.

Porter, C. S.: Grade school children's perceptions of their internal body parts. *Nurs. Res.*, 1974, *23*, 384–391.

Prugh, D. G.: Emotional aspects of the hospitalization of children. In M. F. Shore (Ed.), *Red is the color of hurting*. Washington, D.C.: Government Printing Office, 1965.

Richardson, S. A.: Handicap, appearance, and stigma. *Soc. Sci. Med.*, 1971, *5*, 621–628.

Schilder, P.: *The image and appearance of the human body*. New York: Wiley, 1964.

Shontz, F. C.: *The psychological aspects of physical illness and disability*. New York: Macmillan, 1975.

Simmel, M. L.: Developmental aspects of the body scheme. *Child Develop.*, 1966, *37*, 83–95.

Smith, E.: Are you really communicating? *Amer. J. Nurs.*, 1977, *77*, 1966–1968.

Spinetta, J. J., D. Rigler, and M. Karon: Anxiety in the dying child. *Pediatrics*, 1973, *52*, 482–494.

Waechter, E. H.: Children's awareness of fatal illness. *Amer. J. Nurs.*, 1971, *71*, 1168–1172.

PERCEPTUAL DEVELOPMENT

Chomsky, C.: *The acquisition of syntax in children from 5 to 10*. Cambridge, Mass.: MIT, 1969.

Gibson, E. J., and H. Levin: *The psychology of reading*. Cambridge, Mass.: MIT, 1975.

Levin, H., and A. Turner: Sentence structure and the eye-voice span. In H. Levin, E. J. Gibson, and J. J. Gibson (Eds.), *The analysis of reading skills*. Ithaca, New York: Cornell University Press, 1968.

Pick, H., and A. D. Pick: Sensory and perceptual development. In P. H. Mussen (Ed.), *Carmichael's manual of child psychology*. New York: Wiley, 1970.

GROSS MOTOR DEVELOPMENT

Arnheim, D. D., and R. A. Pestolesi: *Developing motor behavior in children*. St. Louis: Mosby, 1973.

Corbin, C. B.: *A textbook of motor development*. Dubuque, Iowa: Wm. C. Brown, 1973.

Cratty, B. J.: *Perceptual and motor development in infants and children*. New York: Macmillan, 1970.

Gesell, A., and F. L. Ilg: *The child from five to ten*. New York: Harper & Brothers, 1946.

FINE MOTOR DEVELOPMENT

Gesell, A., and F. L. Ilg: *The child from five to ten*. New York: Harper & Brothers, 1946.

Illingworth, R. S.: *The development of the infant and young child—Normal and abnormal*. London: Churchill Livingstone, 1975.

Smart, M. S., and R. C. Smart: *School-age children*. New York: Macmillan, 1973.

COGNITIVE DEVELOPMENT

Church, J. and L. J. Stone: *Children and adolescence* (3d ed.). New York: Random House, 1973.

Flavell, J.: *The developmental psychology of Jean Piaget*. New York: Van Nostrand, 1963.

Mosher, F., and J. Hornsby: On asking questions. In J. Bruner (Ed.), *Studies in cognitive growth*. New York: Wiley, 1966.

Phillips, J. L.: *The origins of intellect: Paiget's theory.* San Francisco: Freeman, 1969.

Piaget, J.: *The child's concept of physical causality.* Totowa, N.J.: Littlefield, Adams, 1965.

Pidgeon, V.: Children's concepts of the rationale of isolation technic. *ANA Clinical Sessions.* New York: Appleton-Century-Crofts, 1967.

———: Characteristics of children's thinking and implications for health teaching. *Matern. Child Nurs. J.*, 1977, 6, 1–8.

———: Child thought and counseling implications in the hospital. *Patient Counseling and Health Education.* Princeton, N.J.: Excerpta Medica, 1978. (To be published.)

Wenar, C.: *Personality development from infancy to adulthood.* Boston: Houghton Mifflin, 1971.

SELF-HELP SKILL DEVELOPMENT

Fishbach, N. D.: Reinforcement patterns of children. In A. Pick (Ed.), *Minnesota symposium on child psychology* (Vol. 7). Minneapolis: University of Minnesota Press, 1973.

Gesell, A., F. Ilg, F. Ames, and J. Rodell: *Infant and child in the culture of today* (2d ed.). New York: Harper & Row, 1974.

Hetherington, E. M., and R. D. Parke: *Child psychology.* New York: McGraw-Hill, 1975.

Lee, P. D., and A. L. Wolinsky: Male teachers of young children: A preliminary empirical study. *Young Child.*, 1973, 28, 342–353.

Osofsky, J. D., and E. J. O'Connell: Parent-child interaction: Daughters' effects upon mothers' and fathers' behavior. *Develop. Psychol.*, 1972, 7, 157–168.

Piaget, J.: *Play, dreams and imitations.* New York: Norton, 1951.

Strommen, E., J. P. McKinney, and H. Fitzgerald: *Developmental psychology: The school-aged child.* Homewood, Ill.: Dorsey, 1977.

Stuart, H. C.: The school age child: Boys 6 to 12 years; girls 6 to 10 years. In H. Stuart and D. Prugh (Eds.), *The healthy child.* Cambridge, Mass.: Harvard, 1964.

Thomes, M. D.: Children with absent fathers. *J. Marr. Family*, 1968, 30, 89–96.

SOCIAL DEVELOPMENT

Bryan, J. H.: Children's cooperative and helping behaviors. In E. M. Hetherington (Ed.), *Review of child development research* (Vol. 5). Chicago: University of Chicago Press, 1975.

Cicirelli, V. G.: Sibling teaching siblings. In V. Allen (Ed.), *Children as teachers: Theory and research on tutoring.* New York: Academic, 1966.

———: The effect of sibling relationships on concept learning of young children taught by child teachers. *Child Develop.*, 1972, 43, 287–294.

———: Effects of sibling structure and interaction on children's categorization style. *Develop. Psychol.* 1973, 9, 132–139.

———: Effects of mother and older sibling on the problem solving behavior of the younger child. *Develop. Psychol.*, 1975, 11, 749–756.

Erikson, E.: *Childhood and society.* New York: Norton, 1963.

Hoffman, M.: Conscience, personality and socialization techniques. *Hum. Develop.* 1970, 13, 90–126.

———: Developmental synthesis of affect and cognition and its implications for altruistic motivation. *Develop. Psychol.*, 1975, 11, 607–622.

Shantz, C.: The development of social cognition. In E. M. Hetherington (Ed.), *Review of child development research* (Vol. 5). Chicago: University of Chicago Press, 1975.

PERCEPTION OF COMPETENCY AND DEVELOPMENT OF SELF-ESTEEM

Arieti, S.: *The intrapsychic self.* New York: Basic Books, 1967.

Brandon, N.: *The psychology of self-esteem.* Los Angeles: Nash, 1969.

Coopersmith, S.: *The antecedents of self-esteem.* San Francisco: Freeman, 1967.

Erikson, E. H.: *Identity: Youth and crisis.* New York: Norton, 1968.

Freud, A.: *Normality and pathology in childhood.* New York: International Universities, 1965.

Harter, S.: Effectance motivation reconsidered: Toward a developmental model. *Hum. Develop.*, 1978, 21, 34–64.

Kohlberg, L.: Development of moral character and model ideology. In M. L. Hoffman and L. W. Hoffman (Eds.), *Review of child development research* (Vol. I). New York: Russell Sage, 1964.

Lidz, T.: *The person.* New York: Basic Books, 1968.

Rosenberg, M.: *Society and the adolescent self-image.* Princeton, N.J.: Princeton, 1965.

Thomas, J. B.: *Self-concept in psychology and education.* Great Britain: NFER, 1973.

Yamamoto, K.: *The child and his image.* Boston: Houghton Mifflin, 1972.

NAME INDEX

Accardo, P. J., 339, 379
Acheson, R. M., 39, 77
Ackerman, B. D., 319
Adam, J. A. J., 221
Adamsons, K., 217, 221, 270, 271, 281
Adler, A., 186
Agunod, M., 318, 369
Ahn, C. I., 318
Ainsworth, M. D., 144, 145, 166, 351, 403, 440
Ainsworth, P., 221
Aiu, P., 335
Alexander, D. P., 260
Alexanderson, B., 62
Allan, D., 326, 454
Allen, R. R., 464, 465
Alpaugh, M., 32
Alpers, D. H., 369
Alpine, W., 169
Alvear, J., 272
Amatruda, C. S., 389, 390, 392, 428, 429, 461
Ames, E., 393
Ames, F., 401
Ames, L. B., 389, 390, 392, 419, 428, 429, 436, 453, 461, 511
Ames, M. D., 318
Andersen, D. H., 369
Anderson, C. M., 418
Anderson, J. E., 454
Andre-Thomas, 349
Andreotti, G., 369
Anthony, E. J., 112
Apgar, V., 261, 294
Appleton, T., 403, 404
Apte, S. V., 265
Arend, R., 440
Arey, L. B., 12, 67, 78, 88, 209, 212, 261

Arieti, S., 514
Aristotle, 205, 331
Arrighi, F. E., 48
Arturson, G. T., 325
Asakawa, T., 37
Asmussen, I., 274
Auld, P. F., 313
Ausubel, D., 452
Avery, G. B., 294, 304
Avery, M. E., 244, 246
Ayer, J. L., 325

Babloyantz, A., 65
Baer, D., 3, 13, 122–123
Bailey, S. M., 272
Baker, T. G., 494
Baldwin, A., 124, 125
Bandura, A., 142
Bard, H., 301
Barden, T., 282
Barnard, K. E., 6–7
Barnes, C., 501
Barnett, H. I., 325
Barnett, H. R., 325
Bartlett, M., 279
Baserga, R., 65
Bayer, L. M., 38, 450
Bayley, N., 13, 38, 155, 351, 440, 450
Beach, F. A., 489
Beebe, B., 397
Bell, S., 402
Benedict, R., 110
Bennett, S. L., 397
Berger, G. S., 269
Bergman, A., 352, 403, 441
Berk, J. E., 319
Bernabeu, E., 500, 501
Bernard, C., 25

Bernfeld, S., 326, 371
Bernstein, B., 464
Berrill, N. J., 12, 13, 56, 205
Berry, L. C., 269
Berstein, P., 393
Bertenthal, B. I., 403
Bertrand, J., 487
Bianchi, D. W., 220
Bierman, E. L., 454
Bijou, S., 3, 13, 122–123
Binzley, V., 337, 374
Birch, H., 5, 116, 142, 174, 193, 437
Birnholz, J. C., 277, 278
Birns, B., 348
Bitsch, V., 318
Blake, F., 4
Blechschmidt, E., 64, 66, 68, 70
Blizzard, R. M., 46
Bloemsma, C. A., 271
Blom, G. E., 456
Bloom, L., 139, 350, 433
Boll, E. S., 147
Bonk, F., 272
Bonner, J., 54, 65
Bossard, J. H., 147
Boué, A., 262
Boué, J., 262
Bower, T. G. R., 129, 337, 423, 424
Bowerman, C. E., 147
Bowlby, J., 45, 109, 145, 165–166, 172, 351, 420, 440
Boyar, R., 488
Boyd, E., 269, 270, 306
Bradley, R. H., 177, 178, 181
Brandon, N., 442, 471, 514
Brandt, I., 364
Branstetter, E., 172
Brasel, J. A., 46, 79, 80, 315

519

NAME INDEX

Brazelton, T. B., 3, 155, 170, 185, 186, 194, 328, 350–352, 399, 438, 467, 468
Brenner, W. E., 267–270, 272
Bridger, W. H., 327, 348
Britten, R. J., 65
Brodie, B., 501
Brook, C. G. D., 364
Brooke, O. G., 272
Brooks, V., 424
Broussard, E., 169–170
Brown, E. V. L., 75
Brown, G. A., 369
Brown, J., 347
Brown, R., 434, 464, 465
Bruner, J., 138, 393, 431
Brunner, G., 65, 66
Bryan, J. H., 144, 146, 402, 470, 513
Bucher, U., 245
Bunge, M. B., 68
Bunge, R. P., 68
Bunney, W. E., Jr., 61
Bustos, J., 496
Butcher, R. E., 263

Caldwell, B. M., 9–11, 117, 176–181
Callender, W. M., 177
Cameron, N., 27, 96
Camp, B. W., 92, 152
Campbell, D., 399
Campbell, F. A., 435
Campbell, J., 498
Campbell, S., 208, 269–271, 273, 274
Campos, J. J., 335–337, 375
Cann, H. M., 220
Cannon, W. B., 25
Caplan, F., 436
Caplan, T., 436
Capute, A. J., 339, 379
Carey, W., 117
Carmichael, L., 12, 16, 266, 276, 280
Carpenter, G., 348
Carpenter, M. B., 227
Carpenter, R. L., 139, 433, 435
Casteneda, A., 143
Castner, B., 389, 390, 392, 428, 429, 461

Centers, L., 496
Centers, R., 496
Cetrulo, C., 284
Challacombe, D. N., 369
Cheek, D. B., 215, 221, 272, 273
Chernich, Y., 244
Chesni, Y., 349
Chess, S., 5, 17, 116, 117, 142, 174, 193–194, 422, 423, 437
Chin, T., 274
Christensen, J. B., 77, 311
Church, J., 118, 125, 507
Cicirelli, V. G., 147
Claireaux, A. E., 261
Cleveland, S., 418, 496
Clifton, R., 403, 404
Coggins, T. E., 139, 433, 435
Cohen, L. J., 145
Cohen, M. H., 66
Cohn, R., 419
Collu, R., 487
Comroe, J. H., 83
Conger, J. J., 12
Cook, L. N., 267, 269–272
Cook, P. R., 66
Coopersmith, S., 351, 441, 442, 472, 473, 514
Copenhaver, W. M., 68
Corliss, C. E., 37, 69, 74, 201, 202, 205, 210, 211, 214, 219, 221, 223, 226, 230, 236, 237, 248, 253
Cratty, B., 487
Crick, F. H., 52, 66
Cumming, E., 147

DaCunha, O., 325
Dale, J. H., 496
Dale, P., 140, 433, 435, 436
Dancis, J., 221
Dargassies, S. S., 349
Davenport, H. T., 172
David, R., 488
Davidson, E. H., 65
Davidson, M., 317
Davies, P. A., 221
Davis, C., 147
Davis, P. W., 54, 63
Dawes, G. S., 266, 267, 277
Dayton, G. O., Jr., 335
Dearden, R., 172
DeFries, J. C., 62

Demirjian, A., 73
De Peretti, E., 487
Dhariwal, A. P. S., 324
Dierstmann, S. R., 65
Dillon, M. S., 452
Dlerker, L. J., 266
Dobash, R. M., 147
Dodds, J. B., 153
Dodson, F., 188–189
Dollard, J., 117
Donnelly, G. F., 119, 121, 128
Dorman, L., 125
Douglas, H. B., 7
Douglas, J. W. B., 420
Dowd, E. L., 419
Downs, M. P., 336
Dreikurs, R., 186–187
Drillien, C. M., 304
Dubignon, J., 399
Dubowicz, L., 297–300, 305
Dubowicz, V., 297–300, 305
Ducharme, J. R., 487
Duenhoelter, J. H., 266, 277
Dunn, E. J., 271

Ebers, D. W., 318
Eckert, H., 437
Edelman, D. A., 267, 269, 270, 272
Edelmann, C. M., Jr., 325
Edelstein, B. B., 66
Edkins, S., 369
Edwards, R. G., 205
Eid, E. E., 31, 95
Eland, J. M., 454
Elardo, R., 181
Elliott, G. B., 279
Elliott, K. A., 279
Ellis, P. P., 374, 451
Ellison, E. H., 318
Enlow, D. H., 71
Epel, D., 65
Erickson, F., 456
Erickson, M. L., 176
Erikson, E., 3, 4, 117, 119–121, 189, 351, 402, 410, 440–442, 454, 467, 471, 472, 512, 514
Escalona, S. K., 142, 395, 401, 440, 469
Espenschade, A., 437
Eveleth, P. B., 488
Exton-Smith, A. N., 488
Eyres, S. J., 7

NAME INDEX 521

Falkner, F., 14, 27, 36, 72, 76, 489
Fallon, J. F., 66
Fanaroff, A., 313
Fantz, R., 393
Farber, B., 175
Faria, M., 277, 278
Farren, F. A., 435
Fein, G., 438
Feinbloom, R. I., 186–187
Feiring, C., 148
Felig, P., 221
Finkelskin, N. W., 435
Finkelstein, J., 488
Finkelstein, M., 45
Fischer, K. W., 403
Fishbach, N. D., 510
Fisher, S., 418, 496, 499
Fitzgerald, H., 510
Fitzgerald, J. D., 278
FitzGerald, M. J. T., 221
Fletcher, B. D., 244
Flynn, J. J., 272
Foley, J., 172
Fomon, S. J., 37, 95, 98, 99, 266, 296
Forbes, G. B., 36, 488, 492
Ford, L. H., 471
Forest, M. G., 487
Forgus, R. H., 131
Foster, J., 301–304
Fraiberg, S., 377, 453, 455
Frank, L. K., 42, 471
Frankenburg, W. K., 92, 152, 153
Franks, D. D., 443, 471
Fraser, R., 81, 83, 244
Freud, A., 370, 419, 453, 454, 456, 471, 472, 498
Freud, S., 4, 113, 117–119, 135–136, 138, 188
Friedlander, B. Z., 152, 424
Friedman, F., 282
Friedman, S., 348
Friis-Hansen, B., 36
Frisancho, A. R., 99, 360, 365
Furman, R. A., 420, 456

Gale, R. F., 471
Gall, J., 48
Gallimore, R., 147
Ganse, G. G., 66
Garn, S. M., 40, 272
Gasser, R. F., 64, 66, 68, 70, 215–218

Gautier, E., 325
Gellert, E., 453, 498
Gennser, G., 266
George, S., 117
Gerber, M., 109
Gersh, I., 260
Gershon, E. S., 61
Gesell, A., 42, 117, 124–125, 389, 390, 392, 401, 419, 428, 429, 436, 453, 461, 506, 507, 511
Gibbs, G. E., 318
Gibson, E. J., 129–130, 132, 336, 375, 377, 424, 458, 459, 503
Gibson, J. J., 130, 424
Gierrer, A., 65–66
Gilbert, D. A., 65
Ginott, H. G., 187–188
Glass, G. B. J., 318, 369
Glass, R. H., 201, 204
Gluck, L., 244–246
Gochman, D., 498
Golbus, M. S., 269
Goldberg, C., 297–300, 305
Goldberg, S., 396, 403, 404
Goldenson, R. M., 471
Goldfarb, W., 45
Goldstein, A. D., 152
Goldstein, H. S., 118, 412
Good, M., 46
Goodlin, R., 284
Gordon, I. J., 13, 16, 389, 391
Gordon, S., 279
Gordon, T., 189–191
Gottlieb, G., 276
Graham, P., 117
Grant, L. D., 263
Grave, G., 487
Gray, M. J., 267, 283
Graystone, J. E., 215, 221
Green, M., 168–169
Greenacre, P., 326, 419, 441
Greenberg, M., 171–172
Greitzer, L. J., 44, 416
Greulich, W. W., 37
Grimwade, J. D., 279
Grobstein, R., 170, 347, 348
Grollman, E. A., 420
Gross, R. L., 315
Groth, T., 325
Grottee, G., 325
Gruen, R. K., 79, 80, 315
Grumbach, M. M., 324, 487, 488

Grunewald, P., 275
Gryboski, J. D., 316, 317, 368
Gryfe, C. I., 488
Gueguen, S., 262
Guignard, J. P., 325
Guyton, A. C., 313, 489, 491

Hadorn, B. G., 418
Haegel, P., 252, 254
Haesslein, H. C., 284
Haith, M. M., 335–337, 375, 376
Halliday, M. A. K., 397
Hallman, M., 244–246
Halverson, H. M., 389, 390, 392, 428, 429, 461
Hamburger, V., 276, 277
Hammill, H. V. V., 29, 30, 32–35, 39–41, 43–46
Hansman, C., 269, 270, 306
Harris, J. A., 4, 24, 26
Harryman, S., 339, 379
Hart, W. R., 494
Harter, S., 441, 471, 473, 514, 515
Hartley, R. E., 471
Hartner, M., 169–170
Harvey, M. A., 411, 416
Hassanein, K., 274
Haverkamp, A., 284
Hayashi, S., 319
Haynes, U., 154
Heider, F., 123–124
Heinicke, C. M., 172
Heller, H., 325
Hellman, L., 488
Henderson, L. J., 17
Hendricks, C. H., 267, 269, 270, 272
Hensleigh, P., 274
Hertz, R. H., 266, 277
Herzenberg, L. A., 220
Herzig, M. E., 5, 142
Hess, R., 464
Hetherington, E. M., 146, 441, 510
Hewer, E. E., 260
Hiernanz, J., 65
Hochberg, J. E., 424
Hoekelman, R. A., 42, 82
Hoffman, L. W., 146

Hoffman, M., 145, 146, 440, 469, 470, 513
Hogg, J. C., 82
Holliday, M. A., 36
Holliday, M. H., 363, 365
Holt, J., 456
Holt, K. S., 172
Holtzer, H., 65
Hsu, T. C., 48
Huang, R. C., 54
Hubel, D., 131
Humphrey, T., 277–279
Hurst, J. W., 240, 241

Ilg, F. L., 42, 124, 389, 390, 392, 401, 419, 428, 429, 436, 453, 461, 506, 507, 510
Iliff, A. 80, 82, 83, 85
Illingworth, R. S., 31, 95, 172
Ireton, H., 154
Irish, D. P., 147
Israel, H., 71
Israel, J., 366
Iverson, G. M., 220
Iyengar, L., 265

Jackson, R. L., 24, 26, 28
Jaffe, J., 397
Jaffe, R. B., 487, 488
Jerauld, R., 169
Johnson, D., 438
Johnson, M., 146, 471
Jones, K. W., 48
Jones, M. H., 335
Jordaan, H. V., 271
Jordan, R., 488

Kagan, J., 12, 393, 396
Kalnins, I., 393
Kant, I., 129
Kaplan, S. L., 324
Karon, M., 501
Karp, G., 12, 13, 56, 205
Kase, N. G., 201, 204
Kastenbaum, R., 456, 501

Katchadourian, H., 489, 491, 496
Katcher, A., 453
Kauffman, S. A., 65, 66
Keen, M. F. L., 260
Keller, A., 471
Keller, F. S., 123
Kendig, E. L., Jr., 244
Kennedy, A. W., 272
Kennell, J., 168–169, 176, 327
Kerenyi, T. D., 269
Kessen, W. H., 335, 376
Kessler, L. R., 61
Kim, Y. J., 318
Kinsey, A. C., 496
Kirschbaum, R. M., 172
Klaus, M., 168–169, 176, 313, 327
Knobloch, H., 15, 155, 437
Knudson, A. G., 420
Kogan, K., 176
Kohlberg, L., 118, 127–128
Kolb, L. C., 326, 371, 453, 496
Korn, S., 117
Korner, A. F., 170, 347, 348
Korones, S. B., 300
Koru, S., 142
Kosson, N., 438
Koupernik, C., 112
Krasilnikoff, P. A., 318
Kreger, N., 169
Krieger, I., 45, 46
Kriegsmann, E., 436
Krout, M. H., 147
Kullander, S., 266
Kupen, S., 488

Lacey, K. A., 73
Lahey, M., 139, 350, 433
Lamb, M., 115, 146, 147, 351, 402, 403, 440, 441
Langford, W., 456
Langley, L. L., 77, 238, 242, 311
Langman, J., 258
Langworthy, O. R., 326
Lauritsen, J. G., 261, 262
Lazar, P., 262
Leblond, C. P., 67, 68
Lee, C. Y., 266
Lee, P. A., 487, 488
Lee, P. D., 511
Lee, V. A., 80, 82, 83, 85
LeMasters, E. E., 163–164

Lemire, R. J., 262
Lenihan, E. A., 172
Levin, H., 117, 400, 503, 504
Levin, M., 453
Levy, D., 453
Lewin, K., 125
Lewis, J. H., 66
Lewis, M., 3, 142, 148, 396
Lidz, T., 514
Lieberman, A., 469
Lieberman, J., 319
Liley, A. W., 221, 277–281
Lillywhite, H., 466
Lindenmayer, A., 66
Linn, L., 419
Lipsitt, L. P., 337, 458
Little, A. B., 267, 283
Locke, J., 129
Lopez, R., 318, 319
Lovell, K., 119, 126, 127
Lubchenco, L., 269, 270, 306
Luciano, D. S., 52, 53, 203
Luhby, A. L., 318, 369
Luria, A., 431
Lybarger, P. M., 365
Lynn, D., 115

McCaffery, M., 419, 454
McCance, R. A., 22, 267
McCann, J. J., 411, 416
McCann, S. M., 324
McClearn, G. E., 62
Maccoby, E. E., 117, 400
McCrory, W. W., 325
MacDonald, A. P., Jr., 398
MacFarlane, A., 334
McFee, J. G., 284
McGraw, M. B., 383–387, 426
McIntyre, I., 418
MacKeith, R., 401, 437
McKeown, T., 215, 269, 273
McKigney, J. I., 28
McKinney, J. P., 510
McKusick, V. A., 59
McLean, F., 270, 271
McMahon, D., 65
McNamara, H., 325
McNeil, D. 139
Maffel, H. V. L., 369
Mahler, M. S., 352, 403, 441

NAME INDEX

Maier, H. W., 119, 121, 127
Malina, R. M., 308
Manning, F. A., 266, 267
Mantell, C. D., 266
Maresh, M. M., 489
Marsal, K., 266
Marshall, R. E., 326
Marshall, T., 215, 269, 273
Marshall, W. A., 80, 485, 486, 488, 491, 497
Martin, C. E., 496
Massler, M., 73
Matas, L., 402, 440
Maurer, A., 372
Mavor, W. O., 22
Mayer, F., 487
Mayne, R., 65
Mazure, C. M., 61
Meacham, J. A., 471
Mead, J., 246
Mead, M., 110, 172
Meadow, R., 401, 437
Medinnus, G. R., 175
Mendel, G., 47, 57
Meredith, H. V., 28
Merrill, J. A., 267, 283
Metcoff, J., 221, 265, 267, 269, 273
Midgley, A. R., 487, 488
Miller, H. C., 274
Miller, N. E., 117
Miner, H., 301
Mittleman, B., 371
Mochan, B., 65
Moffett, A., 393
Moore, K. L., 25, 205, 206, 209–213, 219–222, 244, 259, 263, 264, 269
Morris, N., 171–172
Morrow, C. P., 494
Moss, H. A., 351
Mott, J. C., 325
Mulvihill, J. J., 274
Munroe, R., 437
Murphy, L. B., 347, 395, 441
Murphy, M., 437
Murray, J. F., 81, 84, 244, 314
Mussen, P. H., 12, 146, 351, 403

Nagy, A., 348
Nagy, M., 420, 456, 499, 501
Natterson, J. M., 420
Neal, M., 6

Nellhaus, G., 296
Nelson, K., 433
Nelson, S. E., 266
Nelson, W., 74, 366
Neumann, C. G., 32
Newberry, H., 277
Newman, J., 115
Niall, M., 215, 221
Nightingale, F., 6
Nixon, D. A., 260
Nobrega, F. J., 369
Northern, J. L., 336
Northway, M., 147
Novak, J. C., 419
Nubar, J., 281
Nydick, M., 496

O'Connell, E. J., 511
O'Donnell, A. M., 266
O'Grady, R. S., 419
Ohno, S., 55
Olds, S. W., 117
Oremland, E. K., 326, 327
Oremland, J. D., 326, 327
Osofsky, J. D., 511
Ounsted, C., 221, 267, 269, 270, 272–274
Ounsted, M., 221, 267, 269, 270, 272–274
Owen, G. M., 28

Pajino-Ferrara, F., 369
Papalia, D. E., 117
Papousek, H., 348, 393
Pardue, M. L., 48
Paré, J., 81, 83, 244
Parke, R. D., 170–171, 510
Parmalee, A. H., 332
Parsons, J., 144, 402, 470
Passamanick, B., 15, 155, 437
Pasternack, S. B., 365
Paterson, D. G., 24, 26
Payne, P. R., 488
Pederson, D. R., 376
Peters, B., 499
Piaget, J., 3, 108, 118, 125–127, 130, 135–138, 347–349, 393, 431, 432, 459, 462, 463, 471, 510
Pick, A. D., 375, 377, 459
Pick, H. L., 375, 377, 459

Pill, R., 172
Pine, F., 352, 403, 441
Pipes, P. L., 99
Pitcher, E. G., 456
Pitts, R. F., 260, 325
Pless, I. B., 42
Plumb, N., 168
Polacek, M. A., 318
Polishuk, W. Z., 277
Pomeroy, W. B., 496
Popich, G. A., 308, 366
Porter, C. S., 498
Powell, G. F., 46
Poznanski, E. O., 326
Prader, A., 22, 23, 418, 495
Prechtl, H. F. R., 295, 328, 329
Prelinger, E., 456
Preyer, W., 276
Pritchard, J. A., 266, 277
Prugh, D. G., 172, 371, 454–456, 467, 499
Pyle, S. I., 37

Quilligan, E. J., 267, 283

Raiti, S., 46
Ramey, C. T., 435
Rand, W. M., 492
Rawson, R. H., 335
Rawson, R. W., 496
Rebelsky, F., 125
Record, R. G., 215, 269, 273
Reese, H. W., 337, 458
Reid, L., 244, 245
Reinold, R., 276, 278–281
Rexford, E. N., 176
Reynolds, E. L., 37
Rheingold, H., 396
Rich, E. O., 326
Richardson, S. A., 496
Richmond, J. B., 117
Rigler, D., 501
Riley, P. A., 66
Rimirea, M., III, 143
Ritchie, J. A., 456
Robertson, A., 66

Robertson, J., 172, 420
Robillard, J. E., 325
Robinson, D., 172
Robinson, J. S., 266, 267, 277
Robson, K. S., 351
Rochard, F., 266, 277
Roche, A. F., 28, 76, 368
Rodbro, P., 318
Rodell, J., 401, 436, 511
Roffward, H., 488
Rogers, J. E., 44, 416
Romney, S. L., 267, 283
Ron, M., 278
Root, A. W., 324
Rose, M. H., 172, 335
Rosen, M. G., 277
Rosenberg, M., 515
Rosenblum, L. A., 3
Rosenthal, M. K., 143, 144
Rosso, P., 41
Roy, E. L., 419
Rubenstein, J. E., 339, 379
Rubin, R., 166–168, 176, 352
Rugh, R., 221
Runnstrom, J., 65
Rutter, M., 117, 173, 174

Saayman, G., 393
Sackett, G., 109
Sadovsky, E., 277, 278, 280, 281
Salapatek, P. H., 335, 376
Salk, L., 191–192
Sands, H. H., 172
Sarbin, T. R., 472
Scammon, R. E., 4, 24, 26
Scarpelli, E., 80, 81, 244
Schaeffer, J. P., 78
Schaffer, H. R., 172
Scheer, K., 281
Scheiss, W. A., 325
Schilder, P., 371, 419, 453, 471, 496
Schmerling, D. H., 418
Schneider, D., 147
Schneider, H., 221
Schoenfeld, W. N., 123
Schour, I., 73
Schowalter, J. E., 372, 420

Schreiner, R. L., 301–304
Schröder, J., 220
Schulman, J. L., 172
Schulz, H., 332
Searcy, R. L., 319
Sears, R. R., 117, 121, 400
Selye, H., 25
Sempe, M., 487
Shanklin, D. R., 219, 221
Shantz, C., 146, 440, 470, 513
Shapiro, J. M., 66
Sheehy, G., 4
Sheldon, W. H., 34
Shepard, T. H., 324
Shepard, T. J., 262
Sherman, J. S., 52, 53, 203
Shettles, L. B., 201
Shontz, F. C., 498
Silber, D. L., 438
Silver, H. K., 45
Simandl, B. K., 66
Simmel, M. L., 452, 496
Sinclair, D., 76, 88, 308, 361, 417, 486
Sinqueland, W., 396
Sipowicz, R., 172
Sjoqvist, F., 62
Skinner, A. L., 411, 416
Skinner, B. F., 3, 117
Smart, M., 399
Smart, R., 399
Smith, D. I., 318
Smith, D. W., 222, 261, 262, 272–274, 308, 366, 411, 416, 454
Smith, E., 498
Smith, G. P., 324
Smith, H. T., 347
Smyth, C. N. L., 280
Snell, R. S., 231, 233
Snow, C. E., 465
Solin, M., 369
Solkoff, N., 396
Solnit, A. J., 168–169
Solomon, E. P., 54, 63
Sontag, L. W., 277
Southgate, D. A. T., 269, 270
Spelt, D. K., 277
Spencer, K., 143
Speroff, L., 201, 204
Spicher, C., 372
Spinetta, J. J., 501
Spiro, H. M., 317, 368
Spitz, R. A., 45, 109

Spock, B., 184–186
Sroufe, L. A., 402, 440
Stacey, M., 172
Stander, T., 267, 283
Starr, B. D., 118
Staub, E. M., 172
Steele, B., 335
Steffa, M., 169
Stehbens, J. A., 438
Stephens, J. C., 277, 278
Steptoe, P. C., 205
Stern, D. V., 397
Stevens, T. D., 222
Stevenson, R. E., 273, 274
Steward, C. R., 65
Stickle, G., 261
Stone, L. J., 118, 125, 347, 507
Stork, L., 438
Stott, L. H., 134, 387
Strang, L. B., 244, 245, 247, 313, 314
Streeter, G. L., 208
Striffler, N., 142
Strommen, E., 510
Stuart, H. C., 28
Sullivan, P. G., 71, 72, 485
Sullivan, R., 301–304
Sutterley, D. C., 119, 121, 128
Sutton, W. D., 66
Swafford, L. I., 326, 454

Takaishi, M., 27–29, 31, 412, 488–490
Tanner, J. M., 14, 22, 23, 27–29, 31, 36, 39, 40, 72, 76, 335, 412, 450, 488–491, 493–497
Taqi, Q., 46
Targum, S. D., 61
Telford, I. R., 77, 311
Ter Vrugt, D., 376
Thayer, W. R., Jr., 317, 368
Thomas, A., 5, 17, 116, 117, 142, 174, 193, 422, 423, 437
Thomas, J. B., 351, 352, 472, 473, 514
Thomas, M. D., 511
Thompson, H., 3, 428, 429, 461
Thompson, H. E., Jr., 284, 389, 390, 392
Thompson, J. N., 221
Thompson, S. K., 468
Thwing, E., 154
Timiras, P. S., 35, 36, 317

NAME INDEX

Timor-Tritsch, I. E., 266, 277, 280
Tolpin, M., 403
Torrado, A., 325
Toth, P., 274
Troupkou, V., 325
Truog, W., 411, 416
Tuchmann-Duplessis, H., 252, 254
Tudvad, F. H., 260, 325
Tulkin, S. R., 396
Turner, A., 504
Turner, R. K., 401, 437
Tyson, K. R. T., 319, 369

Usher, R., 270, 271
Užgiris, I., 393

Valpe, J. J., 326
Vandenberg, S. G., 62
Vander, A. J., 52, 53, 203
Van Riper, C., 465
Vaughn, V., 74, 366
Vernon, D. T. A., 172
Vessel, E. S., 62
Vining, E. P. G., 339, 379
von Harnack, G. A., 22, 23

Waechter, E. H., 501
Walker, B. E., 67
Walker, D. W., 279
Walker, W. A., 320, 321

Wallenberg, H. C. S., 271
Wallston, B., 173
Walters, R., 142
Wangenheim, K. H., 65
Wasserman, G. D., 66
Wasserman, L., 438
Waterlon, J., 41
Waters, E., 402
Watson, J. B., 117
Watson, J. D., 47, 52
Wechler, P., 453
Weimer, S. N., 272
Weintraub, H., 65
Weir, R., 424
Weisel, T., 131
Weisner, T. S., 147
Weitzman, E. D., 488
Wenner, W., 332
Werner, H., 136–138
Werry, J. S., 172
Westheimer, I. J., 172
Westman, J. C., 142
Wheeler, E. F., 488
Whipple, D. V., 25
White, B. L., 192–193, 345, 377, 396, 436
White, R. W., 352, 403, 404, 441, 471
Whitehouse, R. H., 27–29, 31, 412, 488–490
Whiting, B., 143
Widdowson, E. M., 22, 36, 267
Wilds, P. L., 266

Windle, W. F., 278
Winick, M., 41
Witken, H. A., 371
Wladimiroff, J. W., 271
Wolff, P. H., 326–328, 334, 347, 348, 399
Wolinsky, A. L., 511
Wolpert, L., 66
Wood, C., 279
Woodward, D. O., 49
Woodward, V. W., 49
Worden, F. G., 131
Wurtman, R. J., 492

Yaffe, H., 278
Yamaguchi, N., 318, 369
Yamamoto, K., 442, 471, 472, 514
Yarrow, L., 116, 172
Yarrow, M. R., 143, 175

Zacharias, L., 492
Zador, I., 266, 277
Zakharov, A. F., 66
Ziegler, E. E., 266
Zoppi, G., 369, 418
Zuckerkandle, E., 66
Zuilkke, S., 166

SUBJECT INDEX

Page numbers in *italic* indicate illustrations or tables.

Abdomen, circumference of, 361, 413–414
Abortion, spontaneous, 261, 265
Accommodation, 126, 135, 137, 430
Achievement motivation, 471
Acid-base balance, 260, 321, 325
   (*See also* Electrolyte balance)
Acrocyanosis, 295, 296
Activities of daily living (*see* Self-help skills)
Adenine, 49, 52, *53*
Adenohypophysis, 250, 321
Adolescence, 120
   (*See also* Puberty)
Adoption, 169
Adrenal gland, 250–251, 321
Adult, developmental tasks of, 120–121
Affective disorders, 61
Age:
   conceptual, 205–207
   dental, 73–74, 77–78
   gestational, 205–207
      estimation of, 297–299, *300*, *305*, 322
   menstrual, 205–207
   skeletal, 37–38, 77–78, 370, 486
Aggression, 122
Aging, 15
Alcohol (beverage), 262, 274
Alleles, 47
Amniocentesis, 208
   effects on fetus, 208, 267, 278
   fetal age for, 208, 265
Amniography, 209
Amnion, 221–222

Amniotic fluid, 221–222, 260, 304
Anal stage of development, 4
Anaphase:
   in meiosis, 55, *56*
   in mitosis, *63*, 64
Anthropometry, 27, 92–95
   (*See also* Abdomen, circumference of; Chest, circumference of; Head, circumference of; Height; Length; Skinfold thickness; Weight)
Anxiety, stranger (*see* Stranger anxiety)
Apgar Newborn Scoring System, 294
Apnea of neonate, 315
Assimilation, 126, 135, 137, 430
Attachment, 145
   father-infant, 170–172
   in infant, 108, 113, 402
   mother-infant, 164–170, 175, 396–397
   in neonate, 351, 352
      hospitalized, 327
   in preschooler, 469
   in toddler, 440
Auditory system:
   of embryo, 232
   of fetus, 279
   hearing problems, screening for, 9, 92
   of infant, 367, 375–376
   of neonate, 307, 336–337
   of preschooler, 459
   of school-age child, 485
   of toddler, 424–425

Autonomy versus shame and doubt, 4, 120, 440, 442
Autosomes, 48

Baby and Child Care (Spock), 184–186
Bayley Scales of Infant Development, 155, 181
Behavior:
   antisocial, 173, 174
   assessment of, 149–157
   development of, 13, 15–16, 107–161
      environmental influences on, 109–117
      genetic influences on, 61–62
   effects on health, 112–113
   as indication of prenatal defect, 263
   and physical development, 13–14, 16–17, 112–113
   prenatal, 274–281
   theories of (*see* Theories, developmental)
   (*See also particular age groups*)
Behavior modification, 3
   (*See also* Behaviorism; Conditioning)
Behavioral state, 294–295, 328–329, 352, 373
   and cognition, 347–348
   and parenting, 329, 403
   and perception, 334–335, 374
   and physical examination, 294–295, 328
   (*See also* Sleep; Temperament)
Behaviorism, 3, 117, 121–124

Between Parent and Child (Ginott), 187–188
Bilirubin, 318–319
Biological clock, 4, 266, 330–334
Birth, 284
   cesarean delivery, 284, 312, 313
   effects on neonate, 294
   expected date of, 205
Birth defects, 261–263
Birth order, 147, 398
Birth weight (*see* Fetus, size at birth; Socioeconomic status, and birth weight)
Birthmarks, 297
Blindness:
   in infancy, 377
   strabismus and, 416–417
Blood, formation of (*see* Hematopoiesis)
Blood gases:
   in neonate, 313–315
   placental transfusion and, 312
   prenatal, 246–247
Blood pressure:
   age differences in, 80, *81*
   of preschooler, 451
   at puberty, 489, *493*
   of school-age child, 482–484
   of toddler, 415
Body composition:
   age differences in, 35–37, 79
   of fetus, 265–266
   of infant, 363–366
   of neonate, 296
   at puberty, 485, 488–489, *492*
   of school-age child, 481, 488
Body image:
   of infant, 370–371
   of neonate, 326
   of preschooler, 452–453
   of school-age child, 496–497, 501
   of toddler, 418–419, 425
Body integrity, 450, 453–454, 457–458, 499
Body proportion, 31, 33–34
   age differences in, 31, *37*, *38*, 76
   of fetus, 265
   of infant, 361
   of preschooler, 451
   of school-age child, 480, *484*
   of toddler, 412–414, *417*
Body surface area, 88
Body temperature (*see* Temperature, body)
Bonding (*see* Attachment)
Bone age, 37–38, 77–78, 370, 486
Bone marrow, 78–79, 235, 243
Boston Children's Medical Center, 186
Brain:
   growth of, 25, 370
      catch-up, 22
   in embryo, 225, *226*, 227–229, *230*
   in undernutrition, 41, 74–75
   role in reproduction, 85, 87
Breast versus bottle feeding, 317, 320, 399
Breast development, 491–492, *494*, 496
Breathing (*see* Respiration; Respiratory rate; Respiratory system)
Breech presentation, 279, 281

Calvarium, 71, 72
   of embryo, 71, 222–224, 235
   of fetus, 264–265, 270–271
   of infant, 366
   of neonate, 307
   at puberty, 485–486
   of school-age child, 485–486
   of toddler, 415–416
   (*See also* Fontanels)
Canalization, principle of, 21–22, 23
Caput succedaneum, 295
Cardiovascular system:
   of embryo, 79–80, 237–243
   of neonate, 308–312
   at puberty, 489, *491*
   (*See also* Circulation, fetal; Heart)
Carnegie stages of embryologic development, 207–208
Cell division (*see* Meiosis; Mitosis)
Cells:
   in embryonic development, 62–66
   population types of, 67–68
Centration of thought, 462
Centromere, 48
Cephalocaudal principle of growth and development, 14, 31, 76
   in infant posture, 362
   in motor control, 133, 345, 381, 385–386, 457
   in neonatal skeletal system, 308
   in prenatal behavior, 277
   in toddler body proportions, 412
Cephalohematoma, 296
Cerebrospinal fluid, 229
Cesarean delivery, 284, 312, 313
Chest, circumference of: age differences in, 94
   of fetus, 271
   of infant, 361
   interpretation of, 94–95
   of neonate, 296
   procedure for measuring, 94
   of toddler, 413
Child, His Parents, and the Nurse, The (Blake), 4
Child abuse, 168, 175
Child Health Encyclopedia (Feinbloom), 186–187
Child rearing:
   autocratic, 186, 187
   books for parents about, 184–194
   cultural variations in, 42–45
   democratic, 186, 187
   permissive, 43, 186
   and socioeconomic status, 177–178
   trends in, 143
Children the Challenge (Dreikus), 186–187
Chorion, 221–222
Chorionic gonadotropin, 221, 250–251
Chromatids, 49
Chromosome banding, 48–49, *50–51*
Chromosome theory of inheritance, 47–48
Chromosomes, 47–49, *50–51*, 62–64
   aberrations of, 48, 262
   sex, 48–49, 55, 60–61
   translocations of, 57
   (*See also* Inheritance)
Cigarette smoking, 274, *275*
Circulation, fetal, 220, 239–243, 308–310, 313
Cleavage, 64, *206*, 209
Cognition, 121, 135–138
   and affect, 138
   and empathy, 146
   of infant, 371, 373, 374, 390, 393–396

SUBJECT INDEX

Cognition *(Cont.)*:
  and language, 140, 142
  of neonate, 327, 333, 347–349
  and perception, 129–132
  of preschooler, 457, 461–464
  of school-age child, 507–510
  of toddler, 424, 429–432
  (See also Thought)
Cognitive theories of development, 3, 108, 124–128, 135–138
Colorado Intrauterine Growth Chart, 299–301, 304, *306*
Competence motivation, 108
Competence of tissue, 25, 66
Conceptual age, 205–207
Conditioning, 3, 117, 123
  of fetus, 277
  of infant, 374, 393–394
  and moral development, 145
  of neonate, 327, 348
  (See also Behaviorism)
Congenital malformations, 261–263
Consanguinity, 59
Conscience *(see* Morality)
Conscious mind, 118
Conservation, concept of, 462, 509
Corpus luteum, 201, *202*
Counterculture, 111
Critical period *(see* Sensitive period)
Crossing-over, chromosomal, 57
Culture:
  and behavioral development, 110–112, 117, 123, 124, 143
  and beliefs about children, 110–112
  and physical development, 42–45
  and sex role, 110
Cutis marmorata, 295
Cystic fibrosis, 59
Cytosine, 49, 52, *53*

DASE (Denver Articulation Screening Exam), 10
DDST (Denver Developmental Screening Test), 9, 152, *152–153*
Deafness, 376, 485
Death:
  concept of: of infant, 372
  of preschooler, 456
  of school-age child, 501
  of toddler, 420
  of parent, 173

Death instinct, 118
Defense mechanisms, 112, 118, 138, 501
Degree of Bother Inventory, 169
Deletions, chromosomal, 57
Delinquency, 173, 174
Dental age, 73–74, 77–78
Denver Articulation Screening Exam (DASE), 10
Denver Developmental Screening Test (DDST), 9, 152, *152–153*
Denver Prescreening Developmental Questionnaire (PDQ), 155
Deoxyribonucleic acid (DNA), 47, 49, 52–55, 57, 64–66
Dependency, 122
  (See also Attachment)
Deprivation:
  maternal, 45–47, 109, 113, 165–166, 327
  oral, 326–327
  stimulus, 109, 327, 377, 416–417
  (See also Stimulation)
Deprivation of Maternal Care: A Reassessment of Its Effects (Ainsworth), 166
Development:
  behavioral *(see* Behavior)
  cognitive, 135–138
    and socioeconomic status, 464
    (See also Cognition)
  definition of, 122
  of language, 139–142, 182
    (See also Language)
  nursing role in promotion of, 3–11, 13, 95
  perceptual, 129–132
    (See also Perception; Sensory system)
  physical, 13–15, 21–105
    assessment of, 90–99
    of infant, 360–372
    of neonate, 294–304
    of preschooler, 450–456
    of school-age child, 478–501
    of toddler, 410–415
  behavioral influences on, 112–113
  environmental influences on, 38–47
    (See also particular age groups)
  principles of, 4–6, 11–16, 21–26, 107–109
    (See also particular principles)

  social, 143–148
    (See also Social development)
  theories of *(see* Theories, developmental)
  (See also Growth)
Developmental Screening Inventory, 154
Developmental stage, 108, 117
Differentiation, 14
  in behavioral development, 107
  cellular, 64–66
  cognitive, 136–137
  gene function in, 53–55, 65
  of tissues and organs, 67–70
Digestion, 369, 418
Diploid number, 47, 55, 57
Disaster, effects on behavioral development, 115
Discipline, 183, 186–187, 189, 191
  for preschooler, 450, 469, 472–473
  for school-age child, 512–515
  for toddler, 440
Divorce, 172–174
DNA (deoxyribonucleic acid), 47, 49, 52–55, 57, 64–66
Dominance, law of, 57, 58
Double helix, 52, *53*
Dressing *(see* Self-help skills)
Drooling, 368
Drugs:
  genetic influence on response to, 62
  as teratogens, 262–263
  (See also particular drugs)
Dysmorphology *(see* Congenital malformations)

Ears:
  embryologic development of, 222–224, 232, 233
  fetal development of, 264, 265
  of infant, 367
  of neonate, 307
  (See also Auditory system; Deafness)
Eating *(see* Feeding)
Ectoderm, 66, 68, 69, 209

Ectomorphy, 33–34
Effect of the Infant on Its Caregiver, The (Rosenblum), 3
Ego, 118, 119, 135–136, 165–166
"Eight stages of man" theory, 4, 119–121
Ejaculation, 204, 496
Electrolyte balance, 35–37, 322
  (*See also* Acid-base balance)
Embryo, 205–263
  age calculations for, 205
  defects of, 261, 263
  differentiation of, genes and, 53–55, 65
  growth and development of, 71, 199–263
    cells in, 62–66
    general concepts of, 205–209
    organogenesis in, 207, 209–215, 222–261
    (*See also particular organ systems*)
  implantation of, 216–219
Empathy, 144–146
  of infant, 402
  of preschooler, 469–470
  of school-age child, 513
  of toddler, 440
En face position, 168, *171*, 396
Endocrine system, 84–85
  of embryo, 85, 250–252, 255–256
  of infant, 370
  of neonate, 321–322, 324, 325
  at puberty, 487–488
  (*See also* Hormones; *particular hormones; particular organs*)
Endoderm, 66, 68, *69*, 209
Endomorphy, 33–34
Engrossment, 171–172
Environment, 16–17, 38–47, 109–117, 144–145
  home, 176–183
  uterine, 25–26
  (*See also* Nature-nurture interaction)
Epstein's pearls, 296
Erythema toxicum neonatorum, 296
Esophagus, 247, 317

Ethnic group, 111
Eyes:
  embryologic development of, 230–232
  fetal development of, 264, 265
  of infant, 366, 367, 374–375
  of neonate, 71, 296, 305–307, 335–336
  of toddler, 415–417, 424
  (*See also* Vision)

Face, 71–72
  of embryo, 222–224
  of fetus, 264–265
  of infant, 366
  at puberty, 485–486
  of school-age child, 485–486
  of toddler, 415
Failure to thrive, 45–46, 168, 365, 366
Familial trait, 47
Family, 111, 172–175
  definition of, in genetics, 47
  one-parent, 7, 143, 173–175
  role in gender identity, 440–441, 471
Father, 170–173, 175
  separation from, 173
  (*See also under* Attachment)
Fear of strangers (*see* Stranger anxiety)
Feeding:
  breast versus bottle, 317, 320, 399
  of infant, 185, 369, 398–400
  of preschooler, 467
  of school-age child, 511
  of toddler, 422, 427–428, 436–437
Fels Research Institute, 170
Fertilization, 204–207
Fetography, 209
Fetoscopy, 209
Fetus, 205–207, 264–284
  age estimation of, 205–207, 297–299, *300*, 305, 322
  anthropometric measurements of, 205, 207, 208, 267–272
  assessment of, 208–209
  behavior of, 274–281
  body composition of, 265–266
  circulation of, 220, 239–243, 308–310, 313

  growth of, 264–274, *264*, *265*, *268*, *270*–272
    (*See also* size at birth *below*; Weight, prenatal)
  heart rate of, 266, 277, 282–284
  hemoglobin in, 246–247
  membranes of, 221–222, 304
  movement of, 267, 274–277, 280–281
  reflexes of, 277–280
  respiratory movements of, 247, 266–267, 277
  response to labor, 282–284
  response to stimulation, 277–280
  size at birth, 265, 267, *268*, 271–274, *275*, 295
  temperature of, 267
Field theory, 125
Figure drawing tests, 156–157
Fine motor development (*see* Motor development, fine)
Fingerprints, 260–261
First Three Years of Life, The (White), 192–193
Fluid, amniotic, 221–222, 260, 304
Fluoridation, 74
Follicle-stimulating hormone (FSH), 86, 201
  in neonate, 324
  at puberty, 494, 495
  in school-age child, 487, 488
Fontanels:
  of infant, 361, 364, 366
  of neonate, 307–308
  of toddler, 415
  (*See also* Calvarium)
Friedman curve of normal labor, 282
Frustration, 122
FSH (*see* Follicle-stimulating hormone)

G staining (Giemsa staining), 48–49, 50–51
Gametes, 47, 55–57, 200–204
  (*See also* Meiosis)
GAS (general adaptation syndrome), 25
Gastrointestinal system, 84–85
  of embryo, 84, 247–249
  of fetus, 264

Gastrointestinal system (Cont.):
　of infant, 368–370
　of neonate, 315–321
　of toddler, 417–418
Gastrula, 65
Gender identity, 144, 146
　of infant, 402–403
　of preschooler, 119, 453, 470–471
　of school-age child, 513–514
　of toddler, 440–441
　(See also Sex role)
General adaptation syndrome (GAS), 25
General-to-specific principle of growth and development, 107
Generativity versus self-absorption or stagnation, 120–121
Genes:
　action of, 49, 52–55
　activation of, 53–55, 65
　arrangement on chromosomes, 49
　and differentiation of embryo, 53–55, 65
　influence on behavior, 61–62
　influence on growth, 411–412, 415, 416
　protein production by, 52–54, 54
　repression of, 53–55, 65
　(See also Inheritance)
Genetic theory of development, 3–4
Genetics, 47–65
　and congenital malformations, 262
　Mendelian laws of, 57–58
Genital stage of development, 119
Genitalia, external, 87, 253–256
　in neonate, 322–323
　prenatal development of, 255–257, 257, 264, 265
　at puberty, 492, 494–497
Genome, 65
Genotype, 47
Gesell Developmental Schedules, 154, 155
Gestalt theory, vision and, 458
Gestational age (see Age, gestational)
Giemsa staining (G staining), 48–49, 50–51
Glands (see particular glands)
Glomerular filtration rate (GFR), age differences in, 87
Gonadotropin-releasing hormone (factor) (GnRF), 86

Goodenough-Harris Drawing Test, 156–157
"Goodness of fit," 116–117, 330
Graafian follicle, 200, 201
Grandparents, 175
Grief work and maternal role, 166
Grooming:
　by preschooler, 468–469
　by school-age child, 511
Gross motor development (see Motor development, gross)
Growth, 21–47
　assessment of: prematurity and, 93
　　recommended schedule for, 30, 92
　of brain (see Brain, growth of)
　catch-up, 22, 23
　　following illness, 39–40
　　in neonate, 22, 274
　　of premature infant, 364
　　in small-for-gestational-age infant, 22, 274
　　following stress, 46–47
　cellular, 62–66
　channelization of, 411–412, 416
　compensatory, 21, 24–25
　definition of, 14, 21
　in deprivation, 113
　directionality of, 14, 31
　disease and, 38–40
　distance curves of, 27–29
　dysharmonic, 22, 24
　genetic influence on, 411–412, 415, 416
　measurements of, 26–37, 92–99
　　head circumference by age, 29, 30
　　height (stature) by age, 34, 35
　　length by age, 32, 33
　　weight by age, 39–41, 43
　　weight by height (stature), 45, 46
　　weight by length, 44
　normative charts for, 29, 30, 32–35, 39–41, 43–46
　sex differences in, 87
　socioeconomic influences on, 28, 41–45
　　(See also Socioeconomic status, and birth weight)
　termination of, 488

　in undernutrition, 40–41, 74, 75, 96, 97
　velocity of, 27, 415
　(See also Body composition; Body proportion; Development; particular age groups)
Growth ambivalence, 108
Growth hormone, 6, 46–47, 85, 250, 364
Growth retardation, 22, 23
　intrauterine, 271, 274
　physiology of, 39–40, 85
Growth spurt, pubertal, 485, 486, 488–497
Guanine, 49, 52, 53
Guide to Normal Milestones of Development, 154
Guilt:
　feelings of, 112, 120
　initiative versus, 120, 450, 467, 469
Gustatory system:
　of embryo, 233–234
　of fetus, 280
　of infant, 376
　of neonate, 307, 337

Habituation, 348, 374
Hair:
　age differences in, 89
　pattern of, 261
　prenatal development of, 261, 265
　sexual, 492, 495–496, 495–497
Handedness, 391, 461
Haploid number, 47, 55, 57
Harvard Medical School, 131
Head:
　circumference of: age differences in, 29–31, 29, 30
　of fetus, 208, 270–271
　of infant, 360, 363
　interpretation of, 94–95, 97, 365
　of neonate, 296
　procedure for measuring, 94, 98
　recommended schedule for assessment of, 30, 92
　of school-age child, 479–480

SUBJECT INDEX **531**

Head: circumference of (Cont.):
   sex differences in, *29–31*
   of toddler, 411, 413, *415*
   molding of, 294, 295, 307
   (See also Calvarium; Face; Fontanels)
Healing and tissue specialization, 67
Health, 7, 38–40, 112–113
Health history, 8–11, 91
   (See also Screening)
Hearing (see Auditory system; Deafness)
Heart, 68, 80, 237–239
   murmurs of, 365
   (See also Cardiovascular system; Circulation, fetal)
Heart rate:
   age differences in, *80*
   of fetus, 266, 277
      during labor, 282–284
   of infant, 365
   of neonate, 296
   of preschooler, 451
   at puberty, 489, *491*, *493*
   of school-age child, 482, *493*
   of toddler, 415
Height, 31
   interpretation of, 94–95, 97–98, 365
   normative charts for, *32–35*
   prediction of, 31, 450
   of preschooler, 450, *452*
   procedure for measuring, 93–94
   at puberty, *480*, *481*, 486–489, *490*
   recommended schedule for measurement of, 30, 92
   of school-age child, 479, *480*, *481*, 489
   sitting, 94, 97
   socioeconomic status and, 42
   of toddler, 411–412, *414*
   weight for, 32, 94, 95, 97
   (See also Height-weight ratio; Length)
Height-weight ratio:
   interpretation of, 32, *44–46*, 95, 99
   procedure for measuring, 94
   use with skinfold thickness, 99

Hemangioma, 297
Hematology values, 80, *82*, 296
Hematopoiesis, 67, 78–79
   in embryo, 212, 235, 243, 249
   in neonate, 318
   at puberty, 489
Hemoglobin:
   fetal, 246–247
   types of, by age, 80
Heredity, definition of, 47
Heterochronism, 21, 22, 24
Histogenesis, 14, 67
Histones, 54–55
Home Observation for Measurement of the Environment (HOME), 9–11, 176–184
Homeostasis, 21, 25–26
Hormones:
   of embryo, 250–252, 255–256
   gonadotropic, 86
   placental, 221, 251–252
   prepubertal changes in, 487–488
   of reproductive cycle, 201–202
   secretion of, during sleep, 488
   (See also particular hormones)
Hospitalization:
   effects of separation during, 172
   of infant, 371–372, 396
   of neonate, 326–327
   of preschooler, 453–456
   of school-age child, 498–501
   of toddler, 419–420
How to Parent (Dodson), 188–189
H-Y antigen, 55
Hyalin membrane disease (see Respiratory distress syndrome)
Hyperplasia, 14
Hypertrophy, 14
Hypoglycemia, 321, 322
Hypophysis, 86, 250, 324
Hypothalamic-pituitary-ovarian axis, 86, 324, 488
Hypothalamic-pituitary-testicular axis, 86, 324
Hypothalamus, 86, 250
Hypothyroidism, 370

ICSH (interstitial cell–stimulating hormone), 86
Id, 118, 119

Identification:
   and moral development, 145
   of mother, with infant, 167
   with parents, 115, 119, 166
   (See also Attachment)
Identity and repudiation versus identity diffusion, 120
Illness:
   and behavioral development, 112
   and infant, 371–372
   mental, 61
   and neonate, 326–327
   and physical growth, 38–40
   and preschooler, 453–456
   and school-age child, 498–501
   and toddler, 419–420
Imitation, 122, 393
Immune system, 321, 370
Implantation, 209, *210*, 216–219
Implanting, 108
Inbreeding, 59
Independent assortment, law of, 57, 58
Index case, 58
Individuation (see Separation-individuation)
Industry versus inferiority, 120, 512, 514
Infant, 3, 359–407
   behavior of, 373–404
      stranger anxiety, 108, 360, 371–372, 402, 403
      temperament and, 117, 329
   body concept of, 370–371
   cognitive development of, 371, 373, 374, 390, 393–396
   feeding of, 185, 369, 398–400
   fine motor development of, 367, 387–393
   gross motor development of, 377–387
   growth of, 6, 113, 360–366
   illness and, 371–372
   individual differences in, 170, 194, 396
   influence on caregiver, 3, 113, 167, 170, 194
   language development of, 376, 377, 396–398
   large-for-gestational-age, 304
   maternal perception of, 169–170
   organ systems of, 366–370

Infant (Cont.):
  parenting of, 166–170, 365–366, 371, 396, 403
  paternal perception of, 170–171
  perceptual development of, 374–377
  physical development of, 360–372
  postmature, 304
  premature, 93, 168–169, 299–301, 302–304
    catch-up growth of, 364
    sleep of, 6–7, 332–333
    stimulation of, 6–7, 109, 396
  self-concept of, 370–371, 403–404
    as separate from environment, 370–371, 393, 394, 403
  self-esteem of, 103–104
  self-help skills of, 398–401
  small-for-gestational-age, 22, 221, 271, 274, 301–304, 364
  social development of, 399–403
  techniques for examination of, 360
  and trust versus mistrust, 3, 4, 119–120
  vital signs of, 365
  (See also Attachment; Feeding; Neonate; particular organ systems)
Infants and Mothers (Brazelton), 194
Inheritance, 47–62
  chromosome theory of, 47–48
  dominant, 57–58, 59
  Mendelian laws of, 57–58
  multifactorial, 61
  polygenic, 61
  recessive, 57–61, 60, 61
  X-linked, 60
Initiative versus guilt, 120, 450, 467, 469
Integrity versus despair, 121
Integumentary system, 67–68, 88–89, 260–261, 265
  (See also Hair; Nails)
Intelligence:
  genetic influence on, 62
  sensorimotor, 126, 393–396, 430
  (See also Cognition)
Intelligence tests, 157, 181
  (See also particular tests)
Interphase:
  in meiosis, 55, 56
  in mitosis, 63, 64

Interstitial cell–stimulating hormone (ICSH), 86
Interviewing, technique for, 180
Intestine:
  of infant, 369–370
  of neonate, 319–320
Intimacy and solidarity versus isolation, 120
Intrusive procedures, 454

Jaundice of neonate, 296, 318–319

Karyotype, 48, 49
Kidneys, 87
  (See also Urinary system)

Labor, 250, 282–284
Language, 123, 139–142, 182, 425, 435–436
  of infant, 376, 377, 396–398
  of neonate, 350
  of preschooler, 457, 458, 461, 464–467
  reading and, 503–504
  of school-age child, 485
  and socioeconomic status, 396, 435
  of toddler, 419, 422, 424–425, 431–436
Latency stage of development, 119
Lecithin, 246
Leiter International Performance Scale, 157
Length:
  crown-heel, 94, 270, 271
  crown-rump, 93–94, 95, 269–270
  of infant, 360, 361
  of neonate, 296
  prenatal, 207, 208, 269–270
  trunk measurement and, 271
  (See also Height)
LH (see Luteinizing hormone)
Libido, 118
Linkage, chromosomal, 57
Liver, 68
  of embryo, 249
  of infant, 361, 362
  of neonate, 296, 310, 318–319
  of toddler, 413, 418

Lungs, 80–84
  assessment of, 82–83
    for prenatal maturity, 246
  (See also Respiratory system)
Luteinizing hormone (LH), 86, 201, 324
  at puberty, 488, 494, 495
Lymphatic system, growth of, 4, 24

MacDonald rule for fundal height, 267
Mandible, 72, 74
MAO (monoamine oxidase), 62
Marriage, quality of, 173
Masturbation, 438, 496
Maternal Care and Mental Health (Bowlby), 165–166
Maturation, 117, 124–125, 142
  as growth process, 15, 21–47, 133
Maxilla, 72, 74
MDI (mental development index), 155
Measurement of Man, The (Harris, Jackson, Paterson, and Scammon), 4
Meiosis, 55, 56, 57
  chromosome distribution during, 47
  deoxyribonucleic acid (DNA) in, 57
  of ovum, 200, 201, 206, 324, 494
Membranes, fetal, 221–222, 304
Menarche, 42, 492
Mendelian laws, 57–58
Menstrual age, 205–207
Menstrual cycle, 86, 201–202, 205
Mental development index (MDI), 155
Mental illness, 61
Merrill-Palmer Scale of Mental Tests, 157
Mesoderm, 66, 68, 69, 209–211
Mesomorphy, 33–34
Metabolic fields, 68–70
Metaphase:
  in meiosis, 55, 56
  in mitosis, 63, 64
Milia, 296

Milk, 317, 320
Mineral balance, 322, 325
Minnesota Child Development Inventory, 154–155
Mitosis, 47, 62, *63*, 64, 202–204
Molding of the head, 294, 295, 307
Mongolian spots, 297
Monoamine oxidase (MAO), 62
Morality, 117–118, 124, 127, 145, 187
    levels of, 128
    of preschooler, 120, 469
    of school-age child, 512–513
    and superego, 118, 119, 165–166
    of toddler, 440
Morphogenesis, 14, 67, 205, 209–215, 264–274
    (*See also* Organogenesis; *particular organ systems*)
Morula, 53–55, 64, *206*, 209
Mother, 166–171, 174–175, 272–274, 275
    employment of, 173, 185, 191
    (*See also under* Attachment; Separation, mother-child)
Motivation, 108, 122, 471
Motor development:
    fine, 134–135, 182, 457
        of infant, 367, 387–393
        of neonate, 345–347
        of preschooler, 461
        of school-age child, 506–507
        of toddler, 427–430
    gross, 42–43, 132–134, 182, 386, 457
        of infant, 377–387
        of neonate, 337–345
        of preschooler, 460–461
        of school-age child, 500–501, 504–506
        of toddler, 425–427
Mouth:
    of neonate, 315–316
    prenatal development of, 222–224, 247, *248*, 265
    of toddler, 417
Müllerian ducts, 252–256
Musculoskeletal system, 40, 75–79, 251, 363

    of embryo, 234–237
    of fetus, 264–265
    of infant, 363, 368
    of neonate, 307–308
    at puberty, 486–489, *491*
    of school-age child, 481, 486–487
    of toddler, 417
Mutilation anxiety, 450, 453–454, 457–458, 499
Myelination, age at completion of, 487, 504

Nagele's rule for expected birth date, 205
Nails:
    of postmature infant, 304
    prenatal development of, 261, 264, 265
Narcotics, abuse of, 262, 274
Nature-nurture interaction, 16–17, 115–128, 328
    developmental theories and, 3, 4, 6, 12
    views of nurse about, 3–4, 6
Neonatal Behavioral Assessment Scale, 155–156, 170, 350
Neonatal Perception Inventories (NPI), 169
Neonate, 75, 294–357
    assessment of, 294–304
        behavioral state and, 294, 328
    behavior of, 328–352
        behavioral state and, 294–295, 328–329, 347–348, 352
    body image of, 326
    cognitive development of, 327, 333, 347–349
    effects on caregivers, 328, 330
    fine motor development of, 345–347
    gross motor development of, 337–345
    growth of, 295–296
    (*See also* Fetus, size at birth)
    illness and, 326–327
    immune mechanisms of, 321
    individuality of, 194, 330
    language development of, 350
    organ systems of, 304–326
    parenting of, 350–351

    perceptual development of, 129, 326–327, 333–337, 347–348, 350–352
    physical development of, 294–327
    reflexes of, 329–330, 338–344, 348
    sleep of, 330–333
    social development of, 350–351
    stimulation of, 327, 348
    techniques for examination of, 294–295
    vital signs of, 295, 296
    (*See also* Temperature, body, of neonate)
    (*See also* Attachment; Feeding; Infants; *particular organ systems*)
Nervous system, 4, 24, 68, 71, 87
    of embryo, 74, 225–229
    of infant, 366–367
    of neonate, 305
    at puberty, 487, *491*, 504
    (*See also* Sensory system)
Neurocranium (*see* Calvarium)
Neurohypophysis, 250, 322
NPI (Neonatal Perception Inventories), 169
Nucleus, 62–65
Nurse, role in promoting child development, 3–11, 13, 95
Nutrition:
    assessment of, 37, 96–99
    (*See also* Skinfold thickness)
    and bone development, 75
    and brain growth, 74–75
    cultural differences in, 43
    of infant, 365
    and physical growth, 40–41, 96, 97
    of pregnant woman, 265, 273

Obesity:
    assessment for, 95, 98–99
    in infancy, 185, 365
Object permanence, concept of:
    by infant, 395, 397
    by toddler, 423, 430–433, 441
Occipital-frontal circumference (OFC), 296
Oedipal stage of development, 119, 120
Olfactory system, 232, 307, 337
Oligohydramnios, 222, 260, 304

One-parent families, 7, 143, 173–175
Oogenesis, 200–202
Oral stage of development, 4
Ordinal position, 147, 171
Organogenesis, 67, 68, 71–89, 200–263
   (*See also* Morphogenesis; *particular organ systems*)
Otitis media, 367, 485
Ovary, 68, 87
   of neonate, 323–324
      prenatal development of, 252–256
   at puberty, 494
Ovulation, 86, 201–202, 205
   endocrine control of, 86
Oxytocin challenge test, 266
Oxytocin from embryo, 250

Pain:
   perception of: by infant, 368, 371
      by neonate, 326
      by toddler, 419
   response to, by preschooler, 454
Pancreas, 251, 319, 321, 370
Parathyroid glands, 251
Parathyroid hormone (PTH), 322
Parent-child relationship, 7, 116, 117, 163–176, 422–423
   assessment of, 175–176
Parent Effectiveness Training (PET), (Gordon), 189–191
Parents, 115–117, 119, 142, 163–196
   adolescent, 175
   effects of child on, 116, 117, 146, 170, 193
   of infant (*see* Infant, parenting of)
   literature for, 184–194
   needs of, 146, 182, 185
   of neonate, 350–351
   of preschooler, 464, 472–473
   of school-age child, 514–515
   single, 7, 143, 173–175
   supports for, 182–183
   of toddler, 422–423, 435–439, 442
   (*See also* Attachment; Child-rearing; Deprivation, maternal; Father; Mother; Parent-child relationship)
Parents in Modern America (LeMasters), 163–164

Passages (Sheehy), 4
PDI (psychomotor developmental index), 155
PDQ (Denver Prescreening Developmental Questionnaire), 155
Peabody Picture Vocabulary Test, 10
Pedigree, 47, 58–61
Peers, 109, 120, 143, 147
   of preschooler, 457, 469, 473
   of school-age child, 510, 513
   of toddler, 440
Perception, 129–132
   in fetus, 277–280
   in infant, 374–377
   methods of studying, 333–334, 374, 423–424
   in neonate, 129, 326–327, 333–337, 347–348, 350–352
   in preschooler, 458–460
   in school-age child, 484–485, 503–504
   in toddler, 423–425
   (*See also* Auditory system; Gustatory system; Olfactory system; Pain, perception of; Sensory system; Stimulation; Vision)
Periodic breathing, 296, 315
PET (*Parent Effectiveness Training*) (Gordon), 189–191
Phallic stage of development, 4
Phenotype, 47, 57, 58
Physical development (*see* Development, physical)
Physiology, relationship to behavior, 13–14, 16–17
Pineal gland, 251
Pituitary, 86, 250, 324
Placenta, 209, 210, 215–221, 251–252, 265
Placental barrier, 219–221, 250
   maternal hormones and, 250, 251
Placental transfusion, 310–312
Play:
   of infant, 397, 403
   of preschooler, 450, 454–456, 460
   of toddler, 441, 442
Pleasure principle, 118
Polar bodies, 62, 64
Polyhydramnios, 222
Polymorphism of chromosomes, 49
Ponderal index, 33

SUBJECT INDEX **535**

Posture:
   of infant, 362–363
   of preschooler, 450
   of toddler, 414–415, 417
Pregnancy, multiple, 209, 273
   (*See also* Twins)
Prematurity, 93, 168–169, 299–301
   (*See also* Infant, premature; Infant, small-for-gestational-age)
Preschooler, 449–475
   behavioral development of, 457–473
   body image of, 452–453
   cognitive development of, 457, 461–464
   feeding of, 467
   growth of, 450–451
   illness and, 453–456
   and initiative versus shame and doubt, 120, 450, 467, 469
   language of, 457, 458, 461, 464–467
   moral development of, 120, 469
   motor development of, 457
      fine, 461
      gross, 460–461
   parenting of, 464, 472–473
   perceptual development of, 458–460
   physical development of, 450–456
   self-concept of (*see* Self-concept, of preschooler)
   self-esteem of, 471–473
   self-help skills of, 457, 467–469
   sex role in, 119, 453, 470–471
   social development of, 469–471
   techniques for examination of, 450
   vital signs of, 451
   (*See also particular organ systems*)
Primordium, 65
Principles of Perceptual Learning and Development (Gibson), 336
Proband, 58
Prophase, 55, 56, 62–64
Propositus, 58
Proprioception:
   in fetus, 278, 279
   in infant, 376

Proprioception *(Cont.):*
  in neonate, 326
  of toddler, 424, 425
Proximodistal principle of growth and development, 14, 277, 362, 412–413
  in fine motor development, 134, 457
  in gross motor development, 133, 345, 386, 457
Psychoanalytic theory, 3–4, 117–121
Psychogenetics, 61–62
Psychomotor developmental index (PDI), 155
Psychosocial theories of development, 119–121
Psychosomatic illness, 113
PTH (parathyroid hormone), 322
Puberty, 86–87
  clinical signs of, 489–497
  delayed, 496
  growth during, 485–497
  nervous system at, 487, *491*, 504
  onset of, 485, 488, 496, *497*
  preparation for, 512
  and psychosocial theory of development, 120
Pulmonary function studies, 82–84
Pulse *(see* Heart rate)
Purines in deoxyribonucleic acid, 49, 52
Pyrimidines in deoxyribonucleic acid, 49, 52

Q staining (quinacrine staining), 48, 50–51
Quickening, 274
Quinacrine staining (Q staining), 48, 50–51

Radiation as a teratogen, 262
Rapid Developmental Screening Checklist, 155
Readiness, 108
  cognitive and psychological, 142
  and fine motor development, 134
  and gross motor development, 133
  and socialization, 144
Reading, 503–504
  (See also Language)
Reality principle, 118, 119
Reflex(es):
  asymmetric tonic-neck, 338, 345, 346
    disappearance of, 377, 381, 384, 385, 387
  Babinski, 278, 343, *346*, 378
    disappearance of, 385, 425
  bite, 316, 399
  body-righting, 379, 383
  corneal, 307
  crossed-extensor, 343–344, 377
  Darwinian, 346
  deep-tendon, 344
  effects of behavior state on, 329, 344
  equilibrium, 380, 384, 425
  extrusion, 368
  of fetus, 277–280
  gag, 316
  Galant's, 342, *344*, 377
  gastrocolic, 320
  Head's paradoxical, 314
  Herring-Breuer, 314
  labyrinthine righting, 379, 381, 383, 425
  Landau, 378, 381, 425
  Moro, 338–339, 377
  neck-righting, 339, *340*, 377–378, 381
  of neonate, 329–330, 338–344, 348
  optical righting, 379, *380–381*
  palmar grasp, 277–278, 345, 346, *348*
  parachute, 380
  placing, 342, *343*, 378
  plantar grasp, 278, 342, *345*, 377
  positive supporting, 340–341, *342*
    disappearance of, 377, 384, 385, 425
  propping, 380, *382*, 385
  protective extension, 380, *382*, 385
  rooting, 278, 346, 347, *349*, 399
  stepping, 342, *343*, 377
  sucking *(see* Sucking)
  swallowing *(see* Swallowing)
  tonic labyrinthine, 340, *341*
    disappearance of, 377, 381, 384, 385, 425
  traction, 339–340, 377
  trunk-incurvation, 342, *344*, 377
  withdrawal, 342, 377
Regeneration and tissue specialization, 67
Reproductive cycle, 86, 201–202, 205
Reproductive system, 4, *24*, 85–87
  of embryo, 55, 215, 252–256, *252–254*, 257
  hormonal control of, 86, 324
  in neonate, 322–324
  at puberty, 485, 488–497
  of school-age child, 487–489
  (See also Genitalia, external)
Respiration:
  initiation of, in neonate, 313
  muscles used in, 82
  prenatal, 247, 266–267, 277
Respiratory distress syndrome, 81, 82, 246, 314–315
Respiratory rate:
  age differences in, 82, *83*
  of infant, 365
  of neonate, 296
  of preschooler, 451
  at puberty, 489
  of school-age child, 484
  of toddler, 415
Respiratory system, 80–84
  of neonate, 312–315
  prenatal, 80–81, 244–247
  of preschooler, 81
  at puberty, 81, *491*, 493
  of school-age child, 81, 484, *491*, *493*
  of toddler, 81
Restraints, responses to, 419–420, 450
Ribonucleic acid (RNA), 47, 53–54, 64
Rites of passage, 110
Rituals, 110
  of toddler, 422, 424, 439
RNA (ribonucleic acid), 47, 53–54, 64
Role theory, 164

Salivary glands, 84
Schema, development of, 108, 126, 130, 131, 137
  by infant, 393–395, *394*
  by neonate, 348, 350
  by toddler, 430

Schizophrenia, 61–62
School, 113–114, 469, 512, 514
School-age child, 477–518
    behavioral development of, 502–515
        school and, 113–114
    cognitive development of, 507–510
    feeding of, 511
    growth of, 478–480
    and industry versus inferiority, 120
    language development of, 485
    motor development of: fine, 506–507
        gross, 500–501, 504–506
    perceptual development of, 484–485, 503–504
    physical development of, 478–501
    self-esteem of, 502, 514–515
    self-help skills of, 510–512
    social development of, 510–514
    techniques for examination of, 478
    vital signs of, 482–484
    (*See also particular organ systems*)
Screening:
    behavioral, 9, 92, 152–155
    compared to diagnosis, 152
    for growth problems, 30
        (*See also* Head, circumference of; Height; Weight)
    for hearing problems, 9, 92
    for inborn problems, 9, 92
    for nutrition problems, 37, 96, 99
    for visual problems, 9, 92
Segregation, law of, 57, 58
Self-concept:
    of ill child, 112
    of infant, 370–371, 403–404
        as separate from environment, 370–371, 393, 394, 403
    of neonate, 351–352
    of preschooler, 452–453
        as separate from environment, 462, 471
    racial minority and, 113
    socioeconomic status and, 113
    of toddler, 418–419, 439, 441–442
        as separate from environment, 419
Self-esteem:
    of infant, 403–404
    of neonate, 351–352
    of preschooler, 471–473

    of school-age child, 502, 514–515
    of toddler, 441–442
Self-help skills, 141–143
    assessment of, 157
    of infant, 398–401
    of preschooler, 457, 467–469
    of school-age child, 510–512
    of toddler, 436–439
Sense organs (*see* Sensory system)
Sensitive period, 21, 25, 108
    in attachment, 113
    in hearing, 377
    maternal, 169
    in personality development, 165–166
    prenatal, 25, *263*
    in sex differentiation, 255
    in visual development, 416–417
Sensory system, 74, 75, 131
    of embryo, 230–234
    of fetus, 277–280
    of infant, 367–368, 374–376
    of neonate, 75, 305–307, 326, 335–337
    of preschooler, 451–452, *454*, 458–460
    of school-age child, 484–485
    of toddler, 416–417, 424–425
Separation, mother-child, 165–166, 168–169, 172–173
    (*See also* Deprivation, maternal)
Separation anxiety:
    of infant, 371–372
    of preschooler, 454
    of toddler, 420
Separation-individuation:
    of infant, 371, 393, 394, 403
    of neonate, 351–352
    of preschooler, 462, 471
    symbiosis and, 352, 403
    of toddler, 419, 441
Sex chromosomes, 48–49, 55, 60–61
Sex differences, 87, 110
    curiosity about, 120, 452, 468
    in dental development, 486
    embryologic development of, 55, 215, 252–256, 252–254, 257
    in musculoskeletal development, 486–487
    in pubertal growth spurt, 485–489
    in response to family discord, 174

    in response of parent to neonate, 170–171
    in size at birth, 272
    and toilet training, 438
Sex education, 120, 191, 468, 512
Sex role:
    culture and, 110
    in infancy, 402–403
    in parent literature, 185, 188, 189
    parenting and, 402–403
    in preschooler, 119, 453, 470–471
    in school-age child, 513–514
    socialization and, 146
    and toilet training, 438
    (*See also* Gender identity)
Sibling relationships, 147–148, 514
Sickle cell disease, 52–53, 59
Simple-to complex principle of growth and development, 107, 133
Skeletal age, 37–38, 77–78, 370, 486
Skin, 67–68, 88–89, 260–261, 265
    (*See also* Hair; Nails)
Skinfold thickness, 37, 95, 98–99
    of infant, 360, 364, 365
Skull (*see* Calvarium)
Sleep, 329–332
    of fetus, 266, 277
    and hormone secretion, 488
    of infant, 6, 373
    of neonate, 330–333
    of toddler, 422
    types of, 6, *330*, 332
    (*See also* Behavioral state)
Smell, sense of, 232, 307, 337
Smiling, 374–375
Snellen E chart, 451, 484
Social development, 109, 122, 143–148
    of infant, 399–403
    of neonate, 350–351
    of preschooler, 469–471
    of school-age child, 510–514
    of toddler, 439–441
Social-learning theory of development, 3–4, 117, 121–124
Socioeconomic status:
    and age at menarche, 42

SUBJECT INDEX

Socioeconomic status (Cont.):
  and birth weight, 41–42, 270, 272, 274, 275
  and child-rearing, 177–178
  and cognitive development, 464
  and height, 42
  and language development, 396, 435
  and mother-infant interaction, 396–397
  and self-concept, 113
Somatotropin, 6, 46–47, 85, 250, 364
Somatotypes, 33–34
Speech (see Language)
Spermatogenesis, 86, 200–204, 495
Sphingomyelin, 246
Spinal cord, embryologic development of, 225, 227, 228–229
Spoiling, 185, 189
Stage formation in behavioral development, 108
Standing, 385, 425
Stanford-Binet Intelligence Scales, 157, 181
Statement on Parental-Infant Attachment (American Nurses Association), 284
Stereotypes, 113, 114, 185
Stimulation, 45–47, 109
  auditory, 109
  fetal responses to, 277–280
  from home environment, 176–183
  and infant development, 368, 373, 376–377
    cognitive, 393, 395–396
  and language development, 140
  methods of providing, 109
  of neonate, 327, 348
  of premature infant, 6–7, 109, 396
  social, 109
  visual, 109
  (See also Deprivation)
Stimuli, novel, 108, 393, 397
Stimulus-response theory (see Behaviorism)
Stomach, 247–249
  of infant, 369
  of neonate, 317–318
  of toddler, 418

Stools of infant, 370
Stork's beak marks, 297
Strabismus, 367, 416–417, 484
Stranger anxiety:
  as behavioral norm, 149
  in infant, 108, 360, 371–372, 402, 403
Substance abuse, 262, 274
Sucking:
  in fetus, 278, 280
  in infant, 368, 398–399
  in neonate, 316–317, 326–327, 347
Superego, 118, 119, 165–166
  (See also Morality)
Surfactant, 80, 83, 84, 244–246, 313–315
Swaddling, 42–43
Swallowing:
  in fetus, 278, 280
  in infant, 368, 399
  in neonate, 316–317, 347
Symbiosis, 352, 403

Tabula rasa, 129
Tactile system:
  of embryo, 234
  of fetus, 277–278
  of infant, 367–368
  of neonate, 307, 326, 337
  of preschooler, 459–460
Taste, sense of (see Gustatory system)
Tay-Sachs disease, 59
Teeth:
  care of, 74, 468, 511
  eruption of, 72–74
  formation of, 72–74, 224
  of infant, 366, 367
  at puberty, 486
  of school-age child, 486
  of toddler, 415–416, *418*
Television, 114–115
Telophase:
  in meiosis, 55, *56*
  in mitosis, *63*, 64
Temper tantrums, 420
Temperament, 5, 116, 174, 193
  assessment of, 117
  of infant, 117, 329
  of toddler, 422–423
  (See also Behavior; Behavioral state)

Temperature, body, 85
  of infant, 365
  of neonate, 295, 296, 322
    cold stress and, 295, 321, 322
  of school-age child, 482
Ten-State Nutritional Survey, 28
Teratogens, 262–263
Testes, 87, 253–256, 322–323, 494–495
Tetany, neonatal, 322
Tetracycline, 224
Theories, developmental, 3–4, 117–128
  behavioristic, 3–4, 117, 121–124
  cognitive, 3, 108, 124–128, 135–138
  field, 125
  genetic, 3–4
  language, 140–141, 425
  maturational, 117, 124–125
  naive, 123–124
  perceptual, 129–130
  psychoanalytic, 3–4, 117–121
  psychosocial, 119–121
  social-learning, 3–4, 117, 121–124
Thought:
  causal, 509–510
  intuitive, 126–127
  logical, 508–509
  operational, 127
  precausal, 463
  preoperational, 126–127, 462
  representational, 126, 430, 432
  symbolic, 424
  syncretic, 136
  undifferentiated, 136–137
  (See also Cognition)
Three Mile Island, 115
Thymine, 49, 52, *53*
Thymus gland, 251
Thyroid gland, 251, 321, 370
Thyroid hormones, 85, 370
Tissue, 25, 66–68, 70
Toddler, 409–446
  autonomy in, 422, 436–442
    versus shame and doubt, 4, 120
  behavioral development of, 422–442
    rituals in, 422, 424, 439
    temper tantrums, 420
  body concept of, 418–419, 425

Schizophrenia, 61–62
School, 113–114, 469, 512, 514
School-age child, 477–518
   behavioral development of, 502–515
      school and, 113–114
   cognitive development of, 507–510
   feeding of, 511
   growth of, 478–480
   and industry versus inferiority, 120
   language development of, 485
   motor development of: fine, 506–507
      gross, 500–501, 504–506
   perceptual development of, 484–485, 503–504
   physical development of, 478–501
   self-esteem of, 502, 514–515
   self-help skills of, 510–512
   social development of, 510–514
   techniques for examination of, 478
   vital signs of, 482–484
   (*See also* particular organ systems)
Screening:
   behavioral, 9, 92, 152–155
   compared to diagnosis, 152
   for growth problems, 30
      (*See also* Head, circumference of; Height; Weight)
   for hearing problems, 9, 92
   for inborn problems, 9, 92
   for nutrition problems, 37, 96, 99
   for visual problems, 9, 92
Segregation, law of, 57, 58
Self-concept:
   of ill child, 112
   of infant, 370–371, 403–404
      as separate from environment, 370–371, 393, 394, 403
   of neonate, 351–352
   of preschooler, 452–453
      as separate from environment, 462, 471
      racial minority and, 113
      socioeconomic status and, 113
   of toddler, 418–419, 439, 441–442
      as separate from environment, 419
Self-esteem:
   of infant, 403–404
   of neonate, 351–352
   of preschooler, 471–473
   of school-age child, 502, 514–515
   of toddler, 441–442
Self-help skills, 141–143
   assessment of, 157
   of infant, 398–401
   of preschooler, 457, 467–469
   of school-age child, 510–512
   of toddler, 436–439
Sense organs (*see* Sensory system)
Sensitive period, 21, 25, 108
   in attachment, 113
   in hearing, 377
   maternal, 169
   in personality development, 165–166
   prenatal, 25, 263
   in sex differentiation, 255
   in visual development, 416–417
Sensory system, 74, 75, 131
   of embryo, 230–234
   of fetus, 277–280
   of infant, 367–368, 374–376
   of neonate, 75, 305–307, 326, 335–337
   of preschooler, 451–452, 454, 458–460
   of school-age child, 484–485
   of toddler, 416–417, 424–425
Separation, mother-child, 165–166, 168–169, 172–173
   (*See also* Deprivation, maternal)
Separation anxiety:
   of infant, 371–372
   of preschooler, 454
   of toddler, 420
Separation-individuation:
   of infant, 371, 393, 394, 403
   of neonate, 351–352
   of preschooler, 462, 471
   symbiosis and, 352, 403
   of toddler, 419, 441
Sex chromosomes, 48–49, 55, 60–61
Sex differences, 87, 110
   curiosity about, 120, 452, 468
   in dental development, 486
   embryologic development of, 55, 215, 252–256, 252–254, 257
   in musculoskeletal development, 486–487
   in pubertal growth spurt, 485–489
   in response to family discord, 174
   in response of parent to neonate, 170–171
   in size at birth, 272
   and toilet training, 438
Sex education, 120, 191, 468, 512
Sex role:
   culture and, 110
   in infancy, 402–403
   in parent literature, 185, 188, 189
   parenting and, 402–403
   in preschooler, 119, 453, 470–471
   in school-age child, 513–514
   socialization and, 146
   and toilet training, 438
   (*See also* Gender identity)
Sibling relationships, 147–148, 514
Sickle cell disease, 52–53, 59
Simple-to-complex principle of growth and development, 107, 133
Skeletal age, 37–38, 77–78, 370, 486
Skin, 67–68, 88–89, 260–261, 265
   (*See also* Hair; Nails)
Skinfold thickness, 37, 95, 98–99
   of infant, 360, 364, 365
Skull (*see* Calvarium)
Sleep, 329–332
   of fetus, 266, 277
   and hormone secretion, 488
   of infant, 6, 373
   of neonate, 330–333
   of toddler, 422
   types of, 6, 330, 332
   (*See also* Behavioral state)
Smell, sense of, 232, 307, 337
Smiling, 374–375
Snellen E chart, 451, 484
Social development, 109, 122, 143–148
   of infant, 399–403
   of neonate, 350–351
   of preschooler, 469–471
   of school-age child, 510–514
   of toddler, 439–441
Social-learning theory of development, 3–4, 117, 121–124
Socioeconomic status:
   and age at menarche, 42

Socioeconomic status *(Cont.):*
   and birth weight, 41–42, 270, 272, 274, 275
   and child-rearing, 177–178
   and cognitive development, 464
   and height, 42
   and language development, 396, 435
   and mother-infant interaction, 396–397
   and self-concept, 113
Somatotropin, 6, 46–47, 85, 250, 364
Somatotypes, 33–34
Speech *(see* Language)
Spermatogenesis, 86, 200–204, 495
Sphingomyelin, 246
Spinal cord, embryologic development of, 225, 227, 228–229
Spoiling, 185, 189
Stage formation in behavioral development, 108
Standing, 385, 425
Stanford-Binet Intelligence Scales, 157, 181
Statement on Parental-Infant Attachment (American Nurses Association), 284
Stereotypes, 113, 114, 185
Stimulation, 45–47, 109
   auditory, 109
   fetal responses to, 277–280
   from home environment, 176–183
   and infant development, 368, 373, 376–377
   cognitive, 393, 395–396
   and language development, 140
   methods of providing, 109
   of neonate, 327, 348
   of premature infant, 6–7, 109, 396
   social, 109
   visual, 109
   (See also Deprivation)
Stimuli, novel, 108, 393, 397
Stimulus-response theory *(see* Behaviorism)
Stomach, 247–249
   of infant, 369
   of neonate, 317–318
   of toddler, 418

Stools of infant, 370
Stork's beak marks, 297
Strabismus, 367, 416–417, 484
Stranger anxiety:
   as behavioral norm, 149
   in infant, 108, 360, 371–372, 402, 403
Substance abuse, 262, 274
Sucking:
   in fetus, 278, 280
   in infant, 368, 398–399
   in neonate, 316–317, 326–327, 347
Superego, 118, 119, 165–166
   (See also Morality)
Surfactant, 80, 83, 84, 244–246, 313–315
Swaddling, 42–43
Swallowing:
   in fetus, 278, 280
   in infant, 368, 399
   in neonate, 316–317, 347
Symbiosis, 352, 403

Tabula rasa, 129
Tactile system:
   of embryo, 234
   of fetus, 277–278
   of infant, 367–368
   of neonate, 307, 326, 337
   of preschooler, 459–460
Taste, sense of *(see* Gustatory system)
Tay-Sachs disease, 59
Teeth:
   care of, 74, 468, 511
   eruption of, 72–74
   formation of, 72–74, 224
   of infant, 366, *367*
   at puberty, 486
   of school-age child, 486
   of toddler, 415–416, *418*
Television, 114–115
Telophase:
   in meiosis, 55, *56*
   in mitosis, *63*, 64
Temper tantrums, 420
Temperament, 5, 116, 174, 193
   assessment of, 117
   of infant, 117, 329
   of toddler, 422–423
   (See also Behavior; Behavioral state)

Temperature, body, 85
   of infant, 365
   of neonate, 295, 296, 322
      cold stress and, 295, 321, 322
   of school-age child, 482
Ten-State Nutritional Survey, 28
Teratogens, 262–263
Testes, 87, 253–256, 322–323, 494–495
Tetany, neonatal, 322
Tetracycline, 224
Theories, developmental, 3–4, 117–128
   behavioristic, 3–4, 117, 121–124
   cognitive, 3, 108, 124–128, 135–138
   field, 125
   genetic, 3–4
   language, 140–141, 425
   maturational, 117, 124–125
   naive, 123–124
   perceptual, 129–130
   psychoanalytic, 3–4, 117–121
   psychosocial, 119–121
   social-learning, 3–4, 117, 121–124
Thought:
   causal, 509–510
   intuitive, 126–127
   logical, 508–509
   operational, 127
   precausal, 463
   preoperational, 126–127, 462
   representational, 126, 430, 432
   symbolic, 424
   syncretic, 136
   undifferentiated, 136–137
   (See also Cognition)
Three Mile Island, 115
Thymine, 49, 52, *53*
Thymus gland, 251
Thyroid gland, 251, 321, 370
Thyroid hormones, 85, 370
Tissue, 25, 66–68, 70
Toddler, 409–446
   autonomy in, 422, 436–442
      versus shame and doubt, 4, 120
   behavioral development of, 422–442
   rituals in, 422, 424, 439
   temper tantrums, 420
   body concept of, 418–419, 425

SUBJECT INDEX

Toddler *(Cont.):*
  cognitive development of, 424, 429–432
  feeding of, 422, 427–428, 436–437
  fine motor development of, 427–430
  gross motor development of, 425–427
  growth of, 411–415
    channelization of, 411–412, *416*
  illness and, 419–420
  language development of, 419, 422, 424–425, 431–436
  moral development of, 440
  organ system development of, 415–418
  parent-child interactions and, 422–423
  perceptual development of, 423–425
  physical development of, 410–421
    assessment of, 410–415
  self-concept of, 418–419, 439, 441–442
  self-esteem of, 441–442
  self-help skills of, 436–439
  social development of, 439–441
  techniques for examination of, 410
  vital signs of, 415
  (See also particular organ systems)
Toddlers and Parents (Brazelton), 194
Toilet training, 185
  of infant, 400–401
  of preschooler, 467–468
  and sex role, 438
  of toddler, 418, 422, 437–438
Touch, maternal, 167–168
Touch, sense of *(see* Tactile system)
Transfusion, placental, 310–312
Transitional object, 403
Translocations, chromosomal, 57
Trunk measurement, 271
Trust versus mistrust, 3, 4, 119–120
Twins, 3, 61, 62, 209, 273

Ultrasonography, 208–209
Umbilical cord, 216, 221, 273, 310–312
Unconscious mind, 118
United Nations, 165
University of Washington, 6
Urinary system, 87–88, 256–260, 324–326

Values, acquisition of, 122
  (See also Morality)
Ventricles of brain, 229, *230*
Ventrodorsal principle of growth and development, 14, 133, 345, 386
Vineland Social Maturity Scale, 157
Viruses as teratogens, 262
Viscerocranium *(see* Face)
Vision, 75
  assessment of, 451
  embryologic development of, 230–232
  fetal capacity for, 280
  of infant, 367, 374–375
  of neonate, 305–307, 335–336
  of preschooler, 451–452, *454*, 458–459
  problems, screening for, 9, 92
  of school-age child, 484–485
  of toddler, 416–417, 424
  (See also Eyes)
Vital signs:
  of infant, 365
  of neonate, 295, 296
  of preschooler, 451
  of school-age child, 482–484
  of toddler, 415
Vitamin K and neonate, 319
Vocabulary, age differences in, 140–141
Vulnerable child syndrome, 168–169

Walking, 385, 425–426
Weaning, 399, 437

Wechsler Intelligence Scale for Children, 157
Weeche's formula for weight gain, 479
Weight, 31–34
  correction for premature infant, 93
  for height, 32, 94, 95, 97
  of infant, 360, *361*, 365
  interpretation of, 94–95, 97–98, 365
  of neonate, *26*, 296
  normative charts for, *39–41, 43–46*
  during pregnancy, 267
  prenatal, *26*, 41–42, 208, 267–269, 270
  of preschooler, 450, 451, 453
  procedure for measuring, 93
  at puberty, *482, 483,* 486, 488–489, *489, 490*
  recommended schedule for measurement of, 30, 92
  of school-age child, 479, *482, 483, 489*
  of toddler, 411–413, *412, 413*
  (See also Height-weight ratio)
Well-child care, 91–99
What Every Child Would Like His Parents to Know (Salk), 191–192
WHO (World Health Organization), 41, 92, 165, 172
Wolffian ducts, 252–256
World Health Organization (WHO), 41, 92, 165, 172

Yale Clinic of Child Development, 155
Your Child Is a Person (Chess, Thomas, and Birch), 193–194

Zygote, 200, 205